THE
MERCK
MANUAL
OF
GERIATRICS

Third Edition

FOREIGN LANGUAGE EDITIONS
of *The Merck Manual of Geriatrics*

Chinese—People's Medical Publishing House, Beijing
French—Editions d'Apres, Paris
Hungarian—Melania Kiadoi Kft, Budapest
Japanese—Medical Book Service, Ltd., Tokyo
Polish—Urban & Partner, Wroclaw

OTHER MERCK BOOKS

THE MERCK MANUAL OF DIAGNOSIS AND THERAPY
Seventeenth (Centennial) Edition, 1999

THE MERCK VETERINARY MANUAL
Eighth Edition, 1998

THE MERCK MANUAL OF MEDICAL INFORMATION—
HOME EDITION
First Edition, 1997

THE MERCK INDEX
Twelfth Edition, 1996

Merck books are published on a nonprofit basis as a service to the scientific community and the public.

THE
MERCK
MANUAL
OF
GERIATRICS

Third Edition

Editors MARK H. BEERS, M.D., and ROBERT BERKOW, M.D.

Senior Assistant Editors ROBERT M. BOGIN, M.D.; ANDREW J. FLETCHER, M.B., B.Chir.; and MIRZA I. RAHMAN, M.D., M.P.H.

Editorial Board Richard W. Besdine, M.D.
Robert N. Butler, M.D.
Christine K. Cassel, M.D.
Terry T. Fulmer, Ph.D., R.N., F.A.A.N.
Edward G. Lakatta, M.D.
John E. Morley, M.B., B.Ch.
Mary E. Tinetti, M.D.

Published by MERCK RESEARCH LABORATORIES
Division of MERCK & CO., INC.
Whitehouse Station, NJ

2000

Editorial and Production Staff

Executive Editor:	Keryn A.G. Lane
Senior Staff Editor:	Susan T. Schindler
Staff Editors:	Julie Kostecky
	Sandra J. Masse
	Debra Share
Contributing Editor:	Roger I. Schreck, M.D.
Textbook Production Coordinator:	Diane C. Zenker
Project Manager:	Diane Cosner-Bobrin
Medical Textbook Coordinator:	Dorothy A. Bailey
Executive Assistant:	Jean Perry
Administrative Assistant:	Marcia Yarbrough
Designer:	Lorraine B. Kilmer
Illustrator:	Michael Reingold
Indexer:	Susan Thomas, Ph.D.
Publisher:	Gary Zelko
Advertising and Promotional Supervisor:	Pamela J. Barnes

Library of Congress Catalog Card Number 89-63495
ISBN 0911910-88-3
ISSN 1527-6708

PREFACE

With this, the third edition of *The Merck Manual of Geriatrics*, we continue the tradition of providing information of clinical relevance on geriatric care. Providing the best geriatric care requires an extraordinarily large base of information—everything from internal medicine to pharmacology and dermatology to rehabilitation medicine and psychiatry. However, it also requires a different approach to care than many other areas of medical practice, one that coordinates care among physicians, nurses, social workers, therapists, pharmacists, and myriad other health professionals. Geriatric care also requires education for patients and caregivers. Therefore, we have attempted to create a truly interdisciplinary textbook that reflects the optimal approach to geriatric care. We realize that not all of the information provided will be of interest to each reader; however, collectively it covers most of what needs to be known about caring for the elderly. Although this book is written primarily for clinicians, we hope that our expanded coverage will make this edition of *The Merck Manual of Geriatrics* even more useful to others involved in geriatric care, to older people, and to their families and friends.

This new edition of *The Merck Manual of Geriatrics* reflects the vast amount of new information that has been learned about geriatric care since our last edition, five years ago. Geriatrics and gerontology continue to be fertile ground for research. New treatments have already helped greatly to prevent, cure, or control conditions that as recently as five years ago were untreatable. We hope that by the next edition, even more of the devastating conditions of late life will be preventable or curable. When prevention, cure, or control cannot yet be achieved, we offer advice on palliation, including care of the dying, an area that we believe needs greater attention.

In creating the major revisions in this edition, we gratefully acknowledge the contributions provided by our distinguished editorial board who reviewed all chapters and the more than 150 experts who provided manuscripts and served as consultants. All of them share the hope that those who use this book will find it useful and, ultimately, of benefit to their patients.

We welcome your comments and will carefully consider all suggestions for improvement.

MARK H. BEERS, M.D.
ROBERT BERKOW, M.D.

DEDICATION

This edition of *The Merck Manual of Geriatrics* is dedicated to our late colleague Dr. William B. Abrams. Dr. Abrams was co-editor of the first two editions of *The Merck Manual of Geriatrics* and was a leader in improving the quality of geriatric care. He contributed greatly to research in aging and to the development of academic geriatric physicians. And these were but a few of his accomplishments in his productive lifetime.

CONTENTS

SECTION 8 METABOLIC AND ENDOCRINE DISORDERS

SECTION 9 HEMATOLOGIC DISORDERS AND CANCER

SECTION 10 PULMONARY DISORDERS

SECTION 11 CARDIOVASCULAR DISORDERS

SECTION 12   KIDNEY AND URINARY TRACT DISORDERS

SECTION 13   GASTROINTESTINAL DISORDERS

SECTION 14   MEN'S AND WOMEN'S HEALTH ISSUES

SECTION 15   DERMATOLOGIC AND SENSORY ORGAN DISORDERS

SECTION 16   INFECTIOUS DISEASE

APPENDIXES

INDEX 1421

■ GUIDE FOR READERS

The **Contents** (p. vii) shows the pages on which readers will find titles of sections and chapters and the Index. **Thumb tabs** with appropriate abbreviations mark each section and the Index.

Each **Section** begins with its own table of contents, listing chapters and subchapters in that section.

Chapters are numbered serially from the beginning to the end of the book.

The **Index** contains many cross-entries; page numbers in boldface type signify a major discussion of a topic. In addition, **cross-references** throughout the book direct readers to specific page numbers for more information.

Running heads carry the section number and title on left-hand pages and the chapter number and title on right-hand pages.

Abbreviations and symbols, used throughout the book as essential space savers, are listed on p. xiii. Other abbreviations in the text are expanded at their first use in the chapter or subchapter.

The **Tables** and **figures** found throughout the text are referenced appropriately in the Index but are not listed in a Table of Contents.

Laboratory values in the book are given in conventional units. In most cases, however, SI units follow in parentheses.

Drugs are designated in the text mainly by generic (nonproprietary) names. In Appendix III, many of the drugs mentioned in the book are listed in a table alphabetically, with each generic term followed by one or more trade names. This table is followed by another table that provides an alphabetical list of many trade names followed by the drug's generic name.

Important: The authors, reviewers, and editors of this book have made extensive efforts to ensure that treatments, drugs, and dosage regimens are accurate and conform to the standards accepted at the time of publication. However, constant changes in information resulting from continuing research and clinical experience, reasonable differences in opinions among authorities, unique aspects of individual clinical situations, and the possibility of human error in preparing such an extensive text require that the reader exercise individual judgment when making a clinical decision and, if necessary, consult and compare information from other sources. In particular, the reader is advised to check the product information provided by the manufacturer of a drug product before prescribing or administering it, especially if the drug is unfamiliar or is used infrequently.

ABBREVIATIONS AND SYMBOLS

AIDS	acquired immunodeficiency syndrome	**lb**	pound
ATP	adenosine triphosphate	**m**	meter
bid	two times a day	**mEq**	milliequivalent
C	Celsius; centigrade	**mg**	milligram
CBC	complete blood cell (count)	**min**	minute
Ch.	chapter	**mL**	milliliter
cm	centimeter	**mm**	millimeter
CO$_2$	carbon dioxide	**mOsm**	milliosmole
CPR	cardiopulmonary resuscitation	**MRI**	magnetic resonance imaging
CT	computed tomography	**ng**	nanogram (= millimicrogram)
dL	deciliter (= 100 mL)	**oz**	ounce
DNA	deoxyribonucleic acid	**pH**	hydrogen ion concentration
ECG	electrocardiogram	**po**	orally
EEG	electroencephalogram	**prn**	as needed
eg	for example	**q**	every
ESR	erythrocyte sedimentation rate	**qid**	four times a day
F	Fahrenheit	**RNA**	ribonucleic acid
FDA	Food and Drug Administration	**sc**	subcutaneous(ly)
g	gram	**SD**	standard deviation
h	hour	**sec**	second
H$_2$	histamine	**sq**	square
Hb	hemoglobin	**tid**	three times a day
Hct	hematocrit	**U**	unit
Hg	mercury	**vs.**	versus
HIV	human immunodeficiency virus	**wk**	week
HLA	human leukocyte antigen	**yr**	year
Hz	hertz (cycles per second)	**μg**	microgram
ie	that is	**μL**	microliter
Ig	immunoglobulin	**μm**	micrometer; micron
IM	intramuscular(ly)	**μU**	microunit
IU	international unit	**/**	per
IV	intravenous(ly)	**<**	less than
kcal	kilocalorie (food calorie)	**>**	more than
kg	kilogram	**≤**	equal to or less than
L	liter	**≥**	equal to or more than
		±	plus or minus

EDITORS AND EDITORIAL BOARD

EDITORS

MARK H. BEERS, M.D.

Senior Director of Geriatrics, Merck & Co., Inc., and Associate Clinical Professor of Medicine, MCP Hahnemann School of Medicine

ROBERT BERKOW, M.D.

Executive Director of Medical Literature, Merck & Co., Inc., and Clinical Professor of Medicine and Psychiatry, MCP Hahnemann School of Medicine

SENIOR ASSISTANT EDITORS

ROBERT M. BOGIN, M.D.

Merck & Co., Inc., Associate Clinical Professor of Medicine, MCP Hahnemann School of Medicine

ANDREW J. FLETCHER, M.B., B.Chir.

Merck & Co., Inc., Adjunct Professor of Pharmaceutical Health Care, Temple University School of Pharmacy

MIRZA I. RAHMAN, M.D., M.P.H.

Merck & Co., Inc., Adjunct Professor of Pharmacoepidemiology, Temple University School of Pharmacy

EDITORIAL BOARD

RICHARD W. BESDINE, M.D.

Professor of Medicine and Director, University of Connecticut Center on Aging

ROBERT N. BUTLER, M.D.

Professor of Geriatrics and Adult Development, Mount Sinai School of Medicine; President, Chief Executive Officer, International Longevity Center

CHRISTINE K. CASSEL, M.D.

Chairman and Professor, Henry L. Schwartz Department of Geriatrics and Adult Development, Mount Sinai School of Medicine

TERRY T. FULMER, Ph.D., R.N., F.A.A.N.

Professor of Nursing, New York University

EDWARD G. LAKATTA, M.D.

Chief, Laboratory of Cardiovascular Science, National Institute on Aging

JOHN E. MORLEY, M.B., B.Ch.

Dammert Professor of Gerontology, Division of Geriatric Medicine, Saint Louis University Health Sciences Center; Geriatric Research, Education and Clinical Center, Saint Louis VA Medical Center

MARY E. TINETTI, M.D.

Professor of Medicine and Epidemiology and Public Health, Yale University

CONSULTANTS AND ACKNOWLEDGMENTS

CONSULTANTS

MARQUETTE CANNON-BABB, Pharm.D.
Assistant Dean for Admissions, Temple University School of Pharmacy

EUGENE P. FRENKEL, M.D.
Professor of Internal Medicine and Radiology, Patsy R. and Raymond D. Nasher Distinguished Chair in Cancer Research, and A. Kenneth Pye Professorship in Cancer Research, Division of Hematology-Oncology, Department of Medicine, The University of Texas Southwestern Medical Center at Dallas

MICHAEL R. JACOBS, Pharm.D.
Professor of Clinical Pharmacy, Temple University School of Pharmacy

DAVID F. POLAKOFF, M.D.
Instructor in Medicine, Harvard Medical School; Chief Medical Officer, Mariner Post-Acute Network

ACKNOWLEDGMENTS

We wish to express our appreciation to the following persons for their expert assistance in reviewing specific chapters:

Laurence Branch, Ph.D.   Professor of Gerontology, Duke University Center on Aging (*Demographics*)

Janice L. Feinberg, Pharm.D., J.D.   Executive Director, American Society of Consultant Pharmacists Research and Education Foundation (*Pharmacy*)

Harvey Lemont, D.P.M.   Professor, Section of Podiatric Medicine, Temple University School of Podiatric Medicine; Director, Laboratory of Podiatric Pathology (*Foot Disorders*)

G. Alec Rooke, M.D., Ph.D.   Associate Professor of Anesthesiology, University of Washington (*Anesthesia Considerations*)

G. Victor Rossi, Ph.D.   Leonard and Madlyn Abramson Professor of Pharmacology, Philadelphia College of Pharmacy, University of the Sciences in Philadelphia (*Clinical Pharmacology*)

CONTRIBUTORS

WENDY L. ADAMS, M.D., M.P.H.
Assistant Professor of Medicine, University of Nebraska Medical Center
Substance Abuse and Dependence

RONALD D. ADELMAN, M.D.
Associate Professor of Medicine, Weill Medical College of Cornell University
Elder Abuse

CATHY A. ALESSI, M.D.
Associate Professor of Medicine, University of California, Los Angeles; Geriatrician, Geriatric Research, Education and Clinical Center, VA Greater Los Angeles Healthcare System
Sleep Disorders

NEIL ALEXANDER, M.D.
Associate Professor of Internal and Geriatric Medicine, University of Michigan; Research Scientist, Ann Arbor VA Medical Center
Falls

W. McDOWELL ANDERSON, M.D.
Associate Professor of Medicine, University of South Florida; Chief, Pulmonary and Critical Medicine, James A. Haley VA Hospital
Aging and the Lungs

WILLIAM B. APPLEGATE, M.D.
Professor and Chairman, Department of Internal Medicine, Wake Forest University School of Medicine
Hypertension

WILBERT S. ARONOW, M.D.
Adjunct Professor of Geriatrics and Adult Development, Mount Sinai School of Medicine; Corporate Medical Director, Hebrew Hospital Home, Bronx and Westchester County
Coronary Artery Disease

MACK N. BARNES III, M.D.
Assistant Professor of Gynecology/Oncology, University of Alabama at Birmingham
Female Genital Disorders

NIR BARZILAI, M.D.
Associate Professor of Medicine, Diabetes Research Center, Albert Einstein College of Medicine
Disorders of Carbohydrate Metabolism

JANE BEAR-LEHMAN, Ph.D.
Assistant Professor of Clinical Occupational Therapy, Columbia University College of Physicians and Surgeons
Occupational Therapy

BARBARA ROE BECK, M.A.
Clinical Audiologist, Department of Communication Sciences and Disorders, Saint Louis University
Hearing Loss

DOUGLAS L. BECK, Au.D.
Clinical Audiologist; President, HearAmerica, Inc., St. Louis
Hearing Loss

RICHARD BECKER, M.D.
Professor of Medicine and Director, Coronary Care Unit and Cardiovascular Thrombosis Research Center, University of Massachusetts Medical School
Hypercoagulability and Anticoagulation

MARK H. BEERS, M.D.
Editor, THE MERCK MANUALS and Senior Director of Geriatrics, Merck & Co., Inc.; Associate Clinical Professor of Medicine, MCP Hahnemann School of Medicine
Behavior Disorders in Dementia

DAVID W. BENTLEY, M.D.
Professor of Internal Medicine, Division of Geriatric Medicine, Saint Louis University School of Medicine; Director, Geriatric Evaluation and Management Unit, Saint Louis VA Medical Center
Human Immunodeficiency Virus Infection

BARBARA BERKMAN, Ph.D.
Helen Rehr/Ruth Fizdale Professor of Health and Mental Health, Columbia University School of Social Work
Geriatric Social Work

RICHARD W. BESDINE, M.D.
Professor of Medicine and Director, University of Connecticut Center on Aging
Quality of Life and Therapeutic Objectives; Hyperthermia and Hypothermia

DAN G. BLAZER, M.D., Ph.D.
J. P. Gibbons Professor of Psychiatry and Behavioral Sciences, Duke University School of Medicine
Depression; Anxiety Disorders; Somatoform Disorders; Psychotic Disorders

MARIE L. BORUM, M.D., M.P.H.
Associate Professor of Medicine, The George Washington University Medical Center
Esophageal Disorders; Gastric Disorders; Malabsorption; Irritable Bowel Syndrome; Fecal Incontinence

CHAD BOULT, M.D., M.P.H.
Professor, Department of Family Practice and Community Health, University of Minnesota Medical School
Comprehensive Geriatric Assessment

RISA BRECKMAN, M.S.W.
Director of Social Work, New York Presbyterian Hospital, Wright Center on Aging
Elder Abuse

DAVID BUCHNER, M.D., M.P.H.
Professor, Department of Health Services, University of Washington, Seattle; Investigator, Northwest Center for Outcomes Research in Older Adults, VA Puget Sound Health Care System, Seattle
Exercise

ROBERT N. BUTLER, M.D.
Professor of Geriatrics and Adult Development, Mount Sinai School of Medicine; President, Chief Executive Officer, International Longevity Center
Sexuality

LOUIS R. CAPLAN, M.D.
Professor of Neurology, Harvard Medical School; Neurologist, Beth Israel Deaconess Medical Center
Cerebrovascular Disease

ANTONI CASTELLS, M.D.
Research Fellow, Massachusetts General Hospital, Harvard School of Medicine
Gastrointestinal Tumors

MELVIN CHEITLIN, M.D.
Professor of Medicine (Emeritus), University of California, San Francisco; former Chief of Cardiology, San Francisco General Hospital
Valvular Heart Disease; Infective Endocarditis

NOEL CHIU, M.D.
Department of Dermatology, Boston University School of Medicine
Aging and the Skin; Common Skin Disorders; Skin Cancers

GENE D. COHEN, M.D., Ph.D.
Director, Center on Aging, Health and Humanities, The George Washington University; Director, Washington DC Center on Aging
Aging and Mental Health

BARRY S. COLLET, D.P.M., M.P.H.
Consultant, Hebrew Rehabilitation Center for Aged, Boston; Consultant, Brockton Hospital
Foot Disorders

BARRY J. CUSACK, M.D.
Associate Professor of Medicine, Division of Gerontology and Geriatric Medicine, University of Washington, Seattle; Chief, Gerontology and Geriatric Medicine, VA Medical Center, Boise
Clinical Pharmacology

NANCY N. DUBLER, LL.B.
Professor of Bioethics, The Albert Einstein College of Medicine; Director, Division of Bioethics, Montefiore Medical Center
Legal and Ethical Issues

THEODORE C. EICKHOFF, M.D.
Professor of Medicine, Division of Infectious Disease, University of Colorado Health Sciences Center
Immunization

W. GARY ERWIN, Pharm.D.
Vice President, Health Systems Program, Omnicare, Inc., Radnor, PA
Pharmacy

WALTER H. ETTINGER, M.D.
Executive Vice President, Virtua Health, Marlton, NJ
Nonmetabolic Bone Disease; Local Joint, Tendon, and Bursa Disorders; Rheumatic Diseases; Vasculitic Syndromes

PAUL FADDEN, M.D.
Resident, Department of Surgery, Division of Urology, University of Wisconsin Medical School
Male Genital Disorders

BRUCE A. FERRELL, M.D.
Associate Professor of Medicine, University of California, Los Angeles; Clinical Director, Geriatric Research, Education and Clinical Center, VA Greater Los Angeles Healthcare System
Pain

HOWARD FILLIT, M.D.
Clinical Professor of Geriatrics and Medicine, The Mount Sinai Medical Center; Executive Director, The Institute for the Study of Aging, Inc.
Managed Care

JEROME L. FLEG, M.D.
Head, Human Cardiovascular Studies, Gerontology Research Center, National Institute on Aging
Diagnostic Evaluation; Arrhythmias and Conduction Disturbances

MARSHAL F. FOLSTEIN, M.D.
Francis Arkin Professor of Psychiatry and Chairman of Psychiatry, Tufts University School of Medicine and New England Medical Center
Mental Status Examination

SUSAN E. FOLSTEIN, M.D.
Professor of Psychiatry, Tufts University School of Medicine and New England Medical Center
Mental Status Examination

MICHAEL L. FREEDMAN, M.D.
The Diane and Arthur Belfer Professor of Geriatric Medicine, New York University School of Medicine; Director, The Diane and Arthur Belfer Geriatric Center, New York University Medical Center
Aging and the Blood; Anemias; Hematologic Malignancies; Lymphomas

SANDOR A. FRIEDMAN, M.D.
Professor of Medicine, State University of New York, Health Science Center at Brooklyn; Chairman, Department of Medicine, Coney Island Hospital
Peripheral Arterial Disease; Peripheral Venous Disease; Aneurysms

TERRY T. FULMER, Ph.D., R.N.
Professor of Nursing, New York University
Geriatric Interdisciplinary Teams; Nursing; Continuity of Care: Integration of Services

TOBIN N. GERHART, M.D.
Clinical Assistant Professor of Orthopaedic Surgery, Harvard University
Fractures

BARBARA A. GILCHREST, M.D.
Professor and Chairman of Dermatology, Boston University School of Medicine; Chief of Dermatology, Boston Medical Center
Aging and the Skin; Common Skin Disorders; Skin Cancers

JACK M. GURALNIK, M.D., Ph.D.
Chief, Epidemiology and Demography Office, National Institute on Aging
Demographics

RICHARD J. HAVLIK, M.D., M.P.H.
Associate Director, Epidemiology, Demography and Biometry Program, National Institute on Aging
Demographics

MICHAEL HOROWITZ, M.D.
Professor of Medicine, University of Adelaide; Director of Endocrine Unit, Royal Adelaide Hospital, Adelaide, South Australia
Aging and the Gastrointestinal Tract

KATHRYN HYER, Dr.P.A.
Faculty, University of South Florida, Department of Gerontology and Geriatric Interdisciplinary Team Training Project Director
Geriatric Interdisciplinary Teams; Home Health Care; Long-Term Care

MASAYOSHI ITOH, M.D., M.P.H.
Associate Professor of Clinical Rehabilitation, New York University; Senior Administrative Consultant, Goldwater Memorial Hospital
Rehabilitation; Rehabilitation for Specific Problems; Speech Disorders

HUGO E. JASIN, M.D.
Professor of Internal Medicine and Director, Division of Rheumatology, University of Arkansas for Medical Sciences
Diffuse Idiopathic Skeletal Hyperostosis

LARRY E. JOHNSON, M.D., Ph.D.
Associate Professor of Family and Community Medicine and Geriatric Medicine, University of Arkansas for Medical Sciences
Vitamin and Trace Mineral Disorders

ROBERT J. JOYNT, M.D., Ph.D.
Distinguished University Professor, University of Rochester; Professor of Neurology and Neurobiology and Anatomy, University of Rochester School of Medicine and Dentistry
Aging and the Nervous System

JAMES O. JUDGE, M.D.
Associate Professor of Medicine, University of Connecticut School of Medicine; Vice President for Medical Affairs, Masonicare
Gait Disorders

PAUL R. KAESBERG, M.D.
Clinical Assistant Professor of Medicine, Hematology/Oncology, University of Wisconsin
Cancer

FRAN E. KAISER, M.D.
Adjunct Professor of Medicine, Saint Louis University School of Medicine; Senior Medical Director, South Central Region, Merck & Co., Inc.
Sexual Dysfunction in Men; Sexual Dysfunction in Women

HOSAM KAMEL, M.D.
Assistant Professor of Medicine, State University of New York at Stony Brook School of Medicine; Chief, Division of Geriatric Medicine, Nassau County Medical Center
Human Immunodeficiency Virus Infection

WILLIAM B. KANNEL, M.D., M.P.H.
Professor of Medicine and Public Health, Boston University School of Medicine; Medical Director (Emeritus), Framingham Heart Study
Atherosclerosis

MARILYN C. KINCAID, M.D.
Clinical Professor of Ophthalmology and Pathology, Saint Louis University Eye Institute
Ocular Disorders

TALMADGE E. KING, JR., M.D.
Constance B. Wofsy Distinguished Professor, University of California, San Francisco; Chief, Medical Services, San Francisco General Hospital
Interstitial Lung Diseases

DALANE W. KITZMAN, M.D.
Associate Professor of Internal Medicine (Cardiology), Wake Forest University School of Medicine; Director of Echocardiography, Wake Forest University Baptist Medical Center
Heart Failure and Cardiomyopathy

HAROLD KLEINERT, M.D.
Clinical Professor of Surgery, University of Louisville School of Medicine
Hand Disorders

HAROLD G. KOENIG, M.D.
Associate Professor of Psychiatry, Duke University; Geriatric Research, Education and Clinical Center, VA Medical Center
Religion and Spirituality

JOYANN KROSER, M.D.
Assistant Professor of Medicine, Gastrointestinal Division, University of Pennsylvania
Gastrointestinal Tumors

MARK LACHS, M.D., M.P.H.
Co-Chief of Geriatric Medicine and Associate Professor of Medicine, Weill Medical College and School of the Graduate Medical Sciences of Cornell University; Medical Director for Geriatric Medicine, The New York Presbyterian Health System
Elder Abuse

EDWARD G. LAKATTA, M.D.
Chief, Laboratory of Cardiovascular Science, National Institute on Aging
Aging and the Cardiovascular System

MATHEW H. M. LEE, M.D.
Howard A. Rusk Professor, Department of Rehabilitation Medicine, New York University School of Medicine; Medical Director, Rusk Institute of Rehabilitation Medicine
Rehabilitation; Rehabilitation for Specific Problems; Speech Disorders

ROSANNE M. LEIPZIG, M.D., Ph.D.
Associate Professor and Vice Chair for Education, Department of Geriatrics and Adult Development, Mount Sinai School of Medicine
Breast Cancer

MYRNA LEWIS, M.S.W.
Assistant Clinical Professor, Department of Community and Preventive Medicine, Mount Sinai School of Medicine
Sexuality

ROBERT D. LINDEMAN, M.D.
Professor (Emeritus) and former Chief, Division of Gerontology, Department of Medicine, University of New Mexico School of Medicine
Aging and the Kidney; Renal Disorders

LEWIS A. LIPSITZ, M.D.
Associate Professor of Medicine, Harvard Medical School; Physician-in-Chief and Vice President of Medical Affairs, Hebrew Rehabilitation Center for Aged
Syncope; Hypotension

ELAN D. LOUIS, M.D.
Assistant Professor of Neurology, Gertrude H. Sergievsky Center, New York
Movement Disorders

BRUCE A. LUXON, M.D., Ph.D.
Associate Professor, Department of Internal Medicine, Saint Louis University School of Medicine
Liver and Biliary Disorders

JOANNE LYNN, M.D.
Professor of Health Care Sciences; Director, The Center to Improve Care of the Dying, George Washington University; President, Americans for Better Care of the Dying
Care of the Dying Patient

BARRY J. MAKE, M.D.
Professor of Medicine, University of Colorado School of Medicine; Director, Emphysema Center, National Jewish Medical and Research Center
Pulmonary Rehabilitation

STAVROS MANOLAGAS, M.D., Ph.D.
Professor of Medicine and Director, Division of Endocrinology and Metabolism, University of Arkansas for Medical Sciences
Aging and the Musculoskeletal System

EDWARD MARCANTONIO, M.D.
Assistant Professor of Medicine, Harvard Medical School; Director of Quality Assurance and Outcomes Research, Hebrew Rehabilitation Center for Aged
Delirium; Dementia

DANIEL McNALLY, M.D.
Associate Professor of Medicine and Acting Head, Division of Pulmonary Medicine, University of Connecticut School of Medicine
Respiratory Failure

JOHN R. MICHAEL, M.D.
Professor of Medicine and Director of Medical Intensive Care Unit, University of Utah
Pulmonary Embolism

JEAN-PIERRE MICHEL, M.D.
Chief, Department of Geriatrics, University of Geneva Medical School, Switzerland
Aging and the Immune System

DOUGLAS K. MILLER, M.D.
Professor of Geriatric Medicine and Associate Director, Division of Geriatric Medicine, Saint Louis University
Laboratory Values

PATRICIA A. MILLER, Ed.D., O.T.R.
Assistant Professor of Clinical Occupational Therapy and Public Health, Columbia University
Occupational Therapy

CHARLES V. MOBBS, M.D.
Associate Professor, Fishberg Center for Neurobiology, Mount Sinai School of Medicine
Biology of Aging

TIMOTHY D. MOON, M.D.
Professor of Surgery, Division of Urology, University of Wisconsin Medical School; Assistant Chief of Surgery, Chief of Urology, Madison VA Medical Center
Male Genital Disorders

JOHN E. MORLEY, M.B., B.Ch.
Dammert Professor of Gerontology, Division of Geriatric Medicine, Saint Louis University Health Sciences Center; Geriatric Research, Education and Clinical Center, Saint Louis VA Medical Center
Protein-Energy Undernutrition; Obesity; Hormonal Supplementation

RICHARD T. MOXLEY III, M.D.
Director, Neuromuscular Disease Center, University of Rochester
Muscular Disorders

DAVID H. NEUSTADT, M.D.
Clinical Professor of Medicine, University of Louisville School of Medicine
Hand Disorders

S. RAGNAR NORRBY, M.D., Ph.D.
Professor and Chairman, Department of Infectious Diseases and Medical Microbiology, University of Lund, Sweden
Antimicrobial Drugs

COLLEEN E. O'LEARY, M.D.
Associate Professor of Anesthesiology, State University of New York Health Science Center at Syracuse
Anesthesia Considerations

TERRENCE E. O'SHEA, B.S. Pharm, Pharm.D.
Regional Clinical Director, Omnicare, Inc., Englewood, OH
Pharmacy

JAMES T. PACALA, M.D.
Associate Professor, Program in Geriatrics and Director, Predoctoral Education, Department of Family Practice and Community Health, University of Minnesota
Prevention of Disease and Disability

MARILYN PAJK, R.N., M.S., M.P.H.
Director, Community Case Management, Beth Israel Deaconess Medical Center
Pressure Sores

LIDIA POUSADA, M.D.
Associate Professor of Clinical Medicine, New York Medical College; Chief, Division of Geriatrics and Gerontology, Sound Shore Medical Center
Hospitalization

CHARLENE M. PRATHER, M.D.
Assistant Professor of Internal Medicine, Saint Louis University Health Sciences Center
Constipation and Diarrhea

JACQUES PROUST, M.D.
Adjunct Professor, Department of Geriatrics, University of Geneva Medical School; Medical Director for Prevention of Aging, Clinique de Genolier, Switzerland
Aging and the Immune System

CHRISTINA M. PUCHALSKI, M.D.
Assistant Professor, Department of Medicine, Division of Geriatrics, The George Washington University Medical Center; Director of Education, National Institute for Healthcare Research
Care of the Dying Patient

LAWRENCE G. RAISZ, M.D.
Professor of Medicine, University of Connecticut School of Medicine; Program Director, Lowell P. Weicker, Jr., General Clinical Research Center
Metabolic Bone Disease; Disorders of Mineral Metabolism

SHOBITA RAJAGOPALAN, M.D.
Assistant Professor of Medicine, Division of Infectious Disease, Charles R. Drew University of Medicine and Science
Pulmonary Infections; Urinary Tract Infections

NEIL M. RESNICK, M.D.
Professor of Medicine and Chief, Division of Geriatric Medicine, University of Pittsburgh Medical Center
Urinary Incontinence

SHELDON M. RETCHIN, M.D., M.S.P.H.
Professor of Internal Medicine; President and Chief Executive Officer MCV Physicians; Associate Vice President for Clinical Enterprises, Virginia Commonwealth University
The Elderly Driver

HOLLY ELIZABETH RICHTER, Ph.D., M.D.
Assistant Professor, Division of Medical Surgical Gynecology, Department of Obstetrics and Gynecology, University of Alabama at Birmingham
Female Genital Disorders

MARK ROLFE, M.D.
Assistant Professor, Department of Internal Medicine, University of South Florida
Lung Cancer

ATENODORO MARCIANO R. RUIZ, JR., M.D.
Senior Fellow, Division of Gastorenterology, The George Washington University
Malabsorption

ANIL K. RUSTGI, M.D.
T. Grier Miller Associate Professor of Medicine and Genetics and Chief of Gastroenterology, University of Pennsylvania
Gastrointestinal Tumors

ARTHUR B. SANDERS, M.D.
Professor of Emergency Medicine, University of Arizona College of Medicine
Emergency Medical Care

ERIC W. SARGENT, M.D.
Director, Otology/Neurotology, Saint Louis University School of Medicine
Ear Disorders

ISAAC SCHIFF, M.D.
Joe Vincent Meigs Professor of Gynecology, Harvard Medical School; Chief, Vincent OB/GYN Service, Massachusetts General Hospital
Menopause; Estrogen Replacement Therapy

JOHN T. SCHULZ III, M.D., Ph.D.
Instructor in Surgery, Harvard Medical School; Burn, Trauma, and General Surgery, Massachusetts General Hospital; Staff Surgeon, Shriners Burns Hospital
Anorectal Disorders; Acute Abdomen and Surgical Gastroenterology

JONATHAN SHIP, D.M.D.
Professor and Vice Chair, Department of Oral Medicine/Pathology/Oncology, University of Michigan School of Dentistry; Director, Geriatric Dentistry/Oral Medicine Program
Dental and Oral Disorders

RAHMAWATI SIH, M.D.
Assistant Professor, Loyola University and Hines VA Medical Center
Lipoprotein Disorders

JEFFREY H. SILVERSTEIN, M.D.
Assistant Professor of Anesthesiology, Surgery, Geriatrics and Adult Development, Mount Sinai School of Medicine
Perioperative Care

DAVID H. SOLOMON, M.D.
Professor (Emeritus) of Medicine/Geriatrics, University of California, Los Angeles; Consultant, The RAND Corporation
Thyroid Disorders

AYALEW TEFFERI, M.D.
Associate Professor of Medicine, Mayo Medical School; Consultant, Division of Hematology and Internal Medicine, Mayo Clinic and Mayo Foundation
Chronic Myeloid Disorders

PETER B. TERRY, M.D.
Professor of Medicine, The Johns Hopkins Medical Institutions
Chronic Obstructive Pulmonary Disease

DAVID THOMAS, M.D.
Professor of Medicine, Saint Louis University Health Sciences Center
Surgery; Preoperative Evaluation

RANDALL C. THOMPSON, M.D.
Associate Professor, Clinical Medicine, University of Missouri, Kansas City; Consulting Cardiologist, Mid-America Heart Institute
Cardiovascular Surgery and Percutaneous Interventional Techniques

MARY E. TINETTI, M.D.
Professor of Medicine and Epidemiology and Public Health, Yale University
Chronic Dizziness and Postural Instability

MELVYN S. TOCKMAN, M.D., Ph.D.
Professor of Medicine, University of South Florida; Director, Molecular Screening Programs, H. Lee Moffitt Cancer Center and Research Institute
Aging and the Lungs; Lung Cancer

RONALD G. TOMPKINS, M.D., Sc.D.
John F. Burke Professor of Surgery, Harvard University; Visiting Surgeon, Massachusetts General Hospital
Anorectal Disorders; Acute Abdomen and Surgical Gastroenterology

NINA TUMOSA, Ph.D.
Associate Professor, Department of Internal Medicine, Division of Geriatrics, Saint Louis University Health Sciences Center; Health Care Education Specialist, Saint Louis VA Medical Center
Aging and the Eye

SHERMEEN B. VAKHARIA, M.D.
Assistant Professor of Anesthesiology, State University of New York Health Science Center at Syracuse
Anesthesia Considerations

ROBERT EDWARD VARNER, M.D.
Professor of Obstetrics and Gynecology, University of Alabama at Birmingham School of Medicine
Female Genital Disorders

ROBERT E. VESTAL, M.D.
Senior Medical Director, Early Clinical Development, Covance Inc., Walnut Creek, CA
Clinical Pharmacology

PANTEL S. VOKONAS, M.D.
Professor of Medicine and Public Health, Boston University School of Medicine; Director, Department of Veterans Affairs, Normative Aging Study
Atherosclerosis

ARNOLD WALD, M.D.
Professor of Medicine and Associate Chief, Gastroenterology and Hepatology, University of Pittsburgh
Lower Gastrointestinal Tract Disorders

BRIAN WALSH, M.D.
Assistant Professor, Obstetrics and Gynecology, Harvard Medical School; Director, Menopause Center, Brigham and Women's Hospital
Menopause; Estrogen Replacement Therapy

PHILIP J. WALTHER, M.D., Ph.D.
Professor of Surgery, Urology, and Pathology, Duke University School of Medicine
Urinary Tract Tumors

JEROME D. WAYE, M.D.
Clinical Professor of Medicine, Division of Gastroenterology and Chief, Gastrointestinal Endoscopy Unit, Mount Sinai Medical Center; Chief, Gastrointestinal Endoscopy Unit, Lenox Hill Hospital
Endoscopic Gastrointestinal Procedures

TERRIE WETLE, Ph.D.
Deputy Director, National Institute on Aging,
National Institutes of Health
Social Issues; Health Care Funding

T. FRANKLIN WILLIAMS, M.D.
Professor of Medicine (Emeritus), University
of Rochester; Attending Physician, Monroe
Community Hospital
History and Physical Examination

WILLIAM R. WILSON, M.D.
Director, Division of Otolaryngology, Head
and Neck Surgery, The George Washington
University Medical Center
Nose and Throat Disorders

THOMAS T. YOSHIKAWA, M.D.
Chairman, Department of Internal Medicine,
Charles R. Drew University of Medicine and
Science
Pulmonary Infections; Urinary Tract Infections

EDWARD T. ZAWADA, JR., M.D.
Freeman Professor and Chairman, Department
of Medicine, University of South Dakota; Med-
ical Director of Geriatrics, Sioux Valley Hospital
*Disorders of Water and Electrolyte Balance;
Disorders of Acid-Base Metabolism*

BASICS OF GERIATRIC CARE

1 BIOLOGY OF AGING

Aging: A process of gradual and spontaneous change, resulting in maturation through childhood, puberty, and young adulthood and then decline through middle and late age.

Senescence: The process by which the capacity for cell division, growth, and function is lost over time, ultimately leading to an incompatibility with life; ie, the process of senescence terminates in death.

Although aging has both the positive component of development and the negative component of decline, senescence refers only to the degenerative processes that ultimately make continued life impossible. Not all of the changes that occur with age—even those that occur in late life—are deleterious (eg, gray hair, baldness), and some may even be desirable (eg, increased wisdom and experience). The age-related increase in insulin levels and body fat that occurs in late life may be beneficial when available nutrition is limited. In contrast, the memory impairment that occurs with age is considered senescence. Senescence has no positive features.

Differentiating between normal aging and successful aging is useful. **Normal aging** refers to the common complex of diseases and impairments that characterize many of the elderly. However, persons age very differently: some acquire diseases and impairments, and others seem to escape specific diseases altogether and are said to have died of old age. The latter may maintain an active healthy life until death.

Successful (healthy) aging refers to a process by which deleterious effects are minimized, preserving function until senescence makes continued life impossible. Persons who age successfully avoid experiencing many of the unwanted features of aging. For example, they may avoid near-total tooth loss, which used to be (and is in some societies) usual and universal among the elderly. The elderly may be able to avoid the complications of vascular disease, even while the circulatory system continues to age, by controlling blood glucose levels and body fat percentage.

The concept of successful aging is that aging is not necessarily accompanied by debilitating disease and disability. Although the percentage of persons > 65 and the proportion of the elderly > 85 have both increased in the USA, the percentage of elderly persons residing in nursing homes has decreased (to 5.2%). Similarly, the percentage of persons aged 75 to 84 who report disabilities has decreased (to < 30%), as has the percentage of persons with debilitating disease. Although there may be alternative explanations for these changes in health status, one viable explanation is an increase in the proportion of persons who are aging successfully.

Disease vs. aging: In both aging and senescence, many physiologic functions decline, but normal decline is not usually considered the same as disease. The distinction between normal decline and disease is often but not always clear and may be due only to statistical distribution. Glucose intolerance is considered normal aging, but diabetes is considered a disease, although a very common one. The incidence and prevalence of type II diabetes increase with age, so that among persons > 75 years of age, > 10% have diabetes. Cognitive decline is nearly universal with advanced age and is considered normal aging; however, cognitive decline consistent with dementia, although common in late life, is considered a disease. Alzheimer's disease is a pathologic process distinct from normal aging, a conclusion supported by analysis of brain tissue at autopsy.

LONGEVITY

The average life span of Americans has been increasing dramatically since the industrial revolution. However, most of the gains resulted from decreasing childhood mortality. The maximum life span, generally determined to be about 125 years for women and somewhat shorter for men, has changed little in recorded history, although some experts suggest that it may be slowly increasing.

Several factors influence longevity. One is heredity. Heredity primarily influences whether an individual will contract a disease. Inheriting a propensity to hypercholesterolemia is likely to result in a short life, whereas inheriting genes that protect against heart disease and cancer helps ensure a long life. Medical treatment contributes to increased survival after diseases are contracted, especially when diseases (eg, infectious diseases, cancer) are curable. Another important influence on longevity is lifestyle; avoiding smoking, maintaining a healthy weight and diet, and exercising appropriately help people avoid disease. Exposure to environmental toxins can shorten life span even among people with the most robust genetic makeup.

CELLULAR AND MOLECULAR AGING

Cells lose their ability to divide over time unless they become cancerous. This limit to cellular replicative capacity (Hayflick's limit or phenomenon) can be demonstrated in fibroblasts removed from the umbilical cord of newborns and cultured in vitro. The fibroblasts divide only until they are dense enough to contact each other—a phenomenon called contact inhibition. If diluted, the fibroblasts divide again until maximum density is reached. This process can be repeated; however, after about 50 divisions, the fibroblasts stop dividing regardless of their density. Hayflick's limit is thought to reflect in vivo processes; fibroblasts removed from elderly persons tend to divide fewer times. Studies have shown that the loss of replicative capacity does not depend on the total amount of time cells are cultured (chronologic age) but on the number of divisions (biologic age).

When cells divide so many times that they cannot divide again, they enlarge and exist for some time before gradually dying. Such cells differ in morphology and function from young cells that are still dividing and from young cells whose division has been arrested by experimental manipulation.

One biologic mechanism for Hayflick's limit is now understood. Telomeres are stretches of DNA at the end of chromosomes that serve as handles by which chromosomes are moved during the telophase of meiosis. Telomeres are irreversibly shortened each time a cell divides. When the telomeres become too short, the cell can no longer divide.

In transformed (eg, cancerous) cells, the enzyme telomerase lengthens telomeres after telophase. The telomeres of transformed cells do not shorten after each division, and thus the cells become immortal, dividing far beyond Hayflick's limit. Normal postmitotic cells (except for fetal and germ cells) express telomerase in very small amounts, and their telomeres become shorter after each cell division.

The relevance of Hayflick's limit to senescence of the whole organism is unclear. Although some cells (eg, intestinal epithelial cells, skin fibroblasts) divide more or less continuously throughout life, they are unlikely to approach the limit of 50 divisions. Even if they did, the cells most likely to cause functional failure during senescence are probably those that divide very little (immune and endocrine cells) or not at all (neurons and muscle cells). Furthermore, senescence in metazoans composed entirely of postmitotic cells is just as predictable and robust as that in metazoans containing mitotic cells.

Mechanisms other than telomerase shortening may be involved in senescence. For example, messenger RNA (mRNA) transferred from senescent cells into young cells stops cell division in the young cells. The mRNA acts as a gerontogene (a gene mutation that increases life span), whose function may resemble that of a tumor suppressor gene (eg, *p53*). Mutations in *p53* lead to uncontrolled cell division, cancer, and often death of the organism. Mutations in gerontogenes extend the number of divisions in cells.

Necrosis and apoptosis: Cell death may occur by necrosis or apoptosis. Necrosis is due to physical or chemical insults (eg, metabolic inhibition, ischemia) that overwhelm normal cellular processes and make the cell nonviable. In necrosis, loss of ion gradients across the cell membrane leads to an influx of calcium and other ions, which triggers proteolysis and rupture of organelle membranes. Necrosis is a purely entropic phenomenon due to loss of the cell's ability to transform external energy.

In contrast, apoptosis is a highly regulated, orderly process by which a cell essentially commits suicide; usually, the stimulus for apoptosis is a physiologic signal or a very mild insult. A defining feature of apoptosis is the fragmentation of the cell's DNA, produced by a regulated activation of deoxyribonuclease. However, several other biochemical processes that also lead to cell death are simultaneously induced. Apoptosis is essential for normal development and remodeling.

Apoptosis has been implicated in several age-related diseases, including Alzheimer's disease. Whether age-related cell death is due primarily to necrosis or to apoptosis affects whether aging is considered the result of entropic processes (if due primarily to necrosis) or of relatively simpler, more regulated processes (if due primarily to apoptosis).

THEORIES OF AGING

There are more theories of aging than facts. Aging clearly occurs at different rates for different species, and even within a species, aging occurs at different rates among different individuals. The only reasonable conclusion is that aging must be genetically controlled, at least to some extent. Both within and between species, lifestyle and exposures may alter the aging process.

Most gerontologists view senescence as a collection of degenerative entropic processes related only by the fact that they occur over time. Some theories of aging address what controls these processes and why the controls exist as they do. Other theories of aging address the issues of whether senescence is more programmed than random entropy, thus offering some advantage for a species. For example, senescence may have evolved because without it, a species would accumulate ill-adapted older members. These members would compete with potentially better adapted younger members, slowing the rate at which adaptive mutations are introduced.

Loose cannon theory: This theory posits that an entropy-producing agent—free radicals or glucose—slowly disrupts cellular macromolecular constituents. Theoretically, free radicals, generated during oxidative phosphorylation, can variously modify macromolecules, primarily through oxidation. Considerable evidence suggests that oxidative damage increases with age. For example, in older organisms, specific amino acids in specific proteins tend to be oxidized residues, leading to decreases in the specific activity of these proteins. Additionally, specific oxidized derivatives of nucleotides from DNA increase in frequency. Experimentally induced simultaneous overexpression of superoxide dismutase and catalase (enzymes that attenuate free-radical damage) increases the life span of fruit flies by about 30%.

Glucose is thought to promote senescence mainly through nonenzymatic attachment to proteins and nucleic acids, through the same process that produces glycated hemoglobin. Glycated protein levels increase with age. Otherwise, there is little direct evidence that glycation has a major role in senescence. However, because dietary restriction increases maximum life span and also reduces blood glucose and the rate of glycation, interest in glycation's role in senescence continues.

Rate of living theory: This theory posits that smaller mammals tend to have high metabolic rates and thus tend to die at an earlier age than larger mammals. Thus, this theory is related to the idea that free radicals and other metabolic by-products play a role in senescence. However, studies of metabolic rates have shown wide variation in the correlation between size and longevity, undermining the credibility of this theory.

Weak link theory: This theory posits that a specific physiologic system—usually the neuroendocrine or immune system—is particularly vulnerable (presumably to entropic processes) during senescence. Failure of the weak system accelerates dysfunction of the whole organism. Failure of the neuroendocrine system would be expected to produce profound impairments in homeostatic systems, including loss of reproductive function and metabolic regulation, which occur with age. Failure of the immune system would be expected to produce an increased susceptibility to infection and a decreased ability to reject tumor cells. However, there is little evidence that failure of either system directly contributes to age-related diseases or to mortality (in contrast, for example, to the direct contribution of a compromised immune system to mortality in patients with AIDS). Furthermore, even if this theory explains some manifestations of aging in higher organisms, it does not explain aging in lower organisms, and little is known about the primary mechanism behind such weakness.

Error catastrophe theory: This theory posits that errors in DNA transcription or RNA translation eventually lead to genetic errors that promote senescence. Although data suggest that older organisms have altered proteins reflective of such genetic changes, this theory does little to explain most observed age-related changes.

Master clock theory: This theory is one of the oldest theories of aging and no longer has high credibility; it states that aging is under direct genetic control. Teleologically, it suggests that the rate of aging within each species has developed for the good of each species. Individual variation develops because of maladaption, exposure, and lifestyle. In the wild, such maladapted individuals tend to die out and the well-adapted ones persist, altering longevity in the best interest of the species.

Exactly what controls the rate of aging is unknown. It could be a gene that controls telomere shortening or some other process of cell division. Or it could be genetic control of another cellular process not involved in division, such as DNA repair, thus resulting in apoptosis.

DISEASES OF ACCELERATED AGING

Progeroid syndromes: In progeroid syndromes, which are rare, children exhibit several features similar to those normally observed in the elderly. These include baldness, osteoporosis, and dry, wrinkled skin. However, progeroid syndromes also include features that differ from normal senescent changes, such as lack of gonadal activity and unusually short stature. Thus, progeria is not exactly a model of accelerated aging.

Werner's syndrome produces sclerodermal skin changes and baldness, which make affected children appear elderly, producing an immediate sense of premature aging. Other features include premature cataracts, muscular atrophy, glucose intolerance, a high incidence of cancers (some of which are rare in unaffected persons), and early death due to atherosclerosis. However, the central nervous system is largely spared. The gene involved in Werner's syndrome codes for a DNA helicase, an enzyme that unwinds DNA to allow replication and possibly transcription. This discovery has led to speculation that during normal senescence, many age-related impairments may result from impairments in the helicase mechanism, although this hypothesis has not been studied systematically.

Wiedemann-Rautenstrauch syndrome and **Hutchinson-Gilford syndrome** also produce premature scleroderma, baldness, and other senile pathologies in children. The genetic basis of these syndromes remains undetermined.

Down syndrome: More common than the progeroid syndromes, Down syndrome also produces pathologies typical of senescence, including glucose intolerance, vascular disease, a high incidence of cancers, hair loss, degenerative bone disease, and premature death. In contrast to Werner's syndrome, Down syndrome greatly impairs the central nervous system, usually producing retardation and accelerating the accretion of neuritic plaques and neurofibrillary tangles characteristic of Alzheimer's disease. Because Down syndrome results from duplication of all or a small part of chromosome 21, its cause was originally thought to be duplication of the gene for β-amyloid. Mutations of this gene, located on chromosome 21, have been implicated in Alzheimer's disease. However, although the duplicated region that produces Down syndrome is near the β-amyloid gene, the best evidence suggests that Down syndrome may occur without duplication of the β-amyloid gene. The specific gene or genes involved in Down syndrome remain undetermined.

2 ■ DEMOGRAPHICS

The statistical characteristics of human populations.

As the geriatric population grows in the USA and worldwide, demographics is an important tool in the development of policies on aging.

U.S. DEMOGRAPHICS

POPULATION CHARACTERISTICS

Between 1900 and 1990, the total U.S. population increased three-fold, while the population of persons ≥ 65 years increased tenfold. In 1990, more than 31 million Americans were ≥ 65, nearly twice as many as in 1960 (see TABLE 2–1). This number is estimated to reach almost 35 million by 2000, > 53 million by 2020, and > 75 million by 2040.

TABLE 2–1.   ACTUAL AND PROJECTED GROWTH OF THE ELDERLY POPULATION*

Year	Total Population (all ages)	≥ 65 Years		≥ 85 Years	
		Number	% of Total	Number	% of ≥ 65
1960	179,323	16,560	9.2	929	5.6
1980	226,546	25,550	11.3	2,240	8.8
1990	248,710	31,079	12.5	3,021	9.7
2000	274,634	34,709	12.6	4,259	12.3
2020	322,742	53,220	16.5	6,460	12.1
2040	369,980	75,233	20.6	13,552	18.0

*Numbers in thousands.
From Day JC: "Population projections of the United States, by age, sex, race, and Hispanic origin: 1995 to 2050." *Current Population Reports* Series P25, No. 1130. Washington, DC, U.S. Government Printing Office, 1996.

The proportion of the total population $\geq$ 65 is projected to grow from about 12.5% in 1996 to about 20% by 2040.

One of the fastest growing segments of the population, the oldest old (persons $\geq$ 85), accounts for about 12% of all elderly and is projected to account for 18% by 2040. The subgroup of centenarians is increasing relatively faster and is expected to increase from 57,000 persons in 1996 to 447,000 in 2040. Per capita costs for acute and long-term health care services are highest for persons $\geq$ 85, so the growth of this population segment will markedly affect health care costs.

Like the total U.S. population, the older U.S. population is more racially diverse than in the past. From 1980 to 1990, the older segment of the population increased by about 20% among blacks and whites, by 57% among Hispanics, and by 150% among Asians. In 1994, 11% of the older population was nonwhite or Hispanic; this proportion is expected to increase to about 31% by 2040.

In the second half of the 20th century, the mortality rate for older women declined more rapidly than that for older men. Among persons $\geq$ 65 in 1950, there were 89 men for every 100 women. By 2000, there will be 70 men for every 100 women. For those $\geq$ 85, there will be 41 men for every 100 women.

The rate of widowhood varies by age, sex, and race. Sixty percent of women aged 75 to 84 are widowed. Of persons $\geq$ 85, black women have the highest rate of widowhood (82%); white men have the lowest (31%).

Living arrangements vary greatly with age and sex among community-dwelling persons $\geq$ 65 (see FIGURE 2–1). At ages 65 to 74, one third of women live alone; after age 75, more than one half of women live alone. Before age 85, the elderly seldom live with nonrelatives or with relatives other than a spouse; after age 85, 18% of men and 28% of women living in the community do so.

As the proportion of older to younger persons increases, less financial and social support will be available for the elderly. The elderly support ratio was 1:5 in 1995 (there were 20.9 persons $\geq$ 65 for every 100 persons aged 18 to 64). This ratio is expected to remain stable through 2010 and then to begin increasing steadily—a result of the baby boom generation's reaching age 65 and the low birth rates of the 1960s and 1970s. Between 2030 and 2040, this ratio is projected to exceed 1:3 (35 persons $\geq$ 65 for every 100 persons aged 18 to 64).

The geographic distribution and migration patterns of the elderly in the USA have important implications for medical and long-term care services. In 1994, more than 3 million persons $\geq$ 65 lived in California, more than 2 million lived in New York and Florida, and more than 1 million lived in Pennsylvania, Texas, Illinois, Ohio, Michigan, and New Jersey. States with the highest proportion of persons $\geq$ 65 ($\geq$ 14%) were, in decreasing order, Florida, Rhode Island, Pennsylvania, North

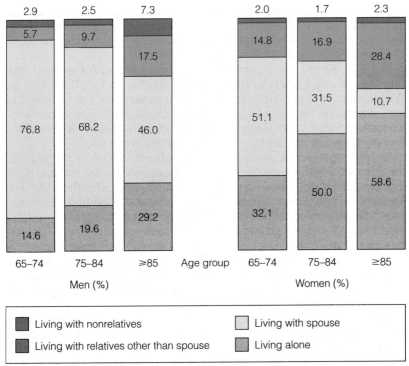

FIGURE 2–1.   **Living arrangements of community-dwelling persons ≥ 65: United States, 1997.** (From Kramarow E, Lentzner H, Rooks R, et al: Health and Aging Chartbook. Health, United States, 1999. Hyattsville, Maryland, National Center for Health Statistics, 1999, pp. 25 and 86.)

Dakota, South Dakota, Nebraska, Iowa, Missouri, Arkansas, Connecticut, and Massachusetts.

The number of elderly persons in all states increased in the 1980s. Between 1980 and 1990, the greatest percentage increases occurred in Nevada (94.1%), Alaska (93.7%), Hawaii (64.2%), Arizona (55.8%), New Mexico (40.7%), and Florida (40.4%). Many elderly persons move to Florida; the high proportion of elderly persons living in the other states results primarily from younger persons moving out of these states. The regional relocation of persons < 75 to the South and West has occurred since the 1960s and that of persons ≥ 75 since the 1970s.

MORTALITY AND MORBIDITY

Life expectancy at all ages has increased dramatically during the 20th century (eg, by 14 years between 1900 and 1940). Gains for persons

≥ 65 have occurred mainly since 1940. Life expectancy at age 65 increased nearly 2 years between 1940 and 1954, remained stable between 1954 and 1968, and increased steadily by 2.9 years between 1968 and 1996—from 14.6 years to 17.5 years.

In 1996, overall life expectancy was 6 years longer for women than for men; among blacks, women lived 8 years longer (see TABLE 2–2). With increasing age, the difference in life expectancy for women and men decreased—to about 1 year at age 85. At birth, life expectancy was about 6 to 8 years longer for whites than for blacks; it was about 2 years longer at age 65 but was nearly equal at age 85.

In 1995, the overall mortality rate for persons ≥ 65 was 5%/year. Of the almost 1.7 million deaths in this age group, 36.3% were due to heart disease, 22.5% to cancer, and 8.2% to cerebrovascular diseases (see TABLE 2–3). However, because multiple chronic conditions are common, the cause of death is often arbitrarily assigned, especially for the oldest old. Physicians should therefore be more specific when completing death certificates. Useful cause-of-death statistics require accurate death certification, including a careful listing of the probable pathologic sequence of events with the underlying or likely cause listed on the certificate. In elderly patients with multiple diseases, other significant causes may need to be added.

Data for 1995 showed that mortality rates for heart disease, cerebrovascular diseases, and pneumonia and influenza increased exponentially after age 55. In contrast, those for cancer and chronic obstructive pulmonary disease increased only modestly after age 65. In persons ≥ 85, deaths from cerebrovascular diseases nearly equaled those from cancer; deaths from pneumonia and influenza surpassed those from chronic obstructive pulmonary disease and were the fourth leading cause of death (see FIGURE 2–2).

The increase in life expectancy for all age groups since the late 1960s is largely attributable to a substantial decrease in the number of deaths from heart disease and stroke. Between 1979 and 1995, the

TABLE 2–2.   LIFE EXPECTANCY IN 1996

Age	Male (years)			Female (years)		
	All	White	Black	All	White	Black
At birth	73.0	73.8	66.1	79.0	79.6	74.2
At 65 years	15.7	15.8	13.9	18.9	19.0	17.2
At 75 years	9.8	9.8	9.0	11.9	12.0	11.2
At 85 years	5.3	5.3	5.3	6.3	6.3	6.2

From Ventura SJ, Peters KD, Martin JA, Maurer JD: "Births and deaths: United States, 1996." *Monthly Vital Statistics Report* vol. 46, no. 12. Hyattsville, MD, Public Health Service, September 11, 1997.

TABLE 2–3.   LEADING CAUSES OF DEATH AMONG PERSONS ≥ 65 YEARS IN 1995

Cause of Death	Number of Deaths	Death Rate (per 100,000 population)	% of All Deaths in Persons ≥ 65 Years
Heart disease	615,426	1,835.3	36.3
Malignant neoplasms, including neoplasms of lymphatic and hematopoietic tissues	381,142	1,136.6	22.5
Cerebrovascular diseases	138,762	413.8	8.2
Chronic obstructive pulmonary disease and associated conditions	88,478	263.9	5.2
Pneumonia and influenza	74,297	221.6	4.4
Diabetes mellitus	44,452	132.6	2.6
Motor vehicle accidents	7,626	22.7	0.4
All other accidents and adverse effects, including therapeutic use of drugs	21,473	64.0	1.3
Alzheimer's disease	20,230	60.3	1.2
Nephritis, nephrotic syndrome, and nephrosis	20,182	60.2	1.2
Septicemia	16,899	50.4	1.0
All other causes, residual	265,359	791.4	15.7
Total	1,694,326	5,052.8	100.0

From Anderson RN, Kochanek KD, Murphy SL: "Report of final mortality statistics, 1995." *Monthly Vital Statistics Report* vol. 45, no. 11, suppl. 2, table 7. Hyattsville, MD, National Center for Health Statistics, 1997.

mortality rate for ischemic heart disease dropped 45% in persons aged 65 to 69, 45% in those 70 to 74, 41% in those 75 to 79, 36% in those 80 to 84, and 25% in those ≥ 85. The mortality rate for cerebrovascular diseases decreased 39 to 43% in persons aged 65 to 84 and 25% in those ≥ 85.

In contrast, the cancer mortality rate increased slightly. Between 1979 and 1995, it increased 5% in persons aged 65 to 69, 9% in those 70 to 74, 13% in those 75 to 79, 12% in those 80 to 84, and 20% in those ≥ 85. This increase may be partly explained by the decrease in heart disease and stroke mortality rates and by the postponement of onset of these diseases until very old age. As a result, more persons die of other diseases, such as cancer.

The incidence of newly diagnosed cancer increases for most cancers through age 75, then decreases for some cancers. At age ≥ 55, prostate cancer is the most common cancer in men and breast cancer is the most

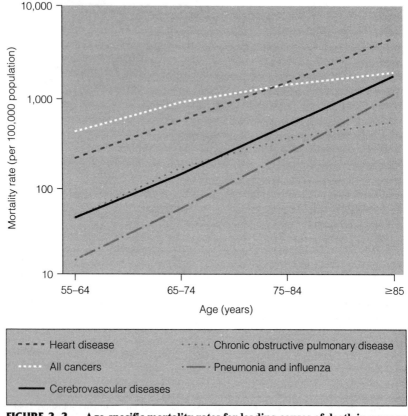

FIGURE 2–2.   **Age-specific mortality rates for leading causes of death in persons ≥ 55 in 1995.** (From National Center for Health Statistics: "Death rates for 72 selected causes, by 10-yr age groups, race, and sex: United States, 1995.")

common cancer in women. Lung cancer has the second highest incidence in men at all older ages and in women aged 55 to 75. Its incidence peaks in men aged 75 to 80 and in women in their early 70s. Historically, the oldest segments of the population have had relatively fewer smokers, because smokers tend to die of cancer or of other smoking-related diseases at younger ages. Thus, the decrease at the oldest ages may be a survival effect. Colon cancer is the third most common cancer in men aged 55 through 85 and in women aged 55 through 75, when its incidence surpasses that of lung cancer.

DISABILITY AND DISEASE

Disability and disease (chronic and/or multiple), which are prevalent in the elderly, greatly affect functioning level, independence, and the

TABLE 2–4.   MOST COMMONLY REPORTED CHRONIC CONDITIONS PER 1000 PERSONS ≥ 65 YEARS IN 1994

Condition	≥ 65 Years	65–74 Years	≥ 75 Years
Arthritis	501.5	476.9	536.6
Hypertension	364.0	347.2	388.0
Heart disease	324.9	281.2	387.3
Hearing impairment	286.4	234.6	360.4
Cataracts	166.2	113.0	242.4
Deformity or orthopedic impairment	165.6	154.1	182.1
Chronic sinusitis	151.2	150.1	152.5
Diabetes	101.2	101.6	100.8
Tinnitus	90.1	90.1	90.0
Visual impairment*	82.2	61.5	111.8

*Blindness or any other trouble seeing with one or both eyes, even with glasses. Corrected cataracts not included.

From Adams PF, Marano MA: "Current estimates from the National Health Interview Survey, 1994." *Vital Health Statistics* 10(193):83–84, 1995. Hyattsville, MD, National Center for Health Statistics.

need for long-term care. Functioning level is determined by the person's ability to perform activities of daily living (ADLs)—such as eating, dressing, bathing, transferring between bed and chair, and using the toilet—and instrumental ADLs (IADLs)—such as preparing meals, performing housework, taking drugs as instructed, going on errands, managing finances, and using a telephone.[1] About 5 to 8% of community-dwelling persons ≥ 65 need assistance with one or more ADLs. With aging, the proportion of the elderly who live at home but need assistance or who live in a nursing home increases markedly to 55% of women and 37% of men ≥ 85.

Chronic conditions that lead to disability include those that also commonly cause death (eg, heart disease, stroke, chronic obstructive pulmonary disease, diabetes) and those that are less likely to cause death but affect functioning (eg, arthritis, osteoporosis, vision and hearing loss). Of persons ≥ 65, one half report having arthritis, and one third report having hypertension, hearing impairment, or heart disease (see Table 2–4).

Comorbidity (the presence of concurrent multiple chronic diseases) becomes more prevalent with age, occurring in most of the oldest old. Disability similarly becomes more prevalent, increasing stepwise with age and with the number of chronic conditions. Developing effective interventions that prevent disease and reduce disability is critical for improving the quality of life of the elderly and controlling health care costs.

[1] see page 42

USE OF HEALTH CARE SERVICES

The demographic changes discussed above will have significant effects on the costs of health care services for the elderly.

HOSPITALIZATION

Persons ≥ 65 accounted for 12 million of the 31 million hospitalizations in the USA in 1995 and spent more than 78 million days in the hospital. Indeed, about 40% of hospital revenue comes from Medicare. In 1995, the leading causes of hospitalization for men and women ≥ 65 were heart disease and cancer. Following close behind were cerebrovascular disease and pneumonia for men and cerebrovascular disease, pneumonia, and fractures for women. For persons ≥ 85, the leading cause of hospitalization was heart disease, followed by pneumonia for men and fractures for women. Dehydration was the sixth leading cause for women ≥ 85.

Hospitalization rates progressively declined for cancer (owing at least partly to more outpatient procedures) and increased for pneumonia between 1981 and 1995. Hospitalization rates for benign prostatic hyperplasia decreased markedly between 1987 and 1995 (again, owing at least partly to more outpatient procedures).

Length of stay decreased dramatically between 1981 and 1995, mostly because of changes in reimbursement for hospitalization of Medicare patients. Decreases occurred in all disease categories for persons ≥ 65 and ≥ 85. A hospital stay that lasted 10 to 14 days in 1981 now lasts about 7 days.

In 1995, cardiac diagnostic and surgical procedures accounted for four of the five most common surgical procedures in the elderly. Based on hospital discharges, per 100,000 persons ≥ 65, there were 1,581 cardiac catheterizations, 954 coronary artery bypass graft surgeries, 762 pacemaker insertions, and 622 angioplasties. The rate for pacemaker insertions in persons ≥ 65 was eight times the rate in persons aged 45 to 64, and the rate for the other procedures was about twice that in the younger group. For persons ≥ 85, the most common procedures were pacemaker implantation (1,624 per 100,000 population) and open reduction of fracture with internal fixation (1,521 per 100,000 population).

OUTPATIENT VISITS

Persons ≥ 65 made more than 167 million visits to physicians' offices in 1995, representing 24% of all visits. Those aged 65 to 74 averaged 4.9 visits per year, and those ≥ 75 averaged 5.9 visits per year. According to the National Ambulatory Medical Care Survey, the most common reasons for visits were the following: general medical examination, postoperative examination, evaluation of vision dysfunction, blood pressure testing and evaluation of hypertension, and evaluation of cough. The most common diagnoses in those ≥ 65 were hypertension, diabetes, cataract, chronic ischemic heart disease, osteoarthritis and associated disorders, and glaucoma.

INSTITUTIONALIZATION

According to 1995 statistics, about 4% of the elderly (1% of those aged 65 to 74; 10% of men and 17% of women ≥ 85) live in nursing homes at any point in time. Of persons reaching age 65, 52% of women and 33% of men will spend some time in a nursing home. Of women who die after age 89, 70% have lived in a nursing home for at least some time. Of all persons living in nursing homes, 45% live there < 1 year, 55% ≥ 1 year, and 21% ≥ 5 years.

About 97% of nursing home residents receive assistance with one or more ADLs, 57% have difficulty controlling bowels or bladder, 65% use a wheelchair, and 25% use a walker. Risk factors for institutionalization include being widowed, living alone, having reduced family and social support, having a reduced income, being mentally disoriented or cognitively impaired, having multiple chronic conditions, and needing assistance with ADLs or IADLs or with ambulation.

Nursing home admission rates are lower for blacks than for whites, suggesting that such factors as cultural preferences and access to care may affect admission. The primary sources of payment for nursing home residents are Medicaid (55.7%); private insurance, personal income, and family support (28.9%); Medicare (12.7%); and other government assistance and charity (2.7%).

LAST YEAR OF LIFE

Of total Medicare expenditures for a given year, > 25% are for services during enrollees' last year of life, with half this amount spent in the last 60 days. Health care expenditures for enrollees during their last year are seven times higher than those for other enrollees; however, Medicare pays for only about one third of these expenses. Importantly, expenditures before death are less among the oldest old than the rest of the elderly population. Expenditures during the last year of life also relate to the cause of death; eg, Medicare expenditures are about twice as high for persons dying of cancer as for those dying of heart or cerebrovascular disease.

WORLD DEMOGRAPHICS

POPULATION CHARACTERISTICS

The world's population is aging. In Italy and Greece, > 22% of the population is ≥ 60, compared with 16.5% in the USA (see FIGURE 2–3). From 1996 to 2025, the percentage of persons ≥ 60 is expected to

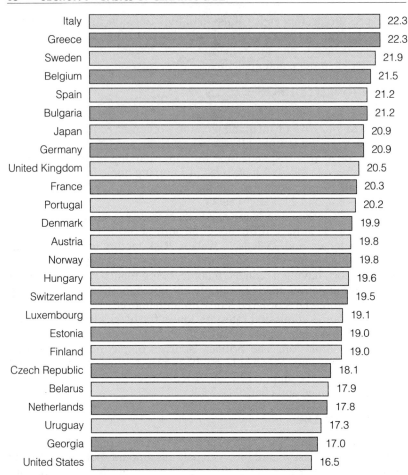

FIGURE 2–3.   The world's oldest countries, with percentage of population ≥ 60 years in 1996. (From U.S. Bureau of the Census, International Programs Center, International Data Base, 1996.)

increase by 17 to 82% in European countries and by about 200% in some developing countries (see TABLE 2–5). By 2025, Italy and Japan are expected to have the highest proportion of persons ≥ 60—nearly one third of the population. However, because developing countries such as China and India have the largest total populations, they have and will continue to have the largest absolute number of elderly persons. In 1996, the greatest number of persons ≥ 75 lived in China, followed by the USA and India. By 2020, the world's population is expected to include more than 1 billion persons ≥ 60, most living in developing rather than in developed countries.

TABLE 2–5.   LIFE EXPECTANCY AND POPULATION ≥ 60 YEARS
IN 1996 AND PROJECTED POPULATION GROWTH THROUGH 2025
FOR SELECTED COUNTRIES

Continent	1996 Life Expectancy at Birth		1996 Population ≥ 60 Years (thousands)	1996 % of Total Population ≥ 60 Years	2025 % of Total Population ≥ 60 Years	1996–2025 % Increase in Population ≥ 60 Years
	Males	Females				
North America						
Canada	76	83	4,765	16.5	28.1	111
Mexico	70	77	6,209	6.5	12.9	198
USA	73	79	43,873	16.5	24.6	88
South America						
Argentina	68	75	4,698	13.6	16.8	59
Brazil	57	67	11,636	7.2	15.5	164
Colombia	70	76	2,514	6.8	16.7	240
Peru	67	71	1,664	6.8	14.1	193
Venezuela	69	75	1,409	6.4	14.2	227
Europe						
France	74	82	11,777	20.3	30.0	55
Germany	73	79	17,423	20.9	31.6	59
Ireland	73	78	541	15.2	24.1	60
Italy	75	81	12,833	22.3	33.0	40
Netherlands	75	81	2,772	17.8	30.8	82
Poland	68	76	6,153	15.9	24.1	60
Romania	66	74	3,953	18.3	23.2	17
Ukraine	62	72	9,677	19.0	23.8	20
Africa						
Egypt	60	63	3,698	5.8	10.0	164
Ethiopia	46	48	2,528	4.4	4.3	92
Morocco	68	72	1,920	6.4	11.8	191
Tanzania	41	44	1,329	4.6	4.3	39
South Africa	57	62	2,782	6.7	10.4	102
Asia						
Bangladesh	56	56	6,296	5.1	9.5	173
China	68	71	115,215	9.5	20.3	152
India	59	60	61,903	6.5	12.2	167
Indonesia	60	64	12,994	6.3	13.1	191
Japan	77	83	26,248	20.9	32.9	51
Pakistan	58	59	7,928	6.1	8.4	123
South Korea	70	77	4,274	9.4	23.4	198
Thailand	65	72	5,130	8.7	20.1	176
Turkey	70	74	5,133	8.2	15.5	171
Australia	76	83	2,931	16.0	26.6	102

From U.S. Bureau of the Census, International Programs Center, International Database, 1996.

The exceptional growth in the percentage of the elderly worldwide is related to the following factors: the substantial decrease in birth rates during the past 20 years in many countries, the migration of younger persons out of certain areas because of economic reasons, and the decrease in overall mortality, including that due to infectious diseases in developing countries and that due to coronary artery disease and stroke in European and other developed countries. In the USA, Canada, and Australia, mortality due to coronary artery disease has decreased by an average of 50% over the past 25 years.

MORTALITY AND MORBIDITY

In the USA, about 70% of all deaths occur after age 65. By 2025, the percentage of deaths postponed to older age is expected to increase for the rest of the world, with > 60% of all deaths occurring after age 65 and > 40% after age 75.

In most countries, the decline in total mortality rate is well documented, but **causes of death,** especially at older ages, vary from country to country. Rates of coronary artery disease, the most common cause of death, vary worldwide. In 1990, the rate was ≥ 2,000 per 100,000 men ≥ 65 in Ireland, Finland, Denmark, the United Kingdom, New Zealand, and the former Soviet Union and was < 700 per 100,000 men in Spain, France, China, Japan, and Hong Kong. Lower rates but similar disparities occurred in women. In Europe, stroke mortality ranged from a low of 494 per 100,000 men ≥ 65 in France to a high of 1,954 per 100,000 men in Portugal, with rates in the Americas and the western Pacific region within this range. Because information on death in the oldest old is relatively rare, cooperation among countries is needed to collect and compare data, so that the causes of extreme longevity can be better understood.

Life expectancy, using mortality data for 1996, is longest for Canadian, Japanese, and Australian women (see TABLE 2–5). In most countries, men have shorter life expectancies. However, in some developing countries (eg, India, Bangladesh), life expectancy for men and women is nearly identical.

In countries such as those of the former Soviet Union, life expectancy decreased by about 4 years in the early 1990s, probably related to an increase in the incidence of fatal diseases that are alcohol- or cigarette-related and to social and economic disruptions. The ramifications for the elderly in these countries are uncertain, but mortality for this group has increased.

Although life expectancy in the USA is not the longest in the world, persons reaching old age in the USA live longer than elderly persons in other countries. By age 80 in women, life expectancy is 9.1 years, which is longer than life expectancy in Japan, Sweden, France, and England (see TABLE 2–6). Life expectancy is longer for older men in

TABLE 2–6.   COMPARISONS OF LIFE EXPECTANCY AT AGE 80*

Birth Cohort or Year	Number of Years				
	USA†	Japan	Sweden	France	England
Women 1880–1884	8.1	6.1	6.8	6.9	6.2
1885–1889	8.6	6.5	7.2	7.1	7.0
1890–1894	9.6	7.0	7.5	7.5	7.3
1987	9.1	8.5	8.3	8.6	8.1
Men 1880–1884	6.8	5.1	6.0	5.6	5.5
1885–1889	9.9	5.4	6.1	5.8	5.6
1890–1894	7.1	5.9	6.1	6.0	5.6
1987	7.0	6.9	6.5	6.7	6.2

*Data for England include data for Wales. Data for Sweden in 1987 represent the average for 1985 to 1989. Data for Japan, Sweden, France, and England are from the Dense Archive of Population Data on Aging, Dense University Medical School, Denmark. Data for U.S. cohorts are from individual death records for 1962 to 1990. The 1987 U.S. data were calculated from period life tables in Actuarial Study 107 of the Social Security Administration. All differences in life expectancies for cohort and cross-sectional comparisons of the USA with the other four countries were significant ($P < 0.01$), except the differences in survival probabilities between U.S. and Japanese men at age 80 in 1987 ($P > 0.10$).
† Whites only.
Adapted from Manton KG, Vaupel JW: "Survival after the age of 80 in the United States, Sweden, France, England, and Japan." *New England Journal of Medicine* 333:1232–1235, 1995.

the USA as well. Cohort life table analyses from earlier birth cohorts, now dead, showed a similar advantage in life expectancy at very old ages in the USA. The absolute life expectancy is shorter for men than for women in the USA, Japan, Sweden, France, and England.

Active or disability-free life expectancy (the average number of years a person is likely to remain in an active or nondisabled state) is calculated using life table techniques that consider all possible transitions in and out of the disabled state. The concept of active life expectancy has expanded to include higher orders of functioning, such as cognitive (eg, dementia-free) life expectancy. The active life expectancy in certain U.S. communities appears to vary from 11.3 to 13.0 years for men and from 15.3 to 17.1 years for women at age 65. Japan appears to have a slightly longer active life expectancy of 14.7 years for men and 17.7 years for women. However, the usual self-reported measures of physical disability can be interpreted differently from country to country, so variability may be due to methodologic differences. For all countries studied, physical disability, as measured by difficulty with ADLs, increases with age. The goal of medical care is to maintain physical functioning as long as possible and to postpone the onset of disability close to the time of death (referred to as compression of morbidity or squaring of the morbidity curve).

USE OF HEALTH CARE SERVICES

As the number of elderly persons increases, the global burden of age-associated chronic conditions, such as cardiovascular disease, hip fracture, and Alzheimer's disease, also increases. Persons with these conditions are likely to need more medical services and home or institutional care. For example, hip fractures commonly cause physical limitation, hospitalization, continuing morbidity, and excess mortality. In a comparison of hip fracture rates in six countries, rates were high but somewhat variable. Rates were based on national hospital discharge data and corrected for national differences in counting transfers between hospitals. The rates increased with age and were higher in women than men. Age-adjusted hip fracture rates were highest in Finland, the USA, and Sweden for men and in Switzerland, the USA, and Scotland for women. The rates were lowest in Venezuela and Chile.

The proportion of all persons hospitalized each year varies widely throughout industrialized countries. In 1996, the highest rates of hospitalization were in Austria, Finland, and Iceland (1 in 4 persons); the lowest rates of hospitalization were in Japan (1 in 10) and in Mexico (1 in 17). The median for industrialized countries was 1 in 6 persons hospitalized (1 in 8 in the USA). The average inpatient stay also varies widely; in 1996, the average was 10.6 days. Japan and the Netherlands had the highest average stay of > 32 days, and Denmark, Ireland, Mexico, New Zealand, Sweden, Turkey, and the USA had the lowest average stay of < 8 days. The average daily hospital expenditures were > $1000 in the USA, $632 in Denmark, and between $300 and $500 in Canada, Spain, Italy, and the United Kingdom. The lowest daily hospital expenditures were between $100 and $200 in Iceland, Luxembourg, Finland, Greece, Norway, Korea, and Austria and < $100 in Japan, the Czech Republic, and Turkey.

INSTITUTIONALIZATION

Hip fractures and physical disabilities affect the need for institutionalization, but the most important factor by far is cognitive disability. The prevalence of institutionalization for those ≥ 65 ranges from about 2 to 8% in various countries (see TABLE 2–7); the prevalence of community living is higher. Sources for nursing home admissions also vary. In the USA, Netherlands, and Italy, most admissions result from previous hospitalizations, possibly because of these countries' reimbursement systems or, more likely, because of social factors.

The U.S. government's Minimum Data Set and Resident Assessment Instrument is used in nursing homes in the USA and is being adapted for other countries. As the use of this instrument expands, it may help determine whether governmental policies, declining acceptance of responsibility by adult children for their parents, or other social factors

TABLE 2–7. COMPARISON OF LONG-TERM CARE USE BY COUNTRY

	% of Persons ≥ 65 Years in		% of Low Care Cases	Source of Nursing Home Admission (%)		
	Nursing home	Community		Home	Other long-term care facility	Hospital
USA	5.0	1.5	30.0	34.9	16.6	41.7
Denmark	4.0	10.5*	42.3	62.2	11.5	14.5
Iceland	8.0	5.0	51.6	68.0	7.1	13.0
Italy	< 2.0	1.0	37.3	51.1	1.9	35.8
Japan	1.5	0.5	51.0	44.5	47.5	4.2
Sweden	2.0	3.0	26.9	—	—	—
Netherlands	2.5	6.5	—	34.6	2.8	49.5
United Kingdom	2.0	3.5†	—	—	—	—
France	2.0‡	4.0	—	—	—	—

* Includes sheltered housing and special dwellings for the elderly.
† Includes some young disabled.
‡ No facilities described as nursing homes; 2% of elderly live in nursing home–like facilities.
Adapted from Ribbe MW, et al: "Nursing homes in 10 nations: A comparison between countries and settings." *Age and Ageing* 26-S2:3–12, 1997; Ikegami N, et al: "Low-care cases in long-term care settings: Variation among nations." *Age and Ageing* 26-S2:67–71, 1997; Frijters DH, et al: "Transitions across various continuing care settings." *Age and Ageing* 26-S2:73–76, 1997.

affect the need for long-term care programs, such as nursing homes and home care.

WORK AND PENSIONS

An indirect but important factor in healthy aging is the financial consequences of retirement. Practices concerning labor force participation, retirement, and pensions vary by country. In 1992, the percentages of persons > 65 participating in the labor force (economically active) were 5.5% in Italy and 3.5% in France; for men only, they were 15.5% in the USA and 16.5% in Ireland. However, although they participated in the potential labor pool, these persons might not have been working at any particular time. Such regional differences in definitions of those who are working make comparisons of the effects of retirement more difficult. Some countries have comprehensive pension programs; others have hardly any coverage. In the USA and United Kingdom, nearly 100% of working persons are covered by Social Security or other pensions, but in China and India, ≤ 20% are covered. Some governments are beginning to understand the importance of pension coverage. For example, in 1989, the government of Japan established the Gold Plan, a legislated program that provides a regular source of revenue that can be used only for evaluating and solving aging-related problems.

HISTORY AND PHYSICAL EXAMINATION

The approach to the history and physical examination sometimes needs to be modified in the assessment of a very old or frail patient. A physician may need to interview the patient and the caregiver separately. The physical examination may have to be performed at a different time than the interview because of patient fatigue; in addition, physical examination may require two sessions. Because a complete history may not be obtainable, the physician may need to focus more on the physical examination.

HISTORY

Physicians often need to spend more time interviewing and evaluating elderly patients than they would younger patients. Elderly patients may present with many nonspecific symptoms, making it difficult to focus the interview. Sensory deficits (eg, hearing or vision loss), common in the elderly, can also interfere with the interview process. Elderly patients may underreport symptoms (eg, dyspnea, hearing or vision loss, problems with memory, incontinence, gait disturbance, constipation, dizziness, falls), which they consider a part of normal aging. However, no symptom should be attributed to normal aging.

In elderly patients, clinical features of diseases may differ from those in younger patients.◼ For example, diseases may manifest solely as functional decline. In such cases, standard questions may not apply (eg, a patient with both arthritis and coronary artery disease whose mobility is severely limited by arthritis may not report dyspnea or chest pain on exertion, even if severe). Questions pertaining to the duration of functional decline can add useful information (eg, "How long have you been unable to do your own shopping?").

Because of cognitive dysfunction, elderly patients may have difficulty recalling all past illnesses, hospitalizations, operations, and drug use; the physician may have to obtain these data from an alternative source (eg, family member, home health aide, medical records). However, the patient's chief complaint may differ from what the family views as the main problem.

Approach to the interview: A physician's knowledge of the everyday concerns, social circumstances, and psychology of elderly persons helps orient and guide the interview. Traditionally, physicians use the chief complaint as the focal point of the interview. However, this highly structured approach may be too limiting for elderly patients. Instead, having the

---

◼ see page 38

patient describe a typical day reveals information about quality of life, liveliness of thought, and physical independence. This approach is especially useful during the first meeting, whether in an emergency room, a hospital, or a nursing home. Allowing the patient to speak with pride about a long life, accomplishments, and things of personal importance leads to physician-patient rapport. A good relationship with the patient helps the physician when communicating with family members or obtaining adherence with treatment.

Often, illness can be detected by verbal and nonverbal clues (eg, the way the story is told, tempo of speech, tone of voice, eye contact). An elderly person may omit or deny symptoms of anxiety or depression, yet betray them with a lowered voice, subdued enthusiasm, or even tears. A patient's comments about sleep and appetite may reveal information about physical and mental health. A change in the fit of clothing or dentures may indicate weight gain or loss. Also important are the patient's personal hygiene and dress, the person who accompanies the patient, and the patient's preference about having that person talk during the interview.

Patients should be fully clothed during the interview. A patient who wears dentures, eyeglasses, or a hearing aid should wear it to facilitate communication. To overcome communication problems due to the patient's hearing or vision loss, the interviewer moves close to the patient, faces the patient directly, and speaks clearly and slowly to allow lipreading. Shouting at the patient does not help because age-related stiffening of the tympanic membrane and ear ossicles distorts high-volume sound. Using a stethoscope in reverse (speaking into the stethoscope like a microphone while the patient wears the earpiece) may be helpful.

A mental status examination may be necessary early in the interview for determining the patient's historical reliability;◪ this examination is conducted tactfully so the patient does not become embarrassed, offended, or defensive, especially if a relative is present. Unless directed by the physician, a person accompanying the patient does not answer the questions.

Some patients prefer to have a relative present; however, unless mental status is impaired, the patient is interviewed alone to encourage the discussion of personal matters. The physician should not invite a relative to be present without asking the patient's permission, because doing so implies that the patient is incapable of providing a complete history. Asking the patient to wait outside while a relative or friend is interviewed can damage the physician-patient relationship.

Past medical history: When reviewing past medical illnesses, the physician asks the patient about diseases that used to be more common (eg, rheumatic fever, poliomyelitis) and about outdated treatments (eg, pneumothorax therapy for tuberculosis, mercury for syphilis). A history of immunizations (eg, tetanus, influenza, pneumococcus), adverse reactions to immunizations, and skin test results for tuberculosis is obtained. If the patient recalls having surgery but does not remember the procedure or its purpose, surgical records can be sought.

Other medical illnesses and complaints are reviewed systematically (see TABLE 3–1).

Drug history: The physician records the drug history—a flow sheet is often useful—and gives a copy to the patient or caregiver. The drug history includes determining which drugs are used, at what dose, how often they are taken, who prescribed them, and for what reason. Topical drugs must be included; eg, eyedrops for treating glaucoma are absorbed systemically, producing cardiovascular, pulmonary, or central nervous system effects that may be comparable to IV dosing. Over-the-counter drugs must be included because their overuse can have serious consequences (eg, constipation from laxative use, salicylism from aspirin use). The precise nature of any drug allergies should be determined.

Sometimes, asking the patient or family members to bring in all of the pills, ointments, or liquids in the patient's medicine cabinet is best. However, possession of current prescription drugs does not guarantee that the patient is complying with treatment. Counting the number of tablets in each vial on the first and subsequent visits may be necessary. If drugs are administered by someone other than the patient, then that person is interviewed.

Patients should demonstrate their ability to read labels (often printed in small type) and open vials (especially the child-resistant type). They should demonstrate their ability to recognize drugs, which may be difficult to differentiate if they have combined them into one vial.

Nutrition history: The type, quantity, and frequency of food eaten, including the number of hot meals per week, are determined. Any special diets (eg, low salt, low carbohydrate) or self-prescribed fad diets are noted. The intake of alcohol, dietary fiber, and prescribed or over-the-counter vitamins is recorded. The amount of money the patient has to spend on food and the accessibility of food stores are important issues. Lack of suitable kitchen facilities may prevent a patient from preparing meals.

The patient's ability to eat (eg, chewing, swallowing) is assessed. It may be impaired by xerostomia (dry mouth), which is common in the elderly. Decreased taste or smell may reduce the pleasure of eating, so the patient may eat less. Patients with decreased vision, arthritis, immobility, or tremors may have difficulty preparing meals and may injure or burn themselves when cooking. Patients who are worried about urinary incontinence may reduce their fluid intake, which may also lead to poor food intake.

Psychiatric history: Psychiatric problems may not be detected as easily in older patients as in younger patients. Insomnia, changes in sleep patterns, constipation, decreased cognition, anorexia, weight loss, fatigue,

TABLE 3-1.   REVIEW OF BODY REGIONS AND ORGAN SYSTEMS

Region or System	Symptom	Possible Problem
Skin	Itching	Dry skin, jaundice, uremia, cancer, hyperthyroidism, allergic reaction, lice, scabies
Head	Headaches	Temporal arteritis, depression, anxiety, cervical osteoarthritis, subdural hematoma
Eyes	Glare from lights at night	Cataracts
	Loss of central vision	Macular degeneration
	Loss of near vision (presbyopia)	None (common with age)
	Loss of peripheral vision	Glaucoma, stroke
	Pain	Glaucoma, temporal arteritis
Ears	Hearing loss	Acoustic neuroma, tumor of the cerebellopontine angle, presbycusis, cerumen, foreign body in the external canal, Paget's disease, trauma from noise, ototoxicity from drugs (eg, aminoglycosides, furosemide, aspirin)
	Loss of high-frequency range (presbycusis)	None (common with age)
Mouth	Burning mouth	Pernicious anemia
	Denture pain	Poorly fitting dentures, oral cancer
	Dry mouth	Drugs (eg, diuretics, antihypertensives, tricyclic antidepressants, psychoactives, antihistamines), salivary gland damage due to infection or radiation therapy of head and neck tumors, autoimmune disorders (eg, rheumatoid arthritis, systemic lupus erythematosus, Sjögren's syndrome), dehydration
	Limited tongue motion	Oral cancer
	Loss of taste	Infection of mouth or nose, adrenal insufficiency, nasopharyngeal tumor, drugs (eg, antihistamines, antidepressants), radiation therapy, smoking
Throat	Dysphagia	Foreign body, Zenker's diverticulum, esophageal stricture, Schatzki's ring, cancer
	Voice changes	Vocal cord tumor, hypothyroidism

Table continues on the following page.

TABLE 3-1.   REVIEW OF BODY REGIONS AND ORGAN SYSTEMS (*Continued*)

Region or System	Symptom	Possible Problem
Neck	Pain	Cervical arthritis, polymyalgia rheumatica
Chest	Dyspnea on exertion	Heart failure, chronic obstructive pulmonary disease, infection
	Pain	Angina pectoris, anxiety, herpes zoster, gastroesophageal reflux, esophageal motility disorders, costochondritis
Cardiovascular	Paroxysmal nocturnal dyspnea	Heart failure, gastroesophageal reflux
Gastrointestinal	Constipation with no other symptoms	Hypothyroidism, hyperparathyroidism, dehydration, hypokalemia, colorectal cancer, inadequate exercise, low-fiber diet, drugs (eg, aluminum-containing antacids, opioids, tricyclic antidepressants, anticholinergics), laxative abuse
	Constipation with pain, vomiting, and diarrhea	Fecal impaction
	Episodic lower abdominal pain and diarrhea	Irritable bowel syndrome
	Fecal incontinence	Cerebral dysfunction, spinal cord lesions, rectal cancer, fecal impaction
	Lower abdominal pain (crampy, sudden onset)	Ischemic colitis, obstruction, diverticulitis
	One bowel movement q 2–3 days	None (may be normal)
	Postprandial abdominal pain (15–30 min after eating, lasting 1–3 h)	Chronic intestinal ischemia
	Rectal bleeding	Hemorrhoids, colon angiodysplasia, ischemic colitis, diverticulosis, colon cancer
Genitourinary	Frequency, dribbling, weak stream, hesitancy	Benign prostatic hyperplasia, prostate cancer, urinary tract infection
	Dysuria with or without fever	Urinary tract infection, prostatitis
	Polyuria	Hyperglycemia, glycosuria
Musculoskeletal	Back pain	Osteoarthritis, compression fractures, Paget's disease, metastatic cancer, infection (tuberculous spondylitis)

TABLE 3-1. (*Continued*)

Region or System	Symptom	Possible Problem
	Proximal muscle pain	Polymyalgia rheumatica
Extremities	Leg pain	Osteoarthritis, radiculopathy (eg, lumbar stenosis, disk herniation), intermittent claudication, night cramps
	Swollen ankles	Heart failure (bilateral swelling), venous insufficiency, hypoalbuminemia .
Neurologic	Change in mental status with fever	Meningitis
	Change in mental status without fever	Depression, decreased cognitive function, paranoia
	Clumsiness in tasks requiring fine motor coordination (eg, buttoning shirt)	Spondylotic cervical myelopathy, arthritis, parkinsonism
	Excessive sweating during meals	Autonomic neuropathy
	Fall without loss of consciousness	Transient ischemic attack, drop attack
	Hesitant gait, intention tremor	Parkinson's disease
	Numbness, tingling in fingers	Spondylotic cervical myelopathy, peripheral neuropathy
	Sleep disturbances	Circadian rhythm disturbances, drugs, sleep apnea, periodic leg movements, depression, anxiety, parkinsonism
	Syncope	Postural hypotension, seizure, cardiac dysrhythmia, aortic stenosis, hypoglycemia
	Transient interference with speech, muscle strength, or sensation	Transient ischemic attack

preoccupation with bodily functions, increased alcohol consumption, and somatic complaints are common symptoms. The patient should be questioned about delusions and hallucinations; past psychiatric care, including psychotherapy, institutionalization, and electroconvulsive therapy; and the use of psychoactive drugs or antidepressants.

Sadness, hopelessness, and crying episodes may indicate depression. Many circumstances (eg, recent loss of a loved one, including pets; hearing loss) may contribute to depression. Irritability may be the primary affective symptom,**1** or patients may present with cognitive loss, often called pseudodementia. **2**

Functional status: Evaluating the patient's functional status is a hallmark of good geriatric care. **3**

Family and social histories: Family history should focus on disorders of later life known to have inherited patterns (eg, Alzheimer's disease, cancer, diabetes). The age of onset in family members is noted.

Social history includes assessment of the patient's living arrangements (number of rooms; plumbing; availability of elevators, heating, and air conditioning), possibly best achieved by a home visit. Home features that can lead to falls (eg, poor lighting, slippery bathtubs, unanchored rugs) are identified and remedies suggested. **4**

Having the patient describe a typical day, including activities such as reading, television viewing, work, exercise, hobbies, and interactions with others, provides valuable information. The patient is asked about the frequency and nature of social contacts (eg, friends, senior citizens' groups), family visits, religious or spiritual participation, and availability of transportation.

Caregivers and support services (eg, church, senior citizens' groups) available to the patient are identified. The ability of family members (eg, their employment status, their health, traveling time to the patient's home) to assist the patient is determined. Other organized support systems (eg, church) may be assisting the patient. The patient's attitude toward the family and the family's attitude toward the patient are explored.

The patient's marital status (single, married, widowed, living in a relationship without marriage) is noted. Questioning about sexual practices and satisfaction must be sensitive and tactful but thorough; the number and sex of sexual partners are elicited**5** and the risk of sexually transmitted diseases assessed.

Economic difficulties due to retirement, a fixed income, or death of a spouse or partner who may have contributed financial support are discussed. Financial or health problems may result in loss of a home, social status, or independence. A longtime relationship with a physician may have been lost because the physician retired or died or because the patient relocated.

Tobacco and alcohol use are recorded; the risk of falling asleep while smoking in bed is increased in the elderly, who should thus be warned against smoking in bed. Patients should be counseled to quit smoking. Alcoholism is also a serious, underdiagnosed problem in the elderly. Signs of alcoholism include confusion, anger, hostility, alcohol odor on the breath, and tremors. The CAGE screening questionnaire identifies patients with a history of drinking problems. **6**

---

1 see TABLE 33–3 on page 313   **2** see page 363   **3** see page 42
4 see TABLE 20–3 on page 200   **5** see page 1157   **6** see page 336

The patient's wishes regarding measures for prolonging life must be documented. The patient is asked what provisions for surrogate decision making have been made in case of incapacity.[1]

PHYSICAL EXAMINATION

Elderly patients may require additional time to undress and transfer to the examining table for the physical examination; they should not be rushed. Examining gowns should be midthigh in length; gowns that are too long may cause the patient to trip. The examining table is adjusted to a height that the patient can easily access; a footstool facilitates mounting. The patient must not be left alone on the table. Portions of the examination may be more comfortable if the patient sits in a chair. The patient may want a relative or aide in the room during the examination.

Preliminary assessment of the patient's functioning can be made by observing personal hygiene. The patient's general appearance is described (eg, comfortable, restless, malnourished, inattentive, pale, dyspneic, cyanotic). If the patient is examined at bedside, use of a water mattress, a sheepskin, bedside rails (partial or full), restraints, a urinary catheter, or an adult diaper is noted.

Vital signs: During measurement of **height and weight,** patients with balance problems may need to grasp grab bars placed near or on the scale.

When the **temperature** is recorded, hypothermia[2] can be missed if the thermometer does not measure low temperatures. The absence of fever does not exclude infection.

Pulses and **blood pressure** (BP) are checked in both arms. The pulse is taken for $\geq$ 30 seconds and any irregularity noted. Because many factors can alter BP, several measurements are taken under resting conditions.[3] BP may be overestimated in elderly patients because of arterial stiffness. This pseudohypertension should be suspected if a patient has elevated systolic and diastolic BP but no end-organ damage. In patients with pseudohypertension, the brachial or radial artery is still palpable after the BP cuff is inflated to a point greater than the systolic pressure (Osler's maneuver).

Orthostatic hypotension may be more common among elderly patients who are not hypertensive. All patients should be checked for it. After BP is measured in the supine position, the patient is observed for $\geq$ 3 minutes in the standing position; a positive result is when systolic BP falls 20 mm Hg or more. Caution is required when testing volume-depleted patients. A postprandial fall in BP with virtually no compensatory increase in pulse rate has been observed in institutionalized patients.[4]

A normal **respiratory rate** in older patients may be as high as 16 to 25 breaths/minute. A rate > 25 breaths/minute may signal a lower respiratory

---

[1] see page 135   [2] see page 663   [3] see also page 836
[4] see also page 848

tract infection, congestive heart failure, or another disorder before other symptoms and signs appear.

Skin: Examination of skin includes a search for premalignant and malignant lesions and tissue ischemia. With pressure sores, the ulceration on the skin surface is smaller than the underlying soft tissue lesion. Unexplained bruises may indicate abuse. Because the dermis thins with age, ecchymoses may occur easily in traumatized skin (eg, on the forearm). Among older persons, uneven tanning may be normal because of progressive loss of melanocytes.

With age, longitudinal ridges may develop on the nails, and the crescent-shaped lunula may disappear. The nail plate becomes thinner and is prone to fracture. Black splinter hemorrhages in the middle or distal third of the fingernail are more likely due to trauma than to bacteremia. In onychomycosis, a fungal infection, the toenail is thickened and yellow. An ingrown toenail (onychocryptosis) has borders that curve in and down. Psoriatic nails are whitish, scale easily, and may have a pitted surface.

Face: Normal age-related changes include the following: The eyebrows may drop below the superior orbital rim, the chin may descend, the angle between the submandibular line and the neck may be lost, and the skin wrinkles and becomes drier. Thick terminal hairs develop on the ears, nose, upper lip, and chin. The temporal arteries should be palpated for tenderness and thickening.

Nose: A normal age-related change is progressive descent of the nasal tip, which may cause the upper and lower lateral cartilage to separate, enlarging and lengthening the nose.

Eyes: A normal age-related change is loss of orbital fat, which may gradually displace the eye backward into the orbit (enophthalmos). Thus, sunken eyes are not necessarily a sign of dehydration in the elderly. Enophthalmos is accompanied by a deepening of the upper lid fold and a slight obstruction of peripheral vision. Pseudoptosis (decrease in size of palpebral aperture), entropion (inversion of lower lid margins), or ectropion (eversion of lower lid margins) may occur. Arcus senilis, a white ring at the limbus, has no pathologic significance. Loss of lens elasticity with age reduces the ability of the lens to change shape when focusing on close objects (presbyopia).

A thorough eye examination includes testing visual acuity and screening for glaucoma and cataracts. ∎ Ophthalmotonometry is performed to check the intraocular pressure to screen for glaucoma, and peripheral vision is tested. Cataracts are best seen with a positive lens of an ophthalmoscope. Despite normal mental function, some elderly persons with decreased visual acuity have visual hallucinations, which are well organized and clearly defined. Such persons are rarely frightened; they quickly recognize that the hallucinations are not real but may not be appropriately concerned.

∎see page 1284

Although signs of hypertension or diabetes may be evident during funduscopic examination, the retina's appearance may not change significantly with age. Because of cortical atrophy, elevated intracranial pressure may not be accompanied by papilledema. Macular degeneration is characterized by areas of black pigment or hemorrhages in and around the macula.

Ears: A normal age-related finding is the presence of tophi, which may be noted during inspection of the pinna. The external auditory canal is examined for cerumen, especially if a hearing problem is noted during the interview. If the patient wears a hearing aid, it is removed and examined; the ear mold and plastic tubing can become plugged with wax. If the battery is dead, no whistle (feedback) is heard when the volume of the hearing aid is turned up.

To assess hearing, the physician, with his face out of view, whispers an easily answered question in each ear of the patient. A patient with presbycusis (hearing loss due to aging[1]), which affects high-frequency hearing, is more likely to report difficulty in understanding speech than in hearing.[2] Evaluation with a portable audioscope, if available, is also recommended.

Mouth: The mouth is examined for bleeding or swollen gums, loose and broken teeth, fungal infections, and signs of cancer (eg, leukoplakia, erythroplakia, ulceration, tumor mass). In patients with xerostomia, the mouth and tongue may be fissured, and the tongue blade may stick to the buccal mucosa. With age, the teeth may darken as a result of extrinsic stains and less translucent enamel. Erythematous, edematous gingiva that bleeds easily can be a sign of gingival or periodontal disease. Bad breath may indicate caries, periodontitis, or other oral diseases.

The dorsal and ventral surfaces of the tongue are examined. Normal age-related changes include varicose veins on the ventral surface, erythema migrans (geographic tongue), and atrophied papillae on the sides of the tongue. In an edentulous patient, the tongue may enlarge to facilitate chewing; however, enlargement may also be a sign of amyloidosis or hypothyroidism. A smooth, painful tongue may indicate vitamin B_{12} deficiency.

Dentures should be removed before examination of the mouth. Denture wearers are at risk of oral candidiasis and of resorption of the alveolar ridges. Improperly fitting dentures can cause inflammation of the palatal mucosa and ulcers of the alveolar ridges.

Edentulous persons who do not wear dentures may have painful, inflamed, fissured lesions at the lip commissures (angular cheilitis), usually caused by fungal infections. Inadequate support of the facial musculature accentuates the grooves at the lip commissures, creating a moist, protected area conducive to fungal growth. The lesions respond promptly to topical therapy.

Temporomandibular joint: A common age-related change is degeneration of the temporomandibular joint (osteoarthrosis), which occurs as teeth are lost and compressive forces in the joint become excessive. Joint crepitus may be felt at the head of the condyle as the patient opens and closes the jaw. Jaw movements may be painful. ∎

Neck: The thyroid gland, which is located low in the neck of elderly persons, often beneath the sternum, is examined for enlargement and nodules. In dehydrated elderly patients with parotitis, the parotid gland is swollen, firm, and tender; pus may be expressed from Stensen's duct.

The significance of carotid bruits in asymptomatic patients is unclear. Arterial bruits due to carotid artery stenosis can be differentiated from those due to transmitted heart murmurs by moving the stethoscope up the neck: A transmitted heart murmur becomes softer, whereas the bruit of carotid artery stenosis becomes louder.

Resistance to passive flexion of the neck occurs in patients with cervical spondylosis or osteoarthritis. This resistance also occurs in patients with meningitis, but the neck can be rotated passively from side to side. Resistance to flexion, extension, and lateral rotation of the neck occurs in patients with cervical spine disease.

Chest and back: All areas of the lungs are examined by percussion and auscultation. Basilar rales may be heard in the lungs of a healthy patient but should disappear after the patient takes a few deep breaths. The extent of respiratory excursions (ie, movement of the diaphragm, ability to expand the chest) should be noted.

The back is examined for scoliosis and tenderness. Spontaneous osteoporotic fractures of the sacrum (characterized by severe low back, hip, and leg pain and marked sacral tenderness) may occur in elderly patients.

Breasts should be examined in men and women for irregularities or nodules. Annual breast examinations by a physician and monthly self-examinations are recommended for elderly women; screening mammography is also recommended, especially in women with a family history of breast cancer. Retracted nipples can be everted with pressure around the nipple when retraction is due to age but not when it is due to an underlying growth.

Cardiovascular system: The size of the heart can usually be assessed by palpating the apex; however, displacement caused by kyphoscoliosis may make assessment difficult. The most common systolic murmur in elderly patients is due to aortic valve sclerosis, which may not be hemodynamically significant. Mitral regurgitation, hypertrophic obstructive cardiomyopathy, and significant aortic valve stenosis also produce systolic murmurs. The murmur of mitral regurgitation is usually soft and heard best along the right sternal border. The murmur of hypertrophic obstructive cardiomyopathy intensifies when the patient performs a Valsalva maneuver. The murmur of aortic valve stenosis peaks late and is transmitted to the carotid arteries, whereas the murmur of aortic valve sclerosis peaks early

---

∎ see also page 1024

and is rarely heard in the carotid arteries. A loud murmur (> grade 2), a dampened second heart sound, and a narrow pulse pressure are classic signs of aortic valve stenosis. However, these signs may not be observed in elderly patients, because with age, the murmur may decrease in loudness, a second heart sound is rarely audible, and narrow pulse pressures are uncommon. The carotid upstroke often does not slow in elderly patients with aortic valve stenosis because vascular compliance is diminished. Fourth heart sounds are common in elderly persons who have no evidence of cardiovascular disease. Diastolic murmurs are abnormal in persons of any age. Heart rates as low as 40 beats/minute may be normal. Unexplained sinus bradycardia in apparently healthy persons may not adversely influence long-term cardiovascular morbidity or mortality; however, sinus bradycardia can be due to abnormal atrioventricular or intraventricular conduction.▯

Patients with pacemakers who develop new neurologic or cardiovascular symptoms are examined for hypotension, heart failure, or variable heart sounds, murmurs, or pulses. These symptoms and signs may be due to the loss of atrioventricular synchrony.

Gastrointestinal system: Elderly persons often have weak abdominal muscles, which may result in hernias. Although most abdominal aortic aneurysms are palpable, only their lateral size can be assessed during physical examination. A mass that is located in front of the aorta and that is transmitting a pulse does not expand laterally. The liver, spleen, and kidneys are palpated for enlargement. Frequency and quality of bowel sounds are checked, and the suprapubic area is evaluated by percussion for tenderness, discomfort, and evidence of urinary retention.

The anorectal area is examined for fissures, hemorrhoids, and strictures. Sensation is tested, and anal winks are elicited. A digital examination to detect a mass or fecal impaction is performed in men and women.

The prostate gland is palpated for nodules. Estimating prostate size by digital examination is inaccurate, and size does not correlate with urethral obstruction; however, digital examination allows a qualitative evaluation.

Female reproductive system: Regular pelvic examinations are recommended, with Papanicolaou (Pap) tests every 2 to 3 years until age 70 years. If an elderly woman has not had regular Pap tests, she should first have at least two tests, 1 year apart. If the results of three consecutive tests performed in a woman > 60 years are normal, the woman can usually stop having tests unless she develops new symptoms or signs of possible disease. For women who have had a hysterectomy, Pap tests are required only if cervical tissue remains.

For pelvic examination, a patient who lacks hip mobility may lie on her left side. Postmenopausal reduction of estrogen leads to atrophy of the vaginal and urethral mucosa, which appears dry and lacks rugal folds. The

▯ see also page 897

ovaries should not be palpable; palpable ovaries suggest malignancy. The patient is asked to cough to check for urine leakage.

Musculoskeletal system: Joints are examined for tenderness, swelling, subluxation, crepitus, warmth, and redness. Heberden's nodes (bony overgrowths at the distal interphalangeal joints) or Bouchard's nodes (bony overgrowths at the proximal interphalangeal joints) can occur in patients with osteoarthritis. Patients with chronic rheumatoid arthritis may have subluxation of the metacarpophalangeal joints with ulnar deviation of the fingers. Hyperextension of the proximal interphalangeal joint and flexion of the distal interphalangeal joint result in a swan-neck deformity; hyperextension of the distal interphalangeal joint and flexion of the proximal interphalangeal joint result in a boutonnière deformity. These deformities may interfere with functioning or usual activities.

Active and passive range of joint motion should be determined. The presence of contractures should be noted. Variable resistance to passive manipulation of the extremities (gegenhalten) sometimes occurs with aging.

Feet: Diagnosis and treatment of foot problems, which are common with age, help the elderly maintain their independence. Common age-related findings include a bunion, a medial prominence of the first metatarsal head with lateral deviation (hallux valgus) and rotation of the big toe, and a bunionette, a lateral prominence of the fifth metatarsal head. Hyperflexion of the proximal interphalangeal joint results in a hammer toe. Hyperflexion of the proximal and distal interphalangeal toe joints results in a claw toe. Patients with foot problems should be referred to a podiatrist for regular evaluation and treatment.

Neurologic status: The neurologic examination for an elderly patient, similar to that for any adult, assesses cranial nerves, motor function, sensory function, and mental status. However, non-neurologic disorders that are common among the elderly may complicate the neurologic examination. For example, diminished sight and hearing may impede the assessment of cranial nerves, and periarthritis of the shoulder due to hemiplegia may interfere with the assessment of motor function.

Signs detected during the examination must be considered in light of the patient's age, history, and other findings. Symmetric findings unaccompanied by functional loss, other neurologic signs, and complaints may be a result of aging. The physician must decide whether these findings justify a detailed evaluation for a neurologic lesion. Patients should be reevaluated periodically for functional changes, asymmetry, or new complaints.

Cranial nerve assessment may be complex. The elderly often have small pupils; their pupillary light reflex may be sluggish, and their pupillary mitotic response to near vision may be diminished. Upward gaze and, to a lesser extent, downward gaze are slightly limited. Eye movements, when tracking a physician's finger during assessment of visual fields, may appear jerky and irregular. Bell's phenomenon (reflex upward movement of the eyes on closure) is sometimes absent.

The elderly often have a diminished sense of smell because they have had numerous upper respiratory infections and have fewer olfactory neurons, but asymmetric loss (ie, loss of smell in one nostril) is abnormal. Taste may be altered because of this diminished sense of smell or because of drugs, some of which decrease salivation. Sight and hearing may be decreased because of difficulties with the end organs.

Motor function assessment includes strength, coordination, gait, and reflexes. The elderly often appear weak during routine testing; during the physical examination, the physician can easily overpower sustained contraction of the extremities. Symmetric weakness that does not bother the patient is likely to be insignificant. Muscle tone, measured by flexing and extending the elbow or knee, may be increased; however, jerky movements during examination and cogwheel rigidity are not normal.

A decrease in muscle bulk is common and is not significant unless accompanied by a loss of function. Hand muscles are particularly affected; the interosseous and thenar muscles of the hands atrophy with age. A patient in a wheelchair may have weak extensor muscles of the wrist, fingers, and thumb due to compression of the upper arm against the armrest, which can injure the radial nerve. Without regular resistance training, muscle strength often deteriorates. Arm function can be tested by having the patient pick up an eating utensil or touch the back of the head with both hands.

With age, motor reaction time often increases, partly because the conduction of signals along the peripheral nerves slows. Motor coordination decreases because of changes in central mechanisms, but usually this decrease is subtle and not disabling.

With age, the muscle strength reflexes (eg, deep tendon reflexes) usually show no or limited changes, although in nearly half of elderly patients, the Achilles tendon reflex is diminished or absent because of decreased tendon elasticity and slowed nerve conduction in the tendon's long reflex arc. This reflex can be elicited with skillful technique in most patients. Achilles tendon reflexes may be asymmetric because of sciatica.

With age, postural reflexes are often impaired, possibly contributing to falls. Postural sway (movement in the anteroposterior plane when the patient remains stationary and upright) may also increase. Cortical release reflexes (known as pathologic reflexes)—the snout, sucking, and palmomental reflexes—occasionally occur in the absence of detectable brain disorders (eg, dementia). The presence of Babinski's reflex (extensor plantar response) in the elderly is abnormal. A common cause for this abnormality is cervical spondylosis with partial cord compression.

Sensory function is largely unaffected by aging. Elderly persons commonly experience a loss of vibratory sensation below the knees due to small-vessel changes in the posterior column of the spinal cord. However, proprioception (joint position sense), which is thought to use a similar pathway, is unaffected.

The fibers in the peripheral nerves, particularly the larger fibers, become smaller. This change may account for the common complaint of numbness, especially in the feet. However, numbness may also be caused by peripheral neuritis, which should be sought. In many cases, no cause can be found. Tremor can be evaluated during handshaking and other simple activities. If tremor is detected, amplitude, rhythm, distribution, frequency, and time of occurrence (at rest, with motion, or with intention) are noted.

Mental status: A patient who resents a mental status examination **1**— a key component of assessment—should be reassured that it is routine. The examiner must ensure that the patient can hear; pure word deafness (an isolated inability to understand speech) may be mistaken for cognitive dysfunction. Assessing the mental status of a patient who has a speech or language disorder (eg, mutism, dysarthria, speech apraxia, aphasia) can be difficult.

Elderly persons process information and retrieve memories more slowly; however, abnormalities of consciousness, orientation, judgment, calculations, speech, language, or praxis cannot be attributed solely to age. The patient should be asked questions that will signal abnormalities in these areas; questions only about orientation fail to indicate dementia in many cases. If abnormalities are noted, further assessment, including a formal test of mental status, is needed.

Nutritional status: Many common measurements of nutritional status may be unreliable in elderly patients. Age can alter height, weight, and body composition (lean body mass and fat content). Arm span is a reliable estimate of original height in the calculation of body mass index in the elderly patient. Skinfold thickness measurements at multiple sites may provide more reliable estimates of fat content than measurement at the triceps only. The nutrition history, **2** including weight loss or possible deficiencies in essential nutrients, may trigger a more thorough evaluation and appropriate laboratory measurements. **3**

UNUSUAL PRESENTATIONS OF ILLNESS

Certain disorders have unusual presentations in elderly patients. Many of the following disorders are covered in more detail elsewhere in this manual.

Hyperthyroidism may not have the classic signs (eg, eye signs, enlarged thyroid gland) in elderly patients. Symptoms and signs may be subtle and may include weight loss, palpitations, weakness, fine skin, tremor, atrial fibrillation, and tachycardia. Patients may appear apathetic rather than hyperkinetic.

Hypothyroidism in elderly patients may be indicated by weight loss rather than weight gain and by cognitive loss, heart failure, constipation, dry skin, delayed reflexes, or hypothermia.

Hyperparathyroidism often does not have the characteristic symptoms in elderly patients. The clinical picture may be nonspecific:

---

1 see page 343   **2** see page 26   **3** see also pages 598–601 fatigue, decreased intellectual capacity, emotional instability, anorexia, constipation, and hypertension.

Giant cell arteritis or **polymyalgia rheumatica** in elderly patients may be indicated by respiratory tract symptoms (eg, cough, sore throat, hoarseness) or mental status changes rather than by the classic manifestations of headache, jaw claudication, and blindness. Patients may report head pain in the frontal, vertex, or occipital area rather than in the temporal area.

Systemic lupus erythematosus in elderly patients is associated with a lower incidence of Raynaud's phenomenon, malar rash, nephritis, and neuropsychiatric disease than in younger patients but with a higher incidence of pneumonitis, interstitial fibrosis, subcutaneous nodules, and discoid lupus. Presenting symptoms may be those of a systemic illness (eg, fever, weight loss, arthritis).

Fibromyalgia in elderly patients is less likely than in younger patients to be manifested by chronic headaches, anxiety, and symptoms aggravated by weather, mental stress, or poor sleep.

Sarcoidosis in elderly patients may be indicated by shortness of breath, blurred vision, myopathy, adenopathy, and fatigue. The clinical manifestations vary.

Bacteremia may not cause an elderly patient to be febrile; instead, the patient may have nonspecific manifestations (eg, general malaise, an unexplained change in mental status).

Urinary tract infections may be present in afebrile elderly patients. These patients may not report dysuria, frequency, or urgency. Dizziness, confusion, anorexia, fatigue, or weakness may occur.

Meningitis in elderly patients may not be associated with symptoms of meningeal irritation. Patients may have fever and a change in mental status without headache or nuchal rigidity.

Pneumonia may be indicated by malaise, anorexia, or confusion in elderly patients. Tachycardia and tachypnea are common, but fever may be absent. Coughing may be mild and without copious, purulent sputum. Coexisting illnesses may alter the presentation of **tuberculosis.** Symptoms may be nonspecific (eg, fever, weakness, confusion, anorexia).

Appendicitis in elderly patients may be indicated by diffuse abdominal pain rather than by pain localized to the right lower quadrant. However, tenderness in this quadrant is a significant early sign.

Biliary disease in elderly patients may be associated with nonspecific mental and physical deterioration (eg, malaise, confusion, loss of mobility) without jaundice, fever, or abdominal pain. Abnormal liver function test results may be the only indication of biliary disease.

Acute bowel infarction may be indicated by acute confusion in elderly patients. Abdominal pain and tenderness may be absent.

Peptic ulcer disease in elderly patients may be indicated by anorexia; nonsteroidal anti-inflammatory drugs can mask the pain. Gastrointestinal bleeding may be painless in the elderly. Slow, unrecognized blood loss may occur, resulting in significant anemia.

Myocardial infarction in elderly patients may manifest as dyspnea, syncope, weakness, vomiting, or confusion rather than as chest pain.

Heart failure in elderly patients may be associated with confusion, agitation, anorexia, weakness, insomnia, or lethargy; patients may not report dyspnea. Orthopnea may cause nocturnal agitation in demented patients with heart failure.

4 ▪ COMPREHENSIVE GERIATRIC ASSESSMENT

A multidimensional process designed to assess an elderly person's functional ability, physical health, cognitive and mental health, and socioenvironmental situation.

Comprehensive geriatric assessment differs from a standard medical evaluation by including nonmedical domains, by emphasizing functional ability and quality of life, and, often, by relying on interdisciplinary teams. ▪ This assessment aids in the diagnosis of health-related problems, development of plans for treatment and follow-up, coordination of care, determination of the need for and the site of long-term care, and optimal use of health care resources.

Geriatric assessment programs vary widely in purpose, comprehensiveness, staffing, organization, and structural and functional components. Most attempt to target their services to high-risk elderly persons and to couple their assessment results with sustained individually tailored interventions (eg, rehabilitation, education, counseling, supportive services).

Comprehensive geriatric assessment of frail or chronically ill patients can improve their care and clinical outcomes. The possible benefits include greater diagnostic accuracy, improved functional and mental status, reduced mortality, decreased use of nursing homes and acute care hospitals, and greater satisfaction with care. However, the cost of comprehensive geriatric assessment programs has limited their use. Although some cost-effectiveness evaluations suggest that these programs can save money, few programs operate in integrated care systems that can track these savings. Wide use of comprehensive geriatric assessment programs has thus been slow to develop. An alternative approach is to conduct less extensive assessments in primary care offices or emergency departments.

▪ see page 74

TABLE 4–1. AN ASSESSMENT INSTRUMENT USED IN PRIMARY CARE SETTINGS

Domain	Item
Daily functional ability	Degree of difficulty eating, dressing, bathing, transferring between bed and chair, using the toilet, controlling bladder and bowel
	Degree of difficulty preparing meals, performing housework, taking drugs, going on errands (eg, shopping), managing finances, using the telephone
Assistive devices	Use of personal devices (eg, cane, walker, wheelchair, oxygen)
	Use of environmental devices (eg, grab bars, shower bench, hospital bed)
Caregivers	Use of paid caregivers (eg, nurses, aides)
	Use of unpaid caregivers (eg, family, friends, volunteers)
Drugs	Name of prescription drugs used
	Name of nonprescription drugs used
Nutrition	Height, weight
	Stability of weight (has the patient lost 4.54 kg [10 lb] in the past 6 mo without trying?)
Preventive measures	Regularity of blood pressure measurements, guaiac test for occult blood in stool, sigmoidoscopy, immunizations (influenza, pneumococcal, tetanus), thyroid-stimulating hormone assessment, and dental care; intake of calcium and vitamin D; regularity of exercise; use of smoke detectors
	For women, regularity of Papanicolaou tests and mammography
Cognition	Ability to remember three objects after 1 min
Affect	Feelings of sadness, depression, or hopelessness
	Lack of interest or pleasure in doing things
Advance directives (see Ch. 14)	Possession of a living will
	Establishment of durable power of attorney for health care
Substance abuse	Use of alcohol determined by the CAGE questionnaire (see Ch. 37)
	Use of cigarettes
Gait, balance	Number of falls in the past 6 months
	Time required to rise from a chair, walk 3.05 m (10 feet), turn around, return, and sit down
	Extent of maximal forward reach while standing
Sensory ability	Ability to report three numbers whispered 0.61 m (2 feet) behind the head
	Ability to read Snellen's chart at 20/40 or better (with corrective lenses, if needed)
Upper extremities	Ability to clasp hands behind the head and back

An assessment instrument designed to help primary care physicians, nurses, and other health care practitioners perform practical, efficient assessment is shown in TABLE 4–1. It includes elements from an instrument recommended by the American College of Physicians and from instruments validated and field-tested in randomized clinical trials.

To identify elderly persons who might benefit from assessment (in a special comprehensive geriatric assessment unit or in a primary care setting), some health care organizations mail multidimensional self-administered health questionnaires to elderly populations. ▯ Responses are scored according to defined algorithms, and reports of high-risk conditions and behaviors are sent to the patients and their primary care physicians to stimulate more detailed follow-up evaluation and treatment. Other organizations identify candidates for assessment by interviewing elderly persons in their homes or meeting places (eg, meal sites, senior centers, places of worship). Family members who are concerned about an elderly relative's health or functional abilities may also arrange referrals for geriatric assessment.

ASSESSMENT DOMAINS

Comprehensive geriatric assessment is most successful when conducted by a geriatric interdisciplinary team, ▯ which typically includes a geriatrician, a nurse, a social worker, and a pharmacist. For most elderly patients, the outpatient clinic is a sufficient and relatively inexpensive setting for evaluation; comprehensive geriatric assessment usually does not require the technology or intense monitoring available in an acute care inpatient setting. However, patients with physical or mental impairments may have difficulty keeping appointments, and chronically ill patients who need to rest during the assessment process may require inpatient assessment.

The principal domains assessed in all forms of geriatric assessment are functional ability, physical health, cognitive and mental health, and the socioenvironmental situation. Standardized instruments make evaluation of these domains more reliable and efficient (see TABLE 4–2). They also facilitate the communication of clinical information among health care practitioners and the monitoring of changes in the patient's condition over time.

Functional ability: Comprehensive geriatric assessment begins with a review of the major categories of functional ability: activities of daily living (ADLs) and instrumental activities of daily living (IADLs). ADLs are self-care activities that a person must perform every day (eg, eating, dressing, bathing, transferring between the bed and a chair, using the toilet, controlling bladder and bowel). Patients unable to perform these activities and

---

▯see page 158   ▯see page 74

TABLE 4–2.   INSTRUMENTS USED IN COMPREHENSIVE GERIATRIC ASSESSMENT

Instrument	Method	Score*	Administration Time (min)
Katz ADL Scale (see TABLE 4–3)	Interview of patient, caregiver, or nurse or self-administered questionnaire	0–12	2–4
Lawton IADL Scale (see TABLE 4–4)	Interview of patient, caregiver, or nurse or self-administered questionnaire	0–16	3–5
Mini-Mental State Examination (see FIGURE 38–1)	Interview of patient	0–30	5–15
Geriatric Depression Scale (short form— see TABLE 33–4)	Interview of patient or self-administered questionnaire	15–0	3–6
Tinetti Balance and Gait Evaluation (see TABLE 21–2)	Observation of patient's performance	0–14	5–15

*From poor to good.
ADL = activities of daily living; IADL = instrumental activities of daily living.

obtain adequate nutrition usually require caregiver support 12 to 24 hours/day. IADLs are activities that enable a person to live independently in a house or apartment (eg, preparing meals, performing housework, taking drugs, going on errands, managing finances, using a telephone). Reliable instruments for measuring patients' abilities to perform ADLs and IADLs and for determining what kind of assistance may be needed include the Katz ADL Scale (see TABLE 4–3) and the Lawton IADL Scale (see TABLE 4–4). Deficits in ADLs and IADLs indicate a need for additional information about the patient's socioenvironmental situation. When elderly persons begin to need help performing these activities, their risk of becoming more dependent increases.

Physical health: The approach to the history and physical examination must be geriatric-specific.[1] In particular, vision, hearing, continence, gait, and balance must be considered. The Tinetti Balance and Gait Evaluation[2] is a useful assessment instrument.

Cognitive and mental health: Several screening tests for cognitive dysfunction have been validated; the Mini-Mental State Examination is popular because it efficiently tests most of the major aspects of cognitive function.[3] Of the several validated screening instruments for depression, the Geriatric Depression Scale and the Hamilton Depression

[1] see page 24   [2] see TABLE 21–2 on page 210
[3] see FIGURE 38–1 on page 346

TABLE 4–3.   KATZ ACTIVITIES OF DAILY LIVING SCALE

Activity	Item	Score
Eating	Eats without assistance	2
	Needs assistance only in cutting meat or buttering bread	1
	Needs assistance in eating or is fed intravenously	0
Dressing	Gets clothes and dresses without assistance	2
	Needs assistance only in tying shoes	1
	Needs assistance in getting clothes or in getting dressed or stays partly or completely undressed	0
Bathing (sponge bath, tub bath, shower)	Bathes without assistance	2
	Needs assistance only in bathing one part of the body (eg, back)	1
	Needs assistance in bathing more than one part of the body or does not bathe	0
Transferring	Moves in and out of bed and chair without assistance (may use cane or walker)	2
	Needs assistance in moving in and out of bed or chair	1
	Does not get out of bed	0
Toileting	Goes to the bathroom, uses toilet, cleans self, arranges clothes, and returns without assistance (may use cane or walker for support and may use bedpan or urinal at night)	2
	Needs assistance in going to the bathroom, using toilet, cleaning self, arranging clothes, or returning	1
	Does not go to the bathroom to relieve bladder or bowel	0
Continence	Controls bladder and bowel completely (without occasional accidents)	2
	Occasionally loses control of bladder and bowel	1
	Needs supervision to control bladder or bowel, requires use of a catheter, or is incontinent	0

Modified from Katz S, Downs TD, Cash HR, et al: "Progress in the development of the index of ADL." *Gerontologist* 10:20–30, 1970. Copyright © The Gerontological Society of America.

Scale ■ are the easiest to use and most widely accepted. However, a two-question screening instrument ("During the past month, have you been bothered by feelings of sadness, depression, or hopelessness? Have you often been bothered by a lack of interest or pleasure in doing things?") is as effective as these longer scales. Specific psychiatric symptoms (eg, para-

■ see TABLES 33–4 and 33–5 on pages 315 and 316

TABLE 4–4.   LAWTON INSTRUMENTAL ACTIVITIES OF DAILY LIVING SCALE*

Activity		Score†
Can you prepare your own meals	without help,	2
	with some help, or	1
	are you completely unable to prepare any meals?	0
Can you do your own housework or handyman work	without help,	2
	with some help, or	1
	are you completely unable to do any housework?	0
Can you do your own laundry	without help,	2
	with some help, or	1
	are you completely unable to do any laundry?	0
Do you or can you take prescribed drugs	without help (ie, correct doses at the correct time),	2
	with some help (ie, someone prepares the drug and/or reminds you to take it), or	1
	are you completely unable to take prescribed drugs without help?	0
Can you get to places beyond walking distance	without help,	2
	with some help, or	1
	are you completely unable to travel unless special arrangements are made?	0
Can you go shopping for groceries	without help,	2
	with some help, or	1
	are you completely unable to do any shopping?	0
Can you manage your own money	without help,	2
	with some help, or	1
	are you completely unable to manage money?	0
Can you use the telephone	without help,	2
	with some help, or	1
	are you completely unable to use the telephone?	0

*Some questions may be sex-specific and can be modified by the interviewer.

†The maximum score is 16, although scores have meaning only for a particular patient (eg, declining scores over time reveal deterioration).

Adapted with permission from M Powell Lawton, PhD, Director of Research, Philadelphia Geriatric Center, Philadelphia.

noia, delusions, behavior abnormalities) are evaluated in the psychologic assessment, but they are less easily quantified and are rarely included in rating scales.

Socioenvironmental situation: Factors that affect the patient's socioenvironmental situation are complex and difficult to quantify. They include the social interaction network, available social support resources, special needs, and environmental safety and convenience, which influence the treatment approach used. Such information can readily be obtained by an experienced nurse or social worker. Several assessment instruments are available, but none is quantitative or clinically useful. A checklist can be used to assess home safety. ▣

▆5▆▆ PREVENTION OF DISEASE AND DISABILITY

For the elderly, prevention focuses mainly on disease, frailty, accidents (ie, unintentional injury), iatrogenic complications, and psychosocial problems. Not all elderly patients benefit from every preventive measure; effectiveness varies depending on the patient's physical health, functional ability, and cognitive status.

The choice of preventive measures is guided by the general condition of patients, ie, healthy (60 to 75% of the elderly), chronically ill (20 to 35%), or frail (2 to 10%). The healthy elderly have minimal or no chronic disease and are functionally independent. Primary and secondary prevention of disease and prevention of frailty are the most beneficial preventive measures for this group. The chronically ill elderly typically have several noncurable disorders, are usually functionally independent or minimally dependent, often take several prescription drugs, and occasionally are hospitalized for exacerbations of their chronic disorders. Tertiary prevention of disease and prevention of frailty are priorities in the chronically ill, followed by primary and secondary prevention of disease and prevention of iatrogenic complications and accidents. The frail elderly typically have many severe chronic disorders, are functionally dependent, and have lost their physiologic reserve. They are frequently hospitalized and institutionalized. Prevention of accidents and iatrogenic complications is most important.

Some preventive measures apply to all elderly persons. Exercise can help prevent frailty. In frail elderly persons, it can help preserve functional ability and reduce the incidence of accidents. Yearly influenza vaccination and pneumococcal vaccination (needed only once, except for patients at highest risk) are effective, inexpensive, and associated with minimal morbidity.

▣ see TABLE 20–3 on page 200

TABLE 5–1.   RECOMMENDED CLINICAL PREVENTIVE SERVICES*

Disorder to be Detected or Prevented	Medical Action	Frequency
Hypertension	Blood pressure measurement	Every 2 years if < 140/85 mm Hg; yearly if diastolic 85–89 mm Hg
Obesity, malnutrition	Height and weight measurement	At least yearly
Cancer (see also TABLE 72–2)		
Breast	Mammography	Every 1–2 years†
Cervical, uterine	Papanicolaou test	At least every 3 years‡
Colon	Fecal occult blood testing	Yearly
	Sigmoidoscopy	Every 3–5 years§
Hearing deficit	Hearing test	Yearly
Visual deficit	Vision test	Yearly
Alcoholism	Alcoholism screening questionnaire	At initial visit and when problem drinking is suspected
Influenza	Influenza vaccination	Yearly‖
Pneumococcal infection	Pneumococcal vaccination	Once at age 65¶
Tetanus	Tetanus booster	Every 10 years#

*Endorsed by the U.S. Preventive Services Task Force and/or the Canadian Task Force on the Periodic Health Examination.

† Should be continued in women > 70 if they have a reasonable life expectancy.

‡ Should be stopped at age 65 in women who have been tested regularly throughout their adult life with no abnormal results; for women who have never been tested, can be stopped after two Papanicolaou tests taken 1 year apart show normal results.

§ Whether fecal occult blood testing or sigmoidoscopy is more effective for colon cancer screening is unclear.

‖ For persons at high risk of influenza A (eg, institutional outbreaks), amantadine or rimantadine may be started at the time of vaccination and continued for 2 weeks.

¶ Recommended for immunocompetent persons ≥ 65, immunocompromised adults at increased risk of pneumococcal infection, and adults with asymptomatic or symptomatic HIV infection. Revaccination with the 23-valent vaccine should be strongly considered for persons who received the 14-valent vaccine if they are at very high risk of fatal pneumococcal infection (eg, asplenic patients). Also, revaccination should be considered for adults at very high risk who received the 23-valent vaccine ≥ 6 years earlier and for those shown to have rapid decline in pneumococcal antibody levels.

#Intervals of 15 to 30 years between boosters are likely to be adequate for patients who received a complete 5-dose series in childhood.

Patient and caregiver issues: Healthy elderly persons should visit their primary care physician at least annually to ensure timely completion of primary and secondary disease prevention activities (see TABLE 5–1). Pursuing regular exercise and a healthy diet (see TABLE 5–2) as

TABLE 5–2. EXERCISE AND NUTRITIONAL RECOMMENDATIONS FOR PREVENTION OF FRAILTY

Measure	Description	Rationale
Aerobic training (eg, brisk walking)	At least 20 min of activity at 50–75% of maximum heart rate 3 times/week	Prevents cardiovascular disease; maintains and builds bone density
Weight (resistance) training	Three sets of 8–15 repetitions at least 2 times/week for all muscle groups	Maintains and builds bone density
Flexibility training	At least 15 sec of static stretching for each muscle group daily	Helps prevent falls
Balance training (eg, dance, tai chi, physical therapy)	At least 3 times/week	Helps prevent falls
Low-fat diet	Fat constituting < 30% of total calories with < 10% from saturated fats	Prevents cardiovascular disease
Low-sodium diet	Recommended limit of 3 g/day, which is difficult to maintain; for most elderly persons, 4–5 g is more reasonable	Lowers blood pressure in some patients
High-calcium diet	For the elderly, 1500 mg/day (most American diets contain only 500–700 mg/day)	Helps maintain bone density
Adequate intake of vitamins and minerals	Adequate intake ensured largely through eating fruits and vegetables; supplementation with vitamin D (400–700 IU/ day), folic acid ($\geq$ 200 µg/day), vitamin E (200–400 IU/day), and selenium (200 µg/day) is recommended by some experts	Prevents bone loss (vitamin D); may prevent coronary artery disease (folic acid); antioxidants (vitamin E and selenium) may prevent a variety of chronic diseases
High-fiber diet	Best obtained through eating fruits, vegetables, and grains	May prevent colon cancer, has a beneficial effect on serum lipids
Moderate alcohol intake	About 1 oz of alcohol/day (more can be harmful)	May prevent cardiovascular disease

well as other disease prevention behaviors (see TABLE 5–3) will help prevent frailty and many individual diseases. Chronically ill patients and their caregivers should learn about their diseases and treatment plans. Regular physician visits and prompt reporting of a change in symptoms can help reduce severe illness exacerbations, which can lead to hospitalization and functional decline.

TABLE 5–3.   LIFESTYLE STRATEGIES FOR PREVENTING COMMON CHRONIC DISEASES

Disease	Preventive Strategy
Atherosclerotic cardiovascular disease (CAD, stroke)	Treatment of hypertension; smoking cessation; weight reduction; dietary saturated fat and cholesterol reduction; increased aerobic exercise
Cancer	Increased aerobic exercise; smoking cessation; dietary fat reduction; reduction in intake of salt- or smoke-cured food; minimized radiation and sun exposure
COPD	Smoking cessation
Diabetes mellitus (type II)	Weight reduction; diet consistent with atherosclerosis prevention
Hypertension	Dietary sodium reduction; weight reduction
Osteoarthritis	Weight reduction
Osteoporosis	Maintenance of dietary calcium; regular exercise; smoking cessation; avoidance of excessive alcohol

CAD = coronary artery disease; COPD = chronic obstructive pulmonary disease.

Caregivers of the frail elderly must work assiduously to prevent accidents through completion of a home safety checklist and other measures. Caregivers should be watchful for even subtle functional changes in elderly patients and promptly report them to health care practitioners. If a patient has multiple unmet needs, especially when coupled with functional decline, a caregiver should consider seeking the care of a geriatric interdisciplinary team.

PREVENTION OF DISEASE

PRIMARY AND SECONDARY PREVENTION

In primary prevention, disease is stopped before it starts, often by reducing or eliminating risk factors. For example, immunoprophylaxis prevents disease through vaccination; chemoprophylaxis, through drug therapy; and counseling, through behavioral change. In secondary prevention, disease is detected and treated at an early stage, thereby minimizing morbidity and mortality.

Screening can be a primary or secondary preventive measure; it can be used to detect risk factors, which may be altered to prevent disease, or to detect disease in asymptomatic persons, who can then be treated early.

Some primary and secondary preventive measures are recommended for all elderly persons (see TABLES 5–1 and 5–3). The effectiveness of other measures, advocated by some organizations, has not been well established (see TABLE 5–4).

TABLE 5–4. POTENTIALLY USEFUL MEASURES FOR DISEASE PREVENTION

Medical Action	Frequency	Disorder to be Detected or Prevented	Comment
Lipid measurement	Every 5 years	Hyperlipo-proteinemia	Treatment of hyperlipoproteinemia is very effective for secondary and tertiary prevention of heart disease; the effectiveness of measuring lipid levels in elderly persons without heart disease is not well established*
Blood glucose testing	Yearly	Diabetic complications	Some experts recommend screening obese persons only
Digital rectal examination	Yearly	Prostate cancer	Effectiveness for preventing death due to prostate cancer is unproved
Prostate-specific antigen testing	Yearly	Prostate cancer	Effectiveness for preventing death due to prostate cancer is unproved
Mental status testing	Yearly	Dementia, delirium	Testing may become more important if early treatment of dementia is shown to change outcomes
Bone density measurement	Once after age 65	Osteoporosis	Measurement is expensive and is commonly recommended for asymptomatic women who have several osteoporosis risk factors or for women and men who take glucocorticoids regularly
Thyroid-stimulating hormone measurement	At least every 5 years	Hypothyroidism	Some experts recommend screening all women
Vitamin B₁₂ deficiency screening	Every 5 years	Pernicious anemia	Early diagnosis may prevent neurologic damage, which is irreversible
Aspirin	81–325 mg po daily	CAD, stroke, colon cancer	Treatment is inexpensive and has few adverse effects
Estrogen replacement therapy	Conjugated estrogen (plus progesterone for women with an intact uterus) daily or cyclically	CAD, osteoporosis	Whether therapy increases the risk of breast cancer is unclear; therapy may reduce the risk of Alzheimer's disease

*Persons with risk factors (eg, smoking, hypertension, diabetes) who are otherwise healthy may benefit from screening.
CAD = coronary artery disease.

TERTIARY PREVENTION

In tertiary prevention, an existing, usually chronic, disease is appropriately managed to prevent further functional loss. Disease management is enhanced by the use of disease-specific practice guidelines and protocols (eg, those published by the Agency for Health Care Policy and Research). Several disease management programs have been developed. In disease-specific case management, a specially trained nurse coordinates protocol-driven care, arranges support services, and teaches patients. In chronic care clinics, patients with the same chronic disease are taught in groups and are visited by a nurse or physician; this approach can help patients with diabetes achieve better control of their blood sugar. A specialty referral involves referring patients with a chronic disease that is difficult to stabilize to a specialist. This approach works best when the specialist and primary care physician work collaboratively.

Patients with the following chronic diseases, which are common among the elderly, can potentially benefit from tertiary prevention:

Arthritis: Osteoarthritis and rheumatoid arthritis, **1** which affect about half of persons $\geq$ 65 years, lead to impaired mobility and increase the risk of developing osteoporosis, aerobic and muscular deconditioning, and pressure sores.

Osteoporosis: Tests to measure bone density can detect osteoporosis before it leads to a fracture. Calcium supplementation, exercise, and avoidance of cigarette smoking can help prevent osteoporosis, and treatment can prevent new fractures. **2**

Diabetes: Hyperglycemia, especially when the glycosylated hemoglobin (Hb A_{1c}) concentration is > 7.9%, increases the risk of retinopathy, neuropathy, nephropathy, and heart disease. The goal of treatment is an Hb A_{1c} concentration of < 8% for frail diabetic patients and an even lower concentration (< 7%) for patients who are not frail. Patient education and foot examinations at each visit can help prevent foot ulcers. **3**

Vascular disease: Elderly patients with a history of coronary artery disease, cerebrovascular disease, or peripheral vascular disease are at high risk of disabling events. Risk can be reduced by management of vascular risk factors (eg, hypertension, smoking, diabetes, atrial fibrillation, hyperlipoproteinemia).

Heart failure: Morbidity due to heart failure is significant among the elderly, and the mortality rate is higher than that of many cancers. Appropriate, aggressive treatment, especially of systolic dysfunction, reduces functional decline, hospitalization, and mortality rates. **4**

Chronic obstructive pulmonary disease (COPD):   Smoking cessation, appropriate use of inhalers and other drugs, and patient education regarding energy-conserving behavioral techniques can decrease exacerbations of COPD leading to hospitalization.

---

1 see pages 489 and 499   **2** see page 478   **3** see page 629
4 see page 904

PREVENTION OF FRAILTY

Frailty refers to a loss of physiologic reserve that makes a person susceptible to disability from minor stresses. Common features of frailty include weakness, weight loss, muscle wasting (sarcopenia), exercise intolerance, frequent falls, immobility, incontinence, and instability of chronic diseases.

Exercise and a healthy diet are recommended for preventing or reducing frailty (see TABLE 5–2), although evidence of effectiveness is limited. Exercise may reduce the risk of becoming frail for young persons and the risk of further functional loss for functionally impaired elderly persons. Older adults who engage in regular aerobic exercise (eg, walking, swimming, running) exhibit up to a 50% reduction in mortality and have less functional decline compared to those who are sedentary. Weight training can aid in increasing bone mass while decreasing the risk of falls and fractures. A healthy diet may prevent or reduce the risk of many disorders that contribute to frailty, including certain cancers (breast and colon), osteoporosis, obesity, and malnutrition, and may reduce morbidity and mortality.

PREVENTION OF ACCIDENTS

Falls: The elderly are vulnerable to injury from falls. A falls prevention program should be implemented for persons who are at high risk of a fall or who have already fallen. ◼

Driving hazards: For the elderly, the risk of injuring themselves and others while driving is higher than that for younger persons because of age-associated conditions such as slowed reaction time, sensory deficits, and dementia. ◻ Management of specific conditions (when possible) and routine driving tests can minimize risks. All elderly persons should be reminded to use lap and shoulder belts and to refrain from driving when under the influence of alcohol or psychoactive drugs. Sensitivity is required when a health care practitioner must recommend cessation of driving because this recommendation threatens autonomy.

Home hazards: The home may have many hazards. For example, persons with peripheral neuropathy are at increased risk of burns from excessively hot water; burns can be prevented by setting the hot water heater temperature at < 49° C (< 120° F). For persons with dementia, using electrical and gas appliances is particularly dangerous; the use of alarms and automatic shut-off features on appliances can help. Smoke detectors should be installed and maintained. Firearms should be safely stored or removed from the home. All patients or their caregivers can complete a home safety checklist to identify hazards. ◼ Physical and occupational therapists may visit a patient's home to assess its safety.

◼ see page 199   ◻ see page 230   ◼ see TABLE 20–3 on page 200

PREVENTION OF IATROGENIC COMPLICATIONS

Risk Factors

The first step in prevention is to identify patients at high risk. Risk factors include the following:

Multiple chronic diseases: The greater the number of chronic diseases, the greater the risk that treatment of one disease will exacerbate others. For example, treatment of arthritis with a nonsteroidal anti-inflammatory drug may exacerbate heart failure or chronic gastritis.

Multiple physicians: Having several physicians can result in uncoordinated care and polypharmacy. Consultation among several physicians every time one of them sees a common patient is difficult. As a result, a patient's therapeutic regimen is frequently changed without the input of the patient's other physicians, thereby increasing the risk of iatrogenic complications.

Multiple drugs (polypharmacy) and use of inappropriate drugs: Taking several drugs concurrently and having several chronic diseases markedly increase the risk of drug-drug or drug-disease adverse interactions. The risk of such interactions is particularly high among patients who are malnourished or who have renal failure. Additionally, certain drugs pose especially high risk of adverse reactions in the elderly. **1**

Hospitalization: Risks due to hospitalization include nosocomial infection, polypharmacy, and transfusion reactions. Hospitalized patients who have dementia or who are immobilized (eg, after surgery) are at high risk of iatrogenic complications.

Medical technology may contribute to iatrogenic complications, including brain damage during CPR, sudden death or myocardial infarction from valvular replacement surgery, stroke from carotid endarterectomy, fluid overload from transfusions and infusions, and unwanted prolongation of life from using feeding tubes.

Interventions

Interventions that can prevent iatrogenic complications include the following:

Case management: Case managers facilitate communication among health care practitioners, ensure that needed services are provided, and prevent duplication of services. Case managers may be employed by physician groups, health plans, or community or governmental organizations. The frail elderly are the greatest beneficiaries of case management.

Geriatric interdisciplinary team: A geriatric interdisciplinary team evaluates all of the patient's needs and develops a coordinated care plan. Because this intervention is resource-intensive, it is best used in very complex cases. **2**

Pharmacist consultation: A pharmacist can help prevent potential complications caused by polypharmacy and inappropriate drug use. **3**

---

1 see page 62   **2** see page 74   **3** see page 84

Acute Care for the Elderly (ACE) units: These units are hospital wards designed to manage the needs of elderly patients.

Advance directives: Patients are encouraged to prepare advance directives, including designation of proxies to make medical decisions.[1] These documents can help prevent unwanted treatment for critically ill patients who cannot speak for themselves.

PREVENTION OF PSYCHOSOCIAL PROBLEMS

Depression screening is recommended because depression is common among the elderly. Screening is relatively easy (several instruments do not require a physician for administration[2]). For patients who feel lonely or isolated, social worker assistance to increase social contacts may prevent morbidity and postpone death.[3] For those who are depressed, appropriate intervention with counseling or drugs is warranted.[4]

A sense of self-worth may contribute to better health. Remaining productive, engaging in leisure activities, and feeling needed by someone enhance self-worth. Obtaining a pet, contributing to household chores, or performing volunteer work or other activities that confirm a sense of social connectedness may help prevent psychosocial problems (and physical disability).

6 ■ CLINICAL PHARMACOLOGY

Safe, effective pharmacotherapy is one of the greatest challenges in clinical geriatrics. Special considerations are necessary when prescribing drugs (see TABLE 6–1). The elderly have many chronic disorders and consequently use more drugs than any other age group. Their diminished physiologic reserves can be further depleted by effects of drugs and acute or chronic disease. Aging alters pharmacokinetics and pharmacodynamics, affecting the choice, dose, and dosing frequency of many drugs. Pharmacotherapy may also be complicated by an elderly patient's inability to purchase or obtain drugs or to comply with drug regimens.

In the USA, about two thirds of persons ≥ 65 years use prescription and over-the-counter (OTC) drugs; this age group accounts for about one third of all prescription drug use. Women use more drugs than men, especially psychoactive and antiarthritic drugs. At any time, an average elderly person uses four to five prescription drugs and two OTC drugs and fills 12 to 17 prescriptions a year. The frail elderly use the most drugs. Drug use is greater in hospitals and nursing homes than in the community; typically, a nursing home resident uses seven or eight drugs.

[1] see page 134   [2] see page 43   [3] see page 80   [4] see page 319

TABLE 6-1.   GUIDELINES FOR EFFECTIVE PRESCRIBING

- Obtain a complete drug history. Have patients bring all drugs to the office visit for review. Ask about allergies; adverse reactions; use of tobacco, alcohol, caffeine, and recreational drugs; and other health care providers.

- Use no drug before its time. Avoid prescribing when no diagnosis has been established, when symptoms are minor or nonspecific, or when the benefit of drugs is questionable.

- Use no drug beyond its time. Review drug lists at each visit and update them. Discontinue any drugs that are no longer indicated. Monitor the use of as-needed and over-the-counter drugs.

- Know the drugs you use. Know the pharmacologic profile of the drugs you prescribe and the potential adverse effects and toxicities. Monitor patients closely for deterioration in functional parameters that could be drug related.

- Start low, go slow. Always use the minimum dosage necessary for efficacy. Use drug levels when available and appropriate.

- Treat adequately. Use dosages sufficient to achieve the therapeutic goal, as tolerated. Do not withhold therapy for treatable diseases.

- Encourage treatment adherence. Clearly communicate with patients about the therapeutic goals and methods to achieve them. Give legible written instructions. Consider complexity of dosing schedules, expense, and potential adverse effects when choosing a drug.

- Use new drugs with particular caution. Most new compounds have not been thoroughly evaluated in the elderly, and the risk/benefit ratio is often unknown.

Modified from Cusack BJ, Parker BM: "Pharmacology and appropriate prescribing." *Geriatrics Review Syllabus: A Core Curriculum in Geriatric Medicine*, ed. 3, edited by DB Reuben, TT Yoshikawa, and RW Besdine. New York, American Geriatrics Society, 1996, p. 35.

The type of drug used most often by the elderly varies with the setting. Community dwellers use analgesics, diuretics, cardiovascular drugs, and sedative-hypnotics most often, whereas nursing home residents use antipsychotics and sedative-hypnotics most often, followed by diuretics, antihypertensives, analgesics, cardiovascular drugs, and antibiotics. According to some surveys, psychoactive drugs are prescribed for 65% of nursing home patients and for 55% of residential care patients; 7% of patients in nursing homes use three or more psychoactive drugs concurrently.

Appropriateness (the potential benefits of a drug outweigh the potential risks) should guide therapy. Determining appropriateness requires an evaluation of such potential benefits and risks. Many drugs benefit the elderly, and some can save lives—eg, antibiotics and thrombolytic therapy for acute illness. Oral hypoglycemic drugs can improve independence and quality of life while controlling diabetes. Antihypertensive drugs and influenza vaccines can help prevent or decrease morbidity. Analgesics and antidepressants can control debilitating symptoms. However, adverse effects of many drugs are more common and serious in the elderly.

Polypharmacy (concurrent use of many drugs) alone is not an accurate measure of appropriateness of therapy because the elderly often have many disorders requiring treatment; however, it may reflect inappropriate prescribing. Many elderly patients in hospitals and nursing homes routinely receive drugs that are not essential (eg, sedative-hypnotics, analgesics, histamine [H_2] blockers, antibiotics, laxatives) and can cause harm, directly or through interactions. A thorough review of drugs can often reduce the number of drugs used and, according to limited data, improve patient outcomes.

Underuse of some drugs is also a significant problem among elderly patients. For example, antidepressant use in nursing homes is low compared with the high prevalence of depression. Also, the dose of antidepressants often is too low and duration of therapy too short. Drugs for incontinence and preventive treatments (eg, glaucoma drugs, influenza and pneumococcal vaccines) are also underused.

Patient and caregiver issues: Increasingly, elderly patients are aware of their diagnoses and the drugs they use for treatment; however, many need to be encouraged to bring health problems and potential drug-related problems to the attention of their physician or caregiver. In particular, patients should be asked to report their use of all drugs (eg, prescription and OTC drugs, vitamins, nutritional supplements) and to report any changes at each visit. Periodically, they should be asked to bring their drugs to the office for review and for comparison with the drug record. The physician should review and update the treatment regimen at each visit. While doing so, the physician can ask about adherence (compliance). When adherence appears to be deficient, efforts should be made to simplify the regimen and to suggest useful aids to enhance adherence (eg, drug calendars, drug dispensers). The physician should also discuss how drugs should be taken (eg, with or without food, route of administration), their mechanism of action, important adverse effects, and appropriate storage. Patients should recognize the role of the pharmacist as a member of the health care team and as a resource for information. The time devoted to communicating with patients about drugs and their usage builds trust and enhances overall patient care.

PHARMACOKINETICS

The time course by which the body absorbs, distributes, metabolizes, and excretes drugs.

Absorption: Despite an age-related decrease in small-bowel surface area and an increase in gastric pH, changes in drug absorption tend to be trivial and clinically inconsequential.

Distribution: Total body water decreases by 10 to 15% between ages 20 and 80 years. ∎ In contrast, the percentage of body weight that is body fat increases from 18 to 36% in men and from 33 to 45% in women. The relative decrease in total body water and thus in sodium space leads to higher blood (and often tissue) concentrations of some water-soluble drugs. Increased body fat increases the volume of distribution for lipophilic drugs and may result in increased elimination half-lives.

With age, serum albumin levels decrease slightly and α_1-acid glycoprotein levels increase, but the clinical effect of these changes on serum drug binding is unclear. In a patient with acute disease or malnutrition, rapid decreases in the serum albumin level may enhance drug effects because serum concentrations of unbound drug are increased until metabolic excretory compensation occurs.

Hepatic metabolism: With age, hepatic mass and hepatic blood flow decrease. Decreased hepatic blood flow significantly affects hepatic elimination of drugs in rare situations—eg, when a drug with high clearance, such as lidocaine, is given IV.

Although expression of drug-metabolizing enzymes in the cytochrome P-450 system does not appear to decrease with age, overall hepatic metabolism of many drugs by these enzymes is reduced. For drugs with reduced hepatic metabolism (see TABLE 6–2), clearance typically decreases 30 to 40%. Theoretically, maintenance drug doses should be reduced by the same percentage; however, the rate of hepatic metabolism of drugs can vary greatly from person to person, and individual titration is required.

In the elderly, presystemic (first-pass) metabolism of some oral drugs (eg, labetalol, propranolol, verapamil) is reduced, increasing their serum concentration and bioavailability. Consequently, initial doses of these drugs should be reduced by about 30%. However, presystemic metabolism of other metabolized drugs (eg, imipramine, amitriptyline, morphine, meperidine) is not reduced.

Hepatic clearance of drugs metabolized by the cytochrome P-450 system (phase I reactions)—eg, diazepam, amitriptyline, chlordiazepoxide—is often reduced in the elderly. Age less often has been shown to affect the clearance of drugs that are metabolized by glucuronate or sulfate conjugation (synthetic or phase II reaction), such as lorazepam, desipramine, and oxazepam.

Many drugs produce active metabolites in clinically relevant concentrations. Examples are some benzodiazepines (eg, diazepam, chlordiazepoxide), tertiary amine antidepressants (eg, amitriptyline, imipramine), antipsychotics (eg, chlorpromazine, thioridazine, risperidone), and opioid analgesics (eg, morphine, meperidine, propoxyphene). Accumulation of active metabolites (eg, *N*-acetylprocainamide, morphine-6-glucuronide) increases the risk of toxicity in the elderly due to age-related decreases in

∎ see page 561

TABLE 6–2. DRUGS WITH REDUCED METABOLISM* OR ELIMINATION IN THE ELDERLY

Class	Reduced Hepatic Metabolism	Reduced Renal Elimination
Analgesics and anti-inflammatory drugs	Dextropropoxyphene Ibuprofen Meperidine Morphine Naproxen	—
Antibiotics	—	Amikacin Ciprofloxacin Gentamicin Nitrofurantoin Streptomycin Tobramycin
Cardiovascular drugs	Amlodipine Diltiazem Lidocaine† Nifedipine Propranolol Quinidine Theophylline Verapamil	N-Acetylprocainamide Captopril Digoxin Enalapril Lisinopril Procainamide Quinapril
Diuretics	—	Amiloride Furosemide Hydrochlorothiazide Triamterene
Psychoactive drugs	Alprazolam† Chlordiazepoxide Citalopram Desipramine† Diazepam Imipramine Nortriptyline Trazodone Triazolam†	Risperidone‡
Others	Levodopa	Amantadine Chlorpropamide Cimetidine Lithium Methotrexate Ranitidine

* According to most studies.
† In men only.
‡ 9-Hydroxyrisperidone is the active metabolite.

renal clearance, particularly in patients with renal disease, unless the maintenance doses are reduced.

Renal elimination: With age, renal mass and renal blood flow (mainly in the renal cortex) decrease significantly. After age 30, creatinine clearance decreases an average of 8 mL/min/1.73 m²/decade in about two thirds of persons but remains the same in the rest. However, serum creatinine levels may remain within normal limits because the elderly have less lean body mass and produce less creatinine. Decreases in tubular function parallel those in glomerular function.

These physiologic changes decrease renal elimination of drugs (see TABLE 6–2). Clinical implications depend on the contribution of renal elimination to total systemic elimination and on the drug's therapeutic index (ratio of the maximum tolerated dose to the minimum effective dose). Creatinine clearance (measured or estimated using computer programs or the Cockcroft-Gault formula) is used to guide drug dose. The Cockcroft-Gault formula uses the serum creatinine concentration to calculate creatinine clearance (Cl_{creat}):

$$Cl_{creat} \text{ (mL/min)} = \frac{(140 - \text{age [yr]) (body wt [kg])}}{(72) \text{ (serum creatinine [mg/dL])}}$$

For women, the calculated values are multiplied by 0.85.

Because renal function is dynamic, maintenance doses of drugs should be adjusted if a patient becomes acutely ill or dehydrated or has recently recovered from dehydration. Also, because renal function may continue to decline with age, the dose of drugs given long-term should be reviewed periodically.

PHARMACODYNAMICS

The time course and effect of drugs on cellular and organ function.

In the elderly, the effects of similar drug concentrations at the site of action may be larger or smaller than those in younger persons (see TABLE 6–3). The difference may be due to changes in drug-receptor interaction, in postreceptor events, or in adaptive homeostatic responses; among frail patients, the difference is often due to organ pathology.

Increased sensitivity due to aging must be considered when drugs that can have serious adverse effects are used. These drugs include morphine, pentazocine, warfarin, angiotensin-converting enzyme inhibitors, diazepam (especially given parenterally), and levodopa. Some drugs whose effects are reduced with normal aging (eg, tolbutamide, glyburide, β-blockers) should also be used with caution in elderly patients because serious dose-related toxicity can occur and signs of toxicity may be delayed.

TABLE 6–3.   EFFECT OF AGING ON DRUG EFFECTS

Class	Drug	Action	Effect of Aging
Analgesics	Aspirin	Acute gastroduodenal mucosal damage	↔
	Morphine	Acute analgesic effect	↑
	Pentazocine	Analgesic effect	↑
Anticoagulants	Heparin	Activated partial thromboplastin time	↔
	Warfarin	Prothrombin time	↑
Bronchodilators	Albuterol	Bronchodilation	↓
	Ipratropium	Bronchodilation	↔
Cardiovascular drugs	Adenosine	Minute ventilation and heart rate response	↔
		Venodilation	↔
	Angiotensin II	Increase in blood pressure	↑
	Diltiazem	Acute antihypertensive effect	↑
	Dopamine	Increase in creatinine clearance	↓
	Enalapril	Acute antihypertensive effect	↑
	Felodipine	Antihypertensive effect	↑
	Histamine	Venodilation	↔
	Isoproterenol	Chronotropic effect	↓
		Ejection fraction	↓
		Venodilation	↓
	Nitroglycerin	Venodilation	↔
	Norepinephrine	Acute vasoconstriction	↔
	Phenylephrine	Acute hypertensive effect	↔
		Acute venoconstriction	↔
	Prazosin	Acute antihypertensive effect	↔
	Propranolol	Chronotropic effect	↓
	Timolol	Chronotropic effect	↔
	Verapamil	Acute antihypertensive effect	↑
Diuretics	Bumetanide	Urine flow and sodium excretion	↓
	Dopamine	Creatinine clearance	↓
	Furosemide	Latency and size of peak diuretic response	↓
Oral hypoglycemics	Glyburide	Chronic hypoglycemic effect	↔
	Tolbutamide	Acute hypoglycemic effect	↓
Psychoactive drugs	Diazepam	Sedation	↑↑
	Diphenhydramine	Psychomotor function	↔

TABLE 6–3.   (*Continued*)

Class	Drug	Action	Effect of Aging
	Haloperidol	Acute sedation	↓
	Midazolam	EEG activity, sedation	↑
	Temazepam	Postural sway, psychomotor effect, sedation	↑
	Thiopental	EEG measure of anesthesia	↔
	Triazolam	Sedation	↔
Others	Atropine	Impairment of gastric emptying	↔
	Levodopa	Dose limitation due to adverse reactions	↑
	Metoclopramide	Sedation	↔

↑ = increased; ↓ = decreased; ↔ = unchanged; EEG = electroencephalogram.
Adapted from Cusack BJ, Vestal RE: "Clinical pharmacology: Special considerations in the elderly," in *Practice of Geriatric Medicine*, edited by E Calkins, PJ Davis, and AB Ford. Philadelphia, WB Saunders Company, 1986, pp. 115–136; used with permission.

Stimulation of β receptors increases intracellular cyclic adenosine monophosphate (cAMP). This activates a protein kinase, an enzyme that phosphorylates proteins, leading to altered cellular function. In elderly persons, the cAMP response to β agonists is decreased in human lymphocytes and cardiac tissue, apparently due to reduced binding affinity of β agonists for the β receptor and to changes in postreceptor response.

Desensitization is not responsible. Up-regulation of receptors in the heart and lymphocytes after β-blockade is unaltered by aging. These changes, however, are tissue-specific and differ in other tissues (eg, adipocytes). Thus, the chronotropic response to bolus administration of the β agonist isoproterenol (isoprenaline) becomes blunted with age. However, sensitivity to isoproterenol is reduced in both the young and old by nonselective β-blockers (eg, propranolol). The effect of propranolol may be due to blockade of β receptors in the peripheral vasculature or in the heart. However, the heart rate response to isoproterenol bolus dosing is largely due to baroreflex responses of vagal withdrawal and sympathetic activation rather than to the direct effect of β receptor activation. Thus, the blunted chronotropic response in the elderly is largely abolished by autonomic blockade by atropine and clonidine, which block the component of the chronotropic response due to baroreceptor reflex activation secondary to isoproterenol-induced vasodilatation. This effect shows that evaluation of drug responses must consider counterregulatory mechanisms.

With age, central nervous system sedation by benzodiazepines is increased. This increase is clinically important. For effective and safe acute sedation, the dose of midazolam should be decreased by 30% in elderly patients because of pharmacodynamic changes with age. The effect of oral triazolam is also increased, but this increase is due to increased drug levels rather than to increased sensitivity. Similar pharmacokinetic and pharmacodynamic considerations apply to long-acting benzodiazepines such as chlordiazepoxide, diazepam, and flurazepam, all of which undergo oxidation to active metabolites that accumulate with chronic dosing and have a prolonged effect. The renal response to furosemide or dopamine is reduced. However, while the acute bronchodilator responses to albuterol (a β_2 agonist) are reduced with age in normal subjects, the responses to albuterol or ipratropium (a muscarinic antagonist) are unaltered with age in patients with asthma or chronic obstructive pulmonary disease.

ADVERSE DRUG REACTIONS

About one third of drug-related hospitalizations and one half of drug-related deaths occur in persons > 60. The elderly are at increased risk of toxicity from certain drugs, especially long-acting benzodiazepines, nonsteroidal anti-inflammatory drugs, warfarin, heparin, aminoglycosides, isoniazid, high doses of thiazides, antineoplastic drugs, and most antiarrhythmics (see TABLE 6–4). Increased risk has not been demonstrated with other drugs (eg, β-blockers, antihypertensives, lidocaine, propafenone).

Increased susceptibility may result from age-associated changes in pharmacokinetics or pharmacodynamics or from disorders aggravated by drugs (eg, prostatism by anticholinergic drugs, postural hypotension by diuretics). The risk of an adverse drug reaction increases exponentially with the number of drugs used, in part because polypharmacy reflects the presence of many diseases and provides an opportunity for drug-disease and drug-drug interactions.

Drug-disease interactions (exacerbation of a disease by a drug) can occur in any age group but are especially important in the elderly because of the increased prevalence of disease and the difficulty in differentiating often subtle adverse drug reactions from the effects of disease (see TABLE 6–5). Anticholinergic drugs are a common cause of such interactions (eg, with glaucoma, benign prostatic hyperplasia, Alzheimer's disease, dry eyes, or xerostomia).

Drug-drug interactions (the altered pharmacokinetics or pharmacodynamics of a drug when taken concomitantly with one or more other drugs) are myriad (see TABLE 6–6). Few prospective studies of drug-drug interactions in the elderly have been conducted. One study showed that 40% of ambulatory elderly patients were at risk of drug-drug interactions; 27% of these interactions were potentially serious (eg, quinidine-digoxin interaction). Inhibition of one drug's metabolism by another does not appear to change with age; eg, cimetidine

TABLE 6–4.   HIGH-RISK DRUGS IN THE ELDERLY

Class	Drug	Prescribing Concern
Analgesics	Indomethacin	Of all available NSAIDs, indomethacin produces the most CNS adverse effects and therefore should be avoided in the elderly
	Meperidine	Meperidine is not an effective oral analgesic and has many disadvantages compared with other opioids. It should be avoided in the elderly
	Pentazocine	Pentazocine is an opioid analgesic that causes more CNS adverse effects (eg, confusion, hallucinations) more commonly than other opioids, and it is a mixed agonist/antagonist. For both reasons, it generally should be avoided in the elderly
	Phenylbutazone	Phenylbutazone may produce serious hematologic adverse effects and should not be used in the elderly
	Propoxyphene and combination products	Propoxyphene has few analgesic advantages over acetaminophen but has the adverse effects of other opioids
Antidepressants	Amitriptyline Doxepin Imipramine	Because of strong anticholinergic and sedating properties, amitriptyline or doxepin is rarely the antidepressant of choice for the elderly
Antihistamines	Bromodiphenhydramine Brompheniramine Chlorpheniramine Cyproheptadine Dexchlorpheniramine Diphenhydramine Hydroxyzine Promethazine Tripelennamine Triprolidine	All OTC and many prescription antihistamines have potent anticholinergic properties. Antihistamines are commonly included with other drugs in cough and cold preparations; however, many cough and cold preparations are available without antihistamines and are safer alternatives for the elderly
Cardiovascular drugs	Digoxin	Because renal clearance of digoxin is decreased in the elderly, doses should rarely exceed 0.125 mg/day, except when used to treat atrial arrhythmias
	Dipyridamole	Dipyridamole frequently causes orthostatic hypotension in the elderly. It has proved beneficial only in patients with artificial heart valves. If possible, it should be avoided in the elderly

Table continues on the following page.

TABLE 6–4.   HIGH-RISK DRUGS IN THE ELDERLY (*Continued*)

Class	Drug	Prescribing Concern
	Disopyramide	Of all antiarrhythmics, disopyramide is the most potent negative inotrope and therefore may induce heart failure in the elderly. It is also strongly anticholinergic. When appropriate, other antiarrhythmics should be used
	Methyldopa Methyldopa/HCTZ	Methyldopa may cause bradycardia and exacerbate depression in the elderly. Alternate treatments for hypertension are generally preferred
	Reserpine Reserpine/HCTZ	Reserpine imposes unnecessary risks in the elderly; it may cause depression, erectile dysfunction, sedation, and orthostatic hypotension. Safer alternatives exist
	Ticlopidine	Ticlopidine is more toxic than aspirin. It should be used only as a second-line drug in the elderly
Gastrointestinal antispasmodics	Belladonna alkaloids Clidinium/ chlordiazepoxide Dicyclomine Hyoscyamine Propantheline	Gastrointestinal antispasmodics are highly anticholinergic and generally produce substantial toxicity in the elderly. Their effectiveness at doses tolerated by the elderly is questionable. All of these drugs are best avoided in the elderly, especially for long-term use
Hypoglycemics	Chlorpropamide	Chlorpropamide has a prolonged half-life in the elderly and can cause prolonged, serious hypoglycemia. It is the only oral hypoglycemic drug that causes SIADH. It should be avoided in the elderly
Muscle relaxants	Carisoprodol Chlorzoxazone Cyclobenzaprine Metaxalone Methocarbamol Oxybutynin	Most muscle relaxants and antispasmodics are poorly tolerated by the elderly, resulting in anticholinergic effects, sedation, and weakness. Their effectiveness at doses tolerated by the elderly is questionable. If possible, they should not be used in the elderly
Sedative-hypnotics	Alprazolam 2 mg* Lorazepam 2 mg Oxazepam 60 mg Temazepam 15 mg Triazolam 0.25 mg Zolpidem 5 mg	Because sensitivity to benzodiazepines is increased in the elderly, smaller doses may be effective and safer. Total daily doses should rarely exceed those listed

TABLE 6–4. (*Continued*)

Class	Drug	Prescribing Concern
	Barbiturates	Barbiturates cause more adverse effects than most other sedative-hypnotics in the elderly and are highly addictive. They should not be started as new therapy in the elderly except to control seizures
	Chlordiazepoxide Chlordiazepoxide/ amitriptyline Clidinium/ chlordiazepoxide Diazepam Flurazepam Nitrazepam	Chlordiazepoxide, diazepam, flurazepam, and nitrazepam have a long half-life in the elderly (often days), producing prolonged sedation and increasing the risk of falls and fractures. Short- and intermediate-acting benzodiazepines are preferred if a benzodiazepine is required
	Diphenhydramine	Diphenhydramine is potently anticholinergic and usually should not be used as a hypnotic in the elderly. When used to treat or prevent allergic reactions, it should be used in the smallest possible dose and with great caution
	Meprobamate	Meprobamate is a highly addictive and sedating anxiolytic. It should be avoided in elderly patients. Those using it for prolonged periods may become addicted, and the drug may need to be withdrawn slowly
Other	Cyclandelate Ergot mesylates	Ergot mesylates and cerebral vasodilators have not been shown to be effective for the treatment of dementia or any other disorder
	Iron supplements > 325 mg	Ferrous sulfate rarely needs to be given in doses > 325 mg/day. With higher doses, total absorption is not substantially increased, but gastrointestinal upset is more likely to occur
	Trimethobenzamide	Trimethobenzamide is one of the least effective antiemetics and can cause extrapyramidal adverse effects. When possible, it should be avoided in the elderly

*Doses may be higher when used to treat panic disorders.
NSAIDs = nonsteroidal anti-inflammatory drugs; CNS = central nervous system; OTC = over-the-counter; HCTZ = hydrochlorothiazide; SIADH = syndrome of inappropriate antidiuretic hormone secretion.

and ciprofloxacin inhibit the metabolic rate of theophylline by about 30% in older and younger healthy persons. Aging's effect on induction of drug metabolism varies; eg, induction of theophylline metabolism by phenytoin is similar in older and younger persons, whereas induction of drug metabolism by dichloralphenazone, glutethimide, and rifampin may be decreased in older persons.

Concurrent use of drugs with similar toxicities can result in serious adverse reactions in the elderly. For example, concurrent use of anticholinergic drugs, such as antiparkinsonian drugs (eg, benztropine), tricyclic antidepressants (eg, amitriptyline, imipramine), antipsychotics (eg, thioridazine), antiarrhythmics (eg, disopyramide), and OTC antihistamines (eg, diphenhydramine, chlorpheniramine) may cause or worsen dry mouth, gum disease, blurred vision, constipation, urinary retention, and delirium.

CONSIDERATIONS FOR EFFECTIVE PHARMACOTHERAPY

The principal clinical concerns include efficacy and safety, dose, complexity of regimen, cost, and patient compliance.

Efficacy and safety are important considerations when prescribing drugs. Because the risk/benefit ratio of drug therapy can be less favorable in the elderly (ie, the risk of adverse effects is increased), it is important to use drugs with documented effectiveness and the lowest toxicity. Drug selection is particularly important for the very old with chronic conditions (eg, hypertension, new-onset diabetes), in whom outcomes are less certain. For example, the benefit of treatment of uncomplicated hypertension in patients $\geq$ 80 is less well established than in those < 80. Therapeutic goals (eg, reduction of blood pressure or glycosylated hemoglobin [Hb A_{1c}]) may have to be modified to minimize the risk of dose-related adverse effects.

Dose must often be reduced in the elderly, although dose requirements vary considerably (up to fivefold) from person to person. In general, starting doses of drugs with a low therapeutic index are about one third to one half the usual adult doses. If a patient has a clinical problem that may be exacerbated by a drug, the usual starting dose should be reduced by about one half, especially if elimination of the drug is reduced with age.

Complexity of drug regimens (eg, multiple drugs, frequent dosing, variable doses) increases the risk of noncompliance. If a patient has more than one disorder (eg, hypertension and angina), it may be possible to treat both conditions with a single drug (eg, a β-blocker or calcium [Ca] channel blocker), thus reducing the number of drugs prescribed. Drugs with once- or twice-daily dosing (long-acting or slow-release preparations) enable better compliance than do those with

TABLE 6–5. SELECTED DRUG-DISEASE INTERACTIONS IN THE ELDERLY

Disease	Drugs	Adverse Reactions
Benign prostatic hyperplasia	α-Agonists, anticholinergics	Urinary retention
Cardiac conduction disorders	β-Blockers, digoxin, diltiazem, tricyclic antidepressants, verapamil	Heart block
Chronic obstructive pulmonary disease	β-Blockers Opioids, sedatives	Bronchoconstriction Respiratory depression
Dementia	Anticholinergics, anticonvulsants, levodopa, benzodiazepines, opioids, antidepressants, antipsychotics	Increased confusion, delirium
Depression	Alcohol, benzodiazepines, β-blockers, centrally acting antihypertensives, corticosteroids	Precipitation or exacerbation of depression
Diabetes	Corticosteroids	Hyperglycemia
Glaucoma	Anticholinergics	Exacerbation of glaucoma
Heart failure	β-Blockers, disopyramide, verapamil	Exacerbation of heart failure
Hypertension	NSAIDs	Increased blood pressure
Hypokalemia	Digoxin	Cardiac arrhythmias
Hyponatremia	Oral hypoglycemics, diuretics, carbamazepine	Decreased sodium concentration
Orthostatic hypotension	Diuretics, levodopa, tricyclic antidepressants, vasodilators	Dizziness, falls, syncope, hip fracture
Osteopenia	Corticosteroids	Fracture
Parkinson's disease	Antipsychotics	Worsening movement disorder
Peptic ulcer disease	Anticoagulants, NSAIDs	Upper gastrointestinal bleeding
Peripheral vascular disease	β-Blockers	Intermittent claudication
Renal impairment	Aminoglycosides, NSAIDs, radiocontrast dyes	Acute renal failure

NSAIDs = nonsteroidal anti-inflammatory drugs.

more frequent dosing. The drug regimen should be discussed with the patient to help form a partnership and to keep the regimen simple.

Cost of drugs can impose a major financial burden, particularly for elderly patients who rely on fixed incomes. Prescribers need to be aware of drug costs and to discuss cost. When cost is a factor, the least

TABLE 6–6. CLINICALLY IMPORTANT DRUG-DRUG INTERACTIONS IN THE ELDERLY

Drug	Interacting Drug	Mechanism	Effect
Pharmacokinetic interactions			
Ciprofloxacin	Sucralfate	Decreased absorption	Decreased antibiotic response
Digoxin	Amiodarone, diltiazem, quinidine, verapamil	Decreased renal or nonrenal clearance	Digitalis toxicity
	Antacids, cholestyramine, colestipol	Decreased absorption	Decreased digoxin effect
Methotrexate	Penicillins, probenecid, salicylate, other organic acids	Decreased active renal tubular secretion	Methotrexate toxicity
Most drugs	Anticholinergic drugs	Altered rate of gastric emptying	Decreased rate of drug absorption
	Metoclopramide	Altered rate of gastric emptying	Increased rate of drug absorption
Phenytoin	Barbiturates, rifampin	Induction of drug metabolism	Loss of seizure control
Theophylline	Carbamazepine, phenytoin, rifampin, smoking	Induction of drug metabolism	Increase in dyspnea
	Cimetidine, ciprofloxacin, disulfiram, enoxacin, erythromycin, mexiletine	Inhibition of drug metabolism	Theophylline toxicity
Warfarin	Aspirin, furosemide	Displacement from plasma protein binding site	Possible increased anticoagulant effect
	Barbiturates, carbamazepine, rifampin	Induction of drug metabolism	Decreased anticoagulation
	Cimetidine, metronidazole, omeprazole, trimethoprim-sulfamethoxazole, amiodarone	Inhibition of drug metabolism	Increased anticoagulation, bleeding
Pharmacodynamic interactions			
Albuterol	β-Blockers	Competitive blockade of β receptors	Decreased bronchodilator response
Aspirin	Warfarin	Effects on platelet function, coagulation, and mucosal integrity	Gastrointestinal bleeding

TABLE 6–6.   (*Continued*)

Drug	Interacting Drug	Mechanism	Effect
Pharmacodynamic interactions (*continued*)			
Benztropine	Other anticholinergics (eg, antihistamines, tricyclic antidepressants, thioridazine)	Additive effect on cholinergic receptors	Confusion, urinary retention
β-Blockers	Digoxin, diltiazem, verapamil	Effects on cardiac conduction	Bradycardia, heart block
Digoxin	Diuretics	Hypokalemia	Digitalis toxicity
Diuretics	Angiotensin-converting enzyme inhibitors, α-blockers, levodopa, phenothiazines, tricyclic antidepressants, vasodilators	Orthostatic hypotension	Falls, weakness, syncope
	Nonsteroidal anti-inflammatory drugs	Reduced renal perfusion	Renal impairment

expensive comparable therapy should first be considered (eg, thiazide diuretics for hypertension).

Compliance (adherence) is affected by many factors, but probably not by age per se. However, about 40% of elderly patients do not take their drugs as directed, usually taking less drug than prescribed.

Patients are more like to comply if they have a good relationship with their physician, in which they are included in the decision making and the physician shows concern that they comply. Clear prescription instructions and explanations of why the treatment is necessary and what to expect (eg, delayed benefits, general adverse effects) also help ensure compliance. Trust in the physician is crucial.

Encouraging patients to ask questions and express their concerns can help them come to terms with the severity of their illness and intelligently weigh the advantages and disadvantages of a treatment regimen. Discussing the unconscious mechanism of denial of illness and how it leads to "forgetting" or otherwise not taking the drug as directed can help patients avoid that pitfall. They should be urged to report any unwanted or unexpected effects to their physician before adjusting or stopping the treatment on their own. Patients often have good reasons for not following a regimen, and their physician can make an appropriate adjustment after a frank discussion of the problem.

Pharmacists and nurses may detect and help solve compliance problems. For example, the pharmacist may note that the patient does not obtain refills or that a prescription is illogical or incorrect. In reviewing prescription directions with the patient, a pharmacist or nurse may uncover a patient's misunderstandings or fears and alleviate them. Communication among all health care practitioners providing care for a patient is important. Support groups for patients with certain disorders can often reinforce treatment plans and provide suggestions for coping with problems.

DRUG CLASSES OF CONCERN

Some drug classes (eg, diuretic, antihypertensive, antiarrhythmic, antiparkinsonian, anticoagulant, psychoactive, hypoglycemic, and analgesic drugs) pose special risks for the elderly. Some individual drugs pose similar risks (see TABLE 6–4), and safer alternatives are often available.

Diuretics: Lower doses of thiazide diuretics (eg, hydrochlorothiazide or chlorthalidone 12.5 to 25 mg) can control hypertension, with less risk of hypokalemia and hyperglycemia than higher doses. Thus, potassium supplements or potassium-sparing diuretics may be required less often. Doses > 25 mg/day have been associated with increased mortality rates.

Antihypertensives: Treatment of hypertension is effective in elderly patients; treatment of only 18 elderly patients for 5 years prevents one cardiovascular event. Different classes of antihypertensives[1] have comparable efficacy in elderly white patients; however, in elderly black patients, β-blockers and angiotensin-converting enzyme inhibitors are generally less effective, whereas diuretics and Ca channel blockers are most effective. Whether any antihypertensives are preferable because they best preserve quality of life in the elderly is unclear. If tolerated, diuretics are the first choice for elderly patients because these drugs reduce cardiovascular morbidity rates and cardiovascular and all-cause mortality rates. Long-acting dihydropyridine-type Ca channel blockers (eg, amlodipine, felodipine, sustained-release nifedipine) also appear to reduce cardiovascular events in the elderly. Short-acting dihydropyridines (eg, nifedipine) should not be used because of an increased mortality risk. The benefits of β-blockers for hypertension in the elderly have been questioned. Contraindications to β-blockers include chronic obstructive pulmonary disease and peripheral vascular disease; to clonidine, depression; and to vasodilators and α-blockers, underlying orthostatic hypotension.

Antiarrhythmics: Antiarrhythmics have the same indications and efficacy in older and in younger patients. However, because of altered pharmacokinetics, the dose of some (eg, procainamide, quinidine, lidocaine) should be reduced in the elderly. In addition, the risk of significant adverse reactions to certain drugs (eg, mexiletine; class IC drugs, such as encainide and flecainide) increases with age. Digoxin clearance decreases an average of 50% in elderly patients with normal serum creatinine levels. Therefore, maintenance doses should be started low (0.125 mg/day) and adjusted according to response and serum digoxin levels.

---

[1] see also TABLE 85–3 on page 839

Antiparkinsonian drugs: Levodopa clearance is reduced in elderly patients, who are also more susceptible to postural hypotension and confusion. Therefore, elderly patients should receive low starting doses of levodopa and should be monitored closely for adverse effects. **1** Patients who become confused while taking levodopa may not better tolerate the newer dopamine agonists (eg, bromocriptine, pergolide, pramipexole, ropinirole). With long-term levodopa treatment, motor complications such as on-off fluctuations and dyskinesias occur. Whether these complications are due to disease progression or to levodopa therapy is unclear. Some neurologists advocate early use of dopamine agonists to reduce exposure to levodopa, thus avoiding or delaying these motor complications. The success of this strategy has not been demonstrated. Because elderly patients with parkinsonism may be cognitively impaired, anticholinergic drugs should be avoided when possible.

Anticoagulants: Aging does not alter the pharmacokinetics of warfarin but may increase sensitivity to its anticoagulant effect (increased prothrombin time or international normalized ratio). Elderly patients generally require lower loading (< 7.5 mg) and maintenance (usually < 5 mg/day) doses of warfarin. **2** If the drug must be stopped (eg, before surgery), the reversal to normal clotting status may be slower in elderly patients than in younger patients.

Psychoactive drugs: In nonpsychotic, demented patients with behavioral disorders, **antipsychotics** control symptoms only marginally better than do placebos. **3** Although antipsychotics can reduce paranoia, they may worsen confusion. Elderly patients, especially women, are at increased risk of tardive dyskinesia, which is often irreversible. Sedation, postural hypotension, anticholinergic effects, and akathisia (subjective motor restlessness) commonly occur in elderly patients using an antipsychotic. Drug-induced parkinsonism can persist for up to 9 months after the drug is stopped. One goal of the U.S. Omnibus Budget Reconciliation Act of 1987 was to reduce the use of antipsychotics as chemical restraints in nonpsychotic elderly patients.

When an antipsychotic is used in the elderly, the starting dose should be about one quarter the usual adult dose and increased gradually. Risk of extrapyramidal dysfunction appears to be less with the new atypical antipsychotics (eg, olanzapine, quetiapine, risperidone)—a potential advantage in the elderly. However, experience with these drugs in the elderly is limited, and initial dose reduction is required (eg, risperidone 2 to 4 mg/day). In frail nursing home patients, a starting dose of 2 mg/day is appropriate. The elderly appear to tolerate olanzapine reasonably well.

The use of **anxiolytics and hypnotics** is problematic. Different benzodiazepines appear equally effective in relieving anxiety symptoms; selection depends on the drug's pharmacokinetics and pharmacodynamics.

---

1 see also page 437   **2** see also page 698   **3** see also page 375

Treatable causes of insomnia should be sought and managed before using hypnotics.[1] In general, short-acting to intermediate-acting benzodiazepines with half-lives < 24 hours (eg, alprazolam, lorazepam, oxazepam, temazepam) are preferable for inducing sedation or sleep. Long-acting benzodiazepines should be avoided because the risk of accumulation and toxicity is increased, leading to drowsiness, impaired memory, and impaired balance with falls and fractures. Drug treatment of anxiety or insomnia should be limited to short-term or occasional use if possible because tolerance and dependence may develop; withdrawal may lead to rebound insomnia and anxiety.

Buspirone, a partial serotonin agonist, is as effective as benzodiazepines in the treatment of general anxiety disorder;[2] elderly patients tolerate doses up to 30 mg/day. Buspirone's slow onset of action (up to 2 to 3 weeks) can be a disadvantage in cases requiring rapid effect. Zolpidem is a nonbenzodiazepine hypnotic that binds mainly to a benzodiazepine receptor subtype; elderly patients with insomnia appear to tolerate doses of 5 to 10 mg. Zolpidem's advantages over benzodiazepines include less disturbance of the sleep profile, fewer rebound effects, and less dependence potential. H_1 blockers (eg, diphenhydramine, hydroxyzine) are not recommended because of their anticholinergic effects.

In general, the **antidepressants** of choice are the selective serotonin reuptake inhibitors (SSRIs—eg, fluoxetine, paroxetine, sertraline, citalopram). SSRIs[3] appear to be as effective as tricyclic antidepressants but produce less toxicity, especially in overdose. One possible disadvantage of fluoxetine is its long elimination half-life, especially of its active metabolite. Paroxetine is more sedating, has anticholinergic action, and, similar to fluoxetine, can inhibit hepatic cytochrome P-450 2D6 enzyme activity, with risk of impairing the metabolism of several drugs (eg, some antipsychotics, antiarrhythmics, and tricyclic antidepressants). Sertraline is more activating, but diarrhea is a common adverse effect. Both sertraline and citalopram appear to have less drug interaction potential. The hepatic clearance of citalopram is reduced in elderly patients. Initial doses of SSRIs should be reduced by up to 50% in the elderly.

Tricyclic antidepressants are effective. Those with the fewest adverse effects are best for the elderly, and those with significant anticholinergic (eg, amitriptyline, imipramine), antihistaminic (eg, doxepin), and antidopaminergic (eg, amoxapine) effects are best avoided. The norepinephrine reuptake inhibitors nortriptyline and desipramine, starting at 10 to 25 mg/day, are most suitable. Both have low anticholinergic potency, and nortriptyline has the least α-blocking (hypotensive) action. However, overdose produces cardiac and neurologic toxicity, precluding the use of these drugs in patients at risk of suicide. Trazodone is now used mainly for sedation in patients with depression and insomnia. It has low anticholinergic potency. Trazodone is less cardiotoxic than tricyclics, but it can produce orthostatic

[1] see also page 452   [2] see page 325   [3] see also page 320

hypotension and priapism. Bupropion is noncardiotoxic but, at higher doses, increases the risk of seizures. Newer drugs (eg, mirtazapine, nefazodone, venlafaxine) are useful for patients not responding to or intolerant of SSRIs. Methylphenidate can be useful in treating some elderly patients with depression who have had a stroke or who have an enervating medical illness. The drug's onset of action is rapid. Monoamine oxidase inhibitors (eg, tranylcypromine, phenelzine) should be prescribed only by psychiatrists with experience in treating elderly patients.

Hypoglycemics: Recent information indicates that treatment of type II diabetes mellitus can improve outcomes, especially microvascular complications. Elderly diabetic patients with reasonable life expectancy deserve careful and aggressive treatment to reduce Hb A_{1c} to about 7%.◘ This reduction may be impossible because of risks of hypoglycemia or resistance to treatment. Oral hypoglycemics remain the mainstay of treatment of type II diabetes. Sulfonylureas increase insulin secretion. They are effective in and well tolerated by elderly patients. However, the incidence of hypoglycemia due to sulfonylureas may increase with age. Chlorpropamide is *not recommended* because elderly patients are at increased risk of hyponatremia and because the drug's prolonged duration of action is dangerous if toxicity or hypoglycemia occurs. Aging can reduce insulin clearance, but the dose of insulin depends on the level of insulin resistance, which varies widely among patients with type II diabetes.

Metformin, a biguanide excreted by the kidney, increases peripheral tissue sensitivity to insulin and can be effective alone or in combination with sulfonylureas. However, long-term efficacy and safety in elderly patients are not well established. Risk of lactic acidosis, a rare but serious complication, increases with the degree of renal impairment and the patient's age. Metformin is contraindicated in patients with renal disease or renal dysfunction (ie, serum creatinine $\geq$ 1.5 mg/dL [$\geq$ 130 μmol/L] in men or $\geq$ 1.4 mg/dL [$\geq$ 120 μmol/L] in women) or in those with an abnormal creatinine clearance.

Thiazolidinediones (eg, rosiglitazone, pioglitazone) improve blood glucose control by increasing peripheral tissue sensitivity to insulin's effects. They are most appropriate as reserve drugs to control blood glucose in patients taking other oral drugs or insulin. Regular monitoring of liver enzymes is advised to detect the development of hepatotoxicity. Hepatic failure with the use of troglitazone led to removal of this drug from the US market. It is not known whether aging increases the risk of hepatotoxicity. Weight gain due to edema can also occur, and for that reason these drugs should not be used in patients with poorly controlled heart failure.

Acarbose, administered with food, reduces postprandial glucose elevations and, in combination with other hypoglycemics, can help improve blood sugar control in some patients. Gastrointestinal intolerance may occur.

◘ see page 630

Analgesics: Nonsteroidal anti-inflammatory drugs (NSAIDs) are among the most widely used drugs, and several are available without prescription. Some data indicate that the clearance of salicylate, oxaprozin, and naproxen is decreased in elderly patients. The risk of peptic ulceration and upper gastrointestinal (GI) bleeding, which can be serious, is greater when an NSAID is begun and when the dose is increased.∎ Ibuprofen, diclofenac, and salsalate may be slightly less likely to cause upper GI bleeding. Aging does not seem to increase the risk of NSAID-induced adverse GI effects; however, these complications, when they occur, increase morbidity and mortality rates in elderly patients. The risk of upper GI hemorrhage increases more than 10-fold when NSAIDs are combined with warfarin. For elderly patients with a high risk of NSAID-induced gastroduodenal complications, misoprostol (a synthetic prostaglandin E_1 analog), a more potent gastric acid inhibitor (eg, omeprazole, lansoprazole), or high-dose H_2 blockers can be added. Such drugs can reduce the risk of peptic ulceration. The risk of NSAID-induced renal impairment may be increased in elderly patients. Monitoring the serum creatinine level is reasonable, especially in patients with other risk factors (eg, heart failure, renal impairment, cirrhosis with ascites, volume depletion, diuretic use). Because elderly persons are at higher risk of poor outcomes due to complications, NSAIDs should be tried only when less toxic analgesics (eg, acetaminophen) have failed. NSAIDs should be used at the lowest effective dose.

NSAIDs nonselectively inhibit cyclooxygenase (COX)-1 (leading to gastrointestinal and renal toxicity) and COX-2 (leading to anti-inflammatory effects). Selective COX-2 inhibitors (eg, celecoxib, rofecoxib) appear to have anti-inflammatory and analgesic properties similar to those of conventional nonselective NSAIDs but cause less GI toxicity. COX-2 inhibitors thus may be safer than NSAIDs for elderly patients, particularly those patients with a history of gastroduodenal ulceration or bleeding. The most suitable COX-2 drug for this age group is unknown.

▆7▆ ▆ **GERIATRIC INTERDISCIPLINARY TEAMS**

An approach to care of the elderly patient in which team members from different disciplines collectively set goals and share resources and responsibilities.

Not all elderly patients need a geriatric interdisciplinary team. However, for patients who have complex medical, psychologic, and social needs, teams are more effective in assessing patient needs and creating an effective care plan than are professionals working alone.

∎ see page 1043

TABLE 7–1.   GERIATRIC INTERDISCIPLINARY TEAMS VS. MULTIDISCIPLINARY TEAMS

Feature	Geriatric Interdisciplinary Team	Multidisciplinary Team
Approach to care	Working in an integrated, cooperative manner with agreed-upon goals	Working in parallel, without integrating care into an overall plan or setting priorities
Training	Attending regular meetings to discuss team goals, structure, process, and communication	Learning to work together on the job, with little or no formal training
Team leaders	Leader changes daily, depending on the patient's needs rather than on the convenience of other team members or the health care system	Leader is assumed to be a physician
Patient's role	Considered a team member and the focus (with the family) of the team	Not considered a team member; informed about the care plan after it has been formulated

Frail elderly patients benefit from interdisciplinary teams, as do caregivers, whose strengths and needs can be incorporated into the care plan.

To create, monitor, or revise the care plan, interdisciplinary teams must communicate openly, freely, and regularly. Core team members must collaborate with trust and respect for the contributions of others and coordinate (ie, delegate, share accountability, jointly implement) the care plan. Some team members work together at the same site, so communication can be informal and expeditious.

Interdisciplinary teams differ from multidisciplinary teams, from which they evolved (see TABLE 7–1); multidisciplinary teams create discipline-specific care plans and implement them simultaneously without explicit regard to their interaction. Interdisciplinary teams also differ from transdisciplinary teams, in which each team member must be so familiar with the roles and responsibilities of other members that tasks and functions become, to some extent, interchangeable.

Core members of a geriatric interdisciplinary team represent geriatric medicine, nursing, social work, and pharmacy (see TABLE 7–2). Other members may represent physical or occupational therapy, home health ("visiting") nursing, psychiatry or psychology, nutritional counseling, or podiatry as needed (on an ongoing basis or for consultation). The roles of these other members are discussed elsewhere in this manual.

To be effective team members, physicians must be knowledgeable about geriatric medicine, familiar with the patient, dedicated to the team process, and have good communication skills. As team members,

TABLE 7–2.   CORE MEMBERS OF THE GERIATRIC INTERDISCIPLINARY TEAM

Team Member	Training	Role
Physician	Undergraduate school (4 years), medical school (4 years), residency in internal medicine or family practice (3 years), geriatric fellowship training (1–2 years)	Performs comprehensive geriatric assessment, diagnosis, and drug regimen review; prescribes drugs; orders laboratory and diagnostic tests; interacts and makes decisions with patients and family members; periodically reassesses, monitors, and treats acute and chronic disease
Nurse	Undergraduate school (4 years); nurse practitioners have in addition graduate school, including certification (2 years)	Provides comprehensive geriatric assessment, diagnosis, and treatment in collaboration with the physician; performs drug regimen review; prescribes drugs; works with patients and family members on health promotion activities, health monitoring, and practical implementation of the care plan; provides information to and consults with family members, caregivers, and home care and nursing home nurses on geriatric care management issues
Social worker	Undergraduate school (4 years), graduate school, including certification (2 years)	Acts as an advocate for the patient and family members; assists in the coordination of services required to meet the patient's health care needs; coordinates community resources; assesses psychologic, social, cultural, environmental, and spiritual needs; provides group and family therapy, relaxation and stress management training, and supportive psychoeducational groups for elderly patients and their caregivers; negotiates with community bureaucracies and resource systems on behalf of elderly persons; serves as resource referral coordinator; helps patients and family members set goals; establishes priorities for care based on cultural or ethnic factors and individual values; liaises between elderly persons and the professional community or health care system
Pharmacist	Undergraduate school (4 years); graduate school ($\geq$ 2 years), with extensive didactic training in biochemistry, medicinal chemistry, anatomy, physiology, pathophysiology, and clinical pharmacology; internship ($\geq$ 1500 hours); clinical clerkship ($\geq$ 6 months)	Dispenses drugs; provides drug information to patients; monitors drug use; liaises between physicians and patients to ensure optimal pharmaceutical care; prevents, rapidly identifies, and resolves any drug-related problems

physicians offer and explain the medical conditions and differential diagnoses that affect care; they then incorporate the team advice into medical orders. In general, physicians must write medical orders agreed on through the team process. The physician should alert the patient, family members, and/or caregivers about team decisions.

A **formal team structure** and **ongoing maintenance** are necessary at all stages. Teams should set deadlines for reaching their goals and have regular meetings to discuss team structure, process, and communication. These meetings are essential to maintain efficiency, continuous improvement, and respect for the process and for other team members, including patients and their caregivers. In general, team leadership should rotate, with the key provider of care reporting on the patient's progress. For example, if the major concern is the medical condition of the patient, a physician should lead the team meeting and introduce the team to the patient and family members. Frequently, the nurse practitioner or social worker updates the team on the patient's progress. Team effectiveness should be defined by specific goals at the outset and monitored by continuous quality improvement measures.

Patient and caregiver issues: Patients and caregivers are part of the team. For example, patients can help the team set goals (eg, advance directives, end-of-life care). They can also discuss drug treatment, rehabilitation, dietary plans, and other forms of therapy. If the team learns that the patient will not take a particular drug or change certain dietary habits, care can be modified accordingly. The team and patient must develop ways to communicate honestly to prevent the patient from suppressing an opinion and agreeing to every suggestion.

Caregivers, including family members, can also enhance the team's goals by identifying realistic and unrealistic expectations based on the patient's habits and lifestyle.

To effectively incorporate patients and caregivers as team members, teams must listen, communicate genuine interest, consider ideas provided by patients and caregivers, respect differing opinions, and follow up with all other members of the team. Methods to better incorporate patients and caregivers should be established at the beginning of every team meeting; the team should later review these methods to determine if they were successful.

8   NURSING

In the USA, nurse generalists (staff nurses) deliver most nursing care in settings ranging from patients' homes to intensive care units. They plan and provide a wide range of geriatric care dealing with problems common in the elderly (eg, skin breakdown, incontinence, eating and feeding problems, falls, confusion, sleep disorders, discomfort and pain). Because they supervise patients round-the-clock, nurse generalists are important members of interdisciplinary teams.∎

Nurses regularly demonstrate self-care procedures (eg, how to irrigate a new colostomy, inject insulin, or care for pressure sores) and then observe the patient performing the procedures. The elderly patient's ability to learn new information or behavior should be evaluated and documented regularly, and the support available to the patient assessed.

In most settings, the nurse explains tests and procedures to the patient and family. Patients undergoing surgery need information about the setting in which surgery will take place and what they may expect during and after surgery.❷ Some patients learn best from written or printed material; others prefer videotaped information. The nurse can determine the best teaching method, which can speed the treatment process dramatically, and tell the interdisciplinary team which method the patient prefers. For example, after a gastroenterologist has used diagrams to explain an endoscopy, the nurse, who is often more familiar with the patient's learning capabilities, can explain the procedure again in simpler language, making sure the patient understands. Nurses may also develop pamphlets containing pertinent information and phone numbers for the patient.

Usually, the nurse communicates with family members of hospitalized patients; continual, open communication lets family members know that their input is valuable. The nurse is likely to obtain useful, accurate information about the patient's home life. Ideally, after the patient is discharged, the nurse is available to the patient and family members to reinforce what the patient has been taught (eg, self-care procedures) and to address new issues. Nurses are also responsible for communicating information to other nurses when patients are transferred to or from a nursing home, home care service, or other care setting.

GERIATRIC NURSE PRACTITIONERS

As of 1996, there were only slightly more than 4,000 certified geriatric nurse practitioners out of more than 70,000 certified nurse practitioners. The curriculum for geriatric nurse practitioners focuses on normal aging, common problems of old age and their management, and detection of complex problems for referral.

Geriatric nurse practitioners perform many functions previously done only by physicians. They conduct physical examinations, diagnose disease, provide long-term monitoring, order laboratory and other diagnostic tests, develop and implement treatment plans for patients with certain acute and chronic illnesses, prescribe certain drugs, teach and counsel patients, consult and collaborate with other professionals, and refer patients to specialists.

Geriatric nurse practitioners work in nursing homes (or for physicians with practices in nursing homes), in acute care settings, and in primary care offices. Community health services (eg, home care agencies, hospices, clinics) are managed primarily by nurse practitioners. Nursing roles have expanded because basic health care services are lacking in certain areas, especially rural areas and inner cities, and because few physicians make home visits. Nurse practitioners help meet the need for primary care in the community.

GERIATRIC NURSE SPECIALISTS

Nurse specialists have substantial clinical experience with patients and their families; they have expertise in formulating health and social policies and in planning, implementing, and evaluating health problems. Unlike nurse practitioners, nurse specialists generally cannot prescribe drugs.

Most geriatric nurse specialists work in hospitals as consultants to interdisciplinary teams. They advise staff nurses about problems common in the elderly and provide continuing education about new research findings. Geriatric nurse specialists also help staff nurses by serving as liaisons between the hospital and nursing homes or community health agencies.

GEROPSYCHIATRIC NURSE SPECIALISTS

Geropsychiatric nursing is the newest geriatric nursing discipline. The number of practicing geropsychiatric nurse specialists is unknown, partly because no certification procedure exists. These specialists often work in hospitals, mental health clinics, and outpatient settings involving elderly patients with mental health impairments, especially cognitive impairment. Geropsychiatric nurse specialists perform physical examinations and psychiatric assessments of elderly patients and work with an interdisciplinary team concerned with the needs, particularly the mental health needs, of the elderly. These specialists are also involved in discharge planning in collaboration with community agencies.

GERIATRIC SOCIAL WORK

Geriatric social work in health care is the fastest growing segment of social work, involving about 49,000 social workers. These health professionals can locate or provide resources, services, and opportunities for the elderly and their families; enhance the problem-solving and coping skills of the elderly and their caregivers; and help develop social policy.

Scope of care: As part of the interdisciplinary team, social workers evaluate patients' cognitive, behavioral, and emotional status and their social support network (see TABLE 9–1). Social workers evaluate a patient's self-assessment of quality of life and the patient's economic resources, which often determine access to medical and personal care and influence options for living arrangements. This information helps the social worker develop a coordinated health care plan for the patient.

Geriatric social workers work directly with the elderly and their families to deal with social support factors that create or exacerbate problems in living. Social support (eg, family, friends, community resources) can maximize the patient's ability to adapt and cope, enhance self-esteem and self-control, reduce hospital admission and readmission rates, and promote recovery. Social workers evaluate the competence of present and potential caregivers, their willingness to provide care, and their acceptability to the patient. They note the caregivers' stress level, support network, and cultural, ethnic, and spiritual values. Family members who care for an elderly relative need support, especially because life span is increasing and more older adults are caring for even older relatives.

Social workers can help defuse the sense of crisis for family members by assisting in health care planning and by ensuring that the elderly person is included in decision making. As care coordinators, social workers can be crucial in maintaining the elderly in their communities.

As counselors, social workers help patients deal with illness, loss, and end-of-life issues. Counseling may take the form of individual counseling for the patient or family counseling. Social workers may also refer patients and family members to group programs to help them cope with the psychosocial effects of a particular disease or life crisis (eg, returning home from the hospital or long-term care facility, being unable to resume previous roles or functioning level, being placed in a long-term care facility).

A major function of social workers is helping the patient with discharge planning and managing the resulting psychosocial elements of care.■ Patients most vulnerable to psychologic, social, and functional stressors during postdischarge recovery must be identified early. Arrangements for appropriate social and health services after hospital discharge can minimize the chances of early or recurrent readmissions. For example, a sick elderly person may require rehabilitation and a range of supportive services,

---

■ see page 103

TABLE 9–1.   THE SOCIAL WORKER'S ROLE IN HEALTH CARE FOR THE ELDERLY

Problem	Role
Functional impairment	Attempts to identify causes of impairment and arranges for appropriate health care services
Psychologic disturbances	Uses standardized assessment tools to screen for psychosocial problems
	Provides counseling for patient and family members
Inadequate social support	Helps the elderly maintain independence by providing information about community resources and helping arrange for services (eg, senior centers, meals-on-wheels, transportation) and obtain government income assistance as needed
	Helps caregivers obtain services such as adult day care and respite care
Environmental obstacles	Makes home visits to assess safety, identify physical barriers, and determine the layout of the home and access to shops (eg, the pharmacy), transportation, and recreation
Grief and loss	Helps the elderly cope with the losses common in old age (eg, death of loved ones, loss of income, loss of self-esteem, loss of health)
Hospitalization	Helps arrange for postdischarge care for patients, eg, provides extra services (social, psychologic, and environmental support) to help the elderly adapt to illness and resultant disability
Legal and ethical issues	Assists in establishing advance directives (eg, living wills, durable power of attorney)
Abuse	Identifies abusive situations and deals with them socially, psychiatrically, and, if necessary, legally
End-of-life issues	Helps the patient adjust to an uncertain prognosis or to imminent death
	Provides case management and advocacy services for dying patients and their family members (eg, helping patients transfer between levels of care and obtain needed services)

including home health care, meal preparation, counseling, adult day care, respite care, and acute and long-term care. Social workers are increasingly involved in the allocation of services offered by federal or state programs to provide a continuum of care.∎

Settings: Social workers practice in a wide variety of settings (see TABLE 9–2). For example, all nursing homes with more than 120 beds must employ a full-time social worker. As hospital stays become shorter, more services are being provided in the home. Home-based social work intervention programs include short-term intensive therapies for distraught patients and family members (eg, due to an unwelcome diagnosis or bereavement).

∎ see page 87

TABLE 9-2.   SETTINGS FOR GERIATRIC SOCIAL WORK

Adult day care and respite programs
Agencies and institutions in substance dependency networks
Agencies in the mental retardation or developmentally disabled
  network
Agencies serving older gay and lesbian persons
Agencies serving persons with HIV or AIDS
Community mental health centers
Department of Public Welfare or Social Services
Employee assistance programs in corporations and in unions
Family service agencies
General and specialized hospitals, including mental hospitals
Geriatric care management agencies
Health care clinics and ambulatory care clinics
Home health care or homemaker service agencies
Independent physicians' and dentists' practices
Independently operated social work practices
Legal service agencies
Managed care companies
Nursing homes and hospices
Nutrition programs
Rehabilitation centers
Senior centers
Senior citizens' apartments, assisted living programs, and public
  housing projects
Social service and health planning agencies (eg, Area Agencies on
  Aging)
Veterans Affairs medical centers

Adapted from Berkman B, Dobrof R, Harry L, Damron-Rodriguez J: "Social work," in *A National Agenda for Geriatric Education: White Papers*, edited by SM Klein. New York, Springer Publishing, 1997.

Referrals: Elderly patients or caregivers who may benefit from social work consultation should be referred to a social worker as early as possible so that a crisis can be prevented. Social workers usually receive referrals from other health care professionals. Local chapters of the National Association of Social Workers are listed in telephone directories and may also offer referral information. In addition, local social work support services can be located by calling the Eldercare Locator at 800-677-1116. The Eldercare Locator, established in 1992, is a nationwide information and referral service sponsored by the Administration on Aging and the National Association of State Units on Aging.

Training: All states and the District of Columbia have licensing or certification laws regarding social work practice and the use of professional titles. Although these licensing requirements may vary, most states rely on

Board examinations by the American Association of State Social Work. Typically, licensing allows a social worker to be employed by a professional clinical practice and to use a title such as Licensed Clinical Social Worker. A social worker with a Master of Social Work degree can also obtain, through the National Association of Social Workers, the credentials of ACSW (Academy of Certified Social Workers) and QCSW (Qualified Clinical Social Worker). There is no specific certification available for geriatric social workers.

10 PHARMACY

Pharmacists not only dispense drugs, they provide drug information to patients, monitor drug use (including adherence), and liaise between physicians (or other health providers) and patients to ensure optimal pharmaceutical care. Pharmaceutical care encompasses the provision of appropriate drug therapy for the purpose of achieving outcomes such as disease prevention, cure or symptom relief, and slower functional decline. A major responsibility of the pharmacist is the prevention, rapid identification, and resolution of drug-related problems (see TABLE 10–1).

Drug-related problems cost over $100 billion annually, exceeding the annual expenditures on the drugs themselves and rivaling the total treatment costs of cancer ($104 billion), Alzheimer's disease ($100 billion), and diabetes ($92 billion). Additionally, adverse drug reactions kill more than 100,000 people annually. The elderly are particularly vulnerable to drug-related problems because they:

- often take several drugs
- have age-related changes in pharmacokinetics and pharmacodynamics that predispose them to adverse drug reactions∎
- frequently do not comply with drug regimens, often overusing or underusing drugs (although the rates of adherence do not change due to age per se but due to other factors common among the elderly)

Training: Pharmacists receive at least 5 years of higher education, with extensive didactic training in biochemistry, medicinal chemistry, anatomy, physiology, pathophysiology, and clinical pharmacology (including pharmacokinetics and clinical therapeutics). They also receive at least 1500 hours of experiential training at internship sites and at least 6 months of clinical clerkship. Many pharmacy colleges offer a 6-year program, which includes 12 months of clinical clerkship.

∎ see page 62

TABLE 10–1.   CATEGORIES OF DRUG-RELATED PROBLEMS

Category	Definition
Untreated medical problem	Patient has a medical problem that requires drug therapy but is not receiving a drug for that problem
Improper drug selection	Patient has a medical problem that requires drug therapy but is taking the wrong drug
Underdosage	Patient has a medical problem that is being treated with too little of the correct drug
Failure to receive drug	Patient has a medical problem but is not receiving the prescribed drug
Overdosage	Patient has a medical problem that is being treated with too much of the correct drug
Adverse drug reaction	Patient has a medical problem that is the result of an adverse drug effect
Drug interaction	Patient has a medical problem that is the result of a drug-drug, drug-food, or drug-disease interaction
Drug use with no indication	Patient is taking a drug for no medically valid reason

Undergraduate training in geriatric pharmacotherapy is slowly being added to curricula, and postgraduate geriatric training programs are becoming increasingly prevalent. Many geriatric residency programs are accredited, and special traineeships in geriatric pharmacotherapy and an examination for geriatric certification are also being offered. Several academic institutions in the USA offer alternative certificate programs in geriatric pharmacy.

PHARMACEUTICAL PRACTICE SETTINGS

COMMUNITY PHARMACIES

The community pharmacist procures and dispenses prescription drugs, provides advice about over-the-counter drugs, and communicates information between the patient and physician as appropriate. The community pharmacist also screens for drug-drug and drug-disease interactions, therapeutic duplication, and adherence with drug regimens. In addition, the community pharmacist provides patient counseling, usually verbal but often enhanced by take-home printed material, which may be in large type for elderly patients.

Some community pharmacists participate in disease management programs, with emphasis on preventive medicine. In this role, the pharmacist must complete a certificate program in one or several disease states that are widely prevalent in the elderly (eg, heart failure, incontinence, diabetes mellitus, osteoporosis, hypertension) and, electively, in areas such as immunization awareness (eg, the importance of vaccination against influenza and pneumococcal pneumonia). Community pharmacists may also offer screening and monitoring programs (eg, for blood pressure and blood glucose).

HOSPITALS

Pharmacists in hospital-based practices have long been involved in geriatric interdisciplinary care teams.■ Upon a patient's admission, a pharmacist is typically involved in obtaining a detailed drug history from the patient or caregiver, focusing on currently prescribed drugs, current or recent over-the-counter drug use, perceived drug effectiveness and adverse effects, and compliance with drug regimens. The pharmacist usually attends patient rounds with physicians and other team members, making drug therapy recommendations and providing drug information when appropriate. When discharge is imminent, the pharmacist provides verbal and written drug-related information to the patient or caregiver.

Hospital pharmacists often participate in collaborative practice agreements, which involve outpatient clinics (eg, anticoagulation, lipid, osteoporosis, pain, asthma, or diabetes clinics). Many of these clinics are managed by pharmacists, who, in collaboration with physicians and other team members, assess, monitor, and adjust drug therapy to optimize drug therapy outcomes and ensure cost-effective care.

LONG-TERM CARE FACILITIES

Consultant pharmacists have adopted a much more proactive approach to the care of the institutionalized elderly patient. They may participate in clinical rounds with physicians and other team members, participate in facility quality-improvement committees, and assess and interview patients. Such activities by pharmacists have been credited with lowering the annual costs of drug-related problems in long-term care facilities from an estimated $7.6 billion to $4 billion. At the same time, these activities are estimated to have improved therapeutic outcomes by 43%.

These pharmacists also procure and dispense drugs. They monitor patients for drug effectiveness; drug-drug, drug-disease, and drug-nutrient interactions; and adverse drug reactions and therapeutic failures. If they identify a problem or a high risk for drug-related problems, they contact the patient's nurse or physician directly.

As required by federal law, long-term care pharmacists conduct a monthly drug regimen review on all patients. The review process is conducted on-site to maximize the pharmacist's access to interdisciplinary team members, patients, and patients' medical records (eg, physician's

■ see page 74

progress notes, nurse's notes, social service notes, dietary progress notes, the Minimum Data Set). The review monitors adherence to federal indicators, ie, that all drug orders have a supporting diagnosis, that the regimen (dosage strength, frequency of use, and route of administration) is appropriate, and that psychoactive drug use is justified and properly monitored. Additional services of consulting pharmacists include formulary and disease management as well as procedural reviews such as inspection of all drugs and biologicals for proper storage, inspection of drug administration policies and procedures, and assessment of all documentation related to drugs. Pertinent findings from clinical reviews are reported to the patient's attending physician and the facility's director of nursing. Findings from procedural and technical reviews are generally reported to the administrator, director of nursing, and medical director.

OTHER SETTINGS

Pharmacists who practice in the **home health care** or **hospice** setting procure, dispense, and deliver drugs and related devices (eg, spacers for inhalers, intravenous therapy supplies) to the patient being cared for at home, especially to patients receiving parenteral therapy. These pharmacists often assess patients, monitor drug therapy, and communicate with physicians on pharmacokinetics-based drug dosing, analgesic dosage adjustments, and other drug-related issues.

Assisted living facilities represent the fastest-growing segment of institutionalized care and are becoming a niche for pharmacists with a particular interest in geriatrics. Because many assisted living facilities use nonlicensed personnel to assist with drug-related issues, frequent staff-education programs by pharmacists are needed. Additionally, residents in assisted living facilities are often appropriate candidates for disease management interventions.

The influx of elderly patients into integrated delivery systems, managed care organizations, group practices, and other types of **organized health systems** has provided pharmacists with new opportunities outside the realm of individual patient care. Pharmacists in organized health systems develop, implement, and manage formularies; participate in the design and implementation of disease-specific critical pathways or therapeutic guidelines; perform pharmacoeconomic evaluations of new or competitive drug products; design, implement, and manage computer-based adverse event tracking systems; design and monitor performance measurement indicators as part of continuous quality improvement initiatives; and establish and manage drug utilization review programs.

![11] CONTINUITY OF CARE: INTEGRATION OF SERVICES

With the advent of managed care organizations and integrated health care systems, more is now known about how to provide the best care across specific settings (eg, the home, hospital, nursing home). A major criticism of the health care system of the recent past was that care in specific settings was compartmentalized—each episode of care was treated as a discrete phenomenon instead of as a part of a larger endeavor, ie, the ongoing provision of health care to the patient. The renewed emphasis on primary vs. specialty care has changed the process of care; patients are now continuously monitored by health care practitioners who can appreciate the continuum of events that contribute to their patients' health status and functional capabilities. Communication among primary care physicians, specialists, other health care practitioners, and patients and their family members is critical to ensuring that patients receive the appropriate care across all settings.

HOME HEALTH CARE

Home health care, the largest component of the home care industry, includes nursing, skilled professional and paraprofessional care, hospice and respite services, durable medical equipment, and infusion services. Nonmedical components include personal emergency response systems, alarm devices and security surveillance, attendant care, homemaker services, and food programs (eg, meals-on-wheels). Patients may need several services, and their needs may change.

Generally, home health care can be classified as postacute, medically complex, or long-term (see TABLE 11–1). For patients who need long-term care, paraprofessional services account for 56% of home health care visits; for those who need medically complex care, they account for 45%. Home health care is being increasingly used to meet the demand for custodial care needs. Home health care, which has been shown to decrease nursing home placement of patients by 23%, is less expensive than institutional care when home health aide and skilled care visits are scheduled appropriately. Diagnostic procedures (eg, x-rays, ECGs, blood tests) and treatments (eg, IV therapy, dialysis, parenteral and enteral nutrition, ventilator support) previously available only in hospitals and skilled nursing facilities can be safely provided in the home.

Physician's role: Physicians are responsible for home health care orders for a patient to receive third-party reimbursement. One third of home care referrals are written for inpatients by hospital personnel to prescribe postdischarge care. Under Medicare regulations, certified home health care agencies report to physicians at least every 62 days, at which

TABLE 11-1. TYPES OF MEDICARE HOME HEALTH CARE

Type	Description	Average Number of Visits	% of Home Care Expenditures
Postacute	Patients are started on home care after hospitalization	47 (2/3 received 30 visits)	22.5
Medically complex	Patients are seriously ill (23 days/year in hospital); 50% use a nursing home every year	91	42.5
Long-term	Patients are generally low-income women who live alone and are medically stable but are severely functionally impaired	81	35

From Leon J, Neuman P, Parente S: (June 1997) Understanding the Growth in Medicare Home Health Expenditures. Project HOPE Center for Health Affairs.

time orders must be rewritten. Physicians who falsely claim that a beneficiary meets Medicare requirements for home health care are subject to fines. Physicians cannot refer patients to or write orders for a home health care program in which they have a financial interest; they cannot recommend a Medicare or Medicaid service in exchange for payment.

Physicians must arrange for emergency coverage when they are unavailable; the patient, caregiver, and home health care agency must be able to reach the referring or covering physician at all times. Physicians must keep records of all necessary Medicare forms and document conversations with home health care practitioners.

Caring for patients at home requires communication among health care practitioners to ensure that the patient is maintaining function and progressing as expected. Changes in the patient's condition need to be promptly reported to nurses or physicians to ensure proper monitoring of the patient.

Reimbursement: Some private insurance companies cover home health care services (eg, infusion services) for patients who are not homebound. However, Medicare does not; it requires patients to meet the following criteria to qualify for home health care benefits:

- The patient must be homebound, except for infrequent, relatively short periods or for medical treatment.

- A physician must initially certify the patient's need for home health care (which must be recertified every 62 days) and develop a care plan.

- The patient must need at least one qualifying service (skilled nursing care, physical therapy, or speech therapy).

- Skilled care must be needed part-time or intermittently. Medicare covers daily care (eg, wound care) only for a limited time, and an end date must be established when the service is begun.
- The home health care agency that provides the service must be certified by Medicare.

Once qualified, a patient is also eligible for ancillary services, which include occupational therapy, medical social work services, limited home health aide services (eg, assistance with bathing, washing hair, using the toilet, dressing), medical supplies and equipment, and prosthetic devices. Occupational therapy can be given only if the patient needs another qualifying service, but once begun, it can be continued even if it remains the sole service. Prescribed services must be reasonable and necessary and must be provided in the patient's home.

Third-party payers are usually billed directly by vendors, although other arrangements exist. Medicare requires home health care agencies to inform patients about which services are reimbursable, and patients can choose, to some extent, which services they want. Third-party payers are increasingly limiting personal services to control costs. If a patient requires skilled care, Medicare allows a limited amount of home health care time, which varies greatly, for personal care. Usually, < 2 hours/day, 5 days/week are reimbursable, but the actual number of visit-hours is often less. However, home health care agencies cannot reduce the care ordered by physicians.

Reimbursement for physician services in home care is considered inadequate because careful documentation is required and reimbursement levels are low. To encourage home care, Medicare provides six codes for home services to allow flexibility in billing. Billable tasks include development and revision of care plans, adjustment of medical therapies, review of patient reports, and discussions with other health care practitioners about the patient. To bill for home health care services, physicians must document the amount of time spent discussing care with the patient or family members, dates and types of services provided, and discussions with visiting nurses and other home health care practitioners.

Fraud and abuse occur in home health care and have been investigated by the federal government. The most common abuses include unnecessary visits and services, care of a patient who is not homebound, absence of valid physician orders, and insufficient documentation.

TYPES OF PROGRAMS

Certified home health care agencies: To be certified, an agency must meet state licensing requirements and federal conditions for participation in Medicare. Such agencies provide skilled care under the direction of physicians. Agencies are directly reimbursed by Medicare, Medicaid, or private insurers.

More than 6500 agencies are certified by the Joint Commission on Accreditation of Healthcare Organizations to provide services at home to Medicare beneficiaries. Home health care agencies vary in ownership, size, location, and services. In 1996, 47% of agencies were proprietary and for-profit; 7% were proprietary and not-for-profit; 28% were affiliated with hospitals, rehabilitation centers, or nursing homes; 12% were publicly (government) sponsored; and 6% were affiliated with the Visiting Nurses Association. About 25% of U.S. agencies are affiliated with chains.

Most agencies arrange for vendors to deliver supplies and durable medical equipment (eg, commodes, wheelchairs, walkers) to the patient's home. Companies specializing in devices and solutions for enteral and parenteral nutrition, IV solutions and equipment, ventilators, or other devices may function as vendors to agencies or as independent home health care services.

Program of All-Inclusive Care for the Elderly (PACE):   This managed care program is designed to keep low-income, frail elderly persons living in the community by providing primary care, adult day care, rehabilitation, and preventive services.∎ An interdisciplinary team develops a treatment plan to meet the needs of the patient and family members. Programs typically provide meals and laundry service at the day care center. Persons who meet the eligibility criteria can join PACE at any time and can disenroll at the end of any month. Enrollees must agree to use PACE physicians and providers. Service packages are comprehensive and very attractive to elderly persons who would receive fewer services from a state Medicaid program.

New York's Nursing Home Without Walls: This capitated program is a prototype for long-term home health care of patients who might otherwise require institutionalization. It provides home health aide services, case management, and limited skilled care at home. Patients receive services as long as they meet state criteria for nursing home placement and the cost does not exceed a percentage of the cost for comparable nursing home care. Unlike Medicare patients in a certified home health care agency program, patients in this program are not required to attain a therapeutic goal or continue to need skilled care to stay in the program.

HOSPICE CARE

Noncurative medical and support services for patients with terminal illnesses (life expectancy ≤ 6 months) and their families.

Every state has at least one certified hospice program, and the care may be provided by home health care agencies, freestanding programs,

∎ see also page 171

hospitals, or skilled nursing homes. Currently, 42 states include hospice care under Medicaid, but hospice accounts for only about 1% of the Medicare budget.

In Medicare-certified hospice programs, core services include nursing and physician services (a physician must be a salaried member of the team); medical social work; counseling (including dietary and pastoral); physical, occupational, and speech therapy; home health aide and homemaker services; short-term inpatient care (including respite care and pain control or management); medical appliances and supplies; and drugs. Bereavement counseling services for family members are provided for up to 12 months after the patient's death.

The team develops and coordinates an individualized care plan together with the patient and family members. Hospice physicians review the care plan, visit the patient regularly, prescribe drugs for palliative care, review the patient's condition and prognosis with hospice personnel, and sign the death certificate. The patient's own physician can retain primary medical responsibility. However, many often willingly relinquish responsibility to the hospice physician because they do not have as much experience in pain management and symptom control and do not have regular contact with hospice team members for home visits and problem solving.■

Patients who elect the Medicare hospice benefit must waive standard Medicare benefits for conditions related to the terminal illness. Eligibility to receive care for other intercurrent problems is not affected (eg, a hospice patient with lung cancer can be treated for injuries sustained in an automobile accident). The Medicare hospice benefit is divided into an initial 90-day period, a subsequent 90-day period, and an unlimited number of subsequent 60-day periods as long as the patient continues to meet eligibility requirements. Physicians must certify at the beginning of each period that the patient's illness is terminal with a life expectancy of ≤ 6 months. The average number of days in hospice has increased from 37 days in 1988 to 59 days in 1995. This increase indicates a greater acceptance of hospice services by patients, their family members, and physicians; however, duration of hospice care is often not long enough to help patients and their family members prepare for death.

Before choosing hospice care, patients and their family members are told that the hospice agency will take only limited action, if any, to prolong life. Hospice patients decide the number and kinds of treatment they will receive. Advance directives, including appointment of a health care proxy and durable power of attorney for health care, ensure that patients' choices are followed.■

■ see also page 115   ■ see page 134

DAY CARE

Day care provides medical, physical, and cognitive services several hours a day, several days a week. Reimbursement for services is limited. In the USA, there are only about 2,900 day care programs compared with more than 16,700 nursing homes. Most day care programs are small, averaging 20 clients.

Medicare does not reimburse for day care services. Funds generally come from the Older Americans Act, Medicaid waiver programs, long-term care insurance, and private funds. Some centers use donated funds to subsidize transportation and a sliding-fee scale to match aid with the patient's financial need.

The **day hospital model** emphasizes rehabilitation or intensive skilled care along with core services (transportation, nutrition, recreational and social activity programs). It is designed for persons recovering from acute events such as a stroke, amputation, or fracture. Day hospital programs are usually limited in duration (6 weeks to 6 months) and are costly, because the ratio of professional staff members to patients is high.

The **maintenance model** combines limited skilled care (screening and monitoring chronic disorders) with core services and physical exercise. Goals are to prevent deterioration and to maintain or improve the patient's functional level for as long as possible; to improve self image; to prevent loneliness, isolation, and withdrawal; to eliminate the monotony of daily life; and to prevent exacerbation of chronic disorders. Maintenance programs provide long-term care and are less costly than day hospital programs.

The **social model** combines counseling, group therapy, and cognitive retraining with core services. It may resemble a typical senior citizens' center, which provides care to elderly persons with varied psychosocial needs, or a mental health center, which provides care to elderly persons with dementia or psychiatric disorders. Programs are increasingly accepting patients who are in wheelchairs and those who are incontinent; however, patients cannot be socially disruptive. Care may be long-term or limited in duration.

RESPITE CARE

Temporary care of a patient by a substitute caregiver to provide relief to the regular caregiver.

Over 50% of U.S. states have respite programs. Medicaid supports almost 50%; grants, 25%; and private funds, 25%.

Programs may be provided in the home by respite care agencies or by home health care agencies; in the community by adult day care centers, respite care cooperatives, or freestanding respite facilities; in a long-term care institution, eg, by board-and-care facilities or nursing homes; or in a hospital. The duration of care may vary (eg, respite care may be limited to 28 days in a calendar year).

EMERGENCY MEDICAL CARE

Most elderly persons need emergency medical care at some time. The elderly use significantly more emergency medical services than do younger adults. In 1995, almost 16% of emergency department visits were made by persons ≥ 65 years. Of elderly patients who go to an emergency department, > 50% receive comprehensive services, with > 70% receiving diagnostic laboratory tests or x-rays. More than 40% of elderly patients seen in an emergency department are admitted to the hospital, 6% to intensive care units. More than 50% are prescribed new drugs.

PREHOSPITAL CARE

The first responder to an emergency may be a basic emergency medical technician (EMT); basic EMTs receive about 150 hours of training and are certified to perform basic extrication and first aid procedures as well as CPR, splinting, spinal immobilization, oxygen support, and transport. Paramedics receive the highest level of training (1000 to 1500 hours); they must pass rigorous state certification examinations and operate under the license of their base station physician. However, specific geriatric training for emergency responders was uncommon in the past.

Because EMTs and paramedics often respond to elderly patients in their homes, they are able to assess the patient's home environment for risks to the patient's health and safety and can report their findings to the appropriate persons. Studies have demonstrated the effectiveness of such reporting when appropriate follow-up is done.

EMERGENCY DEPARTMENT CARE

In the emergency department, there is usually little privacy, long waiting times, few amenities, loud ambient noise, uncomfortable beds, and poor lighting. Staff members may not have enough time to relieve a patient's anxiety, relay test results, or explain necessary procedures. Although most emergency departments have special rooms that focus on the needs of pediatric patients, few provide amenities for geriatric patients, including lower, more comfortable beds; extra pillows; indirect lighting; and a quiet environment.

In many ways, care of an elderly patient is not different from that of other adults. The first priority is determining whether a patient needs treatment for a life- or limb-threatening condition. Once these conditions are reasonably ruled out, other diseases can be further evaluated in an outpatient setting by the primary care physician.

TABLE 11-2. PRESENTATION OF THE ELDERLY PATIENT IN THE EMERGENCY DEPARTMENT

- Manifestations of common diseases may be atypical**1**
- Comorbid diseases and polypharmacy may complicate presentation, diagnosis, and management
- The patient may be cognitively impaired
- Normal values for some diagnostic tests may be different
- The likelihood of decreased functional reserve must be anticipated
- The patient's social support system may be inadequate, necessitating reliance on caregivers
- Baseline functional status must be ascertained so that new complaints can be appropriately evaluated
- Psychosocial adjustment to health problems must be evaluated

Adapted from Sanders AB: *Emergency Care of the Elder Person*. Pasadena, CA, Beverly Cracom Publications, 1996.

Presentation: An elderly patient's presentation to the emergency department is often complex (see TABLE 11–2). Elderly patients often complain of general weakness or "just not feeling themselves." Symptoms and signs may not be as clear as they are in younger patients. For example, < 50% of patients > 80 years with myocardial infarction present with chest pain. In many elderly patients, acute appendicitis does not produce the typical symptoms and signs. Only 50% of elderly patients with surgically proven appendicitis carry that diagnosis at the time of admission to the hospital.

Polypharmacy and adverse drug effects are common in the elderly and may be factors in emergency department presentation, diagnosis, and treatment. Adverse drug effects result in at least 5% of hospital admissions for elderly persons.

Factors that are not apparent may affect an elderly patient's presentation. For example, a fall may result from elder abuse,**2** adverse drug effect (eg, oversedation from diazepam or other drugs), hazards in the home, or physical problems (eg, poor vision), or it may be related to depression or chronic alcoholism. Suicide risk, incontinence, and nutritional and immunization status can be reasonably assessed in the emergency department so that follow-up care can be arranged.

About 30 to 40% of elderly patients seen in emergency departments have not been diagnosed as having dementia but are cognitively impaired; in 10%, cognitive impairment consistent with delirium is unrecognized. Cognitive impairment of recent onset may indicate sepsis, occult subdural hemorrhage, or an adverse drug effect. When indicated, a standardized cognitive assessment should be performed in the emergency department.**3**

1 see page 38   **2** see page149   **3** see page 43

Cognitive impairment affects the reliability of the patient history; it affects diagnosis and must be considered when planning the patient's disposition.

Communication among health care practitioners: Good communication among emergency department physicians and patients, caregivers, primary care physicians, and staff of long-term care facilities greatly enhances the outcome of elderly patients with complicated problems. Advance directives should be promptly and clearly communicated to emergency medicine practitioners.∎ Baseline information from the patient's personal physician facilitates assessment and management planning in the emergency department. For example, knowing whether the onset of cognitive impairment is recent helps determine whether the deficit should be fully assessed in the emergency department. Reports to the patient's primary care physician should describe even simple injuries, such as an ankle sprain or a Colles' wrist fracture, because such injuries can dramatically affect an elderly person's functional ability and independence.

Some elderly patients may be brought to the emergency department by caregivers who need respite care. A social admission to the hospital results when the family caregiver abandons the elderly patient in the hospital, eg, by leaving or refusing to take the patient home.

Disposition: Discharge planning may be complex, because functional ability may be more impaired in the elderly patient by acute illness or injury. Assessment of functional status is essential for planning an elderly patient's disposition. A simple ankle sprain may be incapacitating unless the patient has good support at home. Discharge planning may be improved when nurses, social workers, and primary care physicians are involved. Issues raised during the emergency department assessment must be addressed during follow-up, such as depression, alcoholism, and the patient's cognitive and functional status. Discharge planning should also ensure that the patient is capable of taking drugs appropriately and obtaining the necessary care. An assessment of caregiver capabilities can avoid later problems. For example, providing home health care and meal services might relieve an elderly spouse's or partner's stress.

HOSPITALIZATION

Almost half of adults who occupy hospital beds are $\geq$ 65 years; this proportion is expected to increase as the population ages. Hospitalization can magnify age-related physiologic changes and increase morbidity (see TABLE 11–3).

The outcome of hospitalization appears to be poorer with increasing age, although physiologic age is a more important predictor of outcome than chronologic age. Outcome is also better in patients hospitalized for elective procedures (eg, joint replacement) than in those

∎ see page 134

TABLE 11–3. INTERACTION BETWEEN AGE-RELATED CHANGES AND EFFECTS OF HOSPITALIZATION

Age-Related Changes	Effects of Hospitalization	Potential Primary Risks	Potential Secondary Risks
Vasomotor instability (baroreceptor insensitivity and reduced total body water)	Reduced plasma volume, inaccessibility of fluids	Syncope, dizziness	Falls, fractures
Reduced muscle strength and aerobic capacity	Immobilization due to high bed and rails	Deconditioning, falls	Dependency
Decreased ventilation	Increased closing volume	Reduced arterial oxygen pressure (Pa_{O_2})	Syncope, delirium
Reduced bone density	Accelerated bone loss	Increased fracture risk	Fractures
Fragile skin	Immobilization, shearing forces	Pressure sores	Infection
Tendency toward urinary incontinence	Barriers, tethers (eg, IV lines, catheters)	Functional incontinence	Catheter, family rejection
Altered taste, smell, thirst, and dentition	Barriers, tethers (eg, IV lines, catheters), therapeutic diets	Dehydration, malnutrition	Reduced plasma volume, tube feeding
Tendency toward confusion	Isolation, lost glasses and hearing aids, additional sensory deprivation	Delirium	Improper mental illness diagnosis, need for physical or chemical restraint

Modified from Creditor MC: "Hazards of hospitalization of the elderly." *Annals of Internal Medicine* 118(3):219–223, 1993; used with permission.

hospitalized for serious conditions (eg, multisystem organ failure). The cost of hospital care to Medicare yearly is > \$100 billion, representing 30% of health care expenditures for hospital care in the USA.

About 75% of persons ≥ 75 who are functionally independent when admitted to hospitals from their homes are not functionally independent when discharged; 15% of persons ≥ 75 are discharged to skilled nursing facilities. The trend toward abbreviated acute hospital stays followed by subacute care and rehabilitation in a skilled nursing facility may explain why these percentages are high. However, even when an illness is treatable or appears uncomplicated, patients may not return to prehospitalized functional status. For example, in one study of patients who had hip fracture repair, only 20% returned to their preoperative functional level.

The hospital environment can be designed to reduce significant functional decline among elderly patients. Many successful models for acute care geriatric units have been implemented nationwide over the past decade; each differs in patient mix, targeting, and physical characteristics. A particularly successful model is Acute Care for the Elderly (ACE) intervention, a program of patient-centered care designed to prevent dysfunction.

A geriatric interdisciplinary team can help optimize care of elderly patients. The team members—geriatricians, nurses trained in gerontology, physical and occupational therapists, social workers, pharmacists, and other health care practitioners—work together to meet the complex needs of elderly patients.∎ The clinical nurse specialist typically co-chairs the team along with the geriatrician; facilitates communication; provides assessment, case management, and related interventions for the patient; serves as a teacher and counselor for the staff, patients, and families; identifies ethical and compliance issues and the need for patient and family conferences; and monitors quality improvement in gerontologic nursing.

Some hospitals have implemented primary care nursing, in which one nurse has around-the-clock responsibility for a particular patient, just as an attending physician does. The primary care nurse administers the team's care plan, monitors response to nursing and medical care, supports health promotion, and serves as a teacher and counselor for patients, staff, and family members.

Nurses often make decisions that markedly affect patient outcomes. For example, disruptive patients may be calmed when placed in the hall near the nursing station; this allows for environmental stimulation as well as for close observation. Changing roommates can be critical when a wide functional disparity exists between two acutely ill patients.

Important considerations for the hospitalized elderly patient follow and are summarized by the acronym ELDERS (see TABLE 11–4). Hospitalization is necessary only when the patient cannot receive appropriate treatment in any other environment. The health care practitioner should promptly identify patients who can benefit from medical care in another environment (eg, at home). Acute hospital care should only be of sufficient duration to allow successful transition to home care, a skilled nursing facility, or an outpatient rehabilitation program.

∎ see page 74

TABLE 11–4.   IMPORTANT CONSIDERATIONS FOR THE HOSPITALIZED ELDERLY

Apart from the usual medical problem list addressed by most caregivers in the hospital, the elderly patient's daily problem list should incorporate the following considerations, summarized by the acronym ELDERS.

E = Eating (nutritional status)
L = Lucidity (mental status)
D = Directives for limiting care (eg, do not resuscitate)
      Drug interactions
E = Elimination (incontinence)
R = Rehabilitation needs
S = Skin care (pressure sore prevention and treatment)
      Social issues (discharge planning)

DIRECTIVES

Many elderly persons have strong opinions about health care options, and many have already taken such steps as making funeral arrangements and preparing wills. Patients should be asked to document their choice of health care proxy and other advance directives during routine office visits.◼ It is best when these directives are brought to the hospital as soon as possible. However, if advance directives or assignment of a proxy was not obtained prior to hospitalization for severe illness, the clinician should make every effort to determine the patient's prior wishes. Efforts should also be made to reaffirm patient choices during acute hospitalization.

NUTRITION

Hospitalized elderly patients can become malnourished quickly, or they may have been malnourished on admission. Under the best of circumstances, a patient's appetite and eating habits are markedly affected by an acute hospitalization. Prolonged hospitalization exacerbates this problem and often results in significant nutritional loss. Malnourishment is a serious problem because a malnourished patient cannot fight off infection, maintain skin integrity, heal surgical wounds, or undergo successful rehabilitation.

Many factors contribute to malnutrition in the hospitalized elderly. Meal scheduling, use of medications, and changes in environment may affect appetite and nutritional intake. Hospital food and therapeutic diets (eg, low-salt diets) are unfamiliar and often unappetizing. Eating in a hospital bed with the tray, utensils, and water out of easy reach is difficult, particularly when bed rails and restraints limit movement. Often, by the time someone arrives to help feed a patient, the food has cooled and is even less appetizing. In addition, if dentures are left at

◼ see also page 134

home or misplaced, chewing can be difficult. Labeling dentures helps prevent them from being lost or discarded with the food tray.

Aging is accompanied by a decrease in taste and smell, which can affect appetite and make dietary changes even less tolerable. Also, because thirst perception decreases with age, severe dehydration may occur, leading to stupor and confusion. These states further reduce a hospitalized patient's ability to eat and drink.

Physiologic changes of aging place elderly patients at greater risk of undernutrition, including mild to severe vitamin and trace mineral deficiencies. ◘ Marasmus (a state of borderline nutritional compensation with decreased muscle and fat stores but normal organ function and protein levels) may occur and, with the stress of an acute hospitalization, may rapidly lead to kwashiorkor (hypoalbuminemic protein-energy malnutrition◙).

Patients with preexisting nutritional abnormalities should be identified when admitted and be given appropriate treatment. Physicians and staff members should anticipate nutritional deficiencies in elderly patients. Preventive measures include rescinding restrictive dietary orders as soon as possible and monitoring nutritional intake daily. Hospital staff should confer with the patient and family regarding food preferences and attempt to tailor a reasonable diet specific to each patient's lifelong habits, ethnic food choices, and ability to chew and swallow. Because eating is a social as well as physical activity and because people eat more and better when they eat with others, it is beneficial for family members to join the patient at mealtimes.

Patients should be fed adequately at all times. For patients too sick to swallow, parenteral nutrition or gastrointestinal tube feedings may be given temporarily or permanently. Oral fluid orders should be explicit. If a medical condition does not require fluid restriction, the patient benefits from a fresh and readily accessible bedside water pitcher or other fluids. Family members, friends, and staff members also can regularly offer the patient a drink.

Morbidly obese patients have an entirely different set of problems and present certain challenges, nutrition-related and otherwise. For example, these patients may experience difficulty in undergoing diagnostic tests and procedures, as well as in rehabilitation and independence in activities of daily living. Counseling, along with strict dietary control and behavior modification techniques after hospital discharge, is often the best approach to address a lifetime of habitual overeating.

MENTAL STATUS

Mental status in the aged may be clouded by the proverbial three "D's": dementia, delirium, and depression. A confused and acutely ill

---

◘ see page 588   ◙ see also page 595

elderly patient may show evidence of one or all three of these disorders. Clinicians must always remember that not all ill elderly patients develop confusion, and its presence requires a thorough evaluation and diagnosis. Confusion may be due to a specific disorder; however, age-related changes and acute illness can cause confusion that may be exacerbated by the reduced visual and auditory input in a hospital setting. For example, elderly patients who do not have their eyeglasses and hearing aids may become disoriented in a quiet, dimly lit hospital room. Patients may also become confused by hospital procedures, schedules (eg, frequent awakenings in strange settings and rooms), the effects of psychoactive drugs, and the stress of surgery or illness. In an intensive care unit, the constant light and noise can result in agitation, paranoid ideation, and mental and physical exhaustion for the patient.

Family members can be asked to bring missing eyeglasses and hearing aids. A wall clock and calendar can help to keep patients oriented. The use of physical restraints is discouraged. Tying down agitated patients invariably increases their level of agitation. In addition, the use of physical restraints has been shown to increase the risk of physical injury, including death. Bed rails and chairs sometimes serve as restraints. The use of bed rails increases the risk of falls and injury.🔢 When risk of falling is thought to be significant, beds should be kept low to the ground unless elevation is needed temporarily for examinations or procedures.

DRUGS

Adverse drug reactions occur in up to 36% of hospitalized patients and are usually associated with polypharmacy, which increases as patient age increases. In some cases, the cause may be related to changes in pharmacokinetics and pharmacodynamics that occur with aging.🔢 Drug distribution, metabolism, and elimination vary widely among elderly patients. Therefore, drug doses should be carefully titrated, creatinine clearance of renally excreted drugs calculated for dose adjustment, serum drug levels measured, and patient responses observed.

Important is the number of drugs given to an elderly patient: 6 to 12 different drugs during a single hospitalization are not unusual. Also, nearly half of the drugs given to the elderly by the time of their discharge are new to the patient. Maintaining a daily list of drugs prescribed and received can help prevent adverse drug reactions and interactions.

Patients may have difficulty sleeping in the hospital. However, use of hypnotic drugs should be minimized because of tachyphylaxis and

🔢see page 102   🔢see pages 56 to 62

increased risk of falls and delirium. Short-acting benzodiazepines are generally best. Antihistamines have adverse anticholinergic effects on bladder and bowel function, cognition, and blood pressure and should not be used for sedation.

INCONTINENCE

More than 40% of hospitalized patients ≥ 65 become incontinent of urine or stool, many within a day of hospital admission. The environment may be unfamiliar, the path to the toilet may be unclear, an illness or injury may impair ambulation, the height of the bed may be intimidating, or bed rails may be a barrier. Equipment such as IV lines, nasal oxygen lines, cardiac monitors, and catheters act as restraints. Bedpans may be uncomfortable, especially for postsurgical patients or patients with chronic arthritis. Psychoactive drugs may diminish the perception of a need to void, inhibit bladder or bowel function, and impair ambulation. Patients with dementia or neurologic disease may be unable to use the call bell to request toileting assistance. Anticholinergic drugs, opioids, and constipation may lead to overflow urinary incontinence, and diuretics may precipitate urge incontinence.[1] Fecal impaction, gastrointestinal tract infection (eg, *Clostridium difficile* colitis), adverse effects of drugs, and liquid nutritional supplements may cause uncontrollable diarrhea.

With appropriate diagnosis and treatment, continence can be reestablished, and nursing home placement avoided.

SKIN INTEGRITY

Pressure sores often develop in elderly hospitalized patients.[2] With aging, the epidermis and dermis become thinner, vascularity decreases, epidermal turnover slows, and subcutaneous fat is lost. Direct pressure may cause skin necrosis in as few as 2 hours if the pressure is greater than the capillary perfusion pressure of 32 mm Hg. During a typical emergency department visit, the time elderly patients spend lying on a hard stretcher is often longer than that needed for pressure sores to start developing. After short periods of immobilization, sacral pressures reach 70 mm Hg, and pressure under an unsupported heel averages 45 mm Hg. Shearing forces result when patients sitting in wheelchairs or propped up in beds slide downward. Incontinence, poor nutrition, and chronic illness may contribute to pressure sore development.

Immediately placing patients on a prevention and treatment protocol helps decrease morbidity. Such protocols should be typically initiated upon admission, followed daily by the patient's primary care nurse, and reviewed at least weekly by an interdisciplinary team. Pressure

[1] see also page 965   [2] see also page 1261

sores may be the only reason a patient is discharged to a nursing home rather than to the community.

FALLS

One of the most clinically important manifestations of the change in autonomic function that occurs with age is baroreceptor insensitivity. This insensitivity, combined with age-associated decreases in body water and plasma volume (which can be exacerbated by dehydration), results in a tendency toward orthostatic hypotension.

Bed rest has many pitfalls. It reduces muscle strength and aerobic capacity and accelerates bone loss. Bed rest also decreases plasma volume, peripheral vascular resistance, and baroreceptor sensitivity, all of which increase the risks of orthostatic hypotension and syncope. Sedatives and the intense hypotensive effects of some antihypertensive drugs can further contribute to the possibility of syncope or falls.

Among hospitalized elderly patients, > 60% of falls occur in the bathroom; often, patients strike hard objects.◼ Some patients fall while getting out of high hospital beds, sometimes while climbing over the bed rails. High beds are for the staff's convenience, not the patient's. Patients do not fall out of bed in the hospital any more than they fall out of bed at home. They are injured as they climb in and out of high beds. Because all types of physical restraints pose a significant risk of injury, bed rails should be removed or kept down in most cases. The best alternatives to the use of physical or chemical restraints are careful analysis of risk factors and their modification, diagnosis and treatment of factors contributing to agitation or falling, and close observation by health care practitioners.

REHABILITATION

Rehabilitation is often needed by patients who have become deconditioned because of prolonged bed rest, which is seldom warranted. With complete inactivity, muscle strength decreases by 5% per day, and reduced muscle strength often leads to falls. Even young men on bed rest lose muscle strength at a rate of 1.0 to 1.5% per day (10% per week). Inactivity contributes to muscle shortening and changes in periarticular and cartilaginous joint structure, both of which contribute to limitation of motion and development of contractures. The most rapid changes occur in the legs. Bed rest also markedly decreases aerobic capacity, substantially reducing maximum oxygen uptake.

For an older person who has diminished physiologic reserves but who still can perform daily activities, such as walking, toileting, and bathing, the accelerated losses of muscle strength and aerobic capacity after even a few days of bed rest may result in a prolonged loss of independent function. Even if the loss is reversible, rehabilitation requires extensive and expensive intervention because reconditioning takes longer than deconditioning. In the elderly, bed rest can also cause bony demineralization. Many elderly persons, particularly thin white women, are osteoporotic when admitted, and a prolonged stay accelerates bone loss. In older adults, bed rest can cause vertebral bone loss 50 times faster than in younger adults. The loss incurred from 10 days of bed rest takes 4 months to restore. The loss may be due to lack of weight bearing and the general negative nitrogen balance caused by immobilization.

Unless prohibited for a specific reason, activity, particularly walking, is encouraged; assistance with walking by physicians, nurses, and family members throughout the day is recommended, not only by therapists at scheduled times. Hospital orders should emphasize the need for activity. If immobilization is necessary or results from prolonged illness, procedures to prevent deep vein thrombosis are recommended unless contraindicated.

Realistic goals for rehabilitation at home can be determined by the patient's prehospitalization activity level and current needs.■

SOCIALIZATION

Socialization during treatment for an acute illness promotes recovery. A growing number of hospitals have rooming-in programs, in which a family member sleeps in a reclining chair or bed in the patient's room. These programs may disrupt staff routines and protocols; however, if properly supervised, they provide better one-on-one care and relieve staff members of some caregiving tasks. They also allay patient anxiety, particularly in delirious or demented patients, and allow family members to participate actively in the patient's recovery.

DISCHARGE PLANNING AND TRANSFERS

Early, effective discharge planning shortens the hospital stay, decreases the likelihood of readmission, identifies less expensive care alternatives, facilitates placement of equipment (eg, hospital bed, oxygen) in the patient's home, helps increase patient satisfaction, and may prevent placement in a nursing home.■ As soon as the patient is admitted, all members of the interdisciplinary team begin discharge planning. A social worker or discharge planning coordinator evaluates the patient's needs within 24 hours of admission. Nurses are vital in helping physicians determine when discharge is safe and which setting is most appropriate.

■ see page 265   ■ see also page 140

Patients being discharged to their homes need detailed instructions about follow-up care, and family members or other caregivers may need training to provide care. Failure to teach them how to give drugs, implement treatment, and monitor recovery increases the likelihood of adverse outcomes and of readmission. Writing down follow-up appointments and drug schedules may be helpful for patients and family members. At discharge, a copy of a brief discharge summary plan should be given to patients or family members in case they have questions about care before the primary care physician receives the official summary plan.

When patients are discharged to a nursing home or to another hospital, it is recommended that a written summary be sent with the patient and a copy faxed to the receiving institution. The summary must include information about the patient's mental and functional status, the times the patient last received drugs, known drug allergies, advance directives, and family contacts. The summary should contain complete, accurate information, including resuscitation status, cognitive and physical function, drugs, follow-up appointments and studies, and the names and phone numbers of a nurse and physician who can provide additional information. It is helpful when the patient's nurse calls the receiving institution to review the information shortly before the patient is transferred.

Likewise, when a patient is transferred to the hospital from a nursing home, important transfer information includes the patient's cognitive and physical function, resuscitation status, drugs, drug allergies, and family support. A written copy of the patient's medical and social history should accompany the patient during transfer and may be sent via fax to the receiving hospital to ensure that no information gaps occur. Written confirmation of advance directives is often required by the receiving hospital.

Effective communication between staff members of institutions helps ensure continuity of care. For example, a nurse caring for a hospitalized patient can call the nurse who will care for the patient after discharge.

LONG-TERM CARE

The setting in which long-term care is provided is best determined by the patient's wishes and medical, social, emotional, and financial needs; by the family's ability to meet the patient's needs; and by the provider's ability to achieve the goals established for the patient by the referring physician. The availability, accessibility, and affordability of community-based long-term care services (see TABLE 11–5) often determine whether placement in a nursing home is necessary.

TABLE 11-5.   COMMUNITY-BASED SERVICES

Type of Service	Estimated Number in USA	Services Provided	Reimbursement	Regulation
Independent housing (senior-citizen designated)	600,000 units of subsidized housing and market-rate housing	On-site social services (sometimes)	Private pay, subsidies from federal and state governments	U.S. Department of Housing and Urban Development, state housing authorities
Board-and-care-facilities	70,000	Room, congregate meals, personal care	Private pay, Supplemental Security Income program	State government, varies widely
Assisted living	Difficult to determine because definitions vary widely	Meals, personal care, housekeeping, transportation, 24-hour oversight	Private pay, long-term care insurance, Supplemental Security Income program	State government, varies widely
Life-care communities	1200	Personal care, skilled nursing care, as needed	Private pay, some long-term care insurance, Medicare for covered health care	State government

NURSING HOMES

A general term covering a wide variety of short- and long-term care facilities that provide medical and nursing care and other services.

A skilled nursing facility (SNF) is a term defined by the Health Care Financing Administration as an institution that provides persons ≥ 65 years (and younger disabled persons) with daily skilled nursing care, skilled rehabilitation services, and other medical services. Many also provide additional community-based services (eg, day care, respite care). For patients with functional disabilities resulting from injury or illness, many SNFs provide short-term postacute care services, including skilled nursing care and intensive physical, occupational, respiratory, and speech therapy. SNF beds may be located in hospitals (including rural hospitals with swing-beds) or in freestanding facilities that may or may not be affiliated with a hospital.

To be able to receive reimbursement from Medicare for skilled care, SNFs must be certified. To be certified, SNFs must have the following: a licensed charge nurse on site 24 hours/day, certified nurse assistants, a full-time social worker if the facility has > 120 beds, a medical director and licensed nursing home administrator, a qualified recreational therapist, a rehabilitative therapist, and a dietitian. Although not required to be on site, the following must be available as needed: physicians, pharmacists, dentists, and pastoral services. To qualify for Medicare coverage of services in an SNF, beneficiaries must need daily skilled nursing care or daily rehabilitation therapy and must be admitted to the SNF or rehabilitation service within 30 days after a minimum 3-day hospital stay.▮

The number of nursing home beds continues to increase but is not keeping pace with the increase in the elderly population. In 1996, the USA had about 16,800 certified nursing homes with about 1.8 million beds. The number of beds per 1000 persons ≥ 65 ranged from 80.9 in Kansas to 26.1 in Nevada. Average occupancy was 87.4%, ranging from 98% in New York to 77% in Texas.

The probability of nursing home placement within a person's lifetime is closely related to age; for persons aged 65 to 74, the probability is 17%, but for those > 85, it is 60%. Projections indicate that 43% of persons who turned 65 in 1990 will spend some time in a nursing home before they die, and > 50% of those admitted will spend at least 1 year. Other risk factors for nursing home placement are living alone, loss of ability for self-care, impaired mental status, lack of social or informal supports, poverty, and female sex.

SERVICES

The types of medical, nursing, and social services vary considerably among nursing homes. In addition to the basic services described above for certification, ophthalmologic, otolaryngologic, neurologic, psychiatric, psychologic, and other medical specialty services are provided by consultants but may require transport of patients to other facilities. Some nursing homes provide IV therapy, enteral nutrition through feeding tubes, and long-term oxygen treatment or ventilator support.

Recreational services are required in nursing homes, including weekend and evening programs. High-quality activity programs include scheduled group events and provide choices of leisure-time activities for patients, especially those who are cognitively impaired or bedridden. Some homes provide personal services (eg, hairdressing, makeup), which are usually paid for by patients' personal funds.

Social services also vary. Social workers assist patients and family members to improve the quality of care. They can help alleviate transfer trauma for patients and family members, identify social withdrawal and isolation, and actively assist in maintaining the patients' psychosocial well-being. Social workers can also ensure ongoing communication among the patient, family members, and care team, provide assis-

▮ see also page 165

tance when the patient applies for Medicare or Medicaid coverage, plan an appropriate discharge, and inform the patient and family members about other services.

Some nursing homes have special care units that provide services designed to meet specific problems (eg, Alzheimer's disease, ventilator dependence, cancer). Special care units must specify programs and admissions criteria, train staff specifically for the unit, meet regulations and reimbursement requirements, and have an identifiable area or discrete physical space.

ROLE OF NURSING HOME STAFF

Some states set minimum nurse-to-patient ratios that are more stringent than federal rules, but the ratio of other staff members to patients varies considerably. When too few staff members are employed, they rarely have time to adequately care for the sicker or needier patients, particularly those with dementia; substandard care may result.

Physicians must see patients as often as medically necessary but not less than every 30 days for the first 90 days and at least once every 60 days thereafter. During routine visits, patients should be examined, drug status assessed, and laboratory tests ordered as needed. Findings must be documented in the patient's chart to keep other staff members informed. If possible, the physician who cares for a patient in the nursing home should treat that patient if hospitalization becomes necessary.

Some physicians limit their practice to nursing homes. They are available to participate in team activities and to consult with other staff members, thus promoting better care than that given in hurried bimonthly visits. Such full-time practice is enhanced when physicians also can monitor their patients' hospital care and when they can teach medical students and house staff members. House staff members learn more about geriatric care and that not all nursing home patients are obtunded, dehydrated, and febrile—a misconception commonly held by practitioners whose only contact with such patients is in a hospital emergency department.

Some nurse practitioners and physicians collaborate to manage patients' disorders. By administering antibiotics and monitoring IV lines, suctioning equipment, and sometimes ventilators, nurse practitioners may help prevent patients from being hospitalized.

FINANCIAL ASPECTS

Nursing home care is expensive, averaging $46,000 per year in 1995 according to estimates by the Health Care Financing Administration. About 50% of the cost is paid by Medicaid, 37% by the patient, 8% by Medicare, and 5% by private insurance.

Critics claim that prospective case-mix systems reimburse nursing homes at too low a rate and limit patient access to rehabilitation and services that enhance quality of life, especially for patients with dementia. Other criticisms are that these systems offer insufficient financial incentives to provide restorative care and rehabilitation for low-functioning patients and that they may encourage nursing homes to foster dependence or to maintain the need for high-level care to maximize reimbursement.

DETERMINING THE NEED FOR NURSING HOME PLACEMENT

A patient's preferences and needs can be determined most effectively through comprehensive geriatric assessment. **1**

All disorders are identified and evaluated before a patient is institutionalized. Disabling disorders may be the trigger for considering nursing home placement. However, even modest improvement of a disorder may forestall the need for a nursing home. For example, if a patient who depends on family members for care develops urinary incontinence, the family may be overwhelmed. However, if the causes of incontinence can be treated, the patient may be able to remain at home.

Physical Function

Evaluating a patient's ability to perform the activities of daily living and instrumental activities of daily living is crucial in deciding whether nursing home placement is necessary. Severely impaired mobility may make living at home impossible, but patients with other functional impairments may be able to remain at home with the assistance of adaptive devices and durable medical equipment. Physical and occupational therapists and home health nurses can assess patients in their homes and help determine whether placement in a nursing home or in an assisted-living facility is necessary.

Cognitive Function

Dementia commonly leads to nursing home placement, but supportive family members may be taught ways to deal with frustrating or disruptive behavior. For example, using monitoring devices—purchased or rented— can help with behaviors such as nocturnal wandering.

Social Support

Strongly motivated family members usually can perform elaborate and detailed care; however, without support and respite services, they may become resentful or worn out. Physicians can help by listening while caregivers discuss the burdens and by providing information about community caregiving support groups and about options for paid respite care. All practitioners delivering services to the elderly should be familiar with signs of abuse or neglect and be ready to intervene if elder abuse is suspected. **2**

1 see page 40   **2** see page 149

SELECTION OF A NURSING HOME

When matching the needs of a patient with the services of a nursing home, physicians should consider which clinical care practice model the nursing home uses. Models range from private single-physician practices to large networks of primary care practitioners who routinely visit a certain set of nursing homes. Physicians considering an SNF may compare services available on site with those requiring transfers to other facilities. Cognitively impaired patients are easily disoriented and frightened by the shuffling from one facility to another, and severely deconditioned patients may be exhausted by travel for dental care or blood work. Also, physicians should be familiar with the hospitals that have transfer agreements with the nursing home and with the availability of special therapeutic services, palliative care, hospice, and other services. Differences in services and the employment of full-time vs. part-time staff members may help determine the appropriateness of a home and the quality of its care. Patients' medical coverage, particularly if they are in a Medicare capitated program, must be considered when selecting a nursing home. Medicare covers certain aspects of ongoing medical care, although it does not cover long-term custodial care.**1**

Monitoring quality of care in nursing homes is the responsibility of federal and state regulators. The government is legally responsible for ensuring that a facility is providing good care, not merely that it is capable of doing so; therefore, outcome measures are playing an increasing role in quality assessment. Through observation of care, interviews with patients and staff members, and review of clinical records, surveyors attempt to assess a facility's performance and to detect deficiencies (see TABLE 11–6).

HOSPITALIZATION OF NURSING HOME PATIENTS

Hospitalization is avoided whenever possible because patients often return from the hospital with urinary catheters and pressure sores.**2** Hospitalization often causes patients to become confused or severely deconditioned, and they are often given psychoactive drugs in hospitals. Many patients also prefer to avoid hospitalization because treatment in hospitals can be dehumanizing and impersonal.

When patients are transferred to a hospital, their medical records should accompany them. A phone call from a nursing home nurse to a hospital nurse is useful to explain the diagnosis and reason for transfer and to describe the patient's baseline functional and mental status, drugs, and advance directives.**3** When patients are discharged to a nursing home from the hospital, communication among hospital nurses and nursing home nurses is critical.

1 see page 164   **2** see page 101   **3** see page 134

TABLE 11–6.   MOST COMMON DEFICIENCIES IN NURSING HOMES*

Deficiency	% of Certified Homes Cited
Failure to ensure sanitary food	24
Failure to remove accident hazards	18
Failure to ensure quality of care	17
Failure to provide treatment for pressure sores	17
Failure to prepare comprehensive resident care plans	15
Failure to conduct comprehensive resident assessment	15
Failure to prevent accidents	15
Failure to provide sanitary housekeeping	14
Failure to provide care that protects the dignity of patients	14
Failure to use physical restraints properly	13

*For 1998.
From Harrington C, et al: Nursing Facilities, Staffing, Residents and Facility Deficiencies, 1992–1998. Department of Social and Behavioral Sciences, University of California San Francisco, January 2000, p. 76.

ABUSE AND NEGLECT OF NURSING HOME PATIENTS

Patients are vulnerable and unable to leave the facility, they may have infrequent visitors, and their complaints may not be believed. Subtle types of abuse (eg, using drugs and physical restraints inappropriately) to manage disruptive behavior are still too common. Pinching, slapping, or yanking may be hard to prove, because ecchymosis and skin tears occur easily in the elderly, even without abuse. Detecting, stopping, and preventing abuse is a primary function of physicians, nurses, and other health care practitioners. A public advocacy system exists, and nursing homes can be cited by regulatory agencies.

BOARD-AND-CARE FACILITIES

(Adult Care Homes; Domiciliaries; Rest Homes)

Facilities for elderly persons who cannot live independently but who do not need the constant supervision provided in nursing homes.

Board-and-care facilities typically provide shelter, meals, minimal assistance with personal care, and sometimes supervision of drug administration (see TABLE 11–5). The program costs ≥ $8 billion annually. The number of facilities is increasing because they offer an economic, federally funded means of accommodating the increasing number of elderly persons who would otherwise require nursing home care paid for with state Medicaid funds.

Minimally regulated and sometimes unlicensed, the facilities principally serve two groups, often cared for together—the elderly and the deinstitutionalized mentally ill. Although excellent homes exist, many facilities tend to warehouse the disabled in substandard buildings and to employ few skilled staff members. At least one study uncovered widespread misuse of drugs in board-and-care facilities.

Physicians should try to ensure that their patients in board-and-care facilities are safe and are receiving appropriate care. Physicians may need to visit the facility or send a nurse or social worker to evaluate it.

ASSISTED-LIVING PROGRAMS

(Supportive Housing; Enriched Housing; Congregate Care)

Programs that enable residents with deficits in activities of daily living to maintain their independence in personalized settings by providing or arranging for the provision of daily meals, personal and other supportive services, health care, and 24-hour oversight as needed.

In some states (eg, New York), assisted-living programs are implemented in existing board-and-care facilities (with supplemental care provided by a home health agency), because supplying services to a group of patients in one location costs less than supplying services to persons throughout the community.

LIFE-CARE COMMUNITIES

(Continuing Care Retirement Communities)

Organizations that offer a contract intended to remain in effect for the resident's lifetime and, at a minimum, guarantee shelter and access to various health care services.

Life-care communities offer different levels of care: for persons who can live independently, for those who need assistance, and for those who need skilled nursing care. Generally, persons pay a substantial entrance fee ($50,000 to $500,000) when moving to the community and monthly fees thereafter. In some communities, residents pay only a monthly fee for rent plus service or health packages. In others, residents can purchase a condominium, cooperative, or membership; service or health packages are purchased separately.

Three types of life-care retirement communities are generally recognized: those covered by an all-inclusive contract, those covered by a modified contract limiting the amount of long-term care provided before the monthly fee is increased, and those covered by a fee-for-service contract with billing for health services as they are used.

The number of life-care communities increased by 50% in the 1980s and continues to increase; > 40% of these communities are in five states (Pennsylvania, California, Florida, Illinois, and Ohio). Resident profiles indicate that the average resident is a wealthy, widowed female aged 81.

If well financed and managed, life-care communities provide a broad range of housing, social, supportive, and health services that enable their residents to live comfortably. However, some are not well regulated and, because of unscrupulous real estate dealers or well-intentioned but inept management, the assets of the residents have been wiped out.

Communities may be housed in a single building or may be spread across multiacre campuses with housing options ranging from efficiency apartments to cottages with several rooms. Many have community buildings for organized social events, dining rooms, clubs, sports facilities, planned outings, and vacation options. Life-care communities are usually affiliated with various home care services, adult homes, day care programs, and nursing homes. Access to physicians is usually provided, and most programs are affiliated with local acute care facilities.

12 ■ QUALITY OF LIFE AND THERAPEUTIC OBJECTIVES

A patient's age should not affect the approach to clinical care (ie, relief of suffering, cure when possible) or the therapeutic objectives (ie, optimal health-related quality of life, independence, outcomes consistent with the patient's personal beliefs and objectives).

Quality of life is an intensely personal and variable concept. Most people are comfortable talking about their own quality of life but become uncertain and reluctant if asked to determine the quality of life of others. Thus, in health care, health-related quality of life is best assessed on the basis of the patient's experience. Frequent frank discussions with the patient about lifetime goals and aspirations, focusing on the patient's preferences (eg, based on religious beliefs or previous experiences with health care) and perception of health-related quality of life, help the physician act on the patient's behalf. Questionnaires and other instruments that measure health-related quality of life (designed for research purposes) are rarely clinically useful.

Therapeutic objectives are best guided by objective measures, such as the presence and severity of mental or physical suffering or pain, and by the likelihood that treatment will restore lifestyle and pleasures or result in suffering. The adverse effects of a proposed diagnostic test or treatment (eg, medical complications, discomfort, inconvenience, the temptation to follow up with additional diagnostic tests or treatments) should be weighed against the potential benefit; coexisting conditions may influence the benefit-to-risk ratio, but the need to modify therapy should be unchanged by a patient's age.

Some ethicists have proposed that age be a criterion for rationing or withholding specific treatment and that only palliation be available for ill patients > 75 years. By ignoring differences in individual characteristics (especially functional status) and health care preferences among elderly patients, such proposals are likely to do more harm than good to patients and to society.[1]

Several phenomena that become more prevalent with increasing age affect therapeutic objectives. Chronic disease accompanied by physical disability, pain and suffering, cognitive impairment, institutional confinement (eg, in a nursing home), reduced life expectancy, heavy use of health care resources, accumulated losses, dependence on family and friends, and social isolation must be considered when planning health care.[2]

Chronic Disease

In the USA, > 80% of noninstitutionalized persons > 65 years have at least one chronic disease, and about 50% have some limitations in performing activities of daily living (> 33% cannot perform major activities independently). About 5% of persons > 65 years, about 15% > 75 years, and about 25% > 80 years are homebound. Chronic disease causes 80% of deaths after age 65 and accounts for > 80% of health care expenditures in the USA.

However, 50% of persons > 40 years also have at least one chronic disease. Therefore, the health care delivery system for older adults should be oriented toward care of chronic disease, regardless of the patient's age, and should emphasize continuing care aimed at improving function, postponing deterioration and disability, and preventing complications.

Pain and Suffering

Pain affects function, ranging from a trivial and virtually unnoticed decline to agonizing incapacity and immobilization. Objective pain scales reliably measure the intensity of pain, both absolutely and relatively, over time. Assessment of the severity of pain as perceived by the patient[3] and of its effects on comfort, activities, and quality of life allows the clinician to determine when the focus of treatment must be relief of pain and suffering. Recent evidence suggests that fear of addiction and other complications (eg, falls, delirium) has led to significant undertreatment of pain in frail and institutionalized patients. Although these concerns are legitimate, they must be balanced against the imperative to relieve pain and suffering. Relief can often be accomplished through a combination of appropriate analgesic drugs given in modified doses and the use of nonpharmacologic measures.

---

[1] see page 127   [2] see page 40   [3] see FIGURE 43–1 on page 387

Cognitive Impairment

Evaluation of the severity and functional effect of cognitive impairment ensures that the patient understands and, if possible, consents to treatment. Explaining risks and benefits to a cognitively impaired patient, although complicated and time-consuming, is essential to high-quality care. When the patient cannot participate in such discussions, family or friends familiar with the patient's lifestyle and preferences may provide information that is useful in making decisions about treatment. Advance directives, written before the patient became cognitively impaired, are helpful. ◻

Institutional Confinement

Among nursing home residents, the prevalence of characteristics that can affect therapeutic objectives is disproportionately high. Reduced life expectancy, poverty, cognitive impairment, physical disability, chronic disease, pain and suffering, accumulated losses, and social isolation are common. Nonetheless, the way in which residents view their health-related quality of life must be considered. Discussing treatment issues with the patient and family or proxy, using terms the patient can understand, and respecting autonomy are crucial, regardless of the patient's age or residence.

Reduced Life Expectancy

When a treatment is considered, a patient must be informed of its potential side effects and other consequences. A patient may choose to forgo treatment if any extension of life will likely be spent in an enervated, nauseated state. When the prognosis is poor, treatment must be planned in light of the short life expectancy; the patient's age is not important. Life expectancy based on predictions related to a cohort (eg, 20 years for a 65-year-old woman, 15 years for a 65-year-old man) cannot be the sole criterion. For example, an 82-year-old has an average life expectancy of "only" 5.3 years; should coronary artery bypass surgery with a high probability of improving function be therefore withheld? Although the average life expectancy for a 75-year-old woman is 12 years, estimation of risks for functional decline and for survival, based on individual clinical and demographic characteristics, is essential for a more accurate prediction of outcome and for decision-making concerning the merit of intervention. Some patients whose life expectancy is reduced and who are severely suffering request euthanasia. ◻

For elderly persons who cherish any additional few days, weeks, or months, preserving life through medical intervention—heroic or ordinary—may be more important. Whether to proceed with major clinical interventions requires analysis of the likely outcomes and sharing of the results of this analysis with the patient. Only then can the patient make an informed decision consistent with personal values and goals. All patients should document their wishes in advance directives. ◻

◻ see page 134   ◻ see page 139   ◻ see page 134

13 ■ CARE OF THE DYING PATIENT

Dying is a natural and inevitable part of living. Helping a patient and family members find comfort with and meaning in the experience of dying is often more important than correcting physiologic abnormalities. The physician should preserve and enhance the dignity of the dying patient by allowing the patient and family members to maintain control and participate in end-of-life care whenever possible. The physician and other members of the health care team must also prevent and relieve distress (whether physical, emotional, or spiritual) as effectively as possible. They should know what local laws and institutional policies say about living wills, durable power of attorney, resuscitation, and specific treatments.∎

When facing death, patients differ in what they consider important (eg, some consider quantity of life more important than quality; some accept pain or disfigurement more readily than others). The patient's preferences are paramount, and care must be planned accordingly. Some patients find an appropriate time and way to bring life to a satisfying close; others do not.

Some dying patients benefit from curative, rehabilitative, or preventive care. For others, however, supportive care is the only realistic choice. Good care of the dying involves more than discontinuing unwarranted treatment; it includes developing a care plan that accounts for the patient's goals and the limits imposed by illness.

SYMPTOM CONTROL

Patients with a terminal illness commonly experience physical discomfort and mental distress. Many fear that their discomfort will be protracted and that no one will control it. Relieving discomfort and reassuring patients that their discomfort will be controlled enables them to live as fully as possible and to focus on the unique issues presented by the approach of death.

When survival is expected to be brief, the severity of symptoms often dictates initial treatment choices. When a symptom is less distressing than the fear that the symptom will worsen, reassurance that effective treatment is available may be all the patient needs. If a symptom is severe, immediate therapy may be required. Whether diagnostic tests are appropriate depends on how burdensome the test is and how useful the findings may be.

Because a symptom can have many causes and because patients may respond differently to therapy as their condition deteriorates, treatments must be closely monitored and continuously reevaluated. During periods of altered drug metabolism, special care must be taken to avoid an inadvertent overdose of drugs.

PHYSICAL SYMPTOMS

Pain

About half of patients dying of cancer have severe pain. Of these patients, only half obtain adequate relief. Severe pain is less common among patients with other terminal conditions. Often, pain persists not because it cannot be controlled but because patients and their physicians have misconceptions about pain and the drugs used to control it. The approach to pain control is the same regardless of what the terminal illness is.

Treatment must be individualized because patients perceive pain differently, depending in part on such factors as fatigue, insomnia, anxiety, depression, and nausea. A supportive environment can help control pain.

The most available and appropriate analgesic given by the least invasive route possible should be chosen.◼ Choice of an analgesic depends largely on pain intensity. Analgesics should be administered regularly rather than as needed; controlling pain after it recurs is more difficult than preventing it, partly because pain generates anxiety. Sustained- or continuous-release formulations make regular administration easier. In hospice units, nurses, patients, and family members become competent at making the necessary dosing or scheduling adjustments.

Pain-modification techniques such as hypnosis, guided mental imagery, counseling for stress and anxiety, and relaxation methods may help relieve pain.◼ In one study, patients with spiritual and religious well-being perceived pain as being less intense.◼

In cases of severe, persistent pain, the ability to sense pain, if it occurs in a suitable location, may be eliminated with neurosurgery or anesthetics.

Dyspnea

For dying patients, dyspnea is one of the most feared and most distressing symptoms. Its cause should be treated if it can be identified— eg, antibiotics for pneumonia or thoracentesis for a pleural effusion. Dyspnea in terminally ill patients should be suppressed when its physiologic origins cannot be relieved. Oxygen may be psychologically comforting to the patient and to family members even when it is not physiologically beneficial.

◼ see page 388   ◼ see page 396   ◼ see also page 146

When breathlessness occurs, an opioid can be used to slow respiration and relieve mild chronic symptoms, enabling the patient to sleep more comfortably. Carbon dioxide retention or decreased oxygen levels often produce dyspnea, even though oxygen levels are still physiologically adequate. In such cases, blunting the medullary response may eliminate symptoms without producing adverse effects. Morphine 2.5 mg IV q 2 to 4 h prn or by continuous drip may be used if the oral route is unavailable or too slow. Benzodiazepines may help relieve anxiety.

Useful nonpharmacologic measures include ventilation from an open window or a fan at bedside, relaxation techniques, and massage. Caregivers with a calming presence can help patients stay calm.

Anorexia

Anorexia, common among dying patients, is usually more distressing to family members than to the patient. Counseling may be needed to help family members accept anorexia and understand the futility of tube feedings or parenteral nutrition.

Some steps can be taken to increase a patient's food intake. For example, if a full meal tray is overwhelming, small portions, specially prepared foods, and a flexible meal schedule are recommended. A small amount of a favorite alcoholic beverage served 30 minutes before meals may help. Foods with strong flavors or smells sometimes stimulate the appetite.

Low-dose corticosteroids (eg, dexamethasone 1 mg po qid, prednisone 5 mg po tid), megestrol acetate, or tricyclic antidepressants may also improve a patient's appetite and sense of taste. Metoclopramide may help because it enhances gastric emptying. However, it may not produce maximum therapeutic effect for 1 or 2 weeks, which may be too slow for patients near death, and it may induce tardive dyskinesia. Methylphenidate can improve appetite, but because it can cause dysphoric agitation, the starting dose must be low and subsequent doses increased gradually, and patients must be monitored closely.

Only rarely should dying patients receive tube feedings or parenteral nutrition. Before starting either, the physician should discuss indications for its discontinuation with the patient and family members. Discontinuation may be difficult to accept, because food and water often symbolize caring and nurturing. However, the patient and family members should be told that dying patients may be more comfortable without the artificial administration of food and water. Sips of water or easy-to-swallow foods (eg, sherbet, gelatin) may be more appropriate.

After the decision to forgo artificial administration of food and water has been made, supportive care is imperative. Such care includes providing good oral hygiene (brushing the teeth, swabbing the oral cavity, applying lip salve, and providing ice chips for dry mouth). Oral hygiene is a physically and psychologically comforting service family members can perform for their loved one.

Nausea and Vomiting

Many dying patients experience nausea, often without vomiting. Nausea and vomiting may be caused by constipation, reduced gastric emptying, bowel obstruction, central opioid effects, increased intracranial pressure, gastritis, peptic ulcer, hypercalcemia, uremia, or toxic drug effects. Specific treatment may be warranted if the cause is easy to treat (as for hypercalcemia or constipation), especially if treatment makes a patient more comfortable. As with analgesics for pain control, antiemetics should be given regularly (not "as needed" when symptoms are severe) to prevent nausea and improve patient comfort.

Nonspecific treatment (eg, with a phenothiazine such as prochlorperazine) is almost always indicated. Phenothiazines are most effective because they act on the chemoreceptor zone in the medulla. However, they may have anticholinergic effects. Prochlorperazine 5 to 10 mg po tid to qid can be given prophylactically. If vomiting precludes oral administration, the drug can be given as a suppository (25 mg bid) or by IM injection (5 to 10 mg q 3 to 4 h; maximum dose, 40 mg/day).

Metoclopramide (10 to 20 mg po q 6 to 8 h or 1 to 2 mg/h continuous sc infusion) can be used when nausea and vomiting are caused by decreased gut motility, because the drug increases peristalsis and relaxes the pyloric sphincter. Other helpful antiemetics include corticosteroids (eg, dexamethasone 4 mg po q 8 h or prednisone 5 mg po tid) and antihistamines (eg, hydroxyzine 10 to 25 mg IM tid or dimenhydrinate 50 mg po q 4 to 6 h). The addition of lorazepam 0.5 to 2 mg sublingually may help relieve nausea due to nonspecific or multiple causes.

Ondansetron (4 to 8 mg IV or po q 6 to 12 h) can control nausea and vomiting due to chemotherapy or surgery. However, this drug is much more expensive than other antiemetics. Cannabinoid, the principal psychoactive substance in marijuana, is used primarily for the treatment of nausea and vomiting due to chemotherapy. This drug produces an altered mental state not tolerated well by many elderly persons.

If vomiting due to obstruction occurs in a patient who is near death, conservative treatment without relief of the obstruction is recommended. Sometimes, slowing peristalsis or slowing the gut with morphine and managing dry mouth with ice chips is preferable to performing continuous gastric suction or surgery. Nasogastric suctioning, except as a short-term measure, is difficult for sentient patients to endure. Octreotide 150 μg IM bid or 300 μg/day as a continuous sc infusion combined with an opioid (with dose adjustment based on patient response) is effective nonsurgical care for bowel obstruction. This combination can stop secretions, reduce distention, and alleviate cramping.

Constipation

Physicians often underestimate how important regular bowel movements are to a dying patient's comfort. Constipation is common among dying patients because they are inactive, consume little dietary fiber, are dehydrated, or are receiving opioids or anticholinergic drugs. Laxatives should be given prophylactically to prevent fecal impaction. A stool softener (soluble or insoluble fiber or docusate sodium) is usually given first. However, most patients receiving opioids also require a stimulant laxative (eg, casanthranol, senna, cascara sagrada, bisacodyl).

If the patient does not have a bowel movement within 48 hours of initiating the above therapy, an osmotic laxative (eg, lactulose, magnesium salts, phosphate enema) can be used.◘ Osmotic laxatives stimulate gastrointestinal function indirectly by increasing the fluid content of feces. Lactulose, a semisynthetic disaccharide that is not hydrolyzed by human intestinal enzymes, is an especially effective osmotic laxative for many bedridden patients; however, it is expensive. Sorbitol is usually as effective and is much less expensive.

If a patient has not had a bowel movement in 3 days and stool is detected during rectal examination, a glycerin or bisacodyl suppository is administered. If no bowel movement occurs, a saline enema is administered.

Diarrhea

If diarrhea occurs, an abdominal examination is performed to rule out impaction. All laxatives, including stool softeners, are discontinued. If diarrhea is severe, the patient should be given clear liquids and bland carbohydrates. Other foods can be added as symptoms permit. For severely dehydrated patients, electrolytes may be given po, IV, or sc to make the patient comfortable more quickly.

Often, diarrhea must be suppressed with nonspecific treatment: opioids, loperamide 4 mg po initially, then 2 mg per diarrheal stool (up to 16 mg/day), or diphenoxylate-atropine 2 tablets (5 mg [2.5 mg each as diphenoxylate]) po after each diarrheal stool, up to qid. However, more specific treatment may be needed: for carcinoid tumors or dumping syndrome after gastrectomy, octreotide 150 to 300 μg sc bid or 300 μg continuous IV infusion/24 h; for fungal infection due to immunosuppression, clotrimazole 10 to 20 mg po tid or fluconazole (first dose is 200 mg po, then 100 mg po once daily for ≥ 14 days); and for pancreatic insufficiency, pancreatic enzymes such as pancreatin 1 to 2 tablets with meals and half the dose with any snack. Zinc oxide helps relieve irritation around the anus, and corticosteroid cream (for as few as 1 to 2 days) helps relieve maceration or inflammation.

◘ see also page 1084

Pressure Sores

Many dying patients are immobile, poorly nourished, and cachectic; therefore, they are at great risk of developing pressure sores.◘ The most important preventive measure is rotating the patient every 2 hours using a specialized mattress or a continuously inflated air-suspension bed. Use of a urinary catheter is justified only when the patient experiences pain with bedding changes or when the patient or family members strongly prefer it.

PSYCHOLOGIC SYMPTOMS AND CONCERNS

Confusion

Confusion is common during the terminal stage of illness. Causes include drug therapy, hypoxia, metabolic disturbances, and intrinsic central nervous system disease. Confusion is treated if the cause can be determined and if treatment enables the patient to communicate more meaningfully with family and friends. If the patient is comfortable and less aware of the surroundings, withholding treatment may be preferable. Sedatives (eg, benzodiazepines) may help agitated patients, and low doses of haloperidol (0.25 to 0.5 mg po or 2.5 mg IM q 4 to 8 h or at bedtime) may help patients who have disquieting dreams or threatening hallucinations. Newer antipsychotics, such as risperidone (0.5 mg po at bedtime or bid) or olanzapine (2.5 mg po at bedtime) may have fewer adverse effects than haloperidol.

Sadness and Depression

Most dying patients experience sadness. Sadness may be due to regrets about life or preoccupation with legal, social, or financial problems. Providing psychologic support and allowing a patient to express concerns and feelings is the best and simplest course of action. Helping a patient and family members settle unresolved matters may decrease anxiety. A skilled social worker, physician, nurse, or chaplain can help with conflicts that separate a patient from family members, friends, church, or God. Vegetative signs, including sleep disturbance, should be evaluated; drug therapy may be warranted.

Antidepressants are reserved for the few patients who have persistent, clinically significant depression.◙ Such patients may benefit from a low dose of an antidepressant (eg, paroxetine 10 mg po) given once daily in the morning or at bedtime. Patients with depression and agitation are usually given a sedating tricyclic antidepressant (eg, amitriptyline 10 to 25 mg po at bedtime), supplemented as needed with another appropriate sedative. During the last weeks of life, a sedating antidepressant sometimes provides restful sleep while allevi-

---

◘ see also page 1261   ◙ see also page 320

ating depression. For patients who are near death, the usual concerns about possible cardiac and neurologic effects are not as important.

Patients with depression and significant insomnia can be given trazodone 25 to 50 mg po daily at bedtime, increased in 25- to 50-mg/day increments every 3 days for inpatients and weekly for outpatients, as tolerated, to a maximum of 300 mg daily. Adverse effects include excessive daytime sedation. Sedating tricyclic antidepressants (eg, amitriptyline, doxepin) are effective alternatives for management of insomnia; however, bothersome anticholinergic effects occur. Selective serotonin reuptake inhibitors, which have fewer adverse effects, are appropriate when depression is not associated with sleeplessness. Paroxetine 10 mg po, fluoxetine 10 mg po, and sertraline 25 mg po— all given once daily in the morning—and venlafaxine 25 mg po bid to tid are most commonly used.

For patients who are withdrawn or who have vegetative signs, methylphenidate, initially 2.5 mg once daily in the morning (with dose adjusted to individual response), may help. This drug has a rapid onset of action and fewer adverse effects than most antidepressants, but it may cause agitation.

Anxiety and Agitation

Anxiety and agitation[1] can result from treatable conditions such as pain, respiratory distress, sleep deprivation, a full bladder, fecal impaction, and nausea or from drug therapy (eg, corticosteroids, opioids).

Supportive therapy, including listening and talking to patients, should precede and supplement drug therapy. Sometimes symptoms of anxiety and agitation can be managed with gentle reassurance. Meditation, guided imagery, prayer, music therapy, and massage are often helpful.

If drug therapy is indicated, benzodiazepines are the drug of choice. Lorazepam 0.5 mg po, sc, or sublingually q 4 h is effective. The dose and interval are adjusted as needed. For psychosis or severe agitation, haloperidol 0.25 mg po or IV q 4 to 6 h or chlorpromazine 10 mg IV or 25 mg po or rectally q 6 to 8 h can be used for acute cases, and the dose increased as needed. For maintenance dose of an antipsychotic, olanzapine (2.5 mg po at bedtime) or risperidone (0.5 mg po at bedtime) may have fewer adverse effects than haloperidol. If a crisis occurs and no intravenous access has been established, an injection of lorazepam 1 to 2 mg IM or diazepam 2 to 5 mg IM can calm a patient while the physician determines what therapy is appropriate for longer-term use. If first-line therapies do not control agitation associated with a terminal illness, a bolus infusion of midazolam 5 mg sc, followed by 1 mg/h,

[1] see also page 322

is effective but expensive. The dose is increased or decreased based on the patient's level of consciousness and the recurrence of symptoms.

Insomnia

Insomnia is a symptom, not a diagnosis.∎ Depression and anxiety are the leading causes of insomnia; other causes include a noisy environment, pain, lack of activity, metabolic disturbances, and drugs. Underlying causes and environmental factors should be determined and treated or altered if possible.

Pharmacologic therapy is useful. Trazodone 25 to 50 mg po at bedtime or a hypnotic (eg, zolpidem 5 mg po at bedtime) may be helpful. Relaxation therapies, such as meditation, progressive muscle relaxation, deep-breathing exercises, and listening to relaxation tapes, may be helpful.

Stress

As death approaches, patients may feel stress due to fear of abandonment and separation, anxiety, feelings of hopelessness, or loss of self-esteem because their body image is altered. Family members who care for a dying patient at home may experience physical and emotional stress. Stress is greatest when death is unexpected or when interpersonal conflicts keep patients and family members from sharing their last moments together. Such conflicts can cause anguish for patients and can lead to excessive guilt or an inability to grieve among family members.

When a spouse or long-term partner dies, the survivor may be overwhelmed by the prospect of making legal or financial decisions or of managing the household. Death of a spouse or partner may reveal cognitive impairment or other deficiencies in the survivor for which the deceased person had compensated. Stress is even greater for the survivor if friends or family members do not help. Physicians and other health care practitioners should identify these high-risk situations so that they can mobilize the resources needed to prevent undue suffering and dysfunction.

Usually, the best treatment for dying patients and family members with stress is compassion, information, counseling, and, occasionally, time-limited psychotherapy. In addition to the physician, members of the health care team, such as social workers, nurses, and chaplains, can offer such help. Sedatives should be used sparingly and only briefly.

The team approach to care helps prevent and relieve stress; no one caregiver can be available 24 hours/day, and skills and perspectives from several disciplines are needed to manage the different aspects of care. Palliative care or hospice teams should anticipate potential problems and make appropriate arrangements, such as ways to obtain sup-

∎ see page 452

plies or opioids in an emergency. When death is impending, an experienced team member can comfort family members and may prevent an inappropriate call to the emergency medical system due to panic. Team members may feel stress and grieve with the patient or family members because they become so involved. This involvement can be mitigated by a nurturing work environment and a staff support group that meets regularly to share responses to dying patients and their families.

Grieving

Grieving is a normal process that usually begins before an anticipated death. For patients, it often starts with denial caused by fears about loss of control, separation from loved ones, an uncertain future, and suffering. Staff members can help patients accept the prognosis by listening to their concerns, helping them understand that they can remain in control, explaining what the future probably holds, and assuring them that their pain and other symptoms will be controlled.

Family members may need support in expressing and dealing with grief. Any member of the health care team who has come to know the patient and family may help them through this process and direct them to professional services if needed. Physicians and other team members, including chaplains, should develop regular procedures that ensure follow-up of grieving family members.

FINANCIAL CONCERNS

Obtaining adequate financial coverage for care of the dying can be difficult. Medicare regulations exclude supportive care except in a hospice setting.[1] To qualify for hospice care, patients must have a 6-month prognosis, which physicians are often reluctant to certify.[2] Terminally ill patients with a prognosis of < 6 months may not be easily admitted to a nursing home, even if they have a certified need for a skilled nursing level of care. Nursing homes do not like to admit dying patients for several reasons, including high costs, nursing needs, and effect on the other residents. Physicians should ensure that a core team member is familiar with local care services, financing options, and the financial effects of choices.

LEGAL AND ETHICAL CONCERNS

In some cases, care of a dying patient seems to be directed more toward hastening death than toward prolonging life. Whether such an approach should be construed as good medical care or as a criminal act

[1] see also page 166   [2] see page 90

(ie, homicide or assisted suicide) is debated. Certain situations require a decision between actions that may hasten death and those that may prolong life. For example, a patient or surrogate may request discontinuation of parenteral hydration and nutrition or refuse treatment expected to yield long disease-free remissions, or a patient may develop suffocating dyspnea that can be relieved only with strong sedation, which can accelerate death. Requests from a patient or surrogates that seem contrary to the patient's interests are referred to consultants within the institution or agency. A request may be honored or denied, or a different action taken.

Most medical actions that may hasten but not directly cause death are necessary for relieving pain or other suffering. When initiating such treatment, the physician must inform the patient and family members that the action may shorten life. The physician should be clear that the treatment is for pain and symptom relief, not for causing death. However, good pain management rarely shortens life and may even extend it. In most cases when treatment has shortened life, the forgone life would have been so brief and so anguished that a slight extension of life would not have been in the patient's best interest. Nevertheless, deciding what constitutes wrongful death is sometimes difficult.

Wrongful death cases are only rarely brought to court, for several reasons:

- Most persons, including prosecutors, judges, and jurors, consider motivation and usually find compassion rather than malice in a situation that could have had no better outcome.

- The means of death are agents ordinarily used in treatment (eg, analgesics, sedatives, anesthetics), not those associated with crime (eg, poisons, guns, knives).

- The means of death are not as certain to result in death as are those typically used in criminal acts.

Assisting with suicide is a criminal act in most states, but the laws vary substantially and are rarely invoked. The U.S. Supreme Court has ruled that states can prohibit physician-assisted suicide but has not ruled that states must prohibit it. Therefore, the state governments must decide. Oregon is the only state that has legalized physician-assisted suicide. However, the American Medical Association and most other medical and professional organizations oppose its legalization. In one survey, only 18.3% of physicians were asked by their terminally ill patients to assist in suicide. Most of the patients who were given a prescription for a lethal dose of drugs were within 5 months of predicted life expectancy, and very few filled their prescriptions.

Physicians have not been charged with homicide or attempted homicide for giving dying patients large doses of opioids for pain relief or for allowing patients to refuse life-sustaining treatment, as long as the plan of care evolved in an appropriate, ethical fashion with informed consent from and open dialogue with patients and family members. Physicians who do not provide life-sustaining treatment for patients with a terminal illness should document the decision process thoroughly, provide care in a reputable setting, and be willing to discuss the issues honestly and sensitively with patients, family members, and other health care practitioners. In all states except Oregon, a physician should not use treatment conventionally considered a means of homicide (eg, lethal injection), even though the physician considers it a means of relieving suffering. Health care providers must always be clear that their plan of care was not intended to cause death.

Most patients with terminal illness should execute an advance directive. Advance directives are legal agreements that allow the patient to establish values and treatment preferences to be honored in the future when competency or capacity has lapsed. Advance directives may be in the form of a living will, which expresses the patient's preferences for medical care, or a durable power of attorney, in which the patient designates another person to make health care decisions. **1**

SPIRITUAL CONCERNS

Patients who are dying often ask what their life means, who they really are, why the illness has affected them, and what will happen to them when they die. Patients may question God's existence and love or may feel abandoned by God. **2** Some feel guilty or worry that their behavior caused their illness. Thus, dying can precipitate a spiritual crisis. Unresolved spiritual distress can lead to despair and hopelessness, which in turn can lead to anxiety, depression, and, for some, a desire to die or to commit suicide. Patients need help working through this distress so that despair can be transformed into hope and serenity. Dying patients do not always need to hope for a cure; instead they can hope for having time to reconcile with loved ones, sharing time with family, finishing a personally important project, or making peace with God or a Higher Power. When spiritual distress is relieved, patients can die more peacefully.

Dying patients may review their lives; this process may elicit positive and negative emotions as they try to resolve past hurts, reexamine relationships, and recount accomplished goals. They need to find meaning and purpose in their lives and in their illness. They often need to reconcile themselves with themselves, with others, and, for some, with God or a Higher Power. Belief in an afterlife and possible reunion with loved ones can comfort patients and family members. Physicians,

---

nurses, social workers, chaplains, family members, and friends can listen and offer support; doing so may help them deal with their own feelings of loss.

Patients who are religious need opportunities for prayer, devotional reading, and religious ritual, such as receiving a chaplain's blessing. Other spiritual resources include meditation, guided imagery, music, and art. Patients may need physical space and privacy for these practices. Hospice provides an excellent environment for spiritual practices. Each hospice team includes chaplains and others who are skilled at helping patients and family members with their spiritual needs.

CONCERNS AT THE TIME OF DEATH

The last moments of life can have a lasting effect on family, friends, and caregivers. Therefore, when death is imminent, health care team members should try to make the death as comfortable and as meaningful as possible and to help family members prepare for it. Family members are told exactly what will happen when the patient dies. If the patient is expected to die at home, family members are told whom to call (eg, the physician) and whom not to call (eg, an ambulance service). They are also told how to obtain legal advice and arrange burial services.

The setting should be peaceful, quiet, and physically comfortable. Stains or tubes on the bed are covered, and odors are masked.

In some patients near death, noisy breathing (known as the death rattle) develops because of bronchial congestion or palatal relaxation. If this breathing distresses the family, scopolamine (0.3 to 0.6 mg sc prn), atropine (0.4 to 0.6 mg IM, sc, or nebulized q 4 h or prn), ipratropium (500 µg nebulized q 6 to 8 h), or glycopyrrolate (0.2 mg IV prn or as a continuous infusion) can dry the patient's secretions and reduce the noise. Central nervous system irritability, including agitation and restlessness, may develop; it can be relieved with a sedative.

Family members are encouraged to touch the patient (eg, hold hands) as well as to talk with the patient, pray, or sing if desired. Depending on the desires of the patient and family members and on feasibility, supporters such as clergy and friends are encouraged to be present, and cultural, spiritual, religious, or ethnic rites of passage are performed.

A physician should make the official determination of death as quickly as possible to lessen family members' anxiety and uncertainty. Family members or funeral directors are given a completed death certificate promptly.

Members of the care team (eg, physicians, nurses, chaplains) ensure that family members' psychologic and spiritual needs are met by providing appropriate counseling and ensure that family members have a comfortable environment where they can grieve together and have adequate time to be with the body. Friends, neighbors, and clergy may also provide psychologic and spiritual support. Care team members should be aware that there are cultural differences in behavior at the time of death.

Often, arranging for someone (eg, a nurse, a volunteer) to be with the body when family members visit is helpful. This person can offer to help notify clergy or funeral directors, can reassure family members that the patient was comfortable and received the best care possible, and can contact the most closely affected survivor a few weeks later to answer questions, note whether the survivor is adjusting appropriately, and offer condolences.

The health care system ensures that death did not result from wrongdoing. Physicians should know when local laws require that a death, even when expected, is to be reported to the coroner or police.

The possibility of an autopsy can be discussed before or shortly after the patient's death. Often, a physician chooses not to raise this issue, but family members may ask about it because they have strong feelings for or against autopsy. This discussion is better handled by the patient's physician, not by a covering physician or house officer unfamiliar with the family. Organ donation, if appropriate, is discussed before death or as soon as possible after death. Usually, the body must be attended to promptly by persons licensed to do so, so that it does not present a risk to public health.

The patient's cultural, religious, and personal preferences should be considered when decisions about preparation of the body, religious rituals, time of burial, autopsy, and organ donation are made.

14 ▬ LEGAL AND ETHICAL ISSUES

The most common legal and ethical issues in geriatric care involve assessment of decisional capacity and competence, identification of decision makers, resolution of conflicts about care, disclosure of information, termination of treatment at the end of life, and decisions about long-term care. Although the approach to resolution of these issues is similar for all age groups, the physiologic, psychologic, and social reserves of the elderly place them at greater risk of adverse outcomes. The fact that the elderly often lack the support of family and friends makes them especially vulnerable to the automatic and sometimes unthoughtful process of the health care system.

Although aging may pose some special challenges, it is unfair to make assumptions about a person's abilities or needs based on age alone. Rather, physicians should assess each elderly patient individually and delineate treatment options accordingly. Physicians must also advocate for their patients' ethical interests and legal rights, especially in the medical context, about which patients are often ill-informed or misled (see TABLE 14–1). Elderly patients are often targets of unscrupulous schemes to defraud them of property or money. Health care practitioners may be the first to recognize such schemes and should offer help and referral for legal assistance. Attorneys knowledgeable about elder law can defeat these schemes with timely and effective legal intervention through services provided by the local agency on aging.

CAPACITY

A clinical determination of a patient's ability to make decisions about treatment interventions or other health-related matters.

Capacity is determined by the health care practitioner or, ideally, by the health care team with the aid of cognitive testing, discussion over time, and observation. Capacity is related to memory but is not extinguished by memory loss.

Persons are considered to have **decisional capacity** if they can understand their health condition; can consider the benefits, burdens, and risks of care options; can weigh the consequences of treatment against their preferences and values; can reach a decision that is consistent over time; and can communicate that decision to others.

Elderly patients with decisional capacity have the same rights as other adults to make choices about their care. Because many elderly patients can make some decisions but not others, capacity is considered decision-specific. Thus, a patient may be capable of choosing between relatively benign alternatives that may have few serious consequences but may not be capable of evaluating and choosing alternatives in a life-threatening circumstance.

For the elderly, who are often deprived of the opportunity to make any decision when they are unable to make some, the notion of **partial capacity** is especially important. Many elderly patients have diminished or fluctuating capacity and can be supported in their exercise of some autonomous decision making. For example, patients who become confused at the end of the day (sundowning) can make health care decisions when they are lucid. These decisions can then be recorded in the patient's medical chart. Patients with short-term memory loss may still be able to judge the appropriateness of a suggested intervention, especially if they have shown a long-standing pattern of stable choices that can be corroborated. If, however, patients must retain current information to choose among treatment options, then short-term memory loss is relevant (eg, if memory is needed for compliance with certain rehabilitation regimens, then it is relevant).

TABLE 14-1. A PATIENT'S BILL OF RIGHTS

1. The patient has the right to considerate and respectful care.

2. The patient has the right to and is encouraged to obtain from physicians and other direct caregivers relevant, current, and understandable information concerning diagnosis, prognosis, and treatment.

Except in emergencies in which the patient lacks decision-making capacity and the need for treatment is urgent, the patient may discuss and request information related to the specific procedures and/or treatments, the risks involved, the possible length of recuperation, and the medically reasonable alternatives and their accompanying risks and benefits.

The patient has the right to know the identity of physicians, nurses, and others involved in his care as well as when those involved are students, residents, or other trainees. The patient also has the right to know the immediate and long-term financial implications of treatment choices, if known.

3. The patient has the right to make decisions about the care plan before and during the course of treatment, to refuse a recommended treatment or care plan to the extent permitted by law and hospital policy, and to be informed of the medical consequences of this action. In the case of such a refusal, the patient is entitled to other appropriate care and services that the hospital provides or transfer to another hospital. The hospital should notify the patient of any policy that might affect the patient's choice within the institution.

4. The patient has the right to have an advance directive (ie, a living will or durable power of attorney for health care) concerning treatment or a surrogate decision maker with the expectation that the hospital will honor the intent of that directive to the extent permitted by law and hospital policy. The health care institution must advise the patient of his rights under state law and hospital policy to make informed medical choices, ask if the patient has an advance directive, and include that information in the patient's record. The patient has the right to timely information about hospital policy that may limit its ability to implement fully a legally valid advance directive.

5. The patient has the right to every consideration of privacy. Case discussion, consultation, examination, and treatment should be conducted so as to protect the patient's privacy.

6. The patient has the right to expect that all communications and records pertaining to his care will be treated as confidential by the hospital, except in cases of suspected abuse or public health hazards, in which case reporting is permitted or required by law. The patient has the right to expect that the hospital will emphasize the confidentiality of this information when it releases it to any other parties entitled to review these records.

7. The patient has the right to review his medical records and to have the information explained or interpreted as necessary, except when restricted by law.

8. The patient has the right to expect that, within its capacity and policies, a hospital will respond reasonably to the patient's request for appropriate and medically indicated care and services. The hospital must provide evaluation, service, and/or referral as indicated by the urgency of the case. When medically appropriate and legally permissible or when a patient has so requested, a patient may be transferred to another facility. The institution to which the patient is to be transferred must first have accepted the patient for transfer. The patient must also have the benefit of complete information and explanation concerning the need for, risks, benefits, and alternatives to such a transfer.

9. The patient has the right to ask about and be informed of any business relationships existing between the hospital, educational institutions, other health care providers, or payers that may influence the patient's treatment and care.

10. The patient has the right to consent to or decline participation in proposed research studies or human experimentation affecting care and treatment or requiring direct patient involvement and to have those studies fully explained before consenting. A patient who declines to participate in research or experimentation is entitled to the most effective care that the hospital can otherwise provide.

11. The patient has the right to expect reasonable continuity of care when appropriate and to be informed by physicians and other health care practitioners of available and realistic care options when hospital care is no longer appropriate.

12. The patient has the right to be informed of hospital policies and practices that relate to patient care, treatment, and responsibilities. The patient has the right to be informed of available resources for resolving disputes, grievances, and conflicts, such as ethics committees, patient representatives, or other mechanisms available in the institution. The patient has the right to be informed of the hospital's charges for services and available payment methods.

Adapted from the American Hospital Association, 1992.

A patient's autonomous right to make health care decisions may be compromised by a physician's finding that the patient lacks capacity. The patient may therefore be at risk of disempowerment, especially in acute care settings. In this setting, the effects of illness, drugs, or post-surgical delirium can exclude patients from discussions about care plans. In addition, hospitalization, which may scare, confuse, or intimidate the patient, can compound common problems of aging (eg, loss of hearing or sight). For the already **incapacitated patient,** hospitalization may precipitate a crisis for which surrogates must be identified, hastily assembled, informed of choices, and helped to sort through care options preferred by or in the best interest of the patient.**1** The burden of making decisions for an incapacitated patient falls heavily on both family and care providers. Therefore, whenever possible, health care professionals should discuss treatment options and preferences while the patient still is capable of making and communicating informed choices. These expressed preferences should be recorded in the patient's medical chart and documented in an advance directive.**2**

COMPETENCE

A legal designation that recognizes that persons beyond a certain age generally have the cognitive ability to negotiate certain legal tasks, such as entering into a contract or making a will.

In most states, persons are declared competent at age 18, at which time they can vote, sign binding contracts, and otherwise make legally binding decisions about their lives. The concept of generic competence reflects a societal determination to include or exclude certain persons from full participation and therefore does not reflect a focused assessment of the abilities or disabilities of an individual.

The concept of competence, however, raises the possibility of **incompetence** (ie, the judgment that a lack of certain abilities limits a person's legal rights). Incompetence can only be decided by a court of law.

Before the 1990s, a person could be deemed incompetent by virtue of belonging to a particular category (eg, the elderly, the mentally ill, the physically addicted). However, most states have since revised the statutes that determine incompetency and now require a functional assessment of the person's abilities and disabilities.**3** This focused review becomes the basis from which a court crafts orders tailored to meet the person's functional deficits and demonstrated needs.

All adult patients who are not mentally retarded or who have not been declared incompetent by a court have the same legal rights. Elderly patients, however, are at greater risk of having their legal rights

---

1 see page 137   **2** see page 134   **3** see page 40

abrogated because they are more likely to be isolated, poor, demented or confused, or institutionalized. They may be less able to advocate for their beliefs and desires and tend to have a smaller support network. Health care practitioners, therefore, need to identify and support the rights and interests of elderly patients and guard against their being accidentally or deliberately disempowered.

When the court declares a person incompetent or functionally unable to act in certain areas, it appoints a **guardian,** who is responsible for making some legally binding decisions for the incompetent person, or **ward.** The areas in which the court has found functional incompetence define the powers given to the guardian. The elderly may be in jeopardy of inappropriate attempts to appoint a guardian because a few states still stipulate that old age itself is an acceptable ground for instituting such actions and for a legal finding of diminished ability.

INFORMED CONSENT

A decisionally capable patient's legally binding treatment decision reached voluntarily and based on information about risks, benefits, and alternative treatments gained from discussion with a health care practitioner.

Several legal principles form the basis for informed consent. The right of knowledgeable self-determination and choice obligates the health care practitioner to inform patients of the risks and benefits of alternative treatments. The constitutional **right to privacy,** as well as the concept of personal liberty and restraints on state interference with independent action and choice, allows capacitated persons to choose individually appropriate medical care from among available treatment options.

Self-determination (the concept that "every adult of sound mind has the right to decide what shall be done with his own body"), or autonomy, is the foundation of the legal and ethical doctrine of **informed consent.** When decision making is preceded by discussion with a health care practitioner who provides the patient with the information necessary for choosing among options, the patient's consent or refusal is said to be informed and is ethically valid and legally binding. All states require that informed consent of the capacitated patient precede medical intervention. The patient has the legal and ethical right to make an informed choice, ie, to consent to or refuse care, even if the likely outcome of the refusal is death. The physician is legally and ethically obligated to promote this right to all patients, even to those who are unsophisticated or difficult to inform.

Informed consent arises from discussion between the patient and physician. The patient asks questions that elicit relevant information, and the physician shares facts and insights along with support and advice. Treatment decisions belong to the patient or surrogate, but the physician has a responsibility to offer guidance.

The process of informed consent may be more arduous for elderly patients than for younger patients because of age-related conditions, such as sensory deficits or impaired cognition. For example, many elderly patients who cannot understand or evaluate alternatives are treated as if they can because they nod in agreement or do not actively question a proposed intervention. Such consent is rarely valid but is rarely questioned. Conversely, patients with hearing deficits are difficult to reach in conversations and thus are sometimes bypassed in the decision-making process. In addition, patients may be overly influenced by family members, by the process of "learned helplessness" during institutionalization (a special problem in long-term care facilities), or by the physician.

One way to augment the patient's voice is to allow sufficient time for discussion of preferences. Another is to talk with the patient alone, although many elderly patients, out of dependence or suspicion, request that a family member be present. If the patient exercises autonomy by delegating decisional authority, then that decision should be respected. For example, if the patient says in response to questions, "Do whatever my daughter wants," then the physician should consult the daughter. Even so, the physician should periodically attempt to inform the patient and include him in discussions.

The right of informed consent carries the implicit right of **informed refusal**. A decision to refuse treatment—even if seemingly senseless—does not mean that the patient is incompetent or insane. The most common reasons for a patient's refusal of care are misunderstanding and miscommunication between the physician and patient. The first sign of reluctance, therefore, should not be taken as a final refusal of care; rather, an initial refusal that seems contrary to the patient's best interest is reason to continue rather than conclude the discussion. Physicians are ethically bound to encourage acceptance of the therapeutic recommendation judged to be in the patient's best interest, and most patients' refusals are reversed with attention, extended discussion, and even some cajoling. Advocacy, however, even in the patient's best interest, must stop short of coercion, duplicity, or deceit. Almost never does a court order intervention over a capable patient's clear and consistent refusal.

A patient's refusal of treatment does not constitute attempted suicide, nor does a physician's compliance with a capacitated patient's decision to refuse or reject life-sustaining treatment constitute physician-assisted suicide.◘ Rather, the subsequent death is considered to

◘ see page 139

result from the underlying disease process rather than from an affirmative action causing death. The patient's right to choose almost always supersedes the physician's responsibility to provide customary and indicated medical care. Intractable conflicts between physicians and patients about appropriate treatment are relatively rare and should be approached first as events to be negotiated or mediated.∎ If these actions fail, the physician may need to help the patient find a new physician and then withdraw from the case. A new physician with a different philosophy, personal ethic, and temperament may be able to relate more easily to the patient.

In some states, an exception to the informed consent process, called **therapeutic privilege,** allows a physician to withhold information when, in the physician's judgment, the patient would suffer *direct and immediate harm as a result of the disclosure.* This doctrine is rarely used, however; mere upset or even anguish over grim news does not qualify. When the doctrine is used, the physician should frequently reevaluate the patient's state of mind to ensure that disclosure is made as soon as the danger of serious adverse effects has abated sufficiently.

CONFIDENTIALITY AND DISCLOSURE

Ethical oaths and specific statutes protect the **confidentiality** of physician-patient communication, an ethical and legal bedrock of the therapeutic relationship. Even well-meaning family involvement without the patient's consent violates the patient's right of confidentiality. Protection of private patient information is essential to encouraging patient candor in revealing symptoms and behaviors relevant to diagnosis and treatment. Protection of a patient's secrets, private thoughts, and feelings is also required by decency.

Patient utterances are also protected by the **doctrine of privilege,** which grants patients the right to exclude otherwise relevant and admissible testimony in a court of law. This privilege can be invoked only by the patient. Additionally, most states have professional licensing statutes that incorporate the ethical and legal confidentiality mandates and make them a clear part of professional practice. All patients are entitled to confidentiality unless they give permission for **disclosure** or they clearly can no longer express a preference (eg, a severely confused, comatose, or decisionally incapacitated patient). Even in these cases, secrets should be guarded, although decisions about care may require discussion with appropriate surrogates. When a patient can no longer make health care decisions, prior expressed preferences should be respected whenever possible.

∎ see page 137

ADVANCE DIRECTIVES

Legal statements that allow persons to articulate values and establish treatment preferences to be honored in the future when capacity has lapsed.

All states have laws permitting and governing advance directives, but there is variability in some of the details, and some states have special rules for certain interventions. New York, for example, requires that the patient specifically address the issue of artificially administered food and fluid if the surrogate is to be able to refuse this care.

The Patient Self-Determination Act of 1990 requires that all patients entering federally funded hospitals, nursing homes, or home health care agencies be afforded the opportunity to execute an advance directive if none exists. In most states, the legal requirements are so simple that an attorney's services are unnecessary. Ideally, the directives should be in writing and signed by the patient. Out-of-hospital advance directive forms are available in many communities. The two types of advance directives are living wills and health care proxy appointments, also called a durable power of attorney for health care decision making.

LIVING WILLS

A living will lists the interventions the patient would request, accept, or reject in the future, usually at the end of life. Physicians often have difficulty accepting a patient's choice to abandon aggressive care and permit death.

Most patients use living wills to refuse life-sustaining care when the prognosis for improvement or recovery is hopeless and the ability to relate to others is severely diminished or destroyed. However, as managed care becomes more pervasive and as patients become concerned about being denied care, living wills that request care are becoming more common.

The living will specifies a set of circumstances followed by a set of consequences (eg, "If I am hopelessly ill and my physicians say that I will not recover, then..." or "If I am not able to recognize and relate to family and friends and my physicians say that I will not recover, then..."). The consequences specify the interventions the patient would or would not want (eg, intubation, resuscitation, dialysis, surgery, antibiotic therapy). The document usually states that, despite these specific refusals, all measures necessary for comfort should be provided. The goal of the most usual type of living will—prospective refusal—is to ensure that invasive, aggressive, and life-sustaining treatments will not be used if they would merely prolong the dying process or support a vegetative state. Some living wills limit their applicability to terminal illness; thus a patient desiring to refuse care if in a vegetative state or deep coma should not use this restricted type of living will.

DURABLE POWER OF ATTORNEY FOR HEALTH CARE

A durable power of attorney for health care differs from a regular power of attorney, which addresses decision making concerning financial matters or property rights (eg, the right to sell a car or manage stocks).

A durable power of attorney for health care, or health care proxy, is a legal document that allows the patient to appoint a person, called a health care agent or proxy, to make health care decisions should the patient become temporarily or permanently incapacitated or be declared legally incompetent. This legal appointment places a loving, concerned, trusted person in a dialogue with the physician to reach an appropriate decision. The agent's decisions are guided by specific instructions from the patient, by notions of substituted judgment (what the patient would likely want under the circumstances), and by the concept of best interest.◻ The agent can discuss the patient's diagnosis, prognosis, treatment alternatives, and likely outcomes with the physician, respond to the patient's changing condition, and base a decision on current circumstances in light of known patient preferences and values.

Prior discussions between patient and agent provide the agent with a richer understanding of the patient's values and preferences, allowing more nuanced decisions to be made later. This opportunity for dialogue generally results in a better decision than could have been reached by following the static directives in a living will.

SURROGATE DECISION MAKING

A surrogate is a statutorily designated health care decider or an informally identified person, such as a close family member or friend. The more informal the appointment, the less likely the surrogate will be able to refuse life-sustaining treatment, especially in states with very restrictive laws. If the patient is incapacitated and no advance directive exists, some other person or persons must provide the direction (either a loved one or the medical staff).

Most hospitals and physicians accept consent to provide care from a spouse, an adult child, a close friend, a clergy member, or even a distant and uninvolved relative, although in most states, none of these persons is legally empowered to consent on a patient's behalf without being appointed by a court. However, accepting the judgment of a

◻ see page 137

close relative or friend over that of a distant relative or total stranger makes practical and ethical sense. Thus, a decision agreed on by hospital, physician, and family almost always constitutes the basis for providing care, although it may not be legally adequate if challenged.

Elderly patients without family or close friends may receive a **court-appointed guardian,** who is often disinterested and serves a perfunctory role. Some institutions and jurisdictions are experimenting with the appointment of public guardians and patient advocates, which may prove appropriate and cost-effective.

When surrogates attempt to refuse treatment by deciding to withhold or withdraw interventions (an often articulated distinction without any substantial legal or ethical difference), legal concerns increase because of the possibility of death. The initial questions in these circumstances are (1) Who decides? (2) On what basis is the decision made? and (3) What possibilities exist for appeal and review? Answers vary widely among the states. In New Jersey hospitals, for example, if an ethics or prognosis committee determines that the prognosis is hopeless (and, in the case of elderly residents in long-term care, the state Office of the Ombudsman determines that the decision does not constitute abuse), a specially appointed guardian may opt to withhold treatment. Conversely, in New York, surrogates who have not been appointed by the patient have very limited ability to withhold care unless the patient has addressed a similar circumstance when capacitated and has left explicit instructions to be followed. The problem is that these practices assume that continued existence is the desired state. Under certain circumstances, however, permitting death is not incompatible with a patient's best interest nor with the state's usual interest in preserving life.

Unless there is a durable power of attorney for health care, the choice of a surrogate may be unclear. Once identified, the surrogate bases a decision on one of three standards, in the following hierarchy:

- Explicit directive, ie, the instructions expressed by the patient when capacitated
- Substituted judgment, ie, inferences about what the patient would likely want in this situation based on what is known about his prior behavior and decision making
- Best interest, ie, what the surrogate and health care team believe is best for the patient

Explicit directive, the first standard, is usually determined by a written document (eg, a living will) but can also be fulfilled by discussions with the patient as reported by the surrogate or others, particularly by close family members. Statements to health care practitioners, especially when documented in the medical chart, can also be important in determining the patient's preferences.

Substituted judgment, used when no explicit directives exist, poses various questions to try to discern what the patient would have wanted. What sort of person was this patient when capacitated? What was his lifestyle and pattern of decision making? What did he find rewarding or unacceptable? How did he evaluate the quality of life and define a meaningful existence? How did he feel about diminished capacity, dependence, and confinement?

Finally, **best interest** is resorted to when the patient's history, wishes, and values are unknown. This judgment is informed by the clinical evaluations of the health care team about prognosis and the likely outcome of treatment, some notion of what a reasonable person in the patient's situation would want, and an evaluation of the benefits and burdens of care in maximizing the patient's comfort and function. Especially when making decisions based on substituted judgment and best interest, the surrogate must not confuse the patient's perspective of quality of life with some arbitrary judgment about the value of the patient's life to others.

In making life-or-death decisions for the incapacitated patient, the proxy or surrogate may feel unsupported or even abandoned by the physician or by family members. Making decisions for another, especially life or death ones, can be anguishing. Ideally, the physician's responsibility of informing and supporting the patient would be transferred to the surrogate. However, the physician-surrogate relationship is sometimes strained, due in part to the physician's notion that family members cause trouble after the patient has died, the complexity and fragmentation of care, and the physician's discomfort with decisions that refuse care and permit death. Even when one member of a family is chosen by the patient to be the legally appointed proxy, the family dynamic has an independent existence. If a parent has appointed one child, that person must still relate to the others in the family and circle of friends. Family dynamics among siblings and between generations may be played out in the context of old grievances and present fears and may require support to resolve conflicts.

Tensions and disagreements between and among physicians, nursing staff, surrogate, and family members may be managed and resolved through **mediation** leading to consensus. The mediator, a bioethics consultant or ethics committee member, informs the surrogate and family of their options, empowers the surrogate to question the health care team's judgment, and ensures that all parties are heard. Once a consensus on the best plan of care is reached, especially if that consensus leads to withdrawing or withholding care, the mediator ensures that everyone is as comfortable as possible with the plan and that the plan is carried out according to the agreement. Finally, the mediator follows up to ensure that the family is comfortable with the outcome and that health care practitioners can use this experience in future cases.

In mediation of bioethical disputes, the process is as important as the ultimate decision. The way in which issues are explored and the fact that the health care team and family members reach a consensus are enormously helpful to everyone involved. As conflict is resolved, the surrogate feels more comfortable with his decision.

DO-NOT-RESUSCITATE ORDERS

A statement in the medical record that cardiopulmonary resuscitation will not be performed.

The do-not-resuscitate (DNR) order, which averts CPR in cases of cardiopulmonary arrest, has been particularly useful in preventing unnecessary and unwanted invasive intervention at the end of life. Currently, resuscitation is attempted except in cases in which it would not be effective or that are not in accordance with the desires or best interests of the patient. This default position evolved slowly over recent decades. There is a question of whether the decision to issue the order not to resuscitate belongs to the physician or patient. The New York statute, for example, permits the patient or surrogate to choose resuscitation even if health care practitioners believe it will result in extremely poor subsequent quality of life. Conversely, interpretation by the New York State Department of Health provides for physicians to write a DNR order over patient or family objections in the rare cases of "DNR futility," referring to the very specific circumstances in which resuscitation would be physiologically ineffective. However, even if the physician claims futility as a basis for overriding the patient's or surrogate's decision, the issue must be raised first with the patient or his guardian. In most other jurisdictions, the policies and procedures related to DNR orders are somewhat less demanding. Most hospitals, nursing homes, and home health care agencies have policies for situations in which the likely benefit of CPR is so slim and the burden on the patient so great that a DNR order is appropriate. Most institutions require that resuscitation be discussed with the patient or family, although not that it be raised as a question open for their decision.

Physicians should discuss the possibility of cardiopulmonary arrest with patients, describe CPR procedures, and elicit patients' preferences about interventions. Ideally, discussion takes place in an outpatient setting or early in hospitalization as part of a discussion of general treatment preferences. Under these circumstances, patients are more likely to be mentally alert and relaxed, which helps ensure understanding and thoughtful participation in the decision-making process. Subsequent periodic discussions can determine if the patient has changed his mind due to changes in his condition or in treatment alternatives.

If a patient is incapable of making a decision about CPR, the surrogate may make the decision based on the patient's previously expressed preferences or, if such preferences are unknown, in accordance with the patient's best interests.

No matter who decides, some system should exist for communicating, recording, and reviewing the decision. There is no widely recognized case in which a physician or institution was found liable for respecting a DNR order that was authorized after being discussed with the patient and family and being recorded in the patient's medical record.

It is essential to clarify that DNR does not mean do not treat. Only CPR will not be performed. Other treatments (eg, antibiotics, transfusions, dialysis, ventilatory support) may and should still be provided if indicated. More specific orders are required to indicate whether the person should be hospitalized, treated in an intensive care unit, or subjected to other interventions.

Many hospitals and long-term care facilities have policies to guide decisions about resuscitation. These policies vary widely; some reserve the decision for the physician, whereas others allow patients or designated surrogates to decide. Hospital medical staffs should periodically review their experience with DNR orders, revise their DNR policies as appropriate, and inform physicians about their role in the decision-making process.

WITHHOLDING OF FOOD AND FLUID

All U.S. courts that have considered the issue have held that the artificial administration of food and fluid is a medical treatment subject to the same strictures that guide other medical decisions. However, some states differentiate this intervention from others. Certain religions also regard artificial administration of food and fluid differently from other medical interventions and have special rules governing whether the surrogate can refuse its initiation or continuation.

EUTHANASIA, ASSISTED SUICIDE, AND PALLIATION

Euthanasia, an action taken by a health care practitioner intended to result in a patient's death, is illegal in the USA. Some patients whose life expectancy is reduced and who are suffering severely request euthanasia. Traditionally, euthanasia has been forbidden in medical practice, and purposeful intervention to end life disturbs most physicians and patients. However, in certain clinical situations involving hopelessness and suffering, death is the end of pain, not of meaningful life.

Assisted suicide, an action taken by a patient intended to cause his own death with drugs supplied by a physician, is illegal in all states except Oregon. Physicians can provide treatment intended to minimize physical and emotional suffering, even if a secondary result is the shortening of life, but they cannot specifically intend to hasten death. The issue of **palliation,** or pain relief, is inextricable from that of assisted suicide for two reasons: (1) many dying patients have unrelieved pain or other intolerable symptoms, and (2) most patients requesting assisted suicide do not want to die; they just want the suffering to stop. The U.S. Supreme Court has emphasized the relevance and importance of the **doctrine of double effect,** which states that an intervention intended to relieve pain but that incidentally hastens death is still appropriate. If the physician's goal is to relieve suffering, then the action is protected.

DISCHARGE AND PLACEMENT

Physicians and family members routinely make decisions about discharge and placement without adequately consulting the patient and often over the patient's objections. Just as capacitated patients have the right to consent to or refuse treatment, they also have the right to choose their living arrangements and outpatient care. This right, however, is not as tied to the singular interests of the patient as are the rights of informed consent and refusal of treatment. The legal, financial, practical, and quality-of-life interests of family and neighbors as well as of the patient may be affected and even compromised by the patient's return home.

Despite the family members' best efforts, they may be unable to meet the safety or health care needs of the elderly person. Whereas the patient's decision to consent to or refuse care is determined by patient autonomy, the decision to accept or refuse care is governed by the notion of accommodation, ie, the rights and interests of others may be directly affected by the patient's discharge choice. For example, a patient wishing to live with his daughter may not be able to do so if the daughter has other demands on her time and energy.

Even if residing with family or residing alone poses a greater risk than living in a long-term care facility, the patient has the right to choose either. Decisionally capacitated patients can assume the risks of discharge options. Many elderly persons choose to return home even when health care practitioners believe that residential treatment is medically and socially preferable. Some patients even choose to return home when the possible result is death. If the patient is decisionally capacitated and appreciates and accepts the consequences, this choice can be legally and ethically supportable. A decisionally capacitated patient cannot be placed in a residential facility over his objection without a court order. Overriding a patient's discharge preferences may require petitioning the court for a general or a limited guardianship. **1**

LONG-TERM CARE

During the 1980s and 1990s, long-term care facilities came under legal scrutiny, spurred primarily by exposés of neglectful and abusive care of elderly, vulnerable, and often demented institutionalized patients. The nature and degree of the abuse offended legal, moral, and civic sensibilities, resulting in a framework of federal and state regulations governing many aspects of institutional practice, such as staffing patterns and record-keeping procedures.

Long-term care facilities are now being challenged about policies that automatically hospitalize residents at the end of life or that impose life-sustaining treatment with no provision for evaluating, preventing, or terminating such treatment. Many facilities are afraid to adopt policies that would allow residents to die in the nursing home because they fear accusations of neglect and abuse, despite assurances by state regulators that they look for evidence of thoughtful decision making responsive to the needs of individual residents. The legal and ethical climate suggests that resident-staff-family discussions about future and, especially, end-of-life care should begin soon after admission to a nursing home and not at a time of crisis. In response to the Patient Self-Determination Act of 1990 and because of concerns about legally supportable care decisions, many facilities are discussing future care, including CPR, with their newly admitted patients. Decisions should be reevaluated periodically based on changes in the resident's physical condition and the goals of care for the resident.

Federal and state laws and regulations also govern long-term care financing. **2** Most elderly patients and their families do not understand the complex rules that require poverty-level status before Medicaid will assume the cost of long-term care. In most states, legal advocates can protect a spouse living in the community from impoverishment by appealing to state regulations that permit the segregation of shared funds for the benefit of the community-dwelling spouse. If such an arrangement is not possible, an attorney can file a suit for support in family court or in another appropriate state forum. Every state has a long-term care ombudsman whose office is funded by Medicare. These offices can provide information about some of the rights and protections available to residents of long-term care facilities.

1 see page 131   **2** see also page 164

Social issues influence an elderly person's risk and experience of illness as well as a health care practitioner's ability to deliver timely and appropriate care. A social history[1] helps members of the interdisciplinary team evaluate care needs and social supports. Questions should be asked about marital or companion status, living arrangements, financial status, work history, education, and caregiving responsibilities. Because health interventions may interfere with caregiving responsibilities, patients with caregiving roles may be reluctant to report their own symptoms. Similarly, availability of caregivers influences care planning. Questions about typical daily activities can provide useful information, including how meals are prepared, what activities add meaning to life, and where problems may be occurring.

FAMILY CAREGIVING

Family caregivers play a key role in delaying and possibly preventing institutionalization of chronically ill elderly persons. Although neighbors and friends may help, about 80% of home health care services (physical, emotional, social, and economic) are provided by family caregivers. When the patient is mildly or moderately impaired, a spouse or adult children often provide care, but when the patient is severely disabled, a spouse (usually a wife) is more likely to be the caregiver. Family caregivers may experience considerable stress and subsequent health problems. In addition, couples in which one partner cares for the other tend to be disproportionately poor.

The amount and type of care provided by a family depend on economic resources, family structure, quality of relationships, and other demands on the family members' time and energy. Family caregiving ranges from minimal assistance (eg, periodically checking in) to elaborate full-time care. On average, family caregiving consumes about 4 hours a day.

Although society tends to view family members as having a responsibility to care for one another, the limits of filial and spousal obligations vary among families and among individual family members. The willingness of family members to provide care may be bolstered by supportive services (eg, technical assistance in learning new skills, counseling services, family mental health services) and supplemental services (eg, personal care [assistance with grooming, feeding, dressing], home health care, adult day care, meals programs). Supplemental services may be provided on a regular schedule or as respite care for a few hours or days.[2]

---

[1] see also page 30   [2] see page 92

Changes in demographics and social values have reduced the number of family members available to care for impaired elderly relatives. Because life span has increased, the population of the very old is increasing; their children, who are potential caregivers, are likely to be old also. Moreover, delayed procreation combined with increased longevity have created a sandwich generation of caregivers who care simultaneously for their children or spouse and their parents. The increasing mobility of U.S. society and the increased divorce rate have contributed to the geographic separation of families and have weakened family ties. Nonetheless, 80% of persons ≥ 65 years live within 20 minutes of one child. There has been a steady growth in single-parent households, most headed by women, and in two-income households. Consequently, increasing numbers of women, who previously may have functioned as caregivers for elderly parents, have entered the workforce. The demands of a job may diminish or eliminate a person's ability to provide informal geriatric care. These factors, combined with the increasing number of dependent and sicker elderly, predict an increasing demand for home health care services provided by someone other than family, friends, and neighbors.

LIVING ALONE

In the USA, about one third of the nearly 30 million community-dwelling elderly live alone; four fifths of those living alone are women. Of the oldest old (≥ 85 years), one half of those living in the community live alone.◘ Men are more likely to die before their wives, and widowed or divorced men are more likely to remarry than are widowed or divorced women.

The elderly who live alone are more likely to be poor, especially with advancing age. Many report feelings of loneliness (60% of those > 75) and social isolation. In those with health problems or sensory deficits, new or worsening symptoms may go unnoticed. Many have problems complying with prescribed treatment regimens. Because of physical limitations and because eating is a social activity, some elderly persons who live alone do not prepare full, balanced meals, making malnutrition a concern.

Despite these problems, almost 90% of those living alone express a keen desire to maintain their independence. Many fear being too dependent on others and, despite the loneliness, want to continue to live alone. To help them maintain their independence, physicians should encourage them and social workers should help them to engage in regular physical activity and social interactions.

Coordination and delivery of services during convalescence are difficult for those living alone. Physicians should ensure that home care is

◘ see also page 10

available and recommend additional services as appropriate. A passive or individually activated emergency response device may reassure a patient that help can be obtained if needed.

ALTERNATIVE LIVING ARRANGEMENTS

Aside from living with a spouse, with an adult child, or alone, other living arrangements and relationships are fairly common among the elderly and may raise considerations in care planning. About 5% of persons $\geq$ 65 years never married. A substantial proportion of those who never married, are divorced, or are widowed may have long-standing and close relationships with siblings, friends, and partners. Understanding the nature of these relationships assists the health care practitioner in planning care that is in keeping with the patient's wishes.

It is estimated that between 6 and 10% of the U.S. population are homosexual adults, including as many as 3 million elderly persons. Elderly persons in homosexual relationships face special challenges. The health care system in which they operate may not be aware of their sexual preference, may not recognize their partner as having a role in caregiving decisions, and may not provide services that are appropriate for their circumstances. For example, a partner may not have legal standing in decision making for a cognitively impaired patient, may not be able to share a room in a nursing home or other congregate living setting, and may not be recognized as being part of the patient's family. Health care practitioners are well advised to ask questions about partners and living arrangements and to try to accommodate patient preferences.

EFFECTS OF LIFE TRANSITIONS

Late life is commonly a period of transitions (eg, retirement, relocation) and adjustment to losses.

Retirement is often the first major transition faced by the elderly. Its effects on physical and mental health differ from person to person, depending on attitude toward and reason for retiring. About one third of retirees have difficulty adjusting to certain aspects of retirement, such as reduced income and altered social role and entitlements. Some persons choose to retire, having looked forward to quitting unpleasant work; others are forced to retire, eg, because of health problems or job loss. Appropriate preparation for retirement and counseling for families and retirees who experience difficulties may help.

Relocation may occur several times in old age, eg, to smaller quarters after selling the family home, to retirement housing to reduce the burden of upkeep, and to a nursing home. Some experts contend that such moves cause relocation trauma; however, recent studies find little or no evidence of increased mortality or other indications of trauma, especially among persons prepared for the move. Physical and mental status are significant predictors of relocation adjustment, as is thoughtful and adequate preparation. Persons who respond poorly to relocation are more likely to be living alone, socially isolated, poor, and depressed. Men respond more poorly than women. The stress of relocation correlates inversely with the degree of perceived control over the move and the predictability of the new environment. Patients should be acquainted with the new setting well in advance. For the cognitively impaired elderly person, a move away from familiar surroundings may exacerbate functional dependence and disruptive behavior.

Bereavement affects many aspects of an elderly person's life. For example, social interaction and companionship decrease and social status changes. The death of a spouse affects men and women differently. In the 2 years after the death of a wife, men tend to have increased mortality rates, especially if the wife's death was unexpected. For women who lose a husband, the data are less clear but generally do not indicate increased mortality rates.

Health care practitioners should look for symptoms of stress and depression after a patient has been bereaved. Hasty treatment with antidepressant drugs should be avoided, because these drugs may interfere with the process of grieving and adjustment; however, caregivers and health care practitioners should be aware of the high risk to the bereaved patient of suicide and potential for declining health status. Counseling and supportive services, such as support groups for widows, may facilitate difficult transitions. Prolonged, pathologic grief usually requires psychiatric evaluation and treatment.

RELIGION AND SPIRITUALITY

Religion and spirituality are similar but not identical concepts. Religion is often viewed as more institutionally based, more structured, and more traditional. Spirituality involves feelings, thoughts, experiences, and behaviors that arise from a search for the sacred (a Divine Being, Ultimate Reality, or Ultimate Truth).

Religion involves accountability and responsibility, whereas spirituality has fewer requirements. Persons may reject traditional religion but consider themselves spiritual. In the USA, > 90% of elderly persons consider themselves religious and spiritual; about 5% consider themselves spiritual but not religious. Most research assesses religion, not spirituality, using measures such as attendance at religious services, frequency of private religious practices, use of religious coping mechanisms (eg, praying, trusting in God, turning problems over to God, receiving support from clergy persons), and intrinsic religiosity (internalized religious commitment).

For most elderly persons in the USA, religion plays a major role in their lives: 96% of persons ≥ 65 years believe in God or a universal spirit, > 90% pray, and > 50% attend religious services weekly or more often. This level of religious participation is greater than that in any other age group. For the elderly, the religious community is the largest source of social support outside of the family, and involvement in religious organizations is the most common type of voluntary social activity—more common than all other forms of voluntary social activity combined.

Benefits

A positive and hopeful attitude about life and illness improves health outcomes and mortality rates. Although organized religions generally emphasize a positive attitude, a positive attitude is not the only factor that accounts for the health benefits of religion. The social aspects of the religious community are also involved, as are the meaning and purpose of life that religious beliefs convey and the effect of those beliefs on health behaviors and on the decisions persons make concerning relationships with friends, family members, and colleagues. Evidence indicates that religion is generally associated with better mental health and a greater ability to cope with illness and disability among the elderly and their caregivers. For example, persons who use religious coping mechanisms are less likely to develop depression and anxiety than those who do not; this inverse association is strongest among persons with greater physical disability. Even the perception of disability appears to be altered by the degree of religiousness. Of elderly women with hip fractures, the most religious had the lowest rates of depression (and were able to walk significantly further when discharged from the hospital than those who were less religious). Religious persons also tend to recover from depression more quickly. In a study of caregivers of patients with Alzheimer's disease or terminal cancer, those with a strong personal religious faith and many social contacts were better able to cope with the stresses of caregiving during a 2-year period.

Many elderly persons report that religion is the most important factor in enabling them to cope with physical health problems and life stresses (eg, declining financial resources, loss of a spouse or partner). In one study, > 90% of elderly patients relied on religion, at least to a moderate degree, when coping with health problems and difficult social circumstances.

Religion that improves mental health may improve physical health, because depression and anxiety may aggravate coronary artery disease, hypertension, stroke, and psychosomatic disorders. Furthermore, having a hopeful, positive attitude about the future helps persons who have physical problems and disabilities remain motivated to recover.

Active involvement in a religious community appears to help elderly persons maintain their physical functioning and health status. Levels of interleukin-6 are significantly lower among persons who attend religious services regularly than among those who do not. Elderly persons who attend religious services are more likely to stop smoking, exercise more, increase social contacts, stay married, and live longer. In one study, the mortality rate of patients with low levels of comfort from religion and of social support was 14 times that of those with higher levels of both.

Some religious groups (eg, Mormons, Seventh-Day Adventists) advocate avoidance of tobacco and heavy alcohol use, which is linked to the development of coronary artery disease, chronic obstructive pulmonary disease, lung cancer, disorders of the liver and pancreas, and, to some extent, multiple other disorders. Members of these groups are less likely to develop these disorders, and they live longer than the general population.

Religious beliefs and practices often foster the development of community and broad social support networks. Increased social contact for the elderly increases the likelihood that disease will be detected early and that elderly persons will comply with treatment regimens, because members of their community interact with them, asking them questions about their health and medical care. As a result, the elderly with such community networks are less likely to neglect themselves.

Disadvantages

Religion is not always beneficial to the elderly. Devout religiousness may promote excessive guilt, narrow-mindedness, inflexibility, and anxiety. Religious preoccupations and delusions may develop among patients with obsessive-compulsive disorder, bipolar disorder, schizophrenia, or psychoses. Certain religious groups discourage necessary mental and physical health care, such as immunization of children, prenatal care, and lifesaving therapies (eg, blood transfusions, treatment of life-threatening infections, taking insulin). Instead, they substitute religious rituals (eg, praying, chanting, lighting candles). Religious cults may isolate and alienate elderly persons from family members and the broader social community and, in some cases, may encourage self-destruction.

ROLE OF THE HEALTH CARE PRACTITIONER

The religious beliefs and practices of the elderly are relevant to geriatric health care practitioners because of the potential effect on their patients' mental and physical health. Most health care practitioners believe that inquiring about religious issues during a medical visit is appropriate under certain circumstances, including

- When a patient is severely ill, under significant stress, or near death and there is a specific request or an implied request to the physician to address religious issues

- When a patient tells the physician that he is religious and that religion helps him cope with illness
- When religious needs are evident and may be affecting a patient's health or health behaviors

The elderly often have distinct spiritual needs that may overlap but are not the same as psychologic needs. Ascertaining a patient's spiritual needs can lead to mobilization of the necessary resources.

Spiritual history: Taking a spiritual history shows elderly patients that the health care practitioner is willing to discuss spiritual topics. Patients may be asked if their faith is an important part of their life, how their faith influences the way they take care of themselves, if they are a part of a religious or spiritual community, and how they would like the health care practitioner to address their spiritual needs.

Alternatively, patients may be asked to describe their most important coping mechanism. If the response is not a religious one, patients may be asked whether religious or spiritual resources are of any help. If the response is no, they may be sensitively asked about barriers to those activities (eg, transportation problems, hearing difficulties, lack of financial resources, depression, lack of motivation, unresolved conflicts). However, forcing religious beliefs or opinions on patients or intruding if patients do not want help may be counterproductive.

Referral to clergy: Many clergy members provide counseling services to the elderly at home and in the hospital, often free of charge. Many elderly persons prefer counseling from a clergy member rather than from a mental health care practitioner, because they are more satisfied with the results and because they believe such counseling does not have the stigma that seeing a mental health care practitioner does. However, many clergy members do not have extensive training in mental health counseling and may not recognize when elderly persons need professional mental health care. In contrast, hospital clergy are more likely to have extensive training in the mental, social, and spiritual needs of the elderly. Thus, including hospital clergy as part of the health care team is helpful. They can often bridge the gap between hospital care and care in the community by communicating with clergy in the community. For example, when a patient is discharged from the hospital, the hospital clergy may call the patient's clergy, so that support teams in the patient's religious community can be mobilized to help during the patient's convalescence (eg, by providing housekeeping services, meals, or transportation or by visiting the patient or caregiver).

Support of patients' religious beliefs and practices: Because most religious beliefs and practices, particularly those rooted in major religious traditions, are not harmful to health and probably are beneficial, health care practitioners should support the patient's religious beliefs as long as they do not interfere with necessary medical care.

Spiritual interventions: Interventions include praying with patients, reading religious scriptures to them, and determining whether patients have the religious materials they need (eg, large-print scriptures, religious audiotapes).

Recommendation of religious activities: Health care practitioners may recommend religious activities that can increase socialization, reduce alienation and isolation, and increase a sense of belonging, of meaning, and of life purpose. These activities may also help the elderly to focus on positive activities rather than on their own problems. However, some activities are appropriate only for more religious patients. Suggesting religious activities to patients who are not already involved in them, if done, requires sensitivity. Patients seek medical care for health-related reasons, not religious ones.

Patient and family information: Health care practitioners can provide information about the health benefits of religious beliefs and practices for the elderly and about local religious resources (eg, support groups at local churches, health promotion programs, volunteer activity programs).

ELDER ABUSE

Physical or psychologic mistreatment, neglect, or financial exploitation of the elderly.

Several types of abuse are common—physical abuse, psychologic abuse, neglect, and financial abuse. Each type may be intentional or unintentional. The perpetrators are usually spouses or adult children but may be other family members or paid or informal caregivers.

Physical abuse is the use of force that results in physical or psychologic injury. It includes striking, shoving, shaking, beating, restraining, and improper feeding. It may include sexual assault (any form of sexual intimacy without consent or by force or threat of force).

Psychologic abuse is the use of words, acts, or other means that cause emotional stress or anguish. It includes issuing threats (eg, of institutionalization), insults, and harsh commands; remaining silent; and ignoring the person. It also includes infantilization (a patronizing form of ageism in which the abuser treats the victim as a child), encouraging the victim to become dependent on the abuser.

Neglect is failing to provide food, medicine, personal care, or other necessities.

Financial abuse is the exploitation of or inattention to a person's possessions or funds. It includes swindling, pressuring a person to distribute assets, and managing a person's money irresponsibly.

Epidemiology and Risk Factors

Although the true incidence is unclear, elder abuse appears to be a growing public health problem in the USA. In a large U.S. urban study of persons $\geq$ 65 years, 3.2% were victims of physical abuse, psychologic abuse, or neglect. Because certain forms of abuse (eg, financial exploitation) were not included, the actual incidence of mistreatment was probably higher. In more recent studies conducted in Canada and western Europe, the incidence of abuse was comparable to that in the USA.

For the victim, risk factors for abuse include impairment (chronic diseases, functional impairment, cognitive impairment) and social isolation. For the abuser, risk factors include substance abuse, psychiatric disorder, history of violence, stress, and dependence on the victim (including shared living arrangements—see TABLE 15–1).

Diagnosis

Abuse is difficult to detect because many of the signs are subtle and the victim is often unwilling or unable to discuss the abuse. Victims may hide abuse because of shame, fear of retaliation, or a desire to protect the abuser. Sometimes, when abuse victims seek help, they encounter ageist responses from health care practitioners, who may, for example, dismiss complaints of abuse as confusion, paranoia, or dementia.

Social isolation of the elderly victim often makes detection difficult. Abuse tends to increase the isolation, because the abuser often limits the victim's access to the outside world (eg, denies visitors, refuses telephone calls).

Symptoms and signs of abuse may erroneously be attributed to chronic disease (eg, a hip fracture attributed to osteoporosis). However, certain clinical situations are particularly suggestive of abuse (see TABLE 15–2).

History: If abuse is suspected, the patient should be interviewed alone, at least for part of the time. Other involved persons may also be interviewed separately. The patient interview may start with general questions about feelings of safety but should also include direct questions about possible mistreatment (eg, physical violence, restraints, neglect). If abuse is confirmed, the nature, frequency, and severity of events should be elicited. Abuse usually becomes more frequent and severe over time. The circumstances precipitating the abuse should also be sought (eg, alcohol intoxication).

Social and financial resources of the patient should be assessed because they affect management decisions, eg, living arrangements or the hiring of a professional caregiver. The examiner should inquire whether the patient has family members or friends able and willing to nurture, listen, and assist. If financial resources are adequate but basic needs are not being met, the examiner should determine why. Assessing these resources can also help identify risk factors for abuse (eg, financial stress, financial exploitation of the patient).

TABLE 15–1.   RISK FACTORS FOR ELDER ABUSE

Factor	Comments
Social isolation of victim	Abuse of isolated persons is less likely to be detected and stopped. Social isolation can intensify stress
Chronic disorder and/or functional impairment of victim	The elderly person's ability to escape, seek help, and defend himself is reduced
Cognitive impairment of victim	Persons with dementia may show aggression toward caregivers and act disruptively, precipitating abuse. The rate of abuse of persons with dementia is high
Substance abuse by abuser	Alcohol or drug abuse may lead to abusive behavior
Psychiatric disorder(s) of abuser	Psychiatric disorders (eg, schizophrenia, other psychoses) may lead to abusive behavior. Patients discharged from an inpatient psychiatric institution may return to their elderly parents' home for care. These patients, even if not violent in the institution, may become violent at home; appropriate follow-up can help prevent elder abuse
History of violence by abuser	A history of violence in a relationship (particularly between spouses) and outside the family may predict elder abuse. The transgenerational violence theory is based on this factor; violence is a learned response to difficult life experiences and a learned method of expressing anger and frustration. Because information about past family violence is difficult to obtain, this theory is unsubstantiated
Dependence of abuser on victim	Dependence on the victim for financial support, housing, emotional support, and other needs can contribute to abuse. A family member's (especially an adult child's) attempts to obtain resources from the elderly person can result in abuse. Dependence can produce resentment, which may lead to abuse
Stress affecting abuser	Stressful life events (eg, chronic financial problems, death in the family) and the responsibilities of caregiving increase the likelihood of abuse
Shared living arrangement of abuser and victim	Elderly persons living alone are much less likely to be abused. When living arrangements are shared, opportunities for the tension and conflict that generally precede abuse are greater

Adapted from Lachs MS, Pillemer K: "Current concepts: Abuse and neglect of elderly persons." *New England Journal of Medicine* 332:437–443, 1995.

TABLE 15-2.   CLINICAL SITUATIONS SUGGESTIVE OF ELDER ABUSE

- When there is a delay between the injury or illness and the seeking of medical attention
- When the accounts of the patient and caregiver do not agree
- When the severity of the injury does not fit the explanation given by the caregiver
- When the explanation of the patient or caregiver is implausible or vague
- When visits to the emergency department for chronic disease exacerbations are frequent despite an appropriate care plan and adequate resources
- When a functionally impaired patient presents to the physician without a designated caregiver in attendance
- When laboratory findings are inconsistent with the history
- When the caregiver is reluctant to accept home health care (eg, a visiting nurse) or to leave the elderly person alone with a health care practitioner

The interview with the family member should avoid confrontation. The interviewer should explore whether caregiving responsibilities are burdensome for the family member and acknowledge the caregiver's difficult role, if appropriate. Inquiries are made about recent stressful events (eg, bereavement, financial stresses), the patient's illness (eg, care needs, prognosis), and the reported cause of any recent injuries.

Physical examination: Signs that aid in the diagnosis of abuse are listed in TABLE 15-3. The patient should be thoroughly examined, ■ preferably at the first visit. The physician may need to seek help from a trusted family member or friend of the patient, state adult protective services, or, occasionally, law enforcement agencies to persuade the caregiver or patient to permit the evaluation. A referral to adult protective services is mandatory in most states.

Cognitive status should be assessed, eg, using the Mini-Mental State Examination. ■ Cognitive impairment is a risk factor for elder abuse and may affect the reliability of the history and the patient's ability to make management decisions. ■

Mood and emotional status should be assessed. If the patient feels depressed, ashamed, guilty, anxious, fearful, or angry, then the beliefs underlying the emotion should be explored. If the patient minimizes or rationalizes family tension or conflict, or is reluctant to discuss abuse, the examiner should determine whether these attitudes are interfering with recognition or admission of abuse.

■ see page 31   ■ see FIGURE 38-1 on page 346   ■ see page 357

TABLE 15–3. SIGNS OF ELDER ABUSE

Item	Sign
Behavior	Withdrawal by the patient, infantilization of patient by caregiver, or caregiver's insistence on providing the history
General appearance	Poor hygiene (unkempt appearance, uncleanliness), inappropriate dress
Skin/mucous membranes	Skin turgor, other signs of dehydration, multiple skin lesions in various stages of evolution, bruises, pressure sores, deficient care of established skin lesions
Head and neck	Traumatic alopecia (distinguished from male-pattern alopecia by distribution)
Trunk	Bruises, welts (shape may suggest implement—eg, iron or belt)
Genitourinary region	Rectal bleeding, vaginal bleeding, pressure sores, infestations
Extremities	Wrist or ankle lesions suggesting use of restraints or immersion burn (ie, in stocking/glove distribution)
Musculoskeletal system	Occult fracture, pain, gait disturbance
Mental and emotional health	Depressive symptoms, anxiety

Functional status, including the ability to perform activities of daily living (ADLs)∎, should be assessed and any physical limitations that impair self-protection noted. If help with ADLs is needed, the examiner should determine whether the current helper has sufficient emotional, financial, and intellectual ability for the task. Otherwise, a new helper needs to be identified.

Coexisting disorders that are being caused or exacerbated by the abuse should be looked for.

Laboratory tests: Imaging studies and other laboratory tests (eg, electrolytes to determine hydration, albumin to determine nutritional status, drug levels to document compliance with prescribed regimens) are performed as necessary, both for diagnosis and for documentation of the abuse.

Documentation: The medical record should contain a complete report of the actual or suspected abuse, preferably in the patient's own words. A detailed description of any injuries should be included, supported by photographs, drawings, x-rays, and other objective documentation (eg, laboratory test results indicating drug or electrolyte levels) where possible. Specific examples of how needs are not being met, despite an agreed-on care plan and adequate resources, should be documented.

∎ see page 42

Prevention and Prognosis

A physician or other health care practitioner may be the only person an abuse victim has contact with other than the abuser and should therefore be vigilant for risk factors and signs of abuse. Recognizing high-risk situations can prevent elder abuse (eg, when a frail or cognitively impaired elderly person is being cared for by someone with a history of substance abuse, violence, psychiatric disorder, or caregiver burden [the degree of stress caused by caregiving]). Physicians should pay particular attention to those situations in which a frail elderly person (eg, a person with a recent history of stroke or a newly diagnosed condition) is discharged into a precarious home environment. Physicians should also keep in mind that abusers and victims may not fit stereotypes.

Elderly persons often agree to share their homes with family members who have drug or alcohol problems or serious psychiatric disorders. A family member may have been discharged from a mental or other institution to an elderly person's home without having been screened for a risk of causing abuse. Physicians should therefore counsel elderly patients considering such living arrangements, especially if the relationships were fraught with tension in the past.

Abused elderly persons are at high risk of death. In a large 13-year longitudinal study, the survival rate was 9% for abuse victims compared with 40% for nonabused controls. Multivariate analysis to determine the independent effect of abuse revealed a threefold higher mortality for abused patients over a 3-year period after the abuse than for controls over a similar period.

Treatment

An interdisciplinary team approach (involving physicians, nurses, social workers, lawyers, law enforcement officials, psychiatrists, and other practitioners) is essential. Any previous intervention (eg, court orders of protection) and the reason for its failure should be investigated to avoid repeating any mistakes.

Intervention: If the patient is in immediate danger, the physician, in consultation with the patient, should consider hospital admission, law enforcement intervention, or relocation to a safe home. The patient should be informed of the risks and consequences of each option. If the patient is not in immediate danger, steps to reduce risk should still be taken but are less urgent. The choice of intervention depends on the abuser's intent to harm. For example, if a family member administers too much of a drug because the physician's directions are misunderstood, the only intervention needed may be to give clearer instructions. However, a deliberate overdose requires more intensive intervention.

In general, interventions need to be tailored to each situation. Interventions may include medical assistance; education (eg, teaching victims about abuse and available options, helping them devise safety plans); psychologic support (eg, psychotherapy, support groups); law enforcement and legal intervention (eg, arrest of the abuser, orders of protection, legal advocacy [including protecting assets]); and alternative housing (eg, sheltered senior housing, nursing home placement). Counseling the victim usually requires many sessions, and progress may be slow. If the victim has decision-making capacity, he should help determine his own intervention. If the victim does not have decision-making capacity, the interdisciplinary team, ideally with a guardian or objective conservator, should make most decisions. Decisions are based on the severity of the violence, the lifestyle choices previously made by the patient, and the legal ramifications. Often, there is no single correct decision, and each case must be carefully followed up.

Nursing and social work issues: As members of the interdisciplinary team, nurses and social workers can play an important role in preventing elder abuse. A nurse and/or a social worker can be appointed as coordinator to ensure that pertinent data are properly recorded, that relevant parties are contacted and kept informed, and that necessary care is available 24 hours/day. In-service education on elder abuse should be offered to all nurses and social workers annually. In some states (eg, New York), education on child abuse (but not yet on elder abuse) is mandatory for physician, nursing, and social work licensure.

Reporting: The reporting of suspected or confirmed abuse is mandatory in all states if the abuse occurs in an institution, and in most states if it occurs in a home. Indeed, all U.S. states have laws protecting and providing services for vulnerable, incapacitated, or disabled adults. In more than three quarters of U.S. states, the agency designated to receive abuse reports is the state social service department (adult protective services). In the remaining states, the designated agency is the state unit on aging. For abuse within an institution, the local long-term care ombudsman office should be contacted. Telephone numbers for these agencies and offices in any part of the USA can be found by calling the Eldercare Locator (800-677-1116) or the National Center on Elder Abuse (202-682-2470) and giving the patient's county and city of residence or zip code. Health care practitioners should know reporting laws and procedures for their own states.

Caregiver issues: Caregivers for elderly persons who have chronic medical and functional problems may not realize that their behaviors sometimes border on being abusive. These caregivers may be so immersed in their caregiving roles that they become socially isolated and lack an objective frame of reference for what constitutes normal caregiving. The deleterious effects of caregiver burden, including depression, an increase in stress-related medical conditions, and a shrinking social network, are well documented. Physicians need to point out these effects to caregivers. Services to help caregivers include adult day care, respite programs,∎ and home health care.

∎ see page 92

MANAGED CARE

A method of integrating the financing and delivery of health care to manage quality, costs, and access to care for an insured population.

Managed care and geriatrics share certain principles, priorities, and goals:

- Both emphasize preventive health care
- Both attempt to proactively identify persons who will require care management
- Both attempt to offer a coordinated continuum of care
- Both attempt to provide care at the most cost-effective site (preferably the home)

Managed care organizations (MCOs) attempt to balance individualized care with population-based care (see FIGURE 16–1), applying the principles of appropriate medical management to populations in an attempt to control costs and improve quality. Although some health policy experts are concerned that managed care's attention to reducing costs may undermine quality of care, others believe it can minimize unnecessary costs while improving quality.

MEDICARE MANAGED CARE ORGANIZATIONS

Medicare Part C offers several options for health care coverage, including MCOs. As of July 1998, about 16% (6 million) of persons eligible for Medicare had enrolled in Medicare MCOs.

Advantages of Medicare MCO plans over traditional fee-for-service programs include full Medicare benefits with lower deductibles and copayments plus other benefits—not usually part of Medicare coverage—that vary among MCOs. These other benefits include preventive care; reimbursement for prescription drugs, eyeglasses, and hearing aids; health education and promotion programs; and discounts on or improved access to transportation, day care, respite care, assisted living, and long-term care insurance. Medicare MCOs do not have fee-for-service restrictions on reimbursement to providers, allowing payments for nontraditional services, such as geriatric assessment by an interdisciplinary team.∎

MCOs may be run by payers (eg, insurers) or by providers (eg, hospital systems). They may offer tightly managed health maintenance organization (HMO) plans or more loosely managed point-of-service plans, preferred provider plans, or managed indemnity plans.

∎ see page 74

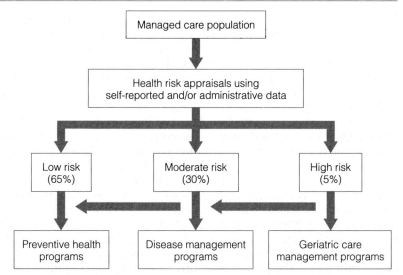

FIGURE 16-1.   A population-based approach to geriatric care management. Patients are directed to appropriate programs on the basis of health risk appraisal. (Adapted from Fillit HM, Hill J, Picariello G, Warburton S: "How the principles of geriatric assessment are shaping managed care." *Geriatrics* 53:76, 1998.)

Relationships between MCOs and providers may follow the staff model, in which MCOs employ physicians; the group model, in which MCOs contract almost exclusively with large multispecialty or primary care groups; or, most commonly, the independent practitioner association (IPA) model, in which MCOs contract with an IPA.

In the IPA model, physicians retain, to varying degrees, ownership of their practices. An MCO may contract with multiple IPAs (network model) or with individual physicians in a single IPA. Geriatric care management∎ is often more difficult in individual IPA models than in the other models because physicians frequently contract with several payers. These physicians typically have an insufficient number of patients from any one payer to commit substantially to that payer's geriatric care management program. However, some IPAs develop their own geriatric care programs, particularly when they have financial incentives for effective medical management.

The method of physician payment affects the ability of an MCO to implement geriatric care management. Physicians may be paid for individual services (fee-for-service programs) or through various capitation models, in which a budget is negotiated between payers and providers that covers health care costs for individuals or groups of

∎see page 161

individuals over a fixed time (usually 1 year). Full or global capitation refers to a contract in which a physician group is responsible for all medical costs, usually including hospitalization. Professional or primary care capitation refers to a contract in which physicians are solely at risk for their own services. Many variations of these contracts exist. In capitation models, physicians are responsible for managing care within a budget, which involves financial risk. Physicians can lose money if patients are not well managed or if medical costs exceed the budget. On the other hand, they can profit if patients are well managed and preventive care is effective, resulting in care being delivered at less than budget. Unburdened by traditional Medicare fee-for-service regulations and restrictions, capitation creates incentives for the redesign of health care in ways that are innovative and cost-effective (eg, payments for geriatric care teams). However, underutilization of needed services is a risk (eg, a physician may be reluctant to hospitalize a patient because of the expense involved). Usually, physicians successfully adjust to capitation, although the transition from fee-for-service may be difficult due to the problems involved in managing a finite medical budget and due to a lack of knowledge concerning population-based medicine.

Various important services, many of which are mandated by the federal government, are provided by Medicare MCOs. Generally, only large MCOs can effectively provide all of the functions listed in TABLE 16–1.

An effective **medical director** is required for the relationship between an MCO and a provider to be successful. The Medicare MCO medical director should be a geriatrician or a physician with experience in geriatric care. Knowledge of geriatric medicine is key in the treatment of frail elderly patients, who account for most health care expenditures in Medicare MCOs. The medical director interacts with other departments of the MCO (eg, government relations, regulatory affairs, network development and contracting, quality improvement, member and physician education). Geriatric care providers (eg, geriatric nurse practitioners, geriatric social workers) can help the medical director in medical management, particularly with regard to supervision and education of care managers.

HEALTH RISK APPRAISAL

A form of screening to identify persons who are likely to need complex health care, who are at risk of adverse health outcomes, and who will benefit from care management programs.

Health risk appraisals are used in managed care as a preventive population-based approach to health screening (see FIGURE 16–1). Tradi-

TABLE 16–1. SOME FUNCTIONS OF MEDICARE MANAGED CARE ORGANIZATIONS

Function	Description
Medical management	Promotes appropriate and consistent care (to avoid overutilization or underutilization of services) by establishing clinical practice guidelines, by providing educational programs for physicians, and by developing physician profiles
	Offers preventive health care programs, technology assessment, pharmacy review, care management, disease management, utilization review (including preauthorization for certain treatments, eg, elective surgery), and discharge planning consistent with Medicare guidelines
Network development and contracting	Develops a coordinated geriatric continuum of care
	Ensures that physicians' credentials meet regulatory standards
	Contracts with physicians for competitive and fair rates
	Ensures that patients have access to the network
Oversight and improvement of quality	Reviews medical records of physicians to ensure appropriate record keeping, to monitor for fraud and abuse, and to ensure patient confidentiality
	Complies with Medicare QISMC (Quality Improvement System for Medicare) regulations and seeks accreditation
Provision of nonmedical services to members	Ensures that patients understand their health benefits and their rights and responsibilities
	Develops and implements policies and procedures for complaints and appeals
	Develops health education and promotion programs

tional fee-for-service programs rarely use these appraisals because of the lack of incentives and reimbursement. Using health risk appraisals with targeted geriatric care management can reduce costs and improve the quality of care. Targeting patients who are too healthy to benefit from the programs results in inefficient utilization of geriatric care management. It is illegal for an MCO to use risk appraisals on persons before they enroll in the MCO. This policy prevents MCOs from "cherry picking," the practice of enrolling only healthy persons.

Health risk appraisals may be based on self-reported health risk data and/or administrative data. **Self-reported health risk data** can be obtained via surveys that assess health status based on various health elements or on screening instruments, which are brief questionnaires used to identify persons at risk of adverse health outcomes (see FIGURE 16–2). Surveys may be conducted by personal interview, by telephone, or by mail. Interviews and telephone surveys are generally more expensive and time consuming than are mailed surveys, although they obtain more reliable and more detailed clinical information. Mailed

What is your sex?   □ Male   □ Female

What is your date of birth? _____

In general, how would you describe your health?

□ Excellent   □ Very good   □ Good   □ Fair   □ Poor

How many drugs do you take each day?

□ None   □ 1–3 Drugs   □ > 3 Drugs

How many times have you seen a physician in the past 6 months?

□ None   □ 1–3 Times   □ > 3 Times

How many times have you seen a physician or visited a clinic in the past 12 months?

□ None   □ 1 Time   □ 2–3 Times   □ 4–6 Times   □ > 6 Times

How many times have you stayed overnight as a patient in a hospital in the past 12 months?

□ None   □ 1 Time   □ 2–3 Times   □ > 3 Times

Have you had diabetes in the past 12 months?   □ Yes   □ No

Have you ever had: Coronary artery disease?   □ Yes   □ No

Angina pectoris?   □ Yes   □ No

Myocardial infarction?   □ Yes   □ No

Is there a friend, relative, or neighbor who would take care of you for a few days if necessary?   □ Yes   □ No

FIGURE 16–2. Example of a typical health risk screening instrument used by Medicare managed care organizations. (Adapted from Picala J, Boult C, Reed RL, Aliberti E: "Predictive validity of the P_{ra} instrument among older recipients of managed care." *Journal of the American Geriatrics Society* 45:614–617, 1997.)

surveys are less expensive, are more efficient, and have relatively high response rates (50 to 60%) in the elderly.

Administrative data include data derived from insurance claims, including medical and pharmacy claims, and data derived from primary care visits. Administrative data are relatively inexpensive to obtain in most Medicare MCOs with sophisticated information systems. However, the quality, timeliness, and availability of such data can be suboptimal.

In general, self-reported health risk data and administrative data equally predict health care use. However, because response rates to self-reported health surveys are generally 50 to 60%, with nonresponders usually having higher health risk, administrative data have advantages because they can be obtained for almost all members and at a much lower cost. For persons newly enrolled in an MCO, self-reported health surveys are more useful for identifying those at high risk because administrative data are generally unavailable. Persons with certain problems (eg, smoking, alcohol use, cognitive impairment, falls, nutritional problems) also cannot generally be identified by administrative data. MCOs often use self-reported health risk data to identify such persons, so that they can be directed to disease management programs.◗ Self-reported health risk data are also useful for promoting wellness (eg, exercise, stress reduction, smoking cessation) in the healthy elderly and for eliciting patient preferences, self-perceived health status, values, and the need for ancillary service (eg, homemaker services, transportation).

Health risk appraisals are the first step in the population-based medical management of health care. Health risk appraisals must be linked to care management programs so that high-risk members can be proactively managed. The proportion of high-risk members (those at risk of adverse health outcomes who are likely to need complex care) in a Medicare MCO profoundly affects the MCO's earnings; typically, 5% of members at the highest risk account for 62% of hospital costs. At present, Medicare pays a fixed capitation (called the average adjusted per capita cost, or AAPCC) for each member, which reflects 95% of the average cost to Medicare under fee-for-service programs for a patient of the same age, sex, and social situation (eg, residence, employment status, financial status). Thus, MCOs with many high-risk members (adverse selection) may lose money, whereas MCOs with few high-risk members (favorable selection) may profit.

Responding to this situation, the Balanced Budget Act of 1997 required that the Health Care Financing Administration (HCFA) institute a health risk–adjusted payment system by January 1, 2000. This system decreases payments to MCOs with favorable selection and increases payments to MCOs with adverse selection, thus potentially increasing the financial incentive to enroll and retain high-risk elderly patients. Consequently, health risk data, primarily from administrative data, will become increasingly important and will be required.

GERIATRIC CARE MANAGEMENT

Frail elderly patients (generally those > 75 years with multiple chronic health problems complicated by significant functional and psychosocial impairments) are generally classified as "high risk." Once identified, high-risk patients are assigned by triage to geriatric care management programs.

Traditional case management and geriatric care management programs differ (see Table 16–2). The content, substance, and emphasis of geriatric care management programs vary greatly, affecting their efficacy. For example, most programs primarily use telephone communication, whereas others may use home visits. Also, some programs

◗ see page 163

TABLE 16–2.   TRADITIONAL CASE MANAGEMENT VERSUS GERIATRIC
CARE MANAGEMENT

Factor	Traditional Case Management	Geriatric Care Management
Primary focus	Acute care (reactive)	Chronic care (proactive)
Primary site	Hospital-based care	Ambulatory care
Primary activity	Utilization review and discharge planning	Prevention of hospital admissions
Knowledge base	Pediatric and adult medicine	Geriatric medicine

depend completely on primary care providers, whereas others focus on patient self-management.∎

Most primary care providers (particularly those in Medicare fee-for-service programs) do not have the financial incentives, time, resources, or, in some cases, knowledge to practice effective geriatric care management. By developing geriatric care management programs that provide knowledge, access to the geriatric continuum of care, and additional personnel and resources, MCOs enable primary care providers to practice better geriatric care. Various risk-sharing capitation arrangements give primary care providers the incentive to prevent iatrogenic problems, functional decline, hospitalization, and institutionalization.

MCOs have the financial incentive and organizational capacity to develop, through contracting, an effective geriatric continuum of care, which is crucial to an MCO's success. An effective geriatric continuum of care enables the MCO to use the site providing the most cost-effective care while maintaining quality. Unnecessary or preventable hospitalization—the most expensive component of health care (generally accounting for about 40% of costs)—is avoided through innovative use of subacute and home care (eg, for community-acquired pneumonia) and through shortening of hospital stays (eg, for hip fractures and strokes).

Most MCO models develop a continuum of care by contracting with preferred physician providers, including geriatricians, and other providers (eg, hospitals, subacute and long-term care facilities, home care agencies). Effective access to the continuum of care may be managed by the geriatric care management program. MCOs that send more patients to a specific facility generally receive better service.

Long-term care is covered by very few MCOs, but it can be incorporated into the continuum of care through network development, facilitating access for Medicare MCO members. In addition, several

∎ see page 163

programs, such as the Program of All-Inclusive Care for the Elderly (PACE), are beginning to create managed care for long-term care. PACE pools Medicaid and Medicare capitation to provide comprehensive geriatric care to nursing home–eligible patients. Other models manage the Medicare portion of long-term custodial care; these models offer medical care primarily through extensive use of nurse practitioners.

DISEASE MANAGEMENT

Preventive care programs that proactively attempt to manage chronic disease.

Disease management programs target high prevalence, costly, chronic illnesses that may be effectively managed with a population-based approach (see FIGURE 16–1). Management of chronic illness between physician visits is an important component of these programs, which typically use nonphysician providers to teach patients self-management and to coordinate care with physician providers.

Carve-outs, case rates, and disease-specific educational programs are sometimes referred to as disease management programs but they are not. With carve-outs, a particular specialty or disease group (eg, mental health) is separated from the contracting model and given to an independent organization or provider group, which becomes responsible for it. Carve-outs for mental health care are common. With case rates, an MCO contracts with a provider for care during an entire episode of illness. This approach is often used for surgical procedures (eg, hip fractures). Finally, programs that are primarily educational are sometimes termed disease management, although they do not actively manage illness.

MCOs often develop disease management programs for classic geriatric problems (eg, heart failure, diabetes, falls, polypharmacy). For example, a typical MCO polypharmacy program includes a direct-to-member and a physician component. Members who use many (eg, $\geq$ 5) drugs within a specified time (polypharmacy∎) are identified through self-reporting or through administrative data obtained from pharmacy records. These members are sent a brown bag with a letter from the MCO medical director describing the risks of taking multiple drugs and asking them to place all their prescription and over-the-counter drugs in the brown bag and take them to their physician. The physician is sent a drug management report that lists and organizes all prescriptions filled by the member, including prescriptions the physician may be unaware of (eg, those obtained from consultants). The report enables the physician to quickly check for drug duplication and

∎ see page 56

drug interactions. Polypharmacy clinical practice guidelines or other educational information (eg, recommendations on improved prescribing) is also sent to the physician. Polypharmacy programs can reduce unnecessary pharmacy costs, improve prescribing, and reduce the number of adverse drug interactions. Occasionally, such programs employ MCO pharmacists to review drug management reports.

17 ▬ HEALTH CARE FUNDING

In the USA, the major sources of funding for elderly health care services are Medicare, Medicaid, other federal programs (eg, Veterans Administration), private insurance, and out-of-pocket payments. In addition, many states offer special benefits and health-related programs for the elderly, ranging from subsidies for transportation, housing, heating, telephone, and food expenses to home help and nutrition services. Health care workers need to assist elderly patients in learning about benefits and entitlements that promote physical and mental health.

MEDICARE

The elderly are eligible for Medicare in every state. The type of physician and hospital visits and the range of services (eg, eyeglasses, prescription drugs, hearing aids) that Medicare covers change regularly with new statutory and regulatory amendments. Physicians should understand basic Medicare rules, supply materials that describe benefits, and make referrals to legal and social services for further counseling and support.

Medicare paid an estimated $216.4 billion in 1997 for elderly health care services. If a patient's Medicare claim is denied, the decision may be reversed by a prompt challenge supported by an appeal in a fair hearing administrative forum, in which the insurance company handling Medicare claims reviews the case. If unsatisfied with the outcome of that review, the patient has the right to a hearing before a judge.

Medicare comprises three parts: hospital insurance (Part A), supplementary medical insurance (Part B), and alternative programs for care (Part C).

PART A

Part A is supported by a payroll tax collected during a person's working years and represents prepaid hospital insurance for Medicare-qualified retirees. Generally, only persons who are eligible to receive monthly Social Security payments are eligible for Part A. Persons who never worked or who did not work enough years to be eligible for Social Security are not eligible for Part A. However, more than 95% of persons ≥ 65 years are enrolled in Part A (many persons receive spousal eligibility, pay part A premiums, or have them paid by Medicaid).

Part A covers inpatient hospital care, inpatient care in a skilled nursing facility, home health care, hospice care, and custodial care under the circumstances discussed below. Care in a hospital or a skilled nursing facility is paid for on the basis of benefit periods. A benefit period begins when a person is admitted to a facility and ends when the person has been out of the facility for 60 consecutive days. If a person is readmitted after the 60 days, a new benefit period begins, and another deductible must be paid.

Inpatient hospital care: Inpatient hospital care, as of 1999, is fully covered for a maximum period of 60 days in any benefit period. The beneficiary pays a deductible, which is established annually ($768 in 1999). If the patient's hospital stay exceeds this maximum period, most of the additional costs are paid up to 90 days, and the beneficiary pays a daily copayment equal to one fourth of the deductible ($192 per day for days 61 to 90 in 1999). Partial coverage is provided for a further 60 hospital days (reserve days) cumulatively during a beneficiary's lifetime. The beneficiary pays a daily copayment of one half of the deductible for reserve days. Part A also provides some coverage for psychiatric hospital stays.

Virtually all medically necessary hospital services are covered (psychiatric care is handled differently), including discharge planning and medical social services, such as identifying eligibility for public programs and referrals to community agencies. Medicare pays for a semiprivate room or, if medically necessary, a private room, but not for such amenities as a television or a telephone.

Payment for inpatient hospital care is determined by the diagnosis-related group, which includes the beneficiary's principal diagnosis with some adjustment for age and comorbidity. The hospital may make or lose money depending on length of admission and costs of diagnosis and therapy. Under this arrangement, the financial pressure for early discharge and limited intervention may conflict with medical judgment. When a patient cannot be discharged home safely or to a nursing home because no bed is available, Medicare pays a relatively low per diem amount for an alternative level of care.

Inpatient care in a skilled nursing facility (skilled nursing care and skilled rehabilitation services) is covered in a similarly complex fashion that can change every year.**1**

The Medicare Prospective Payment System was initiated in 1998, and assigns patients to a resource utilization group system (RUGS III), accord-

---

1 see also page 105

ing to the types and amounts of resources their care is expected to cost. Seven categories—special care, rehabilitation, clinically complex problems, severe behavioral problems, impaired cognition, reduced physical functioning, and a need for extensive services—are subdivided based primarily on the patient's functional dependence. The goal is to increase efficiency and avoid excessive payment for patients who require little care. Prospective per diem rates cover routine, ancillary, and capital costs of care for a patient in a skilled nursing facility.

RUGS III uses data from a version of the Minimum Data Set, the mandated uniform assessment instrument for nursing home patients. Because use of this instrument requires ongoing review of patients, linking patient outcomes with RUGS categories may be possible.

Home health care: Home health care (medical care provided in the home) includes part-time or intermittent skilled nursing care; home health aide services; and physical, speech, and occupational therapy. These services are generally covered if they are part of a physician-approved care plan for a homebound patient. Medical supplies are covered when billed by a home health agency.**1**

Hospice services: Hospice services (medical and support services for a terminal illness) are generally covered if a physician certifies that the patient is terminally ill (estimated life expectancy of ≤ 6 months), the patient chooses to receive hospice care instead of standard Medicare benefits, and a Medicare-certified hospice program provides care.**2**

Custodial care: Custodial care (care of a medically stable patient who needs assistance with activities of daily living [ADLs], such as eating, dressing, toileting, and bathing) is covered in the home only when skilled care (the services of a professional nurse or therapist under a physician-authorized plan of home care) is also required. Custodial care is covered in a skilled nursing facility when it is part of posthospital acute or rehabilitation care.

PART B

Part B is optional and requires the beneficiary to pay a monthly premium ($45.50 in 1999 for persons enrolling promptly after reaching age 65). Premiums generally rise by 10% for each year's delay in enrollment; exceptions are for those currently covered by group insurance through employment of oneself, one's spouse, or a family member. Most state Medicaid programs pay Part B premiums for persons who qualify for both Medicare and Medicaid. Social Security beneficiaries are automatically enrolled in Part B unless they decline the highly subsidized coverage; the federal government pays 75% of Part B costs, and beneficiaries pay 25%. Consequently, 95% of persons aged 65 who retire with Social Security benefits elect Part B coverage and agree to have premiums deducted from their monthly Social Security checks. Persons who decline

1 see also page 89   **2** see also page 90

coverage but later change their minds must pay a surcharge based on how long they delayed enrollment. Participants may discontinue coverage at any time but must pay a surcharge on the premium if they reenroll.

Part B covers part of the cost of physician services; outpatient hospital care (eg, emergency department care, outpatient surgery), with certain restrictions; outpatient physical, speech, and occupational therapy; diagnostic tests, including portable x-ray services in the home; and durable medical equipment for home use. If surgery is recommended, Part B covers part of the cost of an optional second opinion and, if these options differ, a third opinion.

Part B also covers medically necessary ambulance services, certain services and supplies not covered by Part A (eg, colostomy bags, prostheses), drugs and biologicals that cannot be administered by the patient, spinal manipulation by a licensed chiropractor for subluxation demonstrated on x-ray, drugs and dental services if deemed necessary for medical treatment, optometry services related to lenses for cataracts, and the services of physician assistants, nurse practitioners, clinical psychologists, and clinical social workers. Outpatient mental health care, with certain limitations, is covered. As of 1999, Medicare does not cover intermediate or long-term nursing care (with the exception of Part A services noted above) and several health services (eg, routine eye examinations). However, Medicare recently added several preventive services, including prostate cancer screening, physical examinations, and prostate-specific antigen tests; mammograms every 2 years; and Papanicolaou smears every 3 years. Unless the patient is enrolled in a managed care program, Medicare does not generally cover outpatient drugs, although it does cover drugs that cannot be administered by the patient (eg, drugs given IV), some oral anticancer drugs, and certain drugs for hospice patients. A complete description of Part B services and other provisions is available in *Medicare And You 2000* (available on the internet at http:www.medicare.gov or by calling 800-633-4227).

Under Part B, physicians may elect to be paid directly by Medicare (assignment), receiving 80% of the allowable charge directly from the program, once the deductible has been met. Patients are responsible for the remaining 20%. A physician who does not accept assignment of Medicare payments (or does so selectively) may bill the patient up to 115% of the allowable charge; the patient receives reimbursement (80% of the allowable charge) from Medicare. Physicians are subject to fines if their charges exceed the maximum allowable Medicare fees described above. A physician who does not accept assignment from Medicare must give the patient a written estimate for elective surgery if it is > $500. Otherwise, the patient can later claim a refund from the physician for any amount paid over the allowable charge.

Medicare payments to physicians have been criticized as inadequate for the time involved in giving physical and mental status examinations and obtaining the patient history from family members. A Medicare fee schedule based on a resource-based relative value scale for physician services became effective in January 1992 to correct this problem. The effects of the fee schedule on patient care and on the practice of geriatric medicine remain to be determined.

PART C

This program (also called Medicare+Choice) offers several alternatives to the traditional fee-for-service programs, such as Medicare managed care organizations.

MEDICAID

Funded by a federal-state partnership, Medicaid pays for health services for certain categories of the poor (including the aged poor, those who are blind or disabled, and low-income families with dependent children). The federal government contributes between 50 and 83% of the payments made under each state's program; the state pays the remainder. About 10% of the elderly receive services under Medicaid, accounting for about 40% of all Medicaid expenditures. Medicaid is the major public payer for long-term care; it contributed about 47.8% of the $78.5 billion spent for nursing home services in 1996.

Services covered under federal guidelines include inpatient and outpatient hospital care, laboratory and x-ray services, physician services, and skilled nursing care and home health services for persons > 21 years. States may cover certain other services and items, including prescription drugs, dental services, eyeglasses, and intermediate-level nursing home care. Each state determines eligibility requirements, which therefore vary, but persons receiving funds from cash-assistance programs (eg, the Supplemental Security Income program) must be included. Several states offer enriched packages of Medicaid services under waiver programs, which are intended to delay or prevent nursing home admission by providing additional home and community-based services (eg, day care, personal care, respite care).

In most states, persons qualify for Medicaid benefits if their income minus medical expenses is at poverty level. In some states, eligibility depends on income level without offsetting medical expenses. Assets, excluding equity in a home and certain others, are also considered. If the remaining assets exceed the limit, the person is not eligible for Medicaid, even if income is low. Thus, the elderly may have to spend down (ie, pay for care from personal savings until stringent state eligibility requirements are met) to qualify for Medicaid. Spouses of nursing home patients may keep some income (up to $1,718 per month in some states) and half of the couple's assets (up to about $69,000). The extent to which elderly middle-

1 see page 156

class persons give away assets to qualify for Medicaid coverage of nursing home care is unknown. State Medicaid programs cannot attach such assets, but divestment of assets during the 30 months before entrance into a nursing home may delay eligibility for Medicaid benefits. Medicaid denies coverage for a period of time that is determined by the amount of improperly divested funds divided by the average monthly cost of nursing home care in the state. For example, if a person gives away $10,000 in a state where the average monthly cost of care is $3,500, Medicaid coverage is delayed by 3 months.

OTHER FEDERAL PROGRAMS

The **Department of Veterans Affairs** (VA), which operates 171 hospitals, 35 domiciliary facilities, and 127 nursing homes, provides free health care to veterans with disabilities related to military service and, on a complicated priority basis, to those with other conditions. The VA also contracts to provide care in community hospitals and nursing homes. Several innovative geriatric programs, including geriatric assessment units; Geriatric Research, Education, and Clinical Centers; and hospital-based home health care programs, have been developed within the VA system.

The **Older Americans Act** (OAA), enacted in 1965, has evolved from a program of small grants and research projects into a network of 57 state, territorial, and Indian tribal units on aging; 670 area agencies on aging; and thousands of community agencies. The primary purpose of the OAA is to develop, coordinate, and deliver a comprehensive system of services for elderly persons at the community level, including information and referral, outreach, transportation, senior centers, nutritional programs, advocacy, protective services, senior employment, ombudsman programs, and supportive services. The OAA also funds research and training. In 1999, the total appropriation for OAA programs was about $882 million.

Although not usually considered a health program, **Social Security** provides basic pension payments that the elderly use for health care services. The elderly receive two types of payments: Old Age and Survivors Insurance, which is financed by Social Security trust funds and provides payments to retirees, surviving spouses, or qualified dependents, and Supplementary Security Income, which is financed from general revenues and provides a guaranteed minimum income to aged, blind, and disabled persons.

Title XX of the Social Security Act authorizes reimbursements to states for social services, including various home health services and homemaker services (eg, meal preparation, laundry, light housekeeping, grocery shopping) for the frail elderly. These funds have shifted to the Social Services Block Grant program, which was designed to prevent or reduce inappropriate institutional care by providing for community-based care and other assistance that allows the elderly to maintain autonomy in the community. The program is defined, administered, and implemented by states; it does not support institutional care or any service covered by Medicare or Medicaid. The program covers health services only when they are an "integral but subordinate" component of an overall social service program.

PRIVATE INSURANCE

About 87% of beneficiaries enrolled in fee-for-service Medicare programs have supplemental medical insurance. Many types of private insurance are available to the elderly; most are a form of Medigap insurance, which pays for some or all of Medicare deductibles and copayments. Most Medigap insurance is purchased individually from private insurers, although employers may provide it to retirees.

Congress has restricted Medigap insurance to a basic plan with nine possible expansions. No plan may duplicate Medicare benefits. The basic plan covers hospital copayments, coverage for 100% of Medicare Part A–eligible expenses after Medicare hospital benefits are exhausted (ie, 365 days beyond the total hospital benefits lifetime limit provided by Part A), and Part B copayments. The expansion plans, which have higher premiums than the basic plan, may provide additional coverage in a skilled nursing facility and may cover the Part A and Part B deductibles, a percentage of the cost of outpatient prescribed drugs, preventive medical services, and short-term home-based help with ADLs during recovery from an illness, injury, or surgery.

Very few private insurance policies cover services such as long-term home health care or long-term nursing home care. However, some private insurers offer long-term care insurance. As of 1996, about 5 million long-term care policies had been sold, and estimates indicate that about 10 to 20% of the elderly can afford these policies. In 1996, private insurance paid for about 4% of long-term care expenditures, and the percentage of such expenditures covered by private insurance is expected to slowly increase. However, how long-term care will be financed in the future is unknown: whether the elderly or their families will pay the relatively high premiums required, whether persons will enroll in programs covering long-term care at younger ages when premiums are lower, or whether more services will be covered in new government programs.

Out-of-pocket expenditures constitute about one third of annual long-term care costs (not including informal services provided by family members and friends). A large proportion of these expenditures occur when the elderly person spends down to qualify for Medicaid. ◼

MODELS FOR COMPREHENSIVE COVERAGE

Individually, Medicare, Medicaid, Medigap, and private long-term care insurance have shortcomings in providing comprehensive geriatric

---

◼ see page 168

care. Medicare excludes long-term custodial care and many preventive services; Medicaid belatedly intervenes after the patient is impoverished; Medigap, like Medicare, excludes long-term care and outpatient prescribed drugs; and private insurance is too expensive for most of the elderly, leaves them vulnerable to financial catastrophe, and supports only fragments of long-term care. Collectively, these programs rarely promote integration of acute and long-term care or coordination of health and social services. However, several model projects have demonstrated that, with organized delivery of services using combinations of public funding and private insurance, comprehensive geriatric care, including some long-term care, can be adequately financed.

Social health maintenance organizations (SHMOs) are demonstration programs financed by Medicare. They use Medicare, Medicaid, and private patient payments to cover a wide range of care benefits managed by nurses, social workers, and physicians. Patients not eligible for Medicaid benefits use private payments to cover a limited amount of long-term care, principally in the home. Like an HMO, an SHMO is at financial risk for the cost of services and therefore has an incentive to manage resources carefully.

The **Program of All-Inclusive Care for the Elderly** (PACE), a capitated demonstration program authorized in 1997 as part of Medicare Part C, is designed to keep patients in the community as long as medically, socially, and financially possible. A professional interdisciplinary team assesses patient needs, develops a care plan, integrates primary care and other services, and arranges for implementation of services.

On Lok, the forerunner of PACE, operates in San Francisco's Chinatown and provides prepaid comprehensive care for elderly persons whose level of impairment usually requires admission to a nursing home. Adult day care and coordinated, comprehensive services, including custodial or personal care, drug treatment, dentistry, and housekeeping services, are provided in a community setting. Fewer than 6% of On Lok participants (who enroll for life) have needed nursing home placement, and hospital admissions and lengths of stay are half those for comparable elders.

A **life-care community** or **continuing care retirement community** provides housing, health care, and other services under packaged financing and management. These communities may have a clinic, an infirmary, or even a nursing home on the site, and housing is designed to accommodate disabled persons. Many of these communities serve wealthy retirees willing to sign long-term contracts for their housing and care. Some life-care communities fail because inflation and an aging population cause costs for services to exceed income. Some communities keep costs down by providing housing and minimal services with options to purchase additional services.◨

◨see also page 111

SECTION 2

FALLS, FRACTURES, AND INJURY

18 SYNCOPE

(Fainting)

A sudden, transient loss of consciousness characterized by unresponsiveness and loss of postural control.

Syncope is a symptom—not a disease. Studies suggest that about 25% of institutionalized elderly patients have experienced syncope during the past 10 years and that 6 to 7% experience it each year. Syncope is recurrent in about 33% of patients. About 3% of emergency department visits and 2 to 6% of hospital admissions are for syncope; 80% of these visits involve patients $\geq$ 65. In one study of community-dwelling elderly persons, the prevalence of syncope increased with age (to 56 per 1000 men and 36 per 1000 women aged $\geq$ 75 years).

TABLE 18-1.   CAUSES OF SYNCOPE

Cardiac disorders
  Anatomic/valvular
    Aortic stenosis
    Mitral prolapse and regurgitation
    Hypertrophic cardiomyopathy
    Myxoma
  Electrical
    Tachyarrhythmia
    Bradyarrhythmia
    Heart block
    Sick sinus syndrome
  Functional
    Ischemia and infarct
Situational hypotension
  Dehydration (diarrhea, fasting)
  Orthostatic hypotension
  Postprandial hypotension
  Micturition, defecation, coughing, swallowing
	Abnormal cardiovascular reflexes
	  Carotid sinus syndrome
	  Vasovagal syncope
	Drugs
	  Vasodilators
	  Calcium channel blockers
	  Diuretics
	  β-Blockers
	Central nervous system abnormalities
	  Cerebrovascular insufficiency
	  Seizures
	Metabolic abnormalities
	  Hypoxemia
	  Hypoglycemia or hyperglycemia
	  Anemia
	Pulmonary disorders
	  Chronic obstructive pulmonary disease
	  Pneumonia
	  Pulmonary embolus

Etiology

Many disorders can cause syncope (see TABLE 18-1). Often a cause is neither immediately obvious nor ultimately discovered. Although syncope per se does not increase the risk of death in the elderly, it is associated with physical disability and subsequent functional decline.

Abrupt reduction in cardiac output can cause syncope. This reduction may be caused by a number of cardiac disorders, most of which are more common in elderly than in younger patients. Myocardial infarction accounts for 2 to 6% of syncope among elderly patients; however, unless syncope is accompanied by other cardiac symptoms and ECG changes, myocardial infarction is unlikely. Transient ischemia and arrhythmias are other possibilities.

Orthostatic hypotension is usually asymptomatic, but it can cause syncope. Among institutionalized elderly persons, orthostatic hypotension causes 6% of syncopal episodes. Orthostatic hypotension has many causes, ▮ including age-related physiologic changes; drugs; autonomic insufficiency syndromes, such as pure autonomic failure, multiple systems atrophy, and multiple cerebral infarctions; and dehydration.

Postprandial hypotension can cause syncope and is common among elderly persons. ▮ Nearly all elderly nursing home residents and one third of community-dwelling elderly persons experience some postprandial decrease in blood pressure. Small decreases (< 20 mm Hg) in systolic blood pressure are common within 75 minutes of eating a

▮ see page 845   ▮ see page 848

meal and usually produce no symptoms. Large decreases (> 20 mm Hg) may cause syncope. Patients with hypertension may experience the greatest declines in postprandial blood pressure.

Straining while defecating or urinating (micturition or defecation syncope) and strenuous coughing (cough syncope) can cause syncope by increasing intrathoracic pressure, reducing venous return to the heart, decreasing cardiac output, and thereby reducing blood pressure.

Carotid sinus hypersensitivity can cause syncope when neck movement, a tight collar, or a tumor or other lesion at the carotid bifurcation stimulates baroreceptors in the carotid sinus, resulting in excessive cardiac slowing, vasodilation, or both. Carotid sinus syndrome refers to symptomatic carotid sinus hypersensitivity and is defined by a sinus pause longer than 3 seconds (cardioinhibitory response) or a drop in systolic blood pressure of > 50 mm Hg (vasodepressor response) during carotid sinus massage. Risk factors for carotid sinus hypersensitivity include advanced age, cardiovascular disease, and use of drugs that affect the sinus node, including β-blockers, digoxin, methyldopa, and calcium channel blockers.

Vasovagal syncope, which is caused by stimulation of the vagus nerve, is more common among younger than elderly persons. Causes include the simple act of swallowing (swallow syncope), gastrointestinal conditions (eg, fecal impaction, diarrhea), fright, and pain. Hunger, fatigue, or emotional stress commonly predisposes the patient to vasovagal syncope, and a typical autonomic prodrome (light-headedness, pallor, and cold sweat) usually precedes it.

Anemia may increase susceptibility to syncope. If transient hypotension occurs, a person with anemia may not have sufficient blood oxygen to maintain cerebral function, resulting in syncope.

Cerebrovascular insufficiency is considered the cause of syncope only if accompanied by transient focal neurologic deficits. Vertebrobasilar insufficiency due to severe cervical arthritis or spondylosis may rarely cause syncope when the patient moves his head in certain positions.

Drugs (eg, over-the-counter drugs with anticholinergic properties) may cause tachyarrhythmias, which can precipitate syncope. Prescription drugs, including anticholinergic agents (eg, phenothiazines, tricyclic antidepressants), sympatholytic agents (eg, prazosin, terazosin, guanethidine, reserpine), volume-contracting agents (eg, diuretics), and vasodilators (eg, nitrates, angiotensin-converting enzyme inhibitors, calcium channel blockers), may cause syncope. Syncope may also result from ingesting alcohol, which has vasodilatory properties, or from using eye medications that have systemic effects (eg, topical β-blockers, which can cause bronchospasm, bradycardia, or heart failure). Many other drugs have also been implicated.

Situational stresses that reduce blood pressure can cause syncope, including posture change, meal ingestion, straining while defecating, and taking drugs.

A seizure disorder may cause syncope; however, syncope can also cause seizure activity during the syncopal event.

Pathophysiology

Syncope results from inadequate delivery of oxygen or metabolic substrate to the brain or from disorganized electrical activity in the brain (seizures). Elderly persons are subject to many age-related and disease-related conditions that threaten cerebral blood flow or blood oxygen content and that can reduce oxygen delivery dangerously close to the threshold needed to maintain consciousness. In most elderly persons, who already have compromised cerebral perfusion, any acute insult that further reduces oxygen delivery to the brain (eg, pneumonia, cardiac arrhythmia, a hypotensive drug, situational stress that reduces blood pressure) may cause syncope.

Many cardiovascular and neuroendocrine homeostatic mechanisms that normally maintain blood pressure become impaired with age (eg, baroreflex sensitivity to hypertensive and hypotensive stimuli, heart rate response to postural change). Thus, the ability to maintain adequate cerebral perfusion during hypotensive stress is reduced. Hyperventilation associated with heart failure and dyspnea can further decrease cerebral blood flow by as much as 40%. Other common disorders, such as chronic obstructive pulmonary disease and anemia, can reduce cerebral oxygen delivery even further.

Age-related decreases in basal and stimulated renin levels and in aldosterone production and increases in atrial natriuretic peptide levels predispose the elderly to syncope by impairing renal sodium conservation and intravascular volume maintenance. The elderly are less likely to experience thirst in response to hypertonic dehydration. Therefore, they are more likely to become dehydrated and experience hypotension in response to diuretics, acute febrile illness, or limited salt and water intake.

Diagnosis

Syncope in elderly persons usually results from several interacting abnormalities rather than from a single disease. The evaluation should begin with a thorough history and a physical examination; in most cases, these are sufficient to identify the underlying cause.

History: The patient and family members or other persons close to the patient are asked about recent changes in the patient's condition that may suggest the underlying pathophysiology. The physician ascertains whether any prescription or over-the-counter drugs, including eye medications, are being used. All witnesses are asked to describe what the patient was doing just before fainting.

A seizure disorder is suggested when syncope is preceded by an olfactory or a gustatory aura or is accompanied by tongue biting, fecal incontinence, or postictal confusion.

The nature of recovery from syncope can also provide important clues. For example, slow recovery suggests a seizure disorder, focal neurologic abnormalities suggest a stroke or transient ischemic attack, cardiac symptoms and ECG changes suggest myocardial infarction, nausea or abdominal discomfort suggests a vasovagal mechanism, and a rapid return to baseline suggests an arrhythmia.

Physical examination: To rule out orthostatic hypotension, blood pressure and heart rate are checked with the patient supine after resting for 5 minutes, then after standing for 1 minute and 3 minutes (standing is best, otherwise sitting is okay). A small (< 10 beats/minute) or no increase in heart rate on standing or sitting may indicate baroreflex impairment or a drug effect; tachycardia (heart rate > 100 beats/minute), which is uncommon in response to postural change in elderly persons, may indicate volume depletion.

The carotid arteries are auscultated for bruits to rule out flow abnormalities contraindicating carotid sinus massage.◼ The carotid arteries should also be palpated to determine the quality of the carotid upstroke. With normal aging, the upstroke usually becomes brisker because of increased vascular rigidity. In elderly persons with aortic stenosis, the amplitude of the upstroke may be reduced to a level that is considered normal for younger persons but abnormal for elderly persons.

The heart is auscultated for murmurs of aortic stenosis, mitral regurgitation, or hypertrophic cardiomyopathy. An apical heave; a loud, late-peaking aortic systolic murmur; and a diminished second aortic sound suggest significant aortic stenosis. A holosystolic murmur at the apex is characteristic of mitral regurgitation but may also occur with aortic stenosis or hypertrophic cardiomyopathy. Accentuation of the systolic murmur during the Valsalva maneuver helps distinguish hypertrophic cardiomyopathy from aortic stenosis or mitral regurgitation.

A neurologic examination is essential for detecting focal abnormalities that may indicate cerebrovascular insufficiency or space-occupying lesions.

Laboratory tests: Screening tests are often useful because disease can present atypically in elderly patients. These tests include a white blood cell count to detect occult infection and a hematocrit to detect anemia. Electrolyte, blood urea nitrogen, and creatinine measurements help in assessing hydration status and in ruling out electrolyte disorders. Serum glucose measurements help exclude hypoglycemia or hyperglycemia; the first sign of hyperosmolar dehydration with hyperglycemia may be syncope. Other, more specialized, tests are only performed if indicated by the history and physical examination. A resting ECG should be performed in all patients and may reveal ischemia. Cardiac enzyme and isoenzyme measurements can help rule out myocar-

◼ see page 178

dial infarction. It is not necessary to admit elderly patients to the hospital to rule out myocardial infarction unless the ECG, creatine kinase isoenzymes, or history suggests the diagnosis.

Drug concentration levels may be helpful if the patient is taking an antiarrhythmic, an anticonvulsant, a bronchodilator, digoxin, or lithium to determine if the drug level is subtherapeutic, therapeutic, or toxic. If it is subtherapeutic, syncope may have resulted from inadequate treatment of a known predisposing condition, such as a seizure disorder. If it is toxic (sometimes even if within the usual therapeutic range), syncope may have resulted from a drug-induced proarrhythmia.

Ambulatory (24-hour) ECG monitoring (with a Holter monitor) is often used to evaluate syncope, but the results can be difficult to interpret because they usually reveal no arrhythmias or so many asymptomatic arrhythmias that their relationship to syncope is uncertain. Also, some patients with arrhythmias are not candidates for antiarrhythmic drugs because of their severe toxic effects. Thus, an ambulatory ECG is helpful only for patients with arrhythmias who will be treated despite the risk of toxic effects; eg, patients who have underlying cardiovascular disease and patients who have had a recent myocardial infarction and are at high risk of sudden death.

Because symptomatic arrhythmias occur sporadically and are often missed during ambulatory ECG monitoring, self-activated loop recorders may be useful when serious arrhythmias are suspected or syncope is recurrent and otherwise unexplained. Recorders can be worn continuously for 1 month or implanted for longer periods and activated when symptoms occur. A memory function records several minutes of cardiac rhythm before the recorder is activated; thus, patients can document an arrhythmia by activating the recorder after recovering from syncope.

Cardiac electrophysiologic studies can detect occult sinus node disorders, conduction disorders, and inducible ventricular arrhythmias in > 50% of patients with unexplained syncope. However, the value of these studies is difficult to determine, because elderly patients who do not have syncope are likely to have electrophysiologic abnormalities and because those who have syncope often spontaneously stop having episodes. Thus, electrophysiologic studies should be reserved for elderly patients with ECG or other clinical evidence of heart disease and recurrent episodes of unexplained syncope.

Ambulatory blood pressure monitoring may help identify hypotensive responses to meals, drugs, or postural change that may cause syncope. Because blood pressure monitors are often heavy and cumbersome, patients may prefer to use a portable automated device and diary to record blood pressure at certain times of day, including early morning after arising from bed, 1 hour after taking drugs and eating, and at the time the syncopal event occurred.

Carotid sinus massage should be performed to detect carotid sinus hypersensitivity when no other cause of syncope is apparent in patients who have no evidence of cerebrovascular disease (a carotid bruit, a previous stroke, or transient ischemic attacks) or cardiac conduction abnormalities. The technique consists of a circular 5-second massage of one carotid sinus at a time while the patient is monitored with an ECG. Blood pressure is measured before and immediately after each massage. Carotid sinus massage is generally a safe procedure when performed for 5 seconds in carefully screened patients. Serious complications, eg, stroke, have occurred in patients with underlying cerebrovascular disease or during vigorous, prolonged massage.

Doppler echocardiography is often used to detect hemodynamically significant valvular heart disease as well as hypertrophic cardiomyopathy in patients with a cardiac murmur.

Tilt tests (with and without isoproterenol infusions) may be used to evaluate unexplained syncope. A 60 to 80° head-up tilt for up to 45 minutes can precipitate vasovagal syncope with associated bradycardia and hypotension. One mechanism for this response is probably the Bezold-Jarisch reflex, which is provoked by vigorous cardiac contraction around a relatively empty ventricular chamber. Using isoproterenol to strengthen cardiac contraction can increase the test's sensitivity. However, isoproterenol is often contraindicated in elderly patients with known or suspected coronary artery disease. The development of vasovagal syncope during the tilt test suggests that it caused the unexplained episode. Usually, vasovagal syncope can be readily diagnosed without the tilt test based on a history of the typical vagal prodrome (nausea, light-headedness, and pale, cold, clammy skin). The tilt test also may help detect delayed orthostatic hypotension as the cause of syncope.

An **EEG** and a **brain CT scan** are often ordered to evaluate syncope, although studies suggest they have little value unless underlying focal abnormalities are identified during the neurologic examination.

Prevention

Syncope often can be prevented by identifying precipitating factors and teaching patients to avoid them. For example, elderly men with micturition syncope can learn to urinate while sitting down, and cardiac patients with nitrate-induced syncope can take other antianginal drugs or sit or lie down after taking a nitroglycerin tablet. Patients with postprandial syncope can eat small frequent meals and lie down after eating. Walking after a meal may prevent postprandial hypotension, but this measure should be undertaken only with supervision. Patients should not rise from bed quickly, particularly in the middle of the night. Patients with orthostatic hypotension should sit on the edge of the bed and flex their feet before standing. Patients should learn to avoid the Valsalva maneuver (ie, straining) during defecation; using stool softeners and altering their diet helps. Drinking ample fluids helps avoid syncope, particularly during hot weather or episodes of acute illness; diuretics are not recommended during these situations.

Physicians and nurses should avoid prescribing potentially hypotensive drugs to elderly patients who may not need them, and patients who need these drugs should be monitored for orthostatic and postprandial hypotension. The use of alcohol is discouraged. Because the judicious treatment of hypertension may ameliorate orthostatic and postprandial hypotension, hypertensive patients should be cautiously treated while blood pressure is monitored. Physical therapists can help patients maintain sufficient muscle tone in the lower extremities to ensure adequate venous blood return to the heart. Nutritionists can advise patients with orthostatic hypotension how to maintain adequate salt and fluid intake.

Treatment

The optimal treatment of syncope in elderly patients requires a multidisciplinary approach. The first steps are to identify and treat all likely causes and predisposing conditions. Even major interventions (eg, aortic valve repair) are relatively well tolerated in otherwise healthy elderly persons and can significantly improve quality of life. Similarly, pacemaker insertion, coronary artery bypass grafting, and carotid endarterectomy can be considered when appropriate. The patient's coexisting conditions, not age, are the deciding factors when determining treatment.

When no primary cause of syncope is identified, potential predisposing conditions are treated. For example, patients with anemia may benefit from vitamins, iron supplements, erythropoietin, or transfusions, depending on the cause of anemia.

For patients with postprandial hypotension, adjusting the time of hypotensive drug administration to avoid a peak effect after a meal may help. Patients with angina should be given antianginal therapy, as long as it does not reduce blood pressure excessively. The drug regimens of patients with carotid sinus hypersensitivity or a cardiac conduction disorder should be evaluated to ensure that cardioinhibitory or hypotensive drugs are not contributing to syncope.

Patients with orthostatic hypotension may benefit from increasing salt intake, wearing support hose, and elevating the head of the bed. If orthostatic hypotension persists despite these measures, pharmacologic therapy can be tried.∎

For patients with carotid sinus syndrome, discontinuing cardioinhibitory or hypotensive drugs (eg, β-blockers, calcium channel blockers, digoxin, methyldopa) usually helps. If discontinuation is not effective or if these drugs are not implicated, patients with a cardioinhibitory response can be treated with cardiac pacing, and patients with associated hypotension may benefit from vasopressors, such as phenylephrine or midodrine.

∎ see page 848

Because syncope is often recurrent, the care plan should include measures to prevent serious injury or accidents during an episode. Driving is not recommended for at least 6 months after the last episode if syncope is unexplained and untreated. Patients should be taught to recognize premonitory symptoms and lie down immediately when they occur.

19 ■ CHRONIC DIZZINESS AND POSTURAL INSTABILITY

Dizziness is a vague term describing various sensations, including a subjective feeling of uncertainty, postural instability, or motion in space. It also encompasses other sensations (eg, light-headedness, wooziness, near fainting). The elderly often use the term even more broadly to include weakness, fatigue, and myriad other symptoms. Dizziness can be classified, somewhat arbitrarily, as acute (present for < 1 month) or chronic (present for > 1 month). Because the causes, diagnosis, and treatment of acute dizziness are similar for all adults, this chapter discusses only chronic dizziness and postural instability. The prevalence of chronic dizziness among the elderly ranges from 13 to 30%.

Dizziness is divided by history of sensation into five categories: (1) **vertigo:** a rotary motion, either of the patient with respect to the environment (subjective vertigo) or of the environment with respect to the patient (objective vertigo), the key element being the perception of motion; (2) **dysequilibrium** (unsteadiness, imbalance, gait disturbance): a feeling (primarily involving the trunk and lower extremities rather than the head) that a fall is imminent; (3) **presyncope** (faintness, light-headedness): a feeling that loss of consciousness is imminent; (4) **mixed dizziness:** a combination of two or more of the above types; and (5) **nonspecific dizziness:** a sensation of instability that does not fit readily into any of the previous categories.

In the standard clinical approach, dizziness is considered a symptom of one or more discrete diseases. It is further assumed that the categories of dizziness correspond to diseases within specific systems (eg, vestibular, proprioceptive, cardiovascular). These assumptions work well for younger patients and for patients of all ages with acute dizziness. However, among elderly patients with chronic dizziness, the relationship between categories and specific systems or etiologies is less consistent. Using the standard approach, many elderly patients with chronic dizziness are left undiagnosed (and untreated), or the diagnoses made by physicians from different specialties are variable and inconsistent. For these reasons, chronic dizziness might better be considered a geriatric syndrome—a condition resulting from multiple diseases and impairments—rather than solely a symptom of discrete diseases.

Etiology and Pathophysiology

Although the reported prevalence for specific causes varies widely, the most commonly reported discrete disorders causing chronic dizziness include peripheral vestibular disorders (eg, benign paroxysmal positional vertigo, neurolabyrinthitis, Meniere's disease); cervical disorders, particularly spondylosis; cerebrovascular disorders, including vertebrobasilar insufficiency and brain stem infarcts; carotid hypersensitivity; and psychiatric disorders, particularly depression and anxiety (see TABLE 19–1).

Chronic dizziness and postural instability most often result from the combined effects of disorders and impairments in the multiple systems contributing to stability and equilibrium. The sensation of equilibrium requires input from complex networks of sensory, motor, and central integrative neurologic systems. These systems are, in turn, influenced by cardiovascular, respiratory, metabolic, and psychologic factors. Chronic dizziness may occur when there is overwhelming dysfunction of one system or, probably more often, when there is impairment or dysfunction within several systems.

The visual, auditory, vestibular, and proprioceptive systems are responsible for orienting a person in space. These systems interact and can have multiple interconnections. Age-related visual changes include decreased acuity, adaptation to darkness, sensitivity to contrast, and accommodation. In addition, ocular diseases, including macular degeneration, glaucoma, and cataracts, are common. Hearing contributes directly to stability through detection and interpretation of auditory stimuli, which help localize and orient a person in space, especially when other senses are impaired. Decreased hearing is also often a marker of vestibular dysfunction, which is difficult to test clinically.

The vestibular system (see FIGURE 19–1) contributes to spatial orientation at rest and during acceleration and deceleration and is responsible for visual fixation during head and body movements. Age-related decline in vestibular function can be due to changes in the otoconia (tiny calciferous granules that form part of the receptor mechanism in the otolith apparatus), perhaps due to osteoporosis or saccular degeneration. Benign paroxysmal positional vertigo (see TABLE 19–1 and FIGURE 19–2) is thought to result from changes in the otoconia.

The vestibular nerve, which connects the vestibular system to the central nervous system (CNS), is particularly sensitive to hypoglycemia and drugs (aminoglycosides, aspirin, furosemide, quinine, quinidine, and perhaps tobacco and alcohol). Head trauma, mastoid or ear surgery, and middle ear infections may also damage the vestibular nerve.

The proprioceptive system (comprised of peripheral nerves, the mechanoreceptors located in apophyseal joints, the posterior columns in the spinal cord, and multiple CNS connections) orients a person in space during position changes and while walking on uneven surfaces. Abnormalities in any component of the system may cause or exacerbate dysequilibrium. Whether age-related changes occur in peripheral nerves is unknown, although peripheral neuropathy is common in the elderly, especially from diabetes or vitamin B_{12} deficiency. The contribution of cervical mechanoreceptors to proprioception is not widely appreciated. The loss of normal afferent input from mechanoreceptors may result in a disturbance of postural sensation (sense of balance) and of kinesthesia (awareness of head and neck movement), on which precise control of voluntary movements such as walking depend. Whiplash injuries and cervical degenerative diseases (eg, spondylosis) may impair functioning of the cervical mechanoreceptors.

The CNS channels input data from the senses to the appropriate efferents in the musculoskeletal system. Given the multiple connections and their complexity, essentially any CNS disorder may contribute to instability or dizziness.

Systemic disorders may contribute to instability or dizziness by affecting the sensory, central, or effector components. In addition, systemic disorders may result in decreased cerebral perfusion or oxygen delivery, fatigue, confusion, or shortness of breath, which, in turn, may result in instability or dizziness. Common examples include electrolyte disorders, anemia, hypothyroidism, and acid-base disturbances. Cardiac arrhythmias or heart failure may compromise cerebral blood flow. Drugs may cause dizziness through several mechanisms, including postural hypotension, fatigue, dehydration, electrolyte disturbance, and disruption of CNS function.

Diagnosis

Diagnosis is best begun by considering, based on history and examination, whether a single cause (see TABLE 19–1) is likely, in which case specific diagnostic testing is warranted. If the history and examination do not suggest a specific cause, it is unlikely that exhaustive diagnostic testing will be helpful. The goal in most patients, therefore, is to identify and eliminate or ameliorate as many contributing factors as possible (see TABLE 19–2). This approach is based on the following assumptions: (1) the relative importance of individual contributors to dizziness often cannot be determined; (2) the presentation often does not permit identification of a specific cause, thus therapeutic trials are often the best way to determine significant contributors; and (3) ameliorating even a subset of contributors may reduce the dizziness.

History: The patient should be asked to describe the nature of the dizziness, including sensation, frequency and duration, any associated symptoms, any precipitating or provoking factors, and any predisposing exposures and diseases (see TABLE 19–2). However, patients often report more than one manifestation or a vague sensation. The patient should be screened for depression and anxiety, which may provoke or exacerbate the dizziness. A thorough review of all drugs, including

TABLE 19–1. SELECTED DISORDERS THAT CAUSE DIZZINESS*

Disorder	Description	Symptoms	Diagnosis	Treatment
Benign paroxysmal positional vertigo	A common peripheral vestibular disorder caused by particles of inner ear debris that produce bursts of neural activity with certain head positions (see also FIGURE 19–2)	Sudden and fleeting episodes of intense vertigo with specific head or body positions (eg, turning over in bed, looking upward); episodes last days to months and are often recurrent	Confirmed by the Hallpike maneuver (see text and FIGURE 19–3)	Vestibular rehabilitation lessens symptoms in most patients. Even without treatment, symptoms resolve within weeks to months but may recur. A short course of a vestibular suppressant (eg, meclizine) may be used for acute episodes
Meniere's disease	A vertiginous disorder of uncertain etiology characterized by excess endolymph within the cochlear and vestibular labyrinth	Variable, but may include sudden episodes of vertigo lasting a few hours; there are no symptoms between episodes	Strongly suspected if vertigo is accompanied by decreased hearing, tinnitus, and/or a feeling of fullness in one ear. An audiogram revealing sensorineural hearing loss (low, more than high, frequencies) is confirmatory	Salt restriction and diuretics. During acute attacks, vestibular suppressants may be used to relieve vertigo. Surgical interventions, including endolymphatic decompression, vestibular nerve section, and labyrinthectomy, should be considered only in severely debilitating cases
Acoustic neuroma	A benign tumor of the 8th cranial nerve	Gradually progressive imbalance and hearing loss on the affected side are typical	Audiometry reveals asymmetric hearing loss, which should be further evaluated by MRI	Surgical excision

Disorder	Description	Clinical Features	Diagnosis	Treatment
Vertebrobas-ilar insufficiency	Obstruction to flow in the vertebrobasilar arteries, most commonly caused by arteriosclerosis, less commonly by cervical compression	Dizzy spells, usually accompanied by dysarthria or visual disturbances	Vestibular tests are nonspecific; arteriography is diagnostic	Depends on the cause and site of the lesion; hypertension should be controlled; anticoagulant therapy may be indicated
Cervical spondylosis (see also Ch. 50)	Any degenerative lesion of the cervical spine; etiology is unknown	Vertigo or other symptoms of dizziness may occur, together with numbness and tingling of the fingers, clumsiness with fine motor tasks, and, eventually, lower extremity findings. Neck pain, which is exacerbated by movement, is usually present. There may be a history of whiplash injury or other arthritic complaints	Neck range of motion is reduced; neurologic examination may reveal motor and sensory changes	Conservative measures such as soft cervical collars may help but should be avoided long term. Physical therapy is used to preserve and improve balance and gait as well as hand function. Surgery is performed only in those with progressive neurologic findings

*Carotid hypersensitivity, postprandial hypotension, and other cardiovascular disorders, which may cause presyncope, are discussed in Ch. 18.

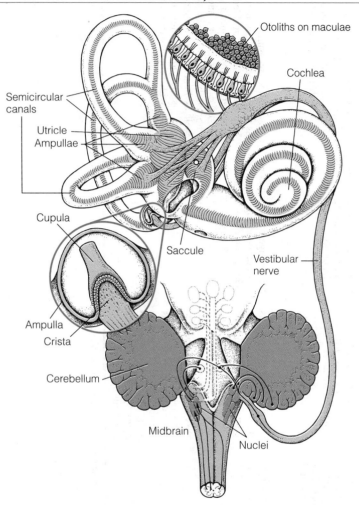

FIGURE 19–1.   The vestibular system. Maintenance of equilibrium depends in part on information provided by hair cells in the inner ear. A crista, located in the ampulla of each of the three semicircular canals, contains hair cells that are connected to fibers of the vestibular nerve. Angular acceleration (eg, rotation of the head) causes the endolymph of the semicircular canal to deflect the cupula of the appropriate canal. Deflection of the cupula increases or decreases (depending on the direction) the firing rate of the hair cells and thus that of the vestibular nerve. Two patches of neuroepithelium (maculae) located in the utricle and saccule contain hair cells embedded in a matrix topped with calciferous particles (otoconia). The mass of the otoconia makes the utricle and saccule sensitive to linear accelerations (eg, up-and-down movements, side-to-side movements, changes in the direction of gravity's pull when the head is tilted). The vestibular nuclei in the brain stem and parts of the cerebellum interpret changes in the firing rate of the vestibular nerve and produce compensatory movements of the eyes to maintain visual fixation and changes in muscle tone to maintain equilibrium.

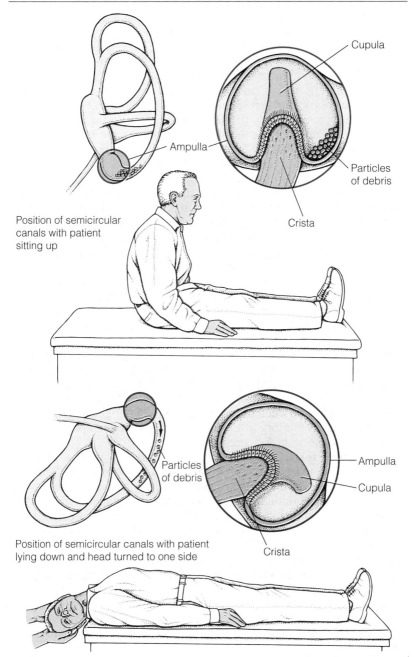

FIGURE 19–2.   Pathophysiology of benign paroxysmal positional vertigo.
Particles of debris in the inner ear produce bursts of neural activity when the head
moves to certain positions.

over-the-counter drugs (especially hypnotics, analgesics, and drugs used for colds and allergies), is also important.

Physical examination: Useful findings of the physical examination are listed in TABLE 19–2. Vestibular system abnormalities are difficult to detect clinically. The examiner should look for nystagmus occurring spontaneously or in response to changes in eye or body position. Because visual fixation can suppress nystagmus, Frenzel glasses (high-diopter lenses in a frame with a light source) are used if available. Two other methods of detecting vestibular dysfunction are checking visual acuity during head shaking and testing balance (eg, one leg or tandem stand) while standing on thick foam with eyes closed. However, the sensitivity and specificity of these two tests have not been determined.

Blood pressure and heart rate measurements should be taken after at least 5 minutes of quiet lying and then at 0 and 2 minutes after standing. A change of $\geq 20\%$ in mean postural blood pressure is most significant.

Neck range of motion, preferably in a standing position, should be determined. Decreased range of motion—with or without symptoms of dizziness or unsteadiness—may be due to a cervical process or, secondarily, to vestibular dysfunction (the sensation of dizziness on head turning can lead to decreased range of motion secondary to prolonged neck immobilization). Decreased head turning can interfere with central compensation; recognizing it is important because vestibular rehabilitation is helpful. [1]

Balance and gait should be evaluated, although most findings are nonspecific. [2] On testing, a performance that is poorer with eyes closed than with eyes open suggests a vestibular or proprioceptive problem. A steppage gait suggests proprioceptive deficits, as does an improvement in gait when the patient touches his fingertip to the examiner's fingertip. Vibratory testing is more sensitive than position sense testing for assessing proprioception.

Provocative tests: Attempts can be made to induce dizziness through various maneuvers. Hyperventilation is not particularly helpful because it may induce dizziness in many elderly patients, with or without a history of chronic dizziness. The Hallpike maneuver involves a rapid change in position from seated to supine with the head hanging 45° to the right or left (see FIGURE 19–3). The occurrence of nystagmus (and often vertigo), which lasts 10 to 30 seconds, after a few seconds of latency indicates a positive response. A positive response in any of the head positions confirms the suspected diagnosis of benign paroxysmal positional vertigo.

Laboratory evaluation and specialized testing: A CBC, thyroid function tests, and glucose and vitamin B_{12} levels should be obtained for all elderly persons presenting with chronic dizziness. Indications for

[1] see page 194   [2] see also page 206

ECG, Holter monitoring, carotid sinus massage, and tilt table testing are discussed in Ch. 18. However, abnormal findings are common among elderly patients with or without dizziness, and abnormal results may or may not correspond to the complaint of dizziness in this age group. Cerebral CT or MRI should be performed only if the history and physical examination suggest a cerebral lesion. Audiometry is useful in identifying the severity and type of hearing loss; specific findings may also indicate Meniere's disease or acoustic neuroma.

Vestibular testing, including caloric testing, electronystagmography, rotational testing, and computerized posturography, can be considered in patients with history or physical examination findings suggestive of vestibular disease.

Caloric testing assesses the symmetry of vestibular function. Each ear is stimulated with 250 mL of first warm (44° C [111° F]) and then cool (30° C [86° F]) water, each instilled over 40 seconds. The ear that shows a shorter duration or lower frequency of nystagmus is presumed to be the diseased ear.

Rotational testing uses a series of well-controlled rotational stimuli to provoke nystagmus. Findings can reveal the degree of peripheral or central vestibular dysfunction; serial measurements can be used to detect worsening of the dysfunction.

Electronystagmography, in which eye movements are recorded on an ECG-like tracing from electrodes placed around the eyes, is used to observe vestibular nystagmus during provocative testing.

In computerized posturography, the patient stands on a platform that is imbedded with four sensors to monitor sway. Testing with the eyes closed or with a moving screen while the platform is synchronized to patient movement eliminates visual and proprioceptive information. This approach examines balance that is principally dependent on vestibular input. Other testing combinations examine visual and proprioceptive inputs to balance. Functional deficits defined by posturography can thus indicate visual, proprioceptive, or vestibular deficits, which require further testing to determine specific diagnoses.

Prognosis and Treatment

Although chronic dizziness may be a symptom of significant disease, it does not per se increase the risk of death. However, it does have adverse physical, psychologic, and social consequences. It increases the risk of falls and fear of falling, decreases performance in activities of daily living, and reduces participation in social activities. The primary goal of treatment is to reduce dizziness sufficiently to minimize the physical, psychologic, and social morbidity.

Treatment is ideally directed toward a specific cause. However, because the etiology is usually multifactorial, the most effective treatment is often to ameliorate one or more contributing factors (see TABLE 19–1). Even partial amelioration of the dizziness may help. Because

TABLE 19–2. POSSIBLE CONTRIBUTORS TO CHRONIC DIZZINESS

Contributor	History	Examination	Possible Causes	Potential Interventions
Vision	Use of bifocals or trifocals	Abnormalities in near/distant acuity; contrast sensitivity; depth perception	Cataract; glaucoma; macular degeneration; perceptual difficulties with glasses	Appropriate refraction; consider avoiding bifocals or trifocals; drugs for glaucoma; surgery; good lighting without glare
Hearing	Deafness in one or both ears; difficulty hearing in social situations	Abnormal findings with Rinne's test, Weber's test, whisper test, or audiometry	Presbycusis; otosclerosis	Hearing aid; surgery (for otosclerosis); hearing rehabilitation; listening devices
Vestibulo-cochlear system	True vertigo; worse in dark or with specific head positions; tinnitus; history of aminoglycosides, furosemide, aspirin use; ear surgery; ear or mastoid infections	Nystagmus (horizontal or rotary nystagmus suggests a peripheral vestibular disorder; vertical nystagmus suggests a central disorder); decreased neck range of motion; decreased hearing; abnormal Hallpike maneuver; abnormal vestibular testing	Drug toxicity; previous infections; tumor (eg, acoustic neuroma); previous surgery; vascular (eg, brain stem infarct); benign positional vertigo; Meniere's disease	Avoid toxic drugs and long-term vestibular suppressants; remove earwax; vestibular rehabilitation; surgery
Peripheral nerves	Worse in dark or on uneven surfaces or inclines	Decreased position sense or vibration; steppage gait; finger-to-finger gait test	Diabetes; vitamin B$_{12}$ deficiency; hypothyroidism; syphilis; most often, unknown etiology	Treatment of underlying disease; appropriate walking aid and footwear; good lighting; balance exercises; gait training
Cervical spine	Same as for peripheral nerves; neck pain; worse with head turning; whiplash injury; other arthritic complaints	Decreased neck range of motion; signs of radiculopathy or myelopathy; clumsiness with fine motor tasks; mild spastic gait; increased tone	Spondylosis; degenerative or inflammatory arthritis	Treatment of underlying disease; cervical or balance exercises; consider surgery

	Symptoms	Signs	Causes	Treatment
Cerebral hypoperfusion	Presyncope; near fainting	Postural hypotension; signs of underlying disease (eg, obstructive pulmonary disease, heart failure)	See causes for syncope in Ch. 18	Treatment of underlying disease
Hypotension				
Postprandial	Symptoms within 1 h of eating	Hypotension after meals	Postprandial hypotension (see Ch. 86)	Small meals; avoid exertion after meals; avoid hypotensive drugs near meals; have caffeine with meals
Postural	Near fainting—worse when getting up, walking, exercising; complaints consistent with predisposing diseases; may be asymptomatic; history of predisposing drugs	Blood pressure and heart rate; signs of predisposing diseases	Drugs, volume/salt depletion; deconditioning; Parkinson's syndrome; diabetes; autonomic dysfunction; vasovagal attack	Treatment of salt and water repletion; reconditioning exercises; ankle pumps or hand clenching; slow rising; elevate head of bed; graduated stockings; lowest effective dosage of essential contributing drugs
Cardiac dysfunction	Variable, depending on specific etiology	Cardiac auscultation, ECG, echocardiography	Cardiac arrhythmias, valvular lesions, myocardial ischemia, myxoma, hypertrophic cardiomyopathy	Variable, depending on specific etiology
Brain stem	Any sensation (eg, vertigo, near fainting, wooziness); transient neurologic symptoms (eg, slurred speech, visual change, one-sided weakness); symptoms on looking up	Findings may be transient or fixed; ataxia	Transient ischemic attack; brain stem infarct; vertebrobasilar insufficiency	Low-dose aspirin; assistive device if ataxic

Table continues on the following page.

TABLE 19–2. POSSIBLE CONTRIBUTORS TO CHRONIC DIZZINESS *(Continued)*

Contributor	History	Examination	Possible Causes	Potential Interventions
Metabolic/respiratory diseases	Symptoms of underlying disease	Signs of underlying disease	Any (especially chronic obstructive pulmonary disease, heart failure, thyroid disorders, diabetes, renal disorders, anemia)	Treatment of underlying disease
Medications Past	Vestibulocochlear symptoms (see above)	See above under vestibulocochlear system	See above under vestibulocochlear system	See above under vestibulocochlear system
Current	Confusion; fatigue; weakness; dizziness often vague, may be constant	May have postural hypotension	Specific: Nitrates, β-blockers, antidepressants, antipsychotics, anticholinergics; vestibular depressants, benzodiazepines, ?others General: Total number and dose of all drugs	Eliminate, substitute, or reduce specific offending drugs if possible; reduce all other drugs to lowest effective dose possible; remember over-the-counter drugs
Depression, anxiety	Constant dizziness; multiple somatic complaints; poor concentration; positive results on anxiety or depression screening; vegetative complaints (sleep, appetite)	See Chs. 33 and 34	Depression, anxiety	Thorough consideration of risks and benefits of antidepressant drug; counseling

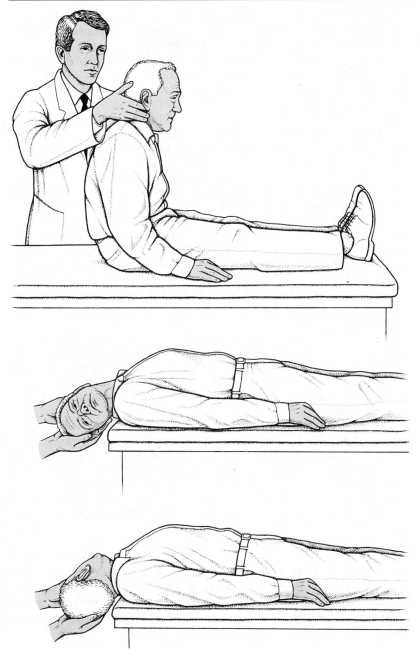

FIGURE 19–3.   **Hallpike maneuver.** Each position is held for at least 10 seconds.

adverse drug effects may contribute to many cases of chronic dizziness, attempts should be made to eliminate as many drugs as possible, to substitute less offending ones, or to reduce the doses.

Drugs: Vestibular depressants (eg, meclizine, diazepam) have little role in the treatment of chronic dizziness. Because of their effects on the CNS and because they may suppress central adaptation, these drugs may even exacerbate dizziness. However, patients with severe unilateral peripheral vestibular dysfunction may benefit from a benzodiazepine.

Rehabilitation and exercise: Vestibular rehabilitation includes combinations of exercises involving head and eye movements while sitting or standing. It also involves various dynamic balance exercises and exercises to improve gait stability during head movement, visual and vestibular interactions, and vestibular spinal responses. Initially, the exercises may worsen the dizziness, but over time (weeks to months) movement-related dizziness improves, likely because of central adaptation. Vestibular rehabilitation has been shown to be effective in most vestibular disorders of central or peripheral origin. Vestibular rehabilitation can be administered in a classroom setting or one to one with a physical therapist. Alternatively, patients can perform the exercises independently at home after being instructed by a physical therapist, who must ensure that the patient can adhere to the program safely and effectively.

Cervical exercises may be effective for patients with cervical spondylosis. Progressive, competency-based balance exercises have proved effective at enhancing the sense of stability and may be useful for patients with dizziness related to sensory and/or motor deficits. When proprioception is impaired, the use of a cane is indicated to provide stability.

Patient education: Patients should be reminded to avoid over-the-counter drugs that may exacerbate dizziness. If postural hypotension is identified, patients should be instructed to rise slowly (the time required for stabilization varies from a few seconds to several minutes). Hand clenching and ankle dorsiflexion exercises performed before standing and the use of support stockings may also help. These patients should also be taught to avoid hot showers or baths and to reduce salt restriction in situations that might lead to dehydration (eg, hot weather, diarrhea, vomiting).

Patients should be instructed on which activities to avoid. Movements such as looking up, reaching up, or bending down are to be avoided, in part by storing items at home strategically. However, patients should be cautioned not to habitually avoid other movements, such as head turning. Avoiding these movements may compromise central adaptation, thereby exacerbating dizziness.

Often, falls go unrecognized by health care practitioners because a specific evaluation for them is not included in the routine history and physical examination and because many persons who fall do not have an obvious injury. Many patients are reluctant to seek assistance because the injury was minimal, because they attribute falling to the aging process, or because they fear being subsequently restricted in their activities or being institutionalized.

Epidemiology

Falls in the elderly are a major public health problem with substantial medical and economic consequences. In 1994, the cost was > $20 billion; in 2020, the cost is projected to be > $32 billion. Annually, about one third of elderly persons living in the community fall. The rate of falls for nursing home residents is about three times higher; the mean is 1.5 falls per bed per year. The rate of falls for elderly hospitalized patients is between the rate for elderly persons living in the community and the rate for elderly nursing home residents. One reason for a higher rate of falls for elderly persons in nursing homes and in hospitals is the greater frailty of these persons; another may be increased reporting in these settings.

In the USA, falls are the leading cause of accidental death and the seventh leading cause of death in persons ≥ 65 years. Seventy-five percent of deaths caused by falls occur in the 12.5% of the population that are ≥ 65. The rate of death due to falls rises exponentially with increasing age for both sexes and for all racial groups ≥ 75.

Most falls occur indoors. No specific time of day or time of year is associated with falling. Among the elderly, most falls occur during usual activities such as walking. Indoor falls occur most often in the bathroom, bedroom, and kitchen. About 10% of falls occur on stairs, with descent being more hazardous than ascent. The first and last steps are the most dangerous. Common sites of outdoor falls are curbs and steps. In institutions, the most common sites of falls are the bedside (during transfers into or out of bed) and the bathroom.

Etiology

By definition, a fall excludes events caused by syncope, ▮ although a person who falls may lose consciousness as a result of the fall. A fall is usually caused by a complex interaction among intrinsic factors (individual disorders—see TABLE 20–1), extrinsic factors (environmental hazards), and situational factors (related to the activity of daily living being performed). For example, an elderly woman with osteoarthritis and Parkinson's disease (intrinsic factors) may trip over the edge of a

---

▮see page 173

TABLE 20–1.   SELECTED DISORDERS CONTRIBUTING TO RISK OF FALLS

Disorder	Function Impaired
Dementia	Central processing
Parkinson's disease, stroke, myelopathy (such as that due to cervical or lumbar spondylosis), cerebellar degeneration, carotid sinus hypersensitivity, peripheral neuropathy, vertebrobasilar insufficiency	Neuromotor
Cataract, glaucoma, age-related macular degeneration	Vision
Acute labyrinthitis, Meniere's disease, benign paroxysmal positional vertigo, hearing loss	Vestibular
Peripheral neuropathy (such as that due to diabetes mellitus), vitamin B_{12} deficiency	Proprioception
Arthritis, foot deformities, corns, calluses, bunions	Musculoskeletal
Postural hypotension, metabolic disorders (eg, thyroid disorders), cardiopulmonary disorders, other acute illness (eg, sepsis)	Systemic

rug (extrinsic factor) while walking to the bathroom at night (situational factor). The main contributor to the risk of falls is the presence of intrinsic factors.

Intrinsic factors include age-related changes and disorders that affect functions needed to maintain balance. These functions include vestibular, proprioceptive, and visual function, which are integrated in the cerebellum; cognition and musculoskeletal function are also important. Thus, arthritis of the legs (with associated pain and limited range of motion and strength) and dementia (with associated lack of judgment, distraction, and confusion) contribute to the risk of falls. Dizziness is common in the elderly.∎

Orthostatic hypotension, which is common among the elderly, is not a common cause of falls, but it often causes affected persons to sit down because of light-headedness. Frequent nocturia is associated with falls, probably because the elderly person has difficulty getting up and walking to the bathroom quickly at night. Metabolic disorders (eg, thyroid, glucose, and electrolyte disorders); anemia and dehydration; and cardiopulmonary disorders (eg, myocardial infarction, arrhythmias, heart failure, pneumonia, emphysema [particularly if acute or decompensated]) may also contribute to increased risk of falls, as may acute illnesses.

Elderly persons who fall in institutions are usually more physically impaired and are exposed to fewer extrinsic factors; thus, intrinsic factors (eg, weakness, balance disorders) contribute the most to the risk of falls and fall-related injury. The use of restraints may increase the risk

∎ see page 181

TABLE 20-2.   DRUGS CONTRIBUTING TO RISK OF FALLS

Mechanism	Drugs
Reduce alertness or retard central processing	Analgesics (especially opioids) Psychoactive drugs (especially antidepressants, long-acting benzodiazepines, phenothiazines)
Impair cerebral perfusion	Antihypertensives (especially vasodilators) Antiarrhythmics Diuretics (especially when the patient is dehydrated)
Contribute to direct vestibular toxicity	Aminoglycosides High-dose loop diuretics
Induce extrapyramidal syndromes	Phenothiazines

of falls because patients struggle to free themselves, and the use of bed rails may increase the risk of falls because patients try to climb over them.

The use of drugs is a major risk factor for falls; the risk of falling increases with the number of prescribed drugs. Psychoactive drugs are the drugs most commonly reported as increasing the risk of falls and hip fractures. Drugs may be categorized by their primary mechanism of effect (see TABLE 20-2).

Extrinsic factors are implicated in up to 50% of falls. Elderly persons living in the community tend to be exposed to greater environmental challenges and more extrinsic factors and tend to be less physically impaired; thus, extrinsic factors contribute the most to risk of falls and fall-related injury. Extrinsic and intrinsic factors interact to contribute to the risk of falls and fall-related injury when extrinsic factors are present, when the environment or tasks performed demand greater postural control and mobility, when situations require changing positions (eg, transferring, turning), when the patient takes risks (eg, walking in stocking feet), and when the patient relocates to a nursing home. Moreover, the faller's tolerance of risk becomes increasingly important.

Situational factors also affect the severity of a fall-related injury. For example, an elderly person is more likely to be seriously injured when falling from an upright position, because more energy is dissipated, or when falling laterally, because impact on the hip is direct.

Complications

Falls may result in injury, including fractures.[1] Up to 2% of falls result in the fracture of a hip; other fractures (eg, in the humerus, wrist,

[1] see page 212

and pelvis) can occur in up to 5% of falls. Serious injuries (eg, head and internal injuries, laceration) can occur in up to 10% of falls. Over 50% of falls among elderly persons result in at least some minor injury.

Quality of life may deteriorate drastically after a fall; at least 50% of elderly persons who were ambulatory before fracturing a hip do not recover their prefracture level of mobility. If elderly persons remain on the floor for a time after a fall, dehydration, pressure sores, rhabdomyolysis, hypothermia, and pneumonia may result.

Elderly persons who fall, particularly those who fall repeatedly, tend to have deficits in activities of daily living and instrumental activities of daily living ◘ and are at high risk of subsequent hospitalization, further disability, institutionalization, and death. Fall-related injuries account for about 5% of hospitalizations in patients ≥ 65. About 5% of elderly persons with hip fractures die while hospitalized; overall mortality in the 12 months after a hip fracture ranges from 12 to 67%.

Falls that do not result in serious injury may still have serious consequences. Elderly persons may fear falling again, which can lead to reduced mobility because of a loss of confidence. Some persons may even avoid certain activities (eg, shopping, cleaning) because of this fear. Decreased activity can increase joint stiffness and weakness, further compromising mobility. Falls are reported to be a contributing factor in 40% of nursing home admissions.

Diagnosis

Because the elderly often do not report falls, they should be asked about them as a routine part of screening. When falls are reported, acute injuries should be evaluated first. Next, the history and physical examination should focus on intrinsic, situational, and extrinsic factors.

History: Open-ended questions are asked during the initial inquiry about the fall, followed by more specific questions about when and where the fall occurred and what the patient was doing. Typical questions include

- Did the patient experience any premonitory or associated symptoms such as palpitations, shortness of breath, chest pain, vertigo, or light-headedness at the time of the fall?
- Were any obvious extrinsic factors involved?
- Did the patient incur an injury and was he able to get up?
- Does the patient have a history of falls?

The history should also include questions about present and past medical problems and drug use. Witnesses to the fall should be questioned.

◘ see also page 42

Physical examination: The physical examination should be comprehensive enough to exclude obvious intrinsic causes of falls. The pattern of injury is useful. Evaluating the cardiovascular system helps exclude arrhythmia, valvular heart disease, and heart failure. Blood pressure is measured with the patient supine and standing to rule out orthostatic hypotension. Vision screening, at least for acuity, is essential. The neck, spine, and extremities should be evaluated for deformities, pain, and limitation in range of motion.

A formal neurologic assessment includes assessment of muscle strength and tone, sensation (including proprioception), coordination (including cerebellar function), and station and gait. [1] Basic postural control and the proprioceptive and vestibular systems are evaluated using the Romberg test (in which the patient stands with feet together and eyes closed). Tests to establish high-level balance function include the one-legged stance and tandem gait. If the patient can stand on one leg for 30 seconds with the eyes open and have an accurate 10-foot tandem gait, the intrinsic postural control deficit is likely to be minimal. Vestibular function should be evaluated. [2] Evaluation of mental status is also indicated. [3] Because falling may be an atypical presentation of an acute illness, occult causes such as infection, myocardial infarction, dehydration, and anemia also are sought.

Performance-based functional assessment: Low scores on these tests [4] may indicate increased risk of falls.

Laboratory testing: Tests such as ECGs, ambulatory cardiac monitoring, measurement of cardiac enzymes, and echocardiograms are recommended only when a cardiac source is suspected. A CBC, blood electrolytes, and tests for occult blood in stool are useful only when systemic disease is suspected. Spine x-rays, CT or MRI of the head, and EEG are only indicated when the history and physical examination detect new neurologic abnormalities.

Prevention and Prognosis

Few data exist regarding the cost-effectiveness of diagnostic evaluation in predicting or preventing falls. Interventions attempt to improve functional capacity, prevent or decrease the number of falls, and minimize fall-related injury. However, the patient's independence is sometimes altered (eg, for safety, ambulating in inclement weather conditions is discouraged). Although falls may not be completely eliminated, severity of injury, hospitalization, and comorbid impairments can be reduced using the interventions discussed below.

Treatment

If falls are caused by intrinsic factors, interventions focus on decreasing disease-related impairment and providing physical therapy. Inter-

---

[1] see page 36   [2] see page 188   [3] see page 343   [4] see Table 21–2 on page 210

TABLE 20-3. HOME ASSESSMENT CHECKLIST FOR FALL HAZARDS

Location	Hazard	Correction	Rationale
General household			
Lighting	Too dim	Provide ample lighting in all areas	Improves visual acuity and contrast sensitivity
	Too direct, creating glare	Reduce glare with evenly distributed light, indirect lighting, or translucent shades	Improves visual acuity and contrast sensitivity
	Light switches inaccessible	Install switches that are immediately accessible when entering room	Reduces risk of falls when walking across dark room
Carpets, rugs	Torn	Repair or replace torn carpet	Reduces risk of tripping and slipping for persons with decreased stepping ability
	Slippery	Provide rugs with non-skid backs; tack down to prevent curling	Reduces risk of tripping and slipping
Chairs, tables	Unstable	Use those stable enough to support weight of person leaning on table edges or chair arms and backs; avoid chairs with wheels; repair legs that are loose	Increases support for persons with impaired balance; aids transfer
	Lack of armrests	Provide chairs with armrests that extend forward enough for leverage when getting up or sitting down	Assists persons with proximal muscle weakness; aids transfer
	Low-back chairs	Provide high-back chairs	Increases support for neck and while transferring weight; prevents patients with parkinsonism from falling backward because of rocking movements
Furniture	Obstructs path	Arrange furnishings so that pathways are not obstructed; avoid cluttered hallways	Helps persons with impaired peripheral vision be more mobile
		Maintain temperature at 22.2° C (72° F) in winter	Reduces risk of falls secondary to hypothermia

TABLE 20–3. (*Continued*)

Location	Hazard	Correction	Rationale
Kitchen			
Cabinets, shelves	Too high	Keep frequently used items at waist level; install shelves, cupboards at accessible height	Reduces risk of falls because of frequent reaching or standing on unstable ladders or chairs
Floors	Wet or waxed	Place rubber mat on floor in sink area; wear rubber-soled shoes in kitchen; use nonslip wax or buff paste wax thoroughly	Reduces risk of slipping, especially for persons with a gait disorder
Gas range	Dial difficult to see	Clearly mark "on" and "off" positions on dials	Reduces risk of gas asphyxiation, especially if sense of smell is impaired
Table	Wobbly, unstable	Install table with sturdy legs of even length; avoid tripod or pedestal tables	Increases support for persons with a gait disorder
Bathroom			
Bathtub	Slippery tub floor	Install skid-resistant strips or rubber mat; use shower shoes or bath seat	Reduces risk of sliding on wet tub floor; reduces risk of falls (eg, persons with impaired balance can sit while showering)
	Side of bathtub used for support or transfer	Use portable grab bar on side of tub; take grab bar on trips	Aids transfers
Towel racks, sink tops	Unstable for use as support while transferring from toilet	Fasten grab rails to wall studs next to toilet	Aids transfer to and from toilet
Toilet seat	Too low	Use elevated toilet seat	Aids transfer to and from toilet
Medicine cabinet	Inadequate lighting	Install brighter lighting	Helps avoid incorrect administration of drugs, especially for persons with visual impairment
	Drugs improperly labeled	Label all drugs according to need for inter-	Helps avoid incorrect administration of

Table continues on the following page.

TABLE 20–3.   HOME ASSESSMENT CHECKLIST FOR FALL HAZARDS (*Continued*)

Location	Hazard	Correction	Rationale
Bathroom (*continued*)		nal or external use; keep magnifying glass in or near cabinet	drugs, especially for persons with visual impairment
Door	Locks	Remove locks from bathroom doors or use locks that can be opened from both sides of door	Enables others to enter if fall occurs
Stairways			
Height	Height of steps too high	Correct step height to < 6 inches	Reduces risk of tripping for persons with decreased stepping ability
Handrails	Missing	Install and anchor well on both sides of stairway; use cylindrical rails placed 1 to 2 inches away from wall	Provides support; enables persons to grasp rail with either hand
	Improper length	Extend beyond top and bottom step, and turn ends inward	Signals that top or bottom step has been reached
Configuration	Too steep or too long	Provide stairways with intermediate landings	Rest stop especially convenient for patients with cardiac or pulmonary disorders
Condition	Slippery	Place nonskid treads securely on all steps	Prevents slipping
Lighting	Inadequate	Install adequate lighting at both top and bottom of stairway; night-lights or bright-colored adhesive strips can be used to clearly mark steps	Outlines location of steps, especially for persons with impaired vision or perception

ventions that may help include the use of dopaminergic drugs if the falls are due to Parkinson's disease and pain management, physical therapy, and surgery if the falls are due to osteoarthritis. Correcting visual impairment may also help. Discontinuation of drugs that may increase the risk of falls or adjustment of their dosage is recommended. Physical therapy or an exercise program that includes balance and gait training and training in the use of canes and walkers may be useful.∎ Interven-

∎ see also pages 294 and 295

tion strategies that include exercise (especially balance training) may reduce the incidence of falls by 10%.

Patient and caregiver issues: Assessing an elderly person's home for fall hazards and correcting them are helpful (see TABLE 20–3). Wheelchair adaptations, removable belts, and wedge seating can sometimes prevent persons from falling but limit mobility less than restraints do. Surveillance by a caregiver or nurse, particularly of patients for whom restraints are being considered, may be useful. Motion detectors may be used, but they require that a caregiver be present to respond to the triggered alarm.

Padding worn over the hip may help protect elderly persons who have fallen and are at risk of a hip injury. Compliant flooring materials can help dissipate the impact force; however, a floor that is too compliant may be destabilizing. A multifactorial approach that combines medical, rehabilitative, environmental, and intervention strategies is often best.

Patients should be taught what to do if they fall and cannot get up. Useful techniques include turning from the supine position to the prone position, getting on all fours, crawling to a strong support surface, and pulling up. Having frequent contact with family or friends, a phone that can be reached from the floor, or a remote alarm system can decrease the likelihood of lying on the floor for a long time after a fall.

21 GAIT DISORDERS

A slowing of gait speed or a deviation in smoothness, symmetry, or synchrony of body movement.

For the elderly, walking, standing up from a chair, turning, and leaning are necessary for independent mobility. Gait speed, chair rise time, and the ability to perform tandem stance (one foot in front of the other) are independent predictors of the ability to perform instrumental activities of daily living (IADLs)—eg, the ability to shop, travel, and cook. Gait speed, chair rise time, and balance are also predictors of the risk of nursing home admission and death.

Walking without assistance requires the effective coordination of adequate sensation, musculoskeletal and motor control, and attention.

Normal Age-Related Changes in Gait

Gait velocity (the speed of walking) remains stable until about age 70; it then declines about 15% per decade for usual gait and 20% per decade for maximal gait. Velocity is lower because elderly people take shorter steps. Several explanations have been proposed for the shortened step length. ∎

∎ see page 205

Cadence (the rhythm of walking) does not change with age. Each person has a preferred cadence, which relates to leg length and usually represents the most energy-efficient rhythm for individual body structure. Tall people take longer steps at a slower cadence; short people take shorter steps at a faster cadence.

Double stance (when both feet are on the ground—also referred to as double support) increases with age—from 18% in young adults to $\geq$ 26% in healthy elderly persons. During double stance, the center of mass is between the feet, which is a stable position. Increased time in the double stance position reduces momentum and therefore reduces time for the swing leg to advance and contributes to short step length. Increased double stance may be needed on uneven terrain or with impaired balance so that step length is sacrificed for stability. Elderly persons with a fear of falling increase their double stance time. Double stance time is a strong predictor of gait velocity and step length.

Walking posture (the body position during walking) changes only slightly with age. Unless elderly persons have diseases such as osteoporosis with kyphosis, they walk upright, with no forward lean. They walk with greater anterior (downward) pelvic rotation, which results in an increase in lumbar lordosis possibly due to a combination of increased abdominal fat, abdominal muscle weakness, and tight hip flexor muscles. Elderly persons also walk with about a 5° greater "toe out," possibly due to a loss of hip internal rotation or to a strategy to increase lateral stability. Foot clearance in swing is the same in elderly as in younger persons.

Joint motion changes with age. Ankle plantar flexion is reduced during the late stage of stance (just before the back foot lifts off), although maximal ankle dorsiflexion is not reduced. The overall motion of the knee is unchanged. Hip motion is unchanged in the sagittal plane but in the frontal plane shows greater adduction. Pelvic motion is reduced in the frontal and transverse planes, and transverse plane rotation is reduced.

Step length is shorter in the elderly. One explanation is that calf muscles are weak and cannot produce sufficient plantar flexion. Another is that elderly persons are reluctant to generate plantar flexion power because of poor balance and poor control of the center of mass during single stance.

Etiology and Symptoms

In health, the movement of the body is usually symmetrical. Step length, cadence, torso movement, and ankle, knee, hip, and pelvis motion are equal on the right and left sides.

Symmetry of motion and timing between left and right sides is often lost, producing regular asymmetry with unilateral neurologic or musculoskeletal disorders. Symmetric short step length usually indicates a bilateral problem. Unpredictable or highly variable gait cadence, step lengths, and stride widths indicate breakdown of motor control of gait due to a cerebellar or frontal lobe syndrome.

Pseudoclaudication symptoms—pain, weakness, and numbness with walking that improves when sitting down—may be caused by spinal stenosis. Spinal stenosis may be due to pressure or tension on portions of the spinal cord in the cervical or lumbar region.∎

Difficulties in initiation of gait may represent isolated gait initiation failure, evidence of Parkinson's disease, or evidence of frontal or subcortical disease. The prevalence of parkinsonian signs (bradykinesia and rigidity) is high in the elderly, increasing sharply after age 75. Once gait is initiated, steps are continuous, with little variability in the timing of the steps. Freezing, stopping, or almost stopping usually suggests a cautious gait, a fear of falling, or a frontal gait disorder.

Gait initiation failure due to high-level sensorimotor (frontal lobe or white matter) disorder may progress to other abnormalities, including stiff posture with short steps, retropulsion (falling backward) in stance, weak or poor corrective responses to perturbations of balance when walking, and a highly variable and unstable gait pattern. Normal-pressure hydrocephalus should be considered if cognitive deficits and urinary incontinence are present in combination with high-level sensorimotor gait disorders. CT or MRI helps determine if lacunar infarcts, white matter disease, or focal atrophy is present and can help determine if normal-pressure hydrocephalus should be considered.

Footdrop secondary to anterior tibialis weakness or reduced knee flexion may cause low foot swing. The cause may be spasticity or lowering of the pelvis due to muscle weakness of the proximal muscles on the stance side (particularly gluteus medius).

Short step length is nonspecific and may represent a fear of falling or a neurologic or musculoskeletal problem. The side with short step length is usually the healthy side, and the short step is usually due to a problem during the stance phase of the opposite leg. For example, a patient with a weak or painful left leg spends less time in single stance on the left leg and develops less power to move the body forward. A shorter swing time for the right leg and a shorter step result. The normal right leg propels the left side forward; a normal single stance duration provides a normal swing time for the left leg, and the forward propulsion of the body by the hip and ankle results in a longer step for the left leg than for the right leg.

Irregular and unpredictable trunk instability can be caused by cerebellar, subcortical, and basal ganglia dysfunction. A consistent or predictable trunk lean to the side of the stance leg may be a strategy with which to reduce joint pain due to hip arthritis or, less commonly, knee arthritis (antalgic gait). In a hemiparetic gait, the trunk may lean to the strong side. In this pattern, the patient leans to lift the pelvis on the

---

∎ see also page 488

opposite side to permit the limb with spasticity (inability to flex the knee) to clear the floor during the swing phase. **Deviations from path** are strong indicators of motor control deficits. Wide stride width can be caused by cerebellar disease, if the width is consistent. Variable stride width suggests poor motor control, which may be due to frontal or subcortical gait disorders.

Diagnosis

Diagnosis is best approached in four parts:

* Discuss the patient's complaints, fears, and goals related to mobility
* Observe gait with and without an assistive device (if safe)
* Assess all components of gait (see TABLE 21–1)
* Observe gait again with a knowledge of the patient's gait components

The goal is to determine as many potential contributing factors to gait disorders as possible. A performance-oriented assessment tool may be helpful (see TABLE 21–2), as may other tests (eg, a screening cognitive examination for patients with gait problems due to frontal lobe syndromes).

Clinical examination: Routine assessment can be performed by a primary care physician; an expert may be needed for complex gait disorders. Assessment requires a straight hallway without distractions and a stopwatch for timing. A measuring tape and a T square or ruler with a right angle may be needed to measure stride length. Measurement of gait kinetics can only be performed reliably in a few laboratories with advanced computer and video technology.

The patient should be prepared for the examination—he should be wearing pants or shorts that reveal the knees. He should be informed that several observations may be needed and should be allowed to rest if fatigued.

Assistive devices provide stability but also affect gait. Use of walkers often results in a flexed posture and discontinuous gait, particularly if the walker has no wheels. If safe to do so, the health care practitioner can instruct the patient to walk without an assistive device, while remaining close. If a patient uses a cane, the health care practitioner can walk with the patient on the cane side or take his arm and walk with him.

Balance is impaired if the patient is unable to perform tandem stance or single leg stance for ≥ 5 seconds.

Proximal muscle strength is tested by having the patient get out of a chair without using his arms.

Gait velocity is measured using a stopwatch. A fixed distance (preferably 6 or 8 meters) is marked. Gait velocity in healthy elderly persons ranges from 1.5 to 1.1 meters/second.

Cadence is measured as steps/minute. Cadence varies with leg length—from about 90 steps/minute for tall adults (72 inches) to about 125 steps/minute for short adults (60 inches).

Step length (the distance from one heel strike to the next) can be measured or observed. Because shorter people take shorter steps and foot size is directly related to height, the easiest way to gauge step length is to measure or calculate the patient's foot length; normal step length is three foot lengths. The following equation calculates average step length in centimeters: $10 \times$ velocity $\times$ time to take 10 steps. An equivalent calculation is $0.16 \times$ velocity $\times$ cadence (steps/minute).

Step height can be assessed by observing the swing foot; if it touches the floor, the patient may trip. Some patients with fear of falling or a cautious gait syndrome will purposefully slide their feet over the floor surface.

Asymmetry or variability of gait rhythm can be detected when the health care practitioner whispers "dum...dum...dum" to himself with each of the patient's foot contacts. Some health care practitioners have a better ear than an eye for rhythm.

Prevention and Treatment

Although no large-scale prospective studies have confirmed the effect of increasing physical activity on gait and independence, prospective cohort studies provide convincing evidence that high levels of physical activity help maintain mobility, even in patients with disease.[1] Walking may be the most important training to prescribe. The importance of deconditioning and the effects of inactivity cannot be overstated. A regular walking program of 30 minutes/day is the best single activity for maintaining mobility. A safe walking course should be recommended. The patient should be instructed to increase gait speed and duration over 4 months. Patients using assistive devices need to be trained by therapists.

Prevention also includes stretching, resistance training, and balance exercises for joint range of motion, muscle power, and motor control. The positive psychologic effects are difficult to measure but are probably just as important.

Although determining why gait is abnormal is important, interventions to alter gait are not always indicated. A slowed, aesthetically abnormal gait may enable the elderly person to walk safely and without assistance.

Frail elderly persons with mobility problems achieve modest improvements with exercise programs. Knee pain lessens in elderly persons with arthritis; gait may improve with regular walking or resistance exercises.

Resistance exercises, implemented by physical therapists, can improve strength and gait velocity, especially in frail patients with

[1] see also page 296

TABLE 21-1. TREATMENT OF GAIT DISORDERS

Component	Common Problem	Treatment	Comment
Bone structure	Kyphosis	Thoracic extension, shoulder rotation, chin tuck exercises; osteoporosis treatment to prevent new compression fractures	Can be diagnosed by measuring bone density
	Leg length differences	Heel lift	
	Severe genu varus or valgus	Orthotics, bracing, quadriceps strengthening	Review knee replacement criteria
	Foot abnormality/pain, hallux valgus (loss of longitudinal arch)	Orthotics, podiatry care, custom shoes	
Joint range of motion	Decreased hip internal rotation	Stretch not usually therapeutic; stretch adductors and strengthen abductors	
	Decreased hip extension	Stretch hip flexors, strengthen hip extensors	
	Decreased ankle dorsiflexion	Stretch calf muscles	
	Hallux rigidus (loss of dorsiflexion of great toe)	Podiatry or orthopedic referral	
Muscle power	Weak hip extension	Chair rise exercises	Chair rise test may be helpful in diagnosis
	Weak knee extension	Chair rise exercises, knee extension with ankle sandbags, squats	Chair rise test may be helpful in diagnosis
	Weak ankle plantar flexion	Heel rises (using body weight)	
	Weak ankle dorsiflexion	Muscle strengthening; ankle foot orthosis for footdrop	
	Weak hip abduction	Hip abduction with ankle weights; side-lying position on the floor	
Sensory systems	Decreased or impaired position sense or balance with eyes closed during Romberg test	Appropriate footwear	Vitamin B_{12} level should be checked

TABLE 21–1.   (*Continued*)

Component	Common Problem	Treatment	Comment
Sensory systems (*continued*)	Decreased or impaired plantar touch sensation or Semmes Weinstein monofilaments	Appropriate footwear	The patient should be assessed for diabetes or alcohol abuse
	Dizziness—vertigo with nystagmus	See Ch. 19	
Motor control	Tandem stance, single leg stance <10 seconds Turn around 360° Forward lean	Balance training involving both static and dynamic balance; tai chi or equivalent	
	Bradykinesia Hypertonia of legs Parkinsonian signs	—	CT or MRI can detect lacunar infarction or white matter disease; vitamin B_{12} level should be checked
Usual physical activity and cardiovascular fitness	Dizziness due to postural hypotension	Review drugs for possible cause; compression stockings; see also Chs. 19 and 86	
	Fatigue, shortness of breath, unable to walk <400 meters at usual pace	Regular walking program	Assessment should be performed for angina, heart failure, pulmonary disease, claudication, and 6-minute walking distance

slowed gait. Two or three training sessions a week are usually needed; resistance exercises consist of three sets of 8 to 14 repetitions during each session. The load is increased every week or two until a plateau of strength is reached.

Leg press machines train all the large muscle groups of the leg and provide back and pelvic support during lifting. However, these machines are not always accessible to elderly patients. Chair rises with weight vests or weights attached to the waist are alternatives. Instructions are required to reduce the risk of back injury due to excess lumbar

TABLE 21–2.   PERFORMANCE-ORIENTED ASSESSMENT OF MOBILITY

Component	Findings	Score*	Clinical Meaning
Initiation of gait (immediately after told to "go")	Any hesitancy or multiple attempts to start	0	Parkinson's disease Isolated gait initiation failure Frontal gait disorder
	No hesitancy	1	
Right step length and height (right swing foot)	Does not pass left stance foot with step or does not clear floor completely with step	0	Arthritis Foot problem Stroke
	Passes left stance foot	1	
	Completely clears floor	1	
Left step length and height (left swing foot)	Does not pass right stance foot with step or does not clear floor completely with step	0	Arthritis Foot problem Stroke
	Passes right stance foot	1	
	Completely clears floor	1	
Step symmetry	Right and left step length not equal (estimate)	0	Unilateral musculoskeletal or focal neurologic deficit
	Right and left step length equal (estimate)	1	
Step continuity	Stopping or discontinuity between steps	0	Frontal gait disorder Fear of falling
	Steps appear continuous	1	
Path (estimated in relation to floor tiles, 12-in. width; observe excursion of one foot over about 10 ft of the course)	Marked deviation	0	Frontal gait disorder
	Mild to moderate deviation or uses walking aid	1	
	Straight without walking aid	2	
Trunk	Marked sway or uses walking aid	0	Cerebellar disease Thalamus, basal ganglia Antalgic gait (hip arthritis)
	No sway but flexion of knees or back pain or spreads arms out while walking	1	

TABLE 21-2.   (*Continued*)

Component	Findings	Score	Clinical Meaning
Trunk (*continued*)	No sway, no flexion, no use of arms, and no use of walking aid	2	
Stride width	Heels apart while walking	0	Hip disease Cerebellar disease Normal-pressure hydrocephalus
	Heels almost touching while walking	1	

*A perfect score is 12. A score <10 is usually associated with limitations in mobility-related function.

Adapted from Tinetti M: "Performance-oriented assessment of mobility problems in elderly patients." *Journal of the American Geriatrics Society* 34:119–126, 1986.

lordosis. Step-ups and stair climbing with the same weights are also useful. Ankle plantar flexion can be performed with the same weights.

Using knee extension machines or attaching sandbag weights to the ankle strengthens the quadriceps. The usual starting weight for frail persons is 3 kg. Resistance for all exercises should be increased every week until the patient reaches a plateau of strength.

Many patients with balance deficits benefit from balance training. Good standing posture and static balance are taught first. Patients are then taught to be aware of the location of pressure on their feet and how the location of pressure moves with slow leaning. Leans forward, backward (with a wall directly behind), and to each side are then practiced. The goal is to stand on one leg for at least 10 seconds.

Dynamic balance training can involve slow movements in single stance, simple tai chi movements, tandem walking, turns, slow forward lunges, and slow dance movements. Multicomponent balance training is probably most effective in improving balance.

Assistive devices can help maintain the patient's mobility and quality of life. New motor strategies must be learned. Ideally, physical therapists should prescribe assistive devices.

Canes are particularly helpful for pain caused by knee or hip arthritis. Canes, especially quad canes, can stabilize the patient. Canes are usually used on the side opposite the painful or weak leg. Many store-bought canes are too long. Although a cane can be purchased in a pharmacy, it should be adjusted to the correct height by cutting a wooden cane or moving the pin settings on an adjustable one. To achieve maximal support, the patient should flex his elbow 20 to 30° when holding the cane.

Walkers can reduce the force and pain at arthritic joints more than a cane, assuming adequate arm and shoulder strength. Walkers provide good lateral stability and moderate protection from forward falls but little or no help preventing backward falls for patients with balance problems. When prescribing a walker, the physical therapist should consider the sometimes competing needs of providing stability and maximizing efficiency (energy efficiency) of walking. Four-wheeled walkers with larger wheels and brakes maximize gait efficiency but provide less lateral stability. These walkers have the added advantage of a small seat to sit on if the patient is fatigued.

22   **FRACTURES**

The incidence of fractures of the distal radius, proximal humerus, proximal tibia, hip, pubic ramus, and vertebrae is low until the 6th and 7th decades of life, when it increases dramatically.

Most fractures in the elderly result from low-energy trauma, often occurring indoors. The elderly are predisposed to fractures because their bones are weakened by osteoporosis (ie, reduced bone mass∎) and thus require less mechanical force to break, because they tend to fall more frequently, and because they have less effective protective reflexes to cushion the impact of a fall. These factors act together to cause fractures in characteristic patterns and anatomic sites.

Pathologic fractures result from underlying disorders that weaken bone, including malignancy, benign bone tumors (eg, endochondroma of the phalanges or metatarsals), metabolic disorders (eg, Paget's disease, hyperparathyroidism), infection, and osteoporosis. The most common malignancies causing pathologic fractures are metastatic lesions originating in the breast, lung, prostate, gastrointestinal tract, kidney, or thyroid gland. Primary bone malignancies occur much less frequently. Multiple myeloma and lymphoma are the most common; osteosarcoma, fibrosarcoma, and chondrosarcoma are rare. However, osteosarcoma is more common in persons with Paget's disease.

Anatomy and Pathophysiology

A typical long bone is divided into the diaphysis (shaft), the epiphysis (the articular region at each end), and the metaphysis (the flared region joining the diaphysis and epiphysis). The diaphysis is composed of cortical bone, whereas the epiphyses and metaphyses are composed primarily of trabecular bone. Cortical bone is histologically dense and thus very strong. Trabecular bone is porous and varies widely in density and strength, depending on age, anatomic site, and associated disorders (eg, osteoporosis).

∎ see page 472

The tensile strength of cortical bone decreases only slightly with age. With age, the diameter of the diaphysis increases as bone is resorbed from the inner (endosteal) surface and is added to the outer (periosteal) surface. This change makes the diaphysis more resistant to bending forces and compensates for the decreased strength of cortical bone in the elderly. Thus, diaphyseal fractures do not occur more frequently with age.

The compressive strength of trabecular bone is proportional to its density. Density decreases with age; trabecular bone is not remodeled, so there is no compensation for the decrease in density. Age-related fractures (of the distal radius, proximal humerus, proximal tibia, proximal femur, pubic ramus, or vertebra) involve predominantly trabecular bone, often in the metaphyses. The fracture threshold (ie, the bone density at which the risk of fracture becomes likely) is estimated to be 0.77 g/cm^3 for the proximal femur; bone density < 0.77 g/cm^3 increases the risk of fracture. In a 70-year-old woman, the average bone density of the proximal femur is 0.70 g/cm^3, usually because of osteoporosis.

Normal healing: Normally, fractures heal in three overlapping phases: inflammation, repair, and remodeling.

The inflammatory phase begins as an immediate response to injury and lasts several days. The trauma that fractures the bone also injures the surrounding blood vessels, muscles, and other soft tissues. Hemorrhage at the fracture site results in a hematoma. Traumatic devascularization of the fracture ends and bony fragments may result in nonviable or necrotic bone, causing immediate acute inflammation. The fracture site becomes swollen and tender.

The reparative phase begins ≤ 24 hours after the fracture and peaks after 1 to 2 weeks. Diaphyseal fractures that are not rigidly stabilized heal by rapid formation of new bone around the fracture site. This new bone, called the external callus, is not visible on x-ray until about 3 to 6 weeks after the fracture. Until the external callus provides sufficient stability (which may take several months for long-bone fractures), the fractured bone can collapse and become displaced.

The remodeling phase may last many months. In diaphyseal fractures, the callus is slowly resorbed and replaced by mechanically stronger bone that is distributed to best resist load-bearing stresses. During remodeling, patients usually feel some activity-related discomfort. Thus, although a fractured wrist may be strong enough for unrestricted use in 2 months, the patient may report pain when gripping forcefully for up to 1 year.

Symptoms and Signs

Most fractures cause swelling, deformity, and pain when movement is attempted. For example, patients with occult subcapital fractures feel pain when the hip is rotated internally, tightening the joint capsule. For patients who cannot speak, refusal to move an extremity may be the only sign of a fracture.

Occasionally, patients present with an impending pathologic fracture (one in which the bone has not broken entirely). The affected area is tender when palpated and painful when the affected limb is used. For example, a patient with an impending femoral fracture may feel pain in the thigh when rising from a chair.

Complications

Compartment syndrome: Compartment syndrome is the most common limb-threatening complication associated with trauma to the extremities. Swelling of injured muscle within a confining envelope (eg, a splint, a dressing, a cast, fascia) increases tissue pressure and blocks normal perfusion. The resulting ischemia leads to further muscle injury and swelling, higher tissue pressures, and, after only a few hours, irreversible injury and necrosis.

The most reliable clinical signs of impending compartment syndrome are progressively increasing pain in an immobilized extremity, pain with passive flexion or extension of the toes or fingers, and numbness in a specific peripheral nerve distribution. The presence of distal pulses in a limb does not exclude compartment syndrome.

Compartment syndrome can be definitively diagnosed using a device that percutaneously measures intramuscular pressure. Treatment consists of removal of all confining envelopes around the swollen muscle. Thus, a splint, dressing, or cast must be thoroughly loosened immediately, or if increased muscle swelling causes the surrounding fascia to become constricting, an emergency fasciotomy must be performed.

Pulmonary embolism: Pulmonary embolism (thromboembolism[1]) is the most common fatal complication due to major hip and pelvic trauma. Of patients with a hip fracture who die, 38% die of pulmonary embolism. Of patients with a hip fracture who are not given anticoagulants, about 50% develop deep vein thrombosis[2]; about 10%, pulmonary emboli; and about 2%, fatal pulmonary emboli. Patients with hip fractures are at high risk because of the combination of trauma to the lower extremity, forced immobilization for several hours or even days, and surgery. The associated clinical findings—pain, swelling, tenderness, Homans' sign (pain on forced dorsiflexion of the foot), fever, leukocytosis—are unreliable criteria for diagnosis. Venography remains the standard diagnostic test; ultrasonography is the most effective noninvasive test for diagnosing deep vein thrombosis.

Warfarin is generally regarded as the most effective prophylaxis against pulmonary embolism for patients with a hip fracture. Warfarin 5 mg may be given up to 24 hours preoperatively because onset of action is delayed. Maintenance doses must be determined by monitoring the prothrombin time; the goal is an international normalized ratio (INR) of 1.5 to 2.0. Advantages of warfarin include once-daily oral administra-

[1] see also page 771   [2] see page 923

tion and low cost; disadvantages include the need for regular monitoring of the prothrombin time, significant bleeding (in 1 to 5% of users), and interaction with many drugs. For example, the combination of warfarin and nonsteroidal anti-inflammatory drugs increases the incidence of hemorrhagic peptic ulcer almost 13-fold in the elderly.

Newer low-molecular-weight heparins have been found to be safe and effective compared with warfarin for patients with a hip fracture. They offer the advantages of subcutaneous fixed dosing (once or twice daily) without the need for laboratory monitoring except for periodic CBC and platelet counts. Preoperative use may increase intraoperative bleeding.

Antiplatelet drugs (eg, aspirin) are easy to administer and provide some prophylaxis against pulmonary embolism but are less effective than warfarin. They are appropriate for patients at lower risk of pulmonary embolism (eg, those with tibial or pubic ramus fractures). Aspirin can be given to patients with a hip fracture if warfarin is contraindicated.

Diagnosis

A pathologic fracture should be suspected when a fracture occurs after minimal trauma or during activities of daily living (eg, walking, getting out of a chair). Usually, a patient with such a fracture has a history of progressively increasing pain in the affected extremity, particularly at night and with weight bearing. Diagnosing a pathologic fracture is important because prognosis and treatment may differ depending on the underlying disorder.

Physical examination may be inadequate for patients who are uncooperative because of pain. For example, a hip fracture makes examination of the contralateral side difficult.

X-rays are the most important tool for diagnosing fractures. Standard x-ray evaluation of suspected fractures should include anteroposterior and lateral views, because on a single view, the characteristic displacement, discontinuity, or altered alignment of a fracture may be hidden by overlap or projection of the broken bone. When a diagnosis cannot be made based on standard views (eg, in minimally displaced spiral fractures), oblique views can help.

Fractures may be missed if only a small area is evaluated. For example, pain in the thigh or knee may be caused by a hip fracture, which may be missed unless x-rays of the entire femur are obtained. A physician should obtain x-rays of both hips and the pelvis for patients with a femoral or pubic ramus fracture because coexisting injuries and preexisting disorders may be present.

Typically, x-rays of pathologic fractures caused by underlying malignancy show multiple lytic lesions, seen as lucencies. X-rays cannot differentiate the disorders that cause abnormally decreased bone density (osteopenia); such disorders include osteoporosis, osteomalacia, hyperparathyroidism, and myeloma. Thus, if a pathologic fracture is caused by osteopenia, laboratory evaluation is required to correctly identify the underlying disorder.

CT, although not routinely needed, can be a useful adjunct to plain x-rays. CT can show occult fractures in areas difficult to image with x-rays because of overlying bony structures (eg, the cervical spine). CT helps determine the extent of articular surface disruption in joint fractures. If a pathologic fracture is suspected, CT may be used to check for bone destruction and soft tissue masses.

MRI readily shows soft tissues and differentiates fat- and water-dense tissues. Within 24 hours, MRI can detect the edema that rapidly accumulates at the fracture site during the initial inflammatory phase, enabling early diagnosis of occult fractures. MRI also helps in the evaluation of pathologic fractures and in the diagnosis of osteonecrosis and osteomyelitis, both of which can mimic fractures. However, MRI cannot directly show calcification or bone mineralization and thus does not image bone structure as well as x-ray or CT does.

Bone scanning, using technetium-99m–labeled pyrophosphate or similar radioactive analogs, can detect focal injury to bone regardless of cause. Uptake occurs wherever new bone forms (eg, in response to infection, arthritis, tumor, or fracture). Occult fractures not visible on x-rays can often be detected on bone scans 3 to 5 days after injury. If a pathologic fracture is suspected, bone scans must be performed to check for metastatic and metabolic bone disease at sites other than the fracture site.

Measurement of the Hct level is the most widely used laboratory test for evaluating blood loss from fractures. Fractures, especially those of the hip, can result in substantial bleeding into soft tissues, which may warrant transfusion.

Measurement of the serum alkaline phosphatase level is the only routinely available laboratory blood test that corresponds directly with fracture healing. The serum alkaline phosphatase level increases when bone turnover (remodeling) increases, which occurs during normal fracture healing, during skeletal growth (in childhood), or when certain malignancies or metabolic disorders (eg, Paget's disease) affect the skeleton. In contrast, the serum calcium level does not change with normal fracture healing. The serum calcium level can increase when one of several endocrine disorders (eg, hyperparathyroidism) or metastatic disease, especially breast cancer, is present and when bone is resorbed very rapidly in bedridden patients with Paget's disease.

Prognosis

The elderly are more adversely affected by the secondary effects of fractures than are younger persons. Immobilization from cast treatment causes joint stiffness. Enforced bed rest predisposes to pulmonary complications, thromboembolism, disorientation, and musculoskeletal weakness. Even minor fractures of the wrist or shoulder may disable formerly independent elderly persons, who may require personal assistance in activities of daily living (eg, eating, dressing, bathing) for many months. More severe injuries have greater impact on the elderly. In the year after a hip fracture, the mortality rate increases by 15%. Of functionally independent patients who lived at home before the fracture, 20% require institutional care for > 1 year, and 30% depend on mechanical aids or assistive personnel.

Treatment

The goal of treatment is rapid return to the activities necessary for independent living rather than restoration of perfect limb alignment and length. The urgency of treatment is frequently mandated by secondary effects of the fracture (eg, pain, loss of function, swelling, uncertainty of outcome) rather than by the fracture itself. For most closed fractures, the application of casts or surgical treatment can be delayed up to 1 week without adversely affecting outcome. Until seen by a physician, the patient should be instructed to immobilize and support the injured limb with a makeshift splint, sling, or pillow; elevate the limb to limit swelling; apply ice to control pain and swelling; and take only acetaminophen to relieve pain. If surgery is a possibility, the patient should drink only small amounts of clear liquids and avoid eating.

When a fracture is suspected, the patient's primary care physician should determine the appropriate facility for treatment. Choice of facility depends on the fracture's severity. For example, patients with displaced hip fractures, who are often immobile and in pain, usually must be transported by ambulance staffed with trained personnel to a hospital with appropriate surgical facilities. Patients with minor wrist and shoulder fractures can be treated in medical offices with x-ray facilities.

Initial immobilization: A fracture is initially immobilized (before definitive stabilization, eg, with casts or surgical stabilization) to prevent further damage. Usually, injuries distal to or at the knee or elbow can be initially immobilized with splints. Splints may be made of preformed aluminum or plastic or inflatable clear plastic, have easily adjustable Velcro closures, or be individually molded of plaster of paris (calcium sulfate hemihydrate), which provides excellent support. Ideally, all splints are applied by one health care practitioner while another holds the injured extremity with gentle longitudinal traction.

Most fractures of the shoulder, upper arm, and elbow can be immobilized with a sling. The arm can be kept close to the body, if necessary, by an elastic wrap or swath. Hip fractures can be immobilized by carefully positioned pillows or by light skin traction.

Casts: Casts keep the fracture aligned while it heals. Because plaster of paris molds and conforms well, it is often used for the initial cast. Subsequent casts may be made of polymeric resins and fiberglass, which are stronger, stiffer, and lighter than plaster of paris. For com-

TABLE 22-1.   CAST CARE GUIDELINES

- When bathing, patients must enclose the cast in a plastic bag and carefully seal the top with rubber bands or tape. Commercially available waterproof covers are convenient to use and are more failproof.

- If a cast becomes wet, the underlying padding may retain moisture. In such cases, the cast must be changed to prevent skin maceration.

- Patients must never push a sharp or pointed object down inside the cast (eg, to scratch the skin).

- Patients must check the skin around the cast every day and apply lotion to any red or sore areas.

- Patients should elevate the cast regularly, as needed, to control swelling. Patients must not push or lean on the cast; it may break.

- When resting, patients must position the cast carefully, possibly using a small pillow or pad, to prevent the edge from pinching or digging into the skin.

- Chafing or pressure sores may develop where the skin is in contact with the edge of the cast. If the edge of the cast feels rough, patients can pad it with soft adhesive tape, moleskin, tissues, or cloth.

- Patients must immediately contact a physician if the cast causes persistent pain or excessive tightness. Pressure sores or unexpected swelling may require urgent removal of the cast.

plete immobilization, the cast must extend one joint above and one joint below the fracture site. For example, the cast for a distal radial fracture should extend from above the elbow to just proximal to the metacarpal joint; however, because joint stiffness is a major problem for the elderly, the cast often ends below the elbow to allow joint motion.

Patients must be taught how to care for the cast (see TABLE 22–1). The extremity should be elevated for 24 to 48 hours after the cast is applied to prevent swelling. Rhythmic flexion and extension of the fingers or wiggling of the toes facilitates venous return. The patient should immediately report progressive or unrelenting pain, pressure, or numbness because muscle swelling under the cast can lead to the compartment syndrome∎.

Surgical stabilization: In the elderly, most fractures, except those of the hip, are treated nonsurgically. However, surgical stabilization can restore function and relieve pain more rapidly. For example, patients with hip fractures can usually begin walking within days after surgery. The risks of immobility or prolonged traction outweigh those of surgery, especially for leg fractures. However, severe osteoporosis, in which bone is very porous and unstable, may make securing the hard-

∎see page 214

ware used in surgical stabilization difficult; the hardware becomes displaced if it does not have a secure hold in the bone.

Surgical stabilization of most fractures should be postponed if the patient has a correctable acute medical problem (eg, fluid and electrolyte imbalance, acute infection, cardiac arrhythmia). Fractures require immediate treatment only if the limb is threatened (eg, if compartment syndrome is impending or if there is neurovascular compromise or an open wound). Some conditions are relative contraindications to surgery; eg, active sepsis can lead to infection of the surgical site and contraindicates the use of metallic implants.

Traction: For the elderly, traction should be used only when application of a cast and surgical stabilization are contraindicated because the fracture is too fragmented or the patient's medical condition is unstable.

Skin traction is applied using foam boots and carefully wrapped moleskin strips, a sash cord, and a pulley with a 2.3-kg (5-lb) weight. *Weights > 2.3 kg should never be used.* This procedure is particularly hazardous for the elderly because of its complications, including pressure sores, deep vein thrombosis, pulmonary embolism, depression, disorientation, loss of appetite, deconditioning, atelectasis, and pulmonary infection. Meticulous, aggressive nursing care with vigilant monitoring is required. Skin traction is used only to provide comfort by temporarily and gently restraining the extremity. If strong, prolonged traction is needed to maintain bone alignment, skeletal traction with pins must be used. The proximal tibia is the most common pin site for femoral and acetabular fractures.

Internal fixation of impending pathologic fractures with metal plates, rods, or prostheses often prevents displacement, relieves pain, and preserves function. If an impending pathologic fracture breaks through completely and becomes displaced, treatment can be more difficult, decreasing function and increasing morbidity.

Joint replacement: Joint (prosthetic) replacement, especially of the hip▉, may be necessary if a fracture damages the joint or the femoral head. Implants made of metal and polyethylene are used to replace the damaged bone fragments. This method restores skeletal strength immediately, unlike alternative treatments that rely on bone fragment healing or bone graft incorporation. Joint replacements, although inappropriate for younger patients, are appropriate for elderly patients because such procedures place fewer demands on the musculoskeletal system and offer other advantages (eg, more rapid return of function and full weight-bearing gait). Other treatments may require patients to use crutches, which the elderly usually cannot use because of diminished muscular strength and coordination.

▉see page 226 and FIGURE 22–5 on page 227

Rehabilitation

Rehabilitation is often prolonged, and recovery is often incomplete. Usually, patients require several months to 1 year to regain their preinjury capabilities. Orthotic and self-help devices may help.∎

Nursing and Caregiver Issues

Elderly persons with fractures are especially vulnerable to certain complications, including stiffness, swelling, pressure sores, and functional impairment. Important nursing and caregiver issues include preventive management of these complications.

Stiffness is managed by daily active and/or passive range-of-motion exercises of joints adjacent to the fracture (eg, the fingers, shoulder, and elbow for patients in a short arm cast). Periodic changes of position can prevent hip and knee flexion contractures caused by unrelieved sitting. Periodic sessions of standing and walking and, in nonambulatory patients, sessions of recumbency promote hip and knee flexibility.

Swelling is managed by elevating the injured extremity to the level of the heart. For upper extremity fractures, elevation uses pillows. For lower extremity fractures, effective elevation requires sessions of recumbency. Daytime use of elastic stockings also helps to control swelling.

Elderly fracture patients with impaired sensation and peripheral circulation are vulnerable to pressure sores when an injured limb rests on a hard surface. Diligent inspection and padding of contact points (especially heels) are mandatory.

Fractures often result in functional impairment in activities of daily living. Diminished muscular strength, flexibility, and balance in elderly fracture patients can impair independence in eating, dressing, bathing, and even walking (if dependent on a walker). Disuse can lead to stiffness, weakness, and further impairment. Nurses and caregivers must help and encourage elderly fracture patients to regain the ability to perform activities of daily living.

DISTAL RADIAL FRACTURES

Distal radial (Colles') fractures are among the most common fractures in the elderly. They occur when the dorsal trabecular bone of the distal radius collapses inward, resulting in angulation and shortening. The cause is usually a fall on an outstretched hand. Patients present with pain, tenderness, and swelling of the wrist.

Prognosis and Treatment

The severity of the fracture and need for reduction are assessed on x-ray. The prognosis is better when the radial styloid has been shortened

< 0.5 cm (< 0.2 inches) compared with the ulna on the anteroposterior view and when dorsal tilting of the distal radius articular surface does not exceed neutral on the lateral view.

Active, fully independent patients should receive aggressive treatment for optimal results. Generally, for less active patients living in an assisted care setting, the fracture is immobilized for a few weeks, after which patients are encouraged to use their hand in daily activities.

Patients who have minimally displaced distal radial fractures or few functional demands are treated with a short arm cast or splint. When a fracture requires closed reduction, anesthesia is necessary. A local injection of lidocaine with hematoma aspiration may be sufficient, but regional (axillary block) or IV general anesthesia is better for relaxation and analgesia. Fractures with significant shortening or intra-articular comminution may require external fixation. The cast is usually worn for 3 to 8 weeks, depending on the fracture's stability and the patient's functional status.

Pain, stiffness, and weakness gradually diminish for 6 to 12 months after the fracture. Moving the fingers, elbow, and shoulder prevents stiffness of the fingers and shoulder, the most common complications. Elevating the hand above heart level minimizes swelling. Symptoms of carpal tunnel syndrome◻ may develop. Physical therapy can help speed recovery.

PROXIMAL HUMERAL FRACTURES

Proximal humeral fractures are most commonly caused by falling on an outstretched arm. Patients present with shoulder pain and inability to move the arm. About 80% of proximal humeral fractures are minimally displaced, with < 45° angulation and < 0.5 cm (< 0.2 inches) displacement of any fragment. Anteroposterior x-ray views of the proximal humerus may show as many as four main fragments—eg, of the humeral head, greater tuberosity, lesser tuberosity, and humeral shaft. These fragments are prone to displacement because of the pull of the rotator cuff, deltoid, and pectoral muscles. If no fracture is apparent on anteroposterior x-ray views, a patient with an acute shoulder injury should be examined for a glenohumeral dislocation and a rotator cuff tear. An axillary or Y-view lateral x-ray shows a dislocation if present. Large rotator cuff tears cause a feeling of painful weakness when the patient elevates and rotates the arm.

The most common complication after a proximal humoral fracture is adhesive capsulitis, which results when the inflamed surfaces of the joint capsule scar and adhere to one another. Capsulitis restricts motion, causing chronic pain and functional disability.

Prognosis and Treatment

Prognosis and treatment depend on the number of fragments and the extent of displacement. Regaining the ability to perform overhead activities (eg, combing hair) may take several months.

If the alignment and position of fragments are satisfactory, the arm may be immobilized in a sling. If they are unsatisfactory, an orthopedist may attempt closed reduction. If closed reduction is unsuccessful, open reduction with internal fixation or insertion of a prosthesis may be indicated. Patients should be told to expect considerable swelling and discoloration, which will spread to the lower arm and hand.

For stable fractures, the patient should be encouraged to use the hand and wrist immediately. Range-of-motion exercises are begun as soon as possible.∎ A physical therapist can teach the patient how to perform range-of-motion exercises and monitors their performance. At 1 week, the patient should begin pendulum exercises in the sling; the patient leans forward and uses the noninjured arm to help swing the injured arm like a pendulum, making circles with the elbow. The sling may be removed daily to allow bathing and elbow motion. By 3 weeks, passive and active arm elevation should be begun.

PROXIMAL TIBIAL FRACTURES

Fractures of the proximal tibia usually result from a lateral bending force (eg, when a car strikes a pedestrian from the side). For elderly persons with severe osteoporosis, a simple fall to the side can fracture the proximal tibia.

Patients present with knee pain and effusion, proximal tibial tenderness, and inability to bear weight. Typically, displaced fractures can be seen on standard anteroposterior and lateral x-ray views, but oblique views may be needed to detect occult fractures. Fat globules in blood aspirated from the knee joint also indicate an occult fracture.

Prognosis and Treatment

Treatment depends on how much of the articular surface is displaced. Stable fractures in which the joint surface is depressed < 5 to 8 mm (< 0.2 to 0.3 inches) can be managed with a cast or brace that holds the knee in full extension. Weight bearing is recommended as tolerated.

For more severe fractures with extensive displacement of the articular surface and structural instability, treatment depends on the patient's activity level and medical condition. Active healthy patients benefit from closed reduction and surgical stabilization of the fracture with metal implants and bone grafting. Patients may need to avoid placing weight on the injured leg for 1 to 2 months. For inactive, debilitated patients, use of a cast or brace with weight bearing as tolerated may be

∎ see page 269

more appropriate. For patients with limited ambulatory ability, function may be satisfactorily restored despite considerable deformity. If pain and dysfunction are unacceptable after the fracture has healed, total knee replacement is an option.

PROXIMAL FEMORAL FRACTURES

According to the U.S. Census, about 340,000 hip fractures occur annually; about 50% occur in persons ≥ 85 years. The annual age-specific incidence of hip fracture increases exponentially with age, doubling every 6 years, reaching 4% per year in women > 90. One in three women and one in six men who reach age 90 will fracture a hip during their lifetime.

Etiology and Pathology

Hip fractures may be intracapsular or extracapsular. Subcapital and femoral neck fractures (see FIGURE 22–1) are intracapsular and frequently disrupt the blood supply to the femoral head (see FIGURE 22–2). Because the femoral head is intra-articular, its sole blood supply comes from vessels traversing the bone of the femoral neck, the surrounding hip capsule, and the ligamentum teres. A displaced fracture completely disrupts the blood vessels of the femoral neck and can tear those of the hip capsule, increasing the risk of osteonecrosis of the femoral head and nonunion of the fracture.

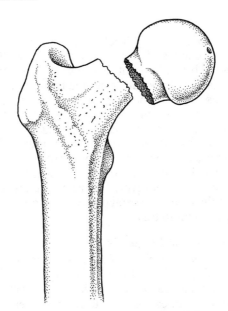

FIGURE 22–1. Subcapital and femoral neck fracture.

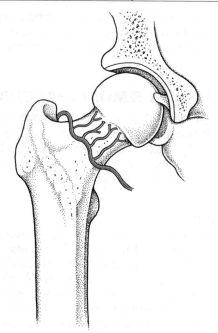

FIGURE 22–2. Blood supply to the femoral head.

Intertrochanteric and subtrochanteric fractures are extracapsular; they expose large areas of well-vascularized cancellous bone surfaces, increasing acute blood loss but favoring callus formation. Osteonecrosis and nonunion rarely occur. In simple two-part fractures, the fracture typically slopes obliquely between the greater and lesser trochanters, as seen on the anteroposterior x-ray view (see FIGURE 22–3). In comminuted fractures, fragments of the greater and lesser trochanters may be present. Subtrochanteric fractures extend below the lesser trochanter.

Acetabular fractures in the elderly occur most frequently as extensions of pubic and ischial rami fractures. Most are minimally displaced and are treated nonoperatively. Central fracture dislocations of the femoral head through the acetabular wall into the pelvis are very rare and are very difficult to treat.

Symptoms, Signs, and Diagnosis

Most patients with displaced fractures of the proximal femur present with obvious diagnostic features: a history of a fall, inability to bear weight, and a fracture easily seen on x-rays. However, occult and insufficiency stress fractures can occur in the elderly without a clearly defined traumatic event. Such patients report persistent pain when

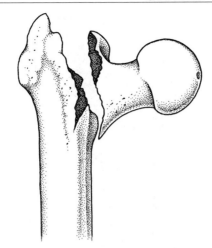

FIGURE 22–3.   Intertrochanteric fracture.

weight is placed on the injured leg. A crack, initially undetectable on x-rays, can continue to propagate through the bone with the stresses of walking, resulting in complete displacement. A bone scan or MRI can detect the fracture earlier than plain x-rays.

During physical examination, patients with displaced fractures typically lie with their injured leg shortened and externally rotated because of the pull of the leg muscles and gravity. Any movement of the leg is painful. Often, patients with impacted or occult fractures can flex their injured hip with only mild discomfort. Passive flexion with internal rotation of the hip, which tightens the joint capsule, is a sensitive test for occult fractures.

Prognosis and Treatment

Most patients benefit from the increased mobility and pain relief provided by surgery, but patients unable to tolerate anesthesia (eg, those who have just had an acute myocardial infarction) may need to delay surgery. A few patients (eg, those who were not ambulatory before the event for reasons unrelated to the affected joint) are candidates for non-surgical management. Rehabilitation is an important aspect of care. ■

For bedridden patients, nursing care must be diligent and meticulous. Complications of enforced bed rest include joint contractures, deconditioning, pressure sores, deep vein thrombosis, pulmonary embolism, pneumonia, osteoporosis, and psychiatric disturbances.

Subcapital and femoral neck fractures: Occult, impacted, or nondisplaced femoral neck fractures are usually managed by internal

■ see page 283

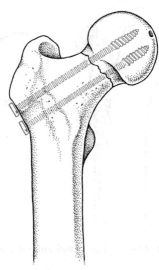

FIGURE 22–4.   Internal fixation of a subcapital fracture with pins.

fixation with multiple pins (see FIGURE 22–4), which allows immediate, full weight bearing and prevents later displacement. Because the blood supply to the femoral head is not severely disrupted, these types of fractures usually heal well.

Displaced fractures can be managed with surgical stabilization or prosthetic replacement. Open reduction with internal fixation is usually reserved for active patients who can comply with a postoperative regimen of limited weight bearing using crutches. The procedure preserves the femoral head, and when healing is successful, the hip is nearly normal. However, if osteonecrosis or nonunion occurs, the result is a painful, nonfunctional joint that requires total hip replacement. Because the need for a second operation is minimized, primary prosthetic replacement of the femoral head (hemiarthroplasty) is often preferred for less active elderly patients with displaced fractures. This procedure also enables the patient to bear weight immediately and fully and to return to independent functioning more quickly.

The simplest prosthesis, the Moore prosthesis, consists of a smooth metal sphere attached to a stem that is wedged into the medullary canal of the femur (see FIGURE 22–5). Disadvantages include a tendency to erode the acetabular articular surface and pain from a loose fit of the stem in the femoral medullary canal. Other prostheses are designed to be stabilized inside the femur and are coated with acrylic cement or with a hydroxyapatite or porous metal, which facilitates direct bone fixation. A bipolar prosthesis with an internal metal-polyethylene bearing can reduce acetabular erosion. Patients who develop acetabular arthritis after hemiarthroplasty may require total hip replacement. Primary total hip replacement is performed for acute femoral neck fractures only when patients have severe preexisting arthritis, because this operation is more extensive and has a higher morbidity rate than does hemiarthroplasty or internal fixation with pins.

Intertrochanteric and many subtrochanteric femoral fractures: Surgical stabilization with a sliding compression screw and side plate (see FIGURE 22–6) provides rigid stabilization while pressing the fracture fragments together, thus helping to ensure healing. Postoperatively, most patients can bear weight immediately, as tolerated with a walker, but some patients with comminuted unstable fractures cannot bear weight fully for several weeks, when healing is sufficient. Patients with good balance and muscle strength can use a cane in 6 to 12 weeks.

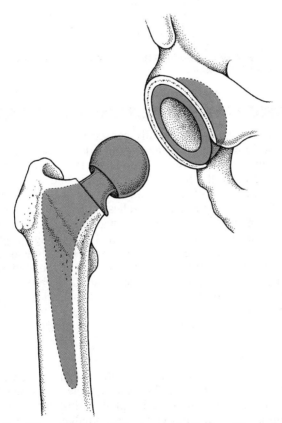

FIGURE 22–5.   Hip replacement. Treatment of a displaced femoral neck fracture may involve use of a Moore solid-stem prosthesis (*left*) or total hip replacement, consisting of a femoral component and a polyethylene bipolar component (*right*).

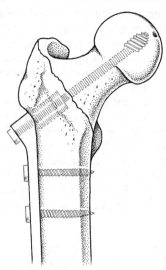

FIGURE 22–6. Fixation of an intertrochanteric fracture with a sliding compression screw and side plate.

PUBIC AND ISCHIAL RAMUS FRACTURES

Pubic ramus fractures are usually caused by a fall on level ground. The pubic and ischial rami on one or both sides of the symphysis pubis may be fractured. Normally, the pelvis bears weight mainly on the strong bony arches in the ilium, with the pubic and ischial rami acting as secondary tie arches. When trauma to the pelvis occurs, the rami tend to fracture first, leaving the iliac arches intact. Patients present with groin pain that may prevent them from walking. However, because the rami are not needed for structural support for walking, weight bearing need not be restricted when the pain eases. The clinical appearance mimics that of a proximal femoral fracture. Localized tenderness in the groin and pain during leg movement suggest the diagnosis; x-rays confirm it. In the presence of osteopenia, an undisplaced pubic ramus fracture may be difficult to diagnose; the fracture can become radiologically visible with callus formation.

Prognosis and Treatment

Pubic ramus fractures typically heal without causing permanent functional disabilities. Most patients feel considerable pain when standing or sitting and should be admitted to a hospital or skilled nursing care facility for monitoring of Hct and vital signs. Analgesics and nonsteroidal anti-inflammatory drugs help relieve pain. To avoid the complications associated with bed rest, patients should begin to walk, bearing weight fully, as soon as possible. Most can walk short distances with a walker by 1 week and are moderately comfortable in 1 to 2 months.

THORACIC AND LUMBAR VERTEBRAL FRACTURES

Thoracic and lumbar vertebral fractures often result from activity that increases the compressive load on the spine (eg, lifting, bending forward, misstepping while walking). However, vertebral fractures occur silently in many elderly persons, who frequently have x-ray evidence of fractures without a history of symptoms or injury.

In thoracic vertebral fractures, the vertebral body is typically compressed into a wedge shape (best seen on lateral x-rays) due to the normal kyphosis of the thoracic region, which concentrates the forces anteriorly. In lumbar vertebral fractures, the vertebral body is generally flattened, sometimes sideways. Collapse may be acute or progressive.

Patients often present with acute pain that is exacerbated by sitting or standing. The primary symptoms are progressive kyphosis and loss of height. Percussion over a specific spinal region reveals localized tenderness. Associated neurologic deficits, manifested by pain radiating into the leg, and bladder or bowel incontinence are rare. Laboratory screening tests for other causes of osteopenia may be indicated.

Prognosis and Treatment

Compression fractures of the vertebral body heal eventually, because the trabecular bone collapses inward and the blood supply is not impaired. Typically, these fractures are relatively stable because the intact posterior elements prevent displacement that is likely to damage the spinal cord. Rarely, a compression fracture that initially appeared benign collapses completely, compromising the spinal canal and leading to neural injury. Surgery may be indicated to decompress the canal.

The goals of treatment include prevention of further collapse, management of symptoms, and resumption of normal function. Initially, institutional care or bed rest may be needed to relieve pain. Physical therapy can help the patient maintain ambulatory ability, improve limb function, and strengthen trunk musculature. Analgesics and nonsteroidal anti-inflammatory drugs help relieve pain. Patients should be encouraged to sit up and walk for short periods as soon as possible to prevent deconditioning and accelerated bone loss. They may be unable to walk independently for up to 1 week and may have considerable back pain for 6 to 12 weeks. Sometimes, after ≥ 1 month, the pain shifts from the fracture site to a higher or lower level, because the deformity alters mechanical stresses.

Use of a brace may not prevent deformity but can help relieve pain and enable the patient to return to daily activities more quickly. A brace is useful only for fractures of the lumbar and lower thoracic spine because adequate support cannot be achieved above these regions.

Although total contact orthoses and hyperextension braces (eg, the Jewett) are most biomechanically effective, they are very confining and not always well tolerated by elderly patients. Hyperextension braces apply three-point stabilization of the spine through an anterior abdominal pad, a chest pad, and a posterior pad at the level of the fracture. Corsets or abdominal binders are effective and better tolerated alternatives for patients with lumbar vertebral fractures.

23 ■ THE ELDERLY DRIVER

For most community-dwelling elderly persons, being able to drive is essential for maintaining autonomy in daily activities (eg, shopping, medical appointments, social visits, church functions). For elderly persons who cannot drive, alternative transportation should be arranged, although such arrangements often involve dependence on family members and friends. The use of public transportation, even if available, is often unacceptable because of inconvenience, cost, or concerns about safety.

Safe driving requires the integration of complex motor, visual, and cognitive tasks, although many drivers with moderate motor, visual, and cognitive deficits can continue to drive safely, probably because these tasks have been consolidated into a learned, instinctive pattern of driving. Performance is usually affected only after considerable loss of function.

To compensate for moderate functional deficits, most elderly persons avoid rush hour and drive fewer miles, shorter distances, and less at night. For instance, average mileage is 64% less for 85-year-old male drivers than for 65-year-old male drivers. Elderly drivers are also more cautious than younger drivers, drive more slowly, and take fewer risks in traffic. Because elderly persons drive less than younger persons and because they are more cautious, they have fewer collisions. Collision rates (per 1000 licensed drivers) decrease steadily with age (see FIGURE 23–1). Thus, it is a myth that elderly drivers are responsible for a disproportionate number of motor vehicle collisions.

However, per mile driven, elderly drivers have higher rates of traffic violations, collisions, and fatalities than all age groups over age 25. Collision rates per mile driven increase after about age 70 and increase more rapidly after age 80 (see FIGURE 23–2). Failure to yield right-of-way and failure to heed a stop sign or red light are the most common violations. Furthermore, elderly drivers have a higher proportion of collisions at intersections. These findings imply that some elderly drivers have difficulty with driving tasks requiring complex decision making.

Elderly drivers involved in collisions fare worse than younger drivers. Collisions involving elderly drivers are more likely to include mul-

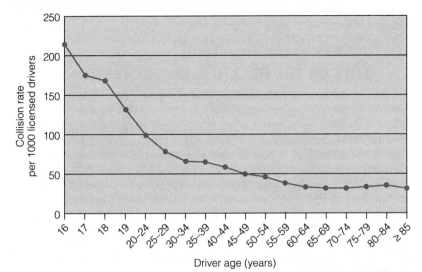

FIGURE 23–1.   Motor vehicle collision rates per 1000 licensed drivers, according to age. From Cerrelli EC. *Crash data and rates for age-sex groups of drivers, 1994.* Research Note. National Highway Traffic Safety Administration Technical Report, October 1995.

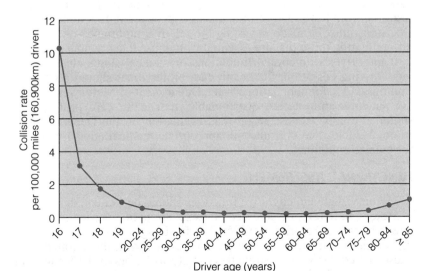

FIGURE 23–2.   Motor vehicle collision rates per 100,000 miles (160,900 km) driven, according to age. From Cerrelli EC. *Crash data and rates for age-sex groups of drivers, 1994.* Research Note. National Highway Traffic Safety Administration Technical Report, October 1995.

tiple vehicles and to result in serious injuries and fatalities, partially because the elderly have different driving patterns and because they have underlying frailties and comorbid disorders.

ROLE OF THE HEALTH CARE PROFESSIONAL

Elderly drivers with important functional deficits or with medical conditions that restrict function may decide to limit or stop driving, or they may continue to drive as usual, denying their limitations. Health care professionals become involved when they detect deficits during a routine examination, when family members seek guidance, or when elderly drivers solicit advice.

Health care professionals should try to preserve a patient's autonomy and quality of life, but after evaluating an elderly driver, they may feel obligated to recommend cessation of driving. Making such a recommendation may be difficult because loss of driving privileges is often the first challenge to an elderly person's autonomy; such a loss may cause major inconvenience and contribute to impaired quality of life and depression.

The first step in assessing an elderly person's ability to drive is to perform a thorough evaluation, including a comprehensive history and physical examination█ with a focus on functional assessment. If any functional deficits are detected or suspected, the health care professional should counsel the elderly driver and family members and discuss issues relevant to the driver's transportation needs. Social isolation resulting from fewer daily trips can lead to worsening functional status. Decisions must be made regarding the relative importance of trips (ie, differentiating those that are essential from those that are nonessential).

If the driver's functional limitations or medical status clearly warrants driving cessation, the health care professional should report the findings and recommendations to the Department of Motor Vehicles. If the patient's abilities are questionable, the health care professional should formally request an on-road evaluation by the Department of Motor Vehicles and consult with appropriate medical advisory boards for precise guidelines.

FUNCTIONAL ASSESSMENT

Motor, visual, and cognitive functions should be evaluated.

Motor function: Decreased **muscle strength,** particularly grip strength, can make driving difficult. Grip strength of < 35 lb (< 15.89 kg) in the dominant hand in men (measured with a dynamometer) is cause for concern. Grip strength is likely to be about 10% lower in women (ie, < 31 lb [< 14.06 kg]). Because power-assisted devices can

█ see page 24

compensate for poor grip strength, other abilities (eg, dexterity, coordination) should be considered.

Reaction time, which increases with the difficulty or number of choices, is important in driving. Reaction time can be classified as "simple," which includes the premotor and movement times, or "choice," which is the time it takes to choose between two or more decisions. However, no reliable measure of reaction time is clinically useful.

Usually, formal evaluation of **range of motion** by an occupational or physical therapist using a goniometer is not required, but the practitioner should perform a qualitative evaluation of joint mobility.

Limited mobility of the neck (eg, in patients with rheumatic disorders) may restrict field of view and is especially worrisome in urgent driving situations. Limited mobility of the shoulder, wrist, or elbow can affect steering, although power-assisted devices may compensate adequately. These devices, available at some automobile body shops, range in cost. For example, spinner knobs are inexpensive. They can be installed on the steering wheel to facilitate control for elderly drivers with limited shoulder or arm mobility (eg, due to stroke or severe arthritis). Driving rehabilitation programs for the elderly, offered by the American Automobile Association (AAA) and the American Association of Retired Persons (AARP), can often refer persons asking about these devices.

Although measurement of **proprioception** is often imprecise, the physician should note proprioceptive difficulties in patients (eg, in disorders such as subacute combined degeneration of the spinal cord caused by vitamin B_{12} deficiency). Patients with obvious deficits may warrant on-road testing or other focused evaluations.

Visual function: Several age-related changes in vision can affect driving performance. Central and peripheral visual acuity commonly declines with age because of physiologic or anatomic changes (eg, opacification of the lens) or specific medical conditions (eg, diabetic retinopathy). The total horizontal peripheral visual field typically decreases from 170° in young adults to 140° in 50-year-olds. Drivers with peripheral visual deficits have collision rates twice as high as those with normal peripheral vision. Because the peripheral retina is very sensitive to decreased light delivery, twilight can be the most difficult time of day for driving.

Age-related decreases in integrated measures of visual performance, such as visual-processing speeds and visual-spatial attention (eg, useful field of view), are associated with higher collision rates. As persons age, they are less able to adapt to changes in light and to accommodate (presbyopia), have reduced depth perception, and are more sensitive to glare. However, the rate and magnitude of age-related deterioration in vision vary greatly among persons. Appropriate medical or surgical intervention can reduce or prevent some functional deficits (eg, treatment of glaucoma or cataracts).

In most states, central visual acuity and peripheral vision are routinely tested at the Department of Motor Vehicles. The frequency of these tests and the minimum acceptable standards vary. However, the most common thresholds are 20/40 in the better eye and a horizontal peripheral vision field of 120°. The useful field-of-view test has established composite scores that assess visual processing speed in fields of view. A patient with a 40% reduction in the useful field of view is considered impaired for driving.

Cognitive function: Many elderly persons with motor or visual impairment drive less frequently because of their condition; however, elderly persons with cognitive impairment may not fully recognize their limitations. The risk of having an accident is estimated to be about five times higher among elderly drivers with mild to moderate dementia than among those without dementia. Of community-dwelling elderly persons, about 3% aged 65 to 74, 14% aged 75 to 84, and > 20% aged > 85 have moderate cognitive impairment.[1] Persons with severe dementia should not continue to drive.

For the assessment of cognition, a short evaluation instrument, such as the Annotated Mini-Mental State Examination,[2] is recommended. Drivers with scores ≤ 23 (of 30 total) should undergo further evaluation (eg, on-road testing). For patients who have moderate cognitive problems or sharp declines in mental performance, the practitioner should recommend on-road testing only when necessary. Unnecessary testing due to injudicious screening can lead to excessive costs. Furthermore, because no evaluation is perfect, unfounded restrictions for capable elderly drivers may result, and such limitations can induce functional decline.

In most elderly drivers with dementia, cognitive impairment is mild; attention deficits in such drivers should be evaluated. The three major types of attention are selective, divided, and sustained. **Selective attention** (the ability to shift focus between competing stimuli) is important in driving because stimuli (eg, a radio, a cellular phone) can be distracting. The driver must selectively disregard noise or other contaminating influences. Selective attention is evaluated with several neuropsychologic tests (eg, dichotic listening test, Stroop test). **Divided attention** is the ability to process two or more stimuli at once and respond appropriately. For example, when the driver is approaching an intersection or merging onto a freeway, he must divide his attention between signaling the turn and accelerating into traffic. **Sustained attention** (endurance in alertness) may be relevant to an elderly driver with a chronic medical condition (eg, fatigue commonly associated with heart failure) or to one taking drugs that can cause fatigue or drowsiness (eg, benzodiazepines, antidepressants). Divided attention and sustained attention are clinically important, yet no reliable test is available for either measure.

[1] see pages 351 and 357   [2] see FIGURE 38–1 on page 346

ASSESSMENT OF MEDICAL CONDITIONS AND DRUG USE

Although functional assessment is usually considered more relevant than a medical diagnosis, certain medical conditions and the use of certain drugs should be considered when a person's ability to drive is evaluated. When beginning treatment with a new drug that could affect motor, visual, or cognitive function, patients should avoid driving for 1 to 2 days to be sure no adverse effects occur.

Heart conditions: The physician should estimate a patient's risk of coronary artery disease, although sudden cardiac events while driving account for < 1/1000 collisions. Patients with unstable angina should not resume driving until symptoms have been treated and the angina has been stabilized or has not recurred for ≥ 1 month. Some antianginal drugs (eg, nitroglycerin) can interfere with driving by causing a precipitous decrease in blood pressure. Many noncardiac drugs (eg, tricyclic antidepressants) have cardiovascular adverse effects, which can affect driving.

Patients should refrain from driving for about 1 month after an uncomplicated myocardial infarction or a coronary artery bypass graft operation or for 3 to 4 days after angioplasty. Some states and provinces have more specific requirements or recommendations for recovery time after these events. Practitioners should consult local Departments of Motor Vehicles or state medical advisory boards for the specific recommendations.

Epilepsy: The incidence of epilepsy increases with age. Drivers who have had one seizure with no detectable underlying neurologic cause are the least likely of all seizure patients to have another seizure. Each state has regulations for drivers with a history of seizures; most states require a seizure-free interval (eg, of 6 months) before reinstating driving privileges. About 70% of patients can adequately control epilepsy with drugs, although relapses may occur when anticonvulsant therapy is withdrawn.

Transient ischemic attacks and strokes: The incidence of transient ischemic attacks and strokes is highest among the elderly. In the absence of comorbid illnesses or other considerations, an elderly driver who has had a transient ischemic attack or stroke should have an event-free interval of ≥ 3 months before resuming driving. Residual disability resulting from a stroke can be evaluated by functional assessment. ◾ One year after a stroke, about 50% of patients have permanently discontinued driving.

Other neurologic diseases: Neurologic diseases such as demyelinating conditions (eg, multiple sclerosis) and Parkinson's disease may affect driving. The degree of disability varies widely. Physicians should

◾ see page 232

perform a functional assessment before deciding on a patient's ability to drive.

Diabetes mellitus: The major issue for patients with insulin-dependent diabetes mellitus is sudden development of hypoglycemia while driving. Patients with diabetes who have autonomic neuropathy or who are taking a β-blocker may have a hypoglycemic event without sufficient warning symptoms. Patients with diabetes who have not had a sudden event affecting consciousness for 3 years can continue to drive. Patients who have had a recent event affecting awareness and those with insulin-dependent diabetes whose insulin levels fluctuate widely (including documented hypoglycemia) should be prohibited from driving for 3 months while they are observed. Diabetic complications (eg, retinopathy) should be evaluated by functional assessment.

Drug use: Elderly drivers should be cautioned about taking **antihistamines** when driving. Antihistamines may produce sedative effects, including somnolence and slower reaction times. Although newer antihistamines (eg, loratadine, cetirizine, acrivastine, fexofenadine) produce fewer sedative effects than the first-generation antihistamines (eg, triprolidine, diphenhydramine, clemastine), they may still affect driving performance, especially if given in higher-than-recommended doses or if combined with alcohol or other drugs that can potentiate their sedative effects (eg, benzodiazepines, antidepressants).

Benzodiazepines, which are among the most frequently prescribed drugs for the elderly, should never be taken before or during driving. Many benzodiazepines have extremely long half-lives and can cause motor dysfunction, visual impairment, cognitive decline, and decreased attention, especially in the elderly. Taking modest doses of frequently used benzodiazepines impairs driving performance in the elderly driver to a level similar to the legal definition of alcohol intoxication.

Similar concerns are relevant when **antidepressants** are prescribed. Single doses of amitriptyline, imipramine, and doxepin, which have sedative effects, can impair many functions involved in driving. Other drugs with sedative effects, including opioid analgesics and antihistamines, may also affect driving performance.

Use of **alcohol,** alone or in combination with other drugs, can have tragic consequences for any driver, regardless of age. In general, the elderly consume alcohol less frequently than any other age group and are involved in fewer alcohol-related fatal crashes. However, elderly drivers should be counseled against alcohol consumption before driving. Smaller amounts of alcohol produce more significant effects in elderly persons than in younger persons because of age-related increases in adipose tissue and decreases in lean body mass, which reduce the amount of tissue distribution. Thus, elderly persons who consume alcohol have higher blood alcohol concentrations than younger persons with similar alcohol intakes. Also, because alcohol can impair cognition if mixed with other drugs, elderly persons taking multiple drugs are especially at risk.

LEGAL IMPLICATIONS

Patient confidentiality presents a dilemma for physicians treating elderly drivers with impairments such as dementia. Disclosure of information about a patient's driving ability, although it may violate patient confidentiality and result in restricted driving privileges that limit the patient's autonomy, is sanctioned when public safety is jeopardized. Physicians who do not notify appropriate authorities about a particular hazard (eg, an impaired driver) may be held liable. About 30% of states have policies that mandate the reporting of impaired drivers; statutes have been established to protect the physician's anonymity.

Foreseeability (the ability to predict a risk or threat to public safety and health) is the principal legal concern for physicians, especially when treating drivers with obvious impairments. Physicians who are uncertain about the significance of an impairment should report the patient to the Department of Motor Vehicles for special testing of driving performance.

SUR/
REH

In the USA, surgical rates are nearly twice as high for persons ≥ 65 years (215 operations per 1000 persons) as for persons < 65 years (120 operations per 1000 persons). Of hospitalized patients ≥ 65 years, 36% underwent a surgical procedure in 1990. About 6,569,000 procedures (or 28% of all procedures) were performed in persons ≥ 65. Also, 50% of all emergency surgical procedures are performed in the elderly; the most common involve the large bowel (25%), abdominal wall (17%), stomach (17%), biliary tract (11%), and small bowel (10%).

Age is generally considered an independent risk factor for surgical complications and death, especially in emergency surgery (see TABLE 24–1). Surgery involving the chest or abdomen increases risk by 20 to 50 times in all age groups. Surgical mortality rates increase nearly linearly with age, and 75% of all postoperative deaths occur in the elderly. Nonfatal complications are also more common in the elderly. Thus, age may be a sufficient reason to avoid surgery. Some operations (eg, extensive reconstructive dental procedures, kidney transplantation, joint replacement when severe pain is absent, cholecystectomy for asymptomatic gallstones) are generally not indicated in the very old except in unusual circumstances.

On the other hand, chronologic and physiologic ages are not necessarily equivalent. The decision to perform surgery should be based on the patient's general health status and the severity of the disorder, not on age alone. Despite chronologic age, the benefits of surgery may outweigh the risks.

Life expectancy◻ can profoundly affect the decision to perform surgery. For example, elective surgery that may be life threatening (eg, aortic aneurysm resection) should be considered if a person's life expectancy is 8 to 10 years but should probably be avoided if life expectancy is 1 to 2 years. Potential benefits must always be weighed against potential risks.

A patient's age can affect the timing of surgery. For elderly patients with cholecystitis, cholecystectomy should be performed early, because the mortality rate increases from 2% when surgery is performed within 12 to 24 hours of diagnosis to 10% when surgery is delayed. In contrast, the mortality rate is lower when certain procedures (eg, for an inguinal hernia or an abdominal aortic aneurysm) are performed as elective surgery rather than as emergency surgery, so delay may be warranted.

Plastic surgery, which can be reconstructive or cosmetic (ie, with no medical indication), is often performed in the elderly. Commonly performed reconstructive surgical procedures include skin tumor removal, flap reconstruction of pressure ulcers and other wounds, head and neck

---

◻see TABLE 2–2 on page 12

surgery, and reconstructive breast surgery. Facial surgery is often erroneously considered cosmetic (thus limiting third-party reimbursement). However, some facial procedures are medically warranted. For example, blepharoplasty often restores vision in patients with sagging skinfolds.

Cosmetic surgery should not be denied solely because of age. Such surgery may improve self-esteem and quality of life and may be affordable for the first time during older age. Indications and risk are essentially the same as for younger persons.

TABLE 24–1.   MORTALITY RATES FOR SOME SURGICAL PROCEDURES IN PATIENTS > 65 YEARS

Surgery	Mortality Rate (%)
Aortic aneurysm excision (elective)	9
Aortic valve replacement	12.1
Appendectomy	
Elective	0.6
Emergency	4–20
Cataract surgery	0.01–0.02
Cholecystectomy	
Elective	5
Emergency	5–16
Colonic resection	12
Coronary bypass	3–7
Hernia surgery	
Elective	0.3
Emergency	1
Internal fixation of a hip fracture (at 1 yr)	15
Knee replacement	1.5
Mastectomy (modified radical)	0.6
Mitral valve replacement	5–50
Partial gastrectomy	24
Percutaneous transluminal coronary angioplasty	5
Peripheral vascular surgery	15
Prostatectomy	0.3
Resection for colorectal carcinoma	4
Transurethral resection of the prostate	0.2–3.5

Adapted from Thomas DR, Ritchie CR: "Progress in geriatrics: preoperative assessment of elderly patients." *Journal of the American Geriatric Society* 43:811–821, 1995.

Preoperative evaluation should include a history, a physical examination, laboratory tests, and an assessment of surgical risk to identify coexisting diseases and complicating conditions and to correct the few that are reversible. Before emergency surgery, complete evaluation and correction of physiologic abnormalities may be impossible, but obtaining as much information as possible helps the surgeon take precautions to prevent complications. Preoperative evaluation may be performed with a geriatric consultation. Additional consultation with social workers, discharge planners, or psychiatrists may be warranted in limited cases; these services may be coordinated through geriatric consultation, in which each member of the health care team is in close communication.

Informed consent and advance directives: Before surgery, the surgeon explains the procedure, including possible complications, to the patient. Then the patient is asked to sign an informed consent agreement.

If a patient has dementia or delirium and cannot understand the surgical risks and benefits, the surgeon must proceed with care based on decisions made by a surrogate (eg, a court-appointed guardian). Advance directives (eg, living wills, durable power of attorney for health care) are written while patients still have the capacity to make health care decisions. **1**

Nursing issues: Nurses should teach patients about what to expect during recovery. As soon as possible, often hours after surgery, patients should get out of bed and be mobile; an active rehabilitation program **2** is developed to help patients quickly regain function. In hospitalized patients, potential postoperative problems include urinary incontinence, sleep problems, and pressure sores. An important concern for patients is pain management. **3** The nurse should interview patients or their caregivers to determine which analgesics they have used in the past and how effective these drugs were. Patients who return home should be given a care plan to optimize function in their home setting. Coordinated and comprehensive preoperative nursing care can help alleviate a patient's fears and enhance intraoperative and postoperative performance.

HISTORY

The surgeon should obtain the patient's history before surgery. The accuracy of the history may be limited by sensory or cognitive deficits, requiring the surgeon to rely on a history given by caregivers. **4** A complete and accurate drug history is especially important. The elderly

---

1 see page 134   **2** see page 264   **3** see page 262
4 see also page 24

often use several drugs concurrently, sometimes leading to adverse drug interactions that may cause problems perioperatively.

In one study, 59% of 178 chronically ill patients made errors reporting their drug use; of these errors, 26% were potentially serious. Therefore, drug use should be verified: patients should be asked to bring all of their prescription and over-the-counter drugs to the physician's office or hospital and to describe exactly how they use them; patients from long-term care facilities should be transferred with an up-to-date drug record; and caregivers should be asked to confirm drug use. When possible, the primary care physician should confirm current therapy.

PHYSICAL EXAMINATION AND LABORATORY TESTS

A complete physical examination should be performed.**1** Examining the skin, oral mucosa, and tongue can provide information about hydration and nutrition. Femoral, popliteal, and pedal pulses should be noted, and evidence of venous disease (eg, varicose veins, postphlebitic ulcers, edema) identified. Mental status should be documented.**2**

Urinalysis, a peripheral blood count, chemistry tests, and measurement of coagulation factors are necessary. A chest x-ray and an ECG are routinely obtained. Perioperative serum electrolyte studies are useful for patients taking diuretics.

ASSESSMENT OF RISK

The percentage of patients with coexisting diseases increases dramatically with age, from < 30% among patients aged 21 to 30 years to 90% among those aged 71 to 80 years. About 30% of elderly patients have three or more coexisting diseases or complicating conditions, and 80% have at least one complicating condition, which increases surgical risk. These diseases or complicating conditions must be systematically evaluated, and a plan must be formulated to manage each during the perioperative period.

Age: Although not a contraindication to surgery, age has been considered an independent risk factor for postoperative death. The risk of death is about 5% for an 80-year-old undergoing major surgery vs. < 2% for a younger patient. In one large multivariate analysis of patients undergoing noncardiac surgery, age > 70 was an independent risk factor for perioperative death. However, in other surgical series, age was not a risk factor for postoperative complications or death. In one such study, the 30-day mortality rate was 6.2% in octogenarians and 8.4% in nonagenarians. Age may be a surrogate for coexisting disease contributing

1 see page 31   **2** see page 343

TABLE 25-1.   AMERICAN SOCIETY OF ANESTHESIOLOGISTS PHYSICAL STATUS CLASSIFICATION*

Class	Preoperative Health Status
I	Healthy
II	Mild systemic disease
III	Severe systemic disease that is not incapacitating
IV	Incapacitating systemic disease that is a constant threat to life
V	Death likely in $\leq$ 24 h with or without surgery

*Assumes an age effect: healthy patients aged > 80 are assigned to class II.

to postoperative death rather than an independent risk factor. Severity of illness predicts outcome better than age does.

General health status: The American Society of Anesthesiologists Physical Status Classification (see TABLE 25-1) is often used to predict surgical outcome based on a patient's preoperative health status. The mortality rate for different age groups varies little among patients in classes I and II and only slightly among those in classes III and IV when grouped by age.

Functional status: All complications, including life-threatening ones, are more common in inactive patients. In one study, surgical risk was 9.7 times higher in men with very limited preoperative activity levels than in those with normal activity levels. Scores on activities of daily living instruments ∎ used preoperatively help predict the 1-year survival of patients who have had a hip fracture.

Nutritional status: The mortality rate is significantly higher in patients who have lost > 20% of body weight before surgery. The incidence of complications is four times higher and the mortality rate is six times higher in patients with a serum albumin level < 35 g/L than in those with a normal level; measurement is warranted when poor nutrition is suspected.

Whether preoperative use of nutritional supplements can improve surgical outcome is controversial. Overall morbidity and mortality rates did not decrease and infection rates increased in elderly patients who received total parenteral nutrition (TPN) preoperatively compared with those who did not. However, in severely malnourished patients who received TPN, infection rates did not increase and fewer complications occurred. Most experts agree that surgery should not be delayed to provide TPN preoperatively, except possibly for severely malnourished patients. However, even in these patients, evidence supporting preoperative use of TPN is inconclusive.

∎ see TABLE 4–3 on page 44 and TABLE 4–4 on page 45

Psychologic status: Social support systems and the will to live, although difficult to quantify, are important predictors of surgical outcome.

Dementia is a major risk factor for a poor outcome; in one series, the postoperative mortality rate was 52% higher in patients with dementia than in those without. Postoperative complications are also more common in demented patients.

Heart disease: Cardiac complications, including myocardial infarction and heart failure, account for 12% of all surgical complications and 20% of potentially reversible deaths. The best predictor of postoperative cardiac complications is the presence of ischemic heart disease. The risk of perioperative infarction or death is 8 to 30% in patients who have had a myocardial infarction in the 3 months before surgery, compared with 3.5 to 5% in patients who have had a myocardial infarction > 6 months before surgery.

The Modified Multifactorial Index (see TABLE 25–2) can be used to assess cardiac risk: 63% of all cardiac complications occur in patients with a score > 15. However, a significant number of cardiac complications occur in patients with a low score, demonstrating that the predictive power of this cardiac index and others is poor in low-risk patients. The exercise tolerance of patients with heart disease should be assessed by asking them what their usual daily activities are and how easily they tire.

The risk of postoperative cardiac complications is increased if any rhythm other than sinus rhythm is present or if premature atrial contractions, often considered a benign finding, are present. An occasional solitary premature ventricular contraction does not require preoperative treatment. Guidelines were developed by the American College of Cardiology and the American Heart Association to help physicians evaluate perioperative cardiac risk and the need for additional evaluation or intervention in patients undergoing noncardiac surgery. The guidelines are based on clinical predictors (see TABLE 25–3), type of surgery to be performed (see TABLE 25–4), and functional assessment.◼ The guidelines include an eight-step algorithm.

Heart failure should be corrected to the degree possible. Patients with preoperative symptoms of heart failure (eg, jugular venous distention, a third heart sound) are more likely to develop postoperative heart failure and frank pulmonary edema than are those who have no symptoms or who have no history of heart failure. Use of digitalis, diuretics, vasodilators, and angiotensin-converting enzyme inhibitors should be considered to improve cardiac performance preoperatively. Potassium depletion due to diuretics should be corrected preoperatively.

◼see page 42

Many cardiac drugs are myocardial depressants and interact with myocardial depressant anesthetics or other vasoactive drugs. Nonetheless, drugs commonly used to treat heart disease should not be withdrawn before surgery; sudden withdrawal, especially of β-blockers, may be dangerous.

Hypertension should be controlled preoperatively, and antihypertensive drugs should not be withdrawn. During anesthesia, absolute reductions in blood pressure are greater in patients with untreated or inadequately controlled hypertension than in those with adequately controlled hypertension.

Carotid artery disease: The influence of carotid artery occlusive disease on perioperative risk of stroke or death is uncertain. The disease appears to increase the perioperative stroke rate in patients undergoing

TABLE 25-2. MODIFIED MULTIFACTORIAL INDEX*

Factor	Points†
Myocardial infarction	
≤ 6 mo before surgery	10
> 6 mo before surgery	5
Angina	
‡Class III (while walking 1–2 blocks on level ground or climbing 1 flight of stairs)	10
‡Class IV (with any activity)	20
Unstable angina ≤ 6 mo before surgery	10
Alveolar pulmonary edema	
≤ 1 wk before surgery	10
> 1 wk before surgery	5
Valvular disease (suspected critical aortic stenosis)	20
Arrhythmia	
Rhythm other than sinus rhythm or sinus rhythm plus atrial premature beats on most recent preoperative ECG	5
> 5 premature ventricular contractions on any preoperative ECG	5
Poor general medical status§	5
Age > 70 years	5
Emergency surgery	10

*Derived from Goldman's index and corrected for disease prevalence.
†The likelihood ratios for cardiac complications are 0.43 for ≤ 15 points, 3.38 for 15–30 points, and 10.60 for > 30 points.
‡Canadian Cardiovascular Society classification.
§Partial pressure of oxygen < 60 mm Hg; partial pressure of carbon dioxide > 50 mm Hg; potassium level < 3 mEq/L, bicarbonate level < 20 mEq/L; blood urea nitrogen > 50 mg/dL (18 mmol/L); creatinine level > 3 mg/dL (260 mmol/L); abnormal aspartate aminotransferase level; signs of chronic liver disease; noncardiac problems requiring bed rest.

Adapted from Detsky AS, Abrams HB, McLaughlin JR, et al: "Predicting cardiac complications in patients undergoing non-cardiac surgery." *Journal of General Internal Medicine* 1:211–219, 1986; used with permission.

TABLE 25-3.   CLINICAL PREDICTORS OF PERIOPERATIVE CARDIOVASCULAR RISK*

Risk Category	Factors
Major	Decompensated heart failure Severe valvular disease Significant arrhythmias (high-grade atrioventricular block, symptomatic arrhythmias with underlying heart disease, supraventricular arrhythmias with uncontrolled ventricular rate) Unstable coronary syndromes (eg, recent myocardial infarction with evidence of ischemic risk, unstable or severe angina)
Intermediate	Compensated or prior heart failure Diabetes mellitus Mild angina pectoris Prior myocardial infarction
Minor	Abnormal ECG Advanced age History of stroke Low functional capacity Rhythm other than sinus Uncontrolled systemic hypertension

*Includes myocardial infarction, heart failure, and death.

myocardial revascularization. However, in patients undergoing other types of surgery, the rate of disease may be increased only in patients who have had transient ischemic attacks or who have severe occlusive disease of both internal carotid arteries and of vertebral arteries.

Pulmonary disease: Pulmonary disease greatly increases the risk of perioperative complications, accounting for 40% of total complications and 20% of deaths. However, preoperative pulmonary function testing is probably unnecessary for most elderly patients. Before nonthoracic surgery, pulmonary screening is most likely to benefit heavy smokers and patients with symptoms and signs of pulmonary disease. Severe chronic obstructive pulmonary disease (forced expiratory volume < 1 to 1.5 L at 1 second) increases the risk of surgery, mainly because the patient has an ineffective cough and cannot clear secretions. Preoperative use of bronchodilators may improve a bronchospastic component. Smokers should not smoke preoperatively; they and other high-risk patients are likely to benefit from a few days of active physical therapy, including percussion and inspiratory exercises, and from the use of broncholytic drugs.

Liver disease: If evidence of impaired liver function is noted on routine liver function tests or by history during preoperative evaluation, a poor surgical outcome is likely. The only consequences of liver diseases that can be corrected preoperatively are coagulation abnormali-

TABLE 25–4.   CARDIAC RISK* FOR NONCARDIAC SURGERY

Risk	Type of Surgery
High	Major emergency surgery Aortic and other major vascular surgery Peripheral vascular surgery Other long procedures in which large fluid shifts or blood loss is likely
Intermediate	Carotid endarterectomy Head and neck surgery Intraperitoneal, intrathoracic, orthopedic, or prostate surgery
Low	Endoscopy Superficial surgery Breast surgery Cataract extraction

*Includes incidence of nonfatal myocardial infarction and heart-related death.

ties, which are managed with vitamin K or protein blood products (eg, fresh frozen plasma, coagulation concentrates).

Renal disease: Renal function is assessed by measuring blood urea nitrogen and serum creatinine levels. In the elderly, the serum creatinine level must be adjusted for age and decreased lean body mass using one of several formulas.[1] Dosages of renally excreted drugs must be adjusted based on renal clearance. Dehydration may lead to prerenal azotemia, which can be corrected by administering fluids. If blood urea nitrogen and serum creatinine levels remain high, peritoneal dialysis or hemodialysis may reverse the uremia and reduce the high surgical risk.

26 ■ PERIOPERATIVE CARE

Elective surgery in the elderly, once considered risky, is now commonly performed with good outcomes, even in centenarians. Surgical risk depends on the patient's overall state of health, not on chronologic age.[2]

INTRAOPERATIVE CARE

The elderly often have multiple disorders or may be frail; they often require special assistance during intraoperative care. Equipment (eg, step stools, grab bars) should be available to help those patients with

[1] see page 59   [2] see page 240

limitations move safely from the bed to a stretcher or from the stretcher to an operating table. Patients who feel pain during movement (eg, those with a hip fracture) should be given an analgesic before they are moved. On the operating table, a bolster can be placed under the knees to relieve stretch on back muscles. Foam padding, available in most operating rooms, can be placed between specific pressure points and the operating table to prevent direct contact, which can lead to pressure sores.∎ Extremities are positioned carefully to avoid injury. Patients with spinal curvature or limited motion need padding placed in a manner that distributes pressure over as large an area as possible, avoiding small pressure points. Arthritic changes can make positioning and intubation difficult. Because the elderly have more fragile skin, they are prone to injury from restraining devices, tape, Bovie pads, and adhesive monitoring devices (eg, ECG electrodes).

MONITORING

Intraoperative monitoring of blood pressure, heart rate and rhythm, ventilation, fluid status, and urinary output is similar in patients of all ages. For frail patients with fragile skin, the blood pressure cuff should be applied with care, using a thin layer of cotton undercast padding to protect the skin if needed.

Oxygen saturation is monitored with a pulse oximeter, typically placed on the finger. However, the signal quality at this site may be inadequate because of decreased pulsatile flow in the elderly. If quality is inadequate, the probe can be placed on the earlobe. Anesthetics or sedatives should be administered only if an accurate pulse oximeter reading is obtained.

Core body temperature is measured and recorded—usually with an esophageal or rectal probe—during long operations, particularly those in which the viscera are exposed. In many elderly patients, core body temperature is lower and more difficult to maintain than in younger patients. For the elderly, the normal mechanisms used to increase body temperature (eg, shivering) can generate excessive oxygen consumption, increasing the metabolic cost of rewarming the body. Therefore, specific intraoperative measures are required to maintain a reasonable body temperature. These measures include using convection warming systems and warmed IV and lavage fluids, maintaining adequate operating room temperature, and minimizing exposure of the abdominal viscera. Despite these measures, elderly patients may lose significant body heat. For elderly patients given general anesthetics, body temperature should be within 0.5° C (0.9° F) of their baseline core body temperature before extubation.

∎ see page 1261

POSTOPERATIVE CARE

After high-risk operations (eg, abdominal aortic surgery, liver resection), most patients, especially elderly ones, are treated in an intensive care unit or recovery room for ≤ 72 hours before being returned to a standard hospital room.

After the acute recovery period, certain preventive measures are important even when convalescence is uncomplicated. Getting out of bed and sitting in a chair may be a first objective. Patients should begin to ambulate soon after surgery; patients who do not do so are more likely to rapidly lose muscle mass and strength and to develop thromboembolism. Elderly patients may need up to two assistants for several days to ambulate and transfer. Elderly patients need assistance because they are likely to have reduced baroreceptor reflexes, causing dizziness or frank loss of consciousness when they assume an upright posture for the first time after surgery.

EARLY POSTOPERATIVE COMPLICATIONS

Many elderly patients experience postoperative complications during the first 2 to 3 days.

Hypoxemia: Analgesics, particularly opioids, may decrease sensitivity to the hypercapnic and hypoxic respiratory drive in elderly patients, predisposing them to arterial desaturation and hypoxemia. Debilitated patients commonly need prolonged intubation and ventilation. Elderly patients are given supplemental oxygen while being transported from the operating room to the recovery room. They should not be discharged from the recovery room until arterial saturation is similar to the preoperative level.

Pain: The elderly are more tolerant of and philosophical about pain than younger persons and, unless asked, may not report pain. However, controlling pain■ is as important as maintaining appropriate blood pressure and body temperature.

Postoperative delirium: Some degree of delirium occurs in up to 25% of elderly patients within 1 week of surgery. Associated with a higher incidence of complications and a poor functional outcome 6 months after surgery, delirium directly contributes to in-hospital morbidity and longer hospital stays. Certain anesthetics, meperidine, and anticholinegics seem to increase the risk of postoperative delirium. The risk of postoperative delirium is similar with general and regional anesthetic techniques; however, most patients who undergo regional anesthesia are also given opioids, benzodiazepines, or other adjuvants that increase risk. Preexisting dementia, fluid and electrolyte imbalance, drugs, sleep deprivation, frequent interruptions for nursing care, altered

■ see page 262

circadian rhythms, and an inability to keep track of time can contribute to confusion and disorientation.

Delirium in surgical patients does not appear to differ from that in other hospitalized patients, and the incidence in the two groups is similar. Postoperative delirium is characterized by difficulty in organizing and coordinating thoughts and by slowed motor function. It ranges from mild confusion to full hallucinations. Patients with delirium may remove vital drains or temporary pacemaker wires, or they may fall and injure themselves when getting out of bed.

No specific treatment is available, although certain measures can help minimize confusion and disorientation.■ When possible, elderly patients are transferred from the intensive care unit or recovery room, both of which are frequently noisy and brightly lit. Patients placed in such units may develop a similar disorder called **intensive care unit psychosis,** which is a diagnosis of exclusion, as is postoperative delirium.

Constant nighttime attendance (eg, by a family member or special aide) is preferable to use of physical or chemical restraints. Unless necessary, physical restraints should not be used in patients with delirium. If sedatives are used, antipsychotics (eg, haloperidol or the newer, atypical antipsychotics) are preferable to benzodiazepines.

Postoperative cognitive dysfunction: Elderly patients are subject to postoperative decreases in cognitive function as measured by psychometric tests. The causes of such decreases are unknown. Although generally thought to be reversible, some cognitive dysfunction may be permanent.

Hypotension: The most common cause of hypotension during the early postoperative period is hypovolemia due to inadequate replacement of intraoperative fluid losses, occult hemorrhage, or internal fluid losses (eg, reaccumulation of ascites, third-space losses). Hypotension due to other conditions is rare during the early postoperative period. It may be due to septic shock, which can develop in patients who had preoperative signs of sepsis (eg, patients with severe intra-abdominal sepsis or massive burns). Factitious causes (eg, faulty blood pressure readings) should also be considered, especially if the patient's history and physical findings do not correlate with the severity of hypotension. Blood pressure monitors must be inspected to be certain they are functioning properly.

The elderly are prone to heart failure postoperatively, and treatment in this setting usually consists of diuretics and inotropic drugs. Diastolic dysfunction develops more rapidly (usually < 1 hour after the operation) than systolic dysfunction and can greatly reduce blood pressure and flow. The most effective immediate treatment is calcium channel blockers.

■ see page 356

Hypothermia: Immediately after a long operation, body temperature may decrease to 32.2° to 35.0° C (90° to 95° F). Treatment includes warming IV and other fluids and using convection warming systems. **1** A vacuum chamber around the forearm and hand may also be helpful; this device creates a low-level vacuum (about 40 mm Hg), thus increasing blood flow to the extremity. A warming pad then efficiently transfers heat to the extremity. Early evidence suggests that this approach may be more efficient than convection blankets for warming elderly patients; however, extra care must be taken to avoid superficial burns.

Respiratory problems: In the elderly, the ability to protect the airway from aspiration is markedly decreased. Therefore, the physician makes sure the patient's airway reflexes (eg, gag reflex, swallowing mechanisms) are adequate before removing an endotracheal tube. Atelectasis is very common among frail elderly patients and predisposes them to pneumonia. In debilitated patients with chronic dehydration, thick copious sputum may develop in the lungs after even minimal hydration. For such patients, percussion and postural drainage must be performed frequently and aggressively.

Sometimes, elderly patients with respiratory problems require prolonged mechanical ventilation, even though it may introduce complications (eg, pneumonia, atelectasis).

Fluid and electrolyte imbalance: In the elderly, the ability to maintain homeostatic levels of fluids and electrolytes is reduced, and the margin between too little and too much fluid is relatively narrow. **2** Overexpansion of the extracellular compartment from excess isotonic fluid administration may be dangerous because cardiopulmonary reserves are limited in the elderly.

During the early postoperative period, the body normally retains water and sodium, and the elderly may have difficulty eliminating the excess fluid.

Initially, the amount of IV fluids can be estimated, but fluid administration should be adjusted to optimize blood pressure, pulse, and urine output (which are closely monitored). Central venous pressure, pulmonary wedge pressure, and urine output measurements help determine fluid requirements. Enough fluids are given to replace insensible fluid losses and measured or estimated external losses and to produce a urine output of 0.5 mL/kg/hour, or about 30 mL/hour.

When external losses are minimal, fluid requirements are usually 1500 to 2500 mL for 24 hours. However, more fluids may be needed if third-space sequestration of fluids is excessive (eg, because of a distended bowel or inflammation of subcutaneous tissues due to burns). The sequestered fluid is usually mobilized on the 3rd to 5th day after surgery.

---

1 see also page 667   **2** see page 561

Electrolyte replacement must include potassium 20 to 100 mEq/day IV or po to replace losses (about two thirds is lost in urine, and the rest from the gastrointestinal tract). If potassium replacement is inadequate, postoperative ileus may be prolonged and resistant metabolic alkalosis may develop. Postoperative ileus delays return to feeding and can prolong hospitalization. Calcium and magnesium may be replaced if serum levels are low.

Hyponatremia is common among elderly patients, particularly among men undergoing transurethral resection of the prostate because hypotonic irrigation solution is absorbed through the open venous sinuses of the prostate. Symptoms appear when the sodium level is < 130 mEq/L, and confusion or a seizure may occur a few days after surgery.

The patient's total body sodium content and total body free water content may be increased, normal, or decreased. Pulmonary edema, excessive peripheral edema, or evidence of major third-space losses suggests increased total body sodium content. Total body free water content may be increased because excess 5% dextrose (in water) is administered postoperatively or because surgery alters the body's responses, resulting in high levels of antidiuretic hormone.

If hyponatremia is due to inadequate sodium intake, 0.9% sodium chloride solution should be given cautiously, avoiding increases in sodium > 10 mEq/L/24 hours. More rapid replacement may result in central pontine myelinolysis. If hyponatremia is due to water overload, 0.9% sodium chloride solution and a diuretic should be given cautiously. In either case, electrolyte levels are monitored frequently. A sodium chloride solution of 3% or 5% is rarely indicated, and its use can result in severe hypernatremia and central nervous system adverse effects.

Nutritional deficiencies: Early, aggressive nutritional support should be given to patients with malnutrition, those with complications (eg, sepsis), and those who have lost > 10% of their premorbid weight. Supplemental oral feedings, tube feedings, or total parenteral nutrition may be given, depending on the patient's condition.∎ If anorexia or dysphagia makes oral feeding difficult but gastric and intestinal motility and absorption are normal, enteral feedings may be given by continuous drip. In such cases, the enteral route is preferable to the parenteral route because it causes fewer complications, costs less, and may have a trophic effect on the intestine. Total parenteral nutrition is used when intestinal motility or absorption is abnormal.

Postoperatively, the metabolic rate, measured by oxygen consumption, briefly increases (usually to 20 to 40% more than the normal basal metabolic rate) unless a complication such as sepsis develops. Age, sex, height, and weight affect the basal caloric requirement, but body tem-

∎ see page 601

perature, protein losses through wounds, and muscular work related to physical activity (eg, ambulation) do not. A total daily caloric requirement of 1.2 to 2 times the basal metabolic rate is generally adequate.

The appropriate mixture of substrates, carbohydrates, proteins, and fats to meet the patient's metabolic needs to produce a positive nitrogen balance must be given. Glucose (a carbohydrate) infused at 5 mg/kg/minute provides enough calories to prevent the breakdown of amino acids as an energy source and suppresses endogenous glucose production via hepatic gluconeogenesis, which requires mobilization of amino acids as gluconeogenic precursors. This infusion rate also approximates the maximum rate of glucose oxidation for a bedridden patient. Any additional glucose is converted to fat.

For most elderly patients, protein infused at 0.5 to 1.0 g/kg/day is sufficient to maintain a positive nitrogen balance. This rate can be increased to 1.5 to 2.5 g/kg/day if needed.

Fats must be given (parenterally or enterally) to meet the patient's total caloric requirement. Fats supply essential fatty acids and enough calories to minimize the mobilization of endogenous proteins for energy and gluconeogenesis.

Other complications: Pressure sores, constipation, and complications from urinary catheters may also occur postoperatively.∎

LATE POSTOPERATIVE COMPLICATIONS

Antibiotic-associated pseudomembranous colitis: This disorder should be considered when diarrhea, which is common after abdominal operations, occurs postoperatively in a patient who has received antibiotics.∎ Antibiotics may alter the balance in normal gut flora, allowing overgrowth of *Clostridium difficile.* Cephalosporins and extended-spectrum penicillins (eg, ampicillin) are most commonly implicated, but clindamycin, lincomycin, tetracycline, chloramphenicol, and trimethoprim-sulfamethoxazole have also been implicated.

Diarrhea usually develops within 1 to 10 days after antibiotics are started. In one study of elderly patients, diarrhea developed an average of 2.7 days after antibiotics were started. If diarrhea occurs postoperatively, stool specimens are obtained immediately for bacterial culture and toxin analysis; up to 75% of patients with postoperative diarrhea have *C. difficile* infections. Sigmoidoscopy may also help make the diagnosis. Treatment is most commonly undertaken with metronidazole 250 mg po qid for 10 days.

Intra-abdominal abscesses: Intra-abdominal abscesses are located deep to the fascia, not within the surgical wound. The elderly may not have the typical symptoms of persistent fever and localized abdominal or flank tenderness, or they may have only vague complaints.

∎ see also page 101   ∎ see page 1066

Intra-abdominal abscesses may be subphrenic, subhepatic, pelvic, or intraloop and may be difficult to localize. CT and ultrasonography are useful in diagnosis and localization and in the percutaneous placement of catheters for drainage. However, surgical drainage is the definitive treatment. During or immediately after surgical drainage, hemodynamic instability due to the distributive shock of sepsis frequently occurs.

27 ANESTHESIA CONSIDERATIONS

The use of anesthetics presents greater risks for the elderly than for younger persons; recovery from the drugs is longer, and complications may be more severe. Also, many age-related anatomic, physiologic, and functional changes (eg, decreases in height, weight, body surface area, and metabolism) affect the use of anesthetics—see TABLE 27–1. ▌ Commonly used measurements of organ function (eg, cardiac index, oxygen consumption, glomerular filtration rate) are decreased in the elderly, but these decreases correlate with an age-related decrease in tissue mass. Also, the function of the liver and kidneys, which are involved in drug metabolism, often decreases in the elderly; as a result, clearance of many drugs, including several commonly used anesthetics (see TABLE 27–2), is decreased.

PREOPERATIVE CONSIDERATIONS

Evaluation: The anesthesiologist must determine whether the patient is in optimal condition for surgery. Medical disorders superimposed on age-related physiologic changes will complicate anesthesiologic management. Consequently, a detailed history and a thorough physical examination ▌ are necessary. The drug history can provide information about disorders that may affect the use of anesthetics (see TABLE 27–3). The patient's primary care physician should be contacted to obtain records of past medical history, functional status, drug use, and allergies. If possible, the results of tests given just before anesthetics are used should be compared with the results of similar tests given earlier by the primary care physician.

Preoperative sedation: Many anesthesiologists do not give sedatives to elderly patients preoperatively because these drugs reduce the already compromised ventilatory response to hypoxia and hypercapnia. Because currently used anesthetics produce fewer respiratory tract secretions, muscarinic anticholinergics (eg, atropine, scopolamine,

TABLE 27-1. AGE-RELATED CHANGES THAT AFFECT THE USE OF ANESTHETICS

Organ System	Anatomic or Physiologic Change	Functional Change	Anesthetic Implications
Cardiovascular	Distensibility decreases	Ventricular filling pressure increases	Control of preload is more difficult
		Contractility decreases	Hemodynamic effect of anesthetics (mostly negative inotropic drugs and vasodilators) is greater than expected
	Compliance decreases	Peripheral resistance increases, peripheral perfusion decreases	Sensitivity to changes in intravascular volume increases
Hepatic	Activity of some hepatic enzymes decreases, number of hepatocytes decreases	Metabolism of some drugs decreases	Patient is predisposed to relative overdosing and drug toxicity
	Perfusion decreases	Metabolism of some drugs decreases	Patient is predisposed to relative overdosing and drug toxicity
Musculoskeletal	Fibrous tissue increases, elasticity decreases	Stiffness increases	Patient is difficult to position for intubation and surgery
	Skeletal calcium decreases	Fragility increases	Risk of fractures increases
	Calcium is deposited	Mobility decreases	Patient is difficult to position for intubation and surgery
Pulmonary	Alveolar air space decreases	Ability to acquire and deliver oxygen decreases, alveolar ventilation decreases	Ventilation/perfusion mismatch increases during positive pressure ventilation and general anesthesia
	Diffusing capacity decreases	Ventilation/perfusion mismatch increases	Uptake of inhaled anesthetics is delayed

System	Physiologic change	Clinical implication
	Compliance of the lungs and chest wall decreases	During regional anesthesia, the function of accessory muscles of respiration may be impaired, predisposing the patient to respiratory insufficiency
	Work of breathing increases	
	Chemoreceptor responsiveness decreases	Administration of sedatives and opioids predisposes the patient to respiratory insufficiency, hypoxia
	Ventilatory response to hypoxia and hypercapnia decreases	
Renal	Number of nephrons decreases	Patient is predisposed to fluid and electrolyte abnormalities
	Water and sodium homeostasis is impaired	
	Renal perfusion decreases	Patient is predisposed to fluid and electrolyte abnormalities
	Water and sodium homeostasis is impaired	
	Creatinine clearance decreases	Patient is predisposed to relative overdosing and drug toxicity
	Elimination of some drugs and their metabolites decreases	
Skin	Subcutaneous tissue decreases	Patient is predisposed to injury from adhesives, monitoring devices, and tape
	Fragility increases	
	Thermal insulation decreases	Patient is predisposed to heat loss and hypothermia
	Protection of bony surfaces decreases	Patient is predisposed to pressure sores

TABLE 27–2.   ANESTHETICS AFFECTED BY AGING

Type	Drug	Mechanism of Elimination
Induction agents	Diazepam	Oxidative metabolism in the liver
	Etomidate	Ester hydrolysis by esterases in the liver and plasma
	Ketamine	N-demethylation in the liver
	Midazolam	Hydroxylation and conjugation in the liver
	Propofol	Glucuronide and sulfate conjugation in the liver
	Thiopental	Oxidative metabolism in the liver
Neuromuscular blockers	Atracurium	Hofmann elimination, ester hydrolysis
	Cisatracurium	Hofmann elimination
	Doxacurium	Excreted unchanged in urine* and bile
	Metocurine	Excreted unchanged in urine
	Mivacurium	Hydrolysis by plasma cholinesterases
	Pancuronium	Excreted unchanged in urine* and metabolized in the liver
	Pipecuronium	Excreted unchanged in urine* and bile
	Rocuronium	Excreted unchanged in bile* and urine
	Succinylcholine	Hydrolysis by plasma cholinesterase
	Tubocurarine	Excreted unchanged in urine* and bile
	Vecuronium	Excreted unchanged in bile* and metabolized in the liver; active metabolites excreted in urine
Opioids	Alfentanil	Oxidative metabolism in the liver
	Fentanyl	Oxidative metabolism in the liver
	Meperidine	Oxidative metabolism in the liver
	Morphine	Glucuronide and sulfate conjugation in the liver
	Remifentanil	Hydrolysis by nonspecific plasma esterases
	Sufentanil	Oxidative metabolism in the liver
Anticholinesterases	Edrophonium	Excreted unchanged in urine
	Neostigmine	Excreted unchanged in urine
	Pyridostigmine	Excreted unchanged in urine

* Major pathway.

glycopyrrolate) are generally not needed to decrease secretions; also, they are particularly problematic in persons with dementia, glaucoma, and benign prostatic hyperplasia. If an anticholinergic is necessary, glycopyrrolate, which is poorly lipid soluble and does not cross the blood-brain barrier, is the drug of choice. Atropine and scopolamine can cause central nervous system adverse effects. Atropine may produce excitement and delirium; scopolamine can cause agitation, restlessness, and hallucinations.

INTRAOPERATIVE CONSIDERATIONS

Monitored anesthesia care: Patients who are given a local anesthetic or no anesthetic should be monitored closely by an anesthesiologist. Monitored anesthesia care consists of monitoring the patient's vital signs and providing sedation as needed. It is often used with procedures such as cataract surgery, pacemaker placement, inguinal hernia repair, and extracorporeal shock wave lithotripsy.

Regional anesthesia: Spinal or epidural anesthetic techniques or blockade of major nerves (eg, of the cervical plexus for carotid endarterectomy or the brachial plexus for arm surgery) may be used to produce regional anesthesia. Spinal or epidural anesthetic techniques can be used for surgery of the lower abdomen, pelvis, or legs; they produce profound sympathetic block, which may cause hypotension, especially in patients who are hypovolemic.◻ Local anesthetics administered epidurally have a faster onset and greater dermatomal spread in elderly persons than in younger persons.

General anesthesia: General anesthesia involves loss of consciousness, amnesia, pain relief,◻ and a variable degree of muscle relaxation depending on the choice of volatile agent or use of a neuromuscular blocker. Most general anesthetics are potent myocardial depressants and vasodilators. Usually, an endotracheal tube is inserted into the patient's airway to control ventilation.

Doses of the induction agents etomidate, midazolam, propofol, and thiopental should be significantly lower for elderly patients than for younger patients. Ketamine and etomidate have minimal effects on the cardiovascular system and thus may be the induction agents of choice for the elderly.

The volatile anesthetics halothane, enflurane, isoflurane, sevoflurane, and desflurane impair the already attenuated chemoreceptor response in the elderly. The minimal alveolar concentration of these drugs decreases linearly with age, so that a smaller dosage is required to achieve anesthetic levels.

Neuromuscular blockers eliminated in urine or bile have a prolonged duration of action in the elderly, whereas the neuromuscular blockers atracurium, cisatracurium, and mivacurium do not. Little information is available about how aging affects succinylcholine activity, but the drug's circulatory time is thought to be longer in the elderly, allowing more time for hydrolysis of the drug. Thus, the initial dose of succinylcholine may need to be larger for elderly patients than for younger patients.

Opioids have a prolonged duration of action and decreased clearance in the elderly, who are more sensitive to them than younger persons are.

◻ see page 251   ◻ see page 262

TABLE 27–3. DISORDERS THAT MAY AFFECT THE USE OF ANESTHETICS

Organ System	Disorder	Effect	Anesthetic Implications
Cardiovascular	Aortic stenosis Arrhythmias Coronary artery disease (especially recent myocardial infarction) Heart failure	Increased incidence of perioperative morbidity (myocardial infarction, pulmonary edema) and mortality	Elective surgery should be postponed Coronary artery surgery or angioplasty should be considered for patients with coronary artery disease Perioperative invasive monitoring may decrease the risk of complications
	Hypertension	Diastolic dysfunction, left ventricular hypertrophy, impaired coronary blood flow, ventricular ectopy, sudden death, end organ damage (heart, brain, kidney)	Poorly controlled hypertension predisposes the patient to intraoperative blood pressure lability, which contributes to myocardial ischemia and to central nervous system and renal complications Elective surgery should be postponed if hypertension is poorly controlled Invasive monitoring for emergency surgery should be considered if hypertension is poorly controlled
Endocrine	Diabetes mellitus	Poor perioperative glucose control, autonomic dysfunction (silent myocardial ischemia, gastroparesis, renal dysfunction, neuropathy)	Oral hypoglycemic drugs should be avoided perioperatively The blood glucose level should be checked frequently Invasive monitoring should be considered The patient is at risk for aspiration The patient may have fluid and electrolyte abnormalities Blood pressure may be labile

Musculoskeletal	Degenerative joint disease	Limited mobility	The patient is difficult to position for surgery, regional anesthetic techniques, and intubation
	Rheumatoid arthritis	Use of NSAIDs	Platelet function is impaired
		High prevalence of atlanto-occipital subluxation and arytenoid involvement	Intubation is hazardous
		Use of corticosteroids	Stress-dose corticosteroid coverage is necessary
Pulmonary	Reactive airways disease (asthma, chronic obstructive pulmonary disease)	Predisposition to decreased airflow, arterial desaturation, increased pulmonary vascular resistance, right-sided heart failure, and ventilation/perfusion mismatch	Pulmonary function must be optimized preoperatively by treating infection, administering bronchodilators, and advising the patient to stop smoking
			Drugs that may cause histamine release should be avoided
			Regional anesthetic techniques should be considered to avoid tracheal intubation
			For perioperative monitoring and respiratory care, ventilation, an intra-arterial catheter, and pulse oximetry are required

NSAIDs = nonsteroidal anti-inflammatory drugs.

The sedative and respiratory depressant effects of opioids may contribute to the postoperative pulmonary complications that frequently occur in the elderly. Remifentanil, a new, potent ultrashort-acting opioid, may be useful intraoperatively for elderly patients, because it is metabolized by nonspecific plasma esterases and, unlike other opioids, its elimination is unaffected by aging.

For elderly patients undergoing hip fracture surgery, regional or general anesthesia is appropriate. The consensus is that regional and general anesthetic techniques do not differ in effect on short-term or long-term survival in these patients and do not alter the incidence of postoperative confusion. Regional techniques provide some protection against deep venous thrombophlebitis but do not improve long-term outcome.

Other age-related operative issues (see TABLE 27–1): Obtaining vascular access to place monitoring devices and to administer drugs, fluids, and blood can be difficult in the elderly. Their veins are fragile, and arthritic changes may make positioning for central line placement difficult. Arthritic changes in the neck and jaw can also make intubation difficult; fiberoptic techniques may offer an advantage.

Because of age-related changes in temperature regulation,❶ the elderly are prone to hypothermia during surgery. During anesthesia, the thermoregulatory center in the hypothalamus is anesthetized; patients are pharmacologically paralyzed and given sympathetic blocking agents. These measures further prevent heat production and promote heat loss.

POSTOPERATIVE PAIN MANAGEMENT

Management of pain,❷ a primary concern after surgery, involves pharmacologic measures (eg, systemic analgesia) and nonpharmacologic measures. Regional analgesia may be used postoperatively. A major goal of pain management is patient comfort; an equally important goal is decreased morbidity and mortality. In the elderly, assessment of pain may be difficult because of cognitive impairment due to acute illness or dementia.

Postoperative pain in the elderly is best managed by a dedicated acute pain service consisting of physicians (generally anesthesiologists) and nurses who specialize in various modalities of postoperative pain control. Hemodynamic parameters and mental status must be closely monitored, and the altered effects of drugs in the elderly must be thoroughly understood. A collaborative approach among surgical, nursing, and acute pain service staff members can result in safe, effective pain management for even the most frail elderly patient.

❶see page 659   ❷see page 387

Pain management in the elderly has been addressed in clinical practice guidelines by the Agency for Health Care Policy and Research and by the American Geriatrics Society and in reports by the American Society of Anesthesiologists and International Association for the Study of Pain. Adequate pain management may improve cardiovascular and pulmonary function and, by preventing the stress response to postoperative pain, may lower the incidence of postoperative myocardial events. Decreased ventilatory function after thoracic or abdominal surgery is caused mainly by surgical trauma and by splinting due to postoperative pain. Pain management cannot restore ventilatory function but can help prevent splinting by enabling patients to breathe deeply and cough, thus improving mucus removal and avoiding atelectasis. Prevention of atelectasis reduces the postoperative risk of pneumonia and hypoxia.

Generally, adequate postoperative pain management helps patients walk sooner and improves functional status, hastening their return to the community. Pain management also enables patients to be discharged earlier, thus reducing medical care costs.

Regional analgesia: Regional anesthetic techniques range in complexity from instillation of a local anesthetic into the surgical incision to specific nerve blocks to continuous epidural infusion of a local anesthetic, an opioid, or both. The technique is chosen based on the surgical site and on the technique's relative complexity and potential advantages or disadvantages.

The primary advantage of using regional anesthetic techniques is that intravenous opioid use can be reduced or eliminated. A regional anesthetic block performed before surgery provides longer pain relief than is expected from a local anesthetic. When the anesthesia wears off and pain recurs, the pain is less intense, and lower opioid doses can be used. The mechanism for this effect involves modulation of impulses sent to the brain; this action appears to occur at the spinal cord level. Disadvantages of regional techniques include the hemodynamic effects of local anesthetics administered epidurally and the potential for intravascular injection, infection, bleeding, and nerve damage.

For **pain after limb surgery,** a single-dose nerve block or continuous opioid infusion is often used. For hand or elbow surgery, the axillary approach is used to block the brachial plexus because of its relative ease and lower incidence of complications compared with other approaches. If prolonged pain relief is needed, a catheter is inserted preoperatively and an infusion of a local anesthetic is begun postoperatively. Often, bupivacaine 0.125% provides complete pain relief. The infusion is usually started at 8 to 10 mL/hour and titrated to desired effectiveness.

For **pain after knee surgery,** a continuous infusion of a local anesthetic solution through a femoral sheath catheter can be effective, even though the sciatic nerve is not blocked. If necessary, femoral catheter infusion may be supplemented by small amounts of intravenous or intramuscular opioid or ketorolac.

For **pain after hip, abdominal, or thoracic surgery,** a continuous epidural infusion is often selected, especially for medically high-risk patients. Infusion of bupivacaine 0.0625% to 0.125% with fentanyl 2 to 4 μg/mL at 8 to 10 mL/hour usually relieves pain, but upward titration may be needed. Ropivacaine, a relatively new local anesthetic, has less cardiovascular toxicity and is used in the same concentrations as bupivacaine.

Insertion of an epidural catheter at the site of perceived discomfort can reduce the amount of local anesthetic and opioid needed, minimizing the possibility of toxicity. For hip surgery, the catheter is inserted in the lumbar region; for abdominal surgery, the lower thoracic region; and for thoracotomy, the midthoracic region. Fentanyl is lipophilic and does not spread widely in the epidural space, so the catheter must be placed near the nerve source of the pain. Epidural morphine spreads more readily; however, the rostral spread of morphine may cause late respiratory depression.

The most common complication of continuous epidural infusion is the inadvertent removal of the catheter during routine nursing care. Meticulous taping of the catheter and nursing education can help solve this problem. Urinary retention due to the local anesthetic and the opioid occurs more commonly among elderly men than among women or younger men. The catheter may migrate to subcutaneous tissues, terminating pain relief. Rarely, the catheter migrates to the spinal space, sometimes resulting in high levels of anesthetic that may be life threatening.

In the elderly, epidural infusion must be titrated precisely, and intravascular volume must be maintained by closely monitoring fluid status and promptly replacing fluids if needed. In an elderly patient with a sympathetic block, blood loss of 300 to 500 mL from a hip wound drain can result in dangerously low blood pressure unless fluids are promptly replaced. **1**

28 REHABILITATION

A combination of physical, occupational, and speech therapy; psychiatric or psychologic counseling; and social work services to help debilitated persons maintain or recover physical capacities.

Rehabilitation is typically needed by patients who, for example, have had a stroke, hip fracture, or limb amputation. **2** It is also commonly

1 see page 251   **2** see page 278

needed by patients, especially elderly patients, who have become deconditioned because of prolonged bed rest (eg, after a myocardial infarction, heart surgery, or a serious illness).

The elderly, even if cognitively impaired, can benefit from rehabilitation. Age alone is not a reason to postpone or deny rehabilitation. However, the elderly may recover slowly because they lack endurance (due to cardiovascular complications), because they have depression or dementia, or because muscle strength, joint mobility, coordination, or agility is diminished.

Programs designed specifically for the elderly are preferable, because the elderly often have different goals, require less intensive rehabilitation, and need different types of care than do younger patients. In age-segregated programs, elderly patients are less likely to compare their progress with that of younger patients and become discouraged, and the social work aspects of postdischarge care can be more readily integrated. Some programs are designed for specific clinical situations (eg, recovery from hip fracture surgery **1**); patients with similar conditions can work together toward common goals by encouraging each other and reinforcing the rehabilitation training.

The rehabilitation team (a specialized type of geriatric interdisciplinary team **2**) coordinates the services needed by debilitated patients and develops and implements a comprehensive treatment plan. Team members may include physicians, nurses, physical therapists, occupational therapists, speech therapists, psychologists, social workers, other health care practitioners, the patient, and family members. Frequently, a physiatrist or a geriatrician coordinates the team. The case manager or the nurse updates the treatment plan as necessary. The nurse augments formal therapy and reinforces the skills learned by patients. The nurse can also help prevent secondary disabilities (eg, contractures, pressure sores), thus helping shorten the hospital stay, improve the quality of life, and accelerate rehabilitation for patients.

Referral: To initiate formal rehabilitation, the physician writes a referral (similar to a prescription) to a physiatrist, therapist, or rehabilitation center. The referral establishes the goals of therapy and therefore should be appropriately detailed, including relevant information (eg, type of illness or injury, date of onset) and initial instructions (eg, indicating the specific therapy needed—see FIGURE 28–1). Although vague instructions (eg, "for physical therapy") are often accepted, they are not adequate to detail a rehabilitation program. Physicians unfamiliar with writing referrals can consult with a senior therapist, physiatrist, or orthopedic surgeon.

Goals of therapy: Establishing goals of rehabilitation helps determine the setting and method of rehabilitation. For the elderly, the goal of rehabilitation is often limited to restoration of the ability to perform

1 see page 283   **2** see page 74

Name of Patient: _John Doe_

Age: _75 years_

Diagnosis and Impairment: _Ischemic stroke, right hemiplegia_

Date of Onset: _February 2, 2000_

Treatment Goal: _Independence in performing activities of daily living_ _at home, including ambulation_

Precaution: _Shortness of breath due to emphysema_

Treatment: _Ambulation training, training in activities of daily living_

FIGURE 28–1.   A sample referral for rehabilitation.

as many activities of daily living (ADLs)[1] as possible. This goal may differ from that for younger patients, whose goal more often is to achieve full, unrestricted function.

The rehabilitation team establishes short-term goals, which are specific, and long-term goals, which are more general. A patient's progress in achieving short-term goals must be followed closely for rehabilitation to be efficient. The treatment plan can be used to track progress; it lists the patient's problems, a short-term goal for each problem, and a method and a deadline for achieving each goal. The patient is encouraged to achieve each short-term goal and is informed of any changes in goals. Improvements in patient performance are noted in the treatment plan.

The goals of therapy may have to be altered if the patient is unwilling or unable (financially or otherwise) to undergo lengthy rehabilitation (eg, complete rehabilitation requires 6 or 8 weeks after a hip fracture and several months after a stroke). Therefore, the duration of rehabilitative therapy should be discussed with the patient and family members before rehabilitation is started. For complete rehabilitation, the patient must reach the premorbid level of functioning. As soon as the patient can transfer with minimum assistance (usually in 5 to 10 days), treatment can be given at home. Family members can be trained to give rehabilitative therapy. If feasible, a visiting physical therapist or occupational therapist can be used.

Discharge planning: Rehabilitation team members must begin discharge planning as soon as the patient is admitted. Discharge planning is based on the patient's wishes, anticipated functional outcome, and

[1] see TABLE 4–3 on page 44

psychosocial history, which includes the patient's premorbid personality, ethnic and religious beliefs, lifestyle (eg, career), coping skills, family relationships, and financial resources. Discharge planning can be hindered if a patient or family member denies physical disability.

Patient and caregiver issues: Patient and family education is an important part of the discharge process, particularly when the patient is discharged into the community. Often, the nurse is the team member primarily responsible for this education. Patients are taught to perform ADLs (including how to walk), to maintain newly regained functions, and to reduce the risk of accidents (eg, falls, cuts, burns) and secondary disabilities. Family members are taught how to help the patient be as independent as possible, so that they do not overprotect the patient (leading to decreased functional status and increased dependence) or neglect the patient's primary needs (leading to feelings of rejection, which may cause depression or interfere with physical functioning).

Emotional support from family and friends is essential. It may take many forms. Spiritual support and counseling by the patient's peers or by religious advisors can be indispensable.

SETTINGS

The setting for rehabilitation varies according to the needs of the patient and, particularly, the level of rehabilitative therapy needed (see TABLE 28–1).

Providing rehabilitation at home by family members is highly desirable, but it can be physically and emotionally taxing for caregivers. The patient's partner may be physically unable to help provide care, adult children may have too many other commitments, and home health aides usually cannot provide 24-hour care. Thus, institutionalization may be necessary for patients with severe disabilities. Nonetheless, creative approaches to home care may be possible, especially for patients with substantial financial resources.

METHODS

The physician or rehabilitation team determines which methods of rehabilitation are appropriate. Most patients require some type of physical therapy. Leisure or recreational therapy is often appropriate for demented or institutionalized patients who need some exercise but not the specialized resources of physical therapy. Occupational therapy for the elderly [1] usually consists of training in ADLs. Specific problems (eg, blindness, heart disease, stroke, hip fracture, leg amputation) may require specialized rehabilitation. [2]

---

[1] see page 287   [2] see page 278

TABLE 28–1. LEVELS OF INPATIENT REHABILITATIVE CARE

Level	CARF Category*	Setting	Physician Contact	Nursing Needs	Extent of Therapy Needed	Expected Outcome
Acute (high risk of medical instability)	1	Hospital	Regular	Multiple, complex rehabilitation nursing, with access to high-acuity skilled nursing intervention	≥ 3 h/day† for 5 days/wk	Return to the community with or without support, or progression to another level of rehabilitative care
Subacute (variable risk of medical instability)	2	Hospital, nursing home‡	As needed	Multiple, complex rehabilitation nursing, with access to high-acuity skilled nursing intervention	1–3 h/day for 5 days/wk	Return to the community, or progression to another level of rehabilitative care
Subacute (low risk of medical instability)	3	Nursing home‡	Occasional	Routine rehabilitation; high-acuity skilled nursing intervention less likely to be needed	1–3 h/day for 5 days/wk	Return to the community
Home care (minimal or no risk of medical instability)	NA	Home	Seldom or never	Caregiver supervision; periodic assessment of progress	Daily or as tolerated	Resumption of activities of daily living and ambulation

NA = not applicable.

* A Certificate of Accreditation of Rehabilitation Facilities (CARF) is granted by the voluntary organization The Rehabilitation Accreditation Commission after completion of an investigation that was requested by the facility.

† Patient needs ≥ 2 therapy sessions daily, one of which must be 2 h.

‡ Hospital-based or freestanding.

PHYSICAL THERAPY

Before prescribing physical therapy, the physician ensures that the patient is medically stable and notes any cardiac, pulmonary, neurologic, or musculoskeletal limitations. Elderly patients may have several problems, and therapy must often be prioritized. After evaluating the patient, the physical therapist, working closely with the physician, develops and implements a prioritized treatment plan, then monitors it, adjusting goals and therapy as needed. Because caloric requirements are increased during rehabilitation, caloric intake must be increased accordingly to prevent weight loss and nutritional deficits.

Range-of-motion exercises: Several physical therapy techniques can help improve range of motion, which commonly becomes restricted after a stroke or prolonged bed rest. Restricted range of motion can cause pain, reduce functional abilities, and predispose patients to pressure sores.

Range of motion should be evaluated with a goniometer before therapy and regularly thereafter. In healthy elderly persons, the range of motion for certain joints is usually lower than would be normal for younger patients (see TABLE 28–2), but this age-related decrease does not usually prevent the elderly from being able to perform ADLs without assistance.

Exercises to increase range of motion are indicated for all elderly patients with restricted motion, unless functional deficits are profound. Range-of-motion exercises may be:

- Active, for patients who can exercise without assistance
- Active assistive, for patients whose muscles are too weak to exercise without assistance (and who also require strengthening exercises) or for patients who experience discomfort during joint movement
- Passive, for patients who cannot actively participate (see FIGURE 28–2)

Active-assistive or passive range-of-motion exercises must be performed very gently. Aggressive movements can easily damage joints with restricted motion or break osteoporotic bones. Movements producing severe pain should be avoided, although some discomfort may be unavoidable. If the affected joint is adjacent to an unfixed fracture, passive exercises should not be performed.

Before beginning therapy, the physical therapist must determine if restricted motion is due to tight ligaments and tendons or to tight muscles; if tight muscles are the cause, the joint can be stretched more vigorously. The affected joint must be moved beyond the point of pain, but the movement should not cause residual pain. Sustained moderate stretching is more effective than momentary forceful stretching. For sustained stretching, 5- to 50-lb (2.3- to 23-kg) weights with pulleys are

TABLE 28-2. NORMAL VALUES FOR RANGE OF MOTION OF JOINTS*

Joint	Motion	Range
Hip	Flexion	0–125°
	Extension	115–0°
	Hyperextension†	0–15°
	Abduction	0–45°
	Adduction	45–0°
	Lateral rotation	0–45°
	Medial rotation	0–45°
Knee	Flexion	0–130°
	Extension	120–0°
Ankle	Plantar flexion	0–50°
	Dorsiflexion	0–20°
Foot	Inversion	0–35°
	Eversion	0–25°
Toes		
Metatarsophalangeal joints	Flexion	0–30°
	Extension	0–80°
Interphalangeal joints	Flexion	0–50°
	Extension	50–0°
Shoulder	Flexion to 90°	0–90°
	Extension	0–50°
	Abduction to 90°	0–90°
	Adduction	90–0°
	Lateral rotation	0–90°
	Medial rotation	0–90°
Elbow	Flexion	0–160°
	Extension	145–0°
	Pronation	0–90°
	Supination	0–90°
Wrist	Flexion	0–90°
	Extension	0–70°
	Abduction	0–25°
	Adduction	0–65°
Fingers	Abduction	0–25°
	Adduction	20–0°
Metacarpophalangeal joints	Flexion	0–90°
	Extension	0–30°
Interphalangeal joints	Flexion	0–120°
	Extension	120–0°
Interphalangeal distal joints	Flexion	0–80°
	Extension	80–0°
Thumb	Abduction	0–50°
	Adduction	40–0°
Metacarpophalangeal joints	Flexion	0–70°
	Extension	60–0°
Interphalangeal joints	Flexion	0–90°
	Extension	90–0°

* Ranges are for persons of all ages. Age-specific ranges have not been established; however, values are typically lower in fully functional elderly persons than in younger persons.
† Extension beyond midline.

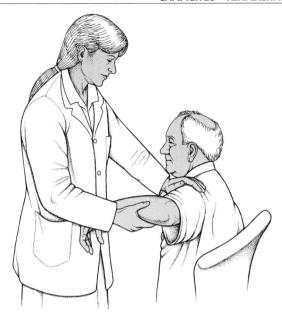

FIGURE 28–2.   Passive range of motion at the shoulder joint. The therapist stabilizes the patient's shoulder with one hand while slowly raising the patient's elbow as high as possible with the other. Over several sessions, the elbow is gradually moved higher, increasing the joint's range of motion.

applied for 20 minutes/day; manual (passive) stretching is time-consuming and fatiguing for therapists. Stretching is usually most effective and least painful when tissue temperature is raised [1] to about 43° C (109° F).

Muscle-strengthening exercises [2]:   For the elderly, the purpose of these exercises is to strengthen muscles enough to perform a given function, not necessarily to regain normal strength for age. Many forms of exercise increase muscle strength; all involve progressively increased resistance. When a muscle is very weak, gravity alone is sufficient. As muscle strength increases, resistance is gradually increased—eg, when muscle strength becomes fair, manual or mechanical resistance (eg, weights) is added (see TABLE 28–3). In this way, muscle mass and strength are increased, and endurance is improved.

Proprioceptive neuromuscular facilitation: This technique promotes useful neuromuscular activity in patients with spasticity due to

---

[1] see page 274   [2] see also page 303

TABLE 28-3. GRADES OF MUSCLE STRENGTH

Grade	Description
5 or N (Normal)	Full range against gravity and full resistance for the patient's size, age, and sex
N− (Normal minus)	Slight weakness
G+ (Good plus)	Moderate weakness
4 or G (Good)	Movement against gravity and moderate resistance at least 10 times without fatigue
F+ (Fair plus)	Movement against gravity several times or mild resistance one time
3 or F (Fair)	Full range against gravity
F− (Fair minus)	Movement against gravity and complete range one time
P+ (Poor plus)	Full range with gravity eliminated but some resistance applied
2 or P (Poor)	Full range with gravity eliminated
P− (Poor minus)	Incomplete range of motion with gravity eliminated
1 or T (Trace)	Evidence of contracture (visible or palpable) but no joint movement
0 (Zero)	No palpable or visible contracture and no joint movement

upper motor neuron damage; it enables them to feel muscle contraction and helps maintain the affected joint's range of motion. For example, in patients with right hemiplegia, strong resistance applied to the left biceps causes the right elbow to flex through contraction of the right (hemiplegic) biceps. The exact mechanism is not clearly understood, but reflex-related proprioception may be involved. Various techniques (eg, Brunnstrom, Rood, Bobath) are widely used.

Coordination exercises: These task-oriented exercises are for patients who need to improve coordination (eg, stroke patients). They involve repeating a meaningful movement that works more than one joint and muscle (eg, picking up an object, touching a body part). The goal is to improve motor skills to the premorbid level.

Transfer training: The patient's ability to transfer must be evaluated, and training provided as needed. Patients who cannot transfer safely and independently from bed to chair, chair to commode, or chair to a standing position generally require 24-hour attendants. Also, patients who cannot transfer safely have a high risk of falling, with risk of fracture or other injury. Such patients may require institutionalization.

Transfer training is particularly important after a hip fracture or stroke.∎ The therapist must patiently and closely supervise the patient.

∎ see page 281

The techniques used depend on whether the patient can bear weight on one or both legs, has sound balance, or has hemiplegia. Assistive devices can sometimes help. For example, persons who have difficulty standing from a seated position may benefit from a chair with a raised seat or a self-lifting chair.

Ambulation exercises: The purpose of these exercises is to improve the patient's ability to walk independently or be assisted by a person or device. Enabling the elderly to walk at the premorbid level is ideal, but enabling them to walk only a few steps (eg, to the toilet or a chair) is often sufficient.

Before starting ambulation exercises, some patients need to improve a joint's range of motion or muscle strength. If a muscle remains weak or spastic, an orthotic device (eg, a brace) may be necessary. Training may begin on parallel bars, especially if the patient's balance is impaired, and progress to walking with aids (eg, walker, crutches, cane). Some patients wear an assistive belt to help prevent falls. Balance training may also be useful. ∎ Persons assisting patients with ambulation should know how to properly support them (see FIGURE 28–3).

As soon as patients can walk safely on level surfaces, they can start training to climb stairs or to step over curbs if either skill is needed. Patients who use walkers must learn special techniques for climbing stairs and stepping over curbs. When climbing stairs, ascent starts with the better leg, and descent with the affected leg (ie, good is up; bad is down). Before the patient is discharged, the social worker or physical therapist should arrange to have secure handrails installed along all stairs in the patient's home.

General conditioning exercises: A combination of the exercises described above is used to counter the effects of debilitation, prolonged bed rest, or immobilization; to reestablish hemodynamic balance; to increase cardiorespiratory capacity; and to maintain range of motion and muscle strength.

Use of a tilt table: For patients with orthostatic hypotension due to paraplegia, quadriplegia, prolonged bed rest, or immobilization, a tilt table may be used to help reestablish hemodynamic balance. The patient, held in place with a safety belt, lies supine on a padded table with a footboard. The table is tilted manually or electrically; the angle is increased very slowly to 85°, if this angle can be tolerated, so that the patient is nearly upright. How long the position is maintained depends initially on the patient's continued tolerance, but it should not exceed 45 minutes. The procedure is performed once or twice daily. Effectiveness depends on the patient's disability and the duration of immobilization.

∎ see page 304

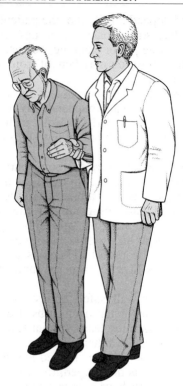

FIGURE 28–3.   Supporting a patient during ambulation. The aide places his arm under that of the patient and gently grasps the patient's forearm while locking his arm firmly under the patient's axilla. In this way, if the patient begins to fall, the aide can provide support at the patient's shoulder. If the patient is wearing a belt around the waist, the aide's left hand grasps it in the back to provide further support.

TREATMENT OF PAIN AND INFLAMMATION

Heat therapy: Heat increases blood flow and the extensibility of connective tissue; decreases joint stiffness, pain, and muscle spasm; and helps inflammation, edema, and exudates resolve. Heat therapy is indicated for acute and chronic traumatic and inflammatory conditions (eg, sprains, strains, fibrositis, tenosynovitis, muscle spasm, myositis, painful back, whiplash injuries, various forms of arthritis, arthralgia, neuralgia). Heat must be applied very carefully to elderly patients because skin sensation or cognitive capacity may be diminished, increasing the risk of burns. The intensity and duration of heat's physiologic effects are determined mainly by tissue temperature, the rate of temperature elevation, and the area treated. When heat does not work, cold can be applied. ∎

Heat application may be superficial or deep. Hot packs, infrared heat, paraffin baths, and hydrotherapy provide superficial heat. Diathermy and ultrasound provide deep heat.

Hot packs, the most common form of heat application, are available as cotton cloth containers filled with silicate gel. They are boiled in water, cooled to a temperature that does not burn the skin, and applied. Wrapping the packs in several layers of towels helps protect against burns. Contraindications include advanced heart disease, peripheral vascular disease, impaired skin sensation (particularly to temperature and pain), and significant hepatic or renal insufficiency.

Infrared heat is applied with a lamp, usually for 20 minutes/day. Contraindications are the same as those for hot packs.

A paraffin bath can be used to apply heat, usually to small joints. Wax heated to 49° C (120° F)—never > 54.4° C (> 130° F)—is applied by dipping or immersing (eg, a hand) or painting (eg, a knee or elbow) and then wrapping with a towel. Because the heating effect is relatively short-lived, infrared heat may be applied immediately afterward. Melted wax should not be applied to open wounds; it is contraindicated in persons allergic to paraffin.

Hydrotherapy, involving agitated warm water, may be used to apply heat or to enhance wound healing by stimulating blood flow and debriding wounds. A Hubbard tank (a large industrial whirlpool) with water heated to 35.5° to 37.7° C (96° to 100° F) is often used. Total immersion in water heated to 37.7° to 40° C (100° to 104° F) may also help relax muscles and relieve pain. For localized pain, the whirlpool and lowboy are used. A lowboy is a small whirlpool with one leg for support, which allows the patient to sit much closer to the water jets than a conventional whirlpool does. It is used primarily for an upper extremity.

Hydrotherapy is particularly useful in conjunction with range-of-motion exercises. Hydrotherapy has no contraindications. However, patients may become fatigued during treatment, and blood pressure may fall.

Short wave diathermy, although less effective than previously thought, is sometimes used to treat inflammation, pain due to urinary calculi, pelvic infections, and acute and chronic sinusitis. Contraindications include malignancy, hemorrhagic conditions, peripheral vascular disease, and loss of sensation. CAUTION: Short wave diathermy is also contraindicated in persons with nonremovable prostheses, electrophysiologic braces, or metallic implants (eg, bars, screws, plates), because the heated metal may absorb heat and cause a burn, and in persons with implanted devices (eg, pacemakers), because the devices may malfunc-

∎see page 276

tion or be destroyed. No metallic substance should be in contact with the skin during the treatment.

Microwave diathermy is simpler and more comfortable to apply than short wave diathermy, and output measurement is more accurate. The heat it provides is deeper and produces less superficial skin damage because microwaves are selectively absorbed into tissues with high water content (eg, muscles). Despite its advantages, microwave diathermy has many adverse effects (eg, burns due to the heating of metallic implants, pacemaker dysfunction) and is not used as widely as short wave diathermy or ultrasound. Indications, contraindications, and precautions are similar to those for short wave diathermy.

Ultrasound involves the use of high-frequency sound waves, which penetrate deep into the tissue (4 to 10 cm [1.6 to 4 inches]) and produce thermal, mechanical, chemical, and biologic effects. This therapy may be used to treat limited range of motion caused by muscle shortening and fibrosis; skin or subcutaneous tissue scarring; bursitis, calcific bursitis, tendinitis, myositis, tenosynovitis, epicondylitis, and spondylitis; pain from postoperative neurofibromas (especially those embedded in scar tissue); myofascial pain syndrome, phantom pain, neuritis; sciatica and other forms of radiculitis; contusions; reflex dystrophies (eg, Sudeck's atrophy, causalgia, shoulder-hand syndrome); and chronic skin ulceration. Ultrasound is contraindicated in patients with ischemic tissue, hemorrhagic diathesis, malignancies, anesthetized areas, or areas of acute infection. Also, it should not be applied over the eyes, brain, spinal cord, ears, heart, reproductive organs, brachial plexus, or healing bone.

Cold therapy (cryotherapy): Application of cold may help relieve muscle spasm, myofascial or traumatic pain, acute low back pain, and acute inflammatory lesions as well as help induce local anesthesia. The choice between heat or cold therapy is often empiric; however, for acute pain, cold therapy seems to be more effective than heat therapy.

Cold may be applied locally using an ice bag, a cold pack, or volatile fluids (eg, ethyl chloride), which cool by evaporation. The spread of cold on the skin depends on the thickness of the epidermis, the thickness of underlying fat and muscle, the water content of the tissue, and the rate of blood flow. Care must be taken to avoid tissue damage (ie, frostbite) and general hypothermia, especially in patients with diminished skin sensation or mental capacity. Cold should not be applied over poorly perfused areas.

Electrical stimulation: Denervated skeletal muscle and innervated muscle that cannot be contracted voluntarily can be stimulated electrically to help alleviate or prevent disuse atrophy and muscle spasticity, especially in patients with hemiplegia due to a cerebrovascular accident, with traumatic paraplegia or quadriplegia, or with peripheral nerve injury. The unipolar technique involves placing a large dispersive electrode on a distant part of the body and a smaller active electrode on the muscle being treated. When this technique produces the desired contractile response, it is preferred to the bipolar technique because it uses a lower current. The bipolar technique involves placing two small electrodes over the ends of the muscle. This technique is useful for severely degenerated muscles caused by gross anatomic or physiologic interruption of the nerve supply and for unusually high skin impedance (eg, when edema exists in the area being treated).

Usually, 10 to 20 muscle contractions per session are sufficient for both the unipolar and bipolar techniques. Overstimulation may cause muscle fatigue and may eventually cause muscle damage. Electrode burns may result from inadequate skin contact or too much current. Areas of skin in contact with electrodes should be closely monitored to prevent burns, especially in elderly patients, who may be prone to burns because of age-related decreases in skin sensation or mental capacity. Electrical stimulation is contraindicated in patients with advanced cardiac disease, because it may precipitate an arrhythmia, and in patients with a pacemaker, because it may interfere with its functioning. Electrical stimulation should not be applied over the eyes.

Transcutaneous electrical nerve stimulation (TENS), which uses low current at low-frequency oscillation, is particularly useful for chronic back pain, rheumatoid arthritis, sprained ankle, contusion, postherpetic neuralgia, causalgia, phantom limb syndrome, and trigger points. It may also promote callus formation in a nonunited fracture. TENS may be applied several times daily for 20 minutes to several hours, depending on the severity of pain. Often, patients are taught to use the TENS device, so that they can decide when to apply treatment. The device produces a gentle tingling sensation without increasing muscle tension.

TENS is generally well tolerated but its effectiveness varies greatly. Advantages include the unit's small size, portability, and low cost. TENS is contraindicated in persons with advanced cardiac disease or a pacemaker because it may precipitate an arrhythmia. It should not be applied over the eyes. If the electrodes are improperly placed on the skin, erythema may develop.

Traction: Spinal traction is used to overcome extrinsic muscle spasm and to keep bony surfaces aligned while fractures heal. A weight and pulley system, the patient's weight, or manual or motorized force can be used. The force may be applied continuously or intermittently.

Cervical traction is often used for chronic neck pain due to cervical spondylosis, disk prolapse, whiplash, or torticollis. A 5- to 10-lb (2.5- to 5-kg) weight is used. Some advocate heavier weights, but sustained traction with > 20 lb (> 10 kg) for more than a few minutes is poorly tolerated; motorized intermittent rhythmic traction is generally well tolerated. Generally, hyperextension of the neck should be avoided, because it may increase root compression in the neuroforamina.

Lumbar traction is rarely used, although it is sometimes recommended for treating patients with painful lumbar osteoarthritis or spondylolisthesis. Its value in treating acute discogenic pain is debated, and it puts the elderly at risk of developing a secondary disability because it requires prolonged bed rest. For patients with severe osteoporosis or osteoarthritis, traction must be carefully and gently applied.

Massage: Massage may relieve pain, reduce swelling and induration due to trauma (eg, fracture, joint injury, sprain, strain, bruise, peripheral nerve injury), and mobilize contracted tissues. Massage may be appropriate for patients with low back pain, arthritis, periarthritis, bursitis, neuritis, fibrositis, hemiplegia, paraplegia, quadriplegia, multiple sclerosis, or cerebral palsy. It should not be used to manage infections or thrombophlebitis.

Acupuncture: Thin needles are inserted through the skin at specific body sites, frequently far from the site of pain. These needles, made of stainless steel, gold, or platinum, are twirled rapidly and intermittently for a few minutes, or a low electric current is applied through the needles. Although the mechanism of action is not fully understood, many practitioners believe that acupuncture stimulates endorphin production, generating analgesic and anti-inflammatory effects. The value of this technique is debated.

Acupuncture should be performed only by trained persons. Sterilized or new needles must be used to avoid infection.

29 ▬ REHABILITATION FOR SPECIFIC PROBLEMS

Rehabilitation can be tailored toward specific problems, such as heart disease, stroke, hip fracture, and leg amputation. The benefits of such rehabilitation can be maximized only after any coexisting disorders (eg, arthritis, cognitive impairment), common in the elderly, are addressed. Speech disorders◾ may also require rehabilitation.

HEART DISEASE

Cardiovascular rehabilitation can benefit some elderly patients who have angina or severe heart failure, who have had a myocardial infarction, or who have undergone bypass surgery or angioplasty. The goal of rehabilitation is to help these patients maintain or regain independence,

---

◾ see page 423

based on their physical capability. For those in poor physical condition because of cardiac disease or physical inactivity, the heart's maximum working capacity (cardiac reserve) may be greatly reduced. Restoration of cardiac reserve through cardiac rehabilitation enables most patients to eventually resume their previous level of physical activity.

Rehabilitation programs typically begin with light activity and gradually progress to moderate activity under the supervision of a trained attendant. However, because patients respond differently to the stress of severe heart disease, rehabilitation programs must be individualized. For some patients (eg, those with heart failure, arrhythmias, or valvular disease), even light activity may increase risk. *Patients with unstable angina should not exercise at all.* High-risk patients should exercise only in a well-equipped cardiovascular rehabilitation facility under the supervision of a trained attendant.

Physical activity is measured in metabolic equivalents (METs), which are multiples of the resting rate of oxygen consumption; 1 MET (the resting rate) equals about 3.5 mL/kg/minute of oxygen. Normal working and living activities (excluding recreational activities) rarely exceed 6 METs. Light to moderate housework is about 2 to 4 METs; heavy housework or yard work is about 5 to 6 METs. **1**

Maximum allowable workloads, established by the New York Heart Association, are based on the patient's functional classification (see TABLE 29–1). For hospitalized patients, physical activity should be controlled so that heart rate remains < 60% of maximum for that age (eg, about 160 beats/minute for persons aged 60); for patients recovering at home, heart rate should remain < 70% of maximum.

For patients who have had an uncomplicated myocardial infarction, a 2-MET exercise test may be performed to evaluate responses as soon as the patient is stable. A 4- to 5-MET exercise test performed before discharge helps guide physical activity at home. Patients who can tolerate a 5-MET exercise test for 6 minutes can safely perform low-intensity (sedentary) activities (eg, light housework) after discharge if they rest sufficiently between each activity.

Unnecessary restriction of activity is detrimental to recovery. **2** The physician and other members of the rehabilitation team can therefore provide psychologic support and explain which activities can be undertaken and which cannot. When discharged, patients can be given a detailed home activity program. Most elderly persons can be encouraged to resume sexual activity, **3** but they will need to stop and rest as necessary to avoid overexertion. Young couples expend 5 to 6 METs during intercourse; whether elderly couples expend more or less is unknown.

---

1 see TABLE 31–4 on page 301   **2** see page 472   **3** see also page 1159

TABLE 29–1. MAXIMUM WORKLOADS BASED ON NEW YORK HEART
ASSOCIATION CLASSIFICATION OF HEART DISEASE

		Maximum Workload (calories/min)		
Class	Functional Limitations	Sustained	Intermittent	Maximum METs
I	Physical activity not limited: ordinary physical activity does not cause undue fatigue, palpitation, dyspnea, or anginal pain	5.0	6.5	6.5
II	Physical activity slightly limited: patient is comfortable at rest, but ordinary physical activity causes undue fatigue, palpitation, dyspnea, or anginal pain	2.5	4.0	4.5
III	Physical activity markedly limited: patient is comfortable at rest, but less-than-ordinary physical activity causes undue fatigue, palpitation, dyspnea, or anginal pain	2.0	2.7	3.0
IV	Physical activity impossible without discomfort: symptoms of cardiac insufficiency or of angina may be present even at rest; any physical activity increases discomfort	1.5	2.0	1.5

METs = metabolic equivalents.

Modified from Karwal SS: "Cardiac rehabilitation," in *Current Therapy in Physiatry, Physical Medicine and Rehabilitation*, edited by AP Ruskin. Philadelphia, WB Saunders Company, 1984, p. 328; used with permission.

STROKE

Rehabilitation can enhance functional performance after a stroke. The success of rehabilitation depends on the patient's general condition, range of motion, muscle strength, bowel and bladder function, premorbid functional and cognitive ability, social situation (eg, likelihood of returning to the community), learning ability, motivation, coping skills, and ability to participate in rehabilitation under the supervision of nurses and physical therapists. Impairment of comprehension often makes rehabilitation very difficult.

Starting rehabilitation early—ie, as soon as patients are medically stable—may prevent secondary disabilities (eg, contractures) and depression. Preventive measures for some complications (eg, pressure sores) must be started even before patients are medically stable.

Patients can safely sit up once they are fully conscious and their neurologic deficits are no longer progressing, usually within 48 hours of the stroke. Early in the rehabilitation period, when the affected extremities are flaccid, each joint is passively exercised through the normal range of motion three to four times daily. [1] For patients with hemiplegia, placing one or two pillows under the affected arm can prevent dislocation of the shoulder. If the arm is flaccid, a well-constructed sling can prevent the weight of the arm and hand from overstretching the deltoid muscle and subluxating the shoulder. A posterior foot splint applied with the ankle in a 90° position can prevent equinus deformity (talipes equinus) and footdrop.

Reeducation and coordination exercises of the affected extremities are added as soon as tolerated, often within 1 week. Active and active-assistive range-of-motion exercises are started shortly afterward to maintain range of motion and, if indicated, to increase muscle strength.

Resistive muscle-strengthening exercises for hemiplegic extremities are controversial because they may increase spasticity, [2] which develops insidiously; if spasticity develops, resistive exercises are stopped. Active exercise of the unaffected extremities must be encouraged, as long as it does not cause fatigue. Various activities of daily living (eg, moving in bed, turning, changing position, sitting up) should be practiced. For hemiplegic patients, the most important muscle for ambulation is the unaffected quadriceps. If weak, this muscle must be strengthened to assist the hemiplegic side.

Regaining the ability to get out of bed and to transfer to a chair or wheelchair safely and independently is important for the patient's psychologic and physical well-being. Ambulation problems, spasticity, visual field defects (eg, hemianopia), incoordination, and aphasia [3] require specific therapy.

Ambulation problems: Before ambulation exercises can be started, [4] patients must be able to stand. Patients first learn to stand from the sitting position. The height of the seat may need to be adjusted. Patients must stand with the hips and knees fully extended, leaning slightly forward and toward the unaffected side. Using the parallel bars is the safest way to practice standing.

The goal of ambulation exercises is to establish and maintain a safe gait, not to restore a normal gait. Most hemiplegic patients have a gait abnormality. During ambulation exercises, patients place the feet ≥ 6 inches apart and grasp the parallel bars with the unaffected hand. Patients take a shorter step with the hemiplegic leg and a longer step with the unaffected leg. Patients who begin walking without the parallel bars may need physical assistance from and, later, close supervision by the therapist. Generally, patients use a cane or walker when first

---

[1] see TABLE 28–1 on page 268   [2] see page 282   [3] see page 425
[4] see also page 273

walking without the parallel bars. The diameter of the cane handle should be large enough to accommodate an arthritic hand.

For stair climbing, ascent starts with the better leg, and descent with the affected leg (good leads up; bad leads down). If possible, patients ascend and descend with the railing on the unaffected side, so that they can grasp the railing. Looking up the staircase may cause vertigo and should be avoided. During descent, the patient should use a cane. The cane should be moved to the lower step shortly before descending with the bad leg.

Patients must learn to prevent falls, **1** which are the most common accident among stroke patients and which often result in hip fracture. Usually, patients explain the fall by saying, "The knees gave way." For hemiplegic patients, who almost always fall on their hemiplegic side, leaning their affected side against a railing (when standing or climbing stairs) can help prevent falls. Performing strengthening exercises for weak muscles, particularly in the trunk and legs, can also help.

For patients with symptomatic orthostatic hypotension, treatment includes support stockings, drugs, and training on a tilt table. Because hemiplegic patients are prone to vertigo, they should change body position slowly and take a moment after standing to establish equilibrium before walking. Comfortable, supportive shoes should be worn, with rubber soles and with heels no higher than 2 cm (3/4 inch).

Spasticity: In some stroke patients, spasticity develops. Spasticity may be painful and debilitating, and it may or may not help ambulation. Slightly spastic knee extensors can lock the knee during standing or cause hyperextension (genu recurvatum), which may require a knee brace with an extension stop. Resistance applied to spastic plantar flexors causes ankle clonus; a short leg brace without a spring mechanism minimizes this problem.

Flexor spasticity develops in most hemiplegic hands and wrists. Unless patients perform range-of-motion exercises several times a day, flexion contracture may develop rapidly in those with flexor spasticity, resulting in pain and difficulty maintaining personal hygiene. Patients and family members are taught and strongly encouraged to perform these exercises. A hand or wrist splint may also be useful, particularly at night. One that is easy to apply and to clean is best.

Heat or cold therapy **2** can temporarily decrease spasticity and allow the muscle to be stretched. Benzodiazepines may be used for hemiplegic patients to minimize apprehension and anxiety, particularly during the initial stage of rehabilitation, but not to reduce spasticity. The effectiveness of long-term benzodiazepine use for reducing spasticity is questionable. Methocarbamol has limited value in relieving spasticity and causes sedation.

---

1 see also page 199   **2** see pages 274–276

Hemianopia: Patients with hemianopia (defective vision or blindness in half the visual field of one or both eyes) should be made aware of it and taught to move their heads toward the hemiplegic side when scanning. Family members can help by placing important objects and by approaching the patient on the patient's unaffected side. Repositioning the bed so that the patient can see a person entering the room through the doorway may be useful. While walking, patients with hemianopia tend to bump into the door frame or obstacles on the hemiplegic side; they may need special training to avoid this problem.

Lack of fine coordination: After a stroke, fine coordination may be absent, causing patients to become frustrated. They may need to modify activities and use assistive devices.

HIP FRACTURE

Rehabilitation after surgery: Rehabilitation is started as soon as possible after hip fracture surgery. The first goals may be to increase strength and to prevent atrophy on the unaffected side. Initially, only isometric exercise of the affected limb while it is fully extended is permitted. Placement of a pillow under the knee is contraindicated because it may lead to flexion contracture of the hip and knee.

Gradual mobilization of the affected limb usually results in full ambulation. The speed of rehabilitation depends partly on the type of surgery performed. For example, after prosthetic hip replacement, rehabilitation usually progresses more rapidly, less rehabilitation is needed, and the functional outcome is better than after nail-and-plate or pin-and-plate fixation. Ideally, full weight bearing starts on the 2nd day after surgery. Ambulation exercises are started after 4 to 8 days (assuming that the patient has achieved full weight bearing and balance), and stair-climbing exercises after about 11 days.

Patients are taught to perform daily exercises to strengthen the trunk muscles and quadriceps of the affected leg. Prolonged lifting or pushing of heavy items, stooping, reaching, or jumping can be harmful. During ambulation, the amount of mechanical stress is about the same whether patients use one or two canes, but using two may interfere with certain activities of daily living. Patients should not sit on a chair, particularly a low one, for a long period and should use the chair arm for support when standing up. While sitting, they should keep their legs uncrossed.

Before the patient is discharged, the therapist should evaluate the patient's home to determine if additional training or assistive devices are needed.

Rehabilitation without surgery: Nonsurgical treatment of hip fracture generally results in a poor functional outcome and is therefore rarely advisable. The hip and leg are usually immobilized for 6 to 8 weeks. During immobilization, prevention of secondary disabilities (eg, pressure sores, muscle atrophy, joint contractures, general deconditioning) is important but often unsuccessful. After immobilization, the rehabilitation program is similar to that for postoperative patients; however, the program begins with general conditioning exercises, and rehabilitation progresses more slowly, in part because patients lose so much muscle mass during the prolonged immobilization.

Some physicians do not allow weight bearing until x-rays show union of the bone, which is rare before 8 weeks and usually occurs 10 to 12 weeks after fracture. Other physicians establish that healing has occurred by comparing x-rays taken under non–weight-bearing and under weight-bearing conditions; if no difference is seen, weight-bearing exercises can proceed. However, patients, even if told not to, often begin weight-bearing activities as soon as they feel no discomfort. The decision to allow weight bearing seems more reasonable when based on the patient's perception rather than solely on x-ray findings.

LEG AMPUTATION

Before amputation, the physician describes to the patient the extensive postsurgical rehabilitation program that will be needed. Psychologic counseling may be indicated. The rehabilitation team and the patient decide whether a prosthesis or a wheelchair will be needed.

Immediately after surgery, measures are taken to prevent secondary disabilities, especially contractures. Flexion contracture of the hip or knee, which may develop rapidly after surgery, can make the fitting and use of a prosthesis difficult. Exercises for general conditioning, stretching of the hip and knee, and strengthening of all extremities are started as soon as the patient is medically stable. Endurance exercises may be indicated.￭ Elderly amputees should begin standing and balancing exercises with parallel bars as soon as possible.

Unilateral amputation: Ambulation requires a 10 to 40% increase in energy expenditure after below-the-knee amputation and a 60 to 100% increase after above-the-knee amputation. To compensate, elderly amputees generally walk more slowly. Gait abnormalities in elderly amputees who can walk safely are not of concern and are often avoidable with a well-fitting prosthesis and good rehabilitation.

Functional prognosis after below-the-knee amputation differs greatly from that after above-the-knee amputation. Elderly patients who have had a below-the-knee amputation and are fitted with a prosthesis usually become functionally ambulatory. Elderly patients who have had an above-the-knee amputation may not have the energy and skills required to deal with the weight of the above-the-knee prosthesis and to control the knee joint.

￭ see page 301

Bilateral amputation: Amputation of both legs is not unusual for diabetic patients or patients with peripheral vascular disease. As with unilateral amputation, functional prognosis depends on whether the amputations are above or below the knee. Bilateral below-the-knee amputees with well-fitting prostheses may be able to walk without canes or crutches. Bilateral above-the-knee amputees with prostheses probably can walk only with two canes or crutches. However, most elderly patients with bilateral above-the-knee amputations do not have the necessary energy or strength to ambulate with prostheses.

For patients who have had a below-the-knee amputation first and can ambulate independently with a prosthesis, ambulation with a second prosthesis is probably possible regardless of the level of the second amputation. Amputees with one below-the-knee and one above-the-knee amputation use the former as the functional leg; a manual knee lock may sometimes be required on the above-the-knee prosthesis.

Regardless of the level of the amputations, walking distance is generally limited, and a wheelchair may be needed, especially outdoors and for long distances.

Stump Conditioning and Prostheses

Stump conditioning promotes the natural process of stump shrinking that must occur before a prosthesis can be used. After only a few days of conditioning, the stump may have shrunk greatly. An elastic stump shrinker or elastic bandages worn 24 hours/day can help taper the stump and prevent edema. The stump shrinker is easy to apply, but bandages may be preferred because they better control the amount and location of pressure. However, application of elastic bandages requires skill, and the bandages must be reapplied whenever they become loose.

Early ambulation with a temporary prosthesis enables the amputee to be active, accelerates stump shrinkage, prevents flexion contracture, and reduces phantom limb pain. ◻ The socket of the pylon, which is made of plaster of paris (calcium sulfate hemihydrate), should fit the stump snugly. Various temporary prostheses with adjustable sockets are available. A patient with a temporary prosthesis can start ambulation exercises on the parallel bars and progress to walking with crutches or canes until a permanent prosthesis is made.

The permanent prosthesis should be lightweight and meet the needs and safety requirements of the patient. If the prosthesis is made before the stump stops shrinking, adjustments may be needed to satisfy the patient and to produce a good gait pattern. Therefore, manufacture of a permanent prosthesis is generally delayed a few weeks to allow shrinkage of the stump. For most elderly patients with a below-the-knee amputation, a patellar tendon-bearing prosthesis with a solid-ankle, cushion-heel foot and suprapatellar cuff suspension is best. Unless

◻see page 286

patients have special needs, a standard below-the-knee prosthesis with thigh corset and waist belt is not prescribed because it is heavy and bulky. For above-the-knee amputees, several knee locking options are available according to the patient's skills and activity level.

Care of the stump and prosthesis: Patients must learn to care for their stump. Because a leg prosthesis is intended only for ambulation, patients should remove it before going to sleep. At bedtime, the stump should be inspected thoroughly (with a mirror if inspected by the patient), washed with mild soap and warm water, dried thoroughly, then dusted with talcum powder. If the skin of the stump is too dry, lanolin or petrolatum may be applied. If the stump sweats excessively, an unscented antiperspirant may be applied. If the skin is inflamed, the irritant must be removed immediately, and talcum powder or a low-potency corticosteroid cream or ointment applied. If the skin is broken, the prosthesis should not be worn until the wound has healed.

The stump sock should be changed daily, and mild soap may be used to clean the inside of the socket. Standard prostheses are neither waterproof nor water-resistant. Therefore, if even part of the prosthesis becomes wet, it must be dried immediately and thoroughly; heat should not be applied. For elderly persons who swim or prefer to shower with a prosthesis, a prosthesis that can tolerate immersion can be made.

Complications

The most common complaint is **stump pain.** Mild to severe pain is felt when the stump is palpated or when a pylon or prosthesis is used. Stump pain is localized and differs from phantom limb pain, from which it must be differentiated. An ill-fitting socket, which may be due to small socket size, an edematous stump, or weight gain, may cause stump pain. However, the most common causes are an amputation neuroma or spur formation at the amputated end of the bone. A neuroma is usually palpable. A spur may be palpable or seen on x-rays. For a neuroma, daily ultrasound treatments for 5 to 10 days are most effective. Alternatives include injection of corticosteroids or analgesics into the neuroma or the surrounding area, use of cryotherapy, or continuous tight bandaging of the stump. Surgical resection of the neuroma often has disappointing results. The only effective treatment of a spur is surgical resection.

Phantom limb pain is more likely to occur if the patient had a painful condition before amputation or if pain was inadequately controlled intraoperatively and perioperatively. Treatments such as simultaneous exercise of both legs, massage of the stump, percussion of the stump with fingers, use of mechanical devices (eg, a vibrator), and ultrasound are effective. Drugs (eg, tricyclic antidepressants, carbamazepine) may help.

Phantom limb sensation is a painless awareness of the amputated limb, sometimes accompanied by mild tingling. Most amputees experience this sensation, which may last several months or years but usually disappears without treatment. Frequently, amputees sense only part of the missing limb, often the foot, which is the last phantom sensation to disappear. Some amputees can even describe the position of the foot, which is often related to its position at the time of amputation. Phantom limb sensation is not harmful; however, amputees, without thinking, commonly attempt to stand with both legs and fall, particularly when they wake at night to go to the bathroom.

Follow-up

Follow-up examinations are performed every 3 to 6 months for the first 2 years for patients who successfully complete a prosthetic rehabilitation program and return to the community. The stump usually continues to shrink with use. An adequate fit of the prosthesis can be achieved by adding layers of socks, although eventually a new socket is needed. Because of continuous use, components of the prosthesis may deteriorate, sometimes altering the gait.

At each visit, the circulatory status of the unaffected leg is checked. Many patients who had a below-the-knee amputation due to vascular disease eventually require an above-the-knee amputation.

An amputee wheelchair, which has wider wheel axles to compensate for the absence of leg weight and to prevent tilting, is eventually needed by all elderly amputees, even those who use a prosthesis. These wheelchairs are needed, for example, when using a prosthesis is bothersome (eg, at night) or impossible (eg, due to the condition of the stump) or when traversing long distances. Properly maintained, wheelchairs last 5 to 10 years.

30 ◼ OCCUPATIONAL THERAPY

Therapy to enhance a patient's ability to perform work and basic and instrumental activities of daily living, productive activities, and leisure activities.

ASSESSMENT

To determine the extent of training needed, occupational therapists assess a patient's functional status and environment. Tasks are classified as **basic activities of daily living** (BADLs), which involve functional mobility and personal self-care; **instrumental activities of daily living** (IADLs); or work and productive activities and leisure. Assessment of BADLs is standardized; assessment of IADLs is often individualized, covering only tasks that a patient needs or wishes to perform. ◼

◼see TABLE 4–4 on page 45

Occupational therapists assess the following dimensions of task performance: skills, habits, personal abilities, and social and physical environmental factors. They monitor the performance of tasks and work with patients to modify any task performance dysfunction. Occupational therapists are in a position to alert physicians when patients cannot perform tasks necessary for survival or independent living and need assistance from family members, neighbors, friends, or health and social services. Assessment data may be used to help determine legal competence.◻ Repeat assessments of task performance are valuable for monitoring the effects of medical interventions on function. For example, deterioration of task performance may signal the need for adjusting the dosage of a psychoactive drug causing adverse effects.

Assessment of Skills and Habits

Occupational therapists must determine whether task performance dysfunction results from a skill or habit deficit. Intervention for patients who lack the skill to perform a task differs from that for patients who lack the will to perform a task or who cannot manage time effectively.

Skill is the ability to initiate, perform, and complete tasks efficiently. Skill is assessed by observing patients performing tasks. Because task performance is influenced by the social environment (eg, a solicitous spouse) and physical environment (eg, a walk-in shower stall that enables a person with impaired mobility to shower), skills are assessed in the setting where the task is performed. If this setting is not available, a simulated home, leisure, or work environment in the occupational therapy clinic may be used.

Skills are rated and recorded for each task assessed. A rating of competence indicates that a patient can perform a task independently, adequately, safely, and within a reasonable time; a rating of disability indicates that a patient cannot. Any need for assistance is classified as minimal ($\leq 25\%$), moderate (26 to 50%), maximal (51 to 75%), or total (76 to 100%). The type of assistance needed is specified (eg, preparation of materials, verbal encouragement, instruction during task performance, manual guidance such as hand-over-hand cueing, physical assistance).

Habits are behaviors that are performed automatically without premeditation. Habits are often assessed by interviewing patients and their caregivers. Observation during skill assessment can also provide valuable information; for example, dentures caked with food particles, dirty clothes scattered on the bedroom floor, or spoiling food in the refrigerator indicates a habitual, functional deficit. No uniform system for describing habit deficits exists. Competency in performing a task does not indicate competency in daily living. For example, a depressed patient may be able to prepare meals but may not do so because of loss of appetite or lack of inter-

◻ see page 130

est; a patient with cardiopulmonary disease may competently prepare a meal in the morning but be too fatigued to do so in the afternoon.

Maladaptive behavior patterns may develop in the elderly; they include inconsistency, activity imbalance, disorganization, inflexibility, and social inappropriateness. Inconsistency is characterized by occasional refusal to perform regular tasks. For example, patients with organic or emotional problems may feed themselves at one meal but refuse to do so at the next. Activity imbalance refers to the performance of too few tasks, tasks that lack diversity, or tasks that are poorly paced (eg, watching television all day and neglecting household chores). Disorganization is characterized by procrastination, haphazard collection of task materials, and progress that is not consistently goal-directed. The inability to anticipate, create, and carry out a plan is a salient feature of organic or emotional disorders. Inflexibility is characterized by an inability to vary routines to accommodate unforeseen or changing circumstances and an inability to adjust emotionally when routines are changed. For example, elderly patients may try to maintain their customary housecleaning schedule even though it now causes exhaustion. Social inappropriateness involves disregard for standards of behavior, particularly for promptness, sociability, independence, cleanliness, and neatness.

Assessment of Personal Abilities

To successfully perform even a simple task (eg, dressing), one must coordinate and integrate many abilities. They include the sensorimotor ability to perform the task, the cognitive ability to create and execute a plan, and the psychologic ability to want to do the task and to persevere until it is completed.

Impairment of one of these abilities may affect task performance; identification of the impairment may permit remediation. **Sensorimotor impairments** include aberrations in sensation, perception, range of motion, muscle strength, muscle tone, endurance, balance, dexterity, or coordination. **Cognitive impairments** include inattention, distractibility, loss of concentration, impaired judgment, indecision, memory deficit, apraxia, cognitive rigidity, and poor problem-solving skills. **Psychologic impairments** include apathy, depression, anxiety, perceived incompetence, frustration, a lack of persistence, and decreased coping skills.

Impairments may be noted during direct observation, by specific testing, and with the aid of information provided by others. For example, the occupational therapist may observe instability as a patient stands, undresses, gets into the bathtub, or reaches overhead to get a towel. Later, a standardized test (eg, the Performance Oriented Assessment of Balance) may be administered to learn more about the extent and nature of the balance disorder. Regardless of how well a patient performs BADLs or IADLs, the patient may be noted to drop objects soon after grasping them. Tests of static and dynamic grip strength (eg, pinch meter, manual muscle test) may be performed to further define the hand impairment. Also, data collected by other health care practitioners (eg, physical therapists, neuropsychologists, speech pathologists) may be useful. Impairments may not be severe enough to hinder performance, or adaptive techniques may compensate for them. Nonetheless, if impairments are identified early, preventive interventions can be started before task performance deteriorates. For example, progressive resistive exercises may be started at the first sign of deteriorating manual strength.

Assessment of Social and Physical Environment

Social factors that affect task performance include the caregivers' attitudes toward functional independence and caregiving and their competence in providing rehabilitative care. The more disabled elderly patients are, the more they depend on their caregivers, and the more important an assessment of patient-caregiver interaction becomes. Social factors are assessed using observation and clinical judgment.

The physical environment includes lighting (eg, focused light on work areas, light switches placed so that lights can be turned on before entering a room), walking surfaces (eg, intact carpeting, no electrical cords in walkways), resting surfaces (eg, stable chairs), and the condition and placement of objects in the environment (eg, unfrayed electrical cords, no clutter). The environment should be free of barriers, especially for persons using wheelchairs or walkers. For cognitively impaired patients, cues that orient (eg, a picture of a toilet on the bathroom door) may enhance safety or function. Objects in the environment (eg, furniture, appliances, tools) should facilitate task performance. For example, many elderly patients have difficulty rising from chairs that are too low; this problem can often be resolved by raising the chair height with chair leg extenders or seat cushions. The physical environment is assessed using standardized protocols. ∎

INTERVENTION

Occupational therapists work in different settings (see TABLE 30–1) and intervene at different levels. **Primary intervention** consists of teaching geriatric interdisciplinary team members, patients, and their family members ways to promote health and prevent functional decline in general. **Secondary intervention** consists of amelioration or stabilization of functional status by identifying task performance dysfunction and starting appropriate therapy. Occupational therapists screen elderly persons at risk of dysfunction, injury, or disability by asking about fear of falling, the physical environment, isolation, and sensory deprivation. **Tertiary intervention** consists of providing direct care to rehabilitate the patient in response to a change in health status (eg, due to myocardial infarction, acute depression, or hip fracture).

∎see TABLE 20–3 on page 200

TABLE 30–1. SETTINGS FOR OCCUPATIONAL THERAPY

Setting	Common Patient Problems	Interventions
Adult day care	Generalized weakness Mild cognitive impairment Depression Impaired BADL skills	Development of appropriate programs (eg, with expressive activities or activities to increase strength and relieve depression) Individual and group problem-solving discussions Discussions and demonstrations on how to reduce or control symptoms Home visits when indicated
Corporation	Detrimental ergonomic environment Anxiety (eg, due to a role change or retirement) Inability to manage time	Education of employers and employees about ergonomic environment with individual assessment and intervention as needed Preretirement and postretirement counseling Time management training
Home health care	Unsafe physical environment Noncompliance with drug regimen	Consultation about improving the environment with appropriate facilitation of changes, recommendation of assistive devices or adaptive techniques, and BADL training
Hospice	Feelings of uselessness Difficulty communicating with family members Restricted mobility	Consultation with staff members or caregivers about the need for purposeful activity Caregiver education to maximize the patient's functional performance and communication of emotional issues Encouragement to achieve individual goals tailored to the patient's capacities and limitations
Outpatient clinic (psychiatric or physical)	Limited social support Pain when performing BADLs Anxiety (eg, due to role performance)	Education of staff, caregivers, and patients about community resources Encouragement of patient self-advocacy for senior volunteer programs Recommendations of group activities to promote health or socialization Simplification of work

Table continues on the following page.

TABLE 30–1.   SETTINGS FOR OCCUPATIONAL THERAPY   *(Continued)*

Setting	Common Patient Problems	Interventions
Outpatient clinic *(continued)*		BADL training Training in meditation and relaxation
Respite care	Depression Regression Motor or cognitive problems	Caregiver education Prioritization of goals for when the patient returns home ADL training Staff, patient, and family member training in communication skills
Senior housing development	Immobility Lack of social interaction Unsafe environment Impaired BADL skills	Advocacy for improved social and physical environment Patient education about sensory loss Training in the use of assistive devices or adaptive techniques
Skilled nursing facility	Poor body mechanics (ie, lack of back or joint protection) Stress Inability to feed self	Staff education about meeting patient needs Individualized training in joint protection and positioning and in self-feeding

BADLs = basic activities of daily living; ADLs = activities of daily living.

The patient and the occupational therapist work together to determine and prioritize intervention goals and select therapeutic tasks. Therapeutic tasks must be meaningful to the patient and commensurate with the patient's ability, and the level of difficulty must increase as performance improves. The therapist reinforces the patient's sense of competence.

Choice of intervention depends on the type of impairment. For example, fine motor activities may be used to reduce incoordination; visual-perceptual tasks, to ameliorate problems in visual scanning; memory retraining, to enhance recognition and recall; and assertiveness training, to better express needs.

Skill acquisition is used when patients need adaptive techniques, healthier movement or behavior patterns, or new skills. Skill acquisition requires practicing tasks under controlled, supervised conditions, using task materials and movement patterns that promote success. For example, if a patient can put a pullover on more easily than a cardigan, training in dressing may begin with the former and progress to the latter. Assistance is given only when needed and only to the extent needed as determined by skill assessment.

Skills learned in occupational therapy must be adapted for home management, leisure, or work. Thus, patients practice tasks using a variety of materials until they can comfortably integrate the tasks into their daily routines.

Patients whose impairments cannot be corrected are taught adaptive techniques, which use the patients' strengths to compensate for dysfunction. Thus, patients with extremity paralysis learn new ways to dress, tie shoes, and fasten buttons. When patients learn new skills, they also learn how to function more effectively in a variety of environments. This process often involves developing effective interpersonal techniques for knowing when and how to ask for help or how to modify the environment.

Habit acquisition provides the incentive, structure, and endurance needed to develop and sustain an ordered, yet flexible, pattern of daily living. For patients with long-standing patterns of maladaptive behavior that may interfere with performance of functional tasks, the occupational therapist designs a socialization experience in which real-life expectations for life tasks are conveyed and practiced. Patients are taught to sequence tasks, link tasks into effective routines, and understand the social norms or expectations regarding task performance. By developing routines, patients can become more efficient and do not have to plan continuously.

Key elements of habit training in occupational therapy include helping patients recognize what is most important to them so that they can prioritize tasks, examining how time is spent, acknowledging maladaptive patterns, exploring and practicing alternative routines, and consolidating new habit structures. Patients are taught time management, ergonomic techniques, and stress management. Tasks are spaced so that labor-intensive ones are distributed over a day or week. Schedules are arranged to provide the best balance of personal self-care, home management, leisure, and work, approximating the schedule that will be followed at home.

Group activities enable patients to experience many roles (eg, leader, follower, nurturer, friend) and to practice social behaviors. Groups focus on realistic tasks (eg, cooking, playing cards, discussing current events, exercising, listening to music, participating in religious activities). They usually meet in senior centers, day care centers, or nursing homes or as part of religious or fraternal organizations.

Social interventions may be necessary to facilitate task performance. Some elderly persons depend on caregivers to schedule tasks, provide needed materials, and help as needed. Involving caregivers in the patient's rehabilitation program is important. However, when a caregiver lacks the skills, energy, or strength to cope with a patient who has severe task performance dysfunction, the occupational therapist can help determine how much additional assistance is needed, particularly if the patient lives alone.

Physical environmental interventions involve changing the physical environment to support task performance. Auditory, visual, tactile, olfactory, gustatory, vestibular, or social understimulation or overstimulation hinders task performance; appropriate changes should be made.

Safety precautions are taken; for example, assistive devices (eg, grab bars) may be installed, scatter rugs removed, and electrical and telephone cords taped down. Accessibility may be improved by removing or modifying architectural barriers (eg, doors, thresholds), adding ramps, or lowering or raising work surfaces. Accommodating a walker or wheelchair may require rearranging furniture. For some patients with cognitive impairments, signs and pictures indicating the location of rooms and objects are helpful.

Other Considerations

In the elderly, the success of occupational therapy may be affected by the coexistence of multiple clinical problems. Elderly patients with hip fracture may need a walker to reduce stress on the hip joint but may be unable to learn to use it effectively because of cognitive impairment secondary to dementia. Engaging a depressed patient in an activity may be complicated by decreased vision secondary to macular degeneration or by a weak or painful grasp secondary to osteoarthritis.

Learning—the core of occupational therapy interventions—may take longer in the elderly because the mechanisms that receive, process, and act on information are less efficient. However, the extent of these changes varies, and many elderly persons remain highly efficient learners. In general, the elderly learn best when they are involved in tasks that have personal meaning and when they can control the pace of learning. The environment should have adequate ambient and focused lighting and should be free of distracting stimuli. Some elderly persons may have difficulty distinguishing relevant cues from irrelevant ones (eg, distinguishing the start button on a microwave oven from other buttons), so relevant cues should be emphasized orally, visually, or manually. A supportive social environment helps reduce the frustration associated with relearning BADLs and IADLs.

When independence cannot be achieved, occupational therapy may help patients reach a measure of independence that benefits them and their caregivers. For example, physical stress on a caregiver is reduced when patients learn to bear some weight during transfers. Even dependent patients may improve their cooperation with caregivers, particularly during ADLs. For example, in a patient with dementia, violent reactions during dressing may be avoided if the caregiver provides breakfast and shows each garment to the patient beforehand. For an institutionalized patient, occupational therapy is crucial for maintaining dignity and maximum physical independence.

Therapeutic and Assistive Devices

Splints are fitted to prevent deformity (eg, contractures) or to promote function (eg, achieving lateral pinch for holding a utensil). Static hand splints may be applied to maintain the wrist in a neutral position, the fingers in extension, and the thumb in opposition to prevent flexion deformities. A wrist cock-up splint supports the wrist in extension but leaves the fingers free. A footdrop splint helps maintain ankle flexion.

Self-help assistive devices are used to promote safety or to compensate for specific impairments. The most commonly used assistive devices are canes, grab bars on the side and the back of the bathtub or toilet, and shower chairs. Reachers or built-up handles on eating utensils, combs and brushes, and shoehorns compensate for restricted range of motion. Raised toilet seats and chair leg extenders compensate for diminished back or leg mobility; tools with built-up handles or with spring-loaded or electric controls compensate for reduced hand mobility. Weighted tools or utensils may reduce tremors. Cups with lids and swivel spoons may prevent spills.

For patients with sensory impairments, stimuli can be enhanced (eg, larger dials can be added to telephones) or changed (eg, for the hearing impaired, a telephone ring [auditory signal] can be replaced with a flashing light [visual signal]). Memory aids include automatic dialing telephones, drug organizers and reminders, and pocket devices that record and play back messages (reminders, instructions, lists) at the appropriate time.

31 ▌ **EXERCISE**

Sustained physical exertion for the general purpose of maintaining or improving physical fitness or joint function.

Depending on the clinical needs and capabilities of patients, a physician may encourage regular exercise or may specifically prescribe therapeutic exercise. Therapeutic exercise is a defined program of regular exercise with specific objectives.

Exercise levels decline with age for many reasons, most commonly because chronic conditions and intercurrent illnesses in the elderly limit physical activity. About 35 to 45% of the elderly participate in minimal exercise. Only about 20 to 25% participate in regular exercise $\geq$ 30 minutes 5 times/week. Women are less active than men. However, low income and low educational level are stronger predictors of inactivity than older age and female sex. Physical inactivity is the second leading cause (after tobacco use) of premature death in the USA.

Health Benefits

The benefits of exercise far exceed its risks, regardless of the presence of other risk factors: Regular exercise can reduce mortality rates even for smokers and obese persons. Indirect benefits include opportunities for social interaction, an enhanced sense of well-being, and possibly an improved quality of sleep. Direct benefits are myriad and include the following:

Improvement of physical and physiologic factors: Regular exercise can preserve skeletal muscle strength, aerobic capacity, and bone density, contributing to mobility and independence. Exercise is one of the few interventions that can restore physiologic capacity once it has been lost.

Skeletal muscle strength and power (rate of doing work) decline with age. These changes (an annual loss of 1 to 2% in strength and 3 to 4% in power between ages 65 and 85) are accompanied by sarcopenia (loss of muscle fibers, muscle mass, and motor units), **1** which contributes to a loss of independence. All of these changes can be prevented, at least partially, or reversed by appropriate exercise.

Regular exercise also promotes a balanced energy state and reduces the risk of obesity. Regular exercise (> 30 minutes/day of moderate-intensity activity) increases success in initial and long-term weight loss, but weight loss usually requires reduced caloric intake as well.

Improvement of functional ability: Regular exercise reduces the risk of age-related decline in functional ability, and it appears to improve quality of life by improving physical functioning and enhancing psychologic well-being.

Prevention and treatment of disease: In the elderly, regular exercise increases insulin sensitivity and glucose tolerance, reduces resting systolic and diastolic blood pressure, normalizes blood lipid levels (including a reduction in circulating triglycerides and an increase in high-density lipoprotein cholesterol), and reduces visceral fat content. Thus, regular exercise can help prevent cardiovascular disease (eg, coronary artery disease, hypertension), diabetes, osteoporosis, obesity-related disorders, colon cancer, and psychiatric disorders (especially mood disorders such as depression). Regular exercise is also recommended as part of the treatment of these disorders and others (eg, pulmonary disorders). It is part of rehabilitation after a myocardial infarction or after surgery. **2**

Endurance (aerobic) **3** and muscle-strengthening exercises **4** can reduce functional limitations in the elderly. The least fit persons improve the most, presumably because of a nonlinear relationship between physical fitness and functional ability. Improvements can be maintained by continued exercise.

Prevention of falls and fall-related injuries: Regular exercise can help prevent falls and fall-related injuries by improving several risk factors for falls related to poor mobility, including strength, balance, neuromuscular coordination, joint function, and endurance. Exercise provides an overall benefit, despite a modest increased risk of falls during the exercise. Regular exercise, especially a program that includes balance training, **5** is recommended by the U.S. Preventive Services Task Force as a primary preventive measure against falls.

---

1 see also page 471   **2** see page 278   **3** see page 301
4 see page 303   **5** see page 304

Reduction in mortality: Many cohort studies report that regularly active elderly persons have 20 to 50% lower mortality rates, despite a slight (but widely publicized) temporary increase in the risk of sudden death during exercise.

Health Risks

Musculoskeletal injury (eg, torn ligaments, pulled muscles) is the most common risk. Falls◼ and fall-related injuries (eg, hip fractures) can occur during exercise. Physically active young and middle-aged persons probably have a slightly higher fracture rate than does the general population. Physically active adults appear to have an overall lower rate, although the risk of fractures increases rapidly with age. In addition, the risk of sudden death is temporarily increased during exercise, especially when the exercise is vigorous and the exerciser is sedentary and poorly conditioned.

PRE-EXERCISE SCREENING

Screening by interview or questionnaire is recommended for all elderly patients starting an exercise program. Because exercise is inappropriate for only a small percentage of elderly adults, the main purpose of screening is to assign patients by triage to appropriate programs. Community exercise classes and fitness centers commonly screen new participants to identify those with chronic disorders or symptoms of chronic disorders. Participants are asked about a history of chest pain, heart disease, and other disorders. Some organizations use the Physical Activity Readiness Questionnaire (PAR-Q), a screening tool that refers participants to a physician to ensure that the proposed exercise is safe and that any medical conditions are stable and appropriately treated. Generally, exercise is unsafe for patients with unstable medical conditions (see TABLE 31–1).

The need for further pre-exercise screening (ie, full medical screening, including medical examination and, possibly, laboratory tests) of elderly patients with chronic disorders depends on what tests have already been performed and on clinical judgment. When exercise is a recommended treatment for patients with a chronic disorder, medical screening should be part of the initial evaluation. For the ambulatory elderly, a program emphasizing walking does not introduce a new activity, and gradually increasing walking time is probably safe, so full medical screening is usually not required. Comprehensive medical screening is not recommended for healthy patients of any age before starting a moderate-intensity activity program. However, some experts recommend such screening, possibly with an exercise stress test, for patients who have two or more cardiac risk factors (eg, hypertension, obesity). The American College of Sports Medicine recommends full medical screening and fitness testing for men > 40

◼ see page 195

TABLE 31-1. CONDITIONS THAT MUST BE STABILIZED BEFORE PATIENTS BEGIN AN EXERCISE PROGRAM

Unstable angina
Uncompensated heart failure
Uncontrolled cardiac arrhythmias
Severe, symptomatic aortic stenosis
Hypertrophic cardiomyopathy
Cardiomyopathy due to recent myocarditis
Severe pulmonary hypertension
Resting systolic pressure > 200 mm Hg
Resting diastolic pressure > 110 mm Hg
Active or suspected myocarditis or pericarditis
Suspected or known dissecting aneurysm
Thrombophlebitis
Recent systemic or pulmonary embolus

years and for women > 50 years who want to start a high-intensity exercise program.

Fitness Testing

Although fitness testing is usually unnecessary, it may sometimes be useful. Performance on a 6-minute walk test can indicate the level of aerobic fitness and suggest the intensity level at which to start exercise. Fitness testing can also include measures of body build and composition (eg, body mass index, percentage of body fat). When periodic fitness testing is used, providing the patient with feedback on fitness improvements can increase adherence.

FORMULATION OF THE EXERCISE PRESCRIPTION

The exercise prescription may include any combination of four types of therapeutic exercise—endurance exercises, muscle-strengthening exercises, balance training exercises, and flexibility exercises. The activities must be appropriate for a patient's level of fitness and medical condition. For example, patients with emphysema typically have low levels of fitness. Treadmill exercise may need to be performed at a very slow speed to accommodate marked deconditioning. Rehabilitation after a broken ankle may emphasize flexibility exercises to restore range of motion and muscle-strengthening exercises to address muscle wasting at the ankle joint due to immobilization. Patients with difficulty standing and walking can participate in seated exercise programs that use cuff weights for strength training and repeated movements for endurance training. Patients with arthritis may prefer an aquatics exercise program.

To maximize adherence, the physician should allow patients to select the activities they enjoy; ideally, the activities selected by the patient should include endurance, strength, balance, and flexibility exercises as prescribed by the physician. Some patients want to do the same activity every day; others want variety. Many patients prefer to exercise alone; some prefer exercise classes. Some patients require medical supervision during exercise (see TABLE 31–2).

The Centers for Disease Control and Prevention recommends that all adults participate in $\geq$ 30 minutes of moderate-intensity physical activity $\geq$ 5 days/week. Patients do not have to be active for 30 minutes at a time but can accumulate 30 minutes over 24 hours. As little as 10 minutes of exercise has health benefits, and three 10-minute bouts of activity have the same fitness effects as one 30-minute bout. Some elderly patients (eg, those with osteoarthritis) may prefer activity in short bouts.

The elderly can meet the recommended activity goal by integrating activity into daily life (eg, walking to the store rather than driving). The U.S. Preventive Services Task Force recommends that health care practitioners counsel all patients on how to incorporate exercise into their daily

---

TABLE 31–2.   DISORDERS AND CLINICAL CHARACTERISTICS THAT REQUIRE PATIENTS TO BE MEDICALLY SUPERVISED DURING EXERCISE*

Disorder
>   Left main or three-vessel coronary artery disease
>   Acquired valvular heart disease
>   Congenital heart disease
>   Cardiomyopathy not due to recent myocardial infarction or to hypertrophic cardiomyopathy
>   Previous cardiac arrest or episode of ventricular fibrillation not due to an acute ischemic event or cardiac procedure
>   Complex ventricular arrhythmias not controlled by drugs during low- to moderate-intensity activity
>   Two or more previous myocardial infarctions
>   Angina
>   A life-threatening medical problem

Clinical characteristic
>   Ejection fraction < 30%
>   Symptoms of heart disease at rest or during low-intensity activity
>   Exercise capacity < 6 METs
>   Ventricular tachycardia, or ischemic horizontal or down-sloping ST depression $\geq$ 1 mm at a workload of 1 to 6 METs
>   Drop in systolic blood pressure with exercise

MET = metabolic equivalent.
*Because of an increased risk of cardiac complications.

Adapted from Balady JG, et al: "Recommendation for cardiovascular screening, staffing, and emergency policies at health/fitness facilities." *Circulation* 97:2283–2293, 1998.

routines (see TABLE 31–3). Some elderly patients can more easily adhere to this type of activity plan than to a formal exercise program. Exercise need not be high intensity to have health benefits. Moderate-intensity activity (see TABLE 31–4) for only 30 minutes/day produces most of the health benefits of regular exercise. For the weak elderly, the usual moderate-intensity activities may be too strenuous. Therefore, activities that provide moderate intensity should be selected relative to fitness level, based on target heart rate and rating of perceived exertion during activity.

Exercises should be started at a low intensity for a short time, then gradually increased to the recommended intensity level. A program may begin by alternating 2 to 3 minutes of activity with 2 to 3 minutes of rest over 15 minutes. In deconditioned patients, even low-intensity activity can increase fitness.

Patients whose exercise program is interrupted for more than a few weeks (eg, by illness) should resume exercising at about half the intensity

TABLE 31–3. IMPROVING COUNSELING ABOUT EXERCISE

- The counseling message is repeated during several clinic visits rather than during one visit.

- The message is individualized, and the patient's readiness to change is considered. Patients are encouraged to find activities that are fun and feel good, because the effects of activity on health are an important, but secondary, reason for most elderly patients.

- Being specific is important. For example, patients can be advised to walk 5 minutes twice/day, gradually building up over 4 months to 20 minutes twice/day, rather than to "walk more."

- Patients can be asked to sign a contract committing to the mutually agreed-on exercise program.

- Individualized strategies to incorporate exercise into daily life are offered. For example, finding a friend to walk with each day at a specified time can provide social support for exercise. Such regular appointments promote adherence.

- Available community resources (eg, senior centers with inexpensive exercise classes) must be investigated. Exercise classes can be a useful way to start an activity program. Patients can exercise on their own once they are exercising regularly and safely.

- Support from the local health care system must be adequate in terms of collecting risk factor data, providing written materials about community resources, and reinforcing the counseling message through postcard or telephone reminders as needed.

- Counseling is offered as part of a community effort that broadly addresses behavioral, environmental, and policy determinants of activity levels.

TABLE 31–4.   ENDURANCE EXERCISES AND THEIR METABOLIC REQUIREMENT

Activity	Metabolic Requirement		
	Intensity Level	METs*	kcal/h
Walking at 3 to 5 km/h (2 to 3 miles/h) Cycling on level terrain at 10 km/h (6 miles/h) Light stretching exercises Swimming (using a float board) Light to moderate housework	Low	2–4	180–300
Walking at 6 km/h (4 miles/h) Cycling at 13 km/h (8 miles/h) Golf (walking or pulling a cart) Light calisthenics Swimming (treading water) Heavy housework or yard work	Moderate	5–6	300–360
Walking or jogging at 8 km/h (5 miles/h) Cycling at 18 to 19 km/h (11 to 12 miles/h) Swimming (0.8 km [1/2 mile] in 30 min) Recreational tennis Hiking	High	7–8	420–480

METs = metabolic equivalents.
*The oxygen expenditure at rest ($>$ 3.5 mL/min/kg body weight).
Adapted from Hanson PG, et al: "Clinical guidelines for exercise training." *Postgraduate Medicine* 67(1):120–138, 1980. Copyright © McGraw-Hill, Inc.

level. Then they can gradually increase to previous levels. Prolonged inactivity, especially bed rest, is not usually advised during recovery from illness. Each day of strict bed rest causes an incremental loss of muscle mass of about 1.5% and substantial losses in muscular performance and in cardiorespiratory fitness.

ENDURANCE EXERCISES

Of all types of exercise, endurance exercises (eg, walking, cycling, dancing, swimming, low-impact aerobics) provide the most well-documented health benefits for the elderly.

Walking is the most common exercise among the elderly in the USA (about 50% of the elderly walk for exercise) and is the most commonly recommended clinically. In a recent study, the mortality rate was reduced 50% in people who walked an average of $\geq$ 3.2 km/day ($\geq$ 2 miles/day). Walking also reduces the risk of new heart disease and of falls. Jogging is generally inappropriate for elderly persons not already accustomed to it.

During endurance exercise, level of exercise correlates with risk of injury and should be monitored. The target heart rate method of estimating exercise intensity is most useful when maximal heart rate has been determined by an exercise stress test. Otherwise, the rating of perceived exertion method is usually better and is necessary in patients who have atrial fibrillation or frequent ectopic beats or who are being treated with drugs or devices that influence or control heart rate (eg, β-blockers, pacemakers).

The target heart rate method: Patients can monitor their heart rate during exercise by taking their pulse or by using an exercise heart rate monitor. Moderate-intensity endurance exercise is defined as exercise that produces 60 to 79% of maximal heart rate. For example, elderly patients with a maximal heart rate of 150 beats/minute have a target heart rate of about 90 to 120 beats/minute during moderate-intensity activity.

An exercise stress test can determine the maximal heart rate and the target heart rate range. For patients who have not had a recent exercise stress test, maximal heart rate can be estimated using the formula "220 minus age." However, this formula is slightly conservative. For 80-year-old patients, the average maximal heart rate is between 140 and 150 beats/minute.

Patients whose heart rate is below the target range (see TABLE 31–5) while performing activities of 5 to 6 metabolic equivalents achieve most of the health benefits of activity and do not need to increase intensity level. However, if safe, an increase in intensity level to increase heart rate into the target range can increase health benefits.

Rating of perceived exertion method: Perception of exertion appears to be a good way to monitor intensity. The most commonly used scale is the Borg scale, on which activity is rated from 6 (extremely light) to 19 (extremely hard); moderate activity is rated 11 to 13. Actual intensity is linearly related to steady-state exercise heart rate, but not to perceived

TABLE 31–5.   TARGET HEART RATE DURING ENDURANCE EXERCISES BY AGE*

Age	Target Heart Rate (beats/min)
40	126–153
50	119–145
60	112–136
70	105–128
80	98–119
90	91–111

*The target heart rate (60 to 79% of the maximal heart rate) is most useful when the maximal heart rate has been determined by an exercise stress test. The maximal heart rate, when predicted according to the patient's age alone, is not very accurate. Heart rate has a normal distribution; 95% of values occur within ± 2 SD of the mean. In the elderly, 1 SD is about 17 beats/min. Thus, among 80-year-old patients with an average maximal heart rate of 150 beats/min, the maximal heart rate varies from 116 to 184 beats/min.

TABLE 31–6.   GUIDELINES FOR DETERMINING PERCEIVED INTENSITY LEVEL

Intensity Level	Description
Low	Talking is possible Singing is possible Perspiration does not occur, unless environment is hot Muscles feel normal
Moderate	Talking is possible Singing is not possible Perspiration occurs during sustained activity Muscles feel normal
High	Talking is difficult Singing is not possible Perspiration occurs Muscles feel rubbery

intensity. The Borg scale helps patients "calibrate" perceived intensity to actual intensity (see TABLE 31–6), often with the help of a fitness instructor.

MUSCLE-STRENGTHENING EXERCISES

Many experts recommend that the elderly perform muscle-strengthening exercises at least 2 days/week. Normally, the same muscle group is not exercised more often than every other day. Strength training can increase bone density as well as improve muscle mass, strength, balance, and overall level of physical activity.

High-intensity programs can greatly increase strength. These programs use weight machines (eg, at gyms and other fitness centers), which are appropriate for healthy elderly patients. Resistance is set at 60 to 80% of the one-repetition maximum (ie, the maximal weight the patient can lift once). Typically, elderly patients perform two sets of 10 repetitions on 8 to 10 machines. Gains in strength can range from 30 to 150% during at least the first year of exercise. Muscle hypertrophy can also occur.

High-intensity programs are particularly appropriate for frail or near-frail elderly patients with sarcopenia. For these patients, machines that use air pressure rather than weights to provide resistance are more useful because the resistance can be set lower and changed in smaller increments. High-intensity programs are safe even for nursing home residents > 80 years old, for whom strength and mobility can be substantially improved. However, these programs are time-consuming because participants usually require close supervision.

Moderate-intensity programs maintain strength, or increase it 10 to 20% over several months and then maintain it. These programs include cuff weight exercises; calisthenics, which use body weight for resistance; and exercises using various thicknesses of elastic tubing for resistance. In cuff weight exercises, weighted cuffs are strapped to ankles or wrists or are held. They do not require expensive equipment, can be performed at home, and are especially useful in weak elderly patients. The weight can be adjusted in 0.227-kg (1/2-lb) increments by removing or adding small weight sacks. "Exercise: A Guide from the National Institute on Aging" (Publication No. NIH 98-4258) describes a cuff weight program.

BALANCE TRAINING EXERCISES

Balance training exercises are indicated for elderly patients at increased risk of falls.◨ Properly designed exercise programs can reduce the risk of falls (by about 10 to 15% in one meta-analysis), but those that include balance training appear most effective.

Tai chi (a variety of exercises involving sequences of movements originally used in the martial arts) is one type of program for improving balance. Home-based balance training exercise programs are also available.

Usually, balance training exercises are graduated. Patients begin with the simplest exercises and advance as appropriate. For example, level 1 = walking while holding onto a table; level 2 = walking with arms outstretched and ready to grab the table if balance is lost; level 3 = walking with arms crossed at the chest; and level 4 = walking with arms crossed at the chest and extra weight in the hands. Balance training exercises do not count toward the recommended 30 minutes/day of moderate-intensity activity.

FLEXIBILITY EXERCISES

Flexibility exercises increase range of motion. Some elderly patients report that flexibility exercises make their bodies feel better. These exercises are commonly recommended to reduce injury risk; however, this benefit has not been studied in the elderly.

A wide variety of stretching exercises are used. Stretching is recommended after endurance and muscle-strengthening exercises, when muscles are warm. A stretch is held for 10 to 30 seconds, 3 to 5 times per session. It is performed slowly, without jerking or bouncing.

Flexibility exercises are generally low intensity. They do not count toward the recommended 30 minutes/day of moderate-intensity activity.

◨see page 195

DRUG USE AND EXERCISE

Doses of **insulin and oral hypoglycemics** in diabetics may need to be adjusted (according to the amount of anticipated exercise) to prevent hypoglycemia during exercise. Exercisers with non–insulin-dependent diabetes benefit from an exercise-induced increase in insulin sensitivity, facilitating uptake of glucose by muscle.

Doses of **drugs that can cause orthostatic hypotension** (eg, antidepressants, antihypertensives, hypnotics, anxiolytics, diuretics) may need to be lowered to avoid exacerbation of orthostasis by fluid loss during exercise, leading to presyncope or syncope. For patients taking such drugs, adequate fluid intake is essential during exercise.

Some **sedative-hypnotics** may reduce physical performance, either indirectly by decreasing activity levels or directly by inhibiting effects on muscles and nerves. These and other psychoactive drugs increase the risk of falls. Discontinuing such drugs or reducing their dose may be necessary to improve the safety of exercise and to increase patient adherence.

When **β-blockers** are used, endurance intensity cannot be monitored by the target heart rate method. These drugs may mask hypoglycemic symptoms other than sweating.

Drugs with anabolic activity (eg, growth hormone, estrogen, testosterone, vitamins) have long been suggested as a means to build muscle mass in elderly patients with sarcopenia. However, studies with exogenous growth hormone have shown mixed results[1]; some have not found an effect on muscle strength, even when combined with muscle-strengthening exercises. Evidence about the effect of estrogen replacement on muscle strength is limited and inconsistent. Testosterone replacement in hypogonadal men appears to increase muscle strength; however, dose-response information is lacking and adverse effects (eg, prostate cancer) are a concern.[2] There is little evidence for or against a role of vitamins in improving muscle strength, although one study showed that vitamin D has no effect.

---

[1] see also page 658   [2] see also page 655

PSYCHIATRIC DISORDERS

PSY

32 ■ AGING AND MENTAL HEALTH

Aging may variably affect cognition, memory, intelligence, personality, and behavior. However, many changes in mental health are difficult to attribute to aging per se; they are often the result of disease. Decreases in mental capacity or performance (eg, cognition, behavior) that are viewed as age related may instead be due to treatable illnesses (eg, depression, hypothyroidism). A rapid decrease in cognition is almost always due to disease.

The effects of aging on mental health may also be related to socioenvironmental factors, including the care setting. For example, the prevalence of psychiatric disorders is 15 to 25% among persons aged 65 living in the community and 27 to 55% among those in the hospital. Psychiatric disorders are a primary or secondary diagnosis in 70 to 80% of nursing home residents; in one study, 94% of nursing home residents had a psychiatric disorder. Brain disorders causing dementia (most commonly, Alzheimer's disease **1**) affect about 10% of persons aged 65 and at least 25% of those aged 85.

COGNITIVE AND INTELLECTUAL DECLINE

With age, cognitive functions may remain stable or decline. In general, cognitive functions that remain stable include attention span, everyday communication skills, many language skills (eg, syntax), the ability to comprehend discourse, and simple visual perception. Vocabulary can improve even in persons in their 80s. Cognitive functions that decline include selective attention, naming of objects, verbal fluency, complex visuospatial skills, and logical analysis. Learning complex new tasks and foreign languages becomes more difficult with age.

Age-related memory changes vary depending on the type of memory function; the ability to acquire, store, and retrieve new memories may be reduced, whereas the ability to retrieve memories that have been stored and consolidated over long periods remains stable. Reduced memory performance can be improved using adaptive strategies.

Intellectual abilities peak during the 30s, plateau throughout the 50s and 60s, and variably decline during the late 70s. Elderly persons may have difficulty with activities requiring a quick reaction time or high degree of precision, although they maintain the ability to understand their situation and learn from new experiences. Reduced reaction time can be compensated for by allocating more time for tasks.

Depression, anxiety, and other psychiatric disorders can also interfere with cognition. Pseudodementia (eg, depression or psychosis mimicking dementia **2**) is an extreme form of such interference.

CHANGES IN PERSONALITY AND BEHAVIOR

Personality remains stable with age. However, whether behavior also remains stable with age is debated. Usually, behavioral and psychologic adaptiveness continues and does not normally regress or become rigid. Increasingly exaggerated, maladaptive, and unmodifiable behaviors or traits **3** may represent psychologic or neurologic problems and not normal aging.

In general, frail or disabled elderly persons are more cautious than younger persons, especially when risk taking involves a predictable and constant payoff (eg, they may not fly standby for a routine visit to family members, even if it increases savings); however, the elderly are not more cautious if the payoff appears to exceed the degree of risk (eg, they may fly standby if it represents the only chance to visit family members for a special occasion). Excessive cautiousness in elderly per-

---

1see page 365   **2**see page 363   **3**see page 371

sons may signal underlying anxiety or a related physical disorder; however, excessive cautiousness in frail or disabled persons may reflect good judgment.

The elderly usually adapt to the concept of impending death after becoming aware of it (sometimes suddenly) during middle age. Although the elderly often think about death, they fear death less than other age groups. Thoughts or conversations about death are more common among the elderly, who likely have peers and relatives who have died or are dying.

A terminal illness, an underlying depression, or other emotional conflict predisposes certain elderly persons to anxiety about death and, in some cases, can lead to despondency. The ability to cope with such stress is maintained or improved with age.

EFFECTS OF PSYCHOLOGIC DYSFUNCTION ON PHYSICAL HEALTH

Elderly persons who experience significant losses (eg, loss of a spouse or partner, economic status, physical health, or overall independence) often have diminished self-esteem and depression. A loss of control over one's life may be so disturbing that it may result in physical symptoms that represent maladaptive efforts to control other persons, gain attention, or signal for help. Vague physical decline does not always indicate physiologic aging or the subtle progression of underlying physical illness. In one study of depressed men and women > 60 years, physical complaints were reported by > 60%. The nature and rate of physical decline in a patient who is clinically depressed can reflect the will to live or die.

Many elderly persons in the community have the same degree of physical disability as those in nursing homes; the differences appear to be related to the availability of family members, the availability of other types of social support, and coexisting psychiatric disorders.

Psychosocial factors may aggravate existing physical disorders or precipitate latent ones. For example, psychologic disorders (eg, anxiety) may lead to physical discomfort in more than half of elderly persons with gastrointestinal complaints. In the elderly, about half of the cases of gastrointestinal distress (eg, irritable colon, spastic colitis, gastritis, heartburn, nausea, diarrhea, constipation) have a psychogenic component.[1]

Physical disorders may affect psychologic disorders. More than 25% of elderly persons have impaired hearing; in such persons, a sensory-deprivation phenomenon may cause psychotic symptoms (eg, delusions).

[1] see page 327

Coexisting physical and psychologic disorders may precipitate further physical or psychologic decline. A frail elderly person with depression or psychosis may be unable to correctly take drugs to treat physical ailments.

33 ■ DEPRESSION

A disorder characterized by feelings of sadness and despair and ranging in severity from mild to life threatening.

Depression is one of the most common psychiatric disorders among the elderly. The prevalence of clinically significant depressive symptoms ranges from 8 to 15% among community-dwelling elderly persons and is about 30% among the institutionalized elderly. Major depression occurs less often in later life than at younger ages and affects about 3% of elderly persons in the community, 11% in hospitals, and 12% in long-term care settings. The current cohort between ages 70 and 90 years has had fewer severe depressive episodes in adult life than earlier cohorts. The number of cases is expected to increase substantially over the next 20 to 30 years as younger cohorts, who have a higher prevalence of depression than the current elderly cohort, age.

Depression is one of the most common risk factors for suicide (see TABLE 33–1). The highest rates of suicide in the USA occur in persons ≥ 70. For white men, suicide is 45% more common among those aged

TABLE 33–1.   RISK FACTORS FOR SUICIDE

Age > 55 years

Male sex

Painful or disabling physical illness

Solitary living situation

Debt, decreased income, or poverty

Bereavement

Depression, especially associated with agitation, excessive guilt, self-reproach, and insomnia

Persistence of depressed mood toward the end of a depressive illness, even though energy has returned

History of drug or alcohol abuse

History of prior suicide attempts

Family history of suicide

Suicidal preoccupation and talk

Well-defined plans for suicide

TABLE 33-2.   SELECTED MEDICAL DISORDERS THAT MAY CAUSE DEPRESSION IN THE ELDERLY

Type	Disorder
Cancer	Cancer of the breast, kidney, lung, ovary, or pancreas; leukemia; lymphoma
Cardiovascular disorders	Postmyocardial infarction, cardiomyopathy, heart failure
Endocrine disorders	Thyroiditis, hyperthyroidism, hypothyroidism, Cushing's disease, Addison's disease, hypopituitarism
Neurologic disorders	Alzheimer's disease, amyotrophic lateral sclerosis, Huntington's disease, Parkinson's disease, multiple sclerosis, vascular dementia (multi-infarct dementia)
Metabolic or nutritional disorders	Malnutrition, hypokalemia, hyperkalemia, hyponatremia, hypernatremia, hypocalcemia, hypercalcemia, hypomagnesemia, vitamin B_{12} deficiency
Viral infections	Hepatitis, HIV infection, herpes zoster

65 to 69 years, > 85% more common among those aged 70 to 74, and more than three and a half times more common among those ≥ 85 than among white men aged 15 to 19 years. Suicide rates do not increase with age among women. The elderly are less likely than younger patients to seek or respond to offers of help designed to prevent suicide. The elderly make fewer suicide gestures but more often succeed at suicide attempts. As many as 70% of elderly persons who completed suicide visited their primary care physician within the previous 4 weeks.

Etiology

The etiology of depression in the elderly, as in younger persons, is biopsychosocial.

Medical disorders may cause depression in the elderly (see TABLE 33-2) as may abuse of alcohol, some prescription drugs (especially some antihypertensives), cocaine, or other illicit drugs. Psychologic risk factors are similar across age groups and include guilt and negative thought patterns. Cognitive dysfunction is another major risk factor. Social risk factors (eg, loss of a spouse or partner, decreased social support) appear to cause depression more often in men than in women. Persons with lower incomes are at greater risk for depression.

Heredity plays less of a role in depression with first onset in late life than in that with first onset in midlife. However, persons who first experience depression in early or midlife and have a recurrence in late life are just as likely to report a family history as are persons who experience depression in midlife. Structural brain changes, seen on MRI and thought to be secondary to vascular insufficiency, are associated with depression in late life. Such cases are referred to as **vascular depression.**

Symptoms and Signs

Chronic and persistent dysphoria (restlessness, malaise) with a mildly depressed mood, common among the elderly, is not severe enough to warrant a diagnosis of depression. The clinical manifestations of depression in the elderly are listed in TABLE 33–3.

Episodes of **brief depression,** which are also common among the elderly, include moderately severe depressive symptoms that are consistent with the *Diagnostic and Statistical Manual of Mental Disorders, Fourth Edition (DSM-IV)* criteria except for their duration (2 weeks). The symptoms may have no clear cause and may resolve spontaneously, and episodes may occur in increasingly rapid cycles.

Some elderly persons experience a brief period (usually lasting a few days) of severe depressive symptoms that usually can be explained by obvious difficulties in adjustment or by bereavement. Adjusting to a severe or ultimately fatal chronic illness and losing a spouse or partner are common causes of such symptoms. Affected persons recover with time or when the stressor resolves.

Dysthymic disorder, which may be chronic, persistent, and moderately severe, is defined by *DSM-IV* as a depressed mood with two or more additional symptoms (eg, sleep problems, decreased appetite, feelings of hopelessness, lethargy). Symptoms must persist for at least 2 years but are not severe enough to constitute a major depressive episode.

Major depression, with or without melancholia, includes a core symptom of dysphoric mood or loss of interest plus at least four of the following symptoms: sleep disturbance (usually decreased sleep), appetite disturbance, weight loss, psychomotor retardation, suicidal ideation, poor concentration, feelings of guilt, and loss of interest in usual activities (if not the core symptom). **Melancholia** is present if these symptoms are predominated by a lack of interest in the social environment, diurnal variation (ie, feeling significantly worse during one part of the day, usually the morning, compared with the remainder of the day), and psychomotor agitation or retardation.

Sometimes major depression is characterized predominantly by psychotic features, especially delusions of illness or guilt about past actions, thoughts, or events. ■ **Psychotic depression** is more prevalent in late life than in midlife. Generally, psychotic symptoms are similar among elderly and younger patients, although elderly patients usually have more of them and are less likely to experience self-deprecation and guilt.

Bipolar I disorder is characterized by one or more manic episodes, with or without episodes of depression. A manic episode is a distinct

■ see page 329

TABLE 33–3.   CLINICAL MANIFESTATIONS OF DEPRESSION IN THE ELDERLY

Item	Symptoms
Mood	Depressed attitude, irritability, or anxiety (however, the patient may smile or deny subjective mood change and instead complain of pain or other somatic distress) Crying spells (however, the patient may complain of inability to cry or to experience emotions)
Associated psychologic manifestations	Lack of self-confidence; low self-esteem; self-reproach Poor concentration and memory Reduction in gratification; loss of interest in usual activities; loss of attachments; social withdrawal Negative expectations; hopelessness; helplessness; increased dependency Recurrent thoughts of death Suicidal thoughts (rare, but serious when present)
Somatic manifestations	Psychomotor retardation; fatigue Agitation Anorexia and weight loss Insomnia
Psychotic manifestations	Delusions of worthlessness and sinfulness Delusions of ill health (nihilistic, somatic, or hypochondriacal) Delusions of poverty Depressive auditory, visual, and (rarely) olfactory hallucinations

period (lasting ≥ 1 week) during which there is an abnormally and persistently elevated, expansive, or irritable mood. Manic episodes may occur for the first time in late life but most often recur from an earlier age. During a manic episode, a person may experience an inflated self-esteem, decreased need for sleep, increased talkativeness, a subjective sense that thoughts are racing, distractibility, psychomotor agitation, and involvement in activities that are perceived to be pleasurable but that can lead to adverse outcomes, such as unrestrained buying. Elderly persons are less likely to experience inflated self-esteem or grandiosity during an episode and are more likely to experience irritability and psychomotor agitation, thus making it somewhat difficult to distinguish a manic episode from agitated depression. A thorough history, including information from the patient and family, can assist in making this distinction. For example, if the elderly person has had previous episodes of depression associated with psychomotor retardation and, over a short period of time, enters an episode of acute agitation, decreased sleep, and increased talkativeness, a manic episode is likely even if the mood is dysphoric.

Some elderly persons may never experience an acute episode of mania but do have clear episodes of major depression. Between the episodes of depression, however, these persons are more elated or more irritable than usual. Such persons are diagnosed as having **bipolar II disorder.** The periods between episodes of depression may last for days, weeks, or even months. The symptoms, although uncharacteristic of the usual behavior of the elderly person, usually do not significantly interfere with function. Relatives and friends, however, may notice a problem with function.

Diagnosis

A thorough **history and physical examination,** including complete neurologic and mental status assessment, are necessary. A complete review of drug use (including illicit drugs) and alcohol use is also critical. Interaction with family members is helpful, and if the patient is demented or uncommunicative, obtaining a history from family members or other informants is essential. When the diagnosis is complicated by comorbid conditions or by poor communication with the patient, the physician should focus on the symptoms reported by family members and on change in symptoms over time.

The Geriatric Depression Scale (see TABLE 33–4) and the Hamilton Depression Rating Scale (see TABLE 33–5) are useful assessment instruments. However, they are screening devices and should not replace a thorough evaluation and interaction with the patient and family members.

Depressed patients should be asked directly about suicidal thoughts and intentions (eg, "Do you ever feel that life is not worth living? Have you thought of harming yourself?"). Asking about suicide does not increase the risk of suicide. Patients with suicidal thoughts should be asked about plans (eg, "Have you planned how you would do it?"). Those with suicidal plans should be hospitalized immediately.

Sometimes a definitive diagnosis cannot be made on the basis of history and examination alone. Such situations are common when demented patients stop eating or deteriorate in another way that suggests depression. A trial of treatment, usually with an antidepressant, is the best course for these patients.

Laboratory tests have an adjunctive role in the evaluation of depressed patients. However, thyroid function should be assessed for all new cases. A slightly low thyroxine level and an elevated thyroid-stimulating hormone level are common during a depressive episode. Most other tests should be ordered only when clinical findings suggest a concurrent disorder.

An ECG can provide a baseline if concerns arise about the effect of tricyclic antidepressants on cardiac function. Although not diagnostic,

TABLE 33-4.   GERIATRIC DEPRESSION SCALE (SHORT FORM)

1.	Are you basically satisfied with your life?	Yes	No
2.	Have you dropped many of your activities and interests?	Yes	No
3.	Do you feel that your life is empty?	Yes	No
4.	Do you often get bored?	Yes	No
5.	Are you in good spirits most of the time?	Yes	No
6.	Are you afraid that something bad is going to happen to you?	Yes	No
7.	Do you feel happy most of the time?	Yes	No
8.	Do you often feel helpless?	Yes	No
9.	Do you prefer to stay at home rather than go out and do new things?	Yes	No
10.	Do you feel you have more problems with memory than most?	Yes	No
11.	Do you think it is wonderful to be alive now?	Yes	No
12.	Do you feel pretty worthless the way you are now?	Yes	No
13.	Do you feel full of energy?	Yes	No
14.	Do you feel that your situation is hopeless?	Yes	No
15.	Do you think that most people are better off than you are?	Yes	No

Score: ___/15 One point for "No" to questions 1, 5, 7, 11, 13 One point for "Yes" to other questions	Normal Mildly depressed Very depressed	3 ± 2 7 ± 3 12 ± 2

Adapted from Sheikh JI, Yesavage JA: "Geriatric depression scale (GDS): Recent evidence and development of a shorter version," in *Clinical Gerontology: A Guide to Assessment and Intervention,* edited by TL Brink. Binghamton, NY, Haworth Press, 1986, pp. 165–173. © By The Haworth Press, Inc. All rights reserved. Reprinted with permission.

the dexamethasone suppression test may help predict prognosis. A positive test result (ie, a postdexamethasone cortisol level of > 5 μg/dL [140 nmol/L]) suggests that a relapse is likely if the level remains high, even when symptoms improve. Polysomnography, when available, can help identify melancholia; decreased sleep time with shortened rapid eye movement latency supports the diagnosis.

The differential diagnosis of major depression includes many medical and psychiatric disorders that may manifest as depression in later life (see TABLE 33–6).

Prognosis and Treatment

Patients with dysphoria rarely benefit from traditional modes of therapy. The outcome of major depression in late life, if uncomplicated, follows the "rule of thirds." One third of elderly patients get better and stay

TABLE 33–5.   HAMILTON DEPRESSION RATING SCALE*

Item†	Cue	Score
Depressed mood (sad, hopeless, helpless, worthless)	0 Has none 1 Indicates these feelings only on questioning 2 Spontaneously reports these feelings 3 Communicates feelings nonverbally (ie, through facial expression, posture, voice, and a tendency to weep) 4 Reports *virtually only* these feelings in spontaneous verbal and nonverbal communication	
Feelings of guilt	0 Has none 1 Shows signs of self-reproach; feels he has let people down 2 Has ideas of guilt or ruminates over past errors or sinful deeds 3 Feels present illness is a punishment; has delusions of guilt 4 Hears accusatory or denunciatory voices, experiences threatening visual hallucinations, or experiences both	
Suicidal ideation	0 Has none 1 Feels life is not worth living 2 Wishes he were dead or has thoughts of possible death 3 Expresses suicidal ideas or makes gesture 4 Attempts suicide (any serious attempt rates 4)	
Insomnia—early	0 Has no difficulty falling asleep 1 Complains of occasional difficulty falling asleep (ie, takes > 30 min) 2 Complains of nightly difficulty falling asleep	
Insomnia—middle	0 Has no difficulty 1 Complains of being restless and disturbed during the night 2 Wakes during the night (any getting out of bed, except to void, rates 2)	
Insomnia—late	0 Has no difficulty 1 Wakes in early hours of the morning but goes back to sleep 2 Is unable to fall asleep again after getting out of bed	

TABLE 33-5. *(Continued)*

Item†	Cue	Score
Work and activities	0 Has no difficulty 1 Has thoughts and feelings of incapacity, fatigue, or weakness related to work or hobbies 2 Has loss of interest in hobbies or work—as directly reported by the patient, or as indirectly indicated by being listless or indecisive (feels he has to push self to work or perform activities) 3 Spends less time in activities or decreases productivity (eg, in a hospital, patient spending < 3 h/day in activities—hospital job or hobbies—exclusive of ward chores rates 3) 4 Has stopped working because of present illness (eg, in a hospital, patient engaging in no activities except ward chores or failing to perform ward chores unassisted rates 4)	
Retardation (slowness of thought and speech, impaired ability to concentrate, decreased motor activity)	0 Has normal speech and thought 1 Is slightly retarded at interview 2 Is obviously retarded at interview 3 Is difficult to interview 4 Is completely stuporous	
Agitation	0 Has none 1 "Plays with" hands, hair, etc. 2 Wrings hands, bites nails or lips, pulls hair	
Anxiety—psychic (demonstrates physiologic concomitants of anxiety, such as dry mouth, flatulence, indigestion, diarrhea, cramps, belching, palpitations, headaches, hyperventilation, sighing, urinary frequency, sweating)	0 Absent 1 Mild 2 Moderate 3 Severe 4 Incapacitating	
Somatic symptoms— gastrointestinal	0 Has none 1 Has loss of appetite but eats without staff encouragement; has heavy feelings in abdomen	

Table continues on the following page.

TABLE 33–5.   HAMILTON DEPRESSION RATING SCALE* (*Continued*)

Item†		Cue	Score
Somatic symptoms— gastrointestinal (*continued*)	2	Has difficulty eating without staff urging; requests or requires laxatives or medication for bowels or medication for gastrointestinal symptoms	
Somatic symptoms— general	0	Has none	
	1	Has heaviness in limbs, back, or head; backaches, headache, muscle aches; loss of energy and fatigability	
	2	Has any clear-cut symptom	
Loss of libido	0	Has no loss	
	1	Has mild loss	
	2	Has severe loss	
Hypochondriasis	0	Has none	
	1	Is self-absorbed (bodily)	
	2	Is preoccupied with health	
	3	Voices frequent complaints, requests for help	
	4	Has hypochondriacal delusions	
Weight loss	0	Has none	
	1	Has probable weight loss associated with present illness	
	2	Has definite (according to patient) weight loss	
Insight (score 0 if the patient is not depressed)	0	Acknowledges being depressed and ill	
	1	Acknowledges illness but attributes cause to bad food, climate, overwork, virus, need for rest, etc.	
	2	Denies being ill	

Total score‡ _____

*The value of the ratings depends entirely on the interviewer's skill and experience. Questions should be directed to the patient's condition in the past few days or week.

†For each item, select the cue that best characterizes the patient and enter the corresponding score.

‡A score of ≥ 16 indicates significant depressive symptoms. A reduction of the score by 50% indicates significant response to therapy.

Adapted from Hamilton M: "Development of a rating scale for primary depressive illness." *British Journal of Social and Clinical Psychology* 6:278–296, 1967; used with permission.

TABLE 33-6. DIFFERENTIAL DIAGNOSIS OF MAJOR DEPRESSION*

Disorder	Comment
Idiopathic primary sleep disorder	This disorder can mimic sleep problems that occur with depression and can result in a reactive (secondary) depression due to sleep deprivation
Dementia (see Ch. 40)	Major depression and dementia often coexist; usually, depressive symptoms remit, but cognitive deficit persists or worsens
Pseudodementia	Treatment is the only test of whether cognitive dysfunction results only from depression
Hypochondriasis (see Ch. 35)	This disorder is often associated with a depressive effect; the gradual onset of symptoms, coupled with the patient's lack of apparent distress, helps confirm the diagnosis

*Other medical disorders can cause depression (see TABLE 33–2).

better, one third get better but relapse, and one third do not improve or improve only marginally. With time, however, most elderly patients who experience major depression in late life recover. Recovery, however, may take months. The prognosis is worse when depression is complicated by an underlying dysthymic disorder, by a medical disorder, or by cognitive impairment.

The key to the management of depression, especially major depression, in the elderly is early identification and intervention. All caregivers must be alert to the possibility of depression, especially when illness or loss of a loved one occurs. Family members, in particular, must be alert for subtle changes in personality, especially lack of enthusiasm and spontaneity, loss of sense of humor, and new forgetfulness. Loss of interest in sex may be apparent only to a spouse or other sexual partner. Nurses must be alert to loss of appetite, new sleep disturbances, and other signs and symptoms of depression. During treatment, family members and professional caregivers must be trained to monitor for adverse effects of drugs. They must also be alert to warning signs that the depression is worsening or that the patient is considering suicide.

Psychotherapy: Elderly patients with mild, recently established depression may respond to psychotherapy alone and may not need pharmacotherapy. Psychotherapy is often effective in treating depression without significant melancholic symptoms. When combined with antidepressants, it may benefit patients with severe depression. Behavioral and cognitive therapies are considered more effective than nondirected or analytically oriented therapies. Behavioral and cognitive therapies may help reintegrate the patient into a social environment after severe depression and may help prevent relapses, especially for episodic depression. Psychotherapy may be conducted by a psychiatrist, clinical psychologist, or mental health social worker, or it may require an interdisciplinary team.

Pharmacotherapy: Treatment of severe depression with melancholic features is primarily pharmacologic. Choosing a drug depends primarily on which one produces the fewest adverse effects. Although tricyclic antidepressants (eg, nortriptyline, desipramine, amitriptyline) are used often, elderly patients have difficulty tolerating the anticholinergic effects (especially those of amitriptyline) and the postural hypotension these drugs are likely to induce. Monoamine oxidase inhibitors are used less often because they have significant adverse effects and because they are not more effective than other drugs.

Therefore, the drugs of choice are the selective serotonin reuptake inhibitors (SSRIs [eg, fluoxetine, nefazodone, sertraline, paroxetine]), which have relatively few adverse cardiovascular and anticholinergic effects. However, agitation, a common adverse effect with some of these drugs (eg, fluoxetine), can be especially troublesome for elderly depressed patients. Sexual dysfunction is a problem for some persons who take SSRIs. Also, SSRIs can cause akinesthesia and other movement disorders.

Usual starting doses in otherwise healthy elderly patients are typically one half the usual adult doses: eg, fluoxetine 10 mg po daily, nefazodone 100 mg po bid, sertraline 25 mg po daily, or paroxetine 10 mg po daily. A typical starting dose for the tricyclic antidepressant nortriptyline is 10 to 25 mg po at night with gradual increases. Doses should be titrated upward slowly (eg, weekly) and not every 3 to 5 days as for younger adults.

Adjuncts may augment the response to antidepressants. For example, low-dose lithium may augment the effect of tricyclic antidepressants and SSRIs, and carbamazepine may reduce a patient's tendency to cycle in and out of depressive episodes. Methylphenidate has been used independently and as an adjunct to antidepressants, especially for patients in long-term care facilities. Its use may be advantageous for patients who have stopped eating because, if the drug works, it works quickly and also independently stimulates appetite. Methylphenidate may activate the depressed patient, is relatively safe, and rarely leads to dependence.

An acute manic episode may be treated with a mood stabilizer coupled with hospitalization to reduce the likelihood of behavior that can harm the patient or others; lithium carbonate, usually 300 to 600 mg/day, is the treatment of choice. Serum levels for effective therapy in the elderly are usually 0.4 to 0.8 mEq/L; higher levels are often associated with agitation and confusion. Given the toxicity of lithium, many clinicians elect to treat with valproic acid, at an initial dose of 10 to 15 mg/kg/day in 1 to 3 divided doses. Acute symptoms may require that the mood stabilizer be augmented with an antipsychotic drug (eg, olanzapine 2.5 mg daily, haloperidol 0.25 to 0.5 mg daily to bid). In such elderly patients, the doses of both the mood stabilizer and the antipsychotic drug must be increased significantly.

Electroconvulsive therapy (ECT):   ECT is used for severely depressed patients, especially those who have previously responded to ECT, those who demonstrate significant psychotic symptoms or self-destructive behavior, and those who do not tolerate or respond to antidepressants. ECT is safest with multiple-channel monitoring (electroencephalography [EEG], ECG, blood pressure, pulse, and respiratory function); it should be administered by a psychiatrist under the supervision of an anesthetist or anesthesiologist. After rehydration, ECT is the treatment of choice for patients with malnutrition and dehydration due to severe depression.

ECT induces improvement in 80% of elderly patients who did not respond to antidepressants—the same rate as for younger patients. Maintenance ECT on an outpatient basis significantly reduces the likelihood of relapse for patients who responded to ECT. If maintenance ECT is impossible, then the risk of relapse can be reduced by the use of antidepressants, even if the patient did not respond to them initially.

Patients who undergo ECT experience acute amnesia, which is often distressing. Some memory loss can persist after ECT, but the nature and extent of this problem have not been determined.

Treatment of Medically Ill and Hospitalized Patients

Some patients respond to an acute or chronic medical disorder by developing a psychiatric disorder (eg, adjustment disorder with depressed mood). Support and psychotherapy (eg, formal intervention with the patient and family members) are often helpful. Small doses of SSRIs (eg, trazodone, 25 mg at night) can help, especially when sleep problems are present. For patients who are dying, similar measures can be used; however, not every dying patient needs psychotherapy or antidepressants.∎

Pharmacotherapy for major depression in patients with other medical disorders requires special attention. Tricyclic antidepressants and SSRIs (although SSRIs are of less concern) can cause adverse cardiovascular effects in patients with heart disease or unstable blood pressure (eg, a tendency toward orthostatic hypotension). Both classes of drugs are reasonably safe when used properly in patients without serious heart disease.

With longer hospitalization, the inability to respond to rehabilitative efforts and a patient's and family members' fears of chronic invalidism become proportionately greater. Hospitalized patients with depression

∎ see page 120

often view themselves as hopeless; their hopelessness spreads to the staff members, who may pay less attention to them. Modifying the patient's environment may help (eg, involving the patient in group activities), but the depression itself also needs to be treated, usually with pharmacotherapy.

34   ANXIETY DISORDERS

Anxiety disorders are classified as phobic disorders, posttraumatic stress disorder, generalized anxiety disorder, obsessive-compulsive disorder, and panic disorder. All exist in the elderly, although they differ in prevalence and sometimes in symptoms and outcome.

Phobic disorders: These disorders involve persistent, unrealistic, yet intense anxiety that is stimulated by certain situations. Examples include fear of public places (agoraphobia) and fear of confinement (claustrophobia). Phobic disorders affect some elderly persons but are more common among children and younger adults. Few data are available regarding the course of phobic disorders into late life. In the elderly, phobic disorders can severely inhibit social interactions.

Posttraumatic stress disorder: In this disorder, an overwhelmingly traumatic event is reexperienced, causing intense fear, helplessness, horror, and avoidance of stimuli associated with the trauma. The stress may have occurred long ago; the adverse effect of severe stress during childhood or young adulthood on late-life psychologic functioning has long been recognized. Psychologic trauma may also occur in late life, although the incidence of new-onset posttraumatic stress disorder among the elderly is low.

Generalized anxiety disorder: This disorder is characterized by at least 6 months of almost daily anxiety and worry about activities or events. It affects up to 5% of community-dwelling elderly persons, making it one of the more common psychiatric problems among the elderly. Women are more likely than men to experience generalized anxiety disorder.

Obsessive-compulsive disorder: This disorder is characterized by recurrent, unwanted, intrusive ideas, images, or impulses that seem silly, weird, nasty, or horrible (obsessions) and by urges to do something that will lessen the discomfort of the obsessions (compulsions). It is common among the elderly, but the symptoms (eg, compulsive hand washing) are not usually prominent. Women are more likely than men to experience obsessive-compulsive disorder.

Panic disorder: This disorder is characterized by recurrent panic attacks (periods of intense fear or discomfort during which the onset of anxiety symptoms is abrupt). Symptoms typically begin in late adolescence or early adulthood and recede by later life. Thus, panic attacks in the elderly are rare and, when they occur, are usually less severe than those in younger adults.

Etiology

The root cause of most cases of phobic disorders and anxiety states is rarely identified. Posttraumatic stress disorder is easier to trace to an event; most cases are caused by trauma such as accidents, although sexual abuse can also be a cause.

In the elderly, several medical disorders and drugs (see TABLE 34–1) may cause anxiety or similar symptoms that can be easily mistaken for an anxiety disorder. Delirium often produces moderately severe anxiety and agitation, especially if the patient is in unfamiliar surroundings. Major depression may produce symptoms of anxiety and agitation, as

TABLE 34–1.   MEDICAL DISORDERS AND DRUGS THAT MAY CAUSE ANXIETY OR SIMILAR SYMPTOMS

Medical Disorder or Drug	Symptoms
Anticholinergic drugs	Memory impairment, producing secondary anxiety; with acute toxicity, a state similar to a panic attack
Caffeine	Anxiety
Cardiac arrhythmias	Palpitations, shortness of breath, anxiety
Delirium	Moderately severe anxiety and agitation, especially if the patient is in unfamiliar surroundings
Dementia	Anxiety, often with periodic panic attacks
Depression	Anxiety and agitation
Drug withdrawal (eg, alcohol, sedatives, hypnotics)	Anxiety
Hyperthyroidism	Agitation, anxiety, palpitations, eating disorders, confusion
Hypochondriasis	Moderately severe generalized anxiety, which is usually intermittent and less severe than that in other psychiatric disorders
Hypoglycemia	Intermittent anxiety with substantial physical manifestations
Over-the-counter sympathomimetic drugs (eg, ephedrine, pseudoephedrine, appetite suppressants, β-blockers)	Anxiety
Postural hypotension	Anxiety
Pulmonary edema	Shortness of breath, anxiety
Pulmonary emboli	Shortness of breath, anxiety

can hypochondriasis, although the anxiety that hypochondriasis produces is usually intermittent and less severe than that produced by other psychiatric disorders.

Dementia may be the most common cause of anxiety in the elderly. Early signs of cognitive impairment, including memory loss, in socially active persons often progress to generalized anxiety, with periodic panic attacks; the panic attacks, in turn, contribute to social withdrawal and isolation. The anxiety causes severe and traumatic behavioral changes, which frequently mask the underlying dementia.

Occasionally, anxiety reported by patients is due to a legitimate fear, such as fear of being mugged or fear of getting lost. In such cases, anxiety does not occur when situations that trigger these fears are avoided.

Symptoms, Signs, and Diagnosis

In generalized anxiety disorder, the anxiety is associated with at least three of the following symptoms: restlessness or edginess, easy fatigability, difficulty concentrating, irritability, muscle tension, and sleep disturbance. In elderly persons without cerebral disorders, the symptoms of generalized anxiety are similar to those in younger persons. Panic disorder often causes depressive symptoms or physical symptoms (eg, postural hypotension).

Agitation (the physical manifestation of hyperactivity) is important to differentiate from anxiety. Agitation without true anxiety often occurs in demented persons. Elderly persons who are agitated do not always experience the sense of impending doom and dread that characterizes anxiety. Elderly persons frequently report early-morning fear and anxiety that border on panic, especially if they awaken in the dark and other persons in the house are asleep. These symptoms tend to remit as the day progresses.

Psychologic testing is rarely of benefit for diagnosing anxiety disorders in the elderly, although such testing is frequently used for diagnosing dementing disorders[1] and mood disorders.[2]

Treatment

Successful management of anxiety disorders requires a good relationship between the patient and mental health provider. After accurate diagnosis, treatment may begin with one-on-one counseling and family support provided by a physician, mental health nurse, mental health social worker, or psychologist.[3] All potential organic causes should be corrected; drugs that may be contributing to the anxiety should be stopped if possible.

Appropriate intervention for coexisting psychiatric disorders may alleviate symptoms of anxiety. For example, an appropriate antidepres-

[1] see page 360   [2] see page 314   [3] see page 326

sant is usually sufficient to eliminate anxiety and agitation due to depression. Providing a more structured environment may alleviate anxiety in a patient with mild dementia.

Pharmacotherapy: An anxiolytic drug can be prescribed based on the suitability of the drug and, for a patient who is taking other drugs, on the possibility of drug-drug interactions. In general, elderly patients respond satisfactorily but not exceptionally to anxiolytic drugs. Most patients experience relief but not elimination of tension and agitation, and many symptoms persist.

For treating anxiety without depression, benzodiazepines are usually best. In general, elderly persons respond better to and experience fewer adverse effects from shorter-acting drugs (eg, alprazolam, lorazepam) than longer-acting drugs (eg, diazepam, chlordiazepoxide). However, ultra–short-acting benzodiazepines, such as triazolam, should generally not be used. The dosage of benzodiazepines for elderly patients is usually lower (eg, alprazolam 0.125 mg po bid or tid) than that for younger patients. Benzodiazepines are usually best prescribed on a fixed dosage schedule rather than as needed, although patients with occasional anxiety may use the drugs intermittently.

Benzodiazepines are likely to cause sedation and may impair the ability to drive◻ or safely perform physically demanding tasks. Ataxia, slurred speech, impaired coordination, confusion, poor concentration, memory loss, sleep disturbances, and depressive symptoms may occur. Patients should be monitored closely for adverse effects. If adverse effects occur, the dose must be reduced or the drug stopped, even if a patient must be hospitalized to effect withdrawal. Rarely, an elderly patient has a paradoxical reaction to benzodiazepines and becomes more agitated and anxious. Occasionally, short-acting benzodiazepines produce a rebound anxiety effect before the next dose is given. In such cases, a longer-acting drug may be preferred.

Often benzodiazepines are needed for only a limited time (eg, up to 4 to 6 weeks). In such cases, discontinuing the drugs is easier if prescribers clarify from the outset that treatment is for only a brief period.

After continuous use for an extended time, benzodiazepines are difficult to discontinue for psychologic and physical reasons. Nevertheless, periodic efforts should be made to discontinue the drug or at least to reduce the dose. Results are best if the drug is discontinued over 3 to 4 weeks, during which the dose is very gradually tapered every few days.

Buspirone is an alternative to the benzodiazepines. The initial dose is 5 mg bid. Divided doses of 10 mg bid or tid are commonly given. Buspirone is less likely than the benzodiazepines to be addictive and, perhaps because of the sedative effect, may be tolerated by elderly persons who cannot tolerate benzodiazepines. However, buspirone does not

◻ see page 236

effect subjective improvement as quickly as the benzodiazepines do; its anxiolytic effect usually occurs after about 2 weeks of continuous therapy. Persons who have responded to benzodiazepines in the past usually do not respond to buspirone.

Antipsychotic drugs (neuroleptics) should not be prescribed for generalized anxiety disorder, except when symptoms are secondary to delusions or other signs of psychosis. Such drugs may produce adverse effects (eg, tremulousness, restlessness, agitation, especially akathisia) that can complicate the management of generalized anxiety. One of the most serious adverse effects is tardive dyskinesia, which is often irreversible.

Tricyclic antidepressants (eg, imipramine 75 mg po at bedtime, nortriptyline 75 mg po at bedtime) are the best choice for initial treatment of panic disorder. If these drugs are ineffective, alprazolam may be prescribed; although the minimal effective dose is usually 0.5 mg po tid, the physician should initially give 0.25 mg po tid to determine if adverse effects will be problematic.

Nonpharmacologic measures: Psychotherapy sometimes alleviates anxiety. Intensive psychotherapy is not as successful as might be hoped, and psychoanalysis has little to recommend it. Short-term insight-oriented therapy, however, may be of some benefit, particularly for an elderly patient with anxiety secondary to bereavement. Short-term psychotherapy may also be of some benefit for a patient with posttraumatic stress disorder.

Supportive psychotherapy may be an important adjunct for treating isolated and physically impaired elderly patients with generalized anxiety disorder. Behavioral therapy may be indicated for anxiety associated with a phobic or panic disorder.

Biofeedback may enable elderly patients to develop some control over symptoms of anxiety. Patients must be able to concentrate on the procedure. Other patients may benefit from relaxation therapy. A paced exercise program can be especially helpful to patients sensing a loss of control over other areas of life.

Interdisciplinary Care Issues

Elderly persons with anxiety disorders, which commonly occur with comorbid physical illness, are much more likely to present to nonphysician health care practitioners in the managed care environment and in long-term care facilities than to physicians. Thus, professionals from multiple disciplines should be aware of the symptoms of anxiety disorders, especially generalized anxiety disorder and panic disorder.

Nurses frequently encounter elderly patients with anxiety disorders in long-term care facilities. Patients initially transferred from the hospital or from home are at increased risk for anxiety, especially mild to moderate symptoms, which may not be reported to a physician. In these cases, brief supportive psychotherapy, which is informative and nondirective, can be beneficial.

Social workers frequently encounter elderly patients with anxiety disorders in mental health centers, although the elderly are less likely than other age groups to use these centers. Such patients usually present with a psychotic disorder or serious mood disorder, frequently with comorbid anxiety. Social workers can provide supportive therapy to the patient and to family members, who may be concerned as to how to manage the patient. Such therapy may be especially beneficial for patients with panic disorder, in whom symptoms can be severe for short periods.

Social workers or psychologists are most likely to provide psychotherapy to elderly persons with anxiety disorders. They usually collaborate with physicians, who can prescribe drugs. Such interdisciplinary care is most effective if it is well coordinated; active ongoing communication between the social worker or psychologist and the physician is essential. For example, for elderly patients in whom psychotherapy has led to increased anxiety, an increase in drug dosages may not be the best short-term approach.

35 ■ SOMATOFORM DISORDERS

A group of psychiatric disorders characterized by physical symptoms that suggest but are not fully explained by a physical disorder, by the direct effects of a psychiatric disorder, or by drug abuse.

The physical symptoms are distressing enough to make the patient seek medical care and to impair social, occupational, or other areas of functioning. A number of somatoform disorders are included in the *Diagnostic and Statistical Manual of Mental Disorders, Fourth Edition (DSM-IV),* but three are relevant to the elderly: somatization disorder, undifferentiated somatoform disorder, and hypochondriasis.

Somatization disorder, a chronic condition, is rare among the elderly, although it is somewhat more common among women (0.2 to 1.0%) than among men (< 0.2%). Diagnosis requires an extensive history of many physical symptoms without objective findings beginning at least by the age of 30. The patient must complain of symptoms in at least four categories: pain symptoms in at least four different locations (eg, the head, abdomen, back, extremities), at least two gastrointestinal symptoms (eg, nausea, vomiting, diarrhea), at least one sexual or reproductive symptom (eg, erectile dysfunction), and at least one neurologic symptom (eg, impaired coordination, paralysis, difficulty swallowing).

Undifferentiated somatoform disorder, a less severe form of somatization, occurs more often, affecting 3 to 5% of elderly persons. The central feature is one or more physical symptoms without objective findings that persist for ≥ 6 months. The symptoms are fewer and need not fall into the four categories noted above; however, they must cause significant distress or functional impairment for the diagnosis to be made. The most common symptoms are chronic fatigue, loss of appetite, abdominal pain, and genitourinary symptoms.

Hypochondriasis is the preoccupation with the fear of having or the idea that the patient has a serious disease. This concern is based on the elderly person's misinterpretation of normal bodily processes or functions. Although the specific symptoms may vary over time, hypochondriacal concerns last for at least 6 months despite appropriate medical evaluation and assurance. Elderly patients with hypochondriasis may also have one or more medical disorders, but these do not explain the nature or the severity of the reported symptoms.

Differential Diagnosis

Despite significant similarities among the somatoform disorders, differentiation is usually straightforward. Somatization disorder and undifferentiated somatoform disorder differ in the number and types of symptoms and severity. Somatization disorder is characterized by multiple symptoms, whereas somatic pain disorder is focused on pain, usually in one location. Hypochondriasis is distinguished by preoccupation with the underlying cause of the symptoms.

The somatoform disorders must be distinguished from a conscious or intentional attempt to appear physically ill, such as occurs in factitious disorder or malingering. In factitious disorder, which is extremely rare in the elderly, the conscious motivation is to assume the sick role and therefore obtain medical evaluation and treatment. In malingering, which is more common, external gain is experienced by rewards associated with remaining ill, such as financial compensation or avoidance of duty.

Medical disorders are ruled out on the basis of the history, physical examination, and laboratory testing. Although extensive testing should be avoided, the physician must remember that the patient presenting with a somatoform disorder also may develop a serious medical disorder. Depression is ruled out by the chronicity of the somatic symptoms and the absence of depressive symptoms (eg, hopelessness, agitation, confusion).

Treatment

The goal of treatment is to improve the patient's quality of life and to control the use of medical services. Treatment for the three somatoform disorders described above is similar. First, a physician seeks to rule out the possibility of a physical disorder while emphasizing to the patient that making a specific diagnosis is difficult and expressing a willingness to work with the patient despite the complexity involved. For somatization disorder, drugs are largely ineffective, and even if a patient agrees to a psychiatric consultation, psychotherapy is rarely beneficial. Usually, the best treatment is a calm, firm, supportive relationship with a physician who offers symptomatic relief and protects the patient from aggressive diagnostic or therapeutic procedures.

Most patients desire some type of drug, and the selection must be made with care. For example, patients who have difficulty sleeping along with other symptoms may respond positively to occasional use of a mild hypnotic drug. Drugs likely to produce adverse effects, such as tricyclic antidepressants, are to be avoided, as are drugs that can lead to addiction. The prescription of a placebo, if discovered by the patient, usually damages the physician-patient relationship.

Once the diagnosis has been made, the patient should be examined on a regular basis for 4 to 6 weeks. After that, the time between appointments usually can be lengthened. Each appointment with the patient should last a specified period of time, usually 10 to 15 minutes; this limit should be explained to the patient at the beginning of treatment. The physician should terminate the appointment on time, even if the patient communicates what appears to be important information at the end. The patient should be encouraged to discuss concerns only during the scheduled appointment; phone calls and other methods of seeking additional attention should be discouraged.

It is best to avoid commenting positively or negatively about physicians who have treated the somatoform disorder previously. Although defending or criticizing treatment by another physician may be tempting, it is best to focus the patient's attention on the present and on discussing factors other than the physical symptoms.

36 ■ PSYCHOTIC DISORDERS

Suspiciousness, persecutory delusions, and paranoid delusions occur often in cognitively impaired or emotionally distressed elderly persons. Between 2 and 5% of elderly persons living in the community exhibit excessive suspiciousness and persecutory delusions. As many as 4 to 5% have delusions and hallucinations, and these symptoms are often disabling. However, the prevalence of schizophrenia, as defined by the *Diagnostic and Statistical Manual of Mental Disorders, Fourth Edition (DSM-IV)*, is < 1% in the elderly. True schizophrenia begins in adolescence or early adulthood and may persist into late life. Late-onset schizophrenia is called paraphrenia. Identifying psychotic behavior in patients with behavior disorders is discussed in Ch. 41.

Investigators and clinicians generally agree on six relatively distinct clinical entities: abnormal suspiciousness; transitional paranoid reactions; late-life paraphrenia (severe paranoid illness without deterioration of other cognitive or affective processes) or paranoia associated with late-onset schizophrenia; persistence of early-onset schizophrenia; acute paranoid reactions secondary to affective illness; and transient psychoses due to neurologic, toxic-metabolic, or systemic disorders.

Symptoms, Signs, and Diagnosis

Abnormal suspiciousness: Most elderly persons who exhibit abnormal suspiciousness do not have contact with mental health practitioners. However, they often have medical disorders and are seen by a primary care physician or a geriatrician. These patients may have vague complaints of external forces controlling their lives. Occasionally, these beliefs become focal, often directed at their children; eg, they believe their children have deserted them or have plotted to obtain control of their finances or property. Perception of a loss of control, coupled with an inability to evaluate the social milieu, favors the development of abnormal suspiciousness.

Physicians may also encounter suspiciousness associated with dementia and attention deficits. Institutionalized patients with dementia are often suspicious of family and staff members; psychosis due to dementia is, however, uncommon. Their accusations are usually disjointed, unfocused, and unaccompanied by sustained emotional distress. Common complaints concern objects being stolen, medicines being swapped, and attendants misbehaving. Symptoms derive from the patient's inability to organize environmental stimuli and comprehend the often confusing activities of the institution. It is unknown whether an underlying paranoid personality contributes to excessive paranoid behavior in persons with dementia. However, physicians must keep in mind that elderly patients, especially those with dementia, at times are mistreated in long-term care facilities and in hospitals and that suspiciousness may be grounded in fact.

Transitional paranoid reactions: These reactions usually occur in women who live alone; they believe that someone is plotting against them. Social isolation and perceptional difficulties contribute to these reactions. The focus of hallucinations and delusional thinking usually moves gradually from outside the home to inside it, eg, from complaints of noises in the basement and attic to reports of physical abuse or molestation. Hence, a transition can be observed from external threats to violations of property and person.

Paraphrenia: Paraphrenia is not universally accepted as a distinct syndrome. Persons who distinguish the syndrome emphasize that it is primary rather than secondary to an affective illness or to an organic mental disorder. In addition, the gross disturbances of affect, volition, and function characterizing schizophrenia are not prominent. Nevertheless, paranoid delusions and hallucinations almost always occur. Paraphrenia may be chronic, but deterioration to the extent observed in schizophrenia or Alzheimer's disease is not characteristic. The boundaries blur not only between paraphrenia and classic paranoid schizophrenia but also between the transitional paranoid state and paraphrenia.

Patients with paraphrenia often report plots against them, focusing on family members. In contrast with mild suspiciousness, these plots are persistent, extreme, and elaborate. Usually, cognitive impairment is not present. Although the patient is physically independent (ie, diet and hygiene are rarely compromised), social functioning and cooperation with staff members are greatly impaired. Such persons rarely speak for long without referring to the symptoms of concern.

Patients with paraphrenia usually are female, live alone, and have evidence of difficult social interactions earlier in life. In contrast with schizophrenia, these patients are friendly and trusting, especially when they are interviewed in their homes and are not threatened with the diagnosis of a mental disorder. Patients with paraphrenia tend to have a hearing impairment, but the relationship between paraphrenia and hearing impairment is not nearly as strong as some authorities contend.

Early-onset schizophrenia: The symptoms include two or more of the following, each present for most of the time for at least 1 month: delusion, hallucination, disorganized speech, grossly disorganized or catatonic behavior, and negative symptoms (eg, flattening of affect). Overall, the symptoms must be present for at least 6 months and significantly interfere with social and occupational functioning. Typically, the symptoms become less acute, yet social functioning continues to deteriorate gradually over time. Acute paranoid thinking may accompany an episode of major depression◻ or acute mania. Treating the mood disorder usually eliminates the paranoid thinking in these patients and therefore rules out the diagnosis of schizophrenia.

Elderly persons who have been treated for schizophrenia for years are likely to have adverse effects of antipsychotic drugs (eg, tardive dyskinesia).

Psychotic disorders due to neurologic, toxic-metabolic, or systemic disorders: These include suspiciousness and agitation due to drug intoxication, physical illness, and postoperative psychosis (eg, psychosis occurring among patients in intensive care units). Visual hallucinations occur more often (as in delirium), yet the psychosis may be organized and elaborate (unlike delirium). These disorders are usually transient and resolve with treatment of the underlying cause or spontaneously. In the midst of the disorder, however, acute management is necessary.

◻ see also page 312

Treatment

Nonpharmacologic measures: Health care practitioners (physicians, psychiatric nurses, and mental health social workers) caring for the elderly patient with a psychotic disorder must establish a trusting and supportive relationship. Displays of respect, a willingness to listen to complaints and fears, and availability by telephone are essential. Most elderly patients do not abuse telephone privileges and are generally willing to wait for the physician to return a call.

Health care practitioners should not—at least initially—confront the patient about the lack of reason and false assumptions inherent in paranoid ideation. Such a confrontation is of no value and may disrupt the therapeutic relationship. However, the health care practitioner must not deceive the patient by pretending to agree with paranoid beliefs. Rather, an interest should be expressed in wanting to understand what is troubling the patient and in working together despite a disagreement over the source of the problem. A desirable goal is to develop a level of confidence that allows for an examination of the patient's beliefs.

The health care practitioner must also establish a relationship with key persons in the patient's social environment. Family members are often the first to notice a deterioration in the patient's condition and, therefore, the first to contact the physician when a problem arises. Police officers, neighbors, and pharmacists also can serve as valuable allies. By understanding the patient's situation and recognizing deterioration in status, these persons can contact the physician or family members when appropriate and not overreact. However, health care practitioners must maintain standards of privilege and confidentiality when talking to family members, neighbors, and friends.

Pharmacotherapy: For most patients with psychotic disorders, effective management also requires antipsychotic drugs. The new, atypical antipsychotic drugs (eg, risperidone, olanzapine) are preferred for the agitated or suspicious elderly patient primarily because these drugs have fewer adverse effects (including fewer extrapyramidal adverse effects) compared with conventional antipsychotics (eg, haloperidol, thioridazine). Initial daily oral dosages (in divided doses) are 1 mg of risperidone, 5 mg of olanzapine, 1 to 3 mg of haloperidol, and 10 to 25 mg of thioridazine. Daily doses may be increased significantly (eg, risperidone 5 to 10 mg); however, except in the most acute cases, the lower doses usually suffice. The drugs may be given once daily (at bedtime) in less severe cases.

Choice of drug is usually determined by the adverse effects the physician wishes to avoid. Risperidone is somewhat sedating, has very few anticholinergic effects, but leads to moderate orthostatic hypotension. Olanzapine is as sedating as risperidone, has somewhat more anticholinergic effects, but is less likely to lead to orthostatic hypotension. In contrast, thioridazine is especially troublesome for patients with postural hypotension, and haloperidol may cause significant parkinsonian symptoms. In treatment-resistant patients and in those with severe psychosis, clozapine is a possible choice. There has been little cumulative experience with clozapine in the elderly, although evidence indicates a higher incidence of agranulocytosis.

Most elderly patients are willing to take an antipsychotic drug if they are told that the drug will also help improve sleep and alleviate anxiety. Compliance is often problematic but less so in later life than earlier. Even paranoid persons usually trust their physicians and are willing to comply with therapy. If the elderly patient objects, family members may be able to help. A strong objection to drugs or other interventions may suggest the need for hospitalization if symptoms are severe.

Some elderly patients who have had long-standing schizophrenia may no longer need antipsychotic treatment. At least one trial of discontinuation should be attempted but only when close supervision is possible.

37 ■ SUBSTANCE ABUSE AND DEPENDENCE

ALCOHOL ABUSE AND DEPENDENCE

The use of alcohol to such an extent that it causes physical or psychosocial harm. Physiologic dependence implies tolerance (ie, increasing amounts are needed to get the same effect) and withdrawal symptoms when consumption ceases.

Between 2 and 10% of the community-dwelling elderly meet the criteria for alcohol abuse or dependence. In addition, drinking behavior that falls short of a formal diagnosis of alcoholism causes considerable morbidity and mortality among the elderly.

Epidemiology

About 50% of persons $\geq$ 65 years report using alcohol at least occasionally; however, persons > 75 are less likely than younger adults to drink alcohol or to be alcoholic.

There is considerable geographic variation in alcohol consumption among the elderly. For example, in east Boston, 70% of elderly persons surveyed reported drinking alcohol within 1 year; 8.4% reported consuming two or more drinks per day. In contrast, in rural Iowa, only 46% reported drinking alcohol within 1 year; 5.4% reported consuming two or more drinks per day.

The prevalence of alcoholism is higher among elderly persons in health care settings than among the general elderly population: 4 to 10% among patients seen by primary care physicians (an additional 10 to 15% of these patients drink heavily but are not considered alcoholics), 14% among emergency department patients, 10 to 21% among hospital inpatients, and 3 to 49% among nursing home residents. The rate of alcohol-related hospitalizations among the elderly is high; it is slightly higher than that for myocardial infarction.

Populations with a large proportion of chronically ill or disabled persons usually have lower rates of alcohol consumption, although these populations include some persons whose illness or disability has been caused by heavy alcohol consumption. Social interaction may also affect alcohol use; retirement community residents with more active social lives are more likely to drink heavily than those who socialize less.

In up to one third of elderly alcoholics in treatment programs, problem drinking is of relatively recent onset. These late-onset alcoholics often have more intact social resources than their long-term counterparts and may have started drinking because of age-related losses and stresses.

The prevalence of heavy drinking and alcoholism declines after age 65 for several reasons:

- The current elderly population has lower lifelong drinking habits than its predecessors.

- The female-to-male population ratio increases with age, and women are less likely to consume alcohol.

- Declining health or functional impairments, which accompany aging, often lead to a decrease in alcohol intake.

- Alcohol-related illnesses and injuries prevent many alcoholics from surviving to old age.

Physiology

Elderly persons develop higher blood alcohol levels per amount consumed because of age-related changes that alter the absorption and distribution of alcohol, the most important of which are increased body fat and decreased lean body mass and total body water. There may be an age-related decrease in the activity of gastric alcohol dehydrogenase. It is unclear whether this age-related decrease occurs in women, but women have a lower level of gastric alcohol dehydrogenase activity than men.

Most alcohol is metabolized in the liver by alcohol dehydrogenase. The liver's ability to metabolize alcohol declines with age, but this change is not clinically important. Although renal function usually declines with age as well, < 5% of ethanol is excreted renally. Susceptibility to psychomotor effects of alcohol may increase with age.

Pathophysiology

Although light to moderate drinking is associated with better health (especially less cardiovascular disease), consuming more than two drinks per day increases the risk of adverse effects, including hypertension, cancer (particularly of the head, neck, and esophagus), and cirrhosis. For the elderly, who have higher blood alcohol levels per amount consumed, the National Institute on Alcohol Abuse and Alcoholism recommends a limit of one drink per day. Alcoholism is commonly accompanied by nutritional deficiencies, particularly deficiencies of thiamine, folate, pyridoxine, niacin, and vitamin A.∎ Thiamine deficiency can lead to Wernicke's encephalopathy and Korsakoff's syndrome. Other deficiencies, such as hypomagnesemia, hypocalcemia, and hypokalemia, may be important in acute intoxication or withdrawal.

Elderly persons who drink heavily are particularly susceptible to declines in cognitive and physical functioning, although the amount of alcohol required to produce such declines is unknown. The pattern of alcohol use is also important in determining the risk of illness or injury; for example, the number of drinks consumed per occasion is an important risk factor for death from injury, whereas the frequency of such drinking occasions is not.

Many drugs used commonly by the elderly interact adversely with alcohol. Cimetidine, ranitidine, and nizatidine inhibit gastric alcohol dehydrogenase, thereby increasing blood alcohol levels by 30 to 40%. The increased alcohol levels may cause somnolence, imbalance, and delirium. Alcohol taken with drugs that suppress central nervous system function (eg, benzodiazepines) may impair balance and predispose to falls, cause somnolence, and slow reaction time, which may contribute to automobile accidents. Nonsteroidal anti-inflammatory drugs, when taken with alcohol, prolong bleeding time and increase gastric inflammation. Determining correct warfarin dosing can be difficult when a patient is drinking variable amounts of alcohol because of varying rates of metabolism in the liver. Acetaminophen combined with alcohol may lead to liver failure; because the amount required to cause harm is highly individual, people who take acetaminophen daily are advised to abstain from alcohol use.

Symptoms and Signs

Some important symptoms of alcoholism may manifest atypically in the elderly, making the diagnosis challenging. Elderly drinkers are less likely to consume extremely large quantities, because fewer drinks are needed to raise their blood alcohol levels. In addition, loss of control of drinking may be more subtle.

Social decline may present differently in the elderly. Because elderly persons are less likely to be working or driving, they are less likely to be

∎ see TABLE 60–1 on page 589

TABLE 37–1.   AGE-RELATED DISORDERS CAUSED OR EXACERBATED BY ALCOHOLISM OR HEAVY DRINKING

- Urinary incontinence as a result of rapid bladder filling and loss of neuromuscular control of bladder function (alcohol inhibits antidiuretic hormone secretion and affects neuromuscular control)

- Gait disturbances resulting from alcohol-induced cerebellar degeneration, peripheral neuropathy, or acute intoxication

- Depression and suicide

- Sleep disturbances and insomnia

- Dementia or delirium

recognized as alcoholics by employers or the police. Social decline may therefore manifest as poor self-care, malnutrition, failure to thrive, or withdrawal from activities.

Alcoholic elderly persons may present with such medical complications as hypertension or diabetes that is difficult to control, frequent gastrointestinal disturbances, peripheral neuropathy, or unexplained seizures, or with problems related to dose adjustment of drugs such as warfarin and phenytoin. Alcohol-related trauma, however, is less common among elderly alcoholics than among younger alcoholics. Alcoholism or heavy drinking may cause or exacerbate age-related disorders (ie, geriatric syndromes—see TABLE 37–1).

Withdrawal symptoms are similar in elderly and younger patients but are often mistaken for other medical conditions in the elderly. Early symptoms of withdrawal, such as tremulousness, tachycardia, and tachypnea, as well as later symptoms, such as delirium, seizures, and hallucinations, are sometimes attributed to other causes.

Laboratory findings: There is no specific laboratory test for alcoholism. Elevated γ-glutamyltransferase, which indicates induction of liver enzymes, and elevated mean corpuscular volume may suggest alcoholism, although these levels are also commonly elevated in the nonalcoholic elderly. A blood alcohol level > 100 mg/dL (> 21.7 mmol/L) without signs of intoxication is a good indication of tolerance to alcohol and usually signifies alcoholism.

Screening and Diagnosis

One of the most useful screening instruments is the CAGE questionnaire, which asks the following:

- Have you ever felt you should *c*ut down on your drinking?

- Does criticism of your drinking *a*nnoy you?

- Have you ever felt *g*uilty about drinking?

- Have you ever had an "*e*ye opener" (a drink first thing in the morning) to steady your nerves or to get rid of a hangover?

Two or more affirmative answers to these questions indicate a probable diagnosis of alcoholism. However, many persons who are not dependent on alcohol drink heavily enough to cause medical complications; these heavy drinkers are unlikely to be detected by the CAGE questions. Therefore, questions regarding the quantity and frequency of alcohol use should be asked in addition to the CAGE questions. The National Institute on Alcohol Abuse and Alcoholism recommends asking the following three questions:

- On average, how many days per week do you drink alcohol?
- On a typical day when you drink, how many drinks do you have?
- What is the maximum number of drinks you had on any given occasion in the past month?

Questions that specify the type of alcoholic beverage sometimes improve reporting. Also, patients may define "a drink" in various ways, so specifying the quantity of alcohol meant may be necessary. Men who consume more than two drinks per day, women who consume more than one drink per day, and anyone who consumes more than four drinks per occasion are at risk of adverse consequences.

Further questioning should focus on symptoms of alcoholism and on alcohol-related issues (eg, loss of control of drinking, tolerance to alcohol, history of withdrawal symptoms, previous treatment for alcoholism) as well as on adverse effects of drinking (eg, family disturbances, citations for driving while intoxicated, alcohol-related illness or injury). Often, a trusting relationship with the physician must be developed slowly before patients will openly discuss alcohol misuse.

The patient is usually the most reliable source of a drinking history. However, cognitive impairment (common among elderly alcoholics) and denial can impede this process. In such cases, family members, close friends, or caregivers can provide the pertinent history. Information from others can also be very helpful when an alcoholic denies problem drinking, although family members sometimes help the alcoholic avoid detection.

Treatment

Counseling: Even brief counseling by the primary care physician can greatly reduce alcohol consumption. Educational materials to assist with brief intervention are available from the National Institute on Alcohol Abuse and Alcoholism. Essential elements of counseling include informing the patient of the adverse effects of drinking and setting limits on drinking. For persons with severe abuse or dependence, abstinence should be the goal, and formal treatment is often necessary.

Many heavy drinkers do not realize that their drinking is excessive and that it is endangering their health. They are often helped by seeing test results that confirm the adverse consequences of their drinking (eg, elevated liver function test results). Keeping a diary of alcohol consumption is also helpful for many patients. Strategies for coping with the desire to drink should be discussed. If coexisting medical and psychosocial problems may be contributing to the perceived need for alcohol, more effective coping strategies should be suggested or referrals for more lengthy counseling made. For example, chronic pain may lead to increased alcohol use, and effective pain management may lower alcohol intake.[1]

Structured programs: Programs designed specifically for the elderly are rare. Such programs are adapted to medical, cognitive, and psychiatric disorders as well as to social issues common in the elderly (eg, coping with retirement). However, elderly patients in mixed-age programs appear to have the same rate of success as their younger counterparts. About 50% remain abstinent 1 year after treatment. After completing a structured treatment program or in lieu of it, many elderly alcoholics are greatly helped by Alcoholics Anonymous and other nonprofessional treatment programs.

Alcoholics with dementia rarely can maintain abstinence unless their access to alcohol is restricted. Because cognitive impairment may lessen only after several months, a long-term alcohol-free residential program is recommended. However, such programs are uncommon, and nursing home placement is often the only alternative.

Pharmacotherapy: Because alcohol withdrawal predisposes the elderly to medical complications (eg, delirium) and because the elderly may take longer to recover than younger patients, hospitalization during this period is recommended. Short-acting benzodiazepines (eg, lorazepam, oxazepam) are the safest and most effective drugs for ameliorating symptoms of alcohol withdrawal, including minor withdrawal symptoms, such as tremulousness and tachycardia. If seizures, delirium, or other serious withdrawal complications occur or if there is a history of these symptoms during previous alcohol withdrawal, scheduled doses of a benzodiazepine, followed by dosage tapering, are indicated. For all patients experiencing alcohol withdrawal, thiamine 100 mg IM daily for 3 days, then 100 mg po daily, should be administered prophylactically to prevent Wernicke's encephalopathy. A thorough medical evaluation is essential, because nutritional deficiencies,[2] fluid and electrolyte imbalances,[3] and concurrent medical disorders are very common.

Antipsychotic drugs lessen delirium but may increase the risk of seizures during withdrawal. Although magnesium deficiency may con-

[1] see page 387   [2] see page 588   [3] see page 561

tribute to hypertension or seizures during withdrawal, studies do not support the routine use of magnesium sulfate in treating withdrawal symptoms.

Naltrexone, an opiate antagonist, decreases the craving for alcohol. It can reduce relapse rates by 50% when combined with psychosocial intervention. The usual dose of 50 mg/day is well tolerated by most elderly patients. The most common adverse effects are nausea (occurring in 10 to 15% of patients) and headache (occurring in 7%). Disulfiram, which produces unpleasant effects when alcohol is consumed concurrently, is less effective than naltrexone and may cause hypotension in elderly patients, especially in patients with underlying heart disease. Acamprosate, an anticraving drug used in Europe, appears promising and will probably soon be available in the USA.

Palliation: If the patient cannot stop drinking, disease management includes lengthening the periods of abstinence, maximizing function, and minimizing suffering. Continued counseling about the benefits of decreasing alcohol intake, although perhaps not immediately effective, often has long-term benefit. When combined with nursing assessment and care coordination as well as attention to social problems addressed by a social worker, such treatment may lower mortality rates from alcoholism and improve quality of life.

Nursing Issues

The fields of substance abuse and geriatrics both have recognized the benefits of a team approach to care. Nurses are indispensable in every phase of detection and management of substance abuse and dependence among the elderly. Because nurses often spend more time with patients than do physicians, they have a greater opportunity to identify problems with alcohol and other drugs. Home care nurses can observe patients in their homes, where signs of substance abuse may be more evident than in formal medical settings. In geriatric medical settings, nurses often do extensive assessment of physical and cognitive functioning, during which sequelae of substance abuse, such as gait problems or cognitive impairment, may be detected. The same questions recommended for screening are also useful in the realm of nursing, although more subtle clues to substance abuse, such as poor self-care or loss of interest in other activities, may also be valuable. Educating patients and families about adverse effects of the substance use and benefits of cessation as well as offering support through the intervention process is essential.

Nurses are often involved in initiating treatment as well as in the treatment process itself and in aftercare. It is difficult for people to acknowledge their addiction and enter treatment, and emotional support during this phase can make or break the success of treatment. Nurses may be the first to notice signs of withdrawal and work with physicians to manage it. They are often involved in counseling during the active treatment phase. Nurse-managed aftercare programs have been shown to decrease the risk of relapse after active treatment.

Patient and Caregiver Issues

Family members and caregivers as well as patients are often unaware of the adverse effects of heavy drinking. In addition, loved ones may not wish to interfere with drinking if it seems to please the elderly person. Teaching family members and caregivers about the harmful effects of drinking (eg, dementia, incontinence, depression, gait disturbances) and the benefits of abstinence can be helpful. Possible interactions between alcohol and prescription drugs should be discussed.

End-of-Life Issues

Alcoholism can be a terminal disease, in which case physicians, nurses, and social workers can help with concerns about dying❶, getting affairs in order, and making decisions about medical interventions under various circumstances.❷

OTHER SUBSTANCE ABUSE AND DEPENDENCE

Use of **illegal drugs** is uncommon among elderly people, although this may change as the baby boom generation ages. Adverse effects of prescription and over-the-counter drugs, on the other hand, occur quite often. Alcoholics are particularly at risk of misuse of other psychoactive drugs. Benzodiazepines and opiates are the categories of drugs most likely to cause trouble in the elderly.

Up to 20% of older people use **benzodiazepines.** Whereas alcohol use and abuse are more common among men, benzodiazepine use is more common among women. Surveys suggest that most people for whom these drugs are prescribed usually take them either as directed or less than as directed. Even when benzodiazepines are taken as directed, tolerance, dependence, adverse effects, and toxicity may develop. Long-acting benzodiazepines have been shown to markedly increase the risk of falls and hip fracture. Because the half-lives of some benzodiazepines are extremely long in the elderly, the drug gradually accumulates in the body, producing a toxic state. High blood levels of benzodiazepines commonly cause such symptoms as slurred speech, ataxia, and delirium.

❶ see page 115   ❷ see page 134

There are very few studies of **opiate abuse** and dependence among the elderly. Intentional misuse of opiates is probably uncommon, but adverse effects of prescribed doses, such as constipation, urinary retention, delirium, and falling, are often problematic.

Tobacco dependence is the only substance-related disorder more common among the elderly than alcoholism. Tobacco-related illnesses cause tremendous suffering, and the benefits of smoking cessation have been documented. Physician counseling is very effective in helping people quit smoking and should be done at every opportunity.

SECTION 5

DELIRIUM AND DEMENTIA

DEL/
DEM

38   MENTAL STATUS EXAMINATION

Part of the physical examination that assesses current mental capacity through evaluation of appearance, mood, anxiety disorders, perceptions (eg, delusions, hallucinations), and all aspects of cognition (eg, attention, orientation, memory).

Problems with mental status can be suggested by the medical history (by both its content and its manner of delivery by the patient); however, determination and documentation of current mental status require a mental status examination. Identification of the underlying cause of abnormal mental status requires integrating all information from the history, the mental status examination, other components of the physical examination,▯ and laboratory tests.

Mental status examination begins with the clinical assessment of the patient and is followed by use of one or more quantitative assessment instruments (see TABLE 38–1), the most widely used being the Annotated Mini-Mental State Examination (see FIGURE 38–1). Quantitative assessment instruments can be used in screening for cognitive and related disorders and in assessing response to treatment. Serial quantitative measurements of cognition should be considered for any elderly patient suspected of experiencing delirium or progressive changes in cognition.

Mental status examinations can help a court establish a person's legal competence for making a will or for giving informed consent for procedures.▯ When combined with functional assessment, these examinations help the physician select an appropriate environment and level of care for a patient after hospital discharge.

CLINICAL ASSESSMENT

Mental status examination should be performed, to some extent, in all patients, even if only to document that no problem exists. The examiner should explain to the patient the need for a mental status examination and request the patient's consent and cooperation. For example, the examiner can say, "I would like to ask you some questions about your feelings, your thinking, and your memory as a routine part of the examination. Is that all right with you?"

At the outset, the examiner should determine whether the patient can hear, see, and attend because impairments can worsen orientation and other cognitive functions. Impairments should be noted in the interpretation of the mental state. Refusal to respond or cooperate is often a sign that the patient is attempting to hide an impairment.

The examiner's questions and responses to the patient's answers should be sympathetic but direct. Each time a patient cannot answer a question, the examiner should move to the next question. Incorrect responses should not be pointed out or corrected. This approach avoids having the patient respond emotionally to the failure, which can worsen cognitive performance.

Appearance

Inappropriate or unkempt clothing and poor grooming may indicate neglect or inability to dress, perhaps because of apraxia (inability to

---

▯ see also page 31   ▯ see page 130

TABLE 38-1.   SELECTED INSTRUMENTS FOR QUANTITATIVE ASSESSMENT OF MENTAL STATUS

Instrument	Purpose
Annotated Mini-Mental State Examination (MMSE)	To assess cognitive function in a face-to-face interview
Confusion Assessment Method (CAM)	To assess delirium, even in the presence of dementia (see TABLE 39–4)
Telephone Interview for Cognitive Status (TICS)	To assess cognitive function in a telephone interview (based on MMSE)
Cornell Scale for Depression in Dementia	To assess behavior problems
Dementia Symptoms Scale	To assess behavior problems
Psychogeriatric Dependency Rating Scale	To assess behavior problems
Hopkins Competency Assessment Test	To assess the ability to make decisions about medical care
General Health Questionnaire	To assess emotional distress, including depression and anxiety, in patients with normal cognition
Hamilton Depression Rating Scale	To assess depression in patients with cognitive impairment (see TABLE 33–5)

perform learned motor acts despite the physical ability and willingness to do so). The use of hearing aids or glasses is noted.

Mood

Abnormalities of mood (eg, mania, depression) can affect cognitive function and must be thoroughly evaluated. Depression is particularly problematic because it can cause dementia, in which case it may be referred to as dementia of depression or pseudodementia. Patients with this condition improve after their depression is treated. In other cases, depression aggravates dementia, making subtle dementia overt or mild dementia more severe.

Mood is evaluated by observation of the patient (eg, facial expressions, posture, speed of movements and thoughts) and of verbal content. Although patients often spontaneously express feelings of helplessness, hopelessness, worthlessness, shame, or guilt, they should be asked directly about such feelings (eg, "Do you feel that you are a good person?" "Do you feel guilty about things you have done?") and about mood (eg, "How are your spirits?" or "How is your mood?"). Questions such as "How does the future look?" and "Do you feel you have unusual talents or abilities?" may detect excessive optimism or overconfidence. The patient should be asked about changes in energy, appetite, or sleep that are related to mood disturbances.

	Score	Points			Score	Points

Orientation
What is the
Year? _____ 1
Season? _____ 1
Date? _____ 1
Day? _____ 1
Month? _____ 1

Where are we
County/Neighborhood? _____ 1
State? _____ 1
Town/city? _____ 1
Name/address of
building? _____
Floor? _____ 1

Registration
Name three objects,
with 1-sec and pause
between each. Give
1 point for each object
the patient can name.
Repeat the objects until
the patient learns all three.
Score for first trial _____ 3

Attention and Calculation
Ask the patient to
substract 7 from 100
and continue to subtract
7 from the remainder
(ie, serial 7's). Give 1
point for each correct
answer. Stop after
5 answers. _____ 5

Recall
Ask the patient to name
the three objects learned
during registration. Give
1 point for each object
the patient can name. _____ 3

Naming
Point to a pencil and
a watch. Give 1 point
for each object the
patient can name. _____ 2

Repetition
Have the patient repeat
"No ifs, ands, or buts." _____ 1

Comprehension
Have the patient follow
a three-stage command:
"Take the paper in your
right hand. Fold the
paper in half. Put the
paper on the floor." Give
1 point for each stage
the patient can perform. _____ 3

Reading
Have the patient read
and obey the following
written command:
"Close your eyes." _____ 1

Writing
Have the patient write
a sentence of his or
her choice. Give 1 point
if the sentence contains
a subject and an object
and makes sense.
Ignore spelling errors. _____ 1

Drawing
Enlarge the design
printed below to 1 to
5 cm per side and
have the patient copy
it. Give 1 point if all
of the sides and angles
are preserved and if
the intersecting sides
form a quadrangle. _____ 1

Total score _____ 30

FIGURE 38–1. **The Annotated Mini-Mental State Examination form.** NOTE: A score of < 26 may indicate a need for further evaluation. However, cognitive performance as measured by this test varies according to the patient's age and educational level, as described in Crum RM, et al: "Population-based norms for the Mini-Mental State Examination by age and educational level." *Journal of the American Medical Association* 269:2386–2391, 1993. (Adapted from the Mini-Mental State Examination, copyright 1975 and 1998 Mini Mental LLC.)

Depression in the elderly**1** may manifest as a sense of dread or impending doom, as apathy, or as irritability without a specific cause. Depression may also be suggested by complaints of pain, tiredness, or other physiologic changes; by slow speech; by anxiety (sometimes as panic attacks with shortness of breath, palpitations, and sweating); by phobias, obsessions, or compulsions; or by abnormal perceptions (eg, delusions, hallucinations).

Anxiety Disorders

Patients should be asked about phobias (irrational fears of particular places, things, or situations leading to avoidance of the provoking stimulus**2**).

Patients should also be asked about obsessions (recurrent, unwanted ideas that cannot be resisted, although they may seem unreasonable) and compulsions (repeated, unwanted behaviors, such as handwashing or rechecking a locked door). In the elderly, obsessions are usually due to severe depression, whereas compulsions often result from an obsession. Obsessions can be elicited by asking, "Do you have thoughts that keep coming to your mind and are difficult to get rid of? Are the thoughts reasonable, or do they sometimes seem silly?" Compulsions can be elicited by asking, "Must you do certain things (eg, wash your hands) repeatedly, more than you need to?"

Delusions and Hallucinations

Delusions are false, fixed, idiosyncratic ideas. Patients may reveal delusional thoughts when questioned (eg, "Are people treating you kindly? Is anyone trying to harm you?"). Delusions of harm (eg, of food poisoning) or of harassment may occur in elderly persons with paranoid schizophrenia or paraphrenia.**3** Delusions also occur in 40% of persons with dementia. Delusions of poverty or of fatal illness may occur in depressed persons, who may believe that they are behaving badly and that their bad behavior will harm others. Delusions of persecution (eg, belief that someone is stealing from them) or of misidentification (eg, belief that family members are strangers or that persons long dead are alive) may occur in persons with dementia. Delusions should be differentiated from overvalued ideas (emotionally laden preoccupations or hobbies that override other activities or concerns), from culturally determined suspicions, and from religious beliefs.

Hallucinations are false visual, auditory, olfactory, or tactile perceptions. Visual or auditory ones may be elicited by asking, "Do you hear voices or see visions? If you hear voices, are they similar to my voice in your ear?" Further questioning is needed to determine whether the phenomena are really perceived (eg, "Do you hear the voices even when you do not see anyone talking? Do you hear them through your

---

1 see page 310   **2** see page 322   **3** see page 330

ears, or are they in your thoughts? Do you hear them as clearly as you hear me now?"). The examiner should respond with sympathy (eg, "That must have frightened you"), not with surprise or disbelief. Visual and tactile hallucinations are prominent in delirium; auditory hallucinations may occur in dementia and late-life schizophrenia (paraphrenia). Auditory hallucinations (eg, hearing one's name called) also may occur in late-life depression. Hallucinations may also occur in persons with sensory deficits, especially profound blindness, at which time the condition is called the Charles Bonnet syndrome. In addition, hallucinations may occur during bereavement, when the patient sees or hears the deceased person.

Cognition

Cognition (the ability to think and to understand the world) depends on alertness and is therefore impaired by drowsiness, stupor, and coma. However, cognition is impaired in the alert patient with mental retardation, Alzheimer's disease, or stroke. Cognitive functions—attention, orientation, memory, and language function—can be assessed quantitatively (eg, with the Annotated Mini-Mental State Examination).

Attention is the ability to focus and sustain thought and perception (eg, during reading or calculating). Attention can be evaluated by asking patients to subtract 7 from 100 and to keep subtracting 7 from each remainder. Patients with little education can be asked to count backward from 20 or to recite the months of the year backward. The ability to shift attention can be assessed by asking patients to count to 10, say the alphabet from A to J, and then combine the two tasks—alternating between numbers and letters (eg, 1, A, 2, B,...).

Most cerebral diseases and metabolic disorders affect attention. Inattention may suggest a brain lesion of the frontostriatal system, parietal cortex, or basal ganglia. Inattention may also occur in other conditions, including dementia, delirium, developmental disorders (eg, mental retardation, dyslexia), depression, mania, or schizophrenia.

Orientation to time and place is graded; ie, patients with cognitive impairment may know the year but not the day of the week; they may know the state they live in but not the floor of the building they are on. Impaired orientation may suggest delirium or dementia.

Memory involves learning (registration) or recalling what has been learned. Aging reduces the ability to learn but not the ability to recall material once it has been learned; dementia and delirium affect both. Normally, even the oldest old can recall at least two of three named objects. Patients who report memory loss but who can recall all three named objects should be evaluated for depression. Memory for events in the distant past is often retained in depression and dementia.

Language function is assessed by asking patients to name specific objects, repeat a phrase, follow an oral command, and read and write a sentence. Inability to perform these functions may suggest disease of the left hemisphere, which may occur in stroke or in Alzheimer's disease.

Other aspects of speech may give diagnostic clues.∎ Rapid speech may indicate mania; slow speech, depression or dementia; and slurred dysarthric speech, stroke or parkinsonism. Language difficulty, such as an inability to repeat, name objects, follow commands, read, or write, occurs in stroke or Alzheimer's disease.

Praxis is the ability to perform learned motor tasks. It can be evaluated by asking patients to draw intersecting pentagons. Loss of praxis (ie, apraxia) may suggest lesions of the parietal lobes, particularly the right lobe (eg, due to stroke or Alzheimer's disease).

Specific functional abilities (eg, understanding and following instructions on drug labels, managing finances, arranging transportation, using the telephone) should be examined directly, because the mental status examination can predict impairment of functional ability only in severe cases.∎

QUANTITATIVE ASSESSMENT

THE ANNOTATED MINI-MENTAL STATE EXAMINATION

The Annotated Mini-Mental State Examination (MMSE—see FIGURE 38-1) is used to assess the elements of cognition: attention, orientation, memory (registration and recall), language function, and praxis. It can be used to screen for or document cognitive impairment. The MMSE can be administered reliably by any practitioner trained to do so (eg, physician, psychologist, nurse, social worker, occupational therapist, technician).

Education level and age affect MMSE scores, but race and sex do not. The expected score for an 85-year-old with 0 to 4 years of education is 20, with 5 to 8 years is 24, with 9 to 12 years is 26, and with > 12 years is 28. A score lower than expected for age and education level may indicate delirium, dementia, or severe depression. Some patients have low scores because they are in poor physical health and take more drugs than those with higher scores.

OTHER QUANTITATIVE ASSESSMENT INSTRUMENTS

Several other quantitative instruments are available to assess different aspects of cognition—see TABLE 38-1.∎

Cognition can be quantitatively assessed by telephone, using such validated tests as the Telephone Interview for Cognitive Status (TICS).

∎ see page 423   ∎ see also page 42
∎ see also page 353 and TABLE 39–4 on page 355

TICS assesses attention, orientation, recall, calculation, information, verbal praxis, finger tapping, and antonyms.

Patients with cognitive disorders often have behavior problems,**1** including insomnia, anorexia, wandering, incontinence, and violence, that require management by a physician. These behaviors can be assessed by several validated scales, including the Dementia Symptoms Scale and the Psychogeriatric Dependency Rating Scale.

Abnormalities of mental status often contribute to an inability to perform activities of daily living, make a will, or sign contracts. Although legal competency is determined only by the court, physicians and nurses are often asked to submit evidence about a patient's mental abilities.**2** Competence to make decisions affecting medical care can be quantitatively assessed by the Hopkins Competency Assessment Test.

Several short rating scales can help in the assessment of mood. For patients with normal cognition, a self-rated questionnaire such as the General Health Questionnaire can be used to assess depression and anxiety. To test for depression in patients with cognitive impairment, the examiner can use the Hamilton Depression Rating Scale.**3**

39 ■ DELIRIUM

A clinical state characterized by an acute, fluctuating change in mental status, with inattention and altered levels of consciousness.

The term delirium is used in various ways. Some health care practitioners use the terms delirium and acute confusional state synonymously. Some use delirium to describe confusion with hyperactivity. Some use delirium to describe severe confusion and use acute confusional state to describe mild disorientation. THE MERCK MANUAL OF GERIATRICS uses delirium as defined above.

Delirium can be classified on the basis of psychomotor activity (ie, level of arousal). In **hyperactive delirium** (about 25% of cases), psychomotor activity is increased and agitation is prominent; hyperactive delirium may be misdiagnosed as an anxiety state, and the patient merely sedated (ie, a serious underlying etiology may be overlooked). In **hypoactive delirium** (about 25% of cases), psychomotor activity is decreased; hypoactive delirium may be misdiagnosed as depression or may be undetected. In **mixed delirium** (about 35% of cases), psychomotor activity has hyperactive and hypoactive features. In about 15% of cases, psychomotor activity is normal.

---

1 see page 371   **2** see page 130   **3** see TABLE 33–5 on page 316

Epidemiology and Etiology

Delirium is very common among the elderly. Of general medical patients ≥ 70 years admitted to the hospital, 10 to 20% are delirious at admission, and 10 to 20% become delirious during hospitalization. The incidence of postoperative delirium▮ among patients ≥ 70 is 15 to 25% after elective procedures and 35 to 65% after emergency procedures (eg, hip fracture repair). The incidence in other settings (eg, nursing homes, the community) is unknown but is likely to be increasing because patients are being discharged earlier from acute care.

Risk factors include advanced old age, underlying dementia, functional impairment, and medical comorbidity and its treatments. Factors that can precipitate delirium are as follows (using the mnemonic DELIRIUM):

- *D*rug use (especially when the drug is introduced or the dosage is adjusted—see TABLE 39–1)
- *E*lectrolyte and physiologic abnormalities (eg, hyponatremia, hypoxemia)
- *L*ack of drugs (withdrawal)
- *I*nfection (especially urinary tract or respiratory infection)
- *R*educed sensory input (eg, blindness, deafness, darkness, change in surroundings)
- *I*ntracranial problems (eg, stroke, bleeding, meningitis, postictal state)
- *U*rinary retention and fecal impaction
- *M*yocardial problems (eg, myocardial infarction, arrhythmia, heart failure)

Also, almost any acute illness affecting any organ system, or an exacerbation of any chronic illness, may precipitate delirium.

Pathophysiology

The neuropathophysiology of delirium is unknown. Serum anticholinergic activity is often increased, probably due to endogenous factors or to drug therapy. The elderly are particularly vulnerable to decreased cholinergic transmission. Levels of phenylalanine and tryptophan, which are involved in neurotransmitter synthesis, may be abnormal, and levels of leukotrienes and interferons may be elevated.

Symptoms and Signs

The hallmark of delirium is acute cognitive dysfunction with impaired attentiveness, which develops suddenly or over a short time (usually hours to days). A patient with delirium has acute fluctuations in

---

▮see page 250

TABLE 39–1. SELECTED DRUGS THAT MAY PRECIPITATE DELIRIUM

Sedative-hypnotics*
Benzodiazepines, especially long-acting (eg, diazepam, flurazepam, chlordiazepoxide); short-acting benzodiazepines are less problematic, except for triazolam and alprazolam
Barbiturates (severe withdrawal syndrome)
Chloral hydrate
Alcohol

Antidepressants
Especially highly anticholinergic tertiary amines (eg, amitriptyline, imipramine, doxepin)
Selective serotonin reuptake inhibitors (less common)

Anticholinergics
Diphenhydramine, oxybutynin, benztropine, atropine, scopolamine

Opioids
Especially meperidine (highly anticholinergic)

Antipsychotics
Uncommon; most likely with low-potency, highly anticholinergic drugs
Atypical antipsychotics, including clozapine

Anticonvulsants
Especially phenytoin at high serum levels

Antiparkinsonian drugs
Levodopa/carbidopa, bromocriptine, trihexyphenidyl, amantadine

H_2 blockers
Famotidine, cimetidine, ranitidine, nizatidine

*Delirium may result from initiation or withdrawal.

mental status, with varying levels of inattention and altered levels of consciousness. Changes in orientation, memory, and abstract thinking may occur but are not diagnostic. Psychomotor activity (level of arousal) may be variably abnormal. Hallucinations, delusions, tremor, abnormalities in the sleep-wake cycle, and other symptoms (see TABLE 39–2) may be present. In some frail elderly patients, delirium precedes the appearance of another illness and is the only early manifestation of that illness. Delirium may persist for many weeks or months; infrequently, it never clearly resolves, or it modulates into chronic cognitive dysfunction (dementia).

Diagnosis

Diagnosis consists of two elements: establishing the presence of delirium and establishing the underlying cause, if possible. Failure to diagnose or misdiagnosis occurs in up to 80% of cases but is less likely with interdisciplinary input (eg, from physicians, nurses, and persons who know the patient well, such as family members). The diagnostic criteria for delirium are shown in TABLE 39–3.

A thorough **history** is required to determine the frequency and duration of mental status changes and other clinical features. A drug review focuses on changes in the drug regimen (eg, additions, deletions, dose changes) that may have precipitated the delirium. Psychoactive drugs, particularly sedative-hypnotics, antidepressants, anticholinergic drugs, and opioids, are likely precipitants (see TABLE 39–1), but almost any drug may be implicated. Use of over-the-counter drugs and alcohol should also be reviewed.

A **physical examination** can be challenging in a patient with delirium. Vital signs, including pulse, blood pressure, respiratory rate, temperature, and oxygen saturation, may provide important etiologic clues. Cardiac, pulmonary, abdominal, neurologic, and mental status examinations should be performed.

The **Confusion Assessment Method** (CAM) may be the most useful tool for diagnosing delirium (see TABLE 39–4). CAM identifies the criteria necessary for diagnosis; other criteria that are not necessary for diagnosis (although common in delirium) include abnormal psychomotor activity, sleep-wake cycle disturbances, hallucinations, delusions, and tremor. CAM can detect delirium even in the presence of dementia.

Laboratory evaluation is guided by the history, drug review, and physical examination. CBC, serum electrolytes, urinalysis, and cultures

TABLE 39–2.   COMPARISON OF DELIRIUM AND DEMENTIA

Delirium	Dementia
Sudden onset	Insidious onset
Precise time of onset	Uncertain time of onset
Usually reversible	Slowly progressive
Short duration (usually days to weeks)	Long duration (years)
Fluctuations (usually over minutes to hours)	Good days and bad days
Abnormal levels of consciousness	Normal level of consciousness
Typically, an association with drug use or withdrawal or with acute illness	Typically, no association with drug use or acute illness
Almost always worse at night (sundowning)	Often worse at night
Inattention	Attention not sustained
Variable disorientation	Disorientation to time and place
Typically slow, incoherent, and inappropriate language	Possible difficulty finding the right word
Impaired but variable recall	Memory loss, especially for recent events

TABLE 39–3.   DIAGNOSTIC CRITERIA FOR DELIRIUM

Disturbance of consciousness (ie, reduced clarity of awareness of the environment) with reduced ability to focus, sustain, or shift attention

Change in cognition (eg, memory deficit, disorientation, language disturbance) or development of a perceptual disturbance that is not better accounted for by preexisting, established, or evolving dementia

The disturbance develops over a short time (usually hours to days) and tends to fluctuate during the course of the day

For delirium due to a general medical condition:

Evidence from the history, physical examination, or laboratory tests that the disturbance is due to the direct physiologic consequences of a general medical condition

For substance intoxication delirium:

Evidence from the history, physical examination, or laboratory tests that either:

1. Symptoms listed in the first two criteria developed during substance intoxication

2. Drug use is etiologically related to the disturbance

For substance withdrawal delirium:

Evidence from the history, physical examination, or laboratory tests that the symptoms listed in the first two criteria developed during or shortly after a withdrawal syndrome

For delirium due to multiple etiologies:

Evidence from the history, physical examination, or laboratory tests that the delirium has more than one etiology (eg, more than one general medical condition, a general medical condition plus substance intoxication or an adverse drug effect)

Adapted from the American Psychiatric Association: *Diagnostic and Statistical Manual of Mental Disorders,* fourth edition. Washington, DC, American Psychiatric Association, 1994, pp. 129, 131–133.

are the most useful laboratory tests. CT of the head, cerebrospinal fluid analysis, and electroencephalography are less useful but are frequently performed. Patients may have to be sedated during these tests, and the risk of sedation may outweigh the benefit of diagnostic yield. Thus, these tests are probably best reserved for patients at particularly high risk (eg, those who have had head trauma and are taking anticoagulants), those with new focal neurologic abnormalities, or those for whom the history, drug review, and physical examination have not confirmed an etiology. An ECG and a chest x-ray can be obtained if an underlying cardiac or pulmonary disorder is suspected.

Differential diagnosis: The primary differential diagnoses are depression[1] and dementia,[2] both of which may co-exist with delirium (see TABLE 39–2). Hypoactive delirium must be differentiated from

[1] see page 310   [2] see page 357

depression. In one study, one third of hospitalized patients referred for evaluation of depression had hypoactive delirium.

Differentiation between delirium and dementia is not always clear, and the features of the two syndromes sometimes overlap. Onset of delirium is rapid; dementia usually develops slowly, although that caused by a stroke or anoxia may occur acutely. In delirium, the ability to attend is primarily affected. In early stages of dementia, memory rather than attention is affected, although in late stages, attention may be severely impaired. Because delirium is often caused by toxic or metabolic factors that impair brain cell function and because dementia is usually caused by damage or loss of brain cells, delirium is often regarded as potentially reversible and dementia as permanent. Therefore, the duration of cognitive decline is probably the clearest way to differentiate these disorders. Although most persons with delirium recover fully, some never do. In addition, a few persons have dementia due to a reversible cause and may recover. The diagnosis of dementia should not be applied until all appropriate treatments have been tried and several months have passed to allow for recovery.

Complications

Patients with delirium are particularly vulnerable to iatrogenic problems, especially those due to physical or chemical (ie, drug) restraints. Bladder and bowel incontinence or retention is common and can directly contribute to delirium. Bedridden patients with delirium are prone to atelectasis, deconditioning, and pressure sores. Acute malnutrition, related to an inability to attend to eating, may occur.

Prognosis and Treatment

Hospitalized patients with delirium have up to a 10-fold higher risk of medical complications (including death), longer hospitalization, higher hospital costs, and increased need for postacute placement at discharge.

TABLE 39–4.   CONFUSION ASSESSMENT METHOD*

Criteria	Evidence
Acute change in mental status	Observation by a family member, caregiver, or primary care physician
Symptoms that fluctuate over minutes or hours	Observation by nursing staff or other caregiver
Inattention	Patient history Poor digit recall, inability to recite the months backwards
Altered level of consciousness	Hyperalertness, drowsiness, stupor, or coma
Disorganized thinking	Rambling or incoherent speech

*The first three criteria plus the fourth or fifth criterion must be present to confirm a diagnosis of delirium.

Management of delirium includes treatment of underlying disorders, removal of contributing factors, behavioral control, avoidance of iatrogenic complications, and support of the patient and family. A geriatric interdisciplinary team, involving family and friends, can provide the best care.∎ Failure to provide sufficient care may lead to life-threatening (and costly) complications and long-term loss of function.

Behavioral control may be necessary to ensure patient comfort and to promote safety. Usually, social restraint is preferred to physical or chemical restraints. Placement of delirious patients in rooms near the nursing station is recommended, and family members are encouraged to stay with patients. Items that help orient patients (eg, clocks, calendars) should be provided, and patients who need glasses and hearing aids should be encouraged to wear them.

Discontinuation of drugs or treatments known to precipitate delirium is recommended. Less commonly, drugs can be used to treat delirium directly; for example, delirium caused by alcohol withdrawal can be treated with benzodiazepines, and anticholinergic drug toxicity, if severe, can be treated with physostigmine.

Psychoactive drug treatment may be required to treat agitation rather than the delirium itself. If psychoactive drug treatment is required, documentation and assessment of the target symptoms and the response to treatment are necessary. For most patients, low doses of high-potency antipsychotics (eg, haloperidol 0.25 to 1 mg po, IM, or IV) are preferred. Use of risperidone (0.25 to 1 mg) has recently been suggested to treat the agitation of hyperactive delirium. Risperidone may have slightly less extrapyramidal effects than does haloperidol at low doses. Benzodiazepines (eg, lorazepam 0.25 to 1 mg po, IM, or IV) are the treatment of choice for patients with delirium due to alcohol or sedative withdrawal or for patients with parkinsonism who cannot tolerate the extrapyramidal effects of an antipsychotic. All drugs used to treat agitation can produce oversedation, and their use sometimes prolongs delirium and increases the risk of complications.

Risk of atelectasis, deconditioning, and pressure sores can be reduced by mobilization; ie, the patient sits in a chair or ambulates rather than remains bedridden. Close attention to nutritional intake and, sometimes, manual assistance with eating are necessary to avoid malnutrition.

Family and staff members should be informed that delirium is usually reversible but that cognitive deficits often take weeks or months to abate after resolution of the acute illness. Patient support and safety are paramount.

∎ see page 74

A deterioration of intellectual function and other cognitive skills, leading to a decline in the ability to perform activities of daily living.

Dementia is characterized by cognitive decline that occurs with a normal state of consciousness and in the absence of other acute or subacute disorders that may cause reversible cognitive decline (eg, delirium, depression). Dementia is one of the most serious disorders affecting the elderly. The prevalence of dementia increases rapidly with age; it doubles every 5 years after age 60. Dementia affects only 1% of those aged 60 to 64 but 30 to 50% of those > 85. In the USA, about 4 to 5 million persons are affected, and dementia is the leading cause of institutionalization among the elderly. The prevalence among elderly nursing home residents is estimated to be 60 to 80%.

The use of clinician must differentiate dementia from **benign senescent forgetfulness** (ie, age-related memory loss), which results from the slowing of neural processes with age. ◻ Persons with benign senescent forgetfulness learn new information and recall previously learned information more slowly. However, if they are given extra time and encouragement, their intellectual performance is essentially unchanged from their baseline. Daily functioning remains unaffected. Persons with this condition are often more concerned about it than are family members; reassurance and coping strategies are helpful.

Etiology

The causes of dementia (see TABLE 40–1) are difficult to differentiate because they are imprecise; many cases can be confirmed only by postmortem pathologic examination, which is usually not performed. Moreover, mixed dementias may be common (eg, recent research shows an interplay between Alzheimer's and cerebrovascular diseases).

Alzheimer's disease and vascular dementias are probably the two most common types, accounting for up to 90% of cases of established dementia in about a 2:1 ratio. Lewy body dementia may account for a large number of cases, but this entity is not well understood. ◻ Dementias are often divided into those with cortical presentation (ie, primary dementias), of which Alzheimer's disease is the prototype, and those with subcortical presentation, of which vascular dementia is the prototype.

Symptoms and Signs

The natural history varies according to the cause of dementia; however, patients typically experience a steady, inexorable decline in intellectual function over 2 to 10 years, culminating in total dependence and death, often due to infection.

◻ see page 380   ◻ see page 369

TABLE 40-1.   ETIOLOGIC CLASSIFICATION OF DEMENTIA

Primary dementia (cortical dementia)
Alzheimer's disease
Pick's disease
Frontal lobe dementia syndromes
Mixed dementia with an Alzheimer's component

Vascular dementia
Multi-infarct dementia
Strategic infarct dementia
Lacunar state
Binswanger's disease
Mixed vascular dementia

Dementia associated with Lewy body disease
Parkinson's-associated dementia
Progressive supranuclear palsy
Diffuse Lewy body disease

Dementia due to toxic ingestion
Alcohol-associated dementia
Dementia due to heavy metal or other toxin exposures

Dementia due to infection
Viral: HIV-associated dementia, postencephalitis
   syndromes
Spirochetal: neurosyphilis, Lyme disease
Prion: Creutzfeldt-Jakob disease

Dementia due to structural brain abnormalities
Normal-pressure hydrocephalus
Chronic subdural hematomas
Brain tumors

Some potentially reversible conditions mimicking dementia
Hypothyroidism
Depression
Vitamin B_{12} deficiency

The most common symptom in **early dementia** is diminished short-term memory. Patients repeatedly ask the same questions, often after only a few minutes, or forget where belongings were placed. The inability to locate belongings may lead to paranoia that they were stolen.

Word-finding becomes difficult; patients may forget a specific word and use elaborate circumlocution to compensate (eg, a necktie may be called "that thing around the collar"). Formerly mastered activities of daily living (eg, driving, handling finances, housekeeping) may also become difficult. A change in the level of functioning is key to diagnosis.

Other symptoms of early dementia include personality changes, emotional lability, and poor judgment. Family members may report that the patient is "not acting like himself" or is doing uncharacteristic things (eg, a miserly widower gives thousands of dollars to a questionable charity). Mood swings, including depression and euphoria, commonly occur. Although early dementia usually does not affect sociability, patients may become increasingly irritable, hostile, and agitated, especially in circumstances in which they are confronted with their cognitive impairment.

Patients with early dementia can usually compensate reasonably well and follow established routines at home. Acute decline often results from disruption of routine or a change in surroundings. For example, an elderly parent who visits a child's home in a distant state may become disoriented or may manifest behavior disorders❶ and functional disability not present in more familiar surroundings.

As patients progress to **intermediate dementia,** their ability to perform basic activities of daily living (eg, bathing, dressing, toileting) becomes impaired. Patients cannot learn new information. Normal environmental and social cues do not register, thus increasing disorientation to time and place. Patients may become lost even in familiar surroundings (eg, they cannot find their bedroom or bathroom). Patients with intermediate dementia are also at increased risk of falls and accidents due to confusion and poor judgment.

Behavior disorders may develop during early or intermediate dementia and can persist into severe dementia. Significant paranoia (eg, specific delusions, generalized suspicion) occurs in about 25% of patients. One particularly poignant delusion results from the loss of self-recognition in mirrors, leading to a suspicion that strangers have entered the home. Wandering can also be a significant problem, particularly if patients are trying to return to familiar surroundings, which may no longer exist. Physical aggressiveness, inappropriate sexual behavior, and nonspecific agitation may also occur during intermediate dementia.

Patients with **severe dementia** cannot perform activities of daily living and become totally dependent on others for feeding, toileting, and mobilization. Short-term and long-term memory is completely lost, and patients may be unable to recognize even close family members. The ability to ambulate is variably affected in different dementias but is usually lost in the later stages of illness, particularly in Alzheimer's disease.❷ Loss of other reflex motor tasks (eg, ability to swallow) puts patients at risk of malnutrition and aspiration. The combination of poor mobility and malnutrition increases the risk of pressure sores. Late in the course of dementia, the incidence of seizures increases. Complications such as dehydration, malnutrition, aspiration, and pressure sores are ultimately inevitable but may be delayed by excellent nursing care.

❶ see page 371   ❷ see page 365

Total functional dependence usually requires that the patient be placed in a nursing home or that similar support be implemented in the home. The usual cause of death is infection from respiratory, skin, and urinary tract sources.

Diagnosis

The *Diagnostic and Statistical Manual of Mental Disorders, Fourth Edition* (*DSM-IV*) criteria for dementia (see TABLE 40–2) include impairment of memory and impairment of at least one other domain of cognition (eg, language, perception, visuospatial function, calculation, judgment, abstraction, problem-solving ability). Often, many or all of these domains are impaired (see TABLE 40–3). This impairment must lead to deterioration in usual daily functioning.

The key to diagnosis of dementia is a thorough **history;** family members should be interviewed whenever possible because they are more aware of cognitive impairment than are patients. The nature of the impairment, time of onset, and pattern of progression should be elicited. Formal mental status examination◻ is also a key component to evaluation of cognitive impairment. Serial assessments can be useful in determining whether cognition is declining.

Patients with cognitive impairment that affects daily functioning require a more thorough evaluation than a mental status examination. Ruling out correctable factors that contribute to cognitive decline (eg, medical disorders, drugs, mood) is most important. With age, persons become more vulnerable to these correctable factors. The older the patient, the more likely that correctable factors are contributing to cognitive impairment.

A thorough review of the patient's known medical disorders and a search for new disorders may hold the key to reversing cognitive deficits. Many acute medical disorders cause acute cognitive decline in the elderly. Rapid onset of cognitive decline is not consistent with dementia and should trigger a prompt evaluation for delirium◻ and correctable medical disorders. Some medical disorders (eg, hypothyroidism, vitamin B_{12} deficiency) develop slowly and may more closely mimic dementia than delirium, but they are still correctable with treatment.

Drug use may be the most important correctable factor contributing to cognitive impairment. Every patient undergoing evaluation for dementia requires a thorough **drug review,** including over-the-counter drugs and ophthalmic preparations. A history of alcohol use should also be obtained. Before dementia can be diagnosed, all psychoactive drugs should be eliminated or substituted with less psychoactive drugs. Par-

---

◻ see page 343   ◻ see page 350

TABLE 40-2.   DIAGNOSTIC CRITERIA FOR DEMENTIA

Development of multiple cognitive deficits manifested by both:
1. Memory impairment (impaired ability to learn new information)
2. One (or more) of the following cognitive disturbances:
   Aphasia (language disturbance)
   Apraxia (impaired ability to carry out purposeful movements despite intact motor function)
   Agnosia (failure to recognize or identify objects despite intact sensory function)
   Disturbance in executive functioning (ie, planning, organizing, sequencing, abstracting)

Each of the cognitive deficits described above causes significant impairment of social or occupational functioning and represents a significant decline from a previous level of functioning.

The course is characterized by gradual onset and continuing cognitive decline.

The deficits are not caused by delirium.

For Alzheimer's disease:
The cognitive deficits listed in the first criterion (parts 1 and 2) are not due to any of the following:
1. Other central nervous system disorders that cause progressive deficits in memory and cognition (eg, cerebrovascular disease, Parkinson's disease, Huntington's disease, subdural hematoma, normal-pressure hydrocephalus, brain tumor)
2. Systemic disorders known to cause dementia (eg, hypothyroidism, vitamin B_{12} or folic acid deficiency, niacin deficiency, hypercalcemia, neurosyphilis, HIV infection)
3. Substance-induced conditions

For vascular dementia:
Focal neurologic signs and symptoms (eg, exaggeration of deep tendon reflexes, extensor plantar response, pseudobulbar palsy, gait abnormalities, weakness of an extremity) or laboratory evidence indicates cerebrovascular disease (eg, multiple infarctions affecting the cortex and underlying white matter) that is judged to be etiologically related to the disturbance.

For dementia due to other medical disorders:
Evidence from the history, physical examination, or laboratory tests indicates that the disturbance is the direct physiologic consequence of such conditions as Parkinson's disease, Huntington's disease, Pick's disease, Creutzfeldt-Jakob disease, head trauma, HIV infection, normal-pressure hydrocephalus, hypothyroidism, brain tumor, vitamin B_{12} deficiency, or intracranial radiation.

Adapted from the American Psychiatric Association: *Diagnostic and Statistical Manual of Mental Disorders, Fourth Edition.* Washington DC, American Psychiatric Association, 1994, pp. 142–143, 146, 152.

TABLE 40–3. POSSIBLE INDICATIONS OF DEMENTIA

Cognitive Domain	Possible Indication*
Ability to learn and retain information	Increased repetition of conversations Difficulty remembering recent conversations, events, appointments (eg, arriving at the wrong time) Misplacement of objects Difficulty discussing current events in an area of interest
Ability to handle complex tasks	Difficulty following a complex train of thought or performing tasks that require many steps (eg, balancing a checkbook, cooking a meal)
Reasoning ability	Inability to respond with a reasonable plan to solve problems at work or at home (eg, knowing what to do if the bathroom is flooded) Uncharacteristic disregard for rules of social conduct
Spatial ability and orientation	Difficulty driving, organizing objects around the house, or finding the way around familiar places
Language	Difficulty finding words to express self Difficulty following conversations
Behavior	Increased passiveness and reduced responsiveness Increased irritability and suspicion Misinterpretation of visual or auditory stimuli Changed behavior or dress

*Increased difficulty in any of these areas generally indicates the need for further assessment for dementia. Asking the patient or family members relevant questions about areas of concern may help.

Adapted from the *Quick Reference Guide for Clinicians: Early Diagnosis of Alzheimer's Disease and Related Dementias.* U.S. Department of Health and Human Services, Agency for Health Care Policy and Research, 1996.

ticularly potent psychoactive drugs include sedative-hypnotics, antidepressants (especially tertiary amine tricyclics), anticholinergics, and opioids.**1** A reasonable strategy is to repeat the mental status examination 6 weeks after optimization of the drug regimen to determine if cognitive impairment persists.

Every elderly patient with a cognitive problem requires a full **mood assessment,** including a symptom review (using the SIG E CAPS evaluation) and a standardized instrument such as the Geriatric Depression Scale short form.**2** Depression affects up to 40% of patients with dementia, usually in the early to intermediate stage. Cognitive decline resembling dementia in a patient with depression is termed pseudodementia.

1 see TABLE 39–1 on page 352   **2** see TABLE 33–4 on page 315

A complete **physical examination** should focus on identifying acute disorders and exacerbations of chronic disorders that may be contributing to cognitive decline. The examination should screen for evidence of a self-care deficit (eg, poor hygiene) that may confirm functional problems described during the history. On neurologic examination, focal neurologic findings may indicate cerebrovascular disease, extrapyramidal signs may indicate parkinsonism or other neurodegenerative diseases, and neuropathies and myopathies may suggest a treatable systemic disorder.

A **screening set of laboratory tests** (eg, CBC, electrolytes, albumin, renal function, liver function, thyroid function, vitamin B_{12} levels) is routinely obtained. Other laboratory tests (eg, ESR, arterial blood gas, serologic tests for syphilis, drug levels, cerebrospinal fluid examination) should be performed only in targeted high-risk patients.

Routine use of **brain imaging** to evaluate the cause of dementia is controversial. Imaging can identify potentially reversible structural abnormalities, such as normal-pressure hydrocephalus, chronic subdural hematomas, and brain tumors. However, these disorders are rare and usually have characteristic presentations. Moreover, whether treatment of these conditions improves cognition is unclear. In practice, the most common use of imaging is to differentiate Alzheimer's disease from vascular dementia. In several studies, the diagnostic yield of imaging patients presenting with classic Alzheimer's disease did not justify the costs of performing the test. However, in practice, most patients evaluated for dementia undergo brain imaging. Unless there is a need to identify small cerebral infarcts affecting the posterior circulation, CT is usually adequate, as opposed to the much more expensive MRI. One imaging study performed after the onset of cognitive decline is sufficient; serial testing is not justified.

Dynamic imaging of cerebral blood flow by single photon emission computed tomography (SPECT) is used in some specialized centers to differentiate Alzheimer's disease from vascular dementia. Alzheimer's disease produces a classic pattern of reduced blood flow to the temporal and parietal lobes, whereas vascular dementia produces a more "patchy" pattern. The expense and limited diagnostic accuracy of SPECT restrict its use to special cases at referral centers. Likewise, electroencephalography may be used to differentiate types of dementia and rule out complex partial seizure disorders, but it has limited diagnostic accuracy and should be reserved for special situations.

Neuropsychologic testing can help in the evaluation of cognitive impairment but is not required in most routine cases. Detailed testing helps primarily in the differentiation between (1) benign senescent forgetfulness and dementia, particularly in borderline cases or those in which the patient or family members are very concerned and desire additional reassurance; (2) dementia and pseudodementia in unusual cases in which depression is particularly hard to diagnose; and (3) dementia and focal syndromes of cognitive impairment (eg, amnesia, aphasia, apraxia, visuospatial difficulties). It is unclear whether neuropsychologic testing differentiates the causes of dementia better than a thorough history and physical examination.

Differential diagnosis: The differential diagnosis of dementia includes normal age-related memory loss, reversible causes of cognitive decline (eg, delirium, depression), milder cognitive impairment that does not meet the criteria for dementia (recently termed CIND— *C*ognitive *I*mpairment *N*o *D*ementia), and focal cognitive impairment affecting only one domain (eg, amnesia).

Treatment

Treatment or elimination of all correctable factors that impair cognition may significantly improve daily functioning and quality of life and may delay severe disability and institutionalization. Patients with significant depressive symptoms should be treated, even if they do not fulfill all criteria for major depression. Treatment of depression reverses pseudodementia and may significantly reduce disability in patients with true dementia. The drugs of choice are usually the newer selective serotonin reuptake inhibitors (eg, sertraline, paroxetine) started at a low dose and increased into the therapeutic range as tolerated. After 6 to 12 weeks of treatment, mental status examination should be repeated.

The next step is to create a supportive environment in which patients can function optimally. Patients with early to intermediate dementia usually function best in familiar surroundings. A home safety evaluation and appropriate modifications to improve function should be considered for all patients with dementia who live at home. For example, signs can be posted to cue patients for safety, especially in the kitchen and bathroom.

Homemaking services can provide assistance with instrumental activities of daily living; home health aide services, assistance with basic activities of daily living; and visiting nurses, drug supervision.

The balance between safety and independence is important, and decisions must be individualized. The decision to move into a more supportive living situation is determined by many factors, including patient preference, the home environment, availability of family members and caregivers, financial resources, and clinical factors other than the severity of dementia.

Patients with dementia are susceptible to disuse atrophy and must engage in physical exercise, mental activity, adequate nutrition, and socialization. A regular, supervised exercise program is often as simple as 15 to 20 minutes/day of walking. Continued mental activity usually focuses on the patient's interests before the onset of dementia (eg, current events, reading, art). These activities should be enjoyable and not used as tests of mental function. Adequate nutrition is necessary to maintain body weight. Patients may require prepared meals; monitoring ensures that meals are eaten.

Social isolation should be minimized if possible because it contributes to all of the problems cited above. Special effort may be required to ensure continued socialization. In some cases, adult day care or companion services provide socialization when family members or friends are not available.

Behavior disorders **1** are best treated with individualized behavioral interventions, rather than with drugs. However, frank psychotic symptoms (eg, paranoia, delusions, hallucinations) should be treated with antipsychotic drugs, started at a low dose. Patients must be carefully monitored for adverse effects.

Dementia is also a strong risk factor for other geriatric problems (eg, falls, **2** urinary incontinence **3**); prevention and treatment strategies should be implemented.

Health care practitioners must provide support for family members and caregivers of patients with dementia. Educational materials about dementia in general and the specific type (if known) can be very helpful but are no substitute for the specific advice, listening, and empathy of the clinician. Close monitoring for caregiver burnout is important; the threshold for burnout varies among persons. Various caregiver support groups are available.

End-of-Life Issues

Medical and financial planning is imperative before dementia becomes too severe. Patients should appoint a health care proxy and discuss health care wishes with the proxy and primary physician. **4** As dementia worsens, the risk/benefit ratio becomes less favorable for highly aggressive interventions and hospital care. In severe cases, patient comfort may be more appropriate than attempts to prolong life; the physician and health care proxy must collaborate on the care plan. A time may come when decisions must be made about artificial feeding or treatment of acute illness. These decisions are best discussed before such a situation arises and then discussed again when the situation becomes critical. Unlike cancer and some other conditions, dementia has no good prognostic models. In general, patients with Alzheimer's disease who can no longer walk have about $\leq$ 6 months to live.

ALZHEIMER'S DISEASE

Alzheimer's disease (AD) is the most common form of dementia affecting the elderly, accounting for up to two thirds of cases. AD is increasingly common with age. The typical pathologic findings are a loss of neurons in multiple areas of the brain; senile plaques (composed of neurites, astrocytes, and glial cells surrounding an amyloid core); and

---

1 see also page 371   **2** see page 195   **3** see page 965   **4** see page 134

neurofibrillary tangles (consisting of paired helical filaments). The specific pathophysiologic mechanism of neuronal cell loss in AD, as well as the role of plaques and tangles, is unknown. Plaques and tangles also occur in normal aging, **1** but to a much lesser degree than in AD. A protein involved in cholesterol transport, apolipoprotein E (apo E), has been genetically linked with AD. The $\epsilon4$ allele of apo E appears to be a risk factor for the disease, the $\epsilon2$ allele appears protective, and the $\epsilon3$ allele is neither associated nor protective. Persons with the $\epsilon4$ allele develop AD more commonly and at an earlier age than those without the allele. For example, $\epsilon4$ homozygotes have a > 50% risk of developing AD by age 70, whereas $\epsilon2/\epsilon3$ persons have only a 12 to 14% risk by age 90. Another important genetic advance has been the localization of the β-amyloid gene to chromosome 21, the same chromosome implicated in some cases of familial AD and AD due to Down syndrome. The finding that $\epsilon4$ binds to β-amyloid may lead to the pathophysiology of the disease. However, none of these findings have yet affected the treatment of AD patients. Moreover, genetic testing for apo E genotype is generally not recommended for most routine cases.

Diagnosis

The diagnosis of AD is based on the clinical features of typical dementia. **2** However, because AD is a common disease, atypical variants, including those with mixed pathophysiology, are also common, and deviations from the classic pattern do not rule out the diagnosis. AD is definitively diagnosed only on postmortem examination of brain tissue.

Treatment

AD is treated the same as dementia of any cause. **3** In addition, treatment involves drugs that improve cognition, given the patient's existing neuronal structure, or drugs that slow progression by reducing the rate of neuronal loss. Of drugs that improve cognition, cholinergic drugs (eg, tacrine, donepezil) are the best studied. Several randomized trials suggest that treatment with these drugs can modestly improve cognitive performance in many patients. This approach "turns the clock back" about 6 to 9 months for the average patient but has no effect on the rate of disease progression. Given the availability of the once-per-day, relatively nontoxic drug donepezil, a closely monitored trial for patients with mild to moderate AD seems reasonable; tacrine is given 4 times per day and is more toxic than donepezil. Donepezil may be started at 5 mg every night and reevaluated after 6 weeks. If improvement does not occur, the drug should be stopped or the dose increased to 10 mg. The 10-mg dose has a much higher incidence of adverse effects than the

---

1 see page 381   **2** see page 357   **3** see page 364

5-mg dose. If the dose is increased, the patient should be reevaluated after another 6 weeks. If improvement still does not occur, the drug should be stopped. If mental status improves (by caregiver impression or formal testing) with either dose, the drug may be continued and the patient reevaluated at 3- to 6-month intervals.

Estrogen, nonsteroidal anti-inflammatory drugs, and vitamin E have all been reported to slow the progression of AD, but more research is needed to determine their efficacy. However, cautious use of these drugs in persons with early dementia is appropriate. Ongoing research is also investigating the use of other antioxidants.

OTHER CORTICAL DEMENTIAS

Pick's disease and frontal lobe dementia syndromes resemble AD. In general, they progress more rapidly than AD and may be associated with more frontal lobe signs and behavioral disturbances earlier in the disease. However, clinical differentiation of these dementias from AD is difficult. The only definitive diagnostic method is pathologic examination of the brain. Because no specific treatments are available for these rare dementias, their diagnosis rarely affects clinical management.

SUBCORTICAL DEMENTIAS

VASCULAR DEMENTIA

A clinical syndrome of intellectual decline caused by ischemic insult to brain tissue.

Vascular dementia causes up to one third of cases of dementia and is likely the second most common cause after AD; it is particularly common among patients with many comorbid diseases. Most of these patients have high-risk factors for stroke (eg, hypertension, diabetes, coronary or peripheral vascular occlusive disease, heart disease, hyperlipidemia) and a history of transient ischemic attacks or sudden-onset neurologic deficits (strokes).

Several distinct patterns exist: classic multi-infarct dementia is caused by two or more major cerebral infarcts in the anterior, middle, or posterior cerebral artery territories; strategic infarct dementia is caused by a single infarct in a crucial area of the brain (eg, the angular gyrus, the thalamus); lacunar state or Binswanger's disease is caused by the buildup of multiple small infarcts, most commonly in the periventricular white matter. CT and MRI show periventricular and white matter abnormalities, which include hypodensities and periventricular lucencies without zones of cortical infarction. Mixed vascular dementia has features of two or more of these patterns.

TABLE 40-4.   MODIFIED HACHINSKI ISCHEMIC SCORE

Feature	Score (points)*
Abrupt onset of symptoms	2
Stepwise deterioration	1
Fluctuating course	2
Nocturnal confusion	1
Relative preservation of personality	1
Depression	1
Somatic complaints	1
Emotional lability	1
History or presence of hypertension	1
History of stroke	2
Evidence of associated atherosclerosis	1
Focal neurologic symptoms	2
Focal neurologic signs	2

*Points are given for each feature that is present. A total score < 4 is consistent with primary dementia (eg, Alzheimer's disease); 4 to 7 is indeterminate; and > 7 is consistent with vascular dementia.

From Rosen WG, Terry RD, Fuld PA, et al: "Pathologic verification of ischemic score in differentiation of dementias." *Annals of Neurology* 7:487, 1980; used with permission.

Symptoms and Signs

The symptoms and signs depend somewhat on which pattern is present; the classic presentation is stepwise cognitive decline, with each step characterized by an ischemic insult. In lacunar state dementia, the steps may be so small as to be indistinguishable from a gradual decline.

Cognitive impairment in vascular dementia, unlike that in AD, is more patchy, and some cognitive domains may be entirely unaffected. Focal, often asymmetric neurologic deficits (eg, weakness, sensory loss, exaggerated reflexes, Babinski's sign, visual field defects, pseudobulbar palsy, incontinence) occur earlier in the course of vascular dementia than in AD. Patients with vascular dementia are thought to be more aware of their deficits than patients with AD, and they may have a higher incidence of depression (although depression is also common in AD).

Diagnosis

Vascular dementia is diagnosed on the basis of a typical clinical history, focal findings on neurologic examination, and evidence of strokes (macro or lacunar) on brain imaging. ■ Several assessment tools, such as the modified Hachinski Ischemic Score (see TABLE 40-4), may help dif-

■ see page 363

ferentiate vascular dementia from AD. Many patients who present with classic vascular dementia ultimately have AD on postmortem examination of the brain, so the true relationship is likely to be complex.

Treatment

The primary treatment is risk reduction for additional cerebrovascular insults, ie, control of hypertension (including isolated systolic hypertension) and treatment with aspirin to prevent cerebrovascular thrombosis or with warfarin to prevent emboli from a cardiac source. Although these treatments prevent stroke, no trials have demonstrated that they slow the rate of progression of vascular dementia.

Vascular dementia does not have the societal stigma of AD, and many patients and family members find this diagnosis easier to accept. However, the prognosis is somewhat worse than AD, because the dementia is associated with concomitant medical disorders.

DEMENTIA ASSOCIATED WITH LEWY BODY DISEASE

Lewy bodies are rounded eosinophilic intracytoplasmic neuronal inclusions classically associated with Parkinson's disease,[1] in which they are found in selected subcortical structures, most notably the substantia nigra. Although Parkinson's disease is primarily an extrapyramidal motor disease, up to 40% of patients have Parkinson's-associated dementia. This "subcortical dementia" has clinical features similar to those of vascular dementia. Treatment focuses on the underlying Parkinson's disease, although levodopa and other treatments for Parkinson's disease seem to have little effect on cognition and may even precipitate psychosis. Dementia is also associated with several other primary extrapyramidal motor system degenerative diseases, including progressive supranuclear palsy.

Dementia due to diffuse Lewy body disease has recently been recognized as a distinct entity: Lewy bodies are found throughout the brain, including the cortex. The importance of diffuse Lewy body disease is under debate; some sources suggest it is the second most common cause of dementia after AD, some claim it is a variant of AD, and some state it is only of minor significance.

The clinical presentation is similar to that of AD, but the psychologic symptoms, particularly paranoia, delusions, and visual hallucinations, are more prominent. Mild parkinsonism may be present. Treatment with antipsychotic drugs usually leads to acute deterioration due to adverse extrapyramidal effects. Further clinical and pathologic studies are needed to better define this entity.

[1]see page 433

DEMENTIA DUE TO TOXIC INGESTION

Acute ingestion of psychoactive drugs may cause acute mental status changes.∎ Rarely, long-term ingestion of these drugs leads to permanent, irreversible cognitive impairment. The most common form, alcohol-associated dementia, is due to heavy ingestion of alcohol for > 10 years. The classic finding is impairment of short-term memory that is disproportionate to the other cognitive domains, although the dementia can be global. Ingestion of other toxic substances (eg, heavy metals) may also cause dementia.

DEMENTIA DUE TO INFECTION

Acute central nervous system infections may cause delirium; chronic infections may cause dementia. The most common, HIV-associated dementia, tends to affect a younger population than most other dementias. Although HIV can directly infect and destroy neurons, dementia usually occurs in the later stages of illness and is rarely a presenting symptom of HIV. Early and sustained antiviral treatment usually prevents dementia. Other viruses that infect the brain may cause acute cognitive dysfunction due to encephalitis or chronic cognitive dysfunction due to a postencephalitis syndrome.

Neurosyphilis and Lyme disease, which are spirochetal infections, can cause dementia-like syndromes. These syndromes are treatable and at least partially reversible, but they are better prevented by early recognition and treatment of the primary infection before it affects the central nervous system. Another dementia having an infectious etiology is Creutzfeldt-Jakob disease, which is caused by a prion. It has no specific treatment.

NORMAL-PRESSURE HYDROCEPHALUS

Normal-pressure hydrocephalus is thought to be caused by a defect in cerebrospinal fluid resorption in the arachnoid granulations. The classic triad of symptoms is gait disturbance ("magnetic" gait, as though the feet are stuck to the floor), urinary incontinence, and dementia. Brain imaging shows ventricular enlargement disproportionate to cortical atrophy. Patients should undergo lumbar puncture with removal of at least 20 mL of cerebrospinal fluid. Improvement in gait, continence, and cognition after large-volume lumbar puncture may predict the response to ventriculoperitoneal shunting. Several case series (although no randomized trials) report significant improvement after ventriculoperitoneal shunting, although gait and continence are more often improved than cognition.

∎ see page 351 and TABLE 39–1 on page 352

DEMENTIA DUE TO STRUCTURAL BRAIN ABNORMALITIES

Chronic subdural hematomas rarely cause dementia. Often, no clear history of head trauma or bleeding diathesis is present. Depending on the duration of the hematoma, drainage may only partially improve cognitive function.

Brain tumors (primary or metastatic) also rarely cause dementia. Treatment includes surgery, radiation, or chemotherapy depending on the location and aggressiveness of the tumor.

41 ■ BEHAVIOR DISORDERS IN DEMENTIA

Intolerable, disruptive actions (eg, wandering, yelling, throwing, hitting) generally occurring in persons with dementia.

Behavior disorders, also called behavior problems, are common among elderly persons with dementia. Elderly persons admitted to hospitals may have or develop a behavior disorder, and behavior disorders are the primary reason for up to 50% of nursing home admissions. As a result, behavior disorders are one of the most costly disorders affecting the elderly. Nevertheless, little research has been done in this area. The epidemiology and natural history of behavior disorders in dementia has not been well characterized, and optimal treatment has not been determined.

Tolerability (ie, what can be tolerated by persons with whom the patient lives) defines whether an action is a behavior disorder. Thus, deciding what constitutes a behavior disorder is highly subjective.

Tolerability depends partly on the patient's living arrangements. For example, wandering at home or sleeping during the day and staying awake all night may be considered eccentric but not intolerable in a person living alone yet problematic in one living with other persons. In a family residence, such behavior may disrupt normal activities. In a nursing home or hospital, staff members may consider such behavior intolerable because it disturbs other patients or interferes with the operation of the institution.

Different persons who interact with the patient may have different tolerance levels. For example, one attendant in a nursing home may readily tolerate frequent, repetitive questioning, but another attendant may become frustrated and annoyed by the constant interruptions. Time of day affects a person's tolerance level. For example, many behaviors of an institutionalized patient with dementia (eg, wandering, repeatedly questioning, being uncooperative) are better tolerated during the day, when many staff members are working and the activity level is high, than during the night, when fewer staff members are working and the activity level is low.

Environmental factors, particularly those related to safety, also affect tolerability. For example, wandering is better tolerated in a safe environment (eg, one in which all doors and gates have locks and alarms). For demented persons, cooking may be considered an intolerable behavior because it is hazardous to them and to others.

Whether **sundowning** (the exacerbation of disruptive behaviors at sundown or early evening in which agitation is prominent) is a matter of tolerability or true diurnal variation is unknown. Indeed, sundowning is a poorly understood phenomenon associated with dementia, and there is little evidence that sundowning is a discrete phenomenon. In nursing homes, 12 to 14% of patients with dementia have more behavior disturbances during the evening than during the day.

Exacerbating Factors

At least four **functional changes** related to dementia may result in behavior disorders. (1) Demented persons may be unable to conform their behavior to sociologic norms. For example, they may yell in an inappropriate environment (eg, in a restaurant) or undress in public. (2) They misunderstand visual and auditory cues. Thus, they may lash out at a nurse whom they perceive as a threat. (3) They have impaired short-term memory, so they cannot remember directions, may repeat questions and conversations, demand constant attention, or ask for things (eg, meals) that they have already received. (4) They cannot express their needs clearly or at all. Thus, they may yell when in pain or short of breath, wander when lonely or frightened, or urinate in public when the bladder feels full.

Institutional living may contribute to behavior disorders because it is highly regimented and restrictive: mealtimes, bedtimes, and toileting times are scheduled, and social and sexual relations are restricted or forbidden. Persons with dementia, who commonly cannot control their frustrations or conform to rules and routines, often adapt poorly to this regimentation. For many elderly persons with dementia, behavior disorders develop or worsen after they are moved to a more restrictive environment.

Physical illness can exacerbate behavior disorders. Pain, shortness of breath, urinary retention, constipation, other physical problems, or physical abuse may cause a change in the pattern or intensity of a behavior disorder. Delirium (acute confusion) superimposed on chronic dementia can also exacerbate behavior disorders; delirium may be the first indication of a new pathophysiologic process.∎

∎see page 350

TABLE 41-1.   TYPES OF BEHAVIOR DISORDERS

Disruptive	Yells or screams Asks questions repeatedly Wanders (not at risk of harm because the environment is safe) Undresses in public Is hypersexual Is uncooperative regarding treatment and care Has insomnia
Physically dangerous	Hits others Harms self Wanders (at risk of harm because the environment is unsafe) Throws objects
Psychologic	Feels anxious Is manic Feels depressed
Psychotic	Has delusions Has hallucinations (auditory or visual) Is paranoid

Classification

Behavior disorders are often collectively referred to as agitation. However, using a term that has so many meanings does not help in planning a management strategy. **Characterizing and classifying the behavior** are more useful (see TABLE 41-1). The specific behaviors (eg, hitting, throwing, refusing treatment, yelling, interrupting staff members, wandering, restlessness, insomnia, crying); the precipitating events (eg, feeding, toileting, drug administration, visits); the time the behavior started and resolved; and the type of, time of, and response to treatment should be recorded. Keeping such a record makes planning a management strategy easier and helps identify changes in pattern or intensity of a behavior. If a change is observed, a physical examination should be performed to exclude physical disorders and physical abuse. Sometimes a change in a patient's behavior reflects a change in the caregiver (eg, nurse, attendant, family member) rather than in the patient.

Identifying psychotic behavior is essential because management differs when psychosis is present. About 10% of demented patients with a behavior disorder show signs of psychosis; this percentage may be slightly higher in nursing homes. Behavior is psychotic if reality testing indicates impairment and if delusions (paranoid or not) or hallucinations are present. Delusions and hallucinations must be differentiated from fearfulness, disorientation, and misunderstanding. The latter three are common among patients with dementia and do not indicate psychosis. Paranoid patients may appear frankly terrified or quietly withdrawn; when questioned, they usually claim that others are trying to harm them, often in a specific way (eg, by poisoning). However, delusions may occur without paranoia; they are particularly difficult to differentiate from disorientation in patients with dementia. Usually, delusional behavior, unlike disoriented behavior, is fixed; ie, it remains the same. For example, delusional patients may repeatedly call the nursing home a prison, whereas disoriented persons may first call the nursing home a prison, then a restaurant, and later a home. Hallucinations usually consist of hearing or seeing something that has no external source, whereas misunderstanding (illusions) involves misinterpreting external sensory stimuli (eg, cellular phones, pagers). Hallucinations may occur in patients with dementia or with paraphrenia.❶

Treatment

Management of behavior disorders associated with dementia is one of the most controversial areas of geriatric medicine. Only a few small, controlled studies have examined the effectiveness of treatments, and no well-designed studies have compared types of drugs.

Nonpharmacologic: A consensus panel on the treatment of elderly persons with a behavior disorder (especially those with psychotic symptoms) recommends including environmental intervention and caregiver education as part of treatment. However, because of traditional training and reimbursement policies, physicians usually prescribe drugs rather than attempt nonpharmacologic management.

Environmental intervention is often the most successful, least expensive, and safest form of treatment. The institutional environment should be safe and flexible to accommodate behaviors that are not dangerous. Doors equipped with locks or alarms and stripes painted on floors (marking areas to avoid) can help ensure the safety of patients who wander. Signs can help patients find their way. Sleeping hours should be flexible to accommodate patients with insomnia, and reorganization of beds (separating noisy from quiet patients) can help reduce intolerable noise levels. Sexual activity should be allowed and facilitated as long as other residents and staff members are protected from unwanted encounters. Couples should room together, in double beds, if they want.

Providing cues about time and place and explaining what is going to happen beforehand (ie, before providing care) often can forestall violent outbursts. Frequent brief visits by staff members can prevent yelling. Physical activity should be encouraged because it often helps patients sleep without the use of drugs and may reduce the incidence of wandering, noisiness, hitting, and throwing. Similar interventions to improve the physical and interpersonal environment can be used at home.

If an institution cannot provide an appropriate environment for a particular patient, the patient should be moved to another institution. For example, if a nursing home cannot provide doors with locks or alarms,

❶ see page 330

transfer to another home for a patient who wanders may be preferable to treatment with drugs.

Nurses and social workers are in the best position to evaluate and implement environmental interventions. With physician support, they can help nursing home administrators design an institutional environment that is appropriate for patients with a behavior disorder.

Pharmacologic: Drugs are used only when nonpharmacologic approaches have failed and when drugs are absolutely necessary to maintain the safety of the patient and others. Drugs should be selected to target the most intolerable behaviors. The need for continued therapy should be reassessed at least every month.

The two classes of drugs most commonly prescribed for behavior disorders are sedative-hypnotics and antipsychotics. Drugs from both classes are commonly used in nursing homes: nearly one third of nursing home residents receive sedative-hypnotics (usually for insomnia), and more than one fourth receive antipsychotics (for other problematic behaviors). Antidepressants should be prescribed only for patients with signs of depression.

Although antipsychotics are widely used to treat behavior disorders, little evidence (worldwide literature on the subject includes only several hundred patients) supports their effectiveness, except perhaps as potent sedatives. No well-designed study has shown statistically significant differences between antipsychotics and placebo in controlling nonpsychotic behaviors associated with dementia. On the other hand, studies have shown that when antipsychotics are withdrawn, behavior does not deteriorate in most patients and improves considerably in many. For patients with psychotic behaviors, however, abundant evidence shows that antipsychotics are usually the drug of choice.

The toxicity of antipsychotics is well documented. At least 40% of elderly patients who use them long-term develop extrapyramidal symptoms. Anticholinergic drugs (eg, diphenhydramine, benztropine) may relieve these symptoms but tend to produce sedation and may worsen confusion. Patients taking antipsychotics may develop tardive dyskinesia or tardive dystonia; often, these disorders do not resolve when the dose is reduced or the drug withdrawn. Informed consent should be obtained from families before antipsychotics are prescribed for long-term use.

Despite concerns about using sedatives and antipsychotics, the frustration of caring for demented patients with behavior disorders often prompts physicians to prescribe them. Many experts prefer to prescribe less toxic sedatives (eg, short-acting benzodiazepines) when drugs are needed (ie, if environmental interventions do not make behavior tolerable). No reliable studies compare the effectiveness of benzodiazepines with that of antipsychotics in patients with a behavior disorder.

The choice of antipsychotic is usually based on relative toxicity. Haloperidol is relatively nonsedating and has less potent anticholiner-

---

TABLE 41–2.   TOPICS FOR CAREGIVER EDUCATION

- What is dementia, and how does it cause behavioral problems?

- What is the best approach to dealing with forgetfulness and repeated questioning, sudden aggressiveness or violence, wandering, noisiness, and eating problems?

- What drugs are available, what can they do and not do, and how should they be used appropriately?

- How can safety in the home be maximized?

- Is an identification bracelet for the patient useful?

- What are the best ways to help the patient maintain good hygiene?

- What are the symptoms and signs of depression and other mood problems?

- How can additional care, including nursing home care, be obtained?

- What are the steps for completing advance medical directives?

- What are the steps for obtaining guardianship?

- What financial planning options are available?

- How can caregiver stress be avoided?

---

gic effects than other conventional antipsychotics, but it is most likely to cause extrapyramidal symptoms. Thioridazine and thiothixene are less likely to cause extrapyramidal symptoms but are more sedating and have more anticholinergic effects than haloperidol.

Although little is known about the comparative efficacy of atypical and conventional antipsychotics in controlling behavior disorders, atypical antipsychotics (eg, risperidone, haloperidol, thioridazine) are generally preferred because they have a better safety profile. They are minimally anticholinergic and produce fewer extrapyramidal symptoms. Despite better safety, the indication for use—psychosis—remains the same. Thus, when an antipsychotic is indicated, an atypical antipsychotic is a reasonable first choice and is often used to treat patients with a behavior disorder.

In elderly patients, antipsychotics should be started at very low doses (eg, risperidone 0.5 mg bid, haloperidol 0.5 to 1 mg once daily or bid, thioridazine 2.5 to 10 mg once daily to tid). If larger doses are appropriate (which is rare for nonpsychotic patients), doses should be increased slowly at 4- to 7-day intervals.

Some evidence suggests that β-blockers can be useful in treating persons with violent physical outbursts. A lipophilic drug (eg, propranolol) may be most effective. The dose should be started low (10 mg bid) initially and, if needed, increased slowly to 40 mg bid; the patient should be monitored for hypotension, bradycardia, and depression. Other drugs such as carbamazepine may be useful in controlling violent outbursts in persons who have not responded to or cannot tolerate β-blockers.

Caregiver Issues

Caregiver education is essential for family members and professional caregivers (eg, staff members in nursing homes, home health care workers) who care for patients with a behavior disorder. Specific topics should be covered (see TABLE 41–2). Nurses and social workers can teach family members and other caregivers how to best meet the patient's needs; this teaching should be ongoing. *The 36-Hour Day,* a guide to caring for patients with dementia, provides invaluable information, including how to deal with daily care, get outside help, and handle financial issues.

Part of caregiver education is learning how to manage stress, which may be considerable and often requires intervention. Stress may be caused by fear of inadequately protecting the patient, frustration from having to repeat directions and restrictions, exhaustion from the intense supervision required by the patient, anger from watching an adult behave like an undisciplined child, and resentment from having to do so much to care for someone. Stress may cause a caregiver, regardless of setting, to punish or abuse the patient. ◨ Physicians and social workers should monitor caregivers for signs of stress.

◨see page 149

NEUROLOGIC DISORDERS

NEU

42   AGING AND THE NERVOUS SYSTEM

CHANGES IN THE BRAIN

In persons who do not have neurologic disease, intellectual performance tends to be maintained until at least age 80. However, tasks may take longer to perform because of some slowing in central processing. Verbal skills are well maintained until age 70, after which, some healthy elderly persons gradually develop a reduction in vocabulary, a tendency to make semantic errors, and abnormal prosody.[1] Other age-related changes in mentation are subtle but can be detected as difficulty learning, especially languages, and forgetfulness in noncritical areas. However, this mild forgetfulness is unlike dementia in that it does not impair recall of important memories or affect function.

The elderly, particularly those with some degree of neurologic disease, are especially susceptible to the actions of drugs. Hypnotics, which may be effective and safe for most persons, may cause confusion or delirium in the elderly. Stress due to medical or psychologic disorders can worsen even minimal brain disease. Depression often produces a dementia-like syndrome (pseudodementia) in elderly persons.[2] New onset of seizures is uncommon in the elderly. The causes of seizures in the elderly are listed in TABLE 42–1.

Loss of nerve cells: With normal aging, the number of nerve cells in the brain decreases. Cell loss is minimal in some areas (eg, brain stem nuclei, supraoptic and paraventricular nuclei) but is as great as 10 to

---

[1] see also page 424   [2] see page 362

TABLE 42–1.   CAUSES OF SEIZURES IN THE ELDERLY

Alzheimer's disease
Cerebrovascular disease
Central nervous system infections (including viral and prion infections)
Drugs (eg, phenothiazine use, benzodiazepine withdrawal)
Head trauma
Renal failure

60% in others (eg, hippocampus). Loss also varies within the cortex (eg, loss is 55% in the superior temporal gyrus but 10 to 35% in the tip of the temporal lobe).

From age 20 or 30 to age 90, brain weight declines about 10%, and the area of the cerebral ventricles relative to the entire brain (as seen on cross section in the coronal view) may increase three to four times. The clinical effects of these changes are difficult to determine because brain weight and ventricular size may not correlate with intelligence; indeed, severe dementia may occur in persons who have normal ventricular size for their age.

Histologic changes: With normal aging, the pigment lipofuscin is deposited in nerve cells, and amyloid in blood vessels. Also, senile plaques and, less frequently, neurofibrillary tangles occur in elderly persons even without clinical evidence of dementia (in Alzheimer's disease, plaques and tangles occur in much greater numbers).

Accumulation of free radicals: Free radicals (atoms or molecules with one unpaired electron), which are produced normally during metabolism, accumulate with age and may have a toxic effect on certain nerve cells.

Changes in neurotransmitter systems: With normal aging, changes in neurotransmitter systems (enzymes, receptors, and neurotransmitters) occur (see TABLE 42–2). For example, choline O-acetyltransferase levels tend to decrease; the number of cholinergic receptors tends to decrease; and γ-aminobutyric acid, serotonin, and catecholamine levels usually decrease. Choline O-acetyltransferase levels and dopamine levels may further decrease in Alzheimer's disease and in Parkinson's disease, respectively. Another age-related change is an increase in monoamine oxidase levels. When this increase is inhibited by monoamine oxidase inhibitors, onset of disability in patients with Parkinson's disease may be forestalled.

Decreased cerebral blood flow: With normal aging, cerebral blood flow decreases by about 20% on average; decreases are even greater in persons with small-vessel cerebrovascular disease due to diabetes and hypertension. Although blood flow in women is usually greater than in men until age 60, the subsequent rate of decrease is slightly more rapid. Decreases are greater in certain areas of the brain (eg, the prefrontal region) and are greater in gray matter than in white matter.

TABLE 42–2. AGE-RELATED CHANGES IN NEUROTRANSMITTER SYSTEMS

Component	Change	Brain Area Affected
Enzymes	Acetylcholinesterase levels decrease	Hippocampus, Meynert's nucleus
	Carbonic anhydrase levels decrease	Cortex
	Catechol O-methyltransferase levels increase	Hippocampus
	Choline O-acetyltransferase levels decrease	Hippocampus, Meynert's nucleus
	Glutamic acid decarboxylase levels decrease	Cortex, thalamus, basal ganglia
	Monoamine oxidase levels increase	Frontal cortex, globus pallidus, substantia nigra, striatum
Receptors	Dopamine 2 receptor levels increase	All
	Muscarinic receptor levels decrease	Cortex, hippocampus
	Serotonin receptor levels decrease	Cortex
Neurotransmitters	Neurotensin levels decrease	Substantia nigra
	Somatostatin levels do not change	All
	Substance P levels decrease	Putamen
	Vasoactive intestinal polypeptide levels increase	Temporal lobe

Adapted from the American Geriatrics Society: *Geriatrics Review Syllabus*, ed. 3, edited by Reuben DB, Yoshikawa TT, Besdine RW. New York, American Geriatrics Society, 1996, p. 17.

Compensatory mechanisms: Certain properties of the brain may reduce the clinical effects of age-related changes. **Redundancy** is a property whereby more nerve cells exist than are needed. For example, diabetes insipidus (due to a lack of antidiuretic hormone) does not appear until > 85% of the nerve cells in the supraoptic and paraventricular nuclei have been destroyed. Furthermore, hydrocephalic patients, who have only a thin cerebral cortical mantle, may have normal intelligence. The number of cells required for certain functions is unknown, so the extent of redundancy is difficult to estimate. However, redundancy probably reduces the effects of age-related neuron loss.

Plasticity at the nerve cell level involves compensatory lengthening and production of dendrites in remaining nerve cells to offset the age-related gradual deterioration and loss of nerve cells. New connections in the dendritic tree may compensate for the fewer nerve cells. Plasticity in the dendritic tree may also occur in Alzheimer's disease, perhaps as a biologic attempt to preserve function.

Other compensatory mechanisms may occur when the brain is damaged. For example, the nondominant hemisphere may compensate when speech centers in the dominant hemisphere are damaged, leading to gradual improvement in speech function. Other motor systems may compensate when large areas of the cerebellum are destroyed by injury, vascular disease, or tumor, often leading to functional recovery. Compensatory mechanisms are more effective in the higher centers. For example, the brain has a greater ability to compensate after injury than does the spinal cord, but the ability to compensate declines with age. The spinal cord does not have the redundancy of the brain to compensate for cell damage.

CHANGES IN THE SPINAL CORD

The number of cells in the spinal cord decreases with age, but actual counts have not been well investigated; the decrease does not appear to affect the functional capacity of the spinal cord. Decreases in nerve conduction are mostly due to changes in the peripheral nerves. A decrease in muscle strength is likely due to a loss of muscle fibers (sarcopenia) rather than to denervation. The principal effect of aging on spinal cord function is due to indirect changes, such as degenerative disease of the spine and intervertebral disks with compression of the spinal cord and entrapment of the nerve roots.

CHANGES IN PERIPHERAL NERVES

Nerve conduction time slows with age, although generally a change in function is not perceptible. In any injury to the peripheral nerves, reparative growth of the axons occurs if the cell body is intact; this reinnervation continues throughout life but is not as effective in elderly persons as in younger persons.

43 ▮ PAIN

A complex subjective and unpleasant sensation derived from sensory stimuli and modified by memory, expectations, and emotions.

Elderly persons who present with pain often have multiple medical problems and many potential sources of the pain. Thus, diagnosis and treatment of pain are more difficult in elderly persons than in younger persons.

Common complications of pain among the elderly include depression, fatigue, decreased socialization, sleep disturbance, impaired ambulation, deconditioning, gait disturbances, polypharmacy, and delayed rehabilitation. Pain management can be complicated by disability, limited resources, and lack of transportation. Pain directly leads to increased health resource utilization and costs. Settings such as nursing homes, assisted-living arrangements, and home care present additional challenges in pain management.

Epidemiology

Pain is one of the most common symptoms reported by the elderly during office visits. However, its precise incidence and prevalence are unknown. In one study, pain prevalence was 25% in persons > 60 years compared with 12.5% in those < 60; in other studies, the prevalence in the elderly ranged from 36 to 88%. A telephone survey found that one fifth of elderly Americans were taking analgesics at least several times per week and two thirds of these persons had been taking prescription analgesics for > 6 months. Among nursing home residents, 49 to 83% reported important pain problems.

Classification

Acute pain is characterized by sudden onset and short duration. The pathology and cause are often obvious (eg, trauma, surgery). Acute pain may be accompanied by autonomic signs (eg, tachycardia, diaphoresis, mild hypertension).

Chronic pain is characterized by a distant onset, long duration beyond the expected time for healing, and long-standing functional and psychologic impairment. The cause is often chronic and disease related (eg, diabetic neuropathy, osteoarthritis, osteoporosis). Autonomic signs are generally absent.

For treatment purposes, most pain can be further classified according to its underlying mechanism (see TABLE 43–1) as nociceptive (caused by specific pain receptors), neuropathic (caused by damage to a nerve or nerve pathway), mixed or unspecified (caused by a mixed or unknown mechanism), or psychologically mediated (caused by psychologic factors that have a major role in onset, severity, exacerbation, or maintenance of the pain).

Etiology

Pain is a universal problem, and its causes are myriad. In the elderly, the most common causes of pain are probably musculoskeletal disorders. In a study of community-dwelling elderly persons, the most prevalent type of pain was joint pain (66%), followed by leg pain at night (56%), back pain (28%), and leg pain while walking (21%). Among nursing home residents, the most prevalent type of pain was joint pain

TABLE 43-1.   CLASSIFICATION OF PAIN

Type	Example
Nociceptive	Pain due to trauma or burns Pain due to infection or inflammation Pain due to ischemia Pain due to mechanical deformity, pressure, or distention Pain due to arthropathies (eg, rheumatoid arthritis, osteoarthritis, gout, posttraumatic arthropathies, mechanical neck and back syndromes) Myalgia (eg, due to myofascial pain syndromes) Pain due to nonarticular inflammatory disorders (eg, polymyalgia rheumatica) Pain of internal organs and viscera

Neuropathic	Peripheral nervous system pain
	    Postherpetic neuralgia
	    Trigeminal neuralgia
	    Pain due to diabetic polyneuropathy
	    Postamputation pain (phantom limb pain)
	Central nervous system pain
	    Pain after stroke ("central pain" or thalamic pain)
	    Myelopathic or radiculopathic pain (eg, due to multiple sclerosis, spinal stenosis, arachnoiditis, or root sleeve fibrosis)
	Sympathetic nervous system pain
	    Reflex sympathetic dystrophy
	    Causalgia-like syndromes (eg, complex regional pain syndromes)

Mixed or unspecified	Chronic recurrent headaches (eg, tension headaches, migraine headaches, mixed headaches—see Ch. 127) Vasculopathic pain syndromes (eg, painful vasculitis)
Psychologically mediated	Somatization disorders Hysterical reactions

(70%), followed by pain at an old fracture site (13%), neuropathic pain (10%), and pain from malignancy (4%).

Elderly persons occasionally present with unusual manifestations of common disorders,∎ such as painless myocardial infarction and painless intra-abdominal catastrophes. Various age-related changes in pain perception have been suggested. These changes are difficult to differentiate from environmental injuries and occult disease. Ultimately,

∎see page 38

changes in pain perception due to age alone are probably not clinically significant.

Diagnosis

Identification of pain and diagnosis of its cause, when possible, are a routine part of patient assessment. In the elderly, assessment may be complicated by concurrent illness, underreporting of symptoms, and cognitive decline. Initial assessment of pain is often difficult in nursing homes and home care settings, in which medical records, consultants, diagnostic procedures, and facilities for other procedures are often unavailable. For some patients, short hospitalization may be required to establish a diagnosis, formulate a plan of care, and establish pain control.

A thorough pain history includes the onset, pattern, duration, location, and character (eg, quality, intensity) of the pain as well as aggravating and palliating factors. Pain may be described in a variety of ways (eg, as hurting, aching, or burning). The effect of pain on mood, sleep, activities of daily living, appetite, and bowel and bladder functions should be determined.

The history should focus on coexisting diseases and current and prior drug use, including analgesic use (eg, the analgesic used, its effectiveness and adverse effects). Coexisting diseases may cause chronic pain or acute pain exacerbations. Trauma or acute inflammatory arthritis (eg, gout, calcium pyrophosphate arthritis) can be easily overlooked as a cause of pain.

Psychiatric and social histories are also important. Depression, anxiety, and decreased socialization often accompany pain and can make management difficult. Several instruments are available to screen for depression. ◻ Health care practitioners should inquire about patients' fears and understanding of pain. For some patients, pain may represent atonement for past transgressions or suggest approaching death. Such emotional issues may complicate diagnosis and management. For most patients, coping skills are crucial and should be discussed; behaviors that are helpful (eg, an optimistic attitude) and harmful (eg, social withdrawal, isolation, exaggeration of minor problems) to pain management should be noted.

Physical examination ◻ should focus on the musculoskeletal system and include palpation for trigger points, swelling, and inflammation. Maneuvers that reproduce pain (eg, range-of-motion testing, straight-leg raising) may help diagnosis. Neurologic examination should include a search for signs of sensory, motor, and autonomic deficits and signs of nerve injuries, which may suggest neuropathic pain. Objective physiologic signs of acute pain may include pallor, sweating, tachycardia, and facial grimacing.

◻ see TABLES 33–4 and 33–5 on pages 315 and 316   ◻ see also page 36

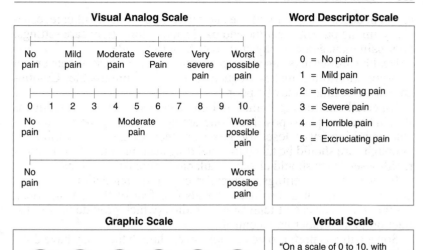

FIGURE 43–1. Examples of pain scales for quantifying pain as it is occurring: a visual analog scale; a word descriptor scale; a graphic scale; and a verbal scale. Adapted from AGS Panel on Chronic Pain in Older Persons: "The management of chronic pain in older persons." *Journal of the American Geriatrics Society* 46:635–651, 1998.

Pain intensity can be measured quantitatively using various pain scales (see FIGURE 43–1). As many as 80% of nursing home patients, including those with significant cognitive impairment, can provide meaningful information using such scales. In general, because the elderly often have impaired memory and difficulty integrating pain experiences over time, recording of pain as it is occurring (eg, in a pain diary) is the most reliable method. This approach may identify pain patterns that are modifiable by drug or dosage adjustments, by nondrug treatment, or by other activities. Several multidimensional pain scales are available (eg, the McGill Pain Questionnaire), but they are complex and often difficult to administer in clinical settings.

Treatment

Several organizations (eg, the Agency for Health Care Policy and Research, the American Pain Society, the American Geriatrics Society) have published clinical practice guidelines for pain management. However, there are few controlled data on pain management strategies in elderly persons, particularly in the oldest old. Information has been largely extrapolated from younger patient populations. Poor pain management decreases quality of life and reflects poor quality of care, especially among patients near the end of life and in long-term care settings; poor pain management may also contribute to suicide.

Health care settings can affect pain management. Lack of convenient transportation often makes frequent clinic visits impossible. Compliance with treatment may be poor.

Especially in nursing homes and home care settings, drug regimens should be as simple as possible. Long-acting drugs are generally preferable, requiring fewer doses for nurses or other caregivers to administer, although care should be taken to avoid drug accumulation. Short-acting rapid-onset drugs should also be available for breakthrough pain.

In institutional settings, overenforcement of regulations, such as excessive limits on use of heating pads (for fear of thermal injuries), visiting hours, or use of television or radios (which provide useful distraction), may hinder pain control.

Some patients prefer to be at home, even though they may have difficulty getting sophisticated pain management in this setting and may experience substantial suffering as a result. Home care can place substantial demands on family caregivers who see their loved ones in pain and do not know what to do. Caregivers often must decide when and how to administer drug treatment, often missing work and interrupting their own sleep to provide such care. They may be further stressed by the conflicting demands of helping the patient control pain while being overly concerned about tolerance and addiction. Consequently, patients with inadequate pain control are often sent to local emergency rooms, risking iatrogenic complications from health care personnel who are unfamiliar with their specific needs and primary goals of care.

Drugs combined with nondrug treatment can result in more effective pain control than either method used alone. Physicians should simplify drug regimens when possible and customize them to each patient's needs and lifestyle. Economic issues may influence treatment choices. Treatment goals, expectations, benefits, and risks should be discussed with the patient. An interdisciplinary approach [1] can be particularly effective.

Analgesics: Oral administration of analgesics is generally preferred, because it is usually convenient and offers relatively steady blood levels. However, onset of action usually does not occur until 30 minutes to 2 hours after administration, which may be a drawback for acute, rapidly fluctuating pain (eg, postoperative pain [2]). Such pain may require IV injection, which provides the most rapid onset and shortest duration of action. Subcutaneous and intramuscular injection, although commonly used, have wider fluctuations in absorption and

[1] see page 74   [2] see page 262

more rapid falloff than does oral administration. Transcutaneous, rectal, and sublingual routes should probably be used only for patients with difficulty swallowing. Chronic pain is generally best treated with long-acting or sustained-release preparations. Usually, it also requires supplemental use of rapid-onset short-acting drugs, especially for breakthrough pain. Pain due to a procedure or activity known to be painful and that can be anticipated can be pretreated.

Placebos should be used as analgesics only in clinical studies in which patients have given informed consent. Although placebo effects often occur, they are neither diagnostically helpful nor reliable indicators of pain relief. If placebos are used surreptitiously, placebo effects are usually short-lived; most patients eventually learn the truth, resulting in a loss of trust and needless suffering.

The elderly are more likely than are younger persons to experience adverse drug reactions from analgesics. Dosing usually requires careful titration ("start low and go slow"), with frequent assessment and dosage adjustments.

Acetaminophen is probably the analgesic of choice for most elderly persons with mild-to-moderate pain, especially those with musculoskeletal disorders. Despite its lack of anti-inflammatory activity, acetaminophen appears to be as effective as ibuprofen for chronic osteoarthritis of the knee. However, acetaminophen may interfere with concomitant administration of warfarin, and chronic use may impair renal function. In dosages of 650 to 1000 mg qid, acetaminophen is safer for most patients than are nonsteroidal anti-inflammatory drugs and other analgesics. The total daily dose should not exceed 4000 mg, because overdose can result in irreversible hepatic necrosis.

Nonsteroidal anti-inflammatory drugs (NSAIDs) are indicated mainly for short-term use in inflammatory arthritic conditions (eg, gout, pseudogout) and acute rheumatic disorders (eg, rheumatoid arthritis). They are also useful in combination with opioids for treating bone pain from cancer.

The anti-inflammatory activity, potency, analgesic efficacy, metabolism, excretion, and adverse effects vary widely among NSAIDs. Failure of response to one NSAID may not predict response to another. One advantage of NSAIDs is their relative lack of sedative or respiratory depressant effects. NSAIDs are not habit-forming. All NSAIDs, whether prescription or over-the-counter, have a ceiling effect (a level at which increased dose results in no increase in analgesia). They can be used alone or in combination with opioids or other analgesics.

NSAIDs, however, should be used with caution. They are no better than acetaminophen for many cases of mild-to-moderate pain (eg, osteoarthritis of the knee and perhaps other chronic pain syndromes). Also, the incidence of adverse reactions is extremely high in the elderly.

For example, the risk of gastrointestinal bleeding due to NSAIDs (which is often life threatening) is about 1% in the general population and 3 to 4% in persons > 60, but almost 10% in persons > 60 who have a history of gastrointestinal bleeding. Risk of gastrointestinal bleeding can be reduced but not eliminated with concomitant use of misoprostol, histamine-2 receptor antagonists, proton pump inhibitors, or antacids. In addition, the adverse effects of these gastroprotective drugs must be weighed against their limited benefits; moreover, these drugs do not reverse other adverse reactions of NSAIDs (eg, renal impairment, sodium retention, bleeding diathesis from platelet dysfunction). For patients with multiple medical problems, NSAID use increases the risk of drug-drug (eg, with antihypertensives or warfarin) and drug-disease interactions.

NSAIDs are contraindicated in patients with a history of gastrointestinal bleeding, renal impairment, or a bleeding diathesis. They should not be used postoperatively (eg, after a craniotomy), when even a small amount of bleeding can be disastrous.

Selective cyclooxygenase (COX-2) inhibitors are a new category of NSAIDs: two are currently available—celecoxib and rofecoxib. Traditional NSAIDs are potent inhibitors of cyclooxygenases (COX-1 and COX-2), which convert arachidonic acid to prostaglandins. COX-1 is synthesized in various organs and modifies gastric mucosal blood flow and barrier function, hepatic blood flow, renal blood flow, and platelet aggregation. COX-2, normally present in lower concentrations, is produced in response to injury or inflammation.

Selective COX-2 inhibitors have similar analgesic and anti-inflammatory activity to traditional NSAIDs (eg, in patients with arthritis). However, they cause less gastrointestinal irritation and bleeding and have less effect on platelet aggregation. Their effects on renal function may not differ substantially from those of traditional NSAIDs.

Opioids act by several mechanisms, including receptor blockade in the central nervous system; they effectively relieve all types of pain. In the elderly, opioids have an increased half-life [1] and possibly a greater analgesic effect than in younger patients. Nonetheless, the most common error in prescribing these drugs is to give them at intervals that allow breakthrough of pain. Many opioids must be dosed every 2 to 3 hours.

Opioids have different potency and adverse effect profiles. The analgesic effect of propoxyphene is similar to that of aspirin or acetaminophen, but dependency and renal impairment may occur; thus, propoxyphene is rarely a drug of choice. Meperidine is a second-line opioid, because it is metabolized to an active form that is prone to accu-

---

[1] see page 259

mulation and may thereby lead to central nervous system excitement and seizures. Because of low oral potency and erratic absorption from muscle, meperidine should only be used intravenously for acute pain, when morphine or other potent opioids are contraindicated. Pentazocine is both an agonist and antagonist of opiate receptors and can cause a high incidence of delirium when used in the elderly. Butorphanol should be used with caution in patients already taking opioids because it has mixed opiate receptor activity and can displace opioids already occupying pain receptors, which can result in immediate withdrawal symptoms including autonomic crisis. Methadone has a long half-life that may be even more prolonged in elderly persons. Fentanyl is perhaps 50 times as potent as morphine; the appropriate dose is less predictable than that of other opioids.

Transdermal preparations of opioids are available. Fentanyl 25 μg/hour transdermal system may be given every 72 hours. The initial dose does not achieve its peak analgesic effect until 18 to 24 hours after application, so a rapid-onset analgesic is required in the meantime. The reservoir for this system is the skin, not the patch, resulting in a 72-hour half-life (or even longer in frail elderly patients). If patients become inadvertently overdosed, removal of the patch does little to abort drug delivery. Thus, transdermal fentanyl should be reserved for patients who cannot take drugs orally and for those who are already accustomed to high-dose opioid drugs.

Continuous opioid infusion, via intravenous, subcutaneous, intrathecal, and epidural routes, provides steady-state analgesic drug levels. It has become the method of choice for perioperative pain management,◪ even in frail elderly patients. It also may be useful if regional techniques and NSAIDs are ineffective or inappropriate in patients near the end of life.

Intramuscular injections produce initially high blood drug levels, which can cause adverse effects. The levels then decrease rapidly, resulting in recurrence of pain.

Patient-controlled analgesia (PCA) allows the patient to increase drug delivery as needed. This technique produces a more stable blood level of drug, avoiding the roller-coaster effects of intramuscular dosing; reduces overall drug use; and causes fewer adverse effects but is more expensive than traditional analgesics. The opioids most commonly used for PCA are morphine and hydromorphone. Confused or demented patients cannot safely or effectively use PCA.

In the elderly, opioids may cause dose-related drowsiness, cognitive impairment, and respiratory depression. Until tolerance to these adverse effects develops (usually within a few days), patients should not drive

◪ see page 262

and should take precautions against falls or other accidents. Physical function often improves once pain relief is adequate and tolerance to these adverse effects has developed.

Opioids frequently cause constipation along with urinary retention. Patients do not develop tolerance to these adverse effects. Constipation should be managed by increasing fluid intake and prescribing stimulant laxatives. **1** Some patients require regular enemas.

Opioids occasionally cause nausea; some patients develop tolerance to nausea within a few days. Nausea may be due to several mechanisms: stimulation of the vestibular system connected to the middle ear; gastric or colonic paresis; or stimulation of midbrain chemoreceptors. If stimulation of the vestibular system causes vertigo, an antihistamine antiemetic (eg, hydroxyzine) may be appropriate, although its anticholinergic effects will worsen constipation; urinary retention and sedating effects will also worsen. If gastroparesis or colonic paresis occurs, drugs that increase gastric propulsion (eg, metoclopramide) may be helpful. For patients with nausea due to stimulation of midbrain chemoreceptors, antipsychotic drugs (eg, low-dose haloperidol, chlorpromazine) can be helpful. However, in the elderly, antipsychotic drugs have a high incidence of adverse effects (eg, movement disorders, delirium, anticholinergic effects).

Tolerance to the analgesic effects of opioids is difficult to predict, occurs much more slowly than tolerance to adverse effects (eg, drowsiness, respiratory depression), and is often insignificant. Indeed, pain in some patients is controlled by stable doses of opioids for many years. Cancer patients tend to develop tolerance to the analgesic effects of opioids, possibly because their pain increases as the cancer advances. **2**

Dependence, characterized by withdrawal effects after abrupt cessation, usually occurs with prolonged use. Nonetheless, fear of dependence should not inhibit the use of opioids when needed; fears about dependence should be addressed so that patients use these drugs appropriately. Dependence requires constant and prolonged drug exposure, although the required dose and duration, as well as the intensity of withdrawal symptoms, vary with the opioid.

Symptoms of opioid withdrawal may include anorexia, nausea, diaphoresis, tachycardia, mild hypertension, and mild fever. Severe symptoms may be accompanied by skin mottling, gooseflesh, and frank autonomic crisis. Withdrawal symptoms can be easily ameliorated by tapering opioids over a few days (in general, a 25% decrease in dose every 24 to 48 hours). Severe autonomic signs due to withdrawal can usually be controlled by short-term use of clonidine in titrated doses.

---

1 see page 1084   **2** see also page 722

True addiction (ie, a psychologic craving and use of opioids for effects other than pain relief) is rare among patients taking opioids for medical reasons. The incidence of opioid addiction appears to be even less among the elderly than among younger patients. Opioids have no ceiling effect with dosage. The maximum dose is whatever is needed to relieve pain, preferably without causing adverse effects. Two unproven dosing rules are useful:

• A dose that severely depresses respiratory function is more than twice the stable, tolerated dose.

• To reestablish pain control after a previously adequate dose becomes inadequate, the previous dose must ordinarily be increased 1.5 times.

Combination analgesic therapy (eg, opioids with acetaminophen or with NSAIDs; NSAIDs with other analgesics) can produce synergistic effects.

Adjuvant analgesic drugs: Adjuvant analgesics include various drugs not formally classified as analgesics that are nonetheless helpful for certain types of pain (see TABLE 43–2). For example, tricyclic antidepressants, anticonvulsants, and local anesthetics are the most frequently used treatment for neuropathic pain but, in general, are less effective for other types of pain. These drugs relieve neuropathic pain (usually only partially) in about 50 to 70% of cases. They are rarely ideal as monotherapy and generally are combined with traditional analgesics or with nondrug strategies.

Antidepressants are the most widely used type of adjuvant analgesic. Their mechanism of action in pain relief is unclear but probably involves interruption of norepinephrine and serotonin-mediated mechanisms in the brain. Their mood-altering capacity may also be helpful, especially in those with concurrent depression. Preliminary data in diabetic neuropathy suggest that desipramine is as effective as amitriptyline in relieving pain and, in the elderly, is better tolerated. Paroxetine may also relieve pain. Other antidepressants generally are less effective for pain relief.

Anticonvulsants such as phenytoin, carbamazepine, and valproic acid may reduce neuropathic pain in diabetic neuropathy. Carbamazepine is probably the drug of choice for trigeminal neuralgia. Gabapentin, when used in relatively high doses (up to 3600 mg/day), is effective in diabetic neuropathy and in postherpetic neuralgia.

Calcitonin, in preliminary studies, appears to reduce chronic pain in osteoporosis.

Local anesthetics, when injected into trigger points, can sometimes relieve pain. They are particularly effective when combined with physical therapy. For example, in myofascial pain syndromes, injection of local anesthetics into trigger points, followed by stretching and recon-

TABLE 43–2. SOME ADJUVANT ANALGESICS

Class and Drugs	Indications	Precautions	Comments
Antidepressants (eg, amitriptyline, desipramine, doxepin, imipramine, nortriptyline)	Neuropathic pain, major depression, sleep disturbance	Elderly persons are more sensitive than younger persons to adverse effects, especially anticholinergic effects; desipramine may be as effective as amitriptyline with fewer adverse effects	Complete relief does not often occur; drugs are more effective as an adjunct to other drug and nondrug treatments for pain; close monitoring for adverse effects is necessary; starting doses are low and are increased slowly every 3–5 days
Anticonvulsants (eg, carbamazepine, clonazepam, gabapentin)	Neuropathic pain only; carbamazepine is probably the drug of choice for trigeminal neuralgia	Carbamazepine may cause leukopenia, thrombocytopenia, and, rarely, aplastic anemia; adverse effects with clonazepam may be similar to those with other benzodiazepines in the elderly; gabapentin may have less severe adverse effects than carbamazepine	Starting doses are low and are increased slowly; blood counts must be checked in patients taking carbamazepine; gabapentin is started at 100 mg tid and titrated slowly while idiosyncratic adverse effects (eg, ankle swelling, ataxia) are monitored; effective gabapentin therapy may require doses as high as 3600 mg/day
Antiarrhythmics (eg, mexiletine)	Neuropathic pain only	The effective dose may be lower for pain than for cardiac disorders; common adverse effects are tremor, dizziness, and paresthesias; blood dyscrasias and hepatic damage occur rarely	Drugs are avoided in patients with preexisting heart disease; starting dose is low (given q 6–8 h) and titrated slowly; ECG monitoring is necessary
Local anesthetics (eg, IV lidocaine)	Diagnostic test	Delirium commonly occurs	The test may be a useful predictor of response to other local anesthetics (eg, mexiletine); local anesthetics should be used as a diagnostic test only in a monitored environment where emergency procedures are readily available to control seizures, cardiac arrest, or other complications

Drug	Use	Comments	
Tramadol	Acute and chronic pain	The drug is primarily a norepinephrine antagonist but is also a partial opioid and serotonin agonist; it may cause drowsiness, nausea, vomiting, and constipation	A ceiling effect is present; doses > 300 mg/24 h are usually not tolerated because of nausea; dosing is q 4–6 h
Muscle relaxants (eg, baclofen, chlorzoxazone, cyclobenzaprine)	Skeletal muscle spasm	Sedation and anticholinergic effects may occur; abrupt withdrawal of baclofen may cause CNS irritability	Mechanism of action is not precisely known; sedation and anticholinergic effects must be monitored; baclofen is tapered on discontinuation
Substance P inhibitors (eg, capsaicin)	Neuropathic and other chronic pain	Burning pain during depletion of substance P may be intolerable for as many as 30% of patients; maximum response may take 14 days; eye contamination must be avoided	Reuptake of substance P is inhibited from primary afferent sensory neuron synapses; starting doses are small; these drugs are available OTC for topical use only; in case of problems, they can be partially removed from the skin with vegetable oil
N-methyl-D-aspartate (NMDA) inhibitors (eg, ketamine)	Surgical anesthesia	—	Only an IV anesthetic drug is available; oral forms are not available

CNS = central nervous system; OTC = over-the-counter.
Adapted from AGS Panel on Chronic Pain in Older Persons: "The management of chronic pain in older persons." *Journal of the American Geriatrics Society* 46:635–651, 1998.

ditioning of the muscles, usually lessens symptoms. These drugs, when administered systemically, can also relieve neuropathic pain. Lidocaine is useful in predicting the response to other systemically administered local anesthetics; however, it is not effective orally and requires continuous IV infusion, which can often cause delirium and other severe adverse effects. Oral mexiletine is sometimes effective against neuropathic pain in diabetic neuralgia. At standard doses, this drug also has a high risk/benefit ratio; some studies have reported response rates using one third to one half of the dose often recommended for cardiac arrhythmias.

Nondrug treatment: Similar benefits to trigger point injections have been obtained using ice massage or vapo-coolant spray followed by muscle stretching and other physical therapy techniques. Pain of muscle spasm can also be relieved by applying heat or cold, immobilizing joints, or using transcutaneous electrical nerve stimulation (TENS**1**). TENS reportedly decreases postoperative use of analgesics and improves mobility but has been shown to have a definite placebo effect.

Endurance and muscle-strengthening exercises,**2** carried out regularly and at a moderate intensity level, can be used to reduce pain due to musculoskeletal disorders and improve functional status.

Cryotherapy involves application of a cryoprobe (an instrument that supplies extreme cold to tissue) to specific peripheral nerves. For example, cryoanalgesia can be applied during surgery to help relieve postthoracotomy pain.

Cognitive-behavioral therapy, particularly when combined with other therapies, may help relieve pain in patients without significant cognitive impairment. This therapy (eg, involving relaxation, biofeedback, or hypnosis) tries to alter beliefs and attitudes about pain and suffering and helps patients develop coping strategies. Caregiver involvement in cognitive-behavioral therapy may enhance its benefits.

Alternative therapies (eg, homeopathy; spiritual healing; vitamin, herbal, and natural remedies) are used by many patients for control of pain. Patients may use alternative therapies with or without their physician's knowledge or recommendation.

Patient and caregiver education: Education programs significantly improve overall pain control. These programs, provided in groups or tailored to individual needs and level of understanding, can address the nature of pain and teach patients and caregivers how to use pain diaries, pain assessment instruments, analgesics, and self-help nondrug strategies.

---

1 see page 277   **2** see pages 301 and 303

44 ■ CEREBROVASCULAR DISEASE

(Cerebrovascular Accident; Stroke)

A heterogeneous group of vascular disorders that result in brain injury.

Each year, about 750,000 Americans have a stroke, and about 150,000 of them die. Stroke is the third leading cause of death in the USA and in most other industrialized countries. At any time, there are about 2 million stroke survivors in the USA. Stroke incidence and mortality rate increase with age, especially after age 65 (see TABLE 44–1). About 72% of persons who have a stroke in a given year are ≥ 65, and > 88% of persons who die of stroke are ≥ 65. Prevalence in the USA is generally higher among men and blacks (see FIGURE 44–1).

More impressive than the mortality rates are the ways in which stroke changes the survivor's quality of life. Daily functioning in the workplace, home, and community is often reduced, and many stroke patients are impaired in their ability to walk, see, and feel. Some cannot read, recall, think, speak, or otherwise communicate as well as they could before the stroke. Dementia may result, especially if multiple lacunar infarcts occur.∎

The complications of stroke may be more devastating than the stroke itself. Strokes activate the body's clotting system, potentially leading to venous thromboembolism and myocardial infarction during the acute period or during convalescence. At times, determining whether the myocardial ischemia or the brain ischemia came first is difficult.

Prevention

Preventing strokes is far better than treating them. Much of prevention is best begun before old age; nonetheless, many preventive measures are still relevant for the elderly (see TABLE 44–2).

Because early treatment of stroke can be beneficial, all patients at risk should be taught about the early symptoms of stroke (see TABLE 44–3). They should be told to seek immediate medical attention if they have such symptoms, with emphasis that treatment should be started within 3 to 6 hours.

Prognosis

Recovery after a stroke has two aspects: neurologic and functional. The extent of neurologic recovery depends on the mechanism, location, and size of the lesion. In general, the smaller the lesion, the better the recovery. About 90% of neurologic recovery usually occurs within 3

∎see page 367

TABLE 44-1.   STROKE DEATH RATES* IN THE USA (1983)

Race	Sex	Age (yr)					
		35-44	45-54	55-64	65-74	75-84	> 84
White	Combined	5.6	18.0	49.1	167.6	643.5	1950.9
	Men	5.5	19.1	56.5	197.1	714.8	1862.9
	Women	5.6	16.9	42.6	144.6	602.0	1986.5
Black	Combined	22.0	64.0	143.0	341.5	807.4	1570.7
	Men	24.3	74.1	163.8	388.0	844.1	1479.4
	Women	20.1	55.7	126.0	308.4	786.7	1603.1

*Per 100,000 population.
Adapted from Caplan LR: "Stroke in African-Americans." *Stroke* 22:558-560, 1991; reproduced with permission. Copyright 1991, American Heart Association.

months. The remaining 10% occurs more slowly. Recovery after hemorrhagic stroke is particularly slow.

Recovery depends on the personal and socioeconomic circumstances of the stroke patient as much as (if not more than) on the injury itself. The patient's physical capabilities and mental health before the stroke are important predictors of subsequent ability to cope and to work toward recovery. Depression, which is common after a stroke, may

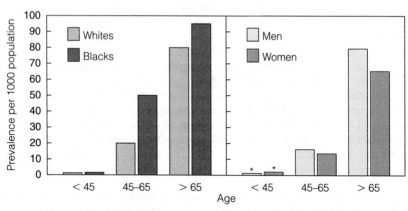

* Unreliable estimate.

FIGURE 44-1.   Prevalence of cerebrovascular disease by age, sex, and race in the USA. Prevalence is higher among men than among women aged ≥ 45. It is much higher among blacks than among whites up to age 75 but may be higher among whites after age 75. (Data by race [1990-1992] based on Gillum RF, Wilson JG: The burden of stroke and its sequelae. Disease Management Health Outcomes 1997; 1:84-94. Data by sex [1995] from the National Center for Health Statistics.)

TABLE 44-2. STRATEGIES TO PREVENT STROKE IN THE ELDERLY

Control of hypertension

Treatment of cardiac disorders (eg, coronary artery disease, heart failure, arrhythmias)

Measurement of serum lipid levels and treatment of hyperlipidemia

Recommendations to stop smoking, to abstain from illicit drug use (eg, amphetamines, cocaine, heroin), to use alcohol only in moderation, and to exercise regularly

Warnings against overeating, undereating, and becoming severely fatigued

Treatment of hematologic disorders (eg, anemia, polycythemia, bleeding diathesis)

impede recovery. Patients are much more likely to return to an active, useful life if they have good resources and a living environment that facilitates independence (eg, a first-floor residence; a car or access to a driver; nearby shopping, recreational, and medical facilities; income for rehabilitation equipment and therapists). A home caregiver is extremely important to recovery.

Treatment and End-of-Life Issues

The health care team must establish an appropriate care plan as soon as possible. Early, aggressive treatment can often effect dramatic improvement. However, aggressive treatment is not warranted for all patients. For some patients, treatment is unlikely to help, because their quality of life is and will remain extremely poor. In such cases, supportive care is the focus. Advance directives (eg, living wills, durable power of attorney∎), if available, can help physicians determine what kind of supportive care to provide for the patient (eg, hydration, nutrition, treatment of infections and pain).

The coexistence of other serious disorders (eg, cancer, incapacitating heart or lung disease, dementia) may affect treatment decisions. Certain treatments may be contraindicated—eg, anticoagulants for patients with severe hypertension or gastrointestinal bleeding. Some treatments (eg, anticoagulants, vascular or brain surgery) have higher risks and complication rates in the elderly; however, age alone is not an absolute contraindication to treatment.

Aggressive diagnostic tests, invasive medical and surgical therapies, and prolonged bed rest often tax the spirit and vigor of elderly patients. Pneumonia, limb contractures, pressure sores, and depression are particularly common and must be prevented or treated if present. Antidepressants are particularly effective in treating the depression caused by

∎see page 134

TABLE 44–3. EARLY SYMPTOMS AND SIGNS OF STROKE

Sudden weakness or numbness on one side of the body (face, arm, or leg)*

Sudden dimness or loss of vision, particularly in one eye*

Sudden slurred speech, loss of speech, or difficulty understanding speech*

Unexplained dizziness, difficulty walking, loss of coordination, or falls*

Sudden, severe headache with no apparent cause*

Difficulty swallowing†

Sudden confusion†

Nausea and vomiting†

*Transient ischemic attacks also produce these symptoms, but the symptoms last ≤ 24 hours.
†These symptoms are less common.

stroke. Certain strategies can help prevent and manage stroke complications (see TABLE 44–4).

If a local institution is not equipped to care for stroke patients with potential for recovery, transfer to a special center is warranted. Similarly, rehabilitation is best performed in special centers. ∎

Nursing Issues

Nurses must be vigilant in preventing sleep problems, problems with eating and feeding, incontinence, confusion, falls, and skin breakdown, which are common among patients with cerebrovascular disease and which can be serious, even fatal. Nurses must also watch for the development of depression, which is common after a stroke. A nurse usually coordinates an interdisciplinary team, ∎ helping organize arrangements for the patient's discharge and helping develop a postdischarge care plan. An interdisciplinary team is needed because cerebrovascular disease is complex and devastating and because team members can follow the patient across care settings.

Developing a postdischarge care plan that is likely to be followed is difficult. Basic issues must be considered; they include transportation to appointments, the patient's willingness to participate in rehabilitation therapy, the patient's ability to adhere to complicated drug regimens, and the patient's willingness and ability to work with caregivers such as nursing attendants in the home. The patient, family members, and home caregivers must attend discharge planning meetings. Consequently, times and locations for the meetings should accommodate these persons.

∎ see page 280   ∎ see page 74

TABLE 44–4.   **STRATEGIES TO PREVENT AND TREAT STROKE COMPLICATIONS**

- Prescribe tight elastic or air-filled support stockings plus frequent active and passive leg exercises
- Turn bedridden patients frequently, giving special attention to pressure sites
- Maintain adequate fluid intake and nutrition
- Use small doses of heparin (5000 U) sc q 8–12 h—so-called miniheparin—or an equivalent amount of low-molecular-weight heparin or heparinoid, when not contraindicated, to prevent thromboembolism
- Encourage early ambulation (as soon as the patient's signs become stable), with close monitoring
- Monitor pulmonary hygiene (eg, smoking cessation, deep breathing exercises, respiratory therapy)
- Observe for and treat infections early, especially pneumonia, urinary tract infections, and skin infections
- Prevent overdistention of the urinary bladder, preferably without using an indwelling catheter
- Prescribe early rehabilitation (eg, active and passive exercises, range-of-motion exercises) and provide education about functional disabilities for patients hospitalized because of acute disease
- Emphasize risk factor control (eg, smoking cessation, weight loss, healthy diet)
- Encourage a positive outlook; all members of the health care team should emphasize that patients can regain a good, active life and that many patients can resume nearly all other previous activities, although return to previous, normal function may be impossible
- Provide early and continuous assistance to family members in preparing for the patient's return home (including instruction about the patient's needs and about necessary changes in the home) or, if the patient is not returning home, assistance in quickly finding a suitable alternative
- Continue in the rehabilitation facility or in the patient's home the preventive measures and treatments begun at the hospital
- Encourage the patient to contact stroke support groups and persons who have overcome similar handicaps

TRANSIENT ISCHEMIC ATTACKS

Focal neurologic abnormalities of sudden onset and brief duration caused by cerebrovascular disease.

Transient ischemic attacks (TIAs) are due to temporary blockage of blood flow to the brain. By definition, they last $\leq$ 24 hours; > 75% last < 5 minutes, but some last several hours.

TIAs can be a warning sign of impending stroke. About one third of persons who have had at least one TIA will have a stroke, and having had a TIA increases the risk of stroke by 9.5. Thus, detection of a TIA and identification of its cause are essential.

Symptoms develop rapidly. They are identical to those of a stroke but are temporary and do not cause permanent damage (see TABLE 44–3). Questioning about TIA symptoms should be systematic and specific; information about temporary prickling or loss of feeling in the arms or legs, temporary limp or other walking problems, sensation of a shade or curtain coming over one eye, and recent new-onset headache should be sought. Treatment depends on the vascular cause, as it does for patients with ischemic stroke.

ISCHEMIC STROKE

A cerebrovascular disorder caused by insufficient blood flow in an area of the brain.

Ischemia accounts for about 80% of strokes. Risk factors include hypertension, heart disease, arrhythmias (eg, atrial fibrillation), hyperlipidemia, and the effects of age on the cerebral vessels.

Brain tissue malfunctions rapidly when deprived of adequate blood flow. Temporary disruption of blood flow may result in ischemia without infarction and thus produce only temporary symptoms. When ischemia is prolonged, infarction occurs and localized brain function is irrevocably lost. However, brain function is plastic, and other, nearby areas may eventually take over the lost function.

Ischemia is caused by an impediment to blood flow, almost always due to a narrowed or occluded artery supplying a local brain region. Arterial occlusion triggers a chain of events; some tend to promote the ischemia and worsen the neurologic deficit, and others (ie, compensatory body reactions) limit the ischemia and the deficit. During the first week after ischemia begins, a thrombus gradually adheres to the arterial wall and becomes organized, diminishing the early tendency of the loosely attached clot to embolize or propagate distally. Similarly, the collateral circulation needs time to become established and stabilized. For these reasons, about one fourth to one half of ischemic strokes are generally presaged by at least one TIA. Strokes may occur days or months after a TIA.

Ischemic strokes are classified on the basis of their site and causes: atherosclerosis of the large arteries in the neck and in the cranium, penetrating artery disease, brain embolization, and systemic hypoperfusion or general circulatory failure.

LARGE-VESSEL ATHEROSCLEROSIS

Atherosclerosis is a major cause of ischemic stroke. Among whites, atherosclerosis of the cerebrovascular bed is most common at the origins of the internal carotid and the vertebral arteries in the neck and in the intracranial vertebral and basilar arteries. The large intracranial arteries (middle, anterior, and posterior cerebral arteries) and their superficial convexal artery branches are affected much less often (see FIGURE 44–2).

Atherosclerosis of the extracranial internal carotid and vertebral arteries is twice as common among white men as among white women; it correlates highly with coronary and peripheral vascular occlusive disease and hyperlipidemia. A history of angina pectoris, myocardial infarction, or leg claudication in patients who have had a TIA strongly suggests extracranial atherosclerosis.

Atherosclerosis of the extracranial internal carotid and vertebral arteries is less common among blacks and Asians than among whites, but atherosclerosis of the major intracranial arteries is more common. Among blacks and Asians, intracranial atherosclerosis does not have a strong male preponderance, does not correlate epidemiologically with coronary or peripheral vascular disease or with hyperlipidemia, and occurs at a younger age than does extracranial atherosclerosis. Among persons with diabetes or hypertension, prevalence of intracranial atherosclerosis is also high.

Sometimes occlusions are caused by hematologic abnormalities, alone or superimposed on a stenotic lumen. Polycythemia and thrombocytosis are major causes of vascular occlusion. A hypercoagulable state◨, which can complicate cancer and other systemic disorders, may lead to obstruction of a narrowed vessel.

Symptoms and Signs

The most common presenting symptom is at least one prior TIA, which is often brief; but TIAs, if untreated, may recur for weeks or months. Some patients present with sudden-onset stroke, probably caused by embolization of intra-arterial clot or plaque material originating in regions of extracranial atherosclerosis and traveling distally to block intracranial recipient arteries. Headache is also common and is probably caused by dilation of collateral arterial channels. Specific symptoms and signs relate to the anatomy of the involved artery and the area it supplies. They may be sensory, motor, or both.

Internal carotid artery in the neck: Transient decreases in arterial flow cause attacks of transient monocular blindness (amaurosis fugax)◨ on the side of the lesion. These attacks are usually described as being like a shade falling or a curtain moving across the eye from the side. They usually last 30 seconds to a few minutes and are sometimes precipitated by sudden standing or bending or by exposure to bright natural light.

Hemispheric ischemia may produce weakness or numbness of the contralateral limbs and the face. The hand and arm are involved more often than the face or leg, but the part affected may vary with each attack. Aphasia◨ is common when the left internal carotid artery is

◨see page 689   ◨see page 1307   ◨see page 425

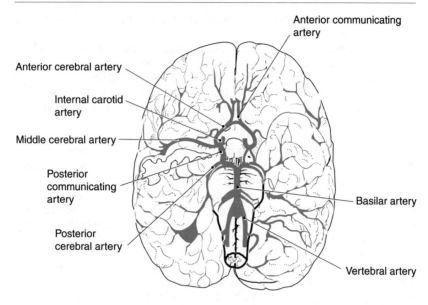

Inferior View

FIGURE 44–2.   Arteries of the brain.

involved. When both transient monocular blindness and attacks of numbness or weakness in the contralateral limbs occur, the diagnosis is internal carotid artery disease in the neck or in the carotid siphon, proximal to the ophthalmic artery branch. Plaque disease and stenosis are most severe at the origin of the internal carotid artery, where it branches from the common carotid artery. TABLE 44–5 lists some signs of internal carotid artery atherosclerosis.

Subclavian artery: Atherosclerosis usually affects the subclavian arteries proximal to the origin of the vertebral artery branches. The left artery is stenosed more often than the right. The most common symptoms involve the ischemic arm, which often aches, is cool, and becomes fatigued easily during exercise. The radial pulse in the ischemic arm is usually weak or delayed, and the blood pressure is lower than that in the opposite arm. At times, a bruit is audible in the supraclavicular fossa. TIAs related to the subclavian arteries are much more common than stroke; they produce evanescent dizziness, blurred vision, diplopia, or staggering; sometimes they are provoked by exercising the ischemic arm. Patients with subclavian artery atherosclerosis usually do well, unless they use the ischemic arm vigorously in sports (eg, golf). Surgery is usually not indicated.

Vertebral artery: Typical characteristics of ischemia related to vertebral artery disease in the neck are evanescent dizziness, vertigo, diplopia,

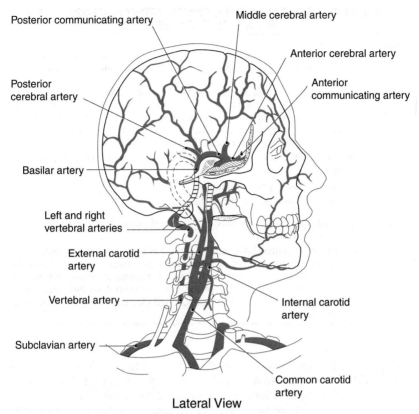

Posterior communicating artery

Middle cerebral artery

Anterior cerebral artery

Posterior
cerebral artery

Anterior
communicating artery

Basilar artery

Left and right
vertebral arteries

External carotid
artery

Vertebral artery

Internal carotid
artery

Subclavian artery

Common carotid
artery

Lateral View

FIGURE 44–2. *Continued.*

and blurred vision. These symptoms may occur when the person moves the head in certain positions. The clinical findings are identical to those of subclavian artery disease, except that the arm is not ischemic and the pulses and blood pressures in the upper limbs are equal. Some patients with a vertebral artery occlusion in the neck present with a sudden posterior circulation stroke; the ischemia is caused by blockage of the intracranial vertebral artery or the posterior cerebral artery or its branches. The blockage results from embolic material originating in the proximal vertebral artery. The most common site of vertebral artery atherosclerosis is the origin and first few centimeters of the artery. The distal portion of the vertebral artery in the neck is vulnerable to tearing or dissection during trauma, sudden movement, or manipulation of the neck.

Occlusion or severe stenosis of an intracranial vertebral artery blocks flow through the posterior inferior cerebellar artery branch and causes ischemia of the lateral medulla and the cerebellum. The most common

TABLE 44–5.   SIGNS OF INTERNAL CAROTID ARTERY ATHEROSCLEROSIS IPSILATERAL TO THE LESION

Site	Signs
Neck	Bruit (long, focal, high-pitched), best heard with a stethoscope bell
Face	Increased pulses in facial, preauricular, and superficial temporal arteries when the common carotid artery is normal and the external carotid artery acts as a collateral vessel; decreased pulses in facial, preauricular, and superficial temporal arteries when the common carotid artery or internal carotid artery and external carotid artery are stenosed
	Increased ABC pulses: A—angular, near medial corner of eye; B—brow, laterally; C—cheek
	Coolness in the supraorbital region
	Reversal of blood flow in the frontal artery
Eyes	Iris: red speckling (rubeosis iridis); fixed, dilated, or irregular pupil; Horner's syndrome
	Retina: white retinal infarcts; Hollenhorst plaques (bright refringent cholesterol crystals usually at bifurcations of retinal arteries); decreased caliber of retinal arteries; asymmetric hypertensive retinopathy that is less prominent on the side of the stenosis; central venous retinopathy (engorged veins, microaneurysms, small-clot hemorrhages, sometimes papilledema)

symptoms and signs of lateral medullary ischemia are listed in TABLE 44–6. Cerebellar ischemia is manifested by staggering gait, ataxia, sensations of disequilibrium, and nausea. Large cerebellar infarcts can increase pressure in the posterior cranial fossa and cause coma due to compression of the brain stem; this potentially fatal complication is treated with surgical decompression of the lesion and removal of infarcted tissue.

Basilar artery: The most common symptoms and signs of basilar artery atherosclerosis are listed in TABLE 44–7. Occlusion can be fatal unless collateral circulation develops. The basilar artery supplies the pons; the region most vulnerable to ischemia is the base of the pons, which contains the long motor tracts. Ischemia causes bilateral weakness of the trunk and limbs with exaggerated reflexes and extensor plantar signs. Sometimes premonitory episodes of dizziness and diplopia occur, especially when the occlusion begins in the vertebral artery and spreads to the basilar artery.

Intracranial carotid artery: When stenosis affects the intracranial carotid artery proximal to the ophthalmic artery branch, the syndrome is similar to that affecting the internal carotid artery origin. No neck bruit is heard, and results of noninvasive studies of the internal carotid artery are normal. Stenosis of the intracranial carotid artery beyond the ophthalmic artery origin is accompanied by attacks of hemispheric ischemia occurring as lateralized weakness, sensory loss, or visual neglect, but transient monocular blindness does not occur. Also lacking are signs and ultrasonographic evidence of decreased ophthalmic artery flow. Aphasia is common among patients with left hemispheric ischemia; defective drawing and copying ability and left-sided visual neglect are common among patients with right hemispheric ischemia.

Middle, anterior, and posterior cerebral arteries: Middle cerebral artery disease is usually most severe in the proximal segment or the upper trunk branch. Anterior cerebral artery disease is less common and usually affects the proximal segment. Posterior cerebral artery disease usually affects the proximal segment.

Middle cerebral artery disease usually causes weakness and numbness of the contralateral limbs, trunk, and especially the face. When the left middle cerebral artery is affected, aphasia usually occurs; when the right middle cerebral artery is affected, visuospatial dysfunction and left-sided neglect (lack of attention to all activity on the left side) occur.

Anterior cerebral artery disease causes weakness and numbness of the contralateral lower extremity and weakness of the contralateral shoulder. At times, the patient may lack spontaneity, be disinterested, or be incontinent.

The cardinal symptoms and signs of posterior cerebral artery atherosclerosis relate to the visual fields. Patients may have transient attacks

TABLE 44-6.   SYMPTOMS AND SIGNS OF LATERAL MEDULLARY ISCHEMIA

Area	Symptoms	Signs
Ipsilateral	Jabbing pain in the eye or face	Decreased sense of pain and temperature along the trigeminal distribution
	Lid droop; decreased facial sweating	Horner's syndrome
	Dizziness and feelings of motion	Nystagmus
	Hoarseness and dysphagia	Decreased movement of ipsilateral palate, pharynx, and vocal cord
	Incoordination of arm and leg	Incoordination, tremor, and rebound of arm and leg
Contralateral	Difficulty with perception of temperature over the arms and legs	Decreased sense of pain and temperature in the arms, legs, and trunk
General	Walking imbalance	Gait ataxia
	Difficulty sitting or standing	Tendency to fall to the side when sitting or standing
		Tachycardia
		Labile blood pressure

TABLE 44–7.   SYMPTOMS AND SIGNS OF BASILAR ARTERY ATHEROSCLEROSIS

Symptoms	Signs
Diplopia	Palsies of extraocular movement (3rd, 4th, and 6th cranial nerves)
Dysphagia	
Dizziness	Internuclear ophthalmoplegia
Dysarthria	Nystagmus—horizontal or vertical
Bilateral weakness in the legs or legs and arms	Bilateral bulbar weakness (face, lips, palate, pharynx, tongue)
Crossed weakness (one side of the face, opposite side of the body and limbs)	Crossed 6th or 7th cranial nerve paralysis and hemiparesis
Bilateral numbness	Decreased hearing
Deafness or tinnitus	Pseudobulbar palsy
Occipital headache	Quadriparesis
	Bilateral extensor plantar reflexes
	Gait ataxia
	Limb ataxia
	Stupor
	Locked-in syndrome
	Bilateral decreased sense of position in the limbs

of hemianopia or scotomata; the hemianopia often develops suddenly. Memory loss, alexia, and agitated delirium also occur when the lesion is large and includes the temporal lobe territory supplied by the posterior cerebral artery.

Diagnosis

A CBC count, prothrombin time test, and platelet count should be performed and the fibrinogen level measured routinely in every patient who has had a TIA or stroke. ECG and echocardiography are also important, especially for patients with heart disease or cardiac symptoms.

CT and MRI: These tests should be routinely performed for all patients who have had a stroke. CT and MRI can delineate the affected vascular territory when an infarct is present and help differentiate ischemia from hemorrhage. Negative results indicate that the ischemia may be reversible; a large infarct indicates a poor prognosis. The distribution of infarction yields clues to the likely location of the vascular lesion. CT and MRI also can show zones of edema and shifts of intracranial contents.

Ultrasonography: Duplex ultrasonography of the internal carotid and vertebral artery origins in the neck has a high sensitivity and specificity for showing severe occlusive lesions. Color-flow Doppler ultrasonography accurately shows occlusive lesions of these arteries. Transcranial Doppler ultrasonography provides useful information about flow velocities in the major intracranial basilar arteries; it can show whether occlusive extracranial lesions reduce intracranial flow, and it can detect severe occlusive disease in the major intracranial arteries.

Angiography: Computed tomography angiography (CTA) and magnetic resonance angiography (MRA) can be used to screen for extracranial and intracranial occlusive disease and aneurysms. The combination of extracranial and intracranial ultrasonography plus CTA or MRA is very effective in showing most important occlusive lesions in large arteries.

Catheterization angiography is the definitive test for imaging extracranial and intracranial arteries and veins. With small amounts of contrast material, computer-generated high-resolution images can be produced.

In younger patients, angiography is warranted only if surgery is planned or considered. In the elderly, angiography is needed when the clinical examination and noninvasive testing cannot provide a clear diagnosis. However, for many patients, ultrasonography, CTA, and MRA provide sufficient information to preclude the need for angiography or to limit standard angiography to one or two vessels.

Angiography has definite risks (eg, stroke, injury to the artery in which the catheter is placed, allergic reactions); the combined morbidity and mortality rate is about 1%. These tests are particularly risky for patients with diabetes or renal failure. Risks can be minimized by providing adequate hydration and using the smallest amount of dye and the least number of injections needed for accurate diagnosis. The expertise of the angiographer and the information supplied by the responsible clinician are vital to reducing risk. The angiographer begins by injecting the artery most likely to harbor the lesion. When sufficient information is obtained to determine treatment, no further angiography should be performed.

Treatment

General treatment considerations are discussed at the beginning of this chapter.

During the relatively unstable period of a few days to 2 weeks after arterial occlusion, any decrease in brain perfusion should be avoided. Blood pressure should not be lowered unless it is ≥ 170/110 mm Hg, and cardiac output should be maximized. Hypovolemia, a common problem among stroke patients who do not eat and drink enough, should be avoided. Because sitting or standing may worsen the ischemia early in its course, patients should be closely observed, and their blood pressure checked when they first sit or stand. Patients whose neurologic signs fluctuate or worsen usually should remain supine to maximize cerebral blood flow until the instability passes.

There are seven specific treatment options:

Endarterectomy is the procedure of choice if an extracranial artery is severely stenotic (ie, residual lumen < 2 mm). The lesion must be surgically accessible. This procedure is not warranted if the patient has had a severe stroke affecting the area of brain tissue supplied by the artery.

Angioplasty (often with stenting) is used mainly for patients with extracranial carotid or vertebral artery occlusive disease when an artery is severely stenotic and the patient is not a surgical candidate or the arterial lesion is not surgically accessible. Angioplasty is also used for patients with intracranial artery disease when symptoms of brain ischemia in the territory of the stenotic artery persist despite maximal medical treatment.

Thrombolysis is an option when patients can be treated soon after the onset of symptoms of brain ischemia and when an arterial occlusion is identified by diagnostic tests (CTA, MRA, extracranial and transcranial ultrasonography, or catheterization angiography) before extensive brain infarction has occurred. IV thrombolysis is used when intracranial branch arteries are occluded, but it is ineffective for carotid artery occlusion. Intra-arterial thrombolysis is often effective for patients with intracranial vertebral, basilar, or middle cerebral artery occlusions. Thrombolysis poses a risk of brain hemorrhage and is contraindicated in patients with uncontrolled hypertension, bleeding disorders, or large infarcts.

Short-term (2- to 3-week) heparin therapy is prescribed for patients with complete occlusion of large arteries. Low-molecular-weight heparins or heparinoids can be used instead of heparin. These drugs prevent propagation and embolization of a clot, allowing the loosely adherent thrombus to become organized on the vascular wall and collateral circulation to become well established.

Low-molecular-weight heparins have a more favorable bioavailability and pharmacokinetic profile than standard heparin. They are thought to cause fewer hemorrhagic complications than standard heparin because they have a less pronounced effect on platelet function and vascular permeability. They also cause fewer cases of thrombocytopenia, skin necrosis, and white-clot syndromes.

Heparins may also be used when the neurologic signs are fluctuating, the occluding lesion is undefined, or definitive information is not yet available. Heparin should be given in a continuous IV infusion, keeping the activated partial thromboplastin time at 1.5 to 2 times the control value. Low-molecular-weight heparins and heparinoids can be given intravenously or subcutaneously.

Warfarin should be started 2 to 4 days after initiation of heparin and is usually continued for 1 to 3 months. Longer-term warfarin therapy should be used when the vascular lesion is severely stenotic and inaccessible (eg, in the internal carotid artery siphon or middle cerebral artery) or the patient is not a candidate for or declines surgery. The international normalized ratio (INR) should be kept between 2 and 3.5. Warfarin is most effective in preventing red clots, composed of erythrocytes and thrombin, which may form in regions of very reduced blood flow (eg, severely stenotic arteries or veins or dilated cardiac chambers). Warfarin is continued as long as the condition that promotes red clots persists.

Antiplatelet drugs, such as aspirin, are prescribed when the vascular lesion is not severely stenotic. The optimal dose is undetermined; 1.3 g/day in divided doses (eg, 325 mg qid, 650 mg bid) has been effective in trials, but 300 to 325 mg/day is probably just as effective. Theoretically, 100 mg/day might work as well, if not better. Clopidogrel, another drug that affects platelet aggregation and function, is given in a dose of 75 mg/day to patients who cannot take aspirin. Clopidogrel is as effective as ticlopidine and has less hematologic toxicity. Aspirin and other antiplatelet drugs are used to prevent white clots, composed of fibrin-platelet clumps that form on irregular surfaces in areas with fast-moving blood flow (eg, craggy plaques in nonstenosed arteries). Dipyridamole alone has not been shown to be effective, but a combination of aspirin 25 mg bid and modified-release dipyridamole 200 mg bid has been shown to be effective. Drugs that inhibit the platelet glycoprotein IIb/IIIa complex and its binding to fibrinogen have been developed; they include abciximab, which consists of monoclonal antibodies to the complex; eptifibatide, which is a cyclic peptide; and lamifiban and tirofiban, which are parenteral nonpeptide mimetics. Platelet glycoprotein IIb/IIIa inhibitors may be able to lyse white clots and to prevent their formation.

Extracranial-intracranial bypass surgery may be performed, but its indications are undetermined. In one major study, the procedure was no better than medical therapy for most patients with an inaccessible occlusive vascular lesion in the anterior circulation. Bypass may be considered for isolated patients who have been thoroughly investigated, who have persistent hypoperfusion and brain ischemia, and who are refractory to medical treatment.

PENETRATING ARTERY DISEASE

(Lacunar Infarcts)

Small, deep infarcts caused by occlusion of penetrating brain arteries.

The small arteries that penetrate deeper brain structures (eg, basal gray nuclei, internal capsule, thalamus, pons) are especially susceptible to degenerative changes caused by hypertension: Medial hypertrophy, fibrinoid changes, and lipohyalinosis gradually narrow the lumens of these arteries, impeding blood flow. Plaques within arteries, blocking or extending into the orifices of penetrating arteries, and microatheromas are more common among patients with diabetes. A high Hct causes increased blood viscosity, which increases the risk of lacunar infarction and large artery occlusion. When a penetrating artery becomes occluded, a small, deep infarct (lacune) results. Lacunes are < 2 cm at their greatest diameter and affect only deeper structures. Microatheromas or microdissections may occlude the origin of the penetrating arteries, causing infarcts in identical distributions. Lacunes are relatively more common in the posterior circulation; prevalence increases with age but does not appear to be correlated with race or sex.

Symptoms and Signs

Because the lesions are small and deep, patients do not have symptoms related to vasodilation or increased intracranial pressure (eg, headache, vomiting, decreased alertness). The clinical syndrome develops over a short period, usually in < 1 week. Although less common in penetrating artery disease than in large-artery atherosclerosis, TIAs are characteristic and brief. The most common syndromes are pure motor hemiparesis and pure sensory stroke (see TABLE 44–8). Often,

TABLE 44–8.   LACUNAR SYNDROMES

Syndrome	Symptoms and Signs
Ataxic hemiparesis	Unilateral combined ataxia and weakness with exaggerated arm or leg reflexes and Babinski's sign
Dysarthria—clumsy hand syndrome	Slurred speech; facial and tongue weakness with ipsilateral clumsiness of the hand; increased reflexes and Babinski's sign
Hemiataxia	Unilateral incoordination, often with abnormal gait
Hemiparkinsonism or hemidystonia	Unilateral abnormal posture, tone, and movement
Pure dysarthria	Dysarthria, sometimes with dysphagia and without other findings
Pure motor hemiparesis	Unilateral weakness of the face, arm, and leg, usually with exaggerated reflexes and Babinski's sign; dysarthria without dysphagia and without cognitive or behavioral abnormalities
Pure sensory stroke	Unilateral paresthesias, dysesthesias, or numbness of the face, arm, leg, and trunk; no accompanying weakness, ataxia, hemianopia, or cognitive or behavioral abnormalities
Sensory stroke limited to the face	Similar to those of pure sensory stroke but limited to the face

the symptoms are subtle, so the patient and family members may not notice every event. Symptoms often result from the cumulative effects of multiple lacunes. Multiple lacunes may lead to dementia❶ or parkinsonism.❷

When lacunes are located deep in the cerebral hemisphere, weakness or numbness is not accompanied by hemianopia, visual field loss or neglect, or abnormal cognitive function or behavior. When the brain stem is involved, the signs are seldom limited to dysfunction of tegmental structures (cranial nerve nuclei and eye movements).

Diagnosis

A typical patient has a history of hypertension or diabetes, rapidly evolving symptoms, and signs characteristic of one of the lacunar syndromes (see TABLE 44–8). CT or MRI shows lacunes or no relevant lesion. With this combination of findings, no further testing is needed. Lacunes may not be visible on CT or MRI scans.

EEGs are rarely helpful, usually showing normal function or minor symmetric abnormalities. Computed tomography angiography and magnetic resonance angiography usually show normal results or unrelated regions of stenosis. Catheterization angiography is usually not indicated for patients with typical lacunar infarcts.

Treatment

Hypertension should be controlled when the patient is no longer vulnerable to ischemia. For the first 1 to (at most) 3 weeks, changes in position, blood pressure, blood volume, and blood flow can increase the ischemic deficit. Because deep penetrating arteries are end vessels, any decrease in flow through adjacent arteries can enlarge the infarct. Blood pressure should be immediately lowered only when it is > 200/120 mm Hg, although several weeks after the acute event, normotension is the goal. Blood glucose levels should be controlled in patients with diabetes. Phlebotomy is important for patients with a Hct of > 45%. Reduction of blood fibrinogen levels may help prevent the development of other lacunes and ischemic damage to white matter. Patients who smoke should be encouraged to stop.

BRAIN EMBOLIZATION

Emboli can arise from the aortic arch or from plaques or dissections in the proximal portions of the large extracranial and intracranial arteries. The heart is also a common source of emboli, especially among the

---

❶ see page 367   ❷ see page 432

elderly. The most important cardiac causes of cerebral embolization are all varieties of valvular heart disease, myocardial ischemia, and atrial fibrillation. (Epidemiologic and clinical findings are the same as those for large-vessel atherosclerosis.■)

Symptoms and Signs

Neurologic symptoms usually begin abruptly, often while the patient is awake and active. Most often, the deficit is maximal at or near onset, because the sudden blockage of a distal artery does not allow adequate time for collateral circulation to become established. When emboli pass distally, the deficit may worsen or improve. Stepwise worsening usually occurs within 48 hours. When angiography is performed > 2 days after the onset of symptoms, emboli are usually no longer visible in intracranial arteries. In the anterior circulation, emboli most often reach branches of the anterior and middle cerebral arteries. In the posterior circulation, emboli most often reach the long circumferential cerebellar arteries and branches of the posterior cerebral arteries. When emboli cause a large infarct, headache and decreased alertness are common. Neurologic signs are identical to those of large-vessel atherosclerosis.■

Diagnosis

CT and MRI usually show superficial wedge-shaped infarcts in the cerebral hemisphere or cerebellum in the territories of the anterior cerebral, middle cerebral, posterior cerebral, or cerebellar arteries. Many infarcts, some unexpected, scattered in different vascular territories, may be detected. Ultrasonography, computed tomography angiography, and magnetic resonance angiography show embolic sources within the proximal extracranial arteries. Angiography shows abrupt distal cutoff of intracranial branch arteries without underlying local atherostenosis, filling defects in the form of thromboemboli, and proximal regions of atherostenosis.

ECG may be useful for detecting myocardial ischemia, chamber hypertrophy, or arrhythmias. Echocardiography detects valvular heart disease, regions of decreased contractility, tumors such as myxomas, and chamber hypertrophy. Holter monitoring can detect intermittent arrhythmias.

Treatment

Specific medical treatment may be available for the cardiac disorder—eg, antiarrhythmic drugs or coronary vasodilators for ischemia. Some cardiac lesions require surgical correction.

■ see page 402   ■ see page 403

Thrombolytic treatment[1] can be given if the patient is seen soon after the embolic event and the thromboembolus is blocking an intracranial artery. **Anticoagulants**[2] are usually indicated when the patient is vulnerable to further emboli. For some patients (eg, those with recent myocardial infarction or reversible arrhythmia), this risk is transient; for others (eg, those with intractable atrial fibrillation), it is lifelong. With heparin, the partial thromboplastin time should be kept to 1.5 to 2 times the control value. Heparin is gradually replaced with warfarin for long-term therapy; the INR should be kept between 2 and 3.5. Anticoagulants are contraindicated if the infarct is large or if the patient is hypertensive, unless blood pressure can be reduced without increasing the neurologic deficit.

If patients with artificial valves develop new emboli while taking warfarin, the addition of dipyridamole (75 to 100 mg po qid) or another antiplatelet drug may be helpful.[3] Investigation of the risk/benefit ratio of prophylactic anticoagulation for patients with potential cardiac embolic sources (eg, atrial fibrillation) has shown that warfarin is indicated for most patients with atrial fibrillation. Warfarin plus dipyridamole may produce less bleeding than warfarin plus aspirin, but dipyridamole may cause orthostatic hypotension in the elderly.

SYSTEMIC HYPOPERFUSION

Brain ischemia due to inadequate cardiac output with systemic hypoperfusion can be caused by acute myocardial infarction, cardiac arrest, and life-threatening ventricular arrhythmias. Less common causes are pulmonary embolism, acute gastrointestinal or systemic bleeding, and shock.

Symptoms, Signs, and Diagnosis

Most often, the patient is pale, sweating, and hypotensive when first examined. Neurologic dysfunction is usually abrupt in onset and follows systemic symptoms related to the underlying disorder. The most prominent findings are decreased alertness and symmetric depression of hemispheric functions.

When ischemia is severe, brain stem function may be abnormal and brain stem reflexes (pupillary, corneal, doll's eye, and pharyngeal) may be absent. Bilateral weakness or decorticate or decerebrate rigidity indicates that the motor system is involved. The arms may be most severely affected, with relative sparing of the face and legs—a distribution described as "a man in a barrel." Severe or prolonged impairment of cerebral perfusion usually results in coma. When stupor lightens, patients may have deficits in visual function and memory. CT results

---

[1] see page 410   [2] see also page 697   [3] see page 411

are usually normal during the acute period in all but the most severely affected patients, but EEGs usually show severe bilateral slowing.

Prognosis and Treatment

Loss of brain stem reflexes for > 24 hours indicates a poor prognosis, as does persistent coma. Treatment is directed at the underlying cardiac or systemic process.

HEMORRHAGIC STROKE

Bleeding into brain tissue or meningeal spaces.

Intracranial hemorrhage accounts for about 20% of strokes. Intracranial hemorrhage is most often caused by aneurysms, vascular malformations, bleeding disorders, hypertension, amyloid angiopathy, and use of illicit drugs.

SUBARACHNOID HEMORRHAGE

Bleeding into the subarachnoid space.

Subarachnoid hemorrhage accounts for about 10% of all strokes but for a much higher percentage of deaths due to stroke. Subarachnoid hemorrhage increases the pressure within the cranium, impairs the drainage of cerebrospinal fluid (CSF), and irritates the arteries at the base of the brain. The blood is usually released quickly into the subarachnoid space at arterial pressure and becomes widely dispersed around the brain and spinal cord. Delayed vasoconstriction of the cerebral arteries, beginning ≥ 48 hours after hemorrhage and possibly continuing for ≥ 1 week, is common. Vasoconstriction with delayed brain ischemia is likely when the hemorrhage is large or produces thick focal collections of blood.

Etiology

The most common causes are vascular malformations, cerebral aneurysms, bleeding disorders (most often due to use of anticoagulants), head trauma, and amyloid angiopathy (degenerative hyalinization of the arteries in the brain and subarachnoid spaces). Vascular malformations rarely cause subarachnoid hemorrhage in elderly patients. Aneurysms occur in the elderly but slightly less commonly than in younger persons. Also, vascular malformations and saccular aneurysms are less likely to be life threatening in persons > 60; dangerous ones have usually ruptured before that age.

Head trauma, common among the elderly because of their tendency to fall, is often undiagnosed. After a fall, patients are often confused or amnesic and cannot clearly describe the event. The physician may incorrectly attribute blood in CSF to a spontaneous subarachnoid hemorrhage rather than to trauma, thus needlessly performing angiography to search for aneurysms. Amyloid angiopathy can cause subarachnoid or intracerebral hemorrhage. Patients often have multiple, recurrent bleeding episodes. Dementia may coexist because of Alzheimer-like changes in the cortex.

Symptoms and Signs

Symptoms and signs of subarachnoid hemorrhage are no different in the elderly than in younger patients. Patients invariably have headache. Headache often begins suddenly, usually during physical activity, and becomes severe almost immediately. The pain is usually diffuse, but at times it is most severe at the back of the head and neck and may radiate down the back or down the lower limbs in a sciatic pattern. Nausea and vomiting, due to the sudden increase in intracranial pressure, are common. Usually, patients cannot perform any activity and often become restless, agitated, and confused.

At presentation, patients are usually not paralyzed and often do not have important focal neurologic signs (eg, hemiparesis, hemisensory loss, hemianopia). During physical examination, the most apparent abnormality is usually a change in the level of consciousness, resulting in restlessness, delirium, sleepiness, stupor, or coma. Stiff neck, difficulty concentrating, impaired short-term memory, and impaired extensor plantar reflexes are also common.

Vasoconstriction may occur after surgical manipulation of the arteries, especially if blood is released into the subarachnoid space during or after the procedure. If vasoconstriction and delayed brain ischemia develop, focal signs (eg, hemiparesis) can occur and are, with headache and decreased alertness, the most common findings.

Cardiac arrhythmias, hydrocephalus, and rebleeding are common complications.

Diagnosis

The approach to diagnosis is the same for elderly and for younger patients. The most important diagnostic tests are CT, lumbar puncture, and angiography. MRI may be used instead of CT. When performed within 24 to 48 hours of hemorrhage, unenhanced CT scans are likely to show blood as hyperdensity in the cisterns, between the cerebral gyri, or in the ventricles. Subarachnoid hemorrhages that are small or that occurred days before may not be visible. CT can also detect small contusions, subdural hematomas, and skull fractures; sometimes, enhanced CT can detect an aneurysm. Restlessness and agitation interfere with the patient's ability to cooperate during cranial CT and thus may compromise quality.

All symptomatic patients have grossly visible blood-stained CSF under increased pressure when lumbar puncture is performed within hours or a few days of the hemorrhage. If patients have severe unexplained headache, CT is usually performed before lumbar puncture. However, if patients have no focal neurologic signs or papilledema and can walk normally, a lumbar puncture can be safely performed without CT.

Computed tomography angiography and magnetic resonance angiography are also useful for finding large aneurysms, but standard catheter angiography is the definitive test for determining their location, size, and shape. If the diagnosis of subarachnoid hemorrhage has been confirmed, angiography is usually delayed until the patient is fit for surgery.

In patients with vasoconstriction, CT scans show no new bleeding but may show a hypodense area of cerebral infarction. Angiography shows general or focal vasoconstriction. Transcranial Doppler ultrasonography, which can measure blood flow velocities in intracranial arteries, is very useful for detecting vasoconstriction and monitoring its severity. CT or lumbar puncture can detect rebleeding.

Treatment

When the cause is an aneurysm or vascular malformation, the involved vessels are clipped or coated before the next bleeding episode. When the cause is use of warfarin, hypoprothrombinemia must be quickly reversed with vitamin K or fresh frozen plasma. When the cause is head trauma, immediate evaluation and treatment of accompanying brain contusions, hematomas, and lacerations are necessary.

All patients should be monitored in a quiet room. Dehydration should be avoided, because it can lead to decreased cerebral blood flow. The sudden increase in intracranial pressure may increase systemic blood pressure; severe hypertension (> 170/110 mm Hg) should be controlled. However, because increased intracranial pressure increases venous pressure in the brain and in the dural venous sinuses, systemic blood pressure must exceed this elevated venous pressure if the brain is to be perfused.

Corticosteroids help control increased intracranial pressure and brain swelling. For example, dexamethasone 10 mg IV may be given, followed by 4 to 20 mg IV or IM q 6 h until response is maximal, then switching to oral corticosteroids. When vasoconstriction is present, both nimodipine and hypervolemic therapy should be considered.

INTRACEREBRAL HEMORRHAGE

Bleeding directly into the brain.

Bleeding destroys brain tissue because of effects of local pressure. Intracerebral hemorrhage accounts for about 10% of all strokes but for a much higher percentage of deaths due to stroke. After age 60, intracerebral hemorrhage is more common than subarachnoid hemorrhage.

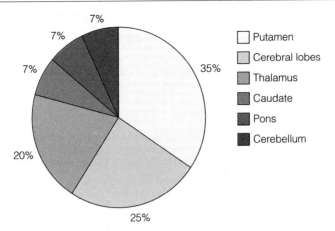

FIGURE 44–3.   Location of intracerebral hemorrhages. Percentages are approximate.

Usually, intracerebral hemorrhage arises from small arteries or arterioles.

Hypertension and coexisting degenerative changes due to aging increase susceptibility to intracerebral hemorrhage in the elderly. Bleeding disorders and use of anticoagulants pose additional risk and more often result in death than does intracerebral hemorrhage due to other conditions. Amyloid angiopathy contributes to up to 20% of intracerebral hemorrhages in patients > 70. Aneurysms and vascular malformations are uncommon causes. Occasionally, bleeding occurs into a previously unsuspected brain tumor, especially if it is metastatic.

Location of hemorrhage varies (see FIGURE 44–3). Warfarin-induced hemorrhages tend to occur in the lobes of the cerebrum and the cerebellum; they begin more insidiously and progress more gradually than hemorrhages due to other conditions. Hemorrhages due to amyloid angiopathy are almost always lobar. Traumatic hematomas are usually multiple. They are located on the surface of the brain, commonly on the orbital frontal lobes and tips of the temporal lobes, which are close to the rough bony ridges at the base of the skull.

Symptoms, Signs, and Diagnosis

The earliest symptoms result from loss of function subserved by the brain region in which the hemorrhage occurs. For example, hemorrhage into the left putamen and internal capsule causes right limb paralysis; hemorrhage in the right occipital lobe causes a left visual field defect; and cerebellar hemorrhage causes an inability to walk. The hemorrhage may expand within minutes, or at most a few hours, and act as a mass, increasing intracranial contents and pressure and causing headache, vomiting, and decreased alertness. However, these symptoms may not

TABLE 44-9. SIGNS OF INTRACEREBRAL HEMORRHAGE

Site	Signs
Putamen	Contralateral hemiparesis, hemisensory loss, and at times hemianopia; conjugate deviation of the eyes to the side of the hemorrhage; normal pupil size and reaction
Left	Aphasia
Right	Left-sided visual neglect
Thalamus	Contralateral hemisensory loss with slight hemiparesis or hemiataxia; deviation of the eyes downward or downward and inward; reduced vertical gaze; small, poorly reactive pupils
Caudate nucleus	Slight transient contralateral hemiparesis; restlessness and confusion; occasionally, ipsilateral Horner's syndrome
Lobe	
Frontal	Decreased spontaneity; contralateral Babinski's sign
Parietal	Contralateral hemisensory loss and hemineglect
Left	Reading and writing deficits; aphasia
Temporal	Agitation and contralateral upper quadrantanopia
Left	Wernicke's fluent aphasia
Occipital	Contralateral hemianopia
Pons	Quadriparesis; reduced alertness; no horizontal gaze; small reactive pupils (some pontine hemorrhages affect the tegmentum or base unilaterally, causing hemiparesis and crossed cranial nerve signs)
Cerebellum	Gait ataxia; vomiting; sometimes ipsilateral conjugate gaze paresis or 6th nerve palsy

occur if the hemorrhage remains small. Nearly 50% of elderly patients with small to moderate intracerebral hemorrhages do not have headache and remain alert because previous atrophy in the brain provides additional space to accommodate the extra contents. On examination, signs of focal abnormality of brain function are apparent (see TABLE 44-9).

If intracerebral hemorrhage progresses, consciousness usually decreases and focal neurologic signs increase. For example, on admission, a patient with a right putamenal hemorrhage may have left hemiparesis, conjugate deviation of the eyes to the right, an extensor left plantar reflex, and normal pupils. If the hematoma expands or the region surrounding the hematoma becomes edematous, the right plantar reflex may become extensor, the eyes may not move horizontally in either direction, the right pupil may become dilated and fixed, and stupor may develop. Without aggressive treatment, patients whose condition worsens in this manner have a high mortality rate.

On CT scans, hematomas appear as white, hyperdense, well-circumscribed lesions. CT can also show location and size, drainage into the ventricles or onto the brain's surface, shifts of intracranial contents, and unsuspected tumors or vascular malformation adjacent to the hematoma. If the patient is anemic, the hematoma may appear hypodense or may have a fluid level. MRI shows the extent and dissection of the hemorrhage in the coronal and sagittal planes better than CT. MRI and magnetic resonance angiography can show vascular malformations. Differentiation between hemorrhage and ischemia is less obvious on routine MRI scans than on CT scans. Fluid-attenuating inversion recovery and gradient-echo susceptibility MRI (sensitive to the presence of iron-containing compounds and calcium) are often required to detect very recent hemorrhages. MRI clearly shows hemosiderin from old hemorrhages.

Treatment

Patients with large hemorrhages usually die before treatment can be initiated. Those with small hemorrhages, which are self-contained and self-limited, require little treatment except preventive measures (eg, controlling hypertension). Although severe hypertension ($>$ 170/100 mm Hg) should be controlled, blood pressure should not be reduced to normal levels, because doing so could compromise cerebral perfusion. Corticosteroids and osmotic drugs (eg, mannitol, glycerol) may help control increased intracranial pressure (see TABLE 44–10). Moderate-sized (2- to 4-cm) hematomas are the most important to treat, especially if the patient's condition is worsening.

Surgical drainage of an expanding hematoma can be lifesaving. However, because surgical drainage substitutes a cavity for the hematoma, it does not diminish the extent of paralysis or other focal abnormalities. For these reasons, neurologic examination should be repeated frequently in patients with new intracerebral hemorrhages. Repeated CT scans often show enlargement of the hematoma and increased pressure effects.

Thalamic and pontine hematomas are not accessible surgically. Surgical decompression is most feasible for cerebellar hemorrhages and lobar hematomas near the brain surface. Some hematomas can be

TABLE 44–10.   **TREATMENT OF INCREASED INTRACRANIAL PRESSURE**

Medical	Surgical
Intubation and mechanical hyperventilation	Drainage of hematoma or large infarct
Dexamethasone 10 mg IV or IM initially, then 4 mg IM, IV, or po q 6 h	Ventricular drainage or shunt
Mannitol (500 g in 500 mL of 5% dextrose in water) 1–2 g/kg over 10–20 min initially, then 50–300 mg/kg IV q 6 h	Excision of bleeding vascular malformation
Glycerin (glycerol) 1–2 g/kg po q 6 h	Repair of aneurysm

drained stereotactically, using a burr hole, rather than by craniotomy. Local instillation of a fibrinolytic drug can make the hematoma more liquid and facilitate stereotactic drainage.

SUBDURAL HEMATOMA

Accumulation of blood between the dura mater and the arachnoid, usually from bleeding of the bridging veins.

Subdural hematomas develop when blunt head trauma causes brain motion within the skull, shearing off the bridging veins between the brain's surface and adjacent dural venous sinuses. The blood leaks and accumulates slowly. The resulting subdural hematoma may be absorbed spontaneously or, after about 2 weeks, may become encapsulated with a liquefied center. The vascular outer membrane of the hematoma may continue to bleed, causing the center to enlarge.

Etiology

Subdural hematomas may be acute (due to severe head trauma) or chronic (usually due to minor trauma). Chronic subdural hematomas typically occur in elderly persons taking anticoagulants or in alcoholics who have some degree of brain atrophy. Other causes include falls, bleeding disorders, and, occasionally, lumbar puncture. Some subdural hematomas occur without previous trauma. Some patients forget a fall or other trauma or consider it too inconsequential to mention. Often, a fall causes retrograde amnesia, and patients may not be fully aware of the injury.

Symptoms and Signs

The most common findings are headache, decreased alertness, and abnormalities of hemispheric function. Headache, usually ipsilateral to the hematoma, may worsen at night. Drowsiness and decreased alertness are due to increased intracranial pressure. Slight weakness, hyperreflexia, and Babinski's sign in the contralateral limbs are common. Patients with a left-sided hematoma may have slight aphasia, and patients with a right-sided hematoma may have right-sided spatial neglect. Usually, neurologic abnormalities are mild. Seizures may occur, probably indicating contusion of underlying brain tissue. As the hematoma enlarges, headache worsens and the level of consciousness often decreases. An ipsilateral Babinski's sign and ipsilateral 3rd-nerve paresis may develop, indicating midbrain compression.

In alcoholic patients with brain atrophy, bleeding often persists, causing headaches, behavioral changes, an altered level of consciousness, and focal neurologic deficits (eg, hemiparesis).

Diagnosis

Elderly patients with behavioral and neurologic abnormalities (including dementia) should be screened for hematomas, a treatable cause of such abnormalities.

For patients with a history of head trauma, the diagnosis is usually obvious. Chronic subdural hematomas, whose symptoms develop insidiously, must be distinguished from vascular dementia, brain tumor, and brain abscess, especially if patients provide no history of trauma. Subdural hematomas can be distinguished from brain infarcts and intracranial hematomas, whose symptoms and signs usually begin more acutely and include more severe focal deficits.

Neuroimaging is necessary to confirm the diagnosis. On a CT scan, an acute subdural hematoma appears as a sickle-shaped, hyperdense lesion over the outer surface of the brain, lying against the inner surface of the skull and dura. A subacute (lasting 7 to 14 days) subdural hematoma appears isodense in relation to the brain, making diagnosis difficult. During the acute period, a T1-weighted MRI can help because it can detect a high-signal-intensity lesion in the subdural space. A chronic subdural hematoma appears hypodense on CT scans.

Prognosis and Treatment

Patients with an acute subdural hematoma have a poor prognosis. The mortality rate for patients treated for an acute subdural hematoma is about 50%. If a chronic subdural hematoma is recognized and treated, the prognosis is good and is related primarily to the degree of associated brain injury.

Subdural hematomas are surgically evacuated. However, small ones may heal spontaneously without medical treatment. In elderly patients and patients with brain atrophy, reexpansion of the compressed brain may be delayed. Because subdural bleeding may recur, a drain must be left in for several days and the patient must be monitored closely for bleeding.

45　SPEECH DISORDERS

Speech is a complex process involving visual and auditory input, central processing, and motor output, not only to the vocal muscles but also to the facial muscles. The facial muscles produce expression and are thus an integral part of vocal communication.

The central processing of speech is also very complex, with input from primary and secondary visual and auditory areas, integration in the association areas (eg, Broca's area for word formation, Wernicke's area for language comprehension), and output through the primary and secondary motor areas. Moreover, the function of the same areas differs between the dominant and the nondominant hemispheres. Nonetheless, it is possible to associate lesions in certain areas with particular speech defects.

AGING AND SPEECH

Speech patterns change with age: The voice becomes deeper and may develop an increasing tremor, speech becomes slower and may develop an abnormal prosody, and enunciation of consonants becomes imprecise. There is a slight increase in laryngeal muscle tension (glottal fold tension), which results in spasmodic dysphonia, and glottal air loss, which results in fewer syllables per breath. As age increases, some healthy elderly persons, even those without cognitive impairment, tend to use fewer words and may make semantic errors. Speech and language disorders affect 3 to 4% of persons > 65 years.

Evaluation of language function (see TABLE 45–1) includes assessment of language production (speaking, writing) and comprehension (listening, reading). In addition, evaluation of word-finding ability should include the use of circumlocutory phrases (eg, "what you use to tell time" for "clock"); nonspecific words (eg, "thing" or "stuff"); incorrect words (paraphasia), including phonemic paraphasia (eg, "trable"

TABLE 45–1. FACTORS ASSESSED DURING EVALUATION OF LANGUAGE FUNCTION

Factor	Manifestation
Mechanical processes of speech	Respiration; phonation; resonance; articulation; prosody
Spontaneous speech	Rate of word output; effort required to initiate speech; length of phrases
Word-finding ability	Ability to name objects and parts of objects
Repetition of words and phrases	Gradual progression from monosyllabic words to multisyllabic words and phrases
Writing ability	Mechanical problems (eg, tremor), which should be differentiated from linguistic difficulties
Oral comprehension	Ability to follow spoken commands, answer yes-or-no questions, and identify named objects
Reading comprehension	Ability to read aloud and to answer questions about the text (history of dyslexia or a learning disorder is noted)

for "table") and semantic paraphasia (eg, "headman" for "president"); or jargon (eg, "gabbagabbahey" for "pin"). If poor auditory or visual function is noted, further testing is required. Impaired respiratory function (eg, shortness of breath) can also interfere with normal speech patterns. Thus, pulmonary function testing and breathing exercises may be indicated.

APHASIA

A defect or loss of language function in which the comprehension or expression of words (or nonverbal equivalents of words) is impaired as a result of injury to or degeneration of the language centers in the cerebral cortex.

Aphasia is the most common speech disorder among the elderly, followed by dysarthria. Aphasia occurs in about 40% of patients with stroke that affects the left hemisphere (where the cortical language centers reside in about 95% of right-handed persons and in about 60% of left-handed persons). Aphasia may be classified as receptive, in which expression is better than comprehension; expressive, in which comprehension is better than expression; or global, in which comprehension and expression are both impaired (see TABLE 45–2). Some authorities use the terms mixed aphasia and global aphasia interchangeably. However, in general, mixed aphasia refers to less severe global aphasia. Other classifications exist, an indication that aphasia is never purely receptive or purely expressive. No classification is completely satisfactory.

Recovery from aphasia, if it occurs, is most pronounced during the first 3 months after brain injury. Rehabilitation focuses on establishing the most effective means of communication. For mildly impaired patients, a context-centered approach that emphasizes ideas and thoughts rather than words is effective. For more impaired patients, the stimulation approach (repetitive presentation of linguistic stimuli) and the programmed stimulation approach (a learning process that uses tactile, visual, and linguistic stimuli for reacquiring language behavior) may be effective. For severely impaired patients, speech-language drills and practice (eg, repetition) are generally ineffective. Patients and caregivers may be able to convey messages by pointing to images in a photography or picture book or by using a communication board or another augmentative device. Bilingual or multilingual aphasic patients are likely to regain their native language first and may not regain their secondary language skills.

Family members and friends usually can provide essential therapy at home (see TABLE 45–3), but they may experience stress, frustration,

TABLE 45–2.   TYPES OF SPEECH DISORDERS

Disorder	Cause	Speech Pattern
Receptive aphasia (sensory, fluent)	Lesion in parietal or temporal lobe due to infarction, tumor, or herpes simplex encephalitis	Fluent speech with jargon and word substitution, poor auditory comprehension, normal (usually) speech production
Expressive aphasia (motor, nonfluent)	Cortical or precortical lesion in prefrontal or frontal region due to hemorrhage, infarction, or tumor	Slow speech (< 50 words/min) with great effort or no speech, use of one- or two-word phrases, poor articulation, difficulty with speech production, abnormal prosody, good comprehension, inability to write sentences verbatim
Global aphasia	Large lesion in dominant frontal, parietal, or superior temporal lobe due to infarction, injury, or tumor	Minimal speech, poor comprehension of written and spoken language
Ataxic dysarthria	Cerebellar lesion (eg, cerebellar atrophy, multiple sclerosis)	Slow, staccato, jerky speech; irregular separation of syllables; imprecise enunciation; poor coordination of speech and respiration
Flaccid dysarthria	Disorder of lower motor neurons or neuromuscular transmission (eg, myasthenia gravis, bulbar palsy, peripheral neuropathies)	A breathy voice and audible inhalation; difficulty with vibratives (eg, "R"); inability to pronounce lingual and labial consonants; nasal quality due to palatal weakness
Hyperkinetic dysarthria	Lesion of the extrapyramidal motor system, possibly in the subthalamic nucleus	Abnormal, random, involuntary movement of muscles used in articulation
Hypokinetic dysarthria	Extrapyramidal disease	Hesitation, loss of vocal inflection, irregular speech, monotonous tone, poor articulation, diminished voice volume
Spastic dysarthria	Lesions along the corticobulbar tract	Slow, labored articulation; imprecise consonants; a strained voice quality; low and monotone pitch; hypernasality
Mixed dysarthria	Degeneration of the upper and lower motor neuron system	Variable symptoms, depending on the dominant type
Verbal apraxia	Lesion in the parieto-occipital area	Difficulty initiating speech, inconsistent articulation errors

TABLE 45-3. GOALS FOR CAREGIVERS OF PATIENTS WITH APHASIA

To be patient at all times

To communicate through simple sentences but not baby talk

To establish safety precautions for patients who may be unable to call for help

To use gestures and pointing to supplement speech

To ask patients questions that require only yes or no answers (patients can nod or shake the head in response)

To avoid interrupting patients who are speaking slowly

and even anger. The physician and speech pathologist can help family members and friends understand that aphasia is a speech disorder, not a mental illness.

DYSARTHRIA

An inability to articulate words properly (eg, incoordinated speech, slow response) due to disturbances in muscular control caused by damage to the central or peripheral nervous system.

Dysarthria is the second most common speech disorder among elderly patients. It may be ataxic, flaccid, hyperkinetic, hypokinetic, spastic, or mixed (see TABLE 45-2). Causes include poor coordination of the lips, tongue, palate, vocal cords, or respiratory muscles due to neurologic diseases (eg, stroke, head trauma, cranial surgery, amyotrophic lateral sclerosis, multiple sclerosis, cranial nerve palsies) and to lesions that affect the speech mechanism (eg, vocal cord tumors).

Despite abnormalities in several or all of the basic mechanical processes of speech (respiration, phonation, resonance, articulation, and prosody), patients produce approximate sounds in the correct arrangement. Because language function is generally intact, patients typically can read and write.

Rehabilitation goals depend on the cause of dysarthria. If the cause is an acute neurologic episode (eg, stroke, head trauma, surgery), the goal is to restore and preserve speech. If the cause is a chronic progressive neurologic disease (eg, amyotrophic lateral sclerosis, multiple sclerosis), the goal is to maintain premorbid function as long as possible. However, as dysarthria worsens, speech must be modified (often through practice) to control rate, consonant emphasis, and articulation. In very severe cases, communication may need to be augmented with devices such as a letter board, picture board, or specially designed electronic devices. If the cause is a lesion affecting the mechanical processes of speech (eg, a vocal cord tumor), specific treatment such as surgery should be considered.

VERBAL APRAXIA

Impairment in the production of phonemes (the basic sound units of spoken language) due to abnormality in initiation, coordination, or sequencing of muscle movements.

Verbal apraxia in the elderly is generally caused by brain damage (eg, as a result of stroke, head injury, or surgery). Patients with verbal apraxia can move the muscles involved in speech but have difficulty speaking due to diminished volitional control of muscles. The patient appears to have forgotten how to make the sounds of language. Inconsistency of phonemic error and groping movements of articulation muscles are characteristic of verbal apraxia. Even when muscle weakness, slowness, or incoordination in reflex and automatic response is insignificant, prosody may be abnormal. Verbal apraxia often occurs with aphasia. ◘ Verbal apraxia must be differentiated from dysarthria and nonspeech oral-facial apraxia. Broca's aphasia is loss of memory of motor pattern, which is necessary for speech, without loss of the muscle movement. Thus, in essence, verbal apraxia is Broca's aphasia.

Rehabilitation for patients with verbal apraxia who also have expressive aphasia ◙ involves melodic intonation therapy (use of natural melodic patterns for common phrases to facilitate speech). However, this method may not help apraxic patients with poor auditory comprehension (eg, those who also have receptive aphasia). An alternative approach for patients with verbal apraxia is intensive practice of sound patterns and speech.

46 ▪ MOVEMENT DISORDERS

(Extrapyramidal Disorders)

Abnormal involuntary movements or postures associated with extrapyramidal pathologic change.

Specific movement disorders include tremor, chorea, dystonia, akathisia, hemiballismus, and myoclonus. Movement disorders may be differentiated by their clinical characteristics, including age of onset, rapidity of onset (eg, sudden vs. insidious), family history (ie, presence or absence of a genetic predisposition), distribution and severity of symptoms (whether localized or generalized, mild or severe), specific characteristics of the abnormal movements (eg, twisting, writhing, jerking), and associated symptoms and signs (eg, depression, dementia).

◘see page 425   ◙see page 425

Movement disorders, a clinical term, is often used synonymously with extrapyramidal disorders, a more anatomic term. These motor disorders are associated with pathology that lies outside of the pyramidal tracts, involving the basal ganglia or cerebellum. Much is known about the clinical aspects of movement disorders, but fundamental anatomic, physiologic, and pathogenetic bases are not well understood. However, information about biochemical alterations in the basal ganglia helps in understanding the mechanisms by which symptoms occur and suggests a rational approach to treatment.

The most prominent biochemical feature of the basal ganglia is a high content of putative neurotransmitters, notably acetylcholine, dopamine, and γ-aminobutyric acid. These neurotransmitters are produced and degraded by substrates and enzyme systems located within the basal ganglia. Some neurotransmitters are produced in the part of the basal ganglia in which their actions occur; others are transported by connecting axons from the area where they are produced to the area where their actions occur. For example, dopamine is produced in the pars compacta of the substantia nigra and is transported via a neuronal tract, the nigrostriatal pathway, to the caudate nucleus and putamen, where it acts.

Normal function appears to depend on an exquisite balance between the various neurotransmitters. Disturbances in production, transport, release, action, or degradation result in symptoms specific to the part of the brain in which the neurotransmitter acts. In general, dopamine deficiency facilitates cholinergic hyperactivity, leading to hypokinetic rigid disorders (eg, parkinsonism). Dopamine hyperactivity, cholinergic hypoactivity, or both result in the hyperkinesia that occurs in disorders such as the choreas. Drug treatment can reestablish neurotransmitter balance by enhancing the production, promoting or inhibiting the release, preventing the degradation, or simulating the effects at receptor sites of the specific neurotransmitters involved.

TREMOR

Rhythmic, sinusoidal, oscillatory movements due to rhythmic contractions of reciprocally innervated antagonistic muscles.

The most common tremors in the elderly are essential tremor, cerebellar tremor, and neuropathic tremor. Other types of tremors due to various causes may also occur (see TABLE 46–1).

ESSENTIAL TREMOR

A 4- to 12-Hz (high frequency, low amplitude) tremor that predominantly affects the upper extremities, may also affect the head and voice, and rarely affects the legs.

TABLE 46-1.   CAUSES OF TREMOR*

Cause	Type of Tremor	Comments
Alcoholism	A permanent, generalized tremor (ie, similar to tremulousness)	—
Alcohol withdrawal	A rapid, coarse tremor that involves the entire body	The tremor is characteristically abolished or diminished by a drink of alcohol
Use of drugs	Depending on the drug used, an action tremor or a resting tremor	Action tremor may be due to theophylline, tricyclic antidepressants, terbutaline, metaproterenol, valproic acid, lithium, or caffeine. Resting tremor may be due to antipsychotic drugs
Withdrawal of narcotics only	A fine tremor of the facial muscles and fingers	The tremor is uncommon in the elderly
Hyperthyroidism	A fine, regular, rapid tremor that is usually confined to the outstretched hands and fingers	—
Poisoning by methyl bromide or heavy metals	Depending on the poison, an action tremor or a resting tremor	Action tremor may be due to methyl bromide, mercury, or lead. Resting tremor may be due to manganese
Metabolic encephalopathy	Asterixis, which is characterized by irregular flapping movements of the outstretched hands	Metabolic encephalopathy may be due to liver failure, uremia, or acidosis

*These tremors are treated by treating the underlying cause.

Essential tremor may affect persons of all ages, although its incidence increases markedly with age. It was once referred to as **senile tremor** because it is most prevalent among persons > 60 years; prevalence is 1.3 to 5% in these persons, although some estimates are as high as 22%. The tremor occurs in men and women, and it is slightly more prevalent among whites than among blacks.

Some forms of essential tremor are also referred to as **familial tremor** because, in these cases, the tremor has a genetic basis and clusters within families. Large kindreds have an autosomal dominant form; in a few kindreds, a linkage to regions on chromosomes 2p and 3q has been shown.

The cause is unknown, although positron emission tomography (PET) studies and functional MRI studies suggest involvement of the cerebellum or cerebellar outflow pathways.

Symptoms and Signs

Essential tremor is a chronic condition. In some elderly persons, the tremor remains mild and affects only the upper limbs; in others, the tremor progresses dramatically. It most often involves the upper limbs (eg, affecting the ability to eat or carry objects), followed by the head (eg, making the head shake when unsupported) and the voice (eg, making speech unsteady). It is an action tremor, meaning that it occurs both with sustained arm extension (postural tremor) and with voluntary movements (kinetic tremor) such as writing, drinking from a glass, or touching finger to nose. No associated weakness or alteration in muscle tone is present.

Essential tremor may be made worse by nervousness, embarrassment (which may be due to the tremor), and handling objects in uncomfortable or strained positions. When embarrassing or debilitating, essential tremor may lead to social isolation. Anxiety may exacerbate the tremor.

Essential tremor may be diagnosed in the setting of a moderate to severe action tremor, providing that other causes (eg, hyperthyroidism; drugs such as levothyroxine, lithium, valproic acid, and prednisone; dystonia) have been excluded.

Treatment

Many patients with mild essential tremor need reassurance that they do not have parkinsonism. ◪ To reduce embarrassment caused by the tremor, patients can be advised to hold objects close to the body so as not to drop them, place napkins between cups and saucers to keep them from rattling during use, avoid eating soup in public, and avoid uncomfortable or awkward positions. Drug treatment is not necessary for mild tremor.

Drug treatment or surgery is required for more severe tremor. Alcohol suppresses the tremor, leading some patients to abuse alcohol. However, small amounts used occasionally may be appropriate.

Tremor often does not respond to drugs as well in the elderly as it does in younger adults. β-Blockers (eg, propranolol 20 to 80 mg tid, nadolol 20 to 40 mg/day) may help, but adverse effects (eg, fatigue, depression) may limit the dose. The anticonvulsant primidone (50 to 100 mg qid) is sometimes helpful but can cause drowsiness and confusion. Some patients may also respond to acetazolamide, gabapentin, or clozapine.

Patients with particularly severe and drug-resistant tremor may be candidates for thalamotomy or for high-frequency deep brain (thalamic) stimulation devices, which are available only at special centers.

◪ see page 432

CEREBELLAR TREMOR

A 3- to 5-Hz (low frequency, high amplitude) coarse, irregular tremor that is present during the finger-to-nose maneuver.

This tremor is the result of cerebellar pathology and represents a problem with the force and timing of motion (ataxia) rather than a true regular tremor or oscillation. It is termed an intention tremor because it tends to worsen when the patient approaches a target using the finger. This intentional component may also be a feature of essential tremor. ∎ However, essential tremor and cerebellar tremor differ in the way in which patients miss their target: Patients with essential tremor who miss their target experience regular oscillation between the right and left sides of the target; those with cerebellar tremor often also experience forward and backward movement (ie, overshoot and undershoot), sometimes causing them to slam into the target with inappropriate force. Those with midline cerebellar disease (ie, of the vermis cerebelli) also experience titubation, in which the head or body rocks back and forth while also rotating or moving side to side.

Some patients have a partial response to buspirone hydrochloride or anticholinergic drugs.

NEUROPATHIC TREMOR

A tremor associated with peripheral nerve pathology.

Neuropathic tremor, which is rare, may be a manifestation of peripheral neuropathy due to porphyria, diabetes, excessive alcohol use, uremia, amyloidosis, vincristine therapy, or relapsing polyneuropathy. The mechanism is unclear, but the tremor may result from impaired sensory input to the motor neuron pool. Alternatively, the tremor may be due to weakened muscle or impaired stretch reflexes. Neuropathic tremor is not responsive to propranolol or other therapy.

PARKINSONISM
(Paralysis Agitans)

A syndrome characterized by tremor (low frequency, low amplitude), muscular rigidity, bradykinesia, and loss of postural reflexes.

Parkinsonism, one of the most frequently encountered disorders of the basal ganglia, is a prominent cause of disability in persons > 50.

∎ see page 429

Most cases of parkinsonism are **Parkinson's disease (primary or idiopathic parkinsonism)**. The crude prevalence of Parkinson's disease among all age groups in the USA is about 100 cases per 100,000; the prevalence is about 50% lower among blacks than among whites. The incidence among all age groups is 10 to 20 cases per 100,000. It increases dramatically with age; among persons in their 70s and 80s, the incidence is about 200 cases per 100,000 in the USA and about 1000 to 2000 cases per 100,000 in other countries (Iceland, India, Scotland, Australia). Parkinson's disease most frequently appears between the ages of 50 and 79. A rare juvenile form has been described in persons < 20, and cases may also occur in adults < 50. The disease affects both sexes and all races. In a few cases, the disease clusters within families and may have a genetic basis; in a small number of these cases, the disease has been linked to a region on the long arm of chromosome 4 that encodes the neuronal protein α-synuclein.

Secondary parkinsonism (parkinsonism due to other causes or nonidiopathic parkinsonism) has a different etiology and pathology from Parkinson's disease. It is the predominant clinical manifestation in many disorders (see TABLE 46–2). It is commonly caused by drugs, especially antipsychotics.

Pathophysiology

Some pathologic features are common to both Parkinson's disease and secondary parkinsonism; the most important is striatal dopamine deficiency. In Parkinson's disease, cell loss occurs in the substantia nigra with formation of an intracellular neuronal inclusion body, the Lewy body. In secondary parkinsonism, nigral cell loss may occur, the nigral striatal pathway may be impaired, or loss of striatal cellular elements may occur. Lewy bodies are not a feature of most secondary forms of parkinsonism. The loss of nigral cells with destruction of the nigrostriatal pathway results in the decreased level of striatal dopamine.

The cause of the selective nigral cell destruction is unknown; however, several pathogenetic mechanisms have been suggested. The most accepted is cellular damage by the oxidative production of toxic free radicals; ie, a relative excess of free radicals develops in nigral cells caused by oxidative stress, leading to increased oxidative degradation of dopamine and the accumulation of toxic metabolic products. The factors that cause oxidative stress are unknown. However, the effect can be counteracted by inhibiting monoamine oxidase (MAO), thereby limiting the catabolism of dopamine and accumulation of toxic metabolic products. Selegiline (L-deprenyl), a selective MAO-B inhibitor, ▮ may protect the brain cells involved in Parkinson's disease.

▮see page 439

TABLE 46–2. CAUSES OF SECONDARY PARKINSONISM

Cause	Comments
Infections	
Viral encephalitis	Can occur during the acute phase or, in rare cases, as a permanent sequela (eg, secondary parkinsonism developed after the epidemic of encephalitis lethargica from 1915 to 1926)
Atherosclerosis of cerebral vessels	Manifests as an akinetic-rigid syndrome that predominantly involves the lower extremities; includes prominent gait disturbance
	Responds only partially to antiparkinsonian drugs
Drugs and toxins	
Antipsychotics	Reversible*
Reserpine	Reversible*; may be dose-dependent or related to the patient's susceptibility (risk factors include older age and female sex)
Metoclopramide	Reversible*; may be dose-dependent or related to the patient's susceptibility (risk factors include older age and female sex)
Methyldopa	Reversible*; may be dose-dependent or related to the patient's susceptibility (risk factors include older age and female sex)
Meperidine analog (MPTP)	Irreversible; occurs in IV drug abusers
Carbon monoxide	Irreversible
Manganese	Includes dystonia and cognitive changes
	Usually occupationally related; occurs with chronic intoxication
Metabolic disorders	
Hypoparathyroidism	Is associated with calcification of the basal ganglia; includes chorea and athetosis
Brain tumors near the basal ganglia	Present as hemiparkinsonism (ie, restricted to one side of the body)
Head trauma	Is often associated with dementia
Degenerative disorders	
Dementing illnesses (eg, Alzheimer's disease, chromosome 17–linked frontotemporal dementias, diffuse Lewy body disease)	Dementia often precedes the parkinsonism
Striatonigral degeneration	Responds poorly to levodopa therapy because of postsynaptic dopaminergic pathology
Progressive supranuclear palsy	Includes supranuclear gaze palsies
Olivopontocerebellar atrophy	Manifests as multisystem atrophy; includes cerebellar features
Shy-Drager syndrome	Includes prominent autonomic dystrophy

*When drugs are withdrawn, symptoms usually disappear within a few days, although they may persist for months or years.

Symptoms and Signs

Parkinsonism begins insidiously; its cardinal manifestations may appear alone or in combination. One of the most common initial symptoms is tremor, usually in one hand but sometimes in both. This tremor classically involves the fingers in a pill-rolling motion. It is present at rest (resting tremor), usually decreases with voluntary movement, and disappears during sleep.

Muscular rigidity, usually evident during passive movement of a limb, may be manifested by smooth resistance or superimposed ratchet-like jerks (cogwheel phenomenon). Other signs include bradykinesia—a paucity of spontaneous movements or movements that are slow—and freezing—sudden interruption of movement. While carrying out routine tasks, patients may find voluntary movement suddenly and unexpectedly frozen or halted, and they may be unable to follow through to complete the action; for example, while walking, patients may suddenly feel their feet are frozen to the ground.

Gait becomes shuffled with short steps, and the arms fail to swing. Tachykinesia, the tendency for movements to become smaller and faster, may affect several functions: Speech tends to become more rapid until words run together into a mumble (tachyphemia). Handwriting tends to involve smaller and tighter loops (micrographia). Gait involves quicker and smaller steps, sometimes breaking into a run (festination). Rapid finger tapping may decrease in amplitude and increase in speed until the fingers seem stuck together.

Postural abnormalities are evident in the erect and sitting positions; an erect posture is not readily assumed or maintained. The head tends to fall forward on the trunk. A loss of postural reflexes causes the body to fall forward (propulsion) or backward (retropulsion) unless supported. Bradykinesia prevents the patient from taking a step or moving the arms to stop the fall. A conspicuous feature of parkinsonism, kyphotic deformity of the spine, causes a stooped posture.

The face can become masklike, with lack of expression and diminished eye blinking. Unsuppressible eye closure can be readily induced when the frontal muscle is tapped (Myerson's sign). Patients have difficulty swallowing and tend to drool. The skin has an oily quality; seborrheic dermatitis may develop.

Mood abnormalities, usually depression or anxiety, are common and may be the heralding symptom. Sometimes bradykinesia and decreased facial expression make a person appear depressed, even when mood is unaffected. Cognitive impairment and dementia commonly occur; whether they are intrinsic to the disease or due to a superimposed but unrelated dementing illness is controversial.

Parkinsonism is invariably progressive. Sometimes the course is extremely rapid, and patients become disabled within 5 years. More often the course is slow and protracted, and patients remain functional for many years.

Diagnosis

Parkinsonism is diagnosed on the basis of the symptoms and signs. However, about 30% of patients may not have tremor initially. Of those who have tremor, the tremor may become less prominent as the disease progresses; this finding should not obscure the diagnosis. Rigidity of some degree usually develops, and its absence makes the diagnosis of parkinsonism suspect.

Patients with essential tremor, ▌ which is the disorder most commonly confused with parkinsonism, have animated facies, normal rates of movement, and normal muscle tone and lack the gait abnormalities associated with parkinsonism. Furthermore, essential tremor is an action tremor rather than a resting tremor, which is most common in parkinsonism. Other disorders that may be confused with parkinsonism include myxedema, normal-pressure hydrocephalus, hepatic encephalopathy, and depression.

A diagnostic challenge in elderly patients may be differentiating mild early parkinsonism from normal aging (eg, slowing down, loss of balance, complaints of stiffness, difficulty walking, stooped posture). However, the bradykinesia and rigidity of Parkinson's disease are usually asymmetric at onset (ie, only one side is slightly affected), and resting tremor and true extrapyramidal rigidity are not features of normal aging.

No serologic or urine test can confirm the diagnosis of parkinsonism. Routine blood, cerebrospinal fluid (CSF), and urine tests yield normal results. The disturbance in cerebral dopamine metabolism may decrease CSF levels of homovanillic acid; however, this finding does not confirm the diagnosis, and testing is not recommended. Neither CT nor MRI scan of the head shows abnormalities in Parkinson's disease but may help diagnose some cases of secondary parkinsonism. Deoxyglucose PET scan of the brain often reveals an abnormal pattern of increased glucose metabolism in the globus pallidus, which is characteristic of Parkinson's disease.

Differentiating between Parkinson's disease and secondary parkinsonism is sometimes impossible, particularly in early cases. The diagnosis is based on neurologic examination findings in combination with MRI and PET scan results.

Treatment

No cure is available for Parkinson's disease or for secondary parkinsonism due to any cause other than drugs (see TABLE 46–2). Most patients require lifelong drug treatment to control symptoms. *Treatment should be individualized* according to the type and severity of symptoms, the degree of functional impairment, the degree of cognitive

▌see page 429

impairment, any associated disease processes, and the risk/benefit ratio. Treatment may require an interdisciplinary team approach, involving the combined efforts of a neurologist, psychiatrist, nurse, physical therapist, occupational therapist, and speech therapist. Drugs that cause or worsen parkinsonism, especially antipsychotics, should be stopped.

Nondrug treatment: A regular exercise program (eg, walking, riding a bicycle) may be helpful. Elderly patients who are limber and active may better adapt to the progressively increasing stiffness and slowness of parkinsonism. Physical therapy ◨ may restore confidence in walking and maintaining balance, may help patients develop simple means of managing unpredictable and disabling freezing episodes (eg, counting out loud while taking steps), and can provide training if a cane or walker is necessary. Occupational therapy ◨ may be indicated to train patients in strategies for carrying out daily tasks (eg, dressing, cooking) and in the use of adaptive equipment to simplify tasks. An occupational therapist may visit the home to help plan the appropriate placement of railings, grab bars, or other assistive devices that may reduce the risk of falling. Continued therapy is warranted, but many patients do without this type of therapy because it is not covered by most insurance plans.

Although treatment of the motor manifestations of parkinsonism is important, many elderly patients also report constipation. Levodopa, a common antiparkinsonian drug; physical inactivity; and parkinsonism itself produce constipation, which is treated by dietary intake of fruit, high-fiber foods, prune and other juices, and other liquids. Drug treatment (eg, senna concentrate, one to six 187-mg tablets/day) is particularly effective when used as part of a regular routine rather than waiting for constipation to become severe.

Drug treatment: Elderly patients with Parkinson's disease tend to develop confusion and toxic psychosis when taking antiparkinsonian drugs (see TABLE 46–3). In general, the therapeutic regimen should be kept simple; the risk of adverse effects is lower when one or two drugs are given at higher doses than when multiple drugs are given at lower doses.

Levodopa provides the most benefit in terms of improving the motor manifestations of Parkinson's disease relative to its central nervous system effects; drugs with stronger anticholinergic properties (eg, anticholinergic drugs, amantadine) provide the least benefit, and the dopamine agonists are in between. Mild toxic psychosis may be treated with clozapine (starting with 6.25 mg/day), which has fewer extrapyramidal effects than do other antipsychotics. Confusion and disorientation can be treated only by lowering the doses of antiparkinsonian drugs or by discontinuing them. Anticholinergic drugs should be discontinued first, followed by selegiline, dopamine agonists, and levodopa.

◨ see page 269   ◨ see page 287

TABLE 46–3. COMMONLY USED ANTIPARKINSONIAN DRUGS

Class	Drug	Starting Dose	Average Daily Dose	Total Daily Dose Range	Major Adverse Effects
Anticholinergic drugs					Sedation, confusion, urinary retention, dry mouth, blurred vision, hallucinations
Antihistamines	Diphenhydramine	25 mg/day	25 mg bid or tid	25 mg tid	
Miscellaneous	Procyclidine	2.5 mg/day	5 mg tid	5 mg tid	
	Trihexyphenidyl	1 mg/day	1 to 2 mg tid	1 to 2 mg tid	
Catechol O-methyltransferase inhibitors	Tolcapone	100 mg/day with levodopa	200 mg tid with levodopa	100 to 600 mg with levodopa	Dyskinesias, nausea, confusion, hallucinations, diarrhea, hepatitis
Dopaminergic drugs					
Dopamine precursors (with decarboxylase inhibitor)	Carbidopa-levodopa 25/100, 10/100, or 25/250 mg	12.5/50 mg tid	25/100 mg qid	75/300 to 200/2000 mg	Nausea, anorexia, confusion, psychotic disturbances, nightmares, dyskinesia
	Carbidopa-levodopa controlled-release 25/100 or 50/200 mg	25/100 mg bid	50/200 mg qid	75/300 to 200/800 mg	
Dopamine agonists	Bromocriptine	1.25 mg/day	2.5 mg qid	10 to 40 mg	Nausea, vomiting, confusion, hallucinations, hypotension, dyskinesia
	Pergolide	0.05 mg/day	0.25 mg qid	1 to 3 mg	
	Pramipexole	0.125 mg/day	0.25 mg qid	1 to 4.5 mg	
	Ropinirole	0.25 mg/day	0.25 mg qid	1 to 3 mg	
Monoamine oxidase-B inhibitor	Selegiline	5 mg bid	5 mg bid	5 to 10 mg	Nausea, insomnia, confusion
Mechanism of action unknown	Amantadine	100 mg/day	100 mg bid	100 to 300 mg	Confusion, urinary retention, elevated intraocular pressure, livedo reticularis

Symptoms of recent onset, especially if tremor predominates and functional impairment is mild, are best treated with drugs that centrally inhibit cholinergic activity. However, in the elderly, anticholinergics often produce sedation, confusion, urinary retention, dry mouth, and blurred vision. These drugs are contraindicated in persons with glaucoma, benign prostatic hypertrophy, and dementia. Diphenhydramine (25 mg bid or tid), an antihistamine with anticholinergic action, may suffice. Trihexyphenidyl (1 to 2 mg tid) is more effective but more toxic and should be administered cautiously, usually below the optimal dosage. ◪

Amantadine (100 mg bid or tid) has mild anticholinergic effects that appear to play a role in its antiparkinsonian effects. It also promotes dopamine release in the corpus striatum.

Selegiline (5 mg bid), an MAO-B inhibitor, may be used in an early stage to prevent or slow disease progression. However, whether selegiline slows the disease progression or just suppresses symptoms is controversial. The drug inhibits oxidative metabolism of dopamine and can delay the need for additional antiparkinsonian drugs. Selegiline is generally well tolerated, although some patients may experience adverse effects (eg, nausea, insomnia, confusion). Although chemically related to other MAO inhibitors, selegiline does not require dietary restrictions.

Patients with severe parkinsonian symptoms should be treated with drugs that can replenish or activate striatal dopaminergic effects. Many studies support delayed use of dopaminergic drugs, and many support early use. Most experts believe that dopaminergic drugs should not be instituted until symptoms cause functional impairment, thus delaying the risk of late adverse effects, which can be distressing.

Dopamine replacement is best accomplished with carbidopa-levodopa. Levodopa is converted to dopamine in the central nervous system and the periphery. Peripheral conversion and systemic effects can be reduced by combining levodopa with carbidopa (a peripheral decarboxylation inhibitor), which does not cross the blood-brain barrier.

Treatment usually begins with a half tablet of the 25/100 combination (25 mg carbidopa to 100 mg levodopa) bid or tid. After 1 week, the dose can be increased to a full tablet tid if needed and if adverse effects are tolerable. After several weeks, the dose can be increased again if needed; it can be increased by a half tablet per day every 5 to 7 days until a maximum dose of 200/2000 mg of carbidopa-levodopa is reached (eg, 8 tablets of carbidopa-levodopa 25/250). For peripheral adverse effects (eg, flushing, abdominal cramping, anorexia), increasing the amount of carbidopa may be helpful; for central adverse effects (eg, nightmares, confusion, hypotension), decreasing the dose of levodopa may be necessary. A controlled-release form (25/100 and 50/200) generally requires a slightly higher total daily dose. Selegiline,

---

◪ see page 446

amantadine, and anticholinergic drugs may also be given with carbidopa-levodopa.

Carbidopa-levodopa is often given with dopamine agonists; dopamine agonists may also be given as monotherapy. Induction requires caution because nausea, orthostatic hypotension, and confusion are common adverse effects. Bromocriptine is begun at 1.25 mg/day and increased by 1.25-mg increments every 2 to 5 days to a total dose of 10 to 30 mg/day. Pergolide is begun at 0.05 mg/day and increased by 0.05-mg increments every 2 to 3 days to a total dose of 1 to 3 mg/day. Newer dopamine agonists include ropinirole, which is begun at 0.25 mg/day and increased as needed to a total dose of 3 mg/day, and pramipexole, which is begun at 0.125 mg/day and increased as needed to a total dose of 4.5 mg/day. Tolcapone, a catechol O-methyltransferase inhibitor, extends the benefit of carbidopa-levodopa by inhibiting the metabolic breakdown of dopamine. It is begun at 100 mg tid and increased to a maximum recommended dose of 600 mg/day.

Depression, a common feature of parkinsonism, is perceived by many elderly patients to be an example of their frailty, mortality, and loss of youth. The adverse effects of many antidepressant drugs, particularly the anticholinergic effects of tricyclic antidepressants, limit their use. The selective serotonin reuptake inhibitors (eg, fluoxetine, sertraline, paroxetine) have fewer adverse effects and are often preferred.

Elderly patients with parkinsonism may also report insomnia; treatment must be individualized. A low dopamine state causes stiffness, malaise, low energy, and a sense of impending doom that are severe enough to awaken some patients from a light sleep during the night. Higher bedtime doses or sustained-release forms of levodopa may be offered to these patients, although some patients prefer to set their alarm clocks to take levodopa in the middle of the night. Insomnia may also result from too much sleep during the day, possibly due to levodopa therapy. The dosage of levodopa may need to be reduced, correcting the reversed sleep-wake cycle. Another cause of insomnia may be frequent awakenings due to urinary frequency, another feature of Parkinson's disease.

Surgical treatment: An approach to replenishing the dopamine deficit involves transplantation or grafting of fetal nigral cells to the corpus striatum. Nigral cells harvested from aborted fetuses are stereotactically inserted in the striatum of patients with Parkinson's disease. These cells remain viable, form neural connections, and can produce dopamine. Because selection criteria have been strict (eg, limiting participants to only those who have developed difficulties with drug treatment), the usefulness of this approach cannot be fully assessed.

Other surgical therapies may be used. Stereotactic pallidotomy primarily reduces severe dyskinesias and improves bradykinesia and rigidity. Thalamotomy or implantation of deep brain (thalamic) stimulator electrodes is used to treat disabling drug-resistant tremors.

Nursing issues: The goal of nursing care for patients with Parkinson's disease is to maintain function and promote quality of life. Clinical care must include systematic assessment with standardized assessment tools (eg, Katz Activities of Daily Living Scale,**❶** Hamilton Depression Scale **❷**) to follow patients as they cope with difficult symptoms and a chronic debilitating disorder. Clinical care also requires astute vigilance for new symptoms resulting from drug treatment or from the sequelae of tremors and musculoskeletal changes. Patient education and family support are the cornerstones to supportive clinical care of patients with Parkinson's disease. Nurses should inform patients and family members about available support groups and societies. Systematic nursing assessment, clinical support in daily functioning (eg, eating, feeding, toileting, mobility, sleeping), and regular communication regarding depression and perceived quality of life are essential.

End-of-life issues: Parkinson's disease is chronic; patients eventually become severely impaired and immobile and are at risk of aspiration. Eating, even with assistance, may become impossible. Many patients also develop dementia. Drugs, although effective for years, may become ineffective as the disease progresses. For all of these reasons, health care practitioners should discuss end-of-life care issues with patients, including whether tube feedings should be given and whether acute illnesses (eg, aspiration pneumonia) should be treated.

PROGRESSIVE SUPRANUCLEAR PALSY
(Steele-Richardson-Olszewski Syndrome)

A rare disorder characterized by parkinsonian symptoms, supranuclear vertical gaze palsy, and square wave jerks.

About 4% of patients with parkinsonism have clinical manifestations of progressive supranuclear palsy. Onset usually occurs during or after age 50, but some patients develop signs in their 40s. The pathogenesis is unknown. Evidence of a transmissible cause is lacking, and familial cases are rare. No ethnic or racial predilection exists, although men are more often affected. Pathologic examination shows degenerative changes in the brain stem, diencephalon, basal ganglia, and cerebral cortex. Microscopic findings include nerve cell loss, neurofibrillary tangles (consisting of unpaired straight filaments 15 to 18 nm in diameter), gliosis, and, occasionally, perivascular cuffing.

Symptoms, Signs, and Diagnosis
The most prominent ophthalmologic manifestation is progressive impairment of voluntary vertical gaze (downward more than upward). Other ophthalmic symptoms include square wave jerks (inability to fix

---

❶see TABLE 4–3 on page 44   **❷**see TABLE 33–5 on page 316 the gaze on a stationary or moving object), blurred vision, diplopia, photophobia, burning, tearing, and retraction of the upper lids leading to a staring, astonished appearance. Other findings are gait unsteadiness with falling (often backwards), dysarthria, dysphagia, rigidity, bradykinesia, deep nasolabial folds, and dystonic neck extension. Resting tremor is often not prominent. Depression and dementia are common late in the course; sleep disturbances (insomnia or hyposomnia), agitation, irritability, apathy, and pseudobulbar affect (emotional lability with a propensity to laugh or cry easily) also occur. Mild to moderate atrophy of the midbrain may be seen on MRI. Sagittal views may show thinning of the quadrigeminal plate. Laboratory findings are normal, except for the CSF protein level, which is occasionally increased. In progressive supranuclear palsy, fluorodopa PET scan often shows reduced mean caudate tracer uptake compared with that in Parkinson's disease.

Prognosis and Treatment

The disease usually progresses rapidly; marked incapacity occurs within 3 to 5 years and death within 10 years, generally due to infection or other complications of immobility. No fully effective treatment is available. Treatment with levodopa, amitriptyline, or anticholinergic drugs may be partially effective. Idazoxan, an α_2 presynaptic inhibitor that increases norepinephrine transmission, may improve motor manifestations. Electroconvulsive therapy is of limited benefit, but transient confusion is a common adverse effect.

SHY-DRAGER SYNDROME

Multisystem degeneration involving the central (preganglionic) autonomic, cerebellar, basal ganglia, pyramidal, and spinal motor neurons.

The major feature differentiating Shy-Drager syndrome from Parkinson's disease is prominent autonomic failure. The mean age of onset is 55 years (range, 37 to 75 years). The syndrome occurs predominantly in males (2:1 or 3:1 ratio). No genetic predisposition has been shown, and familial incidence has been reported in only one case. The pathogenesis is unknown. About 11% of patients with severe orthostatic hypotension have Shy-Drager syndrome.

Symptoms, Signs, and Diagnosis

The major manifestation is autonomic insufficiency with wide swings in blood pressure but no change in pulse rate. Orthostatic hypotension is often the most disabling symptom. Patients report dizziness, light-headedness, or syncope on standing; postexertional weakness; gait unsteadiness; or dimming of vision. Impaired temperature control, reduced sweating, urinary or fecal incontinence, diarrhea, constipation, nocturnal diuresis, erectile dysfunction, iridic atrophy, impaired eye movements, Horner's syndrome, and anisocoria may also occur.

Central neuron degeneration is manifested by parkinsonian features, intention tremor, ataxia, dysarthria, and, in some cases, corticobulbar and corticospinal tract signs. Anterior horn cell degeneration, sometimes seen on electromyography, leads to wasting and fasciculation of distal muscles. Intellectual and emotional function is preserved until late in the disease course. Laboratory findings are usually normal.

Prognosis and Treatment

The syndrome is progressive, and death (usually due to cardiac arrhythmias, aspiration, sleep apnea, or pulmonary emboli) occurs 7 to 10 years after the onset of neurologic symptoms.

Nondrug treatment of autonomic dysfunction includes avoidance of extreme heat, alcohol, large meals, getting up rapidly, and excessive straining at stool. Wearing compressive clothing and elastic stockings, increasing salt and fluid intake, and sleeping in a reverse Trendelenburg's position may ameliorate some orthostatic symptoms. Drugs that may be used to treat the orthostatic hypotension include indomethacin, midodrine, propranolol, and pindolol. Fludrocortisone (0.1 mg/day starting dose) can be used to expand the plasma volume.

CHOREAS

A variety of diseases that, although unrelated etiologically, are manifested primarily by choreiform movements (flowing, continuous, random movements that flit from one part of the body to another).

Chorea can be due to infections, genetic disorders, or other causes (see TABLE 46–4). Many of the pathologic changes, found in various parts of the basal ganglia, influence the motor system via the globus pallidus.

Huntington's disease is an autosomal dominant, cytosine-adenosine-guanosine repeat disorder linked to chromosome 4p. It is characterized by chorea, personality changes, cognitive impairment, and psychiatric signs (eg, psychosis, depression). It may affect persons of all ages, although it tends to progress more slowly in persons whose symptoms begin at age 60 to 70 than in those whose symptoms begin at age 40 to 50.

Senile chorea is characterized by choreiform movements that occur as an isolated symptom in persons > 60; it is not associated with mental disturbance or other causes of chorea. Involuntary complex movements of the face, mouth, and tongue may occur alone or with unilateral or bilateral limb movements. Pathologic findings often include degeneration of the putamen, caudate nucleus, or both.

TABLE 46–4. POSSIBLE CAUSES OF CHOREA

Cause	Example
Central nervous system infections	Encephalitis lethargica (von Economo's disease) Meningoencephalitis secondary to viral infection Parenchymatous neurosyphilis
Autoimmune disorders	Systemic lupus erythematosus Henoch-Schönlein purpura Rheumatoid arthritis Periarteritis nodosa Serum sickness reaction to tetanus antitoxin Lyme disease
Metabolic disorders	Thyrotoxicosis Hyperparathyroidism Hypoparathyroidism Hypocalcemia
Drug intoxication	Atropine and other anticholinergic drugs Anticonvulsants Amphetamines Levodopa Lithium Phenothiazine and related antipsychotic drugs Isoniazid
Genetic disorders	Huntington's disease Acute intermittent porphyria Wilson's disease Acanthocytosis Olivopontocerebellar atrophy, dominant form

Miscellaneous disorders	Pick's disease
	 Alzheimer's disease
	 Senile chorea
	 Benign familial chorea
	 Polycythemia
	 Beriberi
	 Cerebrovascular disease
	     Arteriosclerotic vascular disease
	     Meningovascular syphilis
	 Brain tumor, primary or metastatic
	 Trauma, subdural hematoma

Diagnosis and Treatment

The choreas may be diagnosed on the basis of the identification of choreiform movements. Specific underlying diseases may be identified on the basis of the associated symptoms and signs.

Treatment depends on the underlying disease. In general, choreiform movements are not treated unless they are bothersome (eg, embarrassing, disabling). Treatment includes dopamine receptor blockers, including haloperidol (0.5 mg/day, gradually increased to 1 to 5 mg/day) and chlorpromazine (25 mg/day, gradually increased to 100 to 200 mg/day), and drugs that inhibit the release of dopamine presynaptically, including reserpine (0.25 mg/day, gradually increased to 1 to 5 mg/day). The advantage of these latter drugs is that they do not cause tardive dyskinesias; however, adverse effects include depression and orthostatic hypotension.

DYSTONIA

Twisting movements and abnormal postures due to sustained muscle contractions.

Dystonia may be focal, involving one or more body sites, or generalized, involving all of the limbs and trunk.

Focal dystonia may be idiopathic, due to an underlying genetic predisposition, or the result of focal lesions (eg, brain tumors, arteriovenous malformations). Focal dystonia results in localized dystonic movements or postures that may involve the neck (torticollis), the facial muscles around the eyes (blepharospasm), or the upper limbs (writer's cramp). In adults, focal dystonia is less likely to generalize. *Focal dystonia requires a complete evaluation to determine the cause.*

Generalized dystonia, a progressive syndrome, often evolves from involvement of the foot or leg due to idiopathic torsion dystonia during childhood. It often has a genetic basis; a dystonia gene has been identified on chromosome 9q.

Specific Focal Dystonias

Spasmodic torticollis: This disorder can occur at any age but most often appears in the 3rd to 6th decades. Involuntary activity of the sternocleidomastoid, trapezius, or scalene muscles results in sustained contractions leading to twisting or turning movements of the head. Less often, forward flexion (anterocollis) or forceful extension (retrocollis) may occur. The course varies: in the majority of patients, torticollis remains isolated to the neck muscles, but in 25% of patients, the torticollis spreads beyond the neck to involve other muscles (eg, face, jaw, arms). The severity of the dystonia may remain stable for many years or may increase. Fewer than 10% of patients experience partial remission; relapse occurs eventually.

Cranial dystonias: These disorders usually occur in the 5th or 6th decade; the cause is often unknown. Each is characterized by intermittent spasms of selected groups of muscles, which may markedly interfere with function. Blepharospasm is involuntary spasm of the orbicularis muscle of the eye, causing increased blink rate when mild and forceful sustained closure of the eyes when severe. Oromandibular and orofacial dystonias are involuntary dystonic spasms of the facial muscles, jaw muscles, tongue, and platysma. These dystonias may be provoked by attempts to talk or eat.

Spasmodic dysphonia: This disorder affects the adductor or abductor muscles of the larynx. In adductor dystonia, speech is tight and constricted, with the smooth flow of words broken up. In abductor dystonia, a breathy dysphonia is produced, with the patient speaking in a whispery voice.

Tardive dystonia: Dystonic movements are caused by dopamine receptor blockers (eg, antipsychotics◘). Cranial and cervical dystonias are the most common, but the entire body may be involved.

Diagnosis

Dystonia may be diagnosed by identification of the abnormal muscle contractions or abnormal twisting postures. Depending on the localization of the dystonia, different descriptive terms (eg, blepharospasm, writer's cramp) may be applied. An underlying cause or genetic predisposition should be excluded.

Treatment

Treatment is difficult. Botulinum toxin A is the treatment of choice because it has no central or systemic adverse effects. Injection into the affected muscle produces graded but temporary weakness and relief of dystonic symptoms. It is most effective for torticollis, blepharospasm, and laryngeal dystonias. Additional injections every few months are necessary.

If the dystonia is generalized or not responsive to botulinum toxin A, oral drugs (eg, anticholinergic drugs, baclofen) are the treatment of choice. High doses of anticholinergic drugs may be effective; children may tolerate trihexyphenidyl at doses > 100 mg/day. However, by adulthood, doses > 15 mg/day are rarely tolerated because they cause confusion and disorientation; the elderly rarely tolerate doses > 5 mg/day, which additionally cause hallucinations, constipation and fecal impaction, urinary retention of varying severity, and dry mouth. These adverse effects often place severe restrictions on the use of trihexyphenidyl, which is rarely prescribed to elderly patients who live alone. When trihexyphenidyl is prescribed, the starting dose is often 1 mg at bedtime. If adverse effects do not occur, the dose may be increased slowly and cautiously in 1-mg increments at a rate that is appropriate for the patient (typically every 1 to 3 weeks).

Some patients benefit from baclofen, but somnolence, confusion, and hallucinations may restrict the dose. Typically, the starting dose of 5 mg

◘see also page 447

at bedtime is increased slowly at a rate that allows the patient to acclimatize to each dose adjustment and allows the physician to rapidly reduce the dose to presymptomatic levels if problems arise. Other drugs that may be useful include carbamazepine, clonazepam, diazepam, reserpine, and tetrabenazine.

TARDIVE DYSKINESIA AND TARDIVE AKATHISIA

Tardive dyskinesia is a *syndrome of persistent, stereotyped, repetitive abnormal involuntary movements caused by chronic exposure to dopamine receptor blockers (usually antipsychotic and related drugs such as haloperidol, prochlorperazine, metoclopramide).* Typically, the dyskinesia involves tongue movements and chewing, lip puckering, and lip smacking. The cause relates to dopamine receptor supersensitivity. The prevalence increases with age, and the disorder is more common among elderly women. The incidence in the elderly is about four times that in young adults. Higher drug doses and prolonged treatment increase the likelihood of tardive dyskinesia. Symptoms typically start during drug use and may worsen when the dose is reduced or the drug is discontinued. Reinstituting the drug may alleviate the symptoms.

Tardive akathisia is a *feeling of motor restlessness or an aversion to being still.* This subjective state often results in repetitive movements. The cause is usually drugs, especially antipsychotics. Manifestations include repeatedly rubbing or stroking parts of the body, crossing and uncrossing the arms or legs, picking at clothes, pacing, marching in place, swinging the legs, and moaning, grunting, or shouting. The disorder is frequently misdiagnosed as agitation, which often leads physicians to increase the dose of the drug that is causing the problem.

Treatment

Treatment includes, if possible, discontinuation of the drug that is causing the disorder. Orobuccal dyskinesia, if significant, can be treated with reserpine (0.25 mg/day, gradually increased to 1 to 5 mg/day), although the response is not always good. Other drugs include tetrabenazine (12.5 mg/day, gradually increased to 75 to 150 mg/day) or clozapine (6.25 mg/day, gradually increased to 25 to 75 mg/day), although clozapine may result in agranulocytosis. Opioids, propranolol, and benzodiazepines may also be helpful.

HEMIBALLISMUS

A violent, flinging, flailing movement that is caused by destructive lesions of the contralateral subthalamic nucleus (the corpus luysi) and that resembles large-amplitude proximal chorea.

Hemiballismus occurs when ≥ 20% of the corpus luysi is destroyed, but the substantia nigra, pyramidal tract, and red nucleus must be intact. Most cases are caused by hemorrhagic or ischemic vascular lesions, although some are caused by other pathologic processes (eg, metastatic tumors, cysts, infectious diseases). In the elderly, hemiballismus occurs primarily after a stroke. Symptoms begin soon after the neurologic signs of stroke clear or some time later. They are localized to one side of the body and do not occur during sleep. Forceful throwing of the limbs results from almost continuous activity of the proximal musculature. The arm and leg may be equally involved, but involvement of one is usually more prominent. The neck, tongue, or face may also be affected.

Initially, the violence of these movements may exhaust and incapacitate the patient to such an extent that death ensues. However, the initial intensity often decreases; movements gradually become tolerable and can be somewhat suppressed or briefly interrupted by voluntary action. In about 6 to 10 weeks, the movements may stop spontaneously, particularly when the cause is an ischemic vascular lesion (in 80 to 90% of cases due to an ischemic vascular lesion, recovery occurs spontaneously). The movements persist when the cause is a tumor.

Treatment

Treatment is not very effective, but haloperidol may be tried for postsynaptic dopamine receptor blockade. Valproic acid and reserpine help some patients. Surgery (eg, thalamotomy) is indicated only in life-threatening cases. Paradoxically, hemiballismus has occurred after attempted thalamotomy for other movement disorders, when poor localization led to inadvertent destruction of the corpus luysi.

MYOCLONUS

Sudden, brief, shocklike jerks of a muscle or group of muscles.

Myoclonus can vary in amplitude, frequency, and distribution. The muscle jerks may be induced by sudden noise, movement, light, or visual threat; they are caused by muscular contractions (positive myoclonus) or inhibitions (negative myoclonus) arising from hyperexcitable neurons in the spinal cord, medial reticular formation, or cerebral cortex.

Myoclonus can be classified according to cause. Major causes in the elderly relate to the dementias, metabolic or toxic encephalopathies, or focal central nervous system damage (see TABLE 46–5).

Neurologic disease can cause myoclonus, which may be an early feature of **Creutzfeldt-Jakob disease.** In this case, myoclonus can be elicited

TABLE 46–5. CAUSES OF MYOCLONUS	
Cause	**Example**
Dementias	Alzheimer's disease Creutzfeldt-Jakob disease
Metabolic disorders or conditions	Uremia Long-term hemodialysis Hypercapnia Hepatic failure Renal failure Hypoglycemia Hyponatremia Nonketotic hyperglycemia
Toxic encephalopathies	Drugs (eg, levodopa, tricyclic antidepressants, lithium, valproic acid, carbamazepine, phenytoin, antihistamines, monoamine oxidase inhibitors) Bismuth Heavy-metal poisons Methyl bromide, DDT
Physical encephalopathies	Posthypoxia Posttrauma Heatstroke Electric shock
Degeneration of the basal ganglia	Wilson's disease Torsion dystonia Progressive supranuclear palsy Huntington's disease Parkinson's disease Diffuse Lewy body disease
Viral encephalopathies	Subacute sclerosing panencephalitis Encephalitis lethargica Herpes simplex encephalitis Postinfectious encephalitis

by a stimulus or can occur spontaneously. It is associated with a periodic synchronous discharge on an EEG. Myoclonus can also occur in the later stages of **Alzheimer's disease.** In this case, it is more brief and more focal than in Creutzfeldt-Jakob disease and can occur at rest, with voluntary activity, or with stimulation. Myoclonus after a hypoxic insult is usually precipitated by voluntary motor action.

Metabolic abnormalities (eg, uremia, long-term hemodialysis, hypercapnia, hepatic failure, hypoglycemia, hyponatremia) may be complicated by multifocal, asymmetric, stimulus-sensitive myoclonus. Facial or proximal limb muscles are predominantly involved. If the metabolic abnormality persists, generalized myoclonic jerks and, ultimately, seizures may occur.

Nocturnal myoclonus (periodic limb movements of sleep**❶**) occurs generally at night and affects predominantly the legs.

Drugs, such as long-term levodopa treatment in some patients with parkinsonism, can induce myoclonus characterized by single, abrupt, symmetric jerks of the arms and legs, usually during sleep, during drowsiness, or at rest. A reduction in dose can alleviate the frequency and severity of the myoclonus. Toxic doses of some drugs (eg, tricyclic antidepressants, lithium, valproic acid, carbamazepine, phenytoin, antihistamines, MAO inhibitors) can also induce myoclonus. High-dose penicillin or cephalosporin infusion can induce nonrhythmic, asymmetric, and stimulus-sensitive myoclonus.

Treatment

Whenever possible (eg, in cases of metabolic abnormalities), etiologic factors should be alleviated. Several drugs may be used as the treatment of choice: eg, clonazepam (0.25 mg/day, gradually increased to 1 to 4 mg/day) or valproic acid (125 mg/day, gradually increased to 750 to 1500 mg/day).

47 ■ SLEEP DISORDERS

Disorders that affect the ability to fall asleep or stay asleep, that involve sleeping too much, or that result in abnormal sleep-related behavior.

Up to 50% of elderly persons complain about their sleep, especially difficulty falling and staying asleep. As a result, hypnotic use is more common among the elderly than among younger persons.

There are some age-related changes in sleep. However, sleep disorders in the elderly may be caused by psychologic stressors (eg, bereavement, posttraumatic stress, forced retirement, social isolation, lack of community involvement), medical disorders,**❷** psychiatric disorders (eg, anxiety, dementia, depression), or the adverse effects of drugs (see TABLE 47–1). Several of these conditions may coexist.

A National Institutes of Health Consensus Statement on sleep disorders in the elderly recommends that health care practitioners ask the following questions during screening:

• Is the person satisfied with his or her sleep?

• Does sleep or fatigue intrude on activities?

❶see page 459   **❷**see page 462

• Does the bed partner or other persons notice unusual behavior (eg, snoring, interrupted breathing, leg movements) by the patient during sleep?

CHARACTERISTICS OF SLEEP

Many characteristics of sleep change with age. However, experts disagree on which changes are normal.

The **timing and amount of sleep** change with age. The elderly tend to fall asleep earlier and awaken earlier and to be less tolerant of shifts in the sleep-wake cycle (eg, due to jet lag). Reported changes in the duration of sleep with age appear variable. Although many studies indicate that the elderly sleep less, others report no change or increased sleep time. Daytime napping may compensate for poor nocturnal sleep, but it may also contribute to poor nocturnal sleep.

TABLE 47–1.   DRUGS THAT MAY DISTURB SLEEP

Drug Class or Drug	Effect on Sleep
Antipsychotics	Akathisia may occur, sometimes resulting in behavioral disturbances and awakening. Discontinuation usually resolves the symptoms
β-Blockers	Nightmares may occur. Sleep physiology is altered through CNS effects. Nocturnal wheezing and breathlessness may occur in patients with asthma or chronic obstructive pulmonary disease
Caffeine	Use prior to sleep can prolong sleep latency and interfere with the maintenance of sleep
Carbidopa-levodopa	Nightmares may occur
Centrally acting α agonist antihypertensives (eg, clonidine, methyldopa)	Sleep physiology is altered through CNS effects
Decongestants that contain stimulants (eg, ephedrine, β agonists, methylxanthines)	Nighttime use can prolong initiation of sleep
Diuretics	Nighttime use can produce nocturia, waking patients, who may have difficulty resuming sleep
H_2 blockers	Nocturnal delirium may occur in the elderly
Reserpine	Insomnia and depression may occur. Sleep physiology is altered through CNS effects
Sedative-hypnotics (eg, benzodiazepines)	Discontinuation may lead to rebound insomnia; tolerance (ie, lack of effectiveness) occurs with prolonged use
Sympathomimetic bronchodilators	Stimulation of the CNS occurs, with exacerbation of insomnia

CNS = central nervous system; H_2 = histamine-2.

Sleep efficiency (time asleep vs. time in bed) decreases from 95% during adolescence to < 80% during old age. Nocturnal sleep latency (time to fall asleep) may be prolonged in the elderly. **Sleep structure** describes the stages and cycles during sleep. Sleep can be categorized as nonrapid eye movement (NREM) or rapid eye movement (REM) sleep.

NREM sleep has four stages, ranging in depth from stage 1 (the lightest level, during which waking the sleeper is easy) to stage 4 (the deepest level, during which waking the sleeper is difficult). Stages 3 and 4 are often referred to as slow-wave or deep sleep.

The time spent in stage 1 sleep may increase from 5% in younger adults to 12 to 15% in the elderly, perhaps because the elderly wake more often during the night. The number of transient arousals (2- to 15-second awakenings due to alpha-wave intrusions into sleep) increases with age.

Stage 2 sleep is characterized on EEG by sleep spindles and K complexes; both of these features may decrease with age. The background EEG in stage 2 sleep shows relatively low-voltage mixed-frequency activity.

High-voltage slow (delta)-wave activity, which is characteristic of stages 3 and 4 sleep, decreases with age, possibly beginning as early as age 20; it may cease in extreme old age. Slow-wave activity may be better preserved in elderly women than in elderly men.

Normally, NREM and REM sleep alternate throughout the night in five or six cycles. REM sleep produces characteristic low-voltage mixed-frequency activity on EEG. Bursts of rapid eye movements are a key feature. During REM sleep, the rate and depth of breathing increase, and muscle tone is lower than that during stage 4 NREM sleep. At least 85% of dreaming occurs during REM sleep. Some studies report a decrease in REM sleep time with age; others report no appreciable change. Thus, although the proportion of REM sleep time may be preserved in the elderly, the absolute amount may decrease as a result of reduced total nocturnal sleep time.

INSOMNIA

Difficulty in falling asleep or in staying asleep.

Causes include virtually any medical disorder ∎ and many drugs (see TABLE 47–1). Stress may cause a form of insomnia called adjustment sleep disorder, which may occur in otherwise fair to good sleepers. Insomnia may be transient, short-term, or chronic (see TABLE 47–2). Psychiatric disorders, most commonly depression, can cause insomnia. Winter or seasonal depression (seasonal affective disorder) is char-

∎see page 462

TABLE 47–2.   CLASSIFICATION OF INSOMNIA

Type of Insomnia	Duration	Common Causes
Transient	Several days	Acute stress (eg, due to hospitalization, surgery, bereavement, or retirement); rapid change in the sleep-wake cycle (eg, due to jet lag)
Short-term	1–3 weeks	Prolonged stress; new or discontinued drug use; an acute organic or psychologic disorder
Chronic	> 3 weeks	Aging; chronic stress (eg, due to forced retirement, nursing home placement, bereavement, concurrent illness); use of drugs with sleep-disrupting effects (see TABLE 47–1); poor sleep hygiene (see TABLE 47–3); a psychiatric disorder (in about one third to one half of patients); a primary sleep disorder

acterized by annual recurrent symptoms of depression, daytime fatigue, and increased sleep. The underlying mechanism for this disorder is unknown.

Several aspects of institutional living can contribute to insomnia. In nursing homes, residents are usually required to go to bed based on nursing home routine rather than based on their needs or preferences. This scheduling may not be conducive to good sleep. In hospitals, patients often are awakened throughout the night (eg, to be checked or given drugs), and many find it difficult to resume sleep without a hypnotic. Other factors that can contribute to insomnia in these settings include noise, lack of privacy, uncomfortable beds, rooms that are too warm or too cold, inactivity, lack of daytime light exposure, and excessive daytime napping. After hospital discharge, patients may inappropriately continue taking hypnotics. Thus, sleep hygiene plays an important role in insomnia in the elderly, particularly in these settings.

Symptoms and Diagnosis

Symptoms of insomnia often include the inability to maintain sleep and early morning awakening, which is particularly common in depression. Other symptoms include difficulty falling asleep, frequent nocturnal awakenings, daytime fatigue, irritability, and problems concentrating or performing under stress.

In adjustment sleep disorder, the stress may be a negative or even a positive event, and patients experience similar symptoms.

Diagnosis of the underlying cause of the insomnia should be determined via the history, by asking about the timing and amount of sleep; use of drugs (prescribed and over-the-counter [OTC]); use of hypnotics, alcohol, and tobacco; current illnesses; degree of stress; mood; and level of physical activity. Sleep hygiene must be reviewed, particularly when the insomnia is chronic.

Referral to a sleep specialist is recommended if the insomnia cannot be explained or is refractory to treatment or if periodic limb movements of sleep, sleep apnea, or a circadian rhythm sleep disorder is suspected.

Treatment

Transient or short-term insomnia usually requires no drug treatment. If drug treatment is needed, the lowest effective dose of the safest drug, usually a short- or intermediate-acting benzodiazepine or similar drug (eg, temazepam 7.5 mg or zolpidem 5 mg), should be used. Long-term use of hypnotics should be avoided, but judicious use (for ≤ 2 or 3 weeks, followed by intermittent use and early discontinuation) can help relieve transient insomnia in carefully selected elderly patients.

Chronic insomnia can sometimes be managed through patient education. Informing patients about normal age-related changes in sleep can alter their expectations about a good night's sleep; an occasional sleepless night does not signal poor health. Stimulants (eg, caffeine) should be avoided within several hours of bedtime. Social activities and interaction with friends and family members should be encouraged, because social isolation and daytime inactivity can interfere with the sleep-wake cycle.

Improving sleep hygiene often improves chronic insomnia (see TABLE 47–3). A short (eg, < 30 minutes), refreshing daytime nap, especially when part of a comprehensive treatment plan, usually does not disrupt nocturnal sleep if the nap results from a need for rest rather than from boredom. However, excessive daytime napping can disrupt nocturnal sleep.

Sleep restriction therapy involves limiting the time spent in bed (to increase sleep efficiency) and excluding daytime napping. Patients are instructed to get up at the same time each morning; they determine when to go to bed based on their estimate of usual total sleep time (using a sleep diary). The time spent in bed is gradually increased as sleep efficiency increases.

Other behavioral techniques include progressive muscle relaxation; relaxation methods using a metronome, meditation, or hypnosis; and biofeedback. Referral to a specialist trained in these techniques may be helpful.

Bright light therapy (appropriately timed light exposure) helps reset a person's biologic clock; it can be used to treat seasonal depression, although there are little data for this indication in the elderly. Bright light therapy is usually given from 30 minutes to about 2 hours daily; the duration depends on the brightness of the light. Outdoor light or light from a commercially available light box may be used; usual room lighting is inadequate.

TABLE 47–3.   SLEEP HYGIENE TO IMPROVE SLEEP

Regular sleep schedule: Patients go to bed at the same time each night and, more importantly, get up at the same time each morning, even on weekends.

Bedtime routine: A regular pattern of activities—brushing teeth, washing the face, setting the alarm clock—can set the mood for sleep. This routine is performed every night, at home or away.

Sleep-conducive environment: The bedroom is dark and quiet and not too warm or too cold.

Use of the bedroom primarily for sleeping: The bedroom is not used for eating, reading, watching television, paying bills, or other activities associated with wakefulness.

Avoidance of substances that interfere with sleep: Food and beverages that contain caffeine (eg, coffee, tea, cola drinks, chocolate) or alcohol, smoking, appetite suppressants, and diuretics should be avoided, especially near bedtime.

Use of pillows: Pillows between the knees or under the waist can make a person more comfortable. For persons with back problems, lying supine with a large pillow under the knees may be helpful.

Regular exercise: Exercise can help patients fall asleep naturally. However, exercise in the late evening can stimulate the cardiovascular and nervous systems and keep patients awake.

Relaxation: Stress and worry are major impediments to sleep. Patients who are not sleepy at bedtime can relax by reading or taking a warm bath. Patients can aim to leave problems at the bedroom door.

Adapted from *A to Zzzzz Guide to Better Sleep.* Copyright 1988 by The Better Sleep Council.

Pharmacotherapy: Drug treatment with sedative-hypnotics provides only symptomatic relief. Sedative-hypnotic use increases with age and is more common among women. However, prolonged use of these drugs is not recommended because it often leads to tachyphylaxis, which ultimately results in higher doses being used. Nightly use also can lead to high blood levels, which ultimately impair daytime functioning. Prescription refills must be monitored to ensure compliance with recommended use.

Benzodiazepines are preferred as sedative-hypnotics for the treatment of insomnia because adverse effects are predictable and fatal overdoses are rare. The risk of abuse is low, except for patients with a history of drug or alcohol abuse. Contraindications include sleep apnea, severe depression, and untreated drug or alcohol abuse.

The main differences among benzodiazepines are related to half-life. Short-acting (eg, triazolam) or intermediate-acting (eg, temazepam, estazolam) benzodiazepines are less likely to accumulate in serum and to cause daytime sedation than are long-acting ones. Short-acting benzodiazepines, especially those without active metabolites, pose less risk of drug-drug interactions but are more likely to result in rebound insomnia when discontinued, and the short-acting drug triazolam has been associated with confusion and retrograde amnesia. *Long-acting benzodiazepines (eg, flurazepam, diazepam, chlordiazepoxide, quazepam) should not be used in the elderly.* Patients > 65 who use long-acting benzodiazepines are twice as likely to fracture a hip as those using short- or intermediate-acting benzodiazepines. Long-term use of flurazepam or quazepam in persons > 75 can produce a syndrome mimicking Alzheimer's disease. The lowest effective dose of benzodiazepine should be used. Reasonable choices for the elderly include temazepam (7.5 mg starting dose, 7.5 to 15 mg usual effective dose) or estazolam (0.5 to 1.0 mg starting dose, 0.5 to 1.0 mg usual effective dose). Routine use should be limited to 2 to 4 weeks; if longer-term use is indicated, the drug should be taken no more than 2 or 4 times/week.

Regular nightly use of a benzodiazepine may be less effective than behavioral therapy and may cause the following complications:

- Exacerbation of the dysfunction caused by a sleep disorder such as sleep apnea, due to the depressant effect on the central nervous system

- Risk of harmful drug interactions (eg, with other tranquilizers, alcohol, β-blockers, β agonists, antihistamines, and analgesics)

- Prolonged pharmacologic effects in elderly persons (eg, daytime sedation, cognitive deficits) due to age-related reduction in the rate of metabolization and excretion

- Increased risk of falls, fractures, and death

- Risk of addiction and dependence

- Tolerance, indicating that the drug is no longer effective for promoting sleep

In patients with chronic insomnia who have been using a sedative-hypnotic (or other sleep therapy) long-term, evaluation and treatment are difficult because the drug's adverse effects may be indistinguishable from the symptoms of the insomnia. Patients should therefore be weaned from the hypnotic, giving special attention to withdrawal symptoms and rebound insomnia (which is more likely with abrupt withdrawal). Patients and their family members or caregivers should be warned that hypnotic withdrawal may initially worsen sleep but is necessary for successful treatment. In long-term users who do not want to stop the sedative-hypnotic, education about the above complications is essential, and referral to a specialist may be necessary.

Zolpidem is a short-acting imidazopyridine (not a benzodiazepine) with similar action to that of triazolam. Zolpidem (5 mg starting dose, 5 to 10 mg usual effective dose) reportedly causes little daytime sedation, tolerance, and rebound insomnia. Routine use of zolpidem, like that of benzodiazepines, should be limited to 2 to 4 weeks; if longer-term use is indicated, the drug should be taken no more than 2 or 4 times/week. **Sedating antidepressants** (eg, trazodone, nefazodone) have been used to treat insomnia in elderly persons with or without depression. However, these drugs can have adverse effects (eg, orthostatic hypotension, anticholinergic or gastrointestinal effects) and should thus not be used except when depression is present. For depressed patients who are being treated with a nonsedating antidepressant during the day and who are having sleeping difficulty, physicians may prescribe one of these drugs (at a low dose) for use at night.

Antihistamines and OTC drugs are generally not recommended for insomnia because of their adverse effects. Antihistamines (a common ingredient of OTC sleeping preparations) produce strong anticholinergic effects (eg, confusion, memory loss, dry mouth, blurred vision, constipation, urinary retention).

Barbiturates should not be used as a sleep aid; they have a prolonged duration of action, induce hepatic enzymes, and are highly addictive.

Alcohol used at bedtime initially causes drowsiness, but it disrupts sleep later in the night and should be avoided in persons who have difficulty with nocturnal sleep.

Chloral hydrate may be used for occasional insomnia but can cause delirium, gastrointestinal upset, and serious drug interactions with phenytoin and warfarin; it is contraindicated in severe hepatic or renal impairment.

Melatonin, available as an OTC oral preparation, is controversial. Little data support long-term use of melatonin, and there are virtually no studies in the elderly. Preparations of melatonin are widely available but are unregulated, so their quality is unknown.

CIRCADIAN RHYTHM SLEEP DISORDERS

(Circadian Dysrhythmia)

A group of disorders characterized by sleep and wakefulness that are not in phase with conventional environmental periods.

These disorders are common among the elderly. The usual cause, which may or may not be obvious, is an alteration in the sleep-wake cycle. Types of circadian rhythm sleep disorders are shown in TABLE 47–4.

Persons > 60 are more affected by circadian rhythm sleep disorders than are younger persons, and they take longer to recover. The increased incidence among elderly persons suggests age-related loss of circadian control of the sleeping process. Persons tend to fall asleep earlier and

TABLE 47–4.   TYPES OF CIRCADIAN RHYTHM SLEEP DISORDERS

Type	Description
Jet lag	Transient shift in sleep-wake pattern due to rapid travel across time zones
Shift-work sleep disorder	Shift in sleep-wake pattern due to nighttime shift work
Delayed sleep phase syndrome	Falling asleep later and waking later than desired
Advanced sleep phase syndrome	Falling asleep earlier and waking earlier than desired
Non–24-hour syndrome	Sleep-wake pattern that reflects a circadian cycle that is longer or shorter than 24 hours
Irregular sleep-wake patterns	Falling asleep and waking at irregular times

wake up progressively earlier as they age. However, elderly persons whose sleep is not disturbed may be better able to adapt to external changes in the sleep-wake cycle.

Bright light therapy can be effective, especially for jet lag and for an advanced sleep phase syndrome (ie, going to sleep early and waking early). Melatonin has also been reported to be effective for jet lag, but its use is controversial. Short-term therapy with hypnotics may help restore circadian sleep rhythms; these drugs should be tapered after 7 to 10 days. Gradual alteration of bedtime and awakening time may also be effective.

EXCESSIVE DAYTIME SLEEPINESS

Occasional sleepiness during the daytime is normal, especially among persons deprived of nocturnal sleep. However, daytime sleepiness that is persistent, excessive, and not easily resolved by increased sleep is abnormal and has been linked to automobile and occupational accidents.

Many disorders that interfere with nocturnal sleep (eg, sleep apnea, periodic limb movements of sleep) lead to daytime sleepiness. In addition, many drugs can cause sedation and daytime sleepiness, including antihistamines, some antihypertensives (eg, β-blockers, clonidine), antidepressants, antipsychotics, anticonvulsants, and analgesics. Narcolepsy (a syndrome characterized by daytime sleepiness, overwhelming episodes of sleep, and sudden loss of muscle tone) usually begins at a young age; onset is rare in the elderly.

Patients may report fatigue, lethargy, and problems with memory and concentration. Careful evaluation is needed to identify any treatable causes of excessive daytime sleepiness. A short daytime nap can be helpful for some patients.

PARASOMNIAS

Movements and behaviors that occur during sleep.

Parasomnias that can occur in the elderly include restless legs syndrome and periodic limb movements of sleep. REM sleep behavior disorder is another parasomnia that occurs in the elderly, particularly men. Patients have vivid dreams and vigorous behaviors during sleep that may cause injury. Other parasomnias, such as somnambulism and night terrors, are more common in children than in adults.

RESTLESS LEGS SYNDROME

An uncomfortable sensation in one or both legs (often described as an irresistible urge to move the legs) that is relieved by moving or rubbing the affected limbs.

This syndrome usually occurs immediately before bedtime or while the patient is awake in bed. Relief may occur with movement, and symptoms recur when the legs are stationary. The syndrome leads to difficulty falling asleep and, frequently, to insomnia. Restless legs syndrome differs from idiopathic leg muscle cramps, **1** in which calf pain and muscle spasms may occur at night.

Other than reassurance, treatment is often not needed, although walking, stretching, or rubbing the legs may help. Carbidopa-levodopa or bromocriptine may relieve chronic symptoms; opioids or benzodiazepines may be as effective but are used only for patients with severe symptoms who do not respond to other drugs.

PERIODIC LIMB MOVEMENTS OF SLEEP

(Nocturnal Myoclonus) **2**

Repetitive movements, mainly of the legs, that occur during sleep.

The incidence of periodic limb movements of sleep (PLMS) increases with age; these movements may occur in up to 45% of community-dwelling persons > 65. However, most sufferers are unaware of the movements.

Etiology is unknown. An age-related decrease in dopamine receptors has been suggested as a cause, because carbidopa-levodopa decreases the number of leg movements.

PLMS occurs only during sleep. It typically manifests as unilateral or bilateral flexion of the big toe, rapid flexion of the ankle, and partial

---

1 see page 533   **2** see also page 448

flexion of the knee and hip. Upper extremities may also move. Movement lasts 2 to 4 seconds and occurs throughout the night, sometimes as often as every 20 to 40 seconds. The movement may arouse patients from sleep (although most patients are not aware of having woken) and can cause insomnia and excessive daytime sleepiness.

PLMS is difficult to diagnose and treat; referral to a sleep specialist may be indicated. Some physicians consider carbidopa-levodopa the drug of choice because, when used in low doses, it is safer than the other drugs used to treat this disorder. Carbidopa-levodopa is initially given at night but may also be given during the day if limb movement occurs then. If carbidopa-levodopa is ineffective, a benzodiazepine (eg, clonazepam) or bromocriptine may be used. Opioids are less safe than these other drugs and are restricted to patients with severe symptoms in whom other therapies are ineffective.

SLEEP APNEA

(Sleep-Disordered Breathing)

Sleep apnea, which may be obstructive, central, or mixed, is a temporary interruption of breathing during sleep. Untreated, sleep apnea can cause significant morbidity and mortality.

OBSTRUCTIVE SLEEP APNEA

Temporary interruption of breathing during sleep due to obstruction of the airway.

Obstructive sleep apnea is the most common type of sleep apnea in the elderly. Airway obstruction is caused by temporary collapse of the oropharyngeal wall. Obstructive sleep apnea tends to occur in those who are moderately or severely obese, especially those who sleep supine, and is more common in men than in women. Use of alcohol or hypnotics may precipitate or exacerbate this disorder.

Mild obstructive sleep apnea ($\leq$ 5 episodes per hour) is common among the elderly; it occurs in 24% of those who live independently, in 33% of those in acute care institutions, and in 42% of those in nursing homes.

Symptoms and Signs

Obstructive sleep apnea is characterized by episodes of partial (hypopnea) or complete (apnea) interruption of respiration during sleep. In a hypopneic episode, breathing becomes abnormally slow and shallow. In an apneic episode, breathing stops for > 10 seconds. During these episodes, patients make persistent diaphragmatic efforts to overcome the airway obstruction; nevertheless, periods of profound oxygen desaturation may occur, possibly with systemic and pulmonary hypertension or cardiac arrhythmias (eg, tachycardia, bradycardia, atrial arrhythmias, ventricular arrhythmias). Cacophonous snoring and grunting, usually noticeable by the bed partner, may accompany the airway obstruction.

To resume normal breathing, patients wake (unknowingly) and spend excessive time in the lighter stages of sleep, causing them to be restless and unrefreshed during the day.

Diagnosis

Questionnaires can be used to screen for obstructive sleep apnea. The patient's sleeping partner and/or relatives should be asked about the patient's snoring and other behaviors during sleep. Diagnosis is strongly suggested by observing one or more apneic episodes while the patient is sleeping. Overnight pulse oximetry can detect hypoxemia during apneic episodes.

The diagnosis can be confirmed by overnight polysomnography, which is usually conducted in a sleep laboratory. However, screening with ambulatory (ie, in-home) polysomnography is increasingly available.

Prognosis and Treatment

Obstructive sleep apnea can lead to or exacerbate angina, renal dysfunction, stroke, myocardial infarction, cognitive impairment, impotence, hypertension, and depression. Increased mortality and morbidity occur when episodes are more frequent than 10 times/hour.

Treatment options are complex; treatment begins with common sense measures (eg, weight loss; discontinuation of hypnotics, other drugs, or alcohol use). Nasal continuous positive airway pressure (CPAP) therapy resolves most cases of sleep apnea but must be continued indefinitely. Dental devices to help keep the airway open may be used in some cases. Tracheostomy, which is reserved for the most severe cases, is the only totally successful measure. Uvulopalatopharyngoplasty (enlargement of the pharyngeal airspace through removal of excess tissue) helps < 50% of patients and may not be effective long-term. Laser surgery to reduce or obliterate pharyngeal tissue alleviates snoring but may not reduce the number of apneic episodes.

CENTRAL SLEEP APNEA

Temporary interruption of breathing during sleep due to loss of respiratory effort.

Causes include neurologic disease (eg, stroke), cerebrovascular disease, heart failure, and uremia. Symptoms are typically those of Cheyne-Stokes breathing. The underlying condition should be treated when possible (eg, reducing the severity of heart failure). Other treatments have had mixed results. Nasal oxygen can reduce accompanying hypoxemia. Acetazolamide (a carbonic anhydrase inhibitor) has also been used. The use of antidepressants (eg, clomipramine) and theophylline has also been described but is not well studied.

SLEEP DISORDERS DUE TO DEMENTIA

Changes in sleep with dementia have been described. Alzheimer's disease■ affects the suprachiasmatic nucleus and other neuroanatomic areas involved in the control of sleep (eg, the locus ceruleus, the nucleus basalis of Meynert). Patients with Alzheimer's disease have lower sleep efficiency with more arousals and awakenings and spend a higher percentage of sleep time in stage 1 and proportionately less time in stages 3 and 4 NREM sleep than do elderly persons without dementia. These problems become more pronounced and the percentage of REM sleep decreases as dementia progresses. Studies also suggest that many patients with Alzheimer's disease or multi-infarct dementia also have sleep apnea.

Reversible causes of sleep disorders in patients with dementia (eg, drug-related toxicity, infections, dehydration, drug-drug interactions, painful conditions) should be sought and treated.

A short nap during the day may help provide a needed rest, but a long nap (particularly if due to boredom or routine) may interfere with nocturnal sleep. Other approaches include manipulating the environment (eg, providing adequate daylight exposure and a comfortable nighttime temperature).

SLEEP DISORDERS ASSOCIATED WITH OTHER DISORDERS

Many disorders and their drug treatments can adversely affect sleep, and the symptoms of some may worsen during sleep. Drugs can blunt nocturnal breathing, exacerbate or cause apnea, produce unwanted arousals, and otherwise alter sleep physiology (see TABLE 47–1).

Musculoskeletal disorders: Patients with osteoarthritis may awaken with stiffness and pain, then have difficulty falling asleep again. Fibromyositis, polymyalgia rheumatica, recent fractures, and flexion contractures can cause pain and impair sleep. Treatment consists of managing pain with judicious use of analgesics, exercise, and other forms of physical activity. Behavioral techniques may also help.

Cardiovascular disorders: Heart failure can lead to orthopnea, which interferes with sleep; patients with orthopnea and dementia may

■ see page 365

be unable to explain their complaint, becoming agitated instead. Angina pectoris can prolong sleep latency, reducing the time spent in deep (stages 3 and 4) sleep. This disruption can lead to chronic insomnia and dependency on hypnotics. Improved control of these disorders can benefit sleep.

Pulmonary disorders: Chronic obstructive pulmonary disease can cause frequent awakenings, increase the amount of time spent in lighter (stage 1) sleep, markedly reduce the time spent in stages 3 and 4 and REM sleep, and decrease total sleep time. Sleep may be improved through better control of the respiratory disease.

Gastrointestinal disorders: Because acid secretion increases during the night, patients with peptic ulcer disease have difficulty falling asleep or may awaken. Nocturnal use of H_2 blockers may help, but some (eg, cimetidine) can penetrate the central nervous system and cause adverse effects. Gastroesophageal reflux, which can cause discomfort and thereby insomnia, may be prevented by maneuvers such as elevating the head of the bed and avoiding eating within 2 hours of bedtime. Antacids may also help.

Renal disorders: Patients undergoing renal dialysis experience chronic sleep disturbances. For patients with uremia, long awakenings from all stages of sleep are common, deep sleep time is proportionally decreased, and total sleep time is decreased. Elevated blood urea nitrogen levels correlate with the severity of the disturbance; dialysis alleviates the disturbance, increasing stage 3 and 4 sleep time.

Metabolic disorders: Hypothyroidism results in daytime sleepiness and decreased functional capacity. Stage 3 and 4 sleep time is reduced significantly but returns to normal with thyroid hormone replacement therapy. Hyperthyroidism increases stage 3 and 4 sleep time to almost 70% of total sleep time (25% is normal), but patients with hyperthyroidism often report insomnia. When the euthyroid state is restored, sleep stages become normal.

Neurologic disorders: Parkinson's disease compromises initiation and maintenance of sleep. The effects of levodopa on REM and deep sleep depend on dosage, and the drug can cause nightmares. Amantadine increases the amount of sleep.

SECTION 7

MUSCULOSKELETAL DISORDERS

48 ▌ AGING AND THE MUSCULOSKELETAL SYSTEM

CHANGES IN BONES

From about age 50, bone density (bone mass per unit volume) progressively decreases in both sexes, but more rapidly in women. This process, along with microarchitectural deterioration of the skeleton, leads to enhanced bone fragility and increased risk of fractures, a condition known as osteoporosis. **1** Conventionally, **osteoporosis** is diagnosed when bone density is at least 2.5 SD below the young adult mean; when bone density lies between 1 and 2.5 SD below the young adult mean, the condition is termed **osteopenia.**

A decline in sex hormones and aging itself both contribute to the loss of bone density. In men, testosterone production declines gradually, so bone loss is linear and slow. In women, a rapid phase of bone loss occurs during the first 5 to 10 years after menopause, **2** due to the precipitous loss of estrogen (menopausal bone loss). In addition to this rapid bone loss during early menopause, women, during their growing years and particularly during puberty, accumulate less skeletal mass than men, resulting in smaller, narrower, more fragile bones with thinner cortices. In old age, therefore, the consequences of bone loss are greater among women than among men, and the incidence of bone fractures is twofold to threefold higher. **3**

The loss of bone mass in either sex can be exacerbated by high circulating levels of endogenous or exogenous glucocorticoids and thyroxine, alcoholism, prolonged immobilization, gastrectomy and other gastrointestinal disorders, hypercalciuria, some types of malignancy, and cigarette smoking.

Progressive loss of bone mass that occurs with age affects the axial (primarily cancellous [trabecular]) and appendicular (primarily cortical) skeleton, with observable consequences such as loss of height

1 see page 472   **2** see page 1208   **3** see page 212

(stooping) and dorsal kyphosis (dowager's hump). Two key changes occur in cortical bone: reduced thickness and increased porosity. Women have thinner cortices than men do, so the effect of cortical thinning is more pronounced in women. Two key changes also occur in cancellous bone: thinning of normal trabeculae and destruction of entire trabeculae.

Normal Bone Regeneration

The skeleton undergoes periodic remodeling (ie, replacement of old bone by new), which is responsible for its complete regeneration every 10 years. Remodeling primarily occurs on the internal surfaces of bone and is carried out by a team of juxtaposed osteoclasts (in the front) and osteoblasts (in the rear) that together comprise the basic multicellular unit (BMU).

In cortical bone, BMUs move through the bone, forming a tunnel; in cancellous bone, they move across the trabecular surface, forming a trench. At the leading edge of the BMU, osteoclasts adhere to bone and subsequently remove it by acidification and proteolytic digestion. Osteoclasts then leave the resorption site, and osteoblasts move in and secrete osteoid, which is eventually mineralized into new bone. In healthy adults, 3 to 4 million BMUs are initiated per year, and about 1 million are operating at any moment. Although millions of small packets of bone are constantly being remodeled, bone mass is preserved through a remarkably tight balance between resorption and formation.

Birth of osteoclasts and osteoblasts: Osteoclasts and osteoblasts derive from precursors originating in the bone marrow. Osteoclast precursors are hematopoietic cells of the monocyte/macrophage lineage. Osteoblast precursors are multipotent mesenchymal stem cells, which also give rise to bone marrow stromal cells, chondrocytes, muscle cells, and adipocytes. The development of osteoclasts and osteoblasts is controlled by growth factors and cytokines produced within the bone marrow, by systemic hormones, and probably by mechanical signals.

Death of osteoclasts and osteoblasts: The average life span of the osteoclasts and osteoblasts that constitute the BMU is much shorter than the life span of the BMU itself. After osteoclasts have eroded to a particular distance, either from the central axis in cortical bone or to a particular depth from the surface in cancellous bone, they die by apoptosis and disappear. Fifty percent to 70% of osteoblasts also die by apoptosis once they have completed their bone-forming task. The remaining osteoblasts become elongated lining cells that cover the newly formed bone surface, or they are entrapped in the mineralized matrix and become osteocytes. Osteocytes are stellate cells—reminiscent of the dendritic network of the central nervous system—that constitute about 90% of cells present in bone. Osteocytes are believed to act as sensors, detecting localized need for bone remodeling or repair.

TABLE 48–1.   FEATURES OF BONE LOSS

Menopausal Bone Loss	Senescent Bone Loss
High remodeling (turnover) rate	Low or variable remodeling (turnover) rate
Removal of trabeculae	Thinning of cortices and residual trabeculae (in women)
Increased risk of vertebral and Colles' fractures	Increased risk of vertebral and hip fractures
Increased osteoblast formation	Decreased* osteoblast formation
Increased† osteoclast formation	Decreased osteoclast formation
Bone marrow adiposity unknown	Increased bone marrow adiposity
Increased life span of osteoclasts	Life span of osteoclasts unknown
Decreased life span of osteoblasts	Life span of osteoblasts unknown
Decreased life span of osteocytes	Decreased life span of osteocytes
Probable causes include interleukin-6, interleukin-1, tumor necrosis factor, macrophage colony-stimulating factor, transforming growth factor-β, and removal of direct effects of estrogen on apoptosis	Probable causes include peroxisome proliferator-activated receptor γ_2, prostaglandin J_2, interleukin-11, and insulin-like growth factors

*Undersupply of osteoblasts relative to the need for cavity repair.
†Oversupply of osteoclasts relative to the need for remodeling.

Pathogenesis of Bone Loss

Bone loss that occurs as part of normal aging can be divided into two phases: a rapid one that affects women after menopause (menopausal bone loss) and a slow one that affects both women and men after the age of 50 (senescent bone loss). These two phases have distinct histologic and clinical features (see TABLE 48–1). In women, the two phases eventually overlap and become difficult to differentiate. Senescent bone loss may also overlap with secondary hyperparathyroidism, which may result from the impaired ability of the aging intestine to absorb calcium. Nonetheless, the heterogeneity of underlying conditions in many elderly persons can independently contribute to skeletal deterioration and distort the clinical and histologic picture.

Menopausal bone loss: Before menopause, sex hormones protect the bone, at least in part, by regulating the development and death (apoptosis) of osteoclasts and osteoblasts through altered production of cytokines and altered responsiveness of bone marrow cell progenitors to cytokines. For example, the production of interleukin-6 (IL-6) by osteoblasts is inhibited by estrogen and androgen.

After menopause (or after castration in men), bone loss increases by as much as 10-fold, largely due to overproduction of IL-6. Overproduction of IL-6 seems to play a similar role in several conditions involving increased bone resorption, including multiple myeloma, Paget's disease, rheumatoid arthritis, Gorham-Stout or disappearing bone disease, hyperthyroidism, primary and secondary hyperparathyroidism, and McCune-Albright syndrome.

Estrogen deficiency seems to delay osteoclast apoptosis but promote osteoblast apoptosis, resulting in an imbalance between bone resorption and formation. Furthermore, the delay in osteoclast apoptosis may be responsible for deeper resorption cavities and thereby the trabecular perforation resulting from estrogen deficiency.

Vertebral and Colles' fractures are typical of menopausal bone loss.

Senescent bone loss: The amount of bone formed during remodeling decreases with age in both sexes, indicated by a consistent decrease in wall thickness, especially in trabecular bone. With age, formation of osteoblasts decreases, formation of adipocytes in the bone marrow increases, rate of bone formation decreases, and bone mineral density decreases. These changes may explain the decreased bone formation and the resulting osteopenia and increased adiposity of bone marrow that occur with age.

Vertebral and hip fractures are typical of senescent bone loss.

CHANGES IN CARTILAGE

Nonarticular cartilage grows throughout life; eg, the ears and nose tend to grow larger relative to the face as a person ages. Age-related crystal formation and calcification occur in cartilage, but the effect of these changes on cartilage function is unclear.

In articular cartilage, age-related biochemical changes do not readily correlate with the presence of joint disease. However, an age-related increase in transglutaminase activity in chondrocytes correlates with an increase in anionic protein cross-linkage in the pericellular space and with an increased risk of calcium pyrophosphate dihydrate crystal deposition around chondrocytes. These changes may explain the increased incidence of chondrocalcinosis in the elderly.

Knee cartilage decreases in thickness by about 0.25 mm/year, probably as a result of wear and tear. In some cases, knee cartilage thins more rapidly or remains morphologically normal.

CHANGES IN CONNECTIVE TISSUE

With age, the proliferative capacity and synthetic activity of fibroblasts decrease in vitro. These changes may partially explain diminished healing capacity with age; tensile strength decreases, and the stiffness of connective tissue increases. A demonstrable decrease in the strength of ligaments and tendons, which are largely composed of connective tissue, increases the risk that these structures will fail with age. Other age-related changes in connective tissue affect blood vessel walls, possibly contributing to arteriosclerosis and hypertension.

CHANGES IN MUSCLE

Between ages 30 and 75, lean body mass decreases, primarily due to loss of skeletal muscle mass, and the number and size of muscle fibers progressively decrease. This process is termed **sarcopenia.** The pathogenesis of sarcopenia may involve several age-related factors, such as reduced levels of physical activity; changes in the central or peripheral nervous system, possibly beginning during middle age, that may lead to a loss of motor units; and reduced rate of skeletal muscle protein synthesis. In many elderly persons, loss of muscle mass may be accelerated as a result of greater dietary protein requirements coupled with reduced protein intake. **1**

In healthy young persons, 30% of body weight is muscle, 20% is adipose tissue, and 10% is bone. Muscle accounts for 50% of lean body mass and about 50% of the total amount of body nitrogen. By age 75, about 15% of body weight is muscle, 40% is adipose tissue, and 8% is bone. Thus, half the muscle mass has disappeared because of sarcopenia.

The faster-contracting type II muscle fibers decrease to a greater extent than do the slower-contracting type I muscle fibers. Type II fibers participate in sudden powerful muscle contractions, whereas type I fibers function to maintain posture and to perform rhythmic, endurance-type exercises. The age-related loss of muscle fibers correlates with a loss of maximum isometric contraction force, which decreases 20% by the 6th decade and 50% by the 8th decade.

The reasons for these changes in body composition and isometric contraction force are not completely understood, but contributing factors may include a relative deficiency of anabolic hormones, such as growth hormone, insulin-like growth factor I (IGF-I), testosterone, and dehydroepiandrosterone (DHEA), and a decrease in the routine performance of vigorous muscular work. Patients with such hormone deficits may require hormone supplementation. **2**

In the elderly, the beneficial effects of exercise **3** are usually specific to the task selected as the training activity. For example, if the goal is to achieve greater capability in throwing a ball, then the exercise should involve throwing a ball rather than merely strengthening the muscles involved in throwing. To improve functional ability, elderly persons must incorporate both task-specific training and muscle-strengthening exercises. More studies are needed to determine the optimal frequency,

1 see page 595   **2** see page 655   **3** see page 295

intensity, duration, and types of exercise necessary for maintaining a desirable level of muscular fitness in elderly persons.

Elderly persons whose mobility is restricted because of acute illness, especially elderly persons who are bedridden, are at risk of deconditioning and of accelerated loss of muscle mass and strength. The rate of loss is about 1.5%/day; deconditioning is greatest in the antigravity muscles—those used to sit up, stand up, and pull up—which are essential for performing activities of daily living. Some geriatricians estimate that for 1 day of absolute bed rest, 2 weeks of reconditioning are necessary to return to baseline function. Early intervention with physical therapy and an individualized exercise regimen should be included in the care plan for hospitalized elderly persons, especially those who are bedridden.

Despite age-related reductions in muscle strength, muscle functional ability is similar in older and younger adults. Usually, healthy elderly persons can easily climb stairs, rise from a squatting position, walk along a straight line, hop on either foot, and perform typical activities of daily living.

49 ■ METABOLIC BONE DISEASE

The skeleton is a metabolically active organ that undergoes continuous remodeling throughout life, not only to provide structural integrity and strength to support the body and protect vital organs, but also to store essential minerals, particularly calcium.■ The hematopoietic function of bone also changes with age.■

OSTEOPOROSIS

A disease characterized by low bone mass and microarchitectural deterioration of bone tissue leading to enhanced bone fragility and a consequent increase in fracture risk.

Bone loss in the elderly may be normal, in which bone density is within 1 SD of the young adult mean; osteopenic, in which bone density is between 1 and 2.5 SD below the young adult mean; or osteoporotic, in which bone density is > 2.5 SD below the young adult mean.

In the USA, the estimated prevalence of osteopenia is 15 million in women and 3 million in men. The estimated prevalence of osteoporosis is 8 million in women and 2 million in men. Osteopenia and osteoporo-

■ see page 468   ■ see page 672

sis are major public health problems, resulting in substantial morbidity and estimated health costs of > $14 billion annually.

Classification and Etiology

Primary osteoporosis in the elderly can be classified as type I or II. Type I (menopausal) osteoporosis occurs mainly in persons aged 51 to 75, is six times more common in women, and is associated with vertebral and Colles' fractures. ❶ Type II (senescent) osteoporosis occurs in persons > 60, is two times more common in women, and is associated with vertebral and hip fractures. Overlap between types I and II is substantial, so this classification is of limited clinical use. Primary osteoporosis in premenopausal women and younger men, which is rare, is classified as idiopathic.

Primary osteoporosis is thought to result from the hormonal changes that occur with age, particularly decreasing levels of sex hormones (estrogen in women, testosterone in men). Several other factors are probably contributory.

Secondary osteoporosis accounts for only a small proportion of osteoporosis cases among the elderly, in whom primary and secondary osteoporosis often occur together. It accounts for a much greater proportion of cases among premenopausal women and younger men.

Secondary osteoporosis may be due to many causes, including hyperparathyroidism, hyperthyroidism, malignancy, immobilization, gastrointestinal disease, renal abnormality (eg, idiopathic hypercalciuria), and use of drugs that cause bone loss (eg, anticonvulsants). Mild to moderate vitamin D deficiency, which is common in elderly persons, may give rise to osteoporosis rather than to osteomalacia. ❷ Glucocorticoid-induced osteoporosis is of particular concern in the elderly, who may already have calcium deficiency and impaired bone formation, both of which are worsened by glucocorticoids. Screening for secondary osteoporosis is important in patients of all ages, because many of the causes are treatable or have an important effect on prognosis (see Figure 49–1).

Pathogenesis and Risk Factors

Diminished bone mass can result from failure to reach an optimal peak bone mass in early adulthood, from increased bone resorption, or from decreased bone formation after peak bone mass has been achieved. All three of these factors probably play a role in most elderly persons. Low bone mass, rapid bone loss, and increased fracture risk correlate with high rates of bone turnover (ie, resorption and formation). Presumably, in osteoporosis, the rate of formation is inadequate to offset the rate of resorption and maintain the structural integrity of the skeleton.

---

❶see Table 48–1 on page 469   ❷see page 483

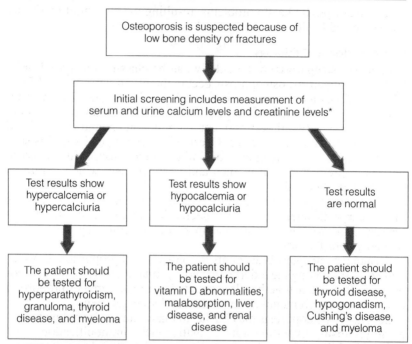

*Measurement of the serum ionized calcium level is preferable. If this test is not possible, the albumin level should be measured. Fasting urine samples are generally adequate, but 24-hour urine samples may be needed.

FIGURE 49–1. **Laboratory tests for secondary osteoporosis.** Adapted from Orlic ZC, Raisz LG: "Causes of secondary osteoporosis." *Journal of Clinical Densitometry* 2:1–14, 1998.

The major risk factors for osteoporosis are increased age, female sex, white or Asian race, positive family history of osteoporosis, and thin body habitus. Other risk factors include decreased lifelong exposure to estrogen, low calcium intake, sedentary lifestyle, and cigarette smoking.

Age: The effect of age on the skeleton is complex. Bone resorption rates appear to be maintained or even to increase with age; bone formation rates tend to decrease. Loss of template due to complete resorption of trabecular elements or to endosteal removal of cortical bone produces irreversible bone loss. Age-related microdamage and death of osteocytes may also increase skeletal fragility. However, osteoporosis is not an inevitable consequence of aging; many persons maintain good bone mass and structural integrity into their 80s and 90s.

Sex: The greater frequency of osteoporotic fractures in women has many causes. Women have lower peak bone mass and lower muscle mass than men. They experience accelerated bone loss at menopause and may also lose bone during the reproductive years, particularly with prolonged lactation. The smaller periosteal diameter of bones in women also increases skeletal fragility. Another reason for female predominance is that women live longer than men.

Race: Although osteoporosis is more prevalent among persons of white and Asian descent than among blacks, the reasons are not well understood; prevalence also varies among ethnic groups. Whites have lower peak bone mass than do blacks, but the difference in fracture risk appears to be independent of the difference in bone density. Differences in body composition, skeletal structure, and bone turnover may play a role.

Heredity: About 50 to 80% of peak bone mass is genetically determined. A positive family history of osteoporosis increases fracture risk, independent of bone density. Genetic studies comparing osteoporotic patients with healthy persons have shown several differences in specific genes for collagen, hormone receptors, and local factors. Many genes probably play a role.

Body habitus: The increased risk of fracture associated with a thin body habitus is probably multifactorial. Thin women produce less estrogen from androgen (this conversion occurs in fat tissue), especially after menopause. Obesity may be associated with increased muscle mass, greater weight-bearing impact on the skeleton, and greater protection of the skeleton, particularly of the hip, by subcutaneous fat.

Systemic hormones: Age-related changes in estrogen levels increase fracture risk. In addition, increased levels of parathyroid hormone and decreased levels of the growth hormone/insulin-like growth factor I system appear to decrease bone mass and increase fracture risk. Although excess glucocorticoids and thyroid hormone can contribute to secondary osteoporosis, they have not been shown to play a role in primary osteoporosis.

Local factors: Animal studies suggest that the interaction of systemic hormones with local regulators of bone remodeling, including cytokines and prostaglandins, plays a critical role in the increase in bone resorption and relative impairment of bone formation that occurs after oophorectomy. However, evidence implicating these local factors in human osteoporosis is limited. Interleukin-1 activity may be increased in osteoporosis; although interleukin-6 activity appears to increase with age, no correlation with osteoporosis has been demonstrated. Inhibition of prostaglandin production by nonsteroidal antiinflammatory drugs (NSAIDs) results in a small increase in bone mass.

Symptoms and Signs

Osteoporosis has been termed a silent disease because, until a frac ture occurs, symptoms are absent.

A loss of height may indicate a vertebral compression fracture, which occurs in many patients without trauma or other acute precipitant. Dor sal kyphosis with exaggerated lordosis (dowager's hump) may result from multiple compression fractures. In some fracture patients, pain may be acute and severe and then subside slowly over several weeks. Chronic back pain in the elderly can be due to vertebral compression from osteoporosis but is as likely to be due to joint or disk disease. Osteoporotic fractures commonly affect the hip because the elderly tend to fall sideways or backwards, landing on this joint. ◻ Younger, more agile persons tend to fall forward, landing on the outstretched wrist, thus fracturing the distal radius ◻. Osteoporosis is also associated with other fractures of the extremities and pelvis and with vertebral fractures, but not with fractures of the head and face.

Diagnosis

The **history** should focus on primary risk factors and secondary causes of osteoporosis. A complete history of menstrual function, pregnancy, and lactation should be obtained in women, and a history of sexual function should be obtained in men, in whom decreased libido and erectile dysfunction may be due to low testosterone levels. Neurologic deficits and drugs that might increase the risk of falls should be analyzed. The family history should include fractures and evidence of endocrinopathy or renal calculi. One of the most important predictors of osteoporotic fractures is a history of a fracture after age 40 due to minimal or moderate trauma. In such persons, the fracture risk may be increased severalfold.

The **physical examination** is often unremarkable. Spinal deformity and tenderness over the lower back should be sought.

X-ray findings are generally insufficient for the diagnosis of primary osteoporosis; x-rays may detect osteopenia only when bone loss is > 30%. Vertebral compression fractures can be seen on x-ray, but anterior wedging may have been present since adolescence (Scheuermann's disease), and some degree of age-related wedging can occur in the absence of marked bone loss. X-ray findings can also suggest other causes of metabolic bone disease, such as the lytic lesions in multiple myeloma and the pseudofractures characteristic of osteomalacia. ◻

Bone densitometry is the only method for diagnosing or confirming osteoporosis in the absence of a fracture. The National Osteoporosis Foundation recommends that bone densitometry be performed routinely in all women > 65, particularly in those who have one or more risk factors. However, such a routine approach is costly. Densitometry can also be used for monitoring the response to therapy.

Currently available densitometric systems have many pitfalls. The relationship between bone density and fracture risk is continuous and graded; with densitometry, diagnostic cutoffs are arbitrary and must be considered in light of other risk factors. In general, a difference of 1 SD

◻ see page 223   ◻ see page 220   ◻ see page 484

from the young adult mean equals a 10 to 12% difference in bone density. There is a 2.7-fold increase in the relative risk of hip fracture for a 1 SD decrease in femoral neck bone density from the young adult mean; the increase in relative risk is somewhat less (about 1.5- to 2.0-fold increase for 1 SD decrease) when density is measured at sites other than the femoral neck. In women > 75, even 1 SD below the age-adjusted norm is highly predictive of fractures.

Furthermore, peripheral densitometry measurement may not reflect central measurement and is subject to artifacts. In the elderly, measurement of the lumbar spine is often complicated by osteoarthritic changes, disk disease, and calcification of the underlying aorta. Another limitation of densitometry is that current criteria are based on data from white postmenopausal women and that appropriate diagnostic criteria for other populations are not established. In addition, bone density values vary with the technique used and the position of the patient.

Dual energy x-ray absorptiometry (DEXA) can be used to measure bone mineral density in the spine, hip, wrist, or total body. Radiation exposure is minimal, and the procedure is rapid. However, the standard apparatus is expensive and not portable. Small DEXA machines that can measure the forearm, finger, or heel are less expensive and are portable. Also, DEXA measures areal density (ie, g/cm^2) rather than true volumetric density.

Quantitative CT measures true volumetric density and can be limited to regions of interest (eg, trabecular bone in the spine); however, the apparatus is expensive, and radiation exposure is somewhat larger than with DEXA.

Ultrasound densitometry can assess the density and structure of the skeleton and appears to predict fracture risk in the elderly. The apparatus is relatively inexpensive, portable, and uses no radiation but can be used only in peripheral sites (eg, the heel), where bone is relatively superficial.

X-ray absorptiometry can be used to measure bone density in the hand in comparison with density in a standardized metal wedge. Its value in predicting fractures is not well established.

Differential diagnosis: To confirm the diagnosis of primary osteoporosis, one must exclude secondary osteoporosis, osteomalacia, and malignancy.

The probability of secondary osteoporosis in an elderly patient, with or without typical osteoporotic fractures, is low, but a limited diagnostic assessment is warranted (see FIGURE 49–1), particularly when serum and urine calcium levels are abnormal. Because vitamin D deficiency usually responds to ordinary supplementation, which is part of the routine care of osteoporotic patients, measurement of 25-hydroxyvitamin D$_3$ levels may be indicated only if malabsorption is evident. The use of biochemical markers of bone turnover in the evaluation of osteoporosis has not been established because, although high turnover is associated with increased bone loss and fracture risk, individual variation is great. However, markers such as collagen cross-links and bone-specific alkaline phosphatase levels can be used to assess the response to therapy.

Prognosis and Treatment

Osteoporosis does not directly cause death. However, an excess mortality of 10 to 20% occurs in patients with established osteoporosis, particularly those with hip fractures.

Prevention of osteoporotic fractures is critical to avoid a worldwide, costly epidemic. Prevention programs should be developed for patients at risk and for patients with diagnosed osteoporosis. Approaches include adequate intake of calcium and vitamin D, regular weight-bearing exercise and other efforts to minimize the risk of falls, smoking cessation, and good general nutrition.

Calcium and vitamin D: The typical diet of elderly Americans provides only about 600 mg/day of calcium and < 200 IU of vitamin D. Supplemental calcium and vitamin D can reduce the risk of fracture by as much as 30% in elderly persons who have relatively low intakes and limited sun exposure, particularly nursing home residents during winter months. Supplementation can be achieved through increased dietary intake of dairy products and other nutrients rich in calcium and vitamin D or through use of supplements. Some calcium supplements and most multivitamin tablets contain vitamin D. The recommended intake for elderly Americans is ≥ 1200 mg/day of elemental calcium and ≥ 400 IU/day of vitamin D; a somewhat larger intake of calcium and vitamin D may be beneficial and is generally considered safe. However, vitamin D intoxication can occur if intake is ≥ 50,000 IU/week. Calcium supplements are generally well tolerated in the elderly, but gastrointestinal complaints, particularly constipation, are common. In these persons, the use of alternative calcium salts (eg, calcium citrate) and efforts to increase dietary calcium are often effective. A good diet should include an adequate amount of vitamin K, because vitamin K deficiency is associated with increased fracture risk. A limited sodium intake may also be helpful, because high sodium intake can result in increased urinary calcium losses.

Exercise: The effects of weight-bearing and muscle-strengthening exercise on bone density are relatively small.∎ However, improved balance and muscle strength decrease the likelihood of falls and improve cardiovascular health.

Antiresorptive therapy: Persons with low bone mass and multiple risk factors, particularly those who have already had an osteoporotic fracture, should be considered for antiresorptive therapy. Antiresorptive

∎ see page 296

drugs include estrogens, bisphosphonates, selective estrogen receptor modulators, and calcitonin.

Estrogen can prevent menopausal bone loss in most women. Estrogen replacement therapy (ERT) is the treatment of choice for post-menopausal women, **1** particularly those who had an early menopause, and for women who have had a hysterectomy. ERT is particularly effective during the first few years after menopause when bone loss is most rapid. **2** Hormone replacement therapy (HRT), which contains a combination of estrogen and progestin, is necessary to prevent endometrial hyperplasia and avoid the increased risk of uterine malignancy in women who have a uterus. Other potential benefits of ERT and HRT include diminished risk of cardiovascular disease and Alzheimer's disease, but these benefits are not as well established. Many women start ERT or HRT during menopause because it provides short-term relief of menopausal symptoms. These women often discontinue therapy after a few years, which leads to resumption of rapid bone loss. The decision to discontinue ERT or HRT might be aided by densitometry. If discontinued, ERT or HRT can be restarted at any age. Estrogen decreases bone resorption and increases bone mass in women in their late 70s and 80s. In these patients, lower doses of estrogen may be effective and produce fewer adverse effects.

Epidemiologic studies and the few prospective clinical trials of estrogen suggest that ERT or HRT decreases the risk of osteoporotic fractures by 30 to 50%. Because other antiresorptive drugs may have an additive effect when given with estrogen, combination therapy should be considered in patients who have very low bone density, continue to lose bone, or incur a fracture while taking ERT or HRT.

Bisphosphonates are potent antiresorptive drugs that directly inhibit osteoclast activity. For women who cannot tolerate estrogen or have contraindications (eg, preexisting breast cancer, risk factors for breast cancer), bisphosphonates are considered the next choice; these drugs increase bone mass and decrease the risk of fractures, particularly in patients taking glucocorticoids. Bisphosphonates, particularly alendronate, have also decreased the incidence of vertebral and nonvertebral fractures by ≥ 50% in large cohorts of postmenopausal women.

Alendronate is used to prevent (5 mg/day) and treat (10 mg/day) osteoporosis. Pamidronate is available IV for treatment of hypercalcemia of malignancy and Paget's disease but has been used in osteoporosis.

A major problem with oral administration of bisphosphonates is poor absorption. Usually < 1% of the drug is absorbed; to achieve optimal absorption, patients must take bisphosphonates without food or other drugs. The major adverse effects with oral use are gastrointestinal,

1 see page 1211   **2** see page 469

particularly esophageal irritation. Bisphosphonates given IV can cause transient hyperpyrexia, which is usually not severe. Because of the gastrointestinal effects, bisphosphonates are often avoided in patients with gastroesophageal reflux disease, but a cautious trial of these drugs may be justified.

Selective estrogen receptor modulators (SERMs) have been developed that are antiestrogenic in the classic target organs (eg, breast, uterus) but have antiresorptive effects on bone. Raloxifene is approved for prevention of postmenopausal bone loss. It is somewhat less effective as an antiresorptive drug than are estrogens or bisphosphonates but can prevent bone loss and decrease the incidence of vertebral fractures.

SERMs have relatively few adverse effects. However, similar to estrogens, they increase the risk of thromboembolism. A possible advantage of SERMs is an apparent ability to reduce the risk of breast cancer.

Calcitonin has been used for many years in the prevention and treatment of osteoporosis. Salmon calcitonin is available in the USA as a nasal spray or subcutaneous injection. Nasal calcitonin 200 IU/day reduces the incidence of vertebral fractures, although the magnitude of the effect is smaller than that seen with estrogens, bisphosphonates, or SERMs. Nasal calcitonin is generally safe; the major adverse effect is local irritation.

Other therapies: Anabolic therapies are under study; none is approved for osteoporosis. Intermittent injections of parathyroid hormone and fluoride stimulate bone formation and inhibit bone resorption, but their safety and efficacy remain to be established. Thiazides can decrease urinary calcium excretion and slow bone loss. They may be particularly useful in patients with hypercalciuria and osteoporosis (eg, those with idiopathic hypercalciuria).

PAGET'S DISEASE OF BONE
(Osteitis Deformans)

A progressive focal disorder of bone remodeling, in which normal bone is removed and replaced with abnormal bone.

The disorder is initiated by the proliferation of abnormally large osteoclasts, which resorb bone at local affected sites. Resorption is followed by a variable, but often marked, increase in the formation of new bone that is architecturally disorganized.

Epidemiology and Etiology

Paget's disease of bone is estimated to occur in 2 to 3% of persons > 60 in the USA. The prevalence varies widely in different regions of the world. The relative risk is increased about sevenfold in first-degree relatives of patients with Paget's disease. The etiology has not been established, but genetic factors and a paramyxovirus infection may be involved. A genetic locus for susceptibility to Paget's disease has been identified on chromosome 18q in some large kindreds of patients, but not all kindreds show this locus, suggesting genetic heterogeneity. Structures resembling viral nucleocapsids have been identified in pagetic osteoclasts, but the results of studies of viral RNA expression in pagetic bone are inconsistent.

Pathology

Pagetic lesions may be single or multiple and can involve any part of the skeleton, most commonly the pelvis, femur, spine, skull, and tibia. Pagetic osteoclasts are large and have many more nuclei than normal. Similarly, the osteoblastic response is exuberant and disorganized, producing "mosaic" bone with a woven pattern of collagen deposition. The adjacent marrow is vascular and often shows fibroblastic proliferation and decreased hematopoiesis. The hypercellularity may diminish, leaving sclerotic bone with little cellular activity, the so-called "burned-out" phase of Paget's disease. Frequently, all phases of the pagetic process occur simultaneously in a patient or even in a single lesion.

Symptoms and Signs

Patients may be asymptomatic for many years. Deformities, neurologic impairment, pathologic fractures, bone pain, hypervascularity, and arthritic changes in adjacent joints may be the initial symptoms. Changes in the skull often lead to impaired central nervous system function, particularly hearing loss due to involvement of the petrous bone. Involvement of the base of the skull may produce platybasia and basilar invagination, which leads to the rare, but serious, complication of brain stem compression. Vertebral deformity may lead to spinal cord compression. Although pagetic long bones often show increased density, their irregular structure leads to skeletal deformity with fragility and increased risk of fracture. The bone deformity can lead to damage to articular cartilage with consequent osteoarthritis, especially in the knee and hip. The hypervascularity of pagetic bone may produce palpable local warmth, increase cardiac output, and aggravate coexisting heart disease. Angioid streaks in the retina may occur but rarely impair vision.

Neoplastic changes in pagetic bone probably occur in < 1% of patients; however, osteosarcoma in the elderly is often associated with Paget's disease. Fibrosarcoma and chondrosarcoma may also occur. Such tumors may result in pathologic fractures. Benign giant cell tumors, which are called reparative granulomas or osteoclastomas, can also occur adjacent to pagetic lesions.

The increased incidence of primary hyperparathyroidism among patients with Paget's disease may be real or may be due to more intense investigation by the metabolic bone disease clinics to which these patients are referred. Hypercalcemia, while uncommon, occurs in immobilized patients with Paget's disease or may be caused by associated hyperparathyroidism; thus, patients with Paget's disease who require immediate bed rest should be monitored. Hypercalciuria, hyperuricemia, and gout occur more frequently in patients with Paget's disease, but the incidence of renal calculi does not seem to be much increased.

Diagnosis

Asymptomatic Paget's disease may be detected incidentally by finding that the serum alkaline phosphatase level is elevated or that a suggestive x-ray abnormality is present. Further evaluation consists of a measurement of bone resorption and a bone scan. Measurement of urinary hydroxyproline can be helpful, but measurement of the new resorption markers, such as the N-telopeptide cross-links of collagen, is equally sensitive and is not affected by collagen in the diet. Increased uptake on bone scan is not diagnostic but indicates the sites at which x-rays should be obtained; it is particularly useful in differentiating degenerative joint disease from pagetic lesions. Serum calcium levels should be measured; hyperparathyroidism appears to be more common in patients with Paget's disease.

X-ray lesions may be largely osteolytic, osteoblastic, or mixed. The initial osteolytic lesion in the skull, termed osteoporosis circumscripta, may be followed by a marked increase in bone formation, ultimately leading to a thickened calvaria with an irregular "cotton wool" appearance. Bowing is common in affected limbs, and kyphosis occurs in patients with vertebral lesions.

Prognosis and Treatment

Patients who develop osteosarcoma, fibrosarcoma, or chondrosarcoma have a grave prognosis and respond poorly to chemotherapy. However, benign giant cell tumors can be sensitive to glucocorticoids and antiosteolytic drugs (eg, bisphosphonates, calcitonin).

Localized asymptomatic disease requires no treatment. Treatment should be given, however, to those at risk of complications, including those with demonstrable osteopenia or osteoporosis and those whose disease affects weight-bearing sites (eg, long bones, vertebrae) or sites where neurologic damage is likely to occur. Severe deformities, neurologic symptoms, and degenerative joint changes in patients with more advanced disease are frequently irreversible. However, treatment can slow or prevent further deterioration.

Patients can be followed with serum alkaline phosphatase measurements for biochemical remission, but measurements of urinary collagen cross-link excretion may be more sensitive for early detection of relapse. In general, treatment should be continued until a biochemical remission has occurred, although remission cannot always be achieved in severe cases.

Hearing loss is common in patients with Paget's disease and should be monitored. The process probably cannot be reversed by treatment, but antiresorptive therapy may prevent progression.

Pharmacotherapy: **Bisphosphonates** are the therapy of choice. Newer bisphosphonates have replaced etidronate, which often produces only partial remissions and, if used in high doses, can impair mineralization, leading to osteomalacia. Pamidronate is available in the USA only for IV therapy. Doses of 30 to 90 mg are given in a single 4- to 6-hour IV infusion, which may be repeated at weekly or monthly intervals until biochemical remission is achieved. In patients with mild or limited disease, a single IV infusion may produce a prolonged remission. Oral alendronate 40 mg/day for 6 months frequently produces a prolonged remission. Shorter courses may be effective in milder cases. Risedronate 30 mg/day po may be given initially for 2 months. This drug produces a prolonged remission more often than etidronate does.

Salmon calcitonin injections 50 to 100 U/day have been widely used. This regimen heals osteolytic lesions, but adverse effects (eg, nausea and vomiting, flushing, local discomfort at the site of injection) are common, and resistance may develop.

Surgery: Patients with severe deformities and irreversible osteo-arthritic changes in the hip or knee joint may be treated surgically. Hip and knee replacements can be successful. Osteotomies can relieve nerve compression.

Ancillary measures: Intake of calcium and vitamin D should be adequate to prevent impairment of mineralization in bone that is turning over rapidly and to help reduce the rate of bone remodeling. Antiarthritic drugs should be used in patients with joint involvement in whom pain often persists despite biochemical remission.

OSTEOMALACIA

A disorder in which the structural and metabolic functions of the skeleton are impaired because of failure of mineralization of newly formed matrix, usually resulting from vitamin D deficiency.

Osteomalacia (analogous to rickets in children) is relatively rare in the elderly, although deficiency of vitamin D and calcium is common.

Vitamin D is really a prohormone. It can be synthesized in the skin in response to specific wavelengths of ultraviolet light or obtained in the diet. Once formed in the skin, vitamin D is converted in the liver to 25-hydroxyvitamin D_3, which is normally present in relatively high concentrations in the circulation, bound to a vitamin D–binding protein. Final activation of vitamin D to 1,25-dihydroxyvitamin D_3 occurs in the kidney; this active hormonal form stimulates intestinal absorption of calcium and phosphorus, thus promoting mineralization of bone.

Etiology

Vitamin D deficiency may be due to inadequate synthesis of vitamin D during the winter months in patients who live in northern latitudes. Impairment of small-bowel absorption of dietary vitamin D occurs in patients with fat malabsorption.

Impairment of conversion to 25-hydroxyvitamin D_3 occurs in patients with severe liver disease and in those taking drugs that alter hepatic hydroxylases, especially anticonvulsants such as phenytoin, barbiturates, or carbamazepine. Impairment of conversion to 1,25-dihydroxyvitamin D_3 is commonly due to loss of renal 1α-hydroxylase activity in renal failure.

Phosphate deficiency (with resulting hypophosphatemia) can cause osteomalacia by impairing bone mineralization. Hypophosphatemia rarely results from inadequate dietary intake, but it can result from impaired absorption (eg, due to malabsorption syndromes or vitamin D deficiency) or from renal losses (eg, due to hyperparathyroidism or congenital disorders of renal phosphate transport). Hypophosphatemia can result from ingestion of large amounts of phosphate-binding antacids (eg, aluminum hydroxide). One form of hypophosphatemic osteomalacia is associated with mesenchymal tumors (neoplastic osteomalacia), but the hypophosphatemia may be due to inhibition of 1α-hydroxylase in the kidney.

Calcium deficiency very rarely causes osteomalacia.

Symptoms and Signs

The major symptoms of osteomalacia are bone pain, deformities, and weakness. Patients may present with vertebral crush fractures, mimicking osteoporosis. Pseudofractures (Looser's zones) may be seen on x-rays of the scapula, pelvis, and long bones. These pseudofractures probably represent localized defects in mineralization. Weakness may be profound in severe osteomalacia and may be attributable to absence of direct stimulatory effects of vitamin D on muscle cell function and to the low levels of calcium and phosphorus.

Diagnosis

Patients with mild to moderate vitamin D deficiency have clinical and pathologic findings characteristic of osteoporosis, ▯ rather than of osteomalacia.

Osteomalacia should be suspected when the serum calcium level is low or low-normal, the serum phosphorus level is low, and the serum alkaline phosphatase level is high. The urine calcium level is usually extremely low in vitamin D deficiency because of impaired absorption,

▯see page 472

but it may not be low when the cause is hypophosphatemia or a renal tubular disorder. Serum calcium levels are often low-normal because of marked secondary hyperparathyroidism. Vitamin D deficiency can be measured directly by assaying the 25-hydroxyvitamin D_3 levels in the serum. 1,25-Dihydroxyvitamin D_3 levels may be normal in vitamin D deficiency, unless impaired 1α-hydroxylase is a contributing cause. Other than pseudofractures, which are pathognomonic, x-ray findings are nonspecific. Vertebral abnormalities are similar to those in osteoporosis. Bowing of the legs may occur in elderly patients, particularly those with congenital hypophosphatemia, which can be readily differentiated from Paget's disease on x-ray. Densitometry is not particularly helpful in diagnosing osteomalacia. Values may be normal or even high because of the accumulation of large amounts of osteoid that are partially mineralized.

In some cases, a bone biopsy is necessary for definitive diagnosis. The biopsy should be processed without demineralization, using tetracycline labeling to identify the defect in mineralization. The wide osteoid seams are also characteristic; however, wide osteoid seams may also occur in other conditions in which bone turnover is high (eg, in hyperparathyroidism).

Treatment

Treatment depends on the underlying cause. The goal is to remineralize the bone safely, without producing hypercalcemia or hypercalciuria. Vitamin D is safe when given at appropriate intervals. In patients with simple vitamin D deficiency, 50,000 or 100,000 U/day for 1 to 2 weeks, followed by a maintenance dose of 400 to 800 U/day, is sufficient. If malabsorption occurs, then doses $\geq$ 50,000 U/week may be needed. Close monitoring of serum and urine calcium levels is critical.

25-Hydroxyvitamin D_3 (calcidiol) 25 to 50 μg can be used in patients with severe malabsorption or with hepatic disease. Calcidiol is better absorbed than is ordinary vitamin D and bypasses any defect in 25-hydroxylation in the liver. In renal disease, the defect is in 1α-hydroxylase, and 1,25-dihydroxyvitamin D_3 (calcitriol) should be administered. Because calcitriol is the potent hormonal form of vitamin D, the margin of safety is the smallest. Replacement doses range from 0.25 to 2 μg/day, and patients should be monitored for hypercalcemia and hypercalciuria. Calcitriol can reverse the bone lesion in neoplastic osteomalacia; finding and removing the tumor also cures the osteomalacia.

In hypophosphatemic disorders, including congenital and renal or gastrointestinal forms, phosphate replacement is critical. However, phosphate tends to cause diarrhea. To minimize this effect, potassium and sodium phosphate should be given in divided doses that are increased gradually to bring the phosphate concentration at least into the low-normal range. Elemental phosphorus 250 mg should be given $\geq$ 4 times/day with a full glass of water. In patients with severe hypophosphatemia, the dosage may be increased to as much as 3 g/day po or 2.5 to 5.0 mg/kg in 0.9% saline solution IV. Excessive phosphate administration or too-rapid repletion may result in hypocalcemia. All patients with osteomalacia need to maintain adequate intakes of calcium (1000 to 1500 mg/day). In cases of malabsorption or severe vitamin D resistance, parenteral calcium may be required.

In patients with the rare autosomal recessive form of osteomalacia in which the vitamin D receptor is defective, the skeletal abnormalities respond to parenteral administration of calcium and phosphorus.

50 ▆ NONMETABOLIC BONE DISEASE

OSTEOMYELITIS

Infection, inflammation, and destruction of bone caused by microorganisms.

The incidence increases in persons > 50. Infection reaches bone via the blood stream (hematogenous osteomyelitis) or by spread from adjoining tissue (contiguous osteomyelitis).

Hematogenous osteomyelitis most often affects the vertebrae but may also affect the long bones (eg, femur, tibia, humerus). About 60% of vertebral osteomyelitis cases occur in persons > 50. Generally, only one organism is isolated, most commonly *Staphylococcus aureus;* however, gram-negative aerobic bacilli, most likely due to genitourinary tract infection or to instrumentation, are also frequently found.

Contiguous osteomyelitis is due to septic foci that usually result from postoperative infections, pressure sores, diabetic ulcers, radiation therapy, or foreign bodies. Mixed bacteria are often found, frequently *S. aureus, S. epidermidis,* gram-negative aerobic bacilli, and anaerobic species.

Vascular insufficiency (eg, due to diabetes, atherosclerosis, or vasculitis) and neuropathy are common contributing factors to osteomyelitis of the foot in elderly patients. The small bones of the feet and toes are most often involved. Mixed bacteria are commonly found, including *S. aureus, S. epidermidis,* streptococci, gram-negative aerobic bacilli, and anaerobic organisms.

Symptoms, Signs, and Diagnosis

Pain is the hallmark symptom of osteomyelitis. However, pain may be absent in debilitated patients with osteomyelitis due to an overlying pressure sore that does not heal and in diabetic patients with osteomyelitis of the foot. Fever may be absent. The ESR is almost always elevated, but leukocytosis is variable. Early-stage osteomyelitis is diagnosed by a technetium bone scan or MRI. Advanced osteomyelitis can be diagnosed by x-ray. Biopsy of bone may be necessary to determine the causative organism and its sensitivity to antibiotics.

Treatment

Antibiotics may be required for weeks to months. Although such treatment is best started in the hospital, it can be provided (orally or intravenously) at home using home health services. The choice of antibiotic should be based on organisms grown from blood cultures or on deep bone biopsy findings; cultures of superficial bone or overlying wounds often produce inaccurate results. While cultures are being processed, before the results are known, broad-spectrum antibiotics covering staphylococci and gram-negative organisms should be given. Debridement is also frequently needed.

CERVICAL SPONDYLOSIS

Narrowing of the cervical canal or neural foramina due to degeneration of the intervertebral disk and the annulus and to formation of bony osteophytes.

Persons with a congenitally narrow cervical canal are at increased risk. Narrowing leads to spinal cord compression, which typically causes a progressive myelopathy, characterized by a spastic gait. If a painful cervical root syndrome predominates, radicular signs often indicate the most involved dermatome, usually one between C-5 and C-6 or between C-6 and C-7. Neural foraminal root compression causes arm weakness and atrophy with segmental reflex loss; spinal cord compression causes hyperreflexia, increased tone, vibratory impairment, and plantar extensor responses in the legs.

Spinal x-rays, including oblique views of the neural foramina, reveal degeneration with osteophytes and disk-space narrowing. If the sagittal diameter of the cervical canal is < 10 mm, spinal cord compression is likely. CT defines the diameter of the canal, and myelography determines the level and extent of the epidural compression, but MRI is rapidly becoming the diagnostic test of choice.

Occasionally, signs improve spontaneously. Conservative therapy includes a soft collar, cervical traction, anti-inflammatory drugs, and mild analgesics. Decompressive laminectomy is used sparingly to halt disease progression or to stabilize the myelopathy.

SPINAL STENOSIS

A narrowing of the spinal canal, causing pressure on the sciatic nerve roots and occasionally on the cord.

The pressure on the spinal cord may result from bony or soft tissue encroachment on the spinal cord or lumbosacral nerve roots. Neurogenic claudication (ie, aching pain with or without paresthesia or numbness in the buttocks, thighs, or calves) is characteristic. Discomfort is caused by prolonged lumbar extension (eg, while walking) and relieved by lumbar flexion (eg, while sitting or leaning forward). Mild to moderate low back pain and symptoms of radicular nerve root compression may be present. Physical findings are often nonspecific. The presence of brisk peripheral pulses helps exclude peripheral vascular disease as a diagnosis.

Diagnosis can be confirmed by CT or MRI. However, many asymptomatic elderly persons have the pathologic changes of spinal stenosis on imaging studies. Thus, careful clinical judgment must be used to determine whether spinal stenosis found on x-ray is the cause of the patient's symptoms.

Treatment for most patients includes an initial course of analgesics and exercise. If a patient does not respond to this approach or if function is severely compromised, spinal decompression by surgery is indicated.

DIFFUSE IDIOPATHIC SKELETAL HYPEROSTOSIS

Widespread calcification and ossification of the anterolateral ligaments of the spine, which may give rise to ankylosis.

The incidence is about 0.5%/year in elderly patients. The male/female distribution is 2:1.

Widespread calcification and ossification of the anterolateral ligaments of the spine are characteristic and may result in bony ankylosis. Peripheral joints may also be involved, with evidence of osteophyte or spur formation and ligamentous calcification (enthesopathy).

The pathogenesis is unknown. Some studies have found a possible link to increases in the plasma concentrations of insulin and growth hormone. Others have postulated a relationship to increases in the concentration of vitamin A and retinoic acid derivatives; this finding is interesting because the x-ray abnormalities of diffuse idiopathic skeletal hyperostosis (DISH) resemble those of chronic hypervitaminosis A.

Symptoms, Signs, and Diagnosis

Typically, patients report stiffness and pain (usually mild) localized mainly to the thoracic spine. Pain may be noted years before x-ray manifestations appear. In about 15% of patients, cervical spine involvement leads to dysphagia. More than one third of patients exhibit peripheral joint manifestations; the most commonly involved sites are the heels (characterized by spur formation), elbows, knees, and shoulders. Spinal stenosis[1] and neurologic manifestations are uncommon.

Physical examination shows few abnormalities. Thoracolumbar and cervical spine mobility may be mildly or moderately decreased, and tenderness may be present over the thoracic spine. Occasionally, anterior cervical osteophytes can be palpated at the posterior aspect of the pharynx. Laboratory findings are usually normal; about 40% of patients have asymptomatic hyperglycemia or overt diabetes mellitus.

Early in the disease, x-rays of the peripheral joints may suggest DISH, but x-rays of the spine may show normal findings. Later in the disease, rheumatic abnormalities are extensive, but pain is often minimal and spinal motion is only moderately limited. X-rays of the peripheral joints show new bone formation (whiskering) and large bone spurs, particularly on the calcaneus and olecranon process. Advanced ligamentous calcification can be seen in the iliolumbar and patellar ligaments. Periarticular osteophytes are usually conspicuous. X-rays of the spine typically show flowing ossification along the anterolateral aspect of at least four contiguous vertebral bodies, preservation of disk height, and the absence of marginal sclerosis and apophysial joint ankylosis.

Treatment

Treatment is symptomatic; physical therapy, massage, and nonopioid analgesics may be sufficient. Painful spurs may be managed by orthotics or local corticosteroid injections. Patients should be reassured that DISH does not cause permanent disability.

51 LOCAL JOINT, TENDON, AND BURSA DISORDERS

OSTEOARTHRITIS

A disorder of hyaline cartilage and subchondral bone, primarily affecting the hand joints, spine, and joints of the lower extremity.

Osteoarthritis is the most common joint disease and is a leading cause of disability in persons > 65 years. It is probably not one disease but several having similar clinical and pathologic features. Thus, the

[1] see page 488

typical changes (eg, cartilage deterioration, bony remodeling) can occur in several diarthrodial joints, but the causes may differ.

Primary (idiopathic) osteoarthritis affects the distal and proximal interphalangeal joints, first carpometacarpal joints, cervical and lumbar spine, hips, knees, and toes. ◻ The metacarpophalangeal joints, wrists, elbows, shoulders, and ankles usually are spared. Secondary osteoarthritis affects any joint that has been damaged by trauma or inflammation.

Aging alone does not cause osteoarthritis, although age-related cellular or matrix alterations in cartilage probably predispose elderly persons to the disease. Other possible predisposing factors include obesity, trauma, congenital abnormalities (eg, hip dysplasia), and primary joint disorders (eg, inflammatory arthritis).

Symptoms, Signs, and Diagnosis

Osteoarthritis is characterized by intermittent or constant joint pain that may be accompanied by limited movement, bone hypertrophy, and joint deformity. Pain is relieved by rest and exacerbated by movement and weight bearing; it is not associated with inflammatory symptoms such as redness and swelling. The disease usually progresses slowly.

In the hands, bony overgrowth of the distal interphalangeal joints (Heberden's nodes) and bony overgrowth of the proximal interphalangeal joints (Bouchard's nodes or nodules) may be present. ◻

The diagnosis is based on a combination of clinical and x-ray findings. Characteristic x-ray findings include osteophytes, subchondral sclerosis and cysts, and asymmetric loss of joint space (implying degeneration of cartilage). However, conventional x-rays are not sensitive for detecting early osteoarthritis because they do not show pathologic changes in cartilage. Moreover, x-ray findings may be present without symptoms. MRI is more sensitive than conventional x-rays but should not be used routinely to diagnose osteoarthritis. The ESR and white blood cell (WBC) count are normal, and no autoantibodies are present. Synovial fluid analysis shows only mild leukocytosis (a WBC count of $< 2000/\mu L$).

Treatment

Comprehensive management involves a balance of cognitive-behavioral, physical, pharmaceutical, and surgical measures. The goals of treatment are to relieve pain and to minimize functional limitations. The patient's functional deficits and preferences for treatment must be considered. The patient should be taught about the chronic nature of the disease; unrealistic treatment expectations can lead to frustration and depression and can impair the patient-physician relationship. Asymp-

---

◻ see also page 557   ◻ see page 535

·tomatic osteoarthritis, diagnosed by x-ray findings, does not require treatment.

Nonpharmacologic measures: Nonpharmacologic measures are the cornerstone of therapy and should be used in all patients. Cognitive-behavioral therapy that is directed toward coping skills and self-efficacy (confidence in performing activities safely) is highly effective in improving function.

A regimen of range-of-motion, strengthening, and endurance exercises is important for pain relief and restoration of function. **1** Adaptive aids (eg, braces, canes, devices to increase hand function) may be indicated to restore function and improve independence. Weight loss is important for obese patients.

Pharmacotherapy: Drugs should be used when nonpharmacologic measures provide insufficient pain relief and restoration of function. In the elderly, the most commonly used drugs are acetaminophen and nonsteroidal anti-inflammatory drugs (NSAIDs—see TABLE 51–1). Acetaminophen is the first choice for pain relief because it is safer than NSAIDs and is effective. It can be prescribed in increasing doses up to 1 g qid (not to exceed 4 g/day) in most patients. Acetaminophen should be used cautiously in patients with liver disease and in those who consume > 2 alcoholic drinks per day because of the increased risk of hepatotoxicity.

For patients who do not adequately respond to acetaminophen, an NSAID should be considered. All NSAIDs appear to be equally effective, but patient responses vary, and several NSAIDs may be tried before relief is obtained. The therapeutic effects of NSAIDs are due to the inhibition of cyclooxygenase (COX), which is required for the synthesis of prostaglandins.

Two COX isoforms exist: COX-1 is expressed in most tissues, including gastric mucosa, and COX-2 is induced in inflammatory cells and synovium during inflammation. COX-2 is also found in the kidney but not in platelets. Most NSAIDs inhibit both COX-1 and COX-2, **2** but newer selective COX-2 inhibitors (eg, celecoxib, rofecoxib) affect only the COX-2 isoform and therefore cause less gastric irritation and ulceration and do not inhibit platelets.

The major adverse effects of older NSAIDs are similar, although the incidence varies by drug and among groups of patients. The most common adverse effect is gastrointestinal upset, which often occurs without evidence of ulceration or bleeding and may require discontinuation of the drug. However, ulceration and gastrointestinal bleeding can occur with all nonselective NSAIDs and are related to dose and frequency of use, but they do not correlate with symptoms, and bleeding can occur without warning. The relative risk for persons > 65 is three to four times greater than that for middle-aged persons. Taking nonselective NSAIDs

1 see pages 269 and 301   **2** see also page 390

TABLE 51–1. NONSTEROIDAL ANTI-INFLAMMATORY DRUGS AND CYCLOOXYGENASE-2 INHIBITORS

Drug	Usual Dosage
NSAIDs	
Aspirin	650–1300 mg q 4–6 hours
Diclofenac	50–75 mg bid
Diflunisal	250–500 mg bid
Etodolac	600–1200 mg/day in 2–4 doses
Fenoprofen	300–600 mg tid or qid
Flurbiprofen	200–300 mg/day in 3–4 doses
Ibuprofen	400–800 mg tid or qid
Indomethacin*	25–50 mg bid or tid
Ketoprofen	25–75 mg tid or qid
Meclofenamate sodium	50–100 mg tid or qid
Nabumetone	1000–2000 mg/day
Naproxen	250–500 mg bid
Naproxen sodium	275–550 mg q 6–8 hours
Nonacetylated salicylates	2–4 g/day
Oxaprozin	600–1800 mg/day
Piroxicam	10–20 mg once/day
Sulindac	150–200 mg bid
Tolmetin sodium	200–600 mg tid
COX-2 Inhibitors	
Celecoxib	100–200 mg daily or bid
Rofecoxib	25–50 mg daily

*Not recommended in the elderly because of central nervous system adverse effects.

with food may help minimize gastrointestinal symptoms, and concomitant use of cytoprotective drugs, such as the prostaglandin misoprostol or proton pump inhibitors, may decrease the incidence of ulcers in high-risk patients.

Older NSAIDs and the newer COX-2 inhibitors can impair renal function and cause sodium and water retention; they should be used cautiously in the elderly, particularly in those who have underlying renal disease, heart failure, volume depletion, or liver disease. Rare toxic effects in the elderly include cognitive dysfunction and personality changes.

In general, indomethacin should not be used as first-line therapy because, compared with other NSAIDs, it has greater toxicity and higher rates of progression of joint space narrowing, as seen on x-ray. It also produces more central nervous system adverse effects. Nonacetylated salicylates may have less renal toxicity and fewer antiplatelet effects than do other NSAIDs, but they are generally less effective.

When necessary, opioid analgesics can be used if they improve function and quality of life. However, given the chronic nature of osteoarthritis, prolonged use of opioid analgesics often causes problems with physical dependency. Sedation and nausea are usually transient with opioids. Constipation may be managed with stimulants or osmotic laxatives.

Intra-articular corticosteroids are indicated for symptomatic large joints unresponsive to the usual treatments. A joint should not be injected more than twice in a 2-week period. Triamcinolone is recommended. Systemic corticosteroids should not be used.

Weekly hyaluronic acid injections for 3 to 5 weeks improve symptoms of osteoarthritis of the knee. Patients > 60 with moderate to severe disease are most likely to benefit from hyaluronic acid.

Topical creams (eg, capsaicin or an NSAID) can be helpful as monotherapy or combined with oral analgesics, especially in patients with osteoarthritis of the hands█ or knees.

A combination of glucosamine sulfate with chondroitin sulfate is available in the USA as a nutritional supplement. Several studies have shown that 500 mg tid is more effective than placebo in relieving pain, but ongoing clinical trials should clarify the role of glucosamine in the treatment of osteoarthritis. This supplement has few adverse effects.

Surgery: Total arthroplasty is highly effective for treating osteoarthritis of the hip and knee, and age alone is not a contraindication. However, treatment goals (eg, pain relief, improved physical function) and the needs and capabilities of the patient must be clearly defined.

Arthroscopy with lavage is useful for osteoarthritis of the knee in patients who do not respond to pharmacologic treatment. The long-term benefits of arthroscopic lavage are unknown. Arthroscopy may also be used for diagnosis and treatment of internal derangements, such as a torn meniscus.

INFECTIOUS ARTHRITIS

(Septic Arthritis)

Inflammation of the joints due to infection of the synovial tissues with pyogenic bacteria or other infectious agents.

The risk of infectious arthritis increases with age. Patients who are immunocompromised as a result of corticosteroid therapy, malignancy, or diabetes are also more likely to develop infectious arthritis.

█ see also page 538

In the elderly, as in younger patients, the most common organism is *Staphylococcus aureus*; however, gram-negative bacteria cause a significant number of cases in elderly patients. Bacterial infection is due to direct inoculation or to bacteremia from a known or unknown source. It most often affects joints with preexisting disease, usually osteoarthritis or rheumatoid arthritis.

Symptoms, Signs, and Diagnosis

The presenting symptom is usually acute febrile illness with monarticular or polyarticular arthritis. Primarily large joints are affected, most commonly the shoulder, elbow, wrist, hip, and knee. Many patients do not look toxemic, particularly elderly persons, who may have a low-grade or no fever and whose peripheral WBC count may be < 14,000/μL.

In febrile patients who cannot give a good history, all of the diarthrodial joints must be examined for a source of infection. Infection is diagnosed by analysis of synovial fluid. A WBC count > 50,000/μL indicates infection unless crystals are present. Infected fluid can have a WBC count of < 50,000/μL, although polymorphonuclear leukocytes predominate in most instances. A synovial fluid glucose level that is 40 mg/dL (2.2 mmol/L) less than the serum glucose level is highly suggestive of infection.

Gram stain and culture identify the infectious organism in up to 50% of cases. Blood cultures should be obtained, because the organism often grows in blood but not in synovial fluid. A specific organism is identified in > 80% of cases when all appropriate sites are cultured.

Other biochemical tests of synovial fluid include lactate level measurement, bacterial antigen detection, and nitroblue tetrazolium test. These tests should be recommended by a rheumatologist, infectious disease specialist, or pathologist.

Treatment

Immediate treatment is required to avoid cartilage destruction and permanent joint damage. Joint fluid should be aspirated repeatedly and as completely as possible. If fever and the signs of arthritis are not substantially reduced in 48 to 72 hours, surgical drainage of the joint may be necessary. Infectious arthritis responds to appropriate systemic antibiotics if the organism is sensitive and the dosage is adequate. Intraarticular antibiotics are not needed.

GOUT

A recurrent acute or chronic arthritis of peripheral joints that results from deposition in and about the joints and tendons of monosodium urate crystals from supersaturated hyperuricemic body fluids.

Gout most often manifests in middle-aged men and postmenopausal women. Gout correlates with hyperuricemia (usually serum urate levels > 7 mg/dL [> 420 μmol/L]), which represents an imbalance between endogenous urate production and renal urate excretion. Most cases of primary and secondary hyperuricemia are characterized by a defect in renal handling of urate. Hyperuricemia may be exacerbated by drugs commonly used by elderly patients (eg, thiazide diuretics and salicylates, even in small doses).

Symptoms, Signs, and Diagnosis

Acute gouty arthritis is characterized by acute onset of inflammatory arthritis, possibly after trauma, illness, or surgery. The metatarsophalangeal joint of the great toe is the typical site of acute pain (podagra). Monarticular or polyarticular pain may also affect the ankle, knee, wrist, elbow, small joints of the hands or feet, or bursae (especially the bursa of olecranon).

Fever (up to 39° C [102.2° F]) often develops. Tenderness is usually so exquisite that the patient cannot move the affected joint or tolerate the weight of bedclothes. Inflammation often extends beyond the joint, suggesting cellulitis in some cases. A history of recurrent acute episodes of arthritis, especially involving the great toe, suggests gout.

Acute gouty arthritis may be accompanied by blood leukocytosis and an elevated ESR. An elevated serum urate level supports the diagnosis but is neither specific nor sensitive. The definitive finding is urate crystals in synovial fluid. If possible, synovial fluid should be analyzed in acute monarticular or oligoarticular arthritis. Microcrystalline disease is important to differentiate from infection. In acute gouty arthritis, the synovial fluid shows typical inflammatory changes with a WBC count of 5,000 to 50,000/μL. In 90% of cases, urate crystals can be seen free in the fluid or engulfed by phagocytes. When viewed with a polarizing microscope, they are negatively birefringent.

Chronic gouty arthritis may cause morning stiffness and achy joints, mimicking rheumatoid arthritis and other chronic polyarticular arthritides. It occurs primarily in patients who have tophaceous gout. Such patients often have x-ray evidence of monosodium urate deposits (tophi) in soft tissue or bone adjacent to the joints. The number of tophi increases with the severity of hyperuricemia. Tophi are commonly found in bursae, the articular cartilage, and bone. Tophi may be confused with rheumatoid nodules when they appear in the bursa of olecranon or over the extensor surface of the forearm.

Treatment

Acute gouty arthritis, if untreated, resolves in a few days to weeks. Treatment begins with an NSAID at the usual dosage (see TABLE 51–1). Relief occurs in 24 hours, and symptoms usually resolve in 3 days, after which the NSAID can be discontinued. If taken at the first sign of a gouty attack, colchicine 0.5 to 1.0 mg daily or bid may prevent the full-blown attack. Alternatively, colchicine relieves acute symptoms when given 1 to 2 mg diluted in 0.9% sodium chloride and injected IV over 3 to 5 minutes to avoid extravasation. *However, severe local and systemic reactions may occur.* Oral colchicine 0.5 mg q 2 h following an initial 1-mg dose also may be given until relief is obtained or gastrointestinal toxicity supervenes. However, because almost all patients must take colchicine until gastrointestinal toxicity occurs, this treatment is used less frequently than in the past. Systemic corticosteroids (prednisone 40 mg/day or equivalent tapered over 5 to 10 days) are effective in treating acute gout, particularly if polyarticular.

Acute gout of the large joints can be treated by withdrawing synovial fluid and injecting a long-lasting corticosteroid (eg, triamcinolone 20 to 40 mg). This treatment is especially effective in patients who cannot take oral drugs nor tolerate NSAIDs or colchicine.

Uricosuric drugs and allopurinol should be *avoided* during the acute attack. Long-term colchicine 0.5 mg bid may lower the incidence of recurrent acute gouty arthritis.

Chronic gouty arthritis may require measures to lower serum urate levels. Such measures may be useful if tophi or renal calculi are present or if long-term colchicine administration does not control acute attacks.

Allopurinol blocks the metabolic pathway of urate production, inhibiting xanthine oxidase. Because allopurinol does not produce its effect through the kidney and reduces the renal urate load, it is indicated in patients with renal calculi. The initial dosage of 100 mg bid may be increased gradually to 600 mg/day if necessary.

Alternatives to allopurinol are the uricosuric drugs. Probenecid (maintenance dosage ranges from 500 mg to 1.5 g po q 12 h) or sulfinpyrazone (100 to 400 mg/day po bid in divided doses) effectively keeps serum urate levels $\leq$ 6.5 mg/dL ($\leq$ 390 μmol/L).

CALCIUM PYROPHOSPHATE DIHYDRATE CRYSTAL DEPOSITION DISEASE

(Pseudogout)

A microcrystalline arthritis associated with calcification of hyaline and fibrous cartilage (chondrocalcinosis).

Calcium pyrophosphate dihydrate (CPPD) crystal deposition disease is rare before the 5th decade and becomes more common with age. The mechanism of cartilage calcification is poorly understood but is likely due to many factors. Hyperparathyroidism, acromegaly, and hypothyroidism are predisposing factors.

Symptoms and Signs

The disease was originally called pseudogout to emphasize the acute, episodic, goutlike attacks of synovitis. However, unlike gout, acute CPPD crystal deposition disease usually occurs in large joints, especially the knee, and may involve the shoulder, hip, wrist, and elbow. This disease may cause a chronic, asymmetric, inflammatory polyarthritis, which may mimic rheumatoid arthritis.

Laboratory Findings and Diagnosis

Hematologic findings are nonspecific. Serum calcium levels are normal unless hyperparathyroidism is present. Hyperuricemia may be present and may play a role in pathogenesis. Chondrocalcinosis of the fibrocartilaginous menisci of the knees, the radial and ulnar joints, the symphysis pubis, and the articular disk of the sternoclavicular joint frequently appears on x-ray and supports the diagnosis. In the acute form of this disease, the synovial fluid has a WBC count of 2,000 to 50,000/μL, which is typical of an inflammatory process. Using polarized light microscopy, intracellular and extracellular CPPD crystals can be identified in 90% of effusions. These crystals are generally rhomboid and, unlike urate crystals, are positively birefringent under polarized light.

The diagnosis is based on a clinical history of recurrent, episodic acute attacks and the demonstration of CPPD crystals in synovial fluid. A search for crystals using polarized light microscopy may be necessary, particularly when the patient has polyarticular chronic disease.

Treatment

NSAIDs or a short course of systemic corticosteroids are effective for an acute attack. Intra-articular corticosteroids may be useful when a large joint is involved; colchicine■ is also effective.

BURSITIS

Acute or chronic inflammation of a bursa.

The causes include acute or chronic trauma, CPPD crystal deposition disease, and infection. Occasionally, bursae are involved in systemic inflammatory diseases such as rheumatoid arthritis.

Symptoms, Signs, and Diagnosis

Before treatment, the cause must be determined. If the history and physical examination do not yield obvious degeneration or trauma, the bursal fluid must be aspirated and examined for crystal deposits or

---

■ see page 496

infection. Aspiration and examination of subdeltoid or trochanteric bursae are rarely necessary before treatment unless signs of infection exist. A bursal fluid WBC count $\geq$ 2000/μL suggests an inflammatory process. The fluid should be examined microscopically for crystals, and a Gram stain should be performed to exclude infection.

Subdeltoid (subacromial) bursitis: The subdeltoid bursa is located between the deltoid muscle and the joint capsule, extending under the acromion and coracoacromial ligament. Subdeltoid bursitis results in painful shoulder movement, particularly abduction and extension. Patients with subdeltoid bursitis tend to awaken at night when they turn on the affected shoulder. The pain often radiates down the arm in the C-5 dermatome. Pain primarily over the anterior shoulder aggravated by forearm supination against resistance is more likely to reflect bicipital tendinitis.

Subdeltoid bursitis is the most common cause of nonarticular shoulder pain. It is often accompanied by inflammation of the supraspinatus tendon, and the two problems may be impossible to differentiate.

Physical examination reveals tenderness over the lateral shoulder and the subacromial space. Pain can be elicited if the arm is abducted and then actively moved toward the body against resistance. Patients report pain on moving the arm downward through the arc of abduction at about 90°.

Trochanteric bursitis: The trochanteric bursa lies between the gluteus maximus and the tendon of the gluteus medius. Trochanteric bursitis usually results in a dull, aching pain or a burning, tingling sensation over the lateral hip. The pain may also be referred to the L-2 dermatome. Pain is worse with activity and after sitting with the affected leg crossed over the other. Sleep disturbances and an inability to lie on the affected side are common.

Physical examination reveals localized tenderness over the bony prominence of the greater trochanter. External rotation with abduction of the hip is often painful, although the range of motion is normal.

Anserine bursitis: The anserine bursa is located about 4 cm (1.6 inches) below the medial aspect of the knee. It lies under the pes anserinus (the combined insertion of the tendinous expansions of the sartorius, gracilis, and semitendinous muscles). Anserine bursitis results in knee pain that is worse at night but may be improved by placement of a pillow between the knees.

Physical examination may reveal point tenderness over the bursa and, occasionally, mild to moderate swelling.

Olecranon bursitis: The bursa of olecranon lies between the skin and the olecranon process. Olecranon bursitis usually results in swelling and tenderness over the most proximal part of the ulna.

Physical examination reveals no tenderness or pain in the elbow, which exhibits full range of motion.

Treatment

If microcrystalline disease and infection are absent, the most successful treatment is fluid aspiration and injection of the bursal sac with a corticosteroid. Aspirin or another NSAID is also effective.

Infection is most commonly due to gram-positive organisms that colonize the skin: *Staphylococcus aureus* and group A streptococci. Antibiotics should be used; they may be given orally if the patient has no systemic symptoms (eg, high fever). An infected bursa should not be drained openly but repeatedly aspirated.

The patient should be encouraged to move the affected area, particularly the shoulder, but should avoid stressful exercise that may irritate it. Limited shoulder movement and frozen shoulder can become severe and long-term if range-of-motion exercises are neglected.

ROTATOR CUFF TEARS

Rotator cuff tears, which are common among the elderly, can be classified as acute or chronic and full or partial thickness. They cause significant upper extremity dysfunction. Pain is usually present and may be severe.

Physical examination reveals signs of supraspinatus tendinitis and weakness on active abduction and external rotation. Rotator cuff tears are best diagnosed by MRI, which has high specificity and sensitivity for this disorder.

Treatment initially should include analgesia, corticosteroid injection, and exercise to improve strength and range of motion. Careful monitoring is necessary because patients often have persistent pain and disability. Patients who do not respond to nonsurgical treatment within 4 to 6 weeks should be referred for rotator cuff repair.

52 ■ RHEUMATIC DISEASES

RHEUMATOID ARTHRITIS

A chronic syndrome of symmetric inflammation of the peripheral joints, resulting in progressive destruction of articular and periarticular structures.

Prevalence of rheumatoid arthritis increases up to age 80. Rheumatoid arthritis is an important cause of disability in elderly persons.

The cause is unknown. Intense inflammation of the synovium of the diarthrodial joints is characteristic. Synovial tissue becomes hyperplastic and infiltrated with lymphocytes and plasma cells. Various inflammatory mediators, including cytokines, prostaglandins, and immunoglobulins, are present in the synovial fluid.

Symptoms and Signs

In many elderly patients, the disease process began during middle age. Some patients have secondary joint deformities and degenerative changes even though the inflammation is inactive. When rheumatoid arthritis develops de novo in an elderly person, the onset may be insidious or acute. In most patients, the arthritis is accompanied by mild or moderate constitutional symptoms (eg, malaise, anorexia). Fever and night sweats occasionally are reported. Rheumatoid arthritis occurs primarily in the joints of the hands (eg, wrists, proximal interphalangeal, and metacarpophalangeal) and feet (eg, metatarsophalangeal and interphalangeal) and in the larger joints (eg, elbows, shoulders, knees). Patients report pain, swelling, and stiffness in these areas, especially in the mornings. Eventually, rheumatoid arthritis becomes a symmetric, additive disease of the joints.

Diagnosis

The diagnosis is based on clinical judgment and requires that the patient exhibit symmetric inflammatory arthritis involving the appropriate joints and prolonged morning stiffness lasting ≥ 1 hour (see TABLE 52–1). The physical examination detects soft tissue swelling, warmth, and tenderness in these areas and, sometimes, nodules along extensor surfaces of the upper extremities and around joints. Other diseases (eg, polymyalgia rheumatica, [1] systemic lupus erythematosus, [2] the arthritis of malignancy) must be excluded.

Patients with rheumatoid arthritis may have normochromic-normocytic anemia, mild leukocytosis, or thrombocytosis. The ESR is elevated in about 80% of cases, and rheumatoid factor is present in about 50%; however, these findings are not specific for rheumatoid arthritis. High titers of rheumatoid factor ($\geq 1:320$) are highly specific; in contrast, low titers are found in patients with other diseases and in up to 25% of elderly patients without evidence of any disease.

Initially, x-rays of involved joints usually show only soft tissue swelling. Characteristic late features include periarticular osteoporosis, joint space narrowing, and marginal erosions.

Prognosis and Treatment

In general, the long-term prognosis is poor. Many patients become progressively disabled despite appropriate treatment, and higher rates

[1]see page 506   [2]see page 503

TABLE 52–1.   REVISED CRITERIA FOR CLASSIFICATION OF RHEUMATOID ARTHRITIS (1987)

Any four of the following criteria must be present to classify patients as having rheumatoid arthritis:

Morning stiffness for ≥ 1 hour*

Arthritis of three or more joints*

Arthritis of hand joints (eg, wrists, metacarpophalangeal or proximal interphalangeal joints)*

Symmetric arthritis*

Rheumatoid nodules

Serum rheumatoid factor (positive in < 5% of healthy persons)

Radiographic changes (hand x-ray changes typical of rheumatoid arthritis must include erosions or unequivocal bony decalcification)

*Must be present for ≥ 6 weeks.

Adapted from Arnett FC, Edworthy S, Block DA, et al: "The American Rheumatism Association 1987, revised criteria for the classification of rheumatoid arthritis." *Arthritis and Rheumatism* 39:723, 1996.

of serious infections and cardiovascular disease increase mortality. Nevertheless, many patients respond to treatment.

Nonpharmacologic treatment: Physical and occupational therapy, exercise, use of assistive devices, and possibly physical modalities for pain relief (eg, locally applied heat or cold) are essential. Rest should be encouraged when symptoms are severe. However, prolonged bed rest in elderly patients exacerbates age-related loss of aerobic capacity and muscle strength and may lead to irreversible immobility; elderly patients can easily cross the threshold at which functional ability is so severely compromised that it cannot be restored.

Nonsteroidal anti-inflammatory drugs: Therapy should include a nonsteroidal anti-inflammatory drug (NSAID) to relieve pain and swelling.▪ Regular use of a full-dose NSAID is often required. The therapeutic effects of NSAIDs are due to the inhibition of cyclooxygenase (COX), which is required for the synthesis of prostaglandins. Two COX isoforms exist: COX-1 is expressed in most tissues, including gastric mucosa, and COX-2 is induced in inflammatory cells and synovium during inflammation. COX-2 is also found in the kidney but not in platelets.

Most NSAIDs inhibit both COX-1 and COX-2, but newer selective COX-2 inhibitors (eg, celecoxib, rofecoxib) affect only the COX-2 isoform and therefore cause fewer gastric ulcers and do not inhibit platelets. Thus, a COX-2 inhibitor should be considered instead of the older NSAIDs because gastrointestinal toxicity and platelet inhibition

▪ see page 389 and TABLE 51–1 on page 492

are less likely. With nonspecific NSAIDs, gastrointestinal toxicity occurs up to four times more frequently among persons > 65 than among younger persons.

Corticosteroids: Low-dose prednisone (eg, 5 to 10 mg/day) may help reduce pain and disability. However, corticosteroids are difficult to discontinue, and their long-term adverse effects (eg, osteoporosis, cataracts, poor wound healing, hyperglycemia, hypertension, hyperlipidemia, reactivation of tuberculosis, increased risk of infection) must be balanced against their therapeutic benefits. Intra-articular injections of corticosteroid esters may temporarily help control local synovitis in one or two particularly painful joints.

Disease-modifying antirheumatic drugs: These drugs slow the disease process, improve function, and reduce mortality. They should be used early in the course of rheumatoid arthritis to prevent joint destruction and disability. These drugs even improve survival. No evidence suggests that elderly patients respond less well to these drugs than do younger patients or that toxicity is different. Therefore, therapy with these drugs should not be withheld because of the patient's age; however, therapy should be managed by a rheumatologist.

Usually, methotrexate is the first choice. The initial oral dosage is usually 7.5 mg/week, which may be increased up to 20 mg/week. Patients receiving methotrexate should be closely monitored for hepatic toxicity, interstitial pneumonitis, bone marrow suppression, and gastrointestinal ulceration and bleeding. Aspirin may increase the toxicity of methotrexate by slowing its excretion rate. Folic acid supplementation (5 mg/week) helps prevent toxicity. Methotrexate is contraindicated in patients with renal insufficiency.

Hydroxychloroquine 6.5 mg/kg/day or 400 mg/day po can be used. Rarely, severe and sometimes irreversible adverse effects, particularly vision loss, occur. Vision should be checked by an ophthalmologist before treatment.

Sulfasalazine 3 to 4 g/day po is an effective disease-modifying antirheumatic drug. The major adverse effects are nausea, vomiting, and upper gastric distress. Patients should be monitored periodically with the use of CBCs and liver function tests.

Combination therapy using methotrexate, hydroxychloroquine, and sulfasalazine has been shown to be more effective than monotherapy. However, high cost and toxicity may limit this approach to therapy.

The biologic response modifier etanercept (10 to 25 mg sc biweekly) is a soluble tumor necrosis factor receptor that blocks the action of the proinflammatory cytokine tumor necrosis factor. The most common adverse effect is a reaction at the injection site. Long-term adverse effects (> 2 years) are unknown. Another biologic response modifier, leflunomide, is given in a loading dose of 100 mg/day po on days 1 to 3, followed by 20 mg/day, to inhibit de novo pyrimidine synthesis. The most common serious adverse effect is hepatic toxicity.

Gold compounds and penicillamine are older drugs that are used less frequently but can be considered for patients who cannot tolerate other drugs. Gold sodium thiomalate and gold thioglucose (aurothioglucose) are injectable (eg, intramuscularly); a test dose of 10 mg for the 1st week is followed by a 25-mg dose 1 week later. All subsequent IM doses of 25 to 50 mg are given weekly until a cumulative dose of 1 g is achieved and a therapeutic response or toxicity occurs. If a therapeutic response occurs, maintenance doses of 25 to 50 mg are continued weekly, then every 2 weeks, then every 3 weeks, then monthly. Monthly therapy should be continued indefinitely to prevent a recurrence. Auranofin, an oral gold compound, may be less effective than the injectable forms; the usual dosage is 3 mg bid or 6 mg/day for 6 months. If no therapeutic response occurs, the dosage may be increased to 3 mg tid.

The most common adverse effects of gold therapy are pruritus, dermatitis, stomatitis, proteinuria, and pancytopenia. Pruritus often precedes diffuse dermatitis, which may cause exfoliation, and stomatitis. When pruritus or even minor dermatitis develops, gold therapy should be discontinued. If the dermatitis resolves, the drug may be restarted at a lower dose. Proteinuria, leukopenia, or thrombocytopenia requires permanent discontinuation of gold therapy. Oral gold therapy causes less mucocutaneous and renal toxicity but more diarrhea and gastrointestinal reactions.

Penicillamine is started at 125 to 250 mg/day po, which is increased at 2- to 3-month intervals by 125- to 250-mg increments to a total of 750 mg/day. Penicillamine should be taken between meals because food decreases absorption. Adverse effects include dermatitis, proteinuria, dysgeusia, and thrombocytopenia; more severe adverse effects (eg, pemphigus, myasthenia gravis, a lupus-like syndrome, severe bone marrow suppression) have also been reported. Patients taking penicillamine must be monitored closely.

Azathioprine, cyclophosphamide, and cyclosporine can be used to treat refractory rheumatoid arthritis. For very advanced cases, a new treatment option consists of apheresis using a staphylococcus protein A immunoadsorption column.

SYSTEMIC LUPUS ERYTHEMATOSUS

A chronic inflammatory connective tissue disorder that occurs mainly in women of childbearing age but also in older persons.

The incidence of systemic lupus erythematosus (SLE) declines in old age. The prevalence is 12% for patients > 50. Furthermore, the female:male ratio declines from 9:1 in younger persons to about 3:1 in elderly persons. Unlike for idiopathic SLE, the incidence and prevalence for drug-induced SLE increases with age, probably because the elderly use many of the causative drugs. Procainamide, hydralazine, chlorpromazine, methyldopa, penicillamine, quinidine, sulfasalazine, and isoniazid are known causes. Captopril, lithium, anticonvulsants, β-blockers, propylthiouracil, levodopa, and nifedipine are strongly suspected. The cause of idiopathic SLE is unknown. The pathogenesis involves the formation of autoantibodies and immune complexes, which damage several organs, especially the kidneys.

Symptoms, Signs, and Diagnosis

The classic malar rash occurs in only about 20% of elderly patients, but other diagnostic symptoms and signs are similar in elderly and younger patients. Arthralgia is prominent, and serositis is common. Dermatitis, asymmetric migratory arthritis, photosensitivity, pleurisy, pericarditis, pneumonitis, and Sjögren's syndrome are typical in idiopathic and drug-induced SLE, but central nervous system and renal manifestations are uncommon in drug-induced SLE. Symptoms of drug-induced SLE can occur up to 2 years after the drug is discontinued.

Some authorities contend that central nervous system, renal, and hematologic manifestations are unusual in elderly patients with SLE. Hypercoagulability may occur due to the presence of the lupus anticoagulant. ∎

Laboratory results for antinuclear antibodies (ANA) are positive in 95% of patients with idiopathic SLE and in 100% with drug-induced SLE. About 50% of patients taking procainamide have positive ANA test results, but only about 5 to 10% develop an SLE-like syndrome. The presence of anti-double-stranded DNA antibodies is considered diagnostic of SLE. Many other autoantibodies are present in patients with SLE but are not usually helpful in diagnosis. Serum complement levels may be depressed, particularly in patients with renal disease. Urinalysis may show proteinuria or cells and casts on microscopic examination; the CBC count may show thrombocytopenia, leukopenia, or anemia. The prothrombin time may be prolonged if the lupus anticoagulant is present.

Treatment

Patients with mild disease, who have primarily arthritis or dermatitis, may respond to NSAIDs. NSAIDs must be used with caution in the elderly, who have an increased risk of renal toxicity. COX-2 inhibitors (eg, celecoxib, rofecoxib) are likely to cause less gastrointestinal toxicity and platelet dysfunction. Hydroxychloroquine may be useful, particularly for patients with dermatitis. Although rare, ocular toxicity may occur with this drug, and an initial eye examination is recommended.

∎see page 689

High-dose corticosteroids are indicated for patients with central nervous system, renal, or severe hematologic manifestations or for those with fever, weight loss, or severe pleurisy or pericarditis. In the elderly, corticosteroid use increases the risk of osteoporosis and subsequent fracture; measurements of bone mineral density may help assess risk. For drug-induced SLE, discontinuing the causative drug and administering an NSAID may be sufficient. However, some patients, particularly those with severe pericarditis, may need prednisone 40 to 60 mg/day po for several weeks.

SJÖGREN'S SYNDROME

A cell-mediated autoimmune disease that results in inflammation, dysfunction, and destruction of the exocrine glands.

This chronic syndrome is characterized by decreased lacrimal and salivary gland activity (sicca syndrome) and a connective tissue disorder.

Symptoms, Signs, and Diagnosis

The most common signs, xerophthalmia (dry eyes) and xerostomia (dry mouth), are reported in up to 25% of elderly patients. However, most persons with such symptoms have atrophic mucus-producing cells rather than an autoimmune disease. Patients with xerophthalmia report a foreign body sensation or grittiness in the eyes. Patients with xerostomia have a need to drink copious amounts of fluids, a loss of taste, and excessive dental caries. Occasionally, Sjögren's syndrome is accompanied by systemic manifestations, including Raynaud's phenomenon, polyarthritis, interstitial pneumonitis, vasculitis, neurologic and psychiatric manifestations, and loss of other exocrine functions.

The diagnosis is based on the symptoms. The Schirmer test, which uses a small strip of filter paper to measure eye moisture, has been advocated as a test for Sjögren's syndrome; however, this test is not standardized. Sjögren's syndrome may be accompanied by autoantibodies, including anti-Ro and anti-La, in the blood. Although rarely needed, biopsy of the minor salivary gland of the lip can confirm the diagnosis. Patients show evidence of focal or diffuse lymphocytic infiltration of the glands.

Treatment

Treatment is symptomatic. Artificial tears and lemon and glycerin mouth rinse are the standard therapies. For the systemic forms of Sjögren's syndrome, corticosteroids and other immunosuppressant drugs have been tried with varied effectiveness.

SYSTEMIC SCLEROSIS
(Scleroderma)

An autoimmune disease characterized by fibrosis of the subcutaneous tissue and thickening of the skin over the fingers, arms, chest, and face.

Systemic sclerosis is rare among elderly persons. The cause is unknown.

Besides the characteristic skin thickening, symptoms and signs include telangiectasis, Raynaud's phenomenon, esophageal dysmotility, pulmonary fibrosis, and, occasionally, vascular involvement of the heart and kidneys. Features of systemic sclerosis sometimes occur with clinical and serologic features of SLE, polymyositis, or rheumatoid arthritis; this overlap syndrome is called **mixed connective tissue disease.** Autoantibodies, especially anticentromere and anti-SCL-70, are often found.

In early stages of systemic sclerosis, treatment is largely symptomatic. For example, Raynaud's phenomenon may be prevented by wearing gloves and using calcium channel blockers. Penicillamine 250 to 500 mg/day po has been advocated, but no randomized clinical trials have shown this drug to be effective. A recent meta-analysis suggests little benefit. Also, penicillamine has significant adverse effects, which may preclude use in elderly patients. Occasionally, patients present with acute renal failure and hypertensive crisis. When such fulminant presentation occurs, it is best treated with angiotensin-converting enzyme inhibitors.

53 ▬ VASCULITIC SYNDROMES

GIANT CELL (TEMPORAL) ARTERITIS AND POLYMYALGIA RHEUMATICA

Giant cell (temporal) arteritis: A chronic inflammatory process involving the extracranial arteries. Polymyalgia rheumatica: A syndrome characterized by pain and stiffness in muscles of the limb girdles.

These disorders occur almost exclusively in the elderly. Although giant cell arteritis and polymyalgia rheumatica may occur separately, 40 to 60% of patients with giant cell arteritis have clinical features of polymyalgia rheumatica, and 10 to 25% of patients with polymyalgia rheumatica have clinical or pathologic features of giant cell arteritis.

The annual incidence, which varies widely among studies, is 0.5 to 4/1000 in persons > 60. The incidence increases strikingly with age:

giant cell arteritis and polymyalgia rheumatica are 10 times more common in patients aged > 80 than in those aged 50 to 59. Both disorders cluster in families and are associated with HLA-DR4. They are twice as common in women than in men and are more common in whites than in blacks.

Etiology and Pathology

In **giant cell arteritis,** round cell infiltration of the intima and inner part of the media is characteristic. Histiocytes, lymphocytes, and monocytes predominate, but the presence of multinucleated Langhans' giant cells is more diagnostic. Many of the lymphocytes are helper T cells. This feature, combined with the rarity of immunoglobulin deposits around elastin fibers, suggests that the arterial lesion results from cellular rather than humoral immunity. Evidence suggests that cytokines from T cells and macrophages are present in unaffected regions of the temporal arteries from patients with both giant cell arteritis and polymyalgia rheumatica, possibly indicating a common pathogenesis for these two disorders.

The inflammatory process involves short segments of the artery and is usually circumferential. Segments of normal artery, which are smooth and often dilated, taper to affected segments, which are smooth and symmetrically stenosed or occluded. Although the superficial temporal artery is most frequently biopsied because it is most accessible, the vertebral, ophthalmic, and posterior ciliary arteries are often concurrently involved. The internal and external carotid and central retinal arteries are less commonly affected, and the intracerebral arteries are rarely affected.

In **polymyalgia rheumatica,** skeletal muscle is histologically normal. Synovitis characterized by round cell infiltration and synovial proliferation are common, although they are less severe than in rheumatoid arthritis. Usually the hips and shoulders are affected; the knees and sternoclavicular joints may also be affected.

Symptoms, Signs, and Diagnosis

Both disorders are often associated with fatigue, weight loss, and fever. Weight loss or fever sometimes is the only finding. In patients with polymyalgia rheumatica, signs or symptoms of giant cell arteritis must be sought; if such signs and symptoms are present, complications may be sudden and serious and the initial dose of corticosteroids used for treatment is higher.

In **giant cell arteritis,** the typical presenting feature is a continuous, throbbing temporal headache. Ischemia of the masseter muscles, tongue, and pharynx causes pain during chewing, talking, or swallowing (jaw claudication). Stenosis of the ophthalmic artery and its branches can cause ocular or orbital pain, transient loss of vision (amaurosis fugax), visual field defects, blurring, or sudden, permanent blindness. Ischemia of the orbital muscle may cause diplopia. Physical examination may reveal characteristic tender, red, swollen, and nodular temporal arteries with diminished pulses. Less commonly, pulses over other head and neck arteries are reduced or absent. Ophthalmic artery involvement generally causes a central scotoma or total blindness; patchy peripheral visual field defects are less common. Ophthalmic artery involvement may produce blockage, which initially results in a pale, swollen optic disk surrounded by pericapillary hemorrhage; the disk later atrophies. Patchy areas of retinal infarction are less common. Patients with orbital muscle damage present with varying degrees of ophthalmoplegia or ptosis.

In **polymyalgia rheumatica,** bilateral pain and stiffness of the shoulders and thighs are most common; these symptoms are often severe and lead to immobility and other functional losses (eg, inability to wash or dress). Pain is most severe in the morning. Nocturnal pain that disturbs sleep is also common. Stiffness after inactivity and morning stiffness lasting > 1 hour are usually present.

Physical examination may elicit some tenderness over the affected muscles and painful limitation of hip and shoulder movements, but the tenderness is mild compared with the severity of symptoms. The wrists, knees, and fingers may be swollen and tender.

Laboratory tests: The most useful laboratory test is the ESR, which is usually > 40 mm/hour and often > 100 mm/hour. Although this test is very sensitive, the results are occasionally normal, particularly with polymyalgia rheumatica. C-reactive protein and interleukin-6 levels are also usually elevated in both disorders; however, neither of these tests has been proven to be more specific or sensitive than the ESR.

Antibody titers (eg, rheumatoid and antinuclear factors) are not elevated. Liver enzyme levels are mildly elevated in one third of patients. Patients often have a normochromic-normocytic anemia.

Temporal artery biopsy: Temporal artery biopsy is the most specific test for giant cell arteritis and should be performed in all patients with clinical features of this disorder. Treatment with corticosteroids can be started up to 1 week before biopsy without affecting biopsy results. Treatment should not be delayed to accommodate biopsy. A 5-cm section of artery should be excised; a shorter section may miss the affected segment. Round cell and Langhans' giant cell infiltration of the media confirms the diagnosis; if the biopsy findings are negative, there is a 5 to 10% chance that the diagnosis has been missed. In exceptional circumstances, a biopsy of the contralateral artery may be justified.

The role of temporal artery biopsy in patients with symptoms of only polymyalgia rheumatica is controversial. A reasonable approach is to forgo biopsy and instead follow the patient's clinical symptoms, ESR, and response to treatment.

Treatment

Corticosteroids are the treatment of choice for both giant cell arteritis and polymyalgia rheumatica; these drugs produce a dramatic response. A patient who was severely crippled may regain mobility and full independence within the first week of treatment.

The starting dosage for giant cell arteritis should be equivalent to prednisone 60 mg/day; for polymyalgia rheumatica, 15 mg/day. Initial dosages should be maintained for ≥ 2 months. When giant cell arteritis is suspected, even before the diagnosis is proven by biopsy of the temporal artery, the physician should start treatment with prednisone 60 mg/day to prevent ocular complications.

Efficacy should be monitored by serial ESR measurements and clinical response. The corticosteroid dosage can be gradually reduced (usually to prednisone 5 to 15 mg/day or equivalent) depending on the ESR and clinical symptoms and signs.

Maintenance therapy should be continued for 1 to 2 years. The corticosteroid dosage should be as low as possible to control symptoms. After corticosteroids are discontinued, the patient should be monitored for ≥ 6 months. If symptoms recur, treatment must be restarted.

Elderly patients started on corticosteroids may experience many adverse effects, including fluid retention, increased appetite, and confusion. Blood sugar must be monitored for hyperglycemia. Dormant tuberculosis should be excluded by history and skin test results. Appropriate preventive treatment for osteoporosis should be implemented. Stress doses of corticosteroids should be given if another medical event occurs.

Nonsteroidal anti-inflammatory drugs have been used for mild polymyalgia rheumatica but are not nearly as effective as corticosteroids.

In addition to drug treatment, physical therapy should be initiated in patients who show muscle weakness or other functional deficits. Restoration and maintenance of muscle function are key to the treatment of elderly persons.

OTHER VASCULITIC SYNDROMES

Although rare, some other vasculitic syndromes, including polyarteritis nodosa and Wegener's granulomatosis, may occur in elderly persons. They are more common among men than among women.

Polyarteritis nodosa (polyarteritis, periarteritis nodosa) is characterized by segmental inflammation and necrosis of medium-sized muscular arteries, with secondary ischemia of tissue supplied by affected vessels. **Wegener's granulomatosis,** which resembles polyarteritis nodosa, usually begins as a localized granulomatous inflammation of upper or lower respiratory tract mucosa and may progress into generalized necrotizing granulomatous vasculitis and glomerulonephritis.

The cause is unknown, but immune mechanisms appear to be involved because immune complexes are occasionally found in vessel walls and glomeruli. One hypothesis suggests that these syndromes are the result of a respiratory tract hypersensitivity reaction.

Symptoms and Signs

Symptoms and signs are nonspecific; fever, malaise, anorexia, weight loss, purpura, arthritis, central nervous system dysfunction, and infarction of various organs are common. Some degree of renal involvement occurs in 70 to 90% of patients; progressive renal failure can be a late manifestation in polyarteritis nodosa. The presentation of these vasculitic syndromes often mimics that of other disorders. Patients with Wegener's granulomatosis often present with upper respiratory complaints, including sinusitis, nasal mucosal ulcerations, and serous or purulent otitis media with hearing loss, cough, hemoptysis, and pleuritis.

Diagnosis, Prognosis, and Treatment

Diagnosis is often difficult because of the varied presentation and because pathologic findings are usually absent. Renal biopsy can confirm the presence of glomerulonephritis. Polyarteritis nodosa may be diagnosed by evidence of organ involvement on biopsy or of multiple aneurysm formation on arteriography. Wegener's granulomatosis may be diagnosed by using pulmonary or respiratory tract biopsy. Some experts recommend the use of antinuclear cytoplasmic antibody (ANCA) as a diagnostic test for Wegener's granulomatosis, but others question ANCA's usefulness because of its poor specificity.

Prognosis is very poor for both disorders, if untreated. Early diagnosis and aggressive treatment are necessary to prevent progression to end-organ damage (eg, end-stage renal disease). High-dose corticosteroids produce remission in some patients with polyarteritis nodosa, but they must be used long-term. Other measures include immunosuppressants, antihypertensive therapy, careful fluid management, attention to renal impairment, and blood transfusion. Cyclophosphamide is the treatment of choice for Wegener's granulomatosis.

Muscular disorders (see TABLE 54–1) are characterized by abnormalities of muscle fibers. In addition, many neurologic disorders (eg, lesions of the central or peripheral nervous system, abnormalities of neuromuscular transmission) can produce symptoms that are primarily muscular—see TABLE 54–2 **1** Other systemic disorders (eg, rheumatic, psychiatric, cardiovascular, respiratory, endocrine) can mimic muscular disorders but do not directly affect muscular function. These systemic disorders account for more than half of muscular complaints.

Approach to the Patient With Muscular Symptoms

History and physical examination (see TABLE 54–3): **Abnormalities in gait 2** and in leg muscle strength that are often symmetric may be due to lesions in the central nervous system (CNS), which can mimic abnormalities of the peripheral nervous system or of muscle fibers. Papilledema, unilateral weakness or sensory loss, and a gait disturbance with the head turned or the neck flexed suggest a CNS cause.

Difficulty in walking, unsteadiness with occasional falls, and joint stiffness with leg pains, especially at night, may also be due to rheumatic diseases (eg, degenerative joint disease, rheumatoid arthritis, polymyalgia rheumatica). Significant degenerative joint disease can limit mobility by producing structural spinal changes and joint symptoms in the limbs and occasionally by damaging the spinal cord, nerve roots, and peripheral nerves.

Muscle weakness in patients with descending motor pathway dysfunction (eg, midline subdural hematoma, midline posterior fossa mass) is frequently greater on functional testing (ie, during performance of common tasks) than on direct muscle strength testing. Muscle weakness in patients with peripheral nerve and muscle damage is similar on functional and direct muscle testing.

Muscle weakness in patients without significant joint or soft tissue disease is suggested by the inability to walk on the heels and toes, rise from a squatting position, rise from a chair without using the arms, or step onto the seat of a chair. A normal person should be able to completely extend the knee against gravity. If the knee tends to remain slightly flexed, the quadriceps of the thigh may be weak, which often causes stumbles and falls. The patient should be able to raise outstretched arms above the head easily and to blanch the knuckles with a forceful grip.

Exercise performance may be limited in patients with anxiety or depression. These patients often do not have intrinsic muscle weakness, yet experience fatigue and lack motivation for activities of daily living.

Pathologic fatigue is characterized by drooping eyelids when a person fixates on a target or by rapid exhaustion during repeated movements

---

1 see also page 488　　**2** see page 203

TABLE 54–1.   ETIOLOGIC CLASSIFICATION OF MUSCULAR DISORDERS

Abnormalities in neuromuscular transmission
Myasthenia gravis
Eaton-Lambert syndrome

Inflammatory muscular disorders
Inclusion body myositis
Dermatomyositis
Polymyositis

Endocrine- and electrolyte-induced muscular disorders
Corticosteroid myopathy
Muscular disorders in hyperthyroidism
Muscular disorders in hypothyroidism
Muscular disorders in osteomalacia
Hypokalemic myopathy

Myopathy due to muscular dystrophy
Myotonic dystrophy
Oculopharyngeal muscular dystrophy

Miscellaneous muscular disorders
Idiopathic muscle cramps
Cervical spondylosis (see Ch. 50)

(eg, elevating the arms above the head, rising from a chair). When due to an abnormality in neuromuscular transmission (eg, myasthenia gravis), pathologic fatigue leads to fluctuations in the ability to chew, keep the eyes open, speak, or smile.

Muscle cramps or pain in the absence of electrolyte or pH disturbance commonly indicates a peripheral nerve disorder and less commonly an abnormality in muscle fibers. Intense pain that is most prominent in proximal muscles in the morning may indicate polymyalgia rheumatica.◨ Pain in localized muscle regions may indicate fibromyalgia. Pain largely restricted to muscle groups and periarticular tissue may indicate diffuse arthritic disease with limited muscle function.

Focal **muscle wasting** indicates an abnormality in muscle fibers or motor nerves. Diffuse muscle wasting can occur after as little as 4 to 6 weeks of absolute bed rest; despite the reduced muscle mass, muscle strength is usually preserved.

Abnormalities in tendon reflexes are important to note on examination. Tendon reflexes are typically increased and plantar extensor responses are present in patients with muscle weakness due to CNS disease. However, ankle or other reflexes are absent in many elderly persons without demonstrable disease. Loss of reflexes with only mild weakness is typical for disease of the peripheral nerve or nerve root, although occasionally cerebellar lesions depress tendon reflexes, sug-

◨ see page 506

gesting muscle weakness. Loss of reflexes in patients with primary myopathy often parallels the degree of weakness. Reflexes are usually maintained in patients with abnormalities of neuromuscular transmission but are frequently lost or hypoactive in patients with Eaton-Lambert syndrome.

Blood tests: Elevation of serum creatine kinase (CK) levels (normal < 130 U/L) is a more sensitive determinant of muscle damage than is elevation of any other serum enzyme level. However, normal exercise, depending on its intensity and the person's conditioning, can elevate CK levels as much as threefold to eightfold. Levels peak several hours after exercise, and maximum levels persist for 24 to 36 hours, partly because of the long plasma half-life of CK (38 to 118 hours). Thus, CK levels should not be measured within 48 hours of vigorous normal exercise. CK levels are also elevated by muscle damage caused by prolonged pressure, which may occur in elderly persons who lie immobile on a hard surface.

CK elevations occur in many disorders affecting the motor unit (the anterior horn cell, motor axon and terminal branches, neuromuscular junctions, and muscle fibers). Mild CK elevations (< 4 times the upper limit of the normal range) occur in some healthy persons with large muscle mass, in healthy persons after minor muscle trauma (eg, after intramuscular injections or needle electromyography), in persons predisposed to malignant hyperthermia, and in persons with certain chronic anterior horn cell diseases such as amyotrophic lateral sclerosis and postpolio syndrome. Moderate to marked CK elevations occur in inflammatory myopathies (eg, polymyositis, dermatomyositis) and after conditions that produce muscle necrosis (eg, hypokalemic myopathy).

CK isoenzymes include CK-MM (found primarily in skeletal muscle), CK-MB (in heart muscle), and CK-BB (in brain tissue); the concentration of CK-MM is > 3 times that of CK-MB and CK-BB. Normal adult skeletal muscle contains about 95% CK-MM and 5% CK-MB. However, regenerating skeletal muscle fibers revert to an embryonic isoenzyme pattern, and CK-MB increases to 10 to 50%. Thus, CK isoenzyme measurements are not useful for diagnosing or monitoring neuromuscular disorders.

Measurements of serum electrolyte and bicarbonate levels (to evaluate for acidosis or alkalosis) are helpful in diagnosing the cause of muscle weakness, particularly muscle weakness accompanied by muscle cramps and pain. Possible causes include hypokalemia, hypophosphatemia, hypocalcemia, hypermagnesemia, and chronic hypofunction or hyperfunction of the thyroid, adrenal, or parathyroid glands. ESR and other blood tests (eg, antinuclear antibody, rheumatoid factor) can be used to screen for collagen vascular diseases; serum and urine immunoelectrophoresis can be used to assess immunoglobulins and Bence Jones protein in multiple myeloma.

TABLE 54–2. CONDITIONS CAUSING MUSCULAR SYMPTOMS IN ELDERLY PATIENTS

Condition	Example	Manifestation
Lesions affecting the descending motor pathways	Intracranial lesions	Midline subdural hematoma Subfrontal or interhemispheral neoplasm Communicating hydrocephalus Midline mass lesion in posterior fossa (eg, metastatic tumor in cerebellum) Degenerative diseases of the central nervous system
	Spinal cord lesions	Compression of spinal cord due to osteoarthritis or disk disease, vertebral collapse (osteoporosis vs. neoplasm), epidural metastasis, or epidural abscess Anterior horn cell disease due to amyotrophic lateral sclerosis or postpolio syndrome Radiation myelopathy Lyme disease
Lesions affecting the motor nerve roots	Comprehensive or infiltrative lesions	Spinal stenosis Infiltration of roots by lymphoma or carcinoma Paget's disease
	Inflammatory lesions	Acute inflammatory polyneuritis Chronic inflammatory demyelinating polyneuropathy
Lesions affecting the peripheral nerve motor fibers	Inflammatory or infectious lesions	Acute inflammatory polyneuritis Chronic inflammatory demyelinating polyneuropathy (idiopathic vs. due to a plasma cell disorder that produces paraprotein) Diphtheria
	Endocrine disease or lesions caused by toxins	Thyroid disease Heavy metal toxicity (lead, mercury)
Lesions affecting neuromuscular transmission	Autoimmune or neoplasm-associated defects	Myasthenia gravis Myasthenia gravis with thymoma Eaton-Lambert syndrome
	Toxin- or drug-induced transmission disorders	Botulism Aminoglycoside, β-blocker, or lithium toxicity Drug-induced myasthenia gravis (eg, penicillamine)

TABLE 54–2. (*Continued*)

Condition	Example	Manifestation
Abnormalities in muscle fibers	Inflammatory or infectious disorders	Inclusion body myositis Dermatomyositis (with or without neoplasm) Polymyositis (many potential causes)
	Endocrine, electrolyte, or drug-induced disorders	Thyroid disease Vitamin D deficiency with osteomalacia Phosphate or magnesium deficiency Corticosteroid, penicillamine, chloroquine, emetine, clofibrate, ethanol, lovastatin, amiodarone, colchicine, or tryptophan toxicity
	Muscular dystrophies (onset late in life is uncommon)	Myotonic dystrophy Oculopharyngeal dystrophy Scapuloperoneal dystrophy

Imaging studies: Plain x-rays of the spine can identify many rheumatic disorders (eg, chronic osteoarthritis, chronic disk herniation with early lumbosacral spinal canal narrowing) and other disorders that might produce muscular symptoms (eg, covert metastatic disease with vertebral collapse). In patients with chronic motor neuropathies, a skeletal survey may help identify the cause (eg, multiple myeloma, osteomalacia).

Ultrasonography, CT, MRI, and radionuclide imaging can quantify muscle atrophy and identify the muscle groups with the most damage before needle biopsy is performed. Ultrasonography can also help identify a muscle abscess. CT and MRI can identify lesions in the brain and spinal cord and occasionally in soft tissues and muscle that other studies cannot identify. Examples include lesions producing symmetric dysfunction in the descending motor pathways, thymoma (in myasthenia gravis), and oat cell carcinoma of the lung (in Eaton-Lambert syndrome). Technetium diphosphonate or pyrophosphate imaging can demonstrate muscle fiber damage in polymyositis.

Electrodiagnosis: Electrodiagnostic testing (see TABLE 54–4) is indicated to identify axonal and demyelinating neuropathies, to demonstrate abnormalities in neuromuscular transmission, and to detect damage to muscle fibers typical of primary muscle diseases. Testing helps confirm the diagnosis of diseases such as chronic inflammatory demyelinating polyneuropathy, Eaton-Lambert myasthenic syndrome,

TABLE 54–3.   DIFFERENTIATING CAUSES OF MUSCULAR SYMPTOMS IN THE ELDERLY

Cause	Site of Involvement	Distribution of Weakness	Sensory Involvement	Tendon Reflexes	Muscular Atrophy	Other Clinical Features	Diagnostic Tests
Chronic subdural hematoma above and between both frontal lobes	Frontal lobes (interhemispheric or subfrontal)	Symmetric leg weakness	None	Normal to slightly increased in legs; variable plantar extensor responses	None	Headache, personality change, drowsiness	MRI or CT of head, clotting profile
Metastasis	Midportion of cerebellum	Gait disturbance; often no true weakness	None	Often decreased; variable plantar extensor responses	None	Unsteady gait, headache	MRI or CT of head with emphasis on posterior fossa
Chronic spinal cord compression caused by C-5 and C-6 osteoarthritis	Cervical spinal cord	Symmetric or slightly asymmetric weakness in hands and legs	Pain and occasional decrease in pinprick sensation and touch response in C-6 and C-7 nerve root distribution	Decreased in arms and increased in legs; plantar extensor responses	Intrinsic hand muscles, mild to moderate	Limited motion of neck, pain with movement, occasional worsening of leg weakness with head flexion or extension	MRI of posterior fossa and cervical and upper thoracic spine; x-rays of cervical spine (flexion and extension views)
Amyotrophic lateral sclerosis	Anterior horn cell	Asymmetric or bulbar weakness	None	Variable	Marked, early development	Fasciculations, cramps, tremor	EMG, nerve conduction studies

Chronic inflammatory demyelinating polyneuropathy	Peripheral nerve	Symmetric, distal, greater than proximal weakness	Distal dysesthesias and loss of vibration greater than pinprick sensation and touch response	Decreased	Mild to moderate	Muscle aches, trouble using stairs, tripping	Nerve conduction studies, EMG, nerve biopsy, CSF analysis
Myasthenia gravis	Neuromuscular junction	Extraocular and bulbar weakness; weakness in the proximal limb muscles	None	Normal	None	Weakness that fluctuates, diurnal variation	Edrophonium test, repetitive nerve stimulation, CT of chest (thymus), measurement of acetylcholine receptor antibody levels
Polymyositis	Skeletal muscle fibers	Symmetric weakness in the proximal limb and bulbar muscles	Aching	Parallel strength	Slight	Slowly progressive weakness over weeks to months	Measurement of creatine kinase levels, ESR, EMG, muscle biopsy

EMG = electromyography; CSF = cerebrospinal fluid.

TABLE 54–4.   ELECTRODIAGNOSTIC FINDINGS IN LESIONS CAUSING MUSCULAR SYMPTOMS

Electro-diagnostic Test	Location of Lesion			
	Descending Motor Pathways	Lower Motor Neuron	Neuromuscular Transmission	Skeletal Muscle
Nerve conduction	Normal	Often normal; abnormal only with demyelination of large nerve fibers	Normal	Normal
Repetitive stimulation	Normal	Normal	Variable; usually abnormal if stimulated muscle is weak	Normal
Electromyography	Reduced firing frequency of motor unit potentials	Signs of acute or chronic denervation	Normal or myopathic in very weak muscles	Myopathic or normal

and inflammatory myopathies. Electrodiagnostic testing is especially useful for evaluating patients who cannot undergo thorough clinical testing because of pain or cognitive impairment. Serial testing is helpful in selected patients for demonstrating improvement and aiding in decisions about treatment.

Nerve conduction assessment uses skin electrodes to stimulate a peripheral nerve at various points and other electrodes to record the motor and sensory action potentials at distal sites, so that conduction velocity of the peripheral nerve can be calculated. In healthy adults, conduction velocity typically ranges from 45 to 75 m/second. (In healthy elderly persons, velocity tends to be in the lower range.) In those with chronic demyelinating polyneuropathies, the velocity may be decreased by ≥ 40%.

Repetitive stimulation testing measures the action potential of the peripheral motor nerve. The nerve is stimulated at a low frequency (3 Hz), usually before and after brief maximal isometric exercise. An incremental decrease in the amplitude of the action potential usually indicates an abnormality in neuromuscular transmission (eg, myasthenia gravis). In contrast, an incremental increase is usually due to Eaton-Lambert syndrome.

Electromyography records electrical activity of muscle at rest (when normally there is none) and during mild and strong contractions. The number and amplitude of motor unit potentials increase as the strength of voluntary contraction increases. In neurogenic disorders that damage the motor axon, electromyographic findings depend on the type and duration of the neuropathy. If the damage produces axonal death, fibrillations (spontaneous activity of single muscle fibers) and positive waves (biphasic action potentials initiated by movement of the recording needle, often occurring in an area of damaged, fibrillating muscle fibers) usually develop after ≥ 3 weeks. Electromyography often differentiates primary myopathy from neuropathy. Typically with myopathy, the test shows a normal number of motor unit potentials, often with decreased amplitude, during maximum contraction. With chronic denervation, the test shows a reduced number of motor unit potentials with very high amplitude. Acute neuropathy may produce fibrillations and positive waves identical to those produced after inflammatory myopathies.

Fasciculations (spontaneous activity of part or all of a motor unit) typically occur with slowly progressive diseases of the anterior horn cell or nerve roots or with electrolyte disturbances; they often do not indicate axonal death. Many normal persons develop fasciculations, especially after exercise.

Muscle biopsy: This test is useful for differentiating myopathy from neuropathy. It is also useful for diagnosing certain connective tissue diseases (eg, polyarteritis nodosa, polymyositis) and disorders such as the muscular dystrophies, congenital myopathies, and specific metabolic diseases of muscle, which are rare in the elderly.

Biopsy is not useful for diagnosing acute generalized weakness, subacute or chronic neurogenic weakness (eg, acute inflammatory polyneuritis, diabetic polyneuropathy), or abnormalities in neuromuscular transmission (eg, myasthenia gravis).

Nerve biopsy: Nerve biopsy is more difficult and traumatic than muscle biopsy and thus has limited use. It can differentiate segmental demyelination from axonal degeneration and identify inflammatory neuropathies. Nerve biopsy also can be used to diagnose uncommon diseases such as amyloidosis, sarcoidosis, leprosy, and certain unusual metabolic and hereditary neuropathies. In elderly patients, the indications are very restricted; the most common indication is diagnosis of chronic inflammatory demyelinating polyneuropathy.

Muscle mass assessment: Measurements of muscle mass are helpful in assessing disease progression or improvement (eg, in patients with chronic slowly progressive neuromuscular diseases). For example, clinical examination may not determine whether weight gain in a patient with inflammatory myopathy is due to treatment with corticosteroids or to an increase in muscle mass. Because a change in muscle strength may not be apparent for several weeks or not at all after a decline in muscle mass, measurements of muscle mass may detect a response to treatment or lack of response that is not evident on clinical examination.

The usual method is a 24-hour urinary creatinine measurement, which varies by < 10%, correlates directly and reliably with total muscle mass, and can be used to determine response to therapy. Normal findings are 1800 to 1700 mg/24 hours (15.8 to 15.0 mmol/24 hours) for persons aged 30 to 50; 1700 to 1500 mg/24 hours (15.0 to 13.2 mmol/24 hours) for those aged 50 to 60; 1600 to 1400 mg/24 hours (14.1 to 12.3 mmol/24 hours) for those aged 60 to 70; and 1400 to 1200 mg/24 hours (12.3 to 10.6 mmol/24 hours) for those aged 70 to 80. Patients must not consume meat for 3 days before urine collection. Specimens collected weeks to months apart are often helpful in documenting sequential changes in muscle mass.

Dual energy x-ray absorptiometry (DEXA) can be used to measure muscle mass and bone density (the usual indication for the test). DEXA is fast (30 minutes) and, unlike urinary creatinine measurement, requires only one session. The x-ray exposure is less than that of a standard chest x-ray. Disadvantages include significantly high cost compared with urinary creatinine measurement and low availability of the equipment required.

MYASTHENIA GRAVIS

An autoimmune disease characterized by episodic muscle weakness caused by loss or dysfunction of acetylcholine receptors at the skeletal muscle motor end plate.

Myasthenia gravis can occur at any age, but the incidence peaks among women in the 3rd and 4th decades and among men in the 6th and 7th decades. Among the elderly, myasthenia gravis is more common in men.

This receptor deficiency is caused by circulating anti-acetylcholine receptor antibodies that block the α-bungarotoxin binding sites to the acetylcholine receptor and accelerate the turnover rate (ie, internalization and destruction) for the receptor. The role of the thymus gland is unknown, but about 65% of patients have thymic hyperplasia, and 10 to 15% have thymoma.

Symptoms and Signs

Muscle weakness and fatigability are characteristic. Symptoms typically fluctuate; they are most pronounced at night and are relieved by rest. Initial symptoms include ptosis, diplopia, or blurred vision in > 50% of patients; generalized weakness and fatigue in about 10%; and dysphagia, facial weakness, or slurred nasal speech in about 5%. In the elderly, symptoms are usually most severe in the extraocular and bulbar muscles. Symptoms remain limited to the extraocular muscles in about 15% of patients and become generalized in 85%, usually within the first year. Symptoms reach maximum severity in the first year in 50% of patients and within 5 years in almost all patients. **Myasthenic crisis** is characterized by the acute onset of respiratory insufficiency, often with difficulty swallowing and speaking, and by increased weakness in the arms and legs. Infection, trauma, or use of aminoglycosides, cardiac drugs, antihistamines, or anxiolytics may precipitate myasthenic crisis.

Diagnosis

The diagnosis is usually based on the history and physical examination. The most sensitive and accurate diagnostic test is a quantitative measurement of anti-acetylcholine receptor antibodies. These antibodies are increased in 85 to 90% of patients with generalized myasthenia gravis and in 50 to 70% of patients with ocular myasthenia. The number of antibodies is also increased in > 90% of patients with thymoma.

Measurement of acetylcholine receptor modulating antibodies is useful in patients with negative results on anti-acetylcholine receptor antibody testing. Patients with thymoma also often have increased numbers of anti–striated muscle antibodies, as do about 55% of patients > 60 with myasthenia gravis alone. Thymoma is diagnosed by CT or MRI; MRI provides more information about the soft tissue and vascular supply.

An anticholinesterase test can temporarily reverse the muscle weakness in those with myasthenia. Edrophonium (a short-acting anticholinesterase) is given IV as a single initial dose of 2 mg and compared with placebo in a double-blind fashion while the patient is monitored by ECG; IV atropine and resuscitative equipment must be available because of the risk of cardiac rhythm disturbance, particularly in elderly persons.

The repetitive stimulation test can identify a pathologic decline in the electrical response to repeated nerve impulses to a specific muscle. A decremental response often occurs 1 to 2 minutes after exercise. As many as 50 to 60% of patients with known myasthenia have positive results when two or three muscles are tested.

Treatment

First-line therapy is often an anticholinesterase drug, such as pyridostigmine bromide at an initial dose of 30 to 60 mg po tid or qid. Some patients require dosing every 2 to 3 hours. Dosage must be carefully adjusted to individual requirements, and mild exacerbations may require an increase in dosage. Concomitant use of ephedrine 25 mg bid or tid with pyridostigmine may have a synergistic effect (the exact mechanism by which ephedrine affects skeletal muscle contraction is unknown).

The elderly usually require additional therapy to these first-line drugs, because their extraocular and bulbar symptoms are especially resistant to anticholinesterase treatment. Immunosuppressants (eg, azathioprine) and corticosteroids (eg, prednisone) are the mainstays of long-term management. Plasmapheresis and IV immune globulin are useful for myasthenic crisis or episodes of severe exacerbation.

Thymectomy is not typically recommended to relieve myasthenia in patients whose myasthenia begins after age 60 because this approach has not been proven to be more effective than immunosuppressants. However, thymoma should be sought and removed because of its potential for malignancy. Surgery has a higher initial risk and often takes 2 to 3 years to achieve maximum benefit for myasthenia. In elderly patients, immunosuppressants offer less long-term risk (eg, for lymphoma, leukemias) because life expectancy is often shorter than the time required to develop malignancy.

Rarely, treatment causes cholinergic crisis, characterized by increasing muscle weakness and increasing cholinergic effects. If cholinergic crisis occurs, treatment consists of withholding drugs, intubating the patient, and providing ventilatory support.

EATON-LAMBERT SYNDROME

An autoimmune disorder affecting muscular function that is frequently associated with small cell carcinoma of the lung (especially in men) and autoimmune diseases (especially in women and younger patients).

This syndrome occurs about five times more often in men than in women. It is an immune-mediated, myasthenia-like syndrome of muscle weakness, characterized by diminished release of acetylcholine from the motor nerve terminal. Serum from patients with Eaton-Lambert syndrome contains circulating IgG antibodies that block the voltage-dependent calcium channels in the terminals of normal motor nerve fibers.

Symptoms, Signs, and Diagnosis

Muscle fatigue with little or no muscle atrophy primarily affects the leg and trunk muscles. Extraocular and bulbar muscles are often unaffected. Hyporeflexia may occur, but contraction of the muscle for a few seconds temporarily restores normal tendon reflex activity.

About 50% of patients have autonomic abnormalities; the most frequent symptom is dry mouth. Impotence, decreased lacrimation and sweating, orthostatic symptoms, and diminished pupillary response to light also occur. Subacute cerebellar degeneration may occur in patients with Eaton-Lambert syndrome of any cause.

Diagnosis requires identification of electrophysiologic responses to repetitive nerve stimulation. Rapid repetitive nerve stimulation (50 Hz) causes a marked increase in the amplitude of the compound muscle action potential. Slow repetitive nerve stimulation (2 to 5 Hz) causes a marked decrease in the amplitude of the muscle response, similar to that of myasthenia gravis. However, slow repetitive nerve stimulation performed immediately after exercise causes a severalfold increase in the amplitude. This increase also occurs in patients with botulism, hypermagnesemia, or hypocalcemia or in those taking certain antibiotics, typically aminoglycosides.

An elevated level of antibodies to the voltage-gated P/Q-type calcium channel confirms the diagnosis. Such elevation occurs in virtually all cases due to lung carcinoma and in about 90% of cases due to other causes.

Treatment

Elderly patients should be evaluated and monitored for carcinoma for at least 2 to 3 years after diagnosis. In some patients, neuromuscular transmission improves after the carcinoma is removed. Patients should also be monitored for the development of other immune-mediated diseases.

Drugs that increase acetylcholine availability and control immune-mediated disease mechanisms are used. Initial treatment usually consists of prednisone in a moderate dose (1 to 1.5 mg/kg every other day) and azathioprine 1.5 to 2 mg/kg/day po. Immune globulin 2 g/kg IV in divided doses is the treatment of choice for patients refractory to immunosuppressive therapy, who may also benefit from plasmapheresis (5 or 6 exchanges) to remove circulating antibodies. Another effective treatment, 3,4-diaminopyridine, is available investigationally in the USA. Guanidine 10 to 35 mg/kg/day po is effective but causes significant adverse effects.

INCLUSION BODY MYOSITIS

A progressive inflammatory myopathy of unknown cause characterized by typical rimmed vacuoles and intracellular amyloid deposits in muscle.

This disorder, which resembles chronic polymyositis, usually occurs in patients > 50; it affects men 3 times as often as women. It is the most common inflammatory myopathy among elderly persons.

The cause is unknown. Autosomal recessive and autosomal dominant inheritance accounts for some cases.

Amyloid deposits and cytoplasmic and intranuclear filamentous inclusions of unknown origin are characteristic. The inherited forms are called inclusion body myopathies, because they do not display the inflammatory infiltrates that characterize inclusion body myositis.

Symptoms, Signs, and Diagnosis

Proximal and distal muscle weakness usually progresses gradually without pain; it is often asymmetric. Weakness of wrist and finger flexors and of knee extensors occurs early and is usually more severe than weakness of other muscles. This pattern of weakness can mislead physicians to suspect motor neuron disease or another neuropathic disorder.

Unlike in polymyositis and dermatomyositis, muscle atrophy develops relatively early in inclusion body myositis. Facial muscles are involved in about one third of cases, but extraocular muscles are spared. Rarely, spinal, respiratory, and abdominal muscles are affected. One recessive form spares the quadriceps femoris muscle, a finding that is atypical. Dysphagia occurs in about 40% of patients. Tendon reflexes are normal or increased and become reduced or absent only with marked muscle wasting. Usually, patients remain ambulatory for many years after symptoms begin.

Diagnosis is based on the clinical findings and elevated CK levels (up to 10-fold above normal). Diagnosis is confirmed by muscle biopsy results, which reveal eosinophilic cytoplasmic inclusion bodies composed of 15- to 18-nm filaments.

Prognosis and Treatment

Prognosis is guarded. No clearly effective treatment is available. The clinical course is slowly progressive over many years. Respiratory compromise due to aspiration pneumonitis is often the cause of death.

Immunosuppressive therapy is usually ineffective. Occasionally, prednisone 1 to 1.5 mg/kg/day po leads to improvement, as does IV immune globulin. Therapeutic trials of β-interferon are ongoing. Supportive care, bracing for occasional footdrop or severe wristdrop, and aquatic physical therapy are helpful.

DERMATOMYOSITIS

A humorally mediated autoimmune disease characterized by vascular lesions and degeneration of the skin and muscle, leading to a typical rash, symmetric weakness, and some muscle atrophy, principally of proximal limb muscles.

Women are affected more often than men. Natural history data for onset after age 40 are not available. This immune disease results from a humorally dependent, antibody-mediated process directed against capillaries and other small blood vessels in muscle. About 10% of patients have a malignancy; breast and lung tumors are the most common, with a disproportionate increase in tumors of the ovary, uterus, and bowel. No consistent relationship exists between tumor discovery and onset of dermatomyositis.

Symptoms, Signs, and Diagnosis

A rash (usually the presenting feature) and muscle weakness are the major clinical signs; the rash can occur without the muscle weakness. The rash is reddish purple (heliotrope) and involves the periorbital regions; a more erythematous rash occurs on the malar regions, neck, shoulders, or extensor surfaces of the arms and legs. Gottron's papules are reddish, raised, scaly lesions over the extensor surfaces of the proximal interphalangeal and distal interphalangeal joints. Thickened, cracked cuticles with dilated capillary loops in the nail beds are also characteristic.

Weakness develops over weeks or months. Proximal limb muscles are typically weaker than distal muscles. Neck flexors are particularly weak. Muscles supplied by cranial nerves are typically spared, except for those involved with swallowing. Dysphagia, myalgia, and muscle tenderness occur in about 50% of patients. Involvement of other organs is not uncommon and includes the joints (arthralgias and arthritis), gastrointestinal tract (delayed gastric emptying and microvasculopathy causing intestinal ulceration or perforation), lungs (interstitial lung disease), and heart (conduction abnormalities and cardiomyopathy).

Blood muscle enzyme levels (especially CK levels) are elevated. The ESR is elevated in about 50% of patients, and the antinuclear antibody titer is elevated in about 25 to 50%.

Diagnosis is suggested by the clinical findings and elevation of muscle enzyme levels. Muscle biopsy shows characteristic perifascicular atrophy of muscle fibers, a decreased number of capillaries, and perivascular infiltrates. Electromyographic findings indicate muscle inflammation.

Prognosis and Treatment

Death may follow severe and progressive muscle weakness accompanied by dysphagia, malnutrition, aspiration pneumonia, or respiratory failure with superimposed pulmonary infection. Prognosis in patients with malignancy-associated myositis is generally determined by the prognosis of the tumor. Prognosis is usually poorer if the rash is necrotizing and muscle weakness is present.

During the acute stages, most patients benefit from immunosuppressive therapy and bed rest. Usually, prednisone is started at 1 to 2 mg/kg/day (60 to 100 mg/day) po. To permit use of the lowest possible dosage of prednisone for the shortest time, another immunosuppressant (eg, azathioprine 2 to 3 mg/kg/day in divided doses) po may be used concomitantly; in many patients, azathioprine is effective as monotherapy after 12 to 18 months of treatment. IV immune globulin therapy is effective and offers an excellent second-choice therapy, even before other immunosuppressants (eg, azathioprine, methotrexate), in patients who cannot achieve full recovery with corticosteroid treatment. Immune globulin can produce headaches, fever, flu-like illness, and, occasionally, meningitis or renal failure. However, these adverse effects are less likely to occur if the drug is given in small infusions (0.4 to 0.5 g/kg/day) to reach a total dose of 2 g/kg. Long-term management includes physical therapy, frequent monitoring of muscle strength, and regular physical activity.

Elderly patients require frequent evaluation for occult tumors, especially in the breast and lung. No predictable relationship exists between tumor removal and resolution of myopathy, but some patients have remarkable recoveries.

POLYMYOSITIS

A systemic autoimmune cellularly mediated inflammatory myopathy characterized by cytotoxic T-cell–mediated attack against muscle fibers, leading to symmetric weakness and some muscle atrophy.

Prevalence is 6 to 8 per 100,000 persons; incidence peaks between 45 and 65 years. Polymyositis is most common in blacks and women.

Although considered an autoimmune connective tissue disease, polymyositis may result from disorders that cause slowly progressive myopathy with muscle fiber damage from cytotoxic lymphocytes (eg, unidentified foreign proteins, viruses, or other illnesses). Polymyositis is cellularly mediated, unlike dermatomyositis, which is humorally mediated. Muscle pathology differs from that of inclusion body myositis and dermatomyositis.

Symptoms, Signs, and Diagnosis

Muscle weakness is generalized but is more prominent in the hips and thighs; it begins as aching pain in about 10% of patients and as tenderness on palpation in 20%. Painless progressive weakness affecting the legs and arms is the presenting complaint in the remaining 70% of patients. Muscle atrophy and loss of tendon reflexes are rare in the early stages. Dysphagia is common. Cardiac involvement (eg, atrioventricular conduction defects, bundle branch block) is relatively common; about 33% of patients have ECG abnormalities. Interstitial lung disease occurs in about 10% of patients.

Polymyositis that occurs with another connective tissue disorder is called an overlap syndrome; as many as 10 to 20% of cases of polymyositis and dermatomyositis can present as overlap syndromes. One example is mixed connective tissue disease, which has elements of scleroderma, lupus, and polymyositis (or dermatomyositis) and is associated with antibodies to ribonucleoprotein.

The diagnosis is based on typical symptoms and signs, a myopathic pattern on electromyography, typical biopsy findings, and elevated CK levels. Anti-Jo-1 antibodies, which are antibodies to histidyl-t-RNA synthetase, are present in about 20% of patients with polymyositis and are positive in about 50% of patients with interstitial lung disease. Arthralgia, fever, an elevated ESR, and a polyclonal hypergammaglobulinemia on electrophoresis may occur.

Prognosis and Treatment

The overall mortality is about four times that of the general population; death is usually due to pulmonary or cardiac complications. Blacks and women have a less favorable prognosis.

Treatment is the same as for dermatomyositis. About 50% of patients recover, and therapy can be discontinued within 5 years of the onset of symptoms. About 20% of patients have persistent active disease requiring continued therapy. The remaining 30% develop inactive disease with permanent residual muscle weakness.

CORTICOSTEROID MYOPATHY

A muscular disorder that results from administered corticosteroids or intrinsic cortisol excess.

Corticosteroid myopathy results from prolonged corticosteroid therapy—often given for conditions that themselves cause muscle weakness (eg, myasthenia gravis, inflammatory myopathy)—or from conditions associated with elevated corticotropin levels (eg, Cushing's disease).

The incidence of muscle weakness ranges from 2 to 20% in persons receiving long-term corticosteroid therapy and from 50 to 80% in those with Cushing's disease.

Critical care quadriparesis is a newly described form of corticosteroid myopathy for which the elderly are at increased risk. It develops acutely, often in a patient with a severe medical disorder that requires large IV doses of corticosteroids, frequently with concomitant use of depolarizing muscle relaxants. Selective dissolution of thick filaments in muscle is characteristic. Recovery often requires many months and is commonly incomplete.

Symptoms, Signs, and Diagnosis

In patients taking long-term systemic corticosteroids and in those with intrinsic cortisol excess (eg, Cushing's disease), muscle weakness usually begins in the hip girdle, especially the quadriceps, and eventually spreads to nearly all muscles. The proximal muscles tend to be most affected; except for the neck flexors, muscles supplied by cranial nerves are spared. Patients often report that they become fatigued more rapidly during activities demanding sudden bursts of power. If the myopathy is long-standing, muscle wasting often becomes apparent, although exercise decreases it. Occasionally, patients experience mild aching in the thigh muscles, but severe pain does not occur. Tendon reflexes remain unchanged, and no fasciculations develop.

A majority of patients have other signs of corticosteroid toxicity (eg, weight gain, cushingoid appearance, hypertension). Typically, serum CK and other muscle enzyme levels, electromyography findings, and nerve conduction studies are normal. Muscle biopsy results often show striking atrophy of type 2 fibers.

Intrinsic cortisol excess can be detected by measurements of plasma cortisol at different times of day. Determination of the underlying cause of the cortisol excess is beyond the scope of this discussion.

Prevention and Treatment

For prevention of iatrogenic disease, switching to alternate-day corticosteroid administration as soon as feasible is often recommended. Maintaining exercise to whatever degree possible is also important.

Treatment of iatrogenic disease is empiric. However, gradually reducing the corticosteroid dosage and closely monitoring the patient are essential. If the weakness is due primarily to an inflammatory myopathy and corticosteroids have slowed but not stopped the progression of weakness, reducing the corticosteroid dose increases creatine excretion and worsens muscle weakness. However, if the weakness is due primarily to corticosteroid therapy, decreasing the corticosteroid dose allows muscle strength to gradually return. Complete recovery usually occurs in 2 to 3 months.

In those in whom the myopathy is due to intrinsic cortisol excess, treatment depends on the underlying cause.

MUSCULAR DISORDERS IN HYPERTHYROIDISM

In elderly patients, hyperthyroidism▯ can cause a subacute proximal myopathy, without the prominent tachycardia or other obvious systemic signs that occur in younger patients. It can also cause myokymia (con-

---

▯ see also page 647

tinuous quivering or undulating movement of muscle surface and overlying skin), acute bulbar myopathy, ocular myopathy, and, rarely, hypokalemic periodic paralysis.

Often, the initial symptoms are weakness of proximal limb muscles and increased muscle fatigue. Usually, the shoulder girdle and upper arm muscles are weaker than the leg muscles. In the legs, the iliopsoas muscle may be primarily affected. Muscle atrophy develops early and occasionally is pronounced. More than 15% of patients have prominent muscle twitches, often with increased tendon reflexes, which may mimic those of amyotrophic lateral sclerosis.

The diagnosis is suspected clinically and confirmed by thyroid function tests.[1] Serum muscle enzyme levels are normal. Electromyography often demonstrates fasciculations and myopathic features in weak muscles. Muscle biopsy results are usually normal.

Prognosis and Treatment

The long-term prognosis is good if the hyperthyroidism is treated and the euthyroid state restored. During the first few weeks of treatment, propranolol 120 to 320 mg/day often reduces proximal muscle weakness. After the euthyroid state has been maintained for several months, muscle bulk and strength typically return to normal.

MUSCULAR DISORDERS IN HYPOTHYROIDISM

Hypothyroidism impairs metabolism in the muscle fiber and decreases contractile force.[2] Repair and replacement of myofibrillar proteins are defective because protein turnover is reduced. Slow muscle contraction and relaxation result from the diminished activity of myosin ATPase and from the impaired uptake of calcium by the sarcoplasmic reticulum. Reduced cardiac output results from β-adrenergic hyposensitivity. The pathophysiology responsible for muscle cramps and muscle fiber enlargement is unknown. Deposition of mucopolysaccharides in muscle occurs inconsistently.

Symptoms and Signs

The primary clinical features are proximal weakness (including pronounced proximal leg muscle weakness and atrophy in some patients), fatigue, slowed movements, stiffness, myalgias, cramps, and, occasionally, enlarged muscles (especially the anterior compartment muscles of the leg). These features generally develop over weeks to months. Tendon reflexes are slowed, with relaxation of the Achilles tendon reflex being markedly prolonged. In about one third of hypothyroid patients,

---

[1] see page 650   [2] see also page 643

myoedema (mounding) lasting $\geq$ 5 seconds can be elicited by direct percussion of muscle. A similar response can occur in malnourished patients.

The severity of symptoms appears to relate more to the total duration of thyroid deficiency and to the percent elevation of the thyroid-stimulating hormone (TSH) level than to the absolute level of free thyroxine or TSH.

Muscle-related symptoms in hypothyroidism may be exacerbated by the use of cholesterol-lowering drugs, which require close monitoring in patients with thyroid deficiency.

Complications include carpal and tarsal tunnel syndromes and a distal, symmetric sensorimotor polyneuropathy. Rarely, marked fatigability of hip girdle and trunk muscles results from impaired neuromuscular transmission.

Diagnosis

The circulating thyroid hormone level is decreased, and (in primary hypothyroidism) the TSH level is elevated. Usually, muscle enzyme levels, especially CK levels, are increased several times the normal values.

Electrodiagnostic testing and muscle biopsy may be needed to rule out other disorders that resemble hypothyroid neuropathy and myopathy. Electromyographic findings may show no abnormality or both neurogenic and myopathic features. Occasionally, muscle membrane hyperirritability is evident. Findings on repetitive nerve stimulation mimic those of Eaton-Lambert syndrome. Electrodiagnostic studies may show compression neuropathies. Muscle biopsy results are usually normal; occasionally the proportion and size of type 2 muscle fibers are reduced.

Prognosis and Treatment

The long-term prognosis is good; however, patients with severe muscle wasting may never fully recover muscle strength and bulk.

Thyroid hormone must be replaced.◱ Once the euthyroid state is achieved, serum CK levels return to normal. Control of muscle pain and fatigue significantly improves in some patients, even those in whom TSH levels are minimally elevated. Surgery rarely is needed to reverse symptoms related to median or tibial nerve compression.

MUSCULAR DISORDERS IN OSTEOMALACIA

Osteomalacia◳ results from vitamin D deficiency. The pathophysiology of the myopathy is unknown.

◱see page 646 ◳see page 483

Symptoms and Signs

About one third of osteomalacia patients have muscle weakness; of these patients, almost all initially report weakness in the pelvic and thigh muscles. Typically, the patient has pain in the back, hip girdle, and legs. Muscle wasting is proportionate to weakness. About half of patients have a waddling gait and use Gowers' maneuver to rise from the supine position (rolling to prone position, kneeling, then rising to standing by pushing with hands against shins, knees, and thighs). About 20% of patients have a marked limp or cannot walk. Tendon reflexes are normal to brisk, and sensation is normal. No cranial nerve abnormalities occur. Bone pain and tenderness are most prominent in the pelvis, femurs, spine, and ribs. Frequently, the vertebrae collapse, sometimes causing skeletal deformities. Occasionally, patients describe total body pain, suggesting a primary psychiatric disorder.

Diagnosis

The serum CK level is normal or slightly elevated. Electromyography may show a myopathic pattern; the results of nerve conduction studies are normal. Muscle biopsy findings are normal or indicate nonspecific changes.

Prognosis and Treatment

For most patients, the long-term prognosis is good. However, if muscle wasting, especially of the quadriceps muscle of the thigh, is marked, patients may never regain full strength despite restoration of normal serum levels of vitamin D and phosphate.

HYPOKALEMIC MYOPATHY

In the elderly, hypokalemia∎ is the most common cause of myopathy due to electrolyte imbalance. A common cause of hypokalemia in this age group is long-term diuretic use. Other conditions that cause hypokalemia include dietary deficiency, alcoholic myopathy, intestinal potassium wastage, Bartter's syndrome, aldosteronism, and licorice intoxication. Acute hypokalemic paralysis may occur after amphotericin B treatment and with diabetic ketoacidosis, renal tubular acidosis, chronic diarrhea, and most conditions that produce chronic hypokalemia.

Hypocalcemia and hypomagnesemia can also produce prominent neuromuscular symptoms, including tetany, irritability, myoclonus, and tremor, but they do not typically produce muscle weakness.

∎ see page 568

Symptoms and Signs

Muscle weakness usually develops slowly over days to weeks. It primarily affects the legs but, in severe cases, affects the arms, trunk, neck, and, occasionally, thoracic and diaphragmatic muscles. Ocular and bulbar muscles are spared. In general, chronic hypokalemic myopathy produces greater weakness in the proximal muscles than in the distal muscles. Patients with diabetic acidosis (in which serum potassium levels fall rapidly over hours) may present with respiratory weakness, and the arms may become weak before the legs. Tendon reflexes become hypoactive and then vanish. The patient has no pain or other sensory complaints. In severe cases, muscle fiber necrosis with myoglobinuria, muscle pain, tenderness, and swelling can develop.

Diagnosis and Treatment

The serum potassium level is usually < 3 mEq/L. The serum CK level may be normal or elevated. Nerve conduction velocities are normal.

Chronic myopathy usually reverses after 1 to 4 weeks of potassium replacement therapy. If myoglobinuria and rhabdomyolysis have occurred, treatment should include vigorous hydration and alkalinization of the urine to avoid renal tubular necrosis and renal failure. Depending on the cause of hypokalemia, long-term potassium replacement may be needed. Occasionally, when hypokalemia is severe, symptomatic, or unresponsive to oral therapy, potassium must be replaced parenterally.

MYOTONIC DYSTROPHY

An autosomal dominant multisystem disorder caused by an abnormality on chromosome 19 that results in slowly progressive muscle atrophy.

Usually, myotonic dystrophy characterized by distal weakness develops in persons in their 20s and 30s; however, the elderly may present with mild forms. In the elderly, the primary symptoms may be frontal baldness and posterior capsular cataracts. Other symptoms include minimal muscle weakness with cardiac conduction defects (eg, atrioventricular block, bundle branch block), gastrointestinal hypomotility, and respiratory insufficiency caused by weakness of the respiratory muscles, primarily the diaphragm. Tendon reflexes are depressed, especially in the legs.

Diagnosis is established by DNA testing. Muscle biopsy findings and mildly to moderately elevated serum CK levels have secondary diagnostic value. The long-term prognosis depends on the severity of muscle weakness and the presence of complications.

Treatment is nonspecific. The goal is to manage complications: respiratory insufficiency; cardiac arrhythmias, particularly conduction block; and gastrointestinal hypomotility. Surgery can be problematic, because patients develop paradoxic rigidity in reaction to succinylcholine and other muscle relaxants; nondepolarizing relaxants (eg, vecuronium, atracurium) are recommended.

OCULOPHARYNGEAL MUSCULAR DYSTROPHY

An autosomal dominant muscular disorder in which the gene defect consists of short GCG expansions in the PABP2 *(poly-A binding protein 2) gene on chromosome 14.*

Onset usually occurs in patients in their 50s and 60s. Patients develop ptosis that is almost always bilateral. Typically, contraction of the occipitofrontal muscle is prominent, and the patient tips the head back to compensate visually for the ptosis. Dysphagia for solid foods usually follows extraocular weakness. Palatal mobility is often diminished, and the gag reflex is impaired. Laryngeal weakness with dysphonia is common.

Oculopharyngeal muscular dystrophy resembles myasthenia gravis.■ However, unlike with myasthenia gravis, tendon reflexes may be diminished or even absent with this disorder. Some patients report cramps in calf muscles despite the absence of significant weakness. Years after onset, the muscles of the limbs, especially of the proximal hip girdle, may become weak.

The diagnosis depends on clinical features and a positive family history. DNA analysis is being developed.

Limb weakness occasionally occurs, but long-term disability results from dysphagia and aspiration pneumonitis. With improvements in care (eg, improved swallowing, supplemental nutrition), patients usually have a normal life span and relatively normal abilities to perform activities of daily living.

No specific treatment is available. However, the use of cricopharyngeal myotomy for dysphagia is helpful.

IDIOPATHIC MUSCLE CRAMPS

These cramps, without significant muscle weakness, frequently occur in healthy middle-aged and elderly patients. They may develop at rest or with minor exercise. Typically, they occur at night during sleep

■ see page 520

and affect the calf or foot muscles, causing forceful plantar flexion of the foot or toes. Diagnosis is based on the history and lack of physical signs or disability.

Prevention and Treatment

Avoiding caffeine and other sympathetic stimulants may be helpful. Stretching the affected muscles for several minutes before sleep is often an effective preventive measure. Stretching immediately after the cramps occur usually relieves them (see FIGURE 54–1). Such exercises improve muscle and tendon flexibility and can reduce the motor unit activity in the stretched muscles.

Stretching is almost always preferable to empiric drug treatment. For example, quinine sulfate 200 to 300 mg at bedtime is not effective for night cramps and can cause a bitter taste, tinnitus, flushing, pruritus, and gastrointestinal disturbances, and it interacts with many other drugs. Calcium supplements (eg, calcium gluconate 1 to 2 g bid) are well tolerated, but their effectiveness is doubtful. Drugs used concomi-

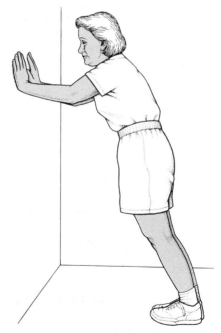

FIGURE 54–1.   To stretch the gastrocnemius and soleus muscles, the patient stands 2 to 3 feet (about 1 meter) from a wall while facing it; leans against the wall with outstretched arms, keeping the heels on the floor, the knees locked, and the body straight; and then stretches the calves for two or three 1-minute intervals with 1-minute rest periods between stretches.

tantly with quinine and calcium include diphenhydramine 50 to 100 mg at bedtime, magnesium carbonate 250 to 500 mg bid, and low-dose benzodiazepines. However, the toxic effects of these drugs are likely to outweigh any benefit. Mexiletine 150 mg tid is sometimes effective when increased irritability of the lower motor neuron is suspected.

55 ▮ HAND DISORDERS

The elderly may report certain nonspecific changes in the hands. For example, many elderly persons describe mild acroparesthesias (ie, "pins and needles" sensation, tingling, and numbness in the hands). Other symptoms and signs indicating a peripheral neuropathy or a nerve entrapment syndrome are absent. The course is frequently intermittent. The majority of patients require reassurance, but they can cope without treatment. Troublesome symptoms may require palliation with pyridoxine (vitamin B$_6$) 50 mg po bid, warm soaks, or topical analgesic creams. Wearing spandex gloves during the night or heated mittens may be helpful.

Some elderly persons are genetically predisposed to develop Heberden's nodes at the distal interphalangeal (DIP) joints and Bouchard's nodules at the proximal interphalangeal (PIP) joints. These large knobby nodules rarely cause pain, although the hands and fingers may feel clumsy and be difficult to close. Warm soaks and flexion-extension exercise of the fingers in warm water followed by a 2- to 3-minute massage with a topical analgesic balm (eg, methyl salicylate) are sometimes useful. Built-up handles on tools or sports equipment help improve grip.

Some patients report unaccountable dropping of objects despite adequate pinch (at the thumb and index finger), grip, and muscle strength. This problem may represent altered proprioceptive sensation, but the cause is unknown. Caution is required when handling valuable objects. Treatment involves reassurance.

Elderly persons may have cold hands for no discernible reason. The palms in particular may feel cool, but color changes and other symptoms are absent. Examination, including vascular evaluation,▮ discloses no abnormalities. Some of these persons also describe a diminished sense of touch, but true numbness or paresthesias are absent. Strong reassurance and smoking cessation may be useful.

Muscle cramps in the hands, similar to writer's cramp, may awaken patients several times during the night. Warm soaks before bedtime

▮ see page 922

ameliorate the cramps; wearing spandex gloves while sleeping may be useful. Occasionally, calcium supplements help prevent the cramps. More elderly persons are reporting overuse syndromes (ie, microtrauma of the hands). This increase is likely due to the widespread use of computers and other technical devices requiring repetitive motion of the hand. Why overuse syndromes affect only some persons is unknown. Treatment includes simple measures such as rest, splinting, and moist heat. Nonsteroidal anti-inflammatory drugs (NSAIDs) and analgesics help control pain, but NSAIDs should be used cautiously in the elderly. The newly available cyclooxygenase-2 (COX-2) inhibitors (eg, celecoxib, rofecoxib) provide increased safety and tolerability. Stretching and isometric strengthening exercises help restore mobility. Recurrence is prevented by avoiding the activity that provokes discomfort and by modifying the work or home environment.

Hand function should be assessed during the physical examination. The presence or absence of hand deformities is not a good indicator of hand function. Rather, the physician should evaluate pinch, grip, and the ability to perform basic skills (eg, opening jars, manipulating zippers or buttons). Consultation with an occupational therapist may be useful.

HAND DEFORMITIES

MALLET FINGER

A flexion deformity of the DIP joint in which the fingertip droops and extension is not possible.

This deformity (see FIGURE 55–1) may result from a tendon injury or an avulsion fracture. Closed injuries may be treated with splinting that holds the DIP joint in extension and leaves the PIP joints free. Pure tendon injuries require about 8 to 10 weeks for the collagen to heal sufficiently, whereas avulsion fractures are usually united after 6 weeks.

SWAN-NECK DEFORMITY

Metacarpal flexion, hyperextension of the PIP joint, and flexion of the DIP joint.

This deformity (see FIGURE 55–2) is a characteristic finding in rheumatoid arthritis. Other causes include untreated mallet finger, volar plate laxity, spasticity, entrapment or rupture of the superficial tendons in the first and second annular pulleys, ligamentous laxity, and malunion of a fracture of the middle phalanx. Inability to overcome hyperextension of the PIP joint makes finger closure impossible and can cause severe disability.

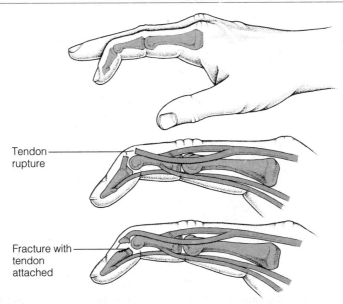

Tendon rupture

Fracture with tendon attached

FIGURE 55–1. **Mallet finger.** A flexion lag at the distal interphalangeal joint results from a tendon injury or avulsion fracture.

True swan-neck deformity does not affect the thumb, which is "missing" a phalangeal joint. However, severe hyperextension of the interphalangeal joint of the thumb with flexion of the metacarpophalangeal (MCP) joint (called a duck bill, Z [zigzag] type, or 90° angle deformity) may occur. If associated with thumb instability, swan-neck deformity can interfere greatly with prehension (pinch). This deformity can usually be corrected surgically. The underlying cause is treated when possible (eg, by correcting the mallet finger or any bony misalignment, by rebalancing the extensor mechanism, or by releasing spastic intrinsic muscles).

BOUTONNIÈRE DEFORMITY

(Buttonhole Deformity)

Fixed flexion of the PIP joint and hyperextension of the DIP joint.

Causes include dislocation, fracture, osteoarthritis, and rheumatoid arthritis. Classically, disruption of the central slip of the middle phalanx extensor tendon creates so-called buttonholing of the proximal phalanx between the lateral bands of the extensor tendon (see FIGURE 55–2). Surgical reconstruction is difficult and may be unsatisfactory.

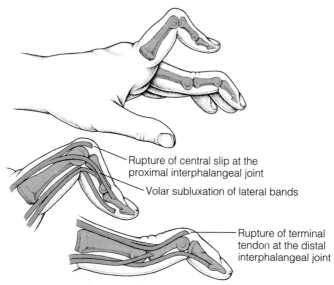

Rupture of central slip at the
proximal interphalangeal joint

Volar subluxation of lateral bands

Rupture of terminal
tendon at the distal
interphalangeal joint

FIGURE 55-2. **Boutonnière deformity of the index finger and swan-neck deformity of the other fingers.** The proximal interphalangeal joint of the index finger is flexed, and the distal interphalangeal joint is hyperextended. The metacarpal and distal interphalangeal joints of the other fingers are flexed, and the proximal interphalangeal joints are hyperextended.

EROSIVE (INFLAMMATORY) OSTEOARTHRITIS

A clinical form of osteoarthritis in the hand in which the DIP joint, some PIP joints, and the first carpometacarpal joints are genetically predisposed to extensive synovitis and cyst formation.

Pain causing disuse or disability of the hands is a major problem among the elderly. Osteoarthritis (OA) of the hands is responsible for much suffering and disability. Bony overgrowth of the DIP joints (Heberden's nodes) and bony overgrowth of the PIP joints (Bouchard's nodules) are present, often without significant soft tissue swelling. Erosive OA does not usually affect the MCP joints or wrists. On x-ray, erosions appear subchondral rather than marginal (as is usually seen in rheumatoid arthritis). The thumb base (carpometacarpal joint) is frequently involved and has a squared-off appearance. The ESR and CBC are usually normal, regardless of disease severity.

Treatment includes range-of-motion exercises in warm water, intermittent splinting to prevent deformity, use of analgesics or NSAIDs, and occasional intra-articular injections of corticosteroid suspension to relieve pain and prevent limited motion in acutely symptomatic joints.

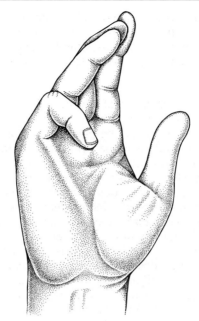

FIGURE 55-3.   **Dupuytren's contracture.** The hand is arched and the fingers flexed due to fibrous contracture of the deep fascia.

DUPUYTREN'S CONTRACTURE

(Palmar Fibromatosis)

Progressive contracture of the palmar fascial bands, producing flexion deformities of the fingers.

Dupuytren's contracture (see FIGURE 55-3) is common; the incidence is higher in men and increases after age 45. This autosomal dominant disorder with variable penetrance occurs more commonly in patients with diabetes, alcoholism, or epilepsy. However, the factor that causes the palmar fascia to thicken and contract is unknown. Some cases are familial.

Symptoms and Signs

The earliest manifestation is usually a tender nodule in the palm (most often at the base of the 3rd or 4th fingers) followed by formation of a superficial pretendinous cord, which leads to contracture of the MCP joints and interphalangeal joints of the fingers. The nodule may initially cause discomfort but becomes painless as it matures. Eventually, the contracture may worsen, and the hand can become arched. The disorder occasionally is associated with fibrous thickening of the dorsum of the PIP joints (Garrod's pads), and Peyronie's disease◼ develops in about 7% of male patients. Rarely, Dupuytren's contracture develops on the plantar surface of the feet (plantar fibromatosis).

Treatment

During the incipient phase, local injection of a corticosteroid suspension into the nodule may delay fibrous thickening. Surgery is usually indicated when the hand cannot be placed flat on a table or when significant contracture develops at the PIP joints, limiting hand function. The PIP joints are particularly recalcitrant to correction, and early surgery is advised when PIP joint contracture occurs. Excision of the diseased fascia must be meticulous because the fascia surrounds neurovascular bundles and tendons. Incomplete excision of new disease results in recurrent contracture, especially among patients with onset at age < 50 or a family history of the disorder, Garrod's pads, Peyronie's disease, or plantar fibromatosis. Otherwise, management consists of watchful waiting. High-dose vitamin E has been recommended to lessen progression of the fibrosis, although data to support this recommendation are lacking. Plantar fibromatosis is treated with corrective footwear; surgery is usually unnecessary.

NEUROVASCULAR SYNDROMES

CARPAL TUNNEL SYNDROME

Constriction of the median nerve as it passes through the carpal tunnel in the wrist.

Carpal tunnel syndrome is common, especially among women aged 30 to 50. Causes include rheumatoid arthritis (sometimes carpal tunnel syndrome is the presenting manifestation), diabetes mellitus, hypothyroidism, acromegaly, amyloidosis, and pregnancy (producing edema in the carpal canal). Carpal tunnel syndrome is more common among elderly persons whose activities or jobs require repetitive flexion and extension of the wrist. The use of crutches or a walker may provoke symptoms. Often, no underlying precipitating cause is identified, although in a large study of workers, an increased association between carpal tunnel syndrome and obesity and tobacco use was statistically significant.

Symptoms, Signs, and Diagnosis

Symptoms include pain of the hand and wrist associated with tingling (paresthesia) and numbness, classically distributed along the

---

◼see page 1161

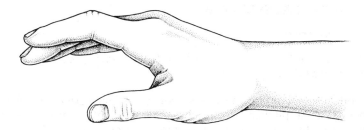

FIGURE 55–4. **Correct positioning of the wrist for splinting.** In patients with carpal tunnel syndrome, a splint should be used to support the wrist at a 15° angle, which keeps the carpal tunnel open to the fullest extent possible. This positioning allows continued use of the wrist with little discomfort.

median nerve (the palmar side of the thumb, the index and middle fingers, and the radial half of the ring finger). Typically, the patient wakes at night with burning or aching pain and with numbness and tingling and shakes the hand to obtain relief and restore sensation. Paresthesia of the 4th and 5th fingers suggests compression of the ulnar nerve.∎ Elderly patients with carpal tunnel syndrome often present with double-level nerve compression (ie, cervical radiculitis and carpal tunnel).

Diagnosis is indicated by a positive Tinel's sign (ie, tingling is elicited by tapping with a reflex hammer at the palmar surface of the wrist over the site of the median nerve in the carpal tunnel). Additional tests include wrist flexion maneuvers, such as Phalen's sign (ie, tingling in the median nerve region is elicited by holding the patient's wrist in acute passive flexion for about 1 minute). Thenar atrophy and weakness of thumb elevation may develop late. Diagnosis is confirmed by electrodiagnostic testing of median nerve conduction velocity, which provides an accurate index of motor and sensory nerve conduction.

Treatment

Treatment includes use of a lightweight wrist splint (see FIGURE 55–4), especially during the night; pyridoxine (vitamin B$_6$) 50 mg bid; and mild analgesics (eg, acetaminophen, NSAIDs). Repositioning the computer keyboard or making other ergonomic corrections may provide relief. If these measures do not control symptoms, a corticosteroid should be locally injected into the carpal tunnel at a site just ulnar to the palmaris longus tendon and proximal to the distal crease at the wrist. If symptoms persist or recur or if hand weakness and thenar wasting progress, surgical decompression of the carpal tunnel using an open technique or arthroscopic approach is recommended.

∎ see page 542

CUBITAL TUNNEL SYNDROME

(Ulnar Neuropathy)

Compression of the ulnar nerve at the elbow, resulting in numbness and paresthesia of the ring and little fingers.

Cubital tunnel syndrome is less common than carpal tunnel syndrome. Baseball pitchers are prone to cubital tunnel syndrome because of the extra twist of the arm required to throw a slider. Symptoms include elbow pain and numbness and paresthesia on the ulnar side of the hand. In advanced stages, weakness of the ring and little fingers may develop. Weakness interferes with pinch of the thumb and index finger. If two or more nerves are simultaneously involved, associated compression invariably occurs at the brachial plexus.

Cubital tunnel syndrome is differentiated from ulnar nerve entrapment at the wrist (ie, in Guyon's canal) by sensory testing, location of Tinel's sign, and electromyography and nerve conduction velocity testing. Treatment involves splinting at night, with the elbow partially extended, and possibly empirical use of pyridoxine (vitamin B_6) 50 mg po bid. Surgical decompression is performed if conservative treatment fails.

REFLEX SYMPATHETIC DYSTROPHY

(Shoulder-Hand Syndrome)

Pain and limited motion of the shoulder and ipsilateral involvement of the hand.

Causes include trauma (eg, falling on the hand, Colles' fracture∎), cardiovascular insult (eg, myocardial infarction), stroke, and possibly certain drugs (eg, barbiturates). An underlying predisposition has been postulated, but the pathogenesis is not completely understood.

Reflex sympathetic dystrophy occurs in three stages: Stage 1 is characterized by the acute onset of diffuse edema and tenderness of the dorsum of the hand and palmar vasomotor phenomena, with shoulder and hand pain, especially during movement. Early x-rays of the involved hands commonly show spotty osteoporosis. Stage 2 is characterized by the abatement of edema and local tenderness; hand pain continues, but less severely. Stage 3 is characterized by resolution of hand swelling, tenderness, and pain, but hand motion is limited because of stiff fingers and fibrotic palmar flexion contractures, which resemble Dupuytren's contracture. X-rays at this stage often show diffuse osteoporosis.

∎ see page 220

Treatment

Precipitating or contributing causes should be treated or eliminated. Contractures can usually be prevented by early rehabilitation and appropriate treatment with sympathetic blockade or a course of corticosteroids. A series of stellate sympathetic ganglion nerve blocks performed every other day or twice weekly followed by physical therapy (exercises) usually relieves pain, permitting return to work or needed activity, but repeated nerve blocks over weeks or months may be required. Alternatively, high-dose corticosteroids can be tried. For example, prednisone 40 to 50 mg/day po can be given initially, then tapered according to response and tolerance. Especially in the elderly, the dose should be reduced to 20 mg within 2 to 3 weeks and to 10 to 15 mg within 4 to 6 weeks.

TENDON DISORDERS

DIGITAL TENDINITIS AND TENOSYNOVITIS

Inflammation of tendons and tendon sheaths of the hand.

Symptoms develop when a tendon cannot glide within its sheath because of a thickening or nodule that catches at the site of the tightened first annular pulley, preventing smooth extension or flexion of the finger. The finger may lock, or "trigger," suddenly extending with a snap. Flexor digital tenosynovitis (trigger finger—see Figure 55–5) occurs commonly in patients with rheumatoid arthritis or diabetes mellitus. In patients with diabetes, trigger finger often coexists with carpal tunnel syndrome and occasionally with fibrotic change of the palmar fascia.

Treatment includes local rest or splinting, moist heat, and NSAIDs. If these measures fail, local injection of a corticosteroid suspension to the flexor tendon sheath is relatively simple and safe and may rapidly relieve pain and triggering. Operative release can be performed if intrasynovial corticosteroid therapy fails.

DE QUERVAIN'S SYNDROME

(Washerwoman's Sprain)

Stenosing tenosynovitis of the short extensor (extensor pollicis brevis) and long abductor tendon (abductor pollicis longus) of the thumb.

This disorder usually occurs after repetitive use (especially wringing) of the wrist, although it occasionally occurs in rheumatoid arthritis. The major symptom is aching pain at the wrist and thumb, aggravated by motion. Tenderness is elicited just distal to the radial styloid process over the site of the involved tendon sheaths.

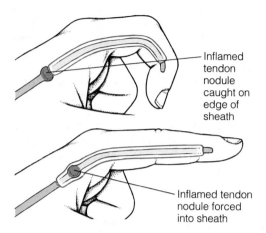

Inflamed
tendon
nodule
caught on
edge of
sheath

Inflamed tendon
nodule forced
into sheath

FIGURE 55–5.   Flexor digital tenosynovitis (trigger finger). Trigger finger occurs when one of the tendons that flex the finger becomes inflamed. The inflamed tendon moves out of the sheath as the finger bends but cannot easily move back in as the finger straightens. To straighten the finger, the patient must force the inflamed area into the sheath, which produces a popping sensation similar to that felt when pulling a trigger.

The Finkelstein test suggests the diagnosis: The patient adducts the thumb on the involved side into the palm and wraps the fingers over the thumb. Passive movement at the wrist is then performed in all ranges of motion; if a forcible ulnar tug of the wrist causes severe pain at the site of the affected tendon sheaths, test results are positive.

Rest, warm soaks, and NSAIDs are effective only in very mild cases. Local intrasynovial injections of corticosteroids are helpful in 80 to 90% of cases. Tendon rupture, a rare complication, can be prevented by careful infiltration of the corticosteroid into the tendon sheath, avoiding the tendon itself.

56 ▬ FOOT DISORDERS

With age, numerous changes occur in the feet (see TABLE 56–1). Foot disorders often begin early in life and are affected by many factors, such as heredity, gait patterns, level of activity, terrain, and improper foot care.

Shoe styles and fit also affect foot disorders. For example, shoes that are tight or ill-fitting may injure the foot, leg, or hip; may cause falls; or may worsen lesions that are difficult to heal because of peripheral vas-

TABLE 56–1.   AGE-RELATED CHANGES IN THE FEET

Type of Change	Comments
Changes in the skin Hair loss Brown pigmentation Dry skin	Usually the initial age-related changes
Hyperkeratotic lesions	Especially common with fixed deformities and bony changes resulting from arthritides
Changes in the toenails Hypertrophy of the nail plate (onychauxis) Curved or hooked nail (onychogryphosis) Fungal infection of the nail (onychomycosis)	Especially common in persons with impaired vascular supply and an increased susceptibility to fungal organisms, such as persons with diabetes or those taking corticosteroids
Contractures	Can cause a change in the gait pattern; may lead to the development of lesions or ulcerations
Claudication, burning, fatigue, paresthesias, cramping	May be due to peripheral vascular or neurologic disease
Edema	May be a sign of cardiac or renal pathology but is also common in elderly persons without disease

cular disease or diabetes mellitus. Shoes should provide adequate support and a roomy toe box to compensate for age-related orthopedic deformities. Proper size and fit should be ascertained at a reliable shoe store.

Elderly persons should avoid shoes that are worn or misshapen, offer no support, or have a narrow or pointed toe box. Oxford-type shoes that have shoelaces are recommended; loafers or slip-ons may be constrictive and do not allow compensation for swelling that may occur as the day progresses. Patients who have lost dexterity in their hands and cannot tie shoelaces may benefit from shoes with Velcro closures or shoes with elastic laces, which can remain tied. Shoe horns are available in extended lengths to allow patients to put on their shoes without bending. Shoes can be custom-made and fitted with special inserts made of polyethylene foam to compensate for painful or pre-ulcerous lesions.

Neglect of the feet throughout a person's active years may eventually result in a foot disorder. Symptoms and signs of various systemic disorders (eg, diabetes, heart disease, arthritis, hypertension, peripheral vascular disease) may initially manifest in the feet. Foot disorders may be particularly problematic for the elderly, who greatly benefit—socially and psychologically—from being able to remain ambulatory. Examination of the feet and treatment of any foot disorders should be part of every health program.

Diagnosis

When evaluating foot pain, the primary symptom of a foot disorder, the physician should record its location, date of onset, duration, and severity. Relevant economic, psychologic, and social factors should be recorded. The physician should attempt to elicit symptoms using palpation and range-of-motion testing while the patient is at rest. The physician should also determine if the patient's shoes are tight or ill-fitting.

Complete inspection of the feet includes noting the size and location of any hyperkeratotic lesions or excrescences; changes in long-standing lesions (eg, bleeding, discoloration); and evidence of a bacterial or fungal infection, dry skin, ulcers, or warts. The feet and legs should be inspected for trophic changes consistent with loss of vasculature (eg, loss of hair growth; red, shiny, atrophic skin; pigmentation changes). The toenails should be inspected for signs of hypertrophy and fungal infection. Missing nails, changes in the color and continuity of the nail plate, foot odor, temperature of the feet, varicosities, and edema should be noted. The pedal pulses (dorsalis pedis, posterior tibial) should be palpated.

Postural deformities, physical limitations, and the position of the foot at heel strike and through the gait cycle are identified by watching the patient walk. ⬛ The degree of pronation or supination should be determined, especially when orthotics are being considered.

Structural foot deformities are usually obvious. The degree of deformity should be noted; x-rays can detect bone changes (eg, osteoporosis, demineralization, previous fractures, arthritis).

Neurologic examination includes evaluation of motor function. The Achilles tendon and superficial plantar reflexes should be elicited (indicating that the spinal pathways are intact), and vibratory sensation should be evaluated, along with sensitivity to pain, temperature, and touch.

Treatment

In the elderly, the choice of treatment depends on the patient's lifestyle, ambulatory ability, and need for an assistive device (eg, cane, walker). The goals of treatment include reduction of pain, restoration and retention of maximum function, increased comfort, and a decreased likelihood of hospitalization or long-term care for a foot disorder caused by a systemic disease (eg, ulceration, infection). Proper foot care is essential (see TABLE 56–2).

⬛see page 206

TABLE 56–2.   FOOT CARE GUIDELINES

- The feet should be washed daily with mild soap in warm water. All soap should be rinsed off. A soft towel can be used to dry the feet thoroughly, especially between the toes.
- Toenails should be trimmed straight across and not too short. Toenails that have sharp edges may cut into the adjacent toes.
- Shoes should be comfortable and worn daily. People should never go barefoot, not even at the beach.
- Clean socks or stockings should be worn daily. Appropriate fit is necessary (ie, not too short, not too tight).
- If the feet are cold, thick warm socks should be worn. The use of heating pads or hot water bottles should be avoided.
- Daily inspection of the feet for cuts, sores, bumps, and color changes is recommended. A mirror may facilitate inspection.
- Dead skin should be removed using a dry towel.
- Lanolin or cold cream should be gently massaged into dry scaly areas of the feet.
- Regular exercise (eg, walking) is important.
- Smoking decreases circulation to the feet and should be avoided.
- Corns or calluses should not be cut, shaved, or treated with over-the-counter drugs (eg, wart removers), which can burn the skin.
- If athlete's foot is a problem, only shoes made of leather or canvas (not synthetics) should be worn. Patients should change their shoes from day to day and wear foot powder.
- Consultation with a physician is necessary if foot problems persist.

SKIN DISORDERS OF THE FEET

CORNS AND CALLUSES

(Clavi; Helomas; Tylomas)

Corn: A conical, concentrated hyperkeratotic lesion most commonly located on the dorsal surface of the proximal interphalangeal joint of the lesser toes. Callus: A diffuse, somewhat rounded hyperkeratotic lesion located on the plantar surface of the foot.

Corns and calluses are usually caused by undue friction and pressure around a bony prominence, often due to tight or ill-fitting shoes. A soft corn (heloma molle), which usually occurs between the toes, is caused by pressure from adjacent toes. Symptoms range from generalized burning to severe pinpoint pain. If not properly treated, a corn can lead to inflammation and infection.

Treatment

Corns and calluses are usually debrided. For corns, aperture or balance padding is applied by cutting an opening in material such as felt or moleskin, which is placed over the lesion. This padding redistributes pressure away from the painful area. For calluses, protective padding (eg, moleskin, lamb's wool, polyurethane) is applied. An emollient cream, preferably one with a urea base, should be applied afterward to reduce keratosis and provide dermal hydration.

If foot vasculature is inadequate, an alternative, more conservative treatment is use of a soft orthotic or modification of a shoe to avoid pressure to the lesion. This approach is combined with routine application of an emollient cream. Excision should be avoided because of subsequent pain and potential scarring.

Corns and calluses due to biomechanical factors require the use of an orthotic.

Many elderly patients with corns attempt to provide self care for a variety of reasons. However, elderly patients with limited limb motion, failing eyesight, and unsteady hands may aggravate an apparently minor problem. Also, over-the-counter preparations (eg, salicylic acid), if used without supervision, can damage already sensitized tissue. This problem is especially of concern in patients with diabetes mellitus or peripheral vascular disease, in whom infection and ulceration are common.

TINEA PEDIS

(Athlete's Foot)

An inflammatory reaction in the foot caused by fungal organisms (dermatophytosis).

Tinea pedis is usually caused by *Trichophyton rubrum, T. mentagrophytes,* or *Epidermophyton floccosum.* The elderly are especially susceptible, because aging and peripheral vascular disease often cause cracks and fissures in the distal tissues of the extremities, providing a portal of entry for invasive organisms.

Symptoms and Signs

Tinea pedis generally occurs in three forms: interdigital, acute vesicular, and dry squamous. The interdigital type is characterized by scaling, pruritus, and fissuring; maceration also occurs and should be debrided. The vesicular type is characterized by bullous lesions, which may rupture, leaving raw and sensitive skin. Secondary bacterial infection may result. Of the three types of tinea pedis, the squamous type has the least amount of inflammation. This type is characterized by a moccasin pattern of scales on the foot.

Diagnosis and Treatment

Tinea pedis may be diagnosed using a dermatophyte-testing medium, in which a simple color change indicates fungal infection. The diagnosis is confirmed by microscopic examination with a potassium hydroxide preparation and by fungal culture.

Treatment consists of soaking the feet in warm water and Epsom salts, then applying a topical antifungal cream (eg, clotrimazole, miconazole). If inflammation and pruritus occur, a preparation combining clioquinol and hydrocortisone or one combining clotrimazole and betamethasone dipropionate can be used.

Oral mycostatic drugs (eg, itraconazole, terbinafine) are effective when blood flow is adequate, but blood flow is inadequate in many elderly patients. Terbinafine is also available in a topical form as a cream or spray.

ERYTHRASMA

A superficial skin infection in the toe webs.

Erythrasma is caused by *Corynebacterium minutissimum*. It resembles tinea pedis. Symptoms include scaling, fissuring, and slight maceration, which are usually confined to the 3rd and 4th interspaces. Diagnosis is established with a Wood's light, under which erythrasma fluoresces a characteristic coral-red color. Treatment includes oral erythromycin and topical antibacterial preparations.

HYPERHIDROSIS

Excessive perspiration due to overactive sweat glands.

Hyperhidrosis may be precipitated or aggravated by tinea pedis, poor foot care (see TABLE 56–2), or metabolic disease. It may also be caused or aggravated by psychogenic factors. In the feet, hyperhidrosis may cause a foul odor (bromhidrosis). The skin may be pink or bluish white and may be macerated, fissured, and scaling. Diagnosis is made through observation of excessive moisture on the foot during clinical examination.

The usual treatment is a 10% formaldehyde solution and routine use of foot powder. Socks should be changed frequently.

XEROSIS

Abnormal dryness of the skin.

Xerosis occurs as a result of diminished hydration of the skin, possibly due to decreased sebaceous activity, endocrine dysfunction, or nutritional deficiency. It may also be due to age. Xerosis is often accompanied by pruritus, which may lead to scratching and bacterial infection. Severe cases may produce painful fissures, which may impair ambulation and require bed rest. Treatment consists of hydration of the affected area with an emollient cream at regular intervals.

TOENAIL DISORDERS

ONYCHIA AND PARONYCHIA

Onychia: Inflammation of the nail matrix. **Paronychia:** *Inflammation of the matrix plus the surrounding and deeper structures.*

The most common cause is trauma (eg, direct injury, pressure from tight or ill-fitting shoes). Skin diseases (eg, psoriasis, eczema) are also common causes. Patients with diabetes mellitus tend to develop onychia and paronychia because of poor circulation and diminished resistance to infection.

The toe becomes inflamed, swollen, and painful. Drainage may occur, with subsequent irritation of the surrounding tissue. Treatment consists of incision and drainage with partial nail avulsion, culture and sensitivity to determine appropriate antibiotic therapy, and warm Epsom salt soaks or compresses followed by an antibiotic ointment and dressing. For chronic onychia or paronychia, permanent correction may be achieved through surgical matrixectomy.

UNGUIS INCARNATUS

(Ingrown Toenail; Onychocryptosis)

Abnormal growth of the lateral nail edge into periungual tissue.

Tight or ill-fitting shoes and improper nail care are the primary causes. Inflammation and sometimes a secondary bacterial infection may result. If the infection does not resolve, painful granulation tissue forms, requiring surgical removal of the ingrown portion of the nail. After the wound is cleaned, a topical antibiotic and a dry, sterile dressing are applied. Soaking the foot in warm water and Epsom salts is recommended twice daily; a new dressing should be applied after each soak. Systemic antibiotics are required in severe cases.

ONYCHOMYCOSIS

A localized fungal infection of the nail or nail bed characterized by degeneration of the nail plate in which the nail becomes brittle, hypertrophic, and granular.

The usual cause is *Trichophyton rubrum, T. mentagrophytes,* or *E. floccosum; Candida* sp also cause some cases. Severe discomfort and disability may result. Onychomycosis may be diagnosed using the appropriate dermatophyte-testing technique.

Treatment

Topical antifungal therapy is rarely effective because of the nail matrix involvement. Also, in the elderly, diminished blood supply in the feet precludes the use of some oral antifungal drugs. Terbinafine has a shorter treatment time, a higher cure rate, and less serious adverse effects than griseofulvin. Newer drugs that cover a broader range of fungi are also available.

If oral drug therapy is not an option, the involved nail plates are trimmed at regular intervals. Patients are instructed about proper foot hygiene and the need for regular podiatric care to keep the nails reduced and smooth. This approach allows more comfortable ambulation, lessens the chance of traumatic injury due to a sharp nail plate, reduces the likelihood of continued shoe irritation due to an enlarged nail, and helps eliminate the risk of traumatic nail avulsion. Proper foot hygiene and regular podiatric care are particularly significant in elderly patients with vascular impairment or diabetes to prevent ulceration, cellulitis, osteomyelitis, and gangrene.

Application of topical antifungal drugs around the nail bed may reduce keratotic buildup that can lead to fissuring and may reduce the chance of developing tinea pedis in the surrounding tissue.

ONYCHAUXIS AND ONYCHOGRYPHOSIS

Onychauxis: Hypertrophy of the nail plate. *Onychogryphosis: Long-standing hypertrophy characterized by a curved or hooked nail (ram's horn nail).*

Hypertrophy of the nail may be caused by many factors, including injury, microtrauma from ill-fitting shoes, infection, peripheral vascular disease, diabetes, and nutritional deficiency.

Symptoms and Signs

Pressure on the nails, even from bedsheets, may produce severe pain. Concomitant onychophosis (callus formation under the tibial and fibular nail grooves) may occur, adding to the pain and disability. Onychogryphosis is almost always associated with changes in the nail matrix and nail bed. A severely hypertrophic nail may penetrate the adjacent toe, causing inflammation and pain.

Treatment

Vascular support stockings, worn by many elderly persons, apply significant pressure to the toes and can worsen this condition. Stockings can be modified by cutting the edges to prevent bunching of the toes.

The use of lamb's wool between the toes may also help. Because the elderly lack the proper flexibility for self-care and may have impaired vision, osteoarthritis, and obesity, professional care is recommended. Treatment involves frequent nail cutting or trimming and instruction in proper foot care (see TABLE 56–2). Occasionally, surgery is necessary.

ORTHOPEDIC AND STRUCTURAL DISORDERS

HALLUX VALGUS

(Bunion)

Deviation of the first metatarsophalangeal joint, which causes the toe to drift laterally and the first metatarsal head to protrude medially.

The cause is usually ill-fitting footwear. Hallux valgus is more common among females than among males. Patients may have a hereditary disposition; the lesser toes are often deformed. Degenerative changes associated with osteoarthritis are common, and a metatarsus primus varus may be present. Hallux valgus is always accompanied by a bunion deformity, indicated by swelling or enlargement, but a bunion is not always accompanied by hallux valgus. An exostosis and an adventitious bursa may form.

Diagnosis

Diagnosis is made by clinical observation of the deformity; by physical examination findings of pain at the medial or dorsomedial aspect of the first metatarsal head, especially if the patient is wearing shoes; and by x-ray findings. Often, the patient's complaints are cosmetic in nature. However, local erythema and skin irritation may occur, and ambulation may be markedly compromised.

Treatment

Local injection of a corticosteroid with an anesthetic relieves inflammation and pain. Oral nonsteroidal anti-inflammatory drugs (NSAIDs) are also effective. When the deformity is severe, a cutout should be made in the patient's shoe and a bunion-last shoe or a custom-made, molded shoe should be considered. A bunion-last shoe provides increased depth in the toe box to conform to the shape of the deformity and to decrease external friction and pressure. It is usually made of soft leather to reduce constriction around the toes. Surgery may be helpful, but the patient's lifestyle and ability to perform self-care postoperatively should be considered.

METATARSALGIA

A generalized ache or soreness directly below the metatarsal heads.

Metatarsalgia results from atrophy of the plantar fat pad that supports the metatarsal heads. It may be accompanied by a plantar callus and, if untreated, may lead to anterior metatarsal bursitis or arthritis of the involved metatarsophalangeal joints. Treatment consists of redistributing the pressure away from the metatarsal heads. Redistribution can be accomplished with an orthopedic shoe, an orthotic, or another device that provides cushioning and shock absorption to this area of the foot.

MORTON'S NEUROMA

A plantar interdigital nerve tumor usually occurring in the 3rd or 4th metatarsal interspace, with pain radiating toward the 3rd and 4th toes.

This deformity is caused by entrapment of the interdigital nerves as they pass between the metatarsal heads. It characteristically occurs in the 3rd interspace, where the metatarsal heads are in closest proximity. Severe, disabling pain may radiate to the toes or legs and is pathognomonic.

Diagnosis and Treatment

Diagnosis is made by physical examination findings of sharp pain in the metatarsal interspaces; the pain may be duplicated clinically by transverse compression of the metatarsals and direct plantar pressure. X-rays may show close juxtaposition of the metatarsal heads.

Foot massage may alleviate the pain. Another nonsurgical option is local injection of a long-acting corticosteroid proximal to the site of pain. Injection is into the interspace at the level of the dorsal aspect of the metatarsophalangeal joints. If symptoms persist, surgical excision is advised.

HAMMER TOE

Malalignment of the toe in a fixed, contracted position at the proximal interphalangeal joint.

Hammer toe may result from years of wearing ill-fitting shoes. When the toe is higher in the shoe than normal, it is exposed to excessive friction, often resulting in a painful corn. In severe cases, the lesion may become inflamed and ulcerated, leading to secondary bacterial infection and ambulatory disability.

Flexion deformity occurs at the proximal interphalangeal joint, with hyperextension of the distal interphalangeal joint. Hammer toe often accompanies hallux valgus. Diagnosis is made by clinical observation of the deformity, by physical examination findings of pain on the dorsal aspect of the proximal interphalangeal joint of the involved toe, and by x-ray findings.

Treatment consists of debriding the lesion. Shoes that irritate the lesion should be avoided. Surgical correction, ranging from simple tenotomy to arthroplasty of the digit, should be considered in severe cases.

SESAMOIDITIS

Inflammation of the tendon and soft tissue structures below the first metatarsal head due to repeated trauma.

The area may be swollen; generally, pain occurs during ambulation and on direct pressure.

Diagnosis is made by physical examination findings of pain on the plantar aspect of the head of the first metatarsal phalangeal joint; by x-ray findings that rule out fracture or show bipartite sesamoids, which are usually bilateral; and by evaluation of shoes or lifestyle. The condition is most common among dancers, joggers, and persons with a history of wearing high heels.

Treatment consists of an aperture pad (dancer's pad) to eliminate pressure on the area. This felt pad is cut to fit around the first metatarsal head. Other treatment modalities (eg, ultrasound, injection of a corticosteroid, oral NSAIDs) are helpful.

HEEL PAIN

The most common cause of heel pain is a heel spur; abnormal pronation causes inflammation by constantly pulling the plantar fascia at its origin in the calcaneus. In the elderly, heel pain may result from gradual age-related atrophy of the fat padding beneath the calcaneus. It also may be due to repetitive activity that increases pressure and irritation in the heel. Systemic conditions such as rheumatoid arthritis, gout, and collagen disease may also cause heel pain. Pain in the longitudinal arch with or without concomitant heel pain is known as plantar fasciitis. Pain generally occurs in the mid arch area; tender nodules may be palpated. Pain usually begins with the first steps in the morning, dissipates, and recurs later in the day.

Haglund's deformity or "pump bump" refers to a calcaneal exostosis most often occurring at the posteromedial aspect of the bone. In **Achilles tendon bursitis,** there is irritation of the bursa lying in front of the tendon and behind the calcaneus. (In other words, the Haglund's deformity is the bony abnormality not the bursitis, but it may lead to the bursitis as it creates abnormal pressure where it is situated.) Pain occurs in the posterior portion of the heel resulting from pressure on the posterosuperior aspect of the calcaneus.

Diagnosis

Diagnosis of heel pain is made by history, including onset; physical examination; and x-ray findings, which show bony spurs and abnormalities. Diagnosis of posterior Achilles tendon bursitis is made by physical examination findings of pain and swelling and thick callus formation at the posterior aspect of the heel and by x-ray findings.

Treatment

Treatment depends on the nature and extent of bone damage as shown on x-ray. Local injections of a corticosteroid and an anesthetic can be given weekly until symptoms subside. Plantar strapping can be used in conjunction with corticosteroid and anesthetic therapy to relieve tension on the plantar fascia. Oral NSAIDs, physical therapy with ultrasound and hydrotherapy, heel cups, and plantar paddings may also reduce heel discomfort. After heel pain diminishes, a biomechanical examination should be performed, and an appropriate orthotic should be made.

For posterior Achilles tendon bursitis, NSAIDs, aspiration (when bursitis is present), heel lifts, aperture padding around the bursal sac, and physical therapy relieve pressure. When pain is acute, slippers should be worn. Ultrasound, hydrotherapy, and surgical excision of the bursal sac and/or exostosis may be necessary.

FOOT FRACTURES

Elderly persons are prone to falls∎ and foot fractures. X-rays using the dorsoplantar, lateral, and oblique views are helpful for diagnosis.

Immediate application of ice to the fracture reduces inflammation; analgesics are given to manage pain. Walking should be restricted; crutches may be necessary. Toe fractures may be treated by splinting the injured toe to an adjacent one to ensure immobilization. Realigning a displaced fracture of the toe requires local anesthesia. More severe fractures, such as those of a metatarsal or tarsal bone, require a plaster or semirigid cast or Unna's boot. Follow-up x-rays should be taken over the next few months to assess healing.

LOCAL NERVE DISORDERS

TARSAL TUNNEL SYNDROME

Compression of the posterior tibial nerve at the ankle that results in severe pain leading to disability and reduced ambulation.

∎see page 195

Presenting symptoms include burning and discomfort, which usually radiate to the toes. Pain increases on ambulation and is relieved by rest. The syndrome may be diagnosed by Tinel's sign (ie, distal tingling produced by tapping on the nerve at the site of compression). Treatment consists of local injections of a corticosteroid (eg, dexamethasone, triamcinolone acetonide) with an anesthetic. Strapping to alleviate pressure on the nerve should also be used. Surgical decompression of the nerve may be necessary.

DORSAL CUTANEOUS NERVE TRAUMA

Injury to the sensory nerves on the dorsum of the foot.

Pain in the dorsolateral aspect of the foot is usually caused by a damaged intermediate dorsal cutaneous nerve. Such damage often results from compression due to ill-fitting shoes and is common after a plantar inversion ankle sprain. Arthritic changes and spur formation may also irritate these nerves. Pain in the dorsomedial aspect may be caused by a defect of the medial dorsal cutaneous nerve due to improper surgical technique or entrapment by fibrosis after bunion surgery.

Treatment consists of local injection of corticosteroids; strapping of the foot or custom-made shoes are also used. Pressure on the injured nerve should be avoided. When the suspected cause is entrapment by severe fibrosis, surgery should be considered.

FOOT PAIN DUE TO SYSTEMIC DISEASE

PERIPHERAL VASCULAR DISEASE

Vascular disease commonly affects the legs and feet.∎ Symptoms include exertional pain, edema, skin color changes, coldness, burning, numbness, loss of hair growth, and ulcers. Nail changes, especially thickening and onychomycosis, occur as vascular disease advances. Poor circulation diminishes the ability to combat infection, and even the slightest cut or bruise may cause ulcers or gangrene.

DIABETES MELLITUS

Patients with diabetes∎ have many of the same symptoms as those with peripheral vascular disease. Diabetes may cause paresthesias, motor weakness, numbness, burning, and cramping. Elderly patients

---

∎ see pages 915 and 923   ∎ see page 624

with diabetes may also have color and temperature changes, dry and scaly skin, and edema that may result from generalized systemic disease or localized infection. Nail changes are similar to those that occur with peripheral vascular disease.

Diabetic patients are prone to ulcers, especially on the weight-bearing surfaces of the foot. Ulcers may be neurotrophic or vascular. A neurotrophic ulcer is usually painless, and the patient may not be aware of it. Ulcers often lead to infection, osteomyelitis, and gangrene. Use of an acidic over-the-counter corn remedy may cause skin sloughing and soft tissue destruction and may precipitate ulceration.

ARTHRITIS AND GOUT

In the elderly, arthritis is the most common cause of foot pain.

Osteoarthritis[1] often involves the ankle and the first metatarsophalangeal joint. Patients have a characteristic walk, with decreased motion at the interphalangeal joint of the hallux. Motion may be limited by exostosis formation. Palpation of the first metatarsophalangeal joint reveals stiffness and pain with severely limited motion. Characteristic x-ray findings include narrowing of the joint space (caused by loss of articular cartilage), osteophyte formation, and increased density of subchondral bone.

Treatment is symptomatic, ranging from NSAID therapy to surgery (if loss of joint function is marked). Local injection of a corticosteroid with an anesthetic may relieve symptoms; exercise of the joint and traction of the toe help increase range of motion. If this approach fails, an orthotic can reduce pain during ambulation.

Rheumatoid arthritis[2] may cause progressive stiffening of the joints, which may lead to deformity and ankylosis. Periods of rest from weight bearing are essential. Shoes must be modified to accommodate painful plantar areas. A custom-made orthopedic shoe is particularly helpful. Local injection of a corticosteroid helps alleviate joint pain, as do oral NSAIDs and analgesics. Surgery should be considered when conservative therapy fails.

Gout[3] causes an inflammatory response, initiated by the urate crystals. This response often begins in the metatarsophalangeal joint of the great toe and is characterized by increasing joint pain, swelling, erythema, and heat. Prevention includes gradual weight reduction, avoidance of alcohol, increased fluid intake, and drug therapy.

---

[1] see page 489   [2] see page 499   [3] see page 494

SECTION 8

METABOLIC AND ENDOCRINE DISORDERS

MET/
END

Thirst, hunger, and renal function control water and electrolyte balance. These systems compensate for losses through the skin, respiratory tract, and gastrointestinal (GI) tract. Hormones and (to a lesser extent) local cell modulatory molecules (eg, eicosanoids) are also critical. With age, all of these functions change, making the elderly more prone to problems with water and electrolyte balance. Imbalances are most likely to occur when acute illness, hospitalization, use of medications, or extremes of weather upset homeostasis.

WATER AND SODIUM METABOLISM

Aging is associated with impaired water conservation and sodium balance—factors that determine extracellular fluid (ECF) volume and tonicity. Thirst and the secretion of antidiuretic hormone (ADH or arginine vasopressin [AVP]) control water balance. The elderly have a delayed and less intense thirst response than do younger persons. The older body tends to secrete ADH despite decreased blood tonicity (the syndrome of inappropriate ADH secretion [SIADH]), especially in a person with chronic cardiac, hepatic, or renal disease. Increased ADH concentration and secretion increase the risk of hyponatremia most intensely when fluid intake increases—a situation common with IV hydration during hospitalization or surgery.

Renal filtration of sodium and water at the glomerulus, renal tubular conservation of sodium, and renal tubular natriuretic substances (eg, atrial natriuretic peptide, renal prostaglandins) control sodium balance. These are all altered with aging (all but atrial natriuretic peptide decrease). Other factors that affect sodium balance include cardiac output, blood pressure, renal blood flow, glomerular filtration rate, and renal sympathetic nerve activity. Again, many of these parameters are altered with age and tend to be severely altered in elderly persons with coexisting cardiovascular or renal disease.

With age, total body water decreases because of an increase in fat and a decrease in lean body mass (from about 60% of body weight in healthy young adults to about 45% of body weight in the elderly). Therefore, the margin of error is reduced for maintaining normal electrolyte balance when water losses occur during acute illness due to fever, because of increased transpiration with tachypnea, or as a result of renal and GI losses.

Serum sodium concentration is determined primarily by body water balance; thus, hyponatremia usually results from excessive water retention and hypernatremia from water loss. With total body sodium and water excess, edema may result. With pure water excess, edema is not present. With a sodium and water deficit, the presentation often includes orthostatic hypotension. With a pure water deficit, vital signs do not change.

The ability to concentrate urine decreases with age in part because of tubular senescence. Many elderly persons also have resistance to the renal action of ADH, ie, a form of acquired partial nephrogenic diabetes insipidus.

The ability to decrease renal sodium excretion is impaired with age and may result partly from an age-related nephron loss, a decrease in circulating renin and aldosterone, and partly from decreased responsiveness to acute stimuli. Elderly persons with an acute illness who are not ingesting sodium develop a negative sodium balance quicker than do younger persons. In the elderly, basal blood levels of atrial natriuretic peptide are increased; atrial natriuretic peptide inhibits aldosterone secretion and may decrease aldosterone blood levels.

DEHYDRATION AND VOLUME DEPLETION

Dehydration: A decrease in total body water without an equal reduction in total body sodium. **Volume depletion:** *A loss of body water and sodium resulting in decreased ECF volume.*

Dehydration is the most common fluid and electrolyte disturbance of the elderly. A history of decreased food or fluid intake, febrile illness, polyuria, vomiting, diarrhea, chronic renal disease, diabetes mellitus, use of diuretics, or nasogastric suction is common. Other factors include impaired renal concentrating ability, reduced thirst, and impaired access to water due to neurologic or orthopedic problems or to deconditioning from medical or surgical conditions. Hot weather is a common contributing factor. Nurses can help prevent dehydration by closely monitoring fluid balance in elderly patients.

Symptoms, Signs, and Diagnosis

The patient may present with altered mental status, lethargy, lightheadedness, or syncope. In general, mild dehydration produces reduced skin turgor, dry mucous membranes, and orthostatic hypotension; moderate dehydration produces these symptoms as well as oliguria or anuria, confusion, and resting hypotension; and severe hypotension produces shock or near shock. However, decreased skin turgor, dry mucous membranes, tachycardia, and orthostatic hypotension may also occur in elderly persons with normal volume status.

Increased Hct, blood urea nitrogen (BUN), and serum creatinine levels may occur. The BUN/creatinine ratio is often elevated because slow urinary flow leads to reabsorption of urea but not of creatinine. The serum sodium concentration may be high, normal, or low, depending on the cause. Urinary sodium concentration is usually < 20 mEq/L when sodium intake has been chronically reduced or when vomiting or diarrhea causes losses. A urinary sodium concentration > 20 mEq/L can occur with volume depletion. In these cases, higher concentrations occur when chronic renal disease impairs the ability to conserve sodium or the patient has been taking diuretics.

Although adrenal insufficiency is less common, it must always be considered. Hypercalcemia, hypokalemia, and hyperglycemia with consequent glycosuria leading to osmotic diuresis must be excluded as causes of the impaired renal ability to conserve water.

Treatment

It is important to estimate the fluid deficit. Elderly persons who are mildly dehydrated have lost fluid equivalent to < 5% of body weight, those moderately dehydrated have lost about 10%, and those severely dehydrated have lost ≥ 15%.

Mild volume depletion can be treated initially with aggressive oral fluid intake (ie, 2 to 3 L of water or clear liquids) followed by continued oral hydration. However, oral hydration may be problematic if a GI disorder or impaired mental status is present. For larger deficits, IV fluid therapy is required, usually with 0.9% sodium chloride, even if the serum sodium concentration is elevated. Free water replacement is not appropriate until the intravascular deficit has been replaced. In general, at least 50% of the loss should be replaced within the first 12 hours (about 1 L/day in nonfebrile patients). For example, in a moderately dehydrated 75-kg woman who has lost 7.5 L of fluid, an appropriate replacement rate is nearly 350 mL/h. Although such rates of replacement are sometimes frightening to clinicians, they can be given safely with adequate monitoring. Inadequate rehydration that is not accomplished quickly can lead to serious complications, including renal failure, heart attack, stroke, and rhabdomyolysis.

Although the initial rate of administration should be high enough to resolve orthostatic hypotension and tachycardia and produce adequate urine output within 24 hours, the remaining deficit should be corrected more slowly. The rate may need to be reduced to replace the calculated deficit and ongoing fluid needs over 2 to 3 days, with monitoring to avoid precipitating heart failure.

HYPONATREMIA

A decrease in the plasma sodium concentration <136 mEq/L caused by an excess of water relative to solute.

An age-related decrease in serum sodium concentration of 1 mEq/L/decade occurs after age 40 (from a mean value of 141 ± 4 mEq/L in younger persons); however, this decrease, especially when mild, often does not produce clinically apparent symptoms. Total ECF volume may be increased, normal, or decreased with hyponatremia.

Etiology and Pathophysiology

In most cases of hyponatremia in the elderly, the concentration of sodium or any other osmotic substance in the plasma is low relative to water content (ie, is hypo-osmolar).

Dilutional hyponatremia is probably the most common type of hyponatremia in the elderly; it is often the most severe hyponatremia, resulting in the greatest morbidity and mortality in the elderly. A common cause of dilutional hyponatremia in elderly patients is the use of nutritional supplements such as Isocal, Ensure, and Osmolite, which are low in sodium. IV fluid administration of hypotonic fluids may also cause dilutional hyponatremia, especially in patients with elevated ADH levels. Primary polydipsia (excessive fluid intake in association with a neuropsychiatric disorder) occurs rarely in the elderly.

Hyponatremia with sodium depletion may occur with vomiting, diarrhea, GI suction, renal disorders, and diuretic therapy. In these cases, volume depletion stimulates ADH release so that excess water is retained in excess of sodium. Hyponatremia resulting from these events is usually mild (rarely < 125 mEq/L).

Hyponatremia in the elderly is rarely caused by the presence of osmotically active solutes in plasma, which draw intracellular water into the extracellular space to dilute the plasma sodium by the shift of water. Although rare, this disorder can occur when plasma osmolality is increased due to ingestion of toxic alcohols (eg, methanol, ethylene glycol). It can also occur when mannitol is administered.

Hyponatremia with total body sodium excess may occur with cirrhosis, nephrosis, and heart failure. These disorders are said to have ineffective circulating volume because they lead to impaired renal ability to create a dilute urine. ADH may also be elevated in these conditions.

Elderly patients with any cause of total body sodium depletion often have normal baseline serum sodium concentrations. However, when fluid intake increases (eg, when IV fluids are given or when oral intake is increased), the increase in body water may lead rapidly to hyponatremia. This condition may occur in institutionalized patients, whose fluid intake is not determined primarily by thirst but by the availability of or access to fluids or by the iatrogenic administration of fluids (as in IV fluids or tube feedings).

Symptoms, Signs, and Diagnosis

The severity of symptoms and signs depends on the degree of hyponatremia and the rapidity with which serum sodium concentration decreases. Hyponatremia is one of the most common causes of delirium in elderly patients.

Severe hyponatremia may be accompanied by depressed sensorium, depressed deep tendon reflexes, hypothermia, Cheyne-Stokes respiration, and pathologic reflexes. Plasma osmolality should be determined. If plasma osmolality is low, the next step is to assess volume status. If hypo-osmolar hyponatremia with edema is present, the diagnosis is cirrhosis, nephrosis, or heart failure. When orthostasis is present with hypo-osmolar hyponatremia, the diagnosis is renal, adrenal, or GI disorders that lead to salt and water loss from GI fluids or urine. When neither edema nor orthostasis is present with hypo-osmolar hyponatremia, the diagnosis is pure water retention due either to excessive oral intake, IV solute administration, or SIADH. A summary of test results is presented in TABLE 57–1.

If plasma osmolality is normal but hyponatremia is present, the diagnosis is pseudohyponatremia, which occurs in patients with marked hyperlipidemia or hyperproteinemia. No mental status changes occur because water does not shift into the brain or other tissues. Pseudohyponatremia may occur in a patient with multiple myeloma with very high protein γ-globulin levels.

Treatment

Usually, restoring the serum sodium concentration to about 120 to 125 mEq/L corrects most symptoms. Both overcorrection and too-rapid correction create worsening neurologic status, which is sometimes irreversible (osmotic demyelination syndrome).

TABLE 57–1.   DIFFERENTIATING FEATURES OF HYPONATREMIA

Type of Hyponatremia	Edema	BUN and Serum Creatinine Levels	Urine Sodium Concentration (mmol/L)	Response to Water Load
Sodium and ECF volume depletion	No	Increased	< 20	Impaired
Decreased effective plasma volume	Yes	Increased	< 20	Impaired
Dilutional + SIADH	No	Normal or decreased	< 20	Impaired
Primary polydipsia	No	Normal or decreased	> 20	Normal
Low-set osmoreceptor*	No	Normal	> 20	Normal

BUN = blood urea nitrogen; ECF = extracellular fluid; SIADH = syndrome of inappropriate antidiuretic hormone secretion.

*Extremely uncommon in the elderly. Patients appear to respond normally to water load but maintain a lower serum sodium concentration and lower serum osmolality. ADH levels are normal.

In patients with severe symptomatic hyponatremia, particularly that resulting from a dilutional state, hypertonic sodium chloride solution is infused carefully until symptoms begin to resolve and the serum sodium concentration reaches 120 mEq/L. For symptomatic hyponatremia, especially when accompanied by seizure or coma, aggressive management consists of giving 100 to 200 mL of 3% sodium chloride solution over 4 to 6 hours, along with simultaneous administration of IV furosemide. For gentler correction of the hyponatremia, 0.9% sodium chloride is given with furosemide. In addition to close monitoring of serum sodium, serum electrolytes must be measured often to allow for potassium and magnesium replacement because of the concomitant diuretic administration.

In hypo-osmolar hyponatremic patients with orthostasis (ie, sodium and ECF volume depletion), the sodium and volume deficit is corrected with 0.9% sodium chloride. Further fluid losses can be prevented with antiemetic therapy and antidiarrheal agents and by stopping diuretics. In hypo-osmolar hyponatremic patients with edema, loop diuretics (eg, furosemide) are used. When hyponatremia is dilutional, it is refractory to treatment. In asymptomatic patients with hypo-osmolar hyponatremia with neither orthostasis nor edema, water restriction of 800 to 1000 mL/day is the treatment of choice.

In patients with hyponatremia due to consumption of nutritional supplements, sodium supplementation starting with 100 mEq/L should be given daily.

In patients with hyperosmolar hypernatremia, osmotically active molecules need to be reduced (eg, through insulin administration to lower hyperglycemia or through urinary elimination or dialysis to eliminate the toxic alcohol).

Management of chronic hyponatremia usually includes restriction of fluid intake (usually 1000 to 1500 mL/day) to maintain a serum sodium concentration > 130 mEq/L. In more refractory or severe cases of chronic dilutional hyponatremia, furosemide may be given along with sodium chloride tablets and restriction of free water. Demeclocycline 600 mg to 1200 mg/day po can induce mild nephrogenic diabetes insipidus with polyuria of 2 to 4 L/24 hours. Patients receiving demeclocycline require close monitoring of fluid balance to avoid excessive fluid loss, elevated serum BUN levels, and drug-induced tubular necrosis.

Patients with pseudohyponatremia require no treatment.

HYPERNATREMIA

An elevation in the plasma sodium concentration > 146 mEq/L caused by a deficit of water relative to solute; total body sodium content is usually normal or nearly normal.

TABLE 57-2.   CAUSES OF HYPERNATREMIA IN THE ELDERLY

Decreased water intake Physical impairment Mental impairment Obtundation Hypodipsia, adipsia **Increased sodium intake** Sodium bicarbonate therapy IV administration of isotonic or hypertonic sodium chloride solution Sodium chloride supplement tablets	**Increased water loss** Increased insensible loss Fever Tachypnea Sweating Diarrhea Dialysis Renal water loss Loop diuretics Osmotic diuresis—glucose, mannitol, sodium, urea Diabetes insipidus Nephrogenic diabetes insipidus Chronic renal disease Polyuria

Excessive loss of body water relative to the loss of sodium underlies hypernatremia (see TABLE 57–2). The prevalence of hypernatremia is about 1% in elderly hospitalized patients and in residents of long-term care facilities. Lower body weight is a risk factor in the elderly. Mortality rate is about 40% in the elderly hospitalized patient and is highest in patients with a rapid onset and in those with serum sodium concentrations >160 mEq/L.

Symptoms and Signs

The symptoms of moderate hypernatremia may be nonspecific; weakness and lethargy are common. More severe hypernatremia (serum sodium concentrations > 152 mEq/L) may cause a focal neurologic deficit (eg, hemiparesis), severe obtundation, stupor, coma, and seizures. CNS manifestations are common and often lead to a depressed sensorium and chronic functional decline in patients who survive the acute episode. Because hypernatremia represents a pure water loss, the signs of volume depletion (eg, decreased skin turgor, dry mucous membranes, orthostatic hypotension) are absent.

In addition to an increased serum sodium concentration, laboratory findings include increased Hct, serum osmolality, BUN, and creatinine levels. Urine osmolality may not be greatly increased because renal ability to concentrate urine is impaired with age.

Treatment

Body water deficits are replaced with hypotonic fluid. A simple way of estimating the deficit is by using the rule of 7's: for every 10 mEq/L the serum sodium is elevated, a 7% deficit of total body water exists.

Either 0.45% sodium chloride solution or 5% dextrose in water should be given at a rate that corrects the water deficit in about 48 hours. The serum sodium concentration should be lowered by ≤ 2 mEq/L/h.

Excessively rapid correction may lead to cerebral edema with permanent brain damage or death. In the elderly patient with coexisting cardiac disease, caution and close monitoring (checking every few hours for symptoms and signs of heart failure) are needed to avoid heart failure from too-rapid administration of hypotonic IV solutions. When the cause of hypernatremia (eg, diabetes insipidus, diuretic therapy, increased sodium intake) is identified, specific treatment should be implemented to correct the cause.

POTASSIUM METABOLISM

With age, total body potassium decreases. This decrease reflects the decrease in lean body muscle mass, which contains about 75% of intracellular potassium. Although aldosterone secretion decreases with age, the kidney's ability to regulate potassium excretion under normal dietary conditions is unaffected. Because most of the total body stores of potassium are within cells, measurement of serum potassium is often inadequate for estimating total body potassium.

HYPOKALEMIA

A decrease in serum potassium concentration < 3.5 mEq/L; total body potassium may be normal or decreased.

Hypokalemia is common in the elderly. Common causes include decreased intake of potassium during acute illness, nausea and vomiting, and treatment with thiazide or loop diuretics. About 20% of patients receiving thiazide diuretics develop hypokalemia, which is dose-dependent but usually mild. Other causes are listed in TABLE 57–3.

Symptoms, Signs, and Diagnosis

Mild hypokalemia rarely produces symptoms. Common symptoms of more severe hypokalemia are fatigue, confusion, and muscle weakness and cramps from impaired skeletal muscle function. Severe hypokalemia (< 2.5 mEq/L) can result in frank paralysis, as occurs with periodic paralysis. Smooth muscle function of the GI tract can also be affected, leading to adynamic ileus. Cardiac function can be affected, resulting in atrial and ventricular ectopic beats, atrial and ventricular tachycardia, ventricular fibrillation, and sudden death, particularly in patients with preexisting heart disease or those taking digitalis preparations. The ECG often shows ST-segment depression, T-wave flattening, and a prominent U wave. With severe hypokalemia, atrioventricular conduction disturbances can develop.

TABLE 57–3.   CAUSES OF HYPOKALEMIA IN THE ELDERLY

Inadequate dietary potassium

Increased gastrointestinal losses
  Vomiting
  Diarrhea
  Laxative use
  Fistulas
  Tube drainage
  Villous adenomatous colon polyps
    (secretory polyps)

Increased renal loss
  Renal tubular acidosis (proximal and
    distal)
  Thiazide diuretic use
  Loop diuretic use (furosemide,
    bumetanide, ethacrynic acid)
  Antibiotic use (gentamicin, penicil-
    lins, amphotericin B)
  Primary hyperaldosteronism
  Secondary hyperaldosteronism (heart
    failure, cirrhosis)

Increased renal loss (*continued*)
  Cushing's syndrome
  Exogenous glucocorticoids
  Exogenous mineralocorticoids
  Hyperreninemic renovascular
    hypertension
  Postobstructive diuresis

Transcellular shift
  Alkalosis
  Insulin administration
  β-agonists

Hypomagnesemia

Hematologic disorders
  Vitamin B_{12} treatment of megalo-
    blastic anemia
  Acute myeloid leukemias

Measuring urinary potassium excretion may help establish if urinary loss is abnormal. Urinary excretion of > 20 mEq/L suggests an excessive loss in a patient with hypokalemia.

Treatment

Treatment consists of correcting the underlying cause (if possible), correcting total body deficits, and restoring normal serum potassium concentrations.

When urgent treatment is not required, potassium chloride 10 to 20 mEq po q 4 to 8 h should be given until the serum potassium concentration is normal. If hypokalemia is caused by a thiazide diuretic, supplemental potassium or a potassium-sparing diuretic such as triamterene, amiloride, or spironolactone may maintain normal blood potassium concentrations once the deficit has been corrected.

When urgent treatment is needed (ie, when the patient has severe symptoms or an arrhythmia), potassium chloride should be given IV. The potassium concentration in the IV fluid usually should not exceed 40 mEq/L, and the administration rate should not exceed 10 to 20 mEq/h with a total dose of 200 mEq/24 h. As long as 10 mEq/h is given each hour, a large deficit can almost always be overcome. Because ongoing additional losses are common, the serum concentration should be measured often (usually every 6 hours). Repeated doses of 10 mEq/h are often needed. If no central venous access is available, the potassium concentration cannot exceed 10 mEq/100 mL of fluid without a high risk of phlebitis and early loss of that access site. If central venous access is available, the potassium concentration can be about 40 mEq/L without risk of central vein scarring, stenosis, or occlusion. Again, the patient should be closely monitored, especially for cardiac function. With IV dosing of substantial amounts of potassium to the elderly, the volume of the IV fluid and the sodium tonicity of that fluid can cause problems.

HYPERKALEMIA

An increase in serum potassium concentration > 5 mEq/L; total body potassium can be high but is more often normal or even low; however, distribution between intracellular and extracellular compartments is abnormal.

Hyperkalemia may be mild (5.0 to 5.5 mEq/L), moderate (5.5 to 6.0 mEq/L), or severe (> 6.0 mEq/L).

Etiology

Hyperkalemia can be caused by a number of disorders or drugs (see TABLE 57–4). A relatively small shift of potassium from the intracellular to the extracellular compartment can result in marked hyperkalemia in patients with metabolic acidosis, especially diabetic ketoacidosis.

TABLE 57–4.   CAUSES OF HYPERKALEMIA IN THE ELDERLY

Pseudohyperkalemia
   Hemolysis in test tube
   Release of potassium from platelets during sample storage

Excessive intake (po or IV)
   Acute renal failure
   Chronic renal failure, especially tubulointerstitial diseases

Transcellular shift
   Metabolic acidosis
   Hyperglycemia (hyperosmolar coma)

Impaired hormone metabolism
   Addison's disease—adrenal insufficiency
   NSAIDs—impaired prostaglandin production

Drug-induced
   Potassium-sparing diuretics—interfere with aldosterone action
   Trimethoprim-sulfamethoxazole—acts as antialdosterone agent
   ACE inhibitors, angiotensin receptor blockers, β-blockers—
      interfere with renin-angiotensin-aldosterone action
   NSAIDs—impaired prostaglandins lead to impairment in renin-
      angiotensin-aldosterone axis

ACE = angiotensin-converting enzyme; NSAIDs = nonsteroidal anti-inflammatory drugs.

Only in patients with renal disease or impaired tubular function does excessive intake lead to hyperkalemia. Patients with acute oliguric renal failure are at especially high risk. Cellular uptake is stimulated by insulin, aldosterone, epinephrine (through β-receptor stimulation), and alkalosis and can modulate the impact of high oral potassium intake on serum levels. Chronic renal disease with hyperkalemia may result from diseases with primary tubular injury (eg, obstructive uropathy) or from chronic analgesic abuse. Primary or secondary adrenal insufficiency must also be considered. Active GI bleeding, especially in a patient with a reduced glomerular filtration rate, can also lead to hyperkalemia.

An elevated serum potassium concentration may result from pseudo-hyperkalemia caused by hemolysis or from the release of potassium from platelets during sample storage.

Symptoms, Signs, and Diagnosis

Hyperkalemia may be asymptomatic until cardiac toxicity develops. Initial ECG changes are a shortened QT interval and tall, narrow T waves. At higher potassium concentrations (usually ≥ 5.5 mEq/L), hyperkalemia can cause nodal and ventricular arrhythmias along with widened QRS complexes and prolonged PR intervals. Ultimately, ventricular fibrillation or asystole can develop. Nonspecific neuromuscular symptoms, including vague weakness and paresthesias, may occur. With severe hyperkalemia, dramatic symptoms (eg, severe weakness, flaccid paralysis) may occur.

Treatment

Severe or rising hyperkalemia may constitute a medical emergency. Atrioventricular block or changes in the QRS complex or P wave on the ECG should be treated with calcium chloride IV using the rule of 10's: 10 mL of 10% calcium chloride every 10 minutes as needed. A glucose-insulin-bicarbonate solution can also be used to shift potassium into cells. If these measures are ineffective, hemodialysis should be initiated promptly.

Moderate hyperkalemia without significant ECG changes should be treated with sodium polystyrene sulfonate 15 to 30 g po dissolved in a 50% oral solution of sorbitol (30 to 60 mL). Sodium polystyrene sulfonate can also be given as a retention enema of 60 g in 120 mL of 50% sorbitol at 4- to 6-hour intervals. Furosemide 40 to 160 mg IV may be used. IV 0.9% sodium chloride is often essential to ensure the maximum renal capacity for excreting potassium. Potassium levels should be checked every 2 to 4 hours.

Mild hyperkalemia may be treated by restricting potassium intake to 40 to 60 mEq/day. Drugs and foods that may contribute to hyperkalemia should be discontinued. Furosemide 40 to 80 mg po bid to qid or fludrocortisone acetate 0.05 to 0.2 mg/day po may be useful in patients with chronic renal disease or hypoaldosteronism.

Disorders of mineral metabolism are increasingly common among the elderly. They include bone diseases (eg, osteoporosis,■ osteomalcia,2 Paget's disease3) and disorders of calcium (hypocalcemia, hypercalcemia), phosphate (hypophosphatemia, hyperphosphatemia), and magnesium (hypomagnesemia, hypermagnesemia).

CALCIUM METABOLISM

The normal range for serum calcium concentration (total calcium) is 8.8 to 10.4 mg/dL (2.2 to 2.6 mmol/L) and is no different in younger and older persons. About 45% of serum calcium is bound to serum proteins, 5% is complexed with anions (eg, phosphate, bicarbonate, citrate), and 50% is ionized. The ionized fraction affects cellular function and is normally between 4.8 and 5.2 mg/dL (between 1.2 and 1.3 mmol/L).

The proportion of ionized calcium to total calcium depends on the concentration of plasma protein (particularly albumin), the concentration of anion bound to ionized calcium, and blood pH (acidosis decreases protein binding, alkalosis increases it). In addition, pH affects the interaction between ionized calcium and the cell membrane. Thus, when the ionized calcium concentration is even moderately decreased, alkalosis can precipitate tetany and acidosis can prevent it. In respiratory alkalosis, tetany can occur even with a normal ionized calcium concentration. Changes in potassium and magnesium concentrations can also alter the response to calcium.

If the ionized calcium concentration is unavailable, total calcium and albumin concentrations should be measured simultaneously, and the total calcium concentration should be corrected to compensate for any albumin deficit. This correction is important in the elderly because hypoalbuminemia is common, particularly in chronically ill and malnourished persons. The correction consists of adding 0.8 mg/dL (0.2 mmol/L) to the total calcium concentration for each 1 g/dL decrease in albumin below its normal concentration of 4 g/dL.

The constancy of serum ionized calcium blood concentrations results from a complex interaction between three major calcium-regulating hormones: parathyroid hormone (PTH), 1,25-dihydroxycholecalciferol, and calcitonin. The PTH concentration needed to maintain a normal serum calcium concentration seems to increase with age, presumably because the elderly have a relative calcium deficiency. With age, the

---

■ see page 472   2 see page 483   3 see page 480

intrinsic capacity of the intestine to absorb calcium decreases, and the response to 1,25-dihydroxycholecalciferol is blunted. Moreover, PTH-mediated renal synthesis of 1,25-dihydroxycholecalciferol may be impaired because renal mass is reduced. Decreased intake of calcium and vitamin D and estrogen deficiency may also contribute to calcium deficiency. No evidence indicates that the increased tubular reabsorption of calcium, the decreased tubular reabsorption of phosphate, or the stimulation of bone resorption by PTH is impaired in the elderly. In fact, the catabolic effects of PTH on bone may be enhanced, because bone resorption is increased and bone formation is decreased with age.

Serum concentrations of 25-hydroxycholecalciferol (the precursor of 1,25-dihydroxycholecalciferol) tend to decrease with age, probably because of decreased dietary intake or decreased sun exposure. Moreover, sunlight in the winter in temperate latitudes is insufficient to activate vitamin D synthesis in the skin. Concentrations of 1,25-dihydroxycholecalciferol are normal, however, in elderly persons who take vitamin D supplements.

HYPOCALCEMIA

A corrected serum calcium concentration < 8.8 mg/dL (< 2.2 mmol/L) or an ionized calcium concentration < 4.8 mg/dL (< 1.2 mmol/L).

Etiology and Pathogenesis

Causes of hypocalcemia are listed in TABLE 58–1. In the elderly, serum calcium tends to decrease for many reasons, including decreased intake of dairy products, lower serum albumin levels, and decreased vitamin D intake or activation. Impaired vitamin D activation is due in part to decreased exposure to sunlight and decreased vitamin D synthesis of the skin. Age-related decreases in hepatic and renal function lead to lower amounts of 25-hydroxycholecalciferol and 1,25-dihydroxycholecalciferol. Drugs may reduce body stores of calcium by increased elimination (eg, the loop diuretics are calciuric) or reduced absorption (eg, anticonvulsants stimulate hydroxylation pathways that produce metabolites of vitamin D that are less effective at absorbing calcium from the gastrointestinal [GI] tract).

A decreased total serum calcium concentration is common among chronically ill elderly patients. However, most of these patients have a normal corrected calcium concentration.

Symptoms and Signs

Mild hypocalcemia may be asymptomatic or accompanied by nonspecific central nervous system (CNS) signs. For example, a patient with chronic hypocalcemia may present with mild diffuse brain disease

TABLE 58-1. CAUSES OF HYPOCALCEMIA IN THE ELDERLY

Primary hypoparathyroidism	Pancreatitis
Surgical (transient or permanent)	Osteoblastic metastases
Idiopathic (autoimmune)	**Parathyroid hormone resistance**
Infiltrative (hemochromatosis or malignancy)	Pseudohypoparathyroidism
Severe hypomagnesemia	**Osteomalacia and rickets**
Relative hypoparathyroidism	Vitamin D deficiency
Inhibition of bone resorption (calcitonin, plicamycin, bisphosphonates)	Vitamin D resistance
Hyperphosphatemia	**False hypocalcemia**
	Decreased serum albumin

mimicking depression, dementia, or psychosis. Chronic hypocalcemia may cause cataracts and calcification of the basal ganglia. Chronic candidiasis may occur in patients with chronic hypocalcemia due to idiopathic hypoparathyroidism.

Tetany develops when hypocalcemia is severe or when an associated alkalosis increases neuromuscular irritability. Tetany is characterized by paresthesias (particularly around the mouth, lips, and tongue) and muscle spasms, particularly of the hands, feet, and face. Without concurrent alkalosis, tetany usually does not occur until the total serum calcium concentration is < 7 mg/dL (< 1.75 mmol/L) or the ionized calcium concentration is < 3 mg/dL (< 0.75 mmol/L). Patients who do not have tetany may still have latent neuromuscular irritability. Latent neuromuscular irritability can be demonstrated by Chvostek's sign (contraction of the facial muscles elicited by tapping the facial nerve) and Trousseau's sign (carpopedal spasm caused by a reduction of the blood supply to the hand when a tourniquet applied to the arm for 3 to 5 minutes exerts pressure that is higher than systolic blood pressure). Severe hypocalcemia can also occasionally cause cardiac arrhythmias and heart block.

Laboratory Findings and Diagnosis

Assessing a low corrected total or ionized calcium concentration requires concomitant measurements of serum creatinine, phosphate, magnesium, potassium, and bicarbonate. When the serum calcium concentration is low, the serum phosphate concentration is usually high. This inversion occurs even in severe vitamin D deficiency, when phosphate reserves are low, possibly because of a physicochemical effect on exchangeable calcium and phosphate in the skeleton. However, mild hypocalcemia can occur with hypophosphatemia, not only in patients with vitamin D deficiency but also in those who have both magnesium and phosphate depletion.

An ECG typically shows a prolonged QT interval.

Differentiation of vitamin D deficiency, pancreatic disease, or renal failure as the cause of hypocalcemia can usually be made based on clinical and laboratory features. The distinction between primary hypoparathyroidism and pseudohypoparathyroidism can be made by measuring immunoreactive PTH concentration; PTH is high only in pseudohypoparathyroidism. The phosphaturic response to PTH administration is also helpful. Human synthetic amino N-terminal 1-34 PTH (teriparatide acetate) is available for diagnosis.

Treatment

Calcitriol (1,25-dihydroxyvitamin D_3) and oral calcium supplements (1 to 2 g/day of elemental calcium) are used to rapidly increase the serum calcium concentration in most patients who have been hypocalcemic for > 1 day. Because of its relatively short half-life, calcitriol is usually given in divided doses of 0.5 to 2.0 μg/day po at 12-hour intervals.

Calcitriol has several advantages over other forms of vitamin D—it is rapidly absorbed, does not require further metabolism to become active, and is rapidly excreted. However, a dose of calcitriol only slightly greater than the physiologic replacement dose can cause severe hypercalcemia and hypercalciuria, although these effects disappear rapidly when the drug is discontinued. Thus, the serum calcium concentration should be monitored closely. With vitamin D itself or with calcidiol (25-hydroxyvitamin D_3), the margin of safety is greater, but these agents require further metabolism to become active; also, toxicity is prolonged, particularly when long-term therapy with large amounts of vitamin D produces accumulations in the liver and adipose tissue.

Calcitriol is also effective for chronic hypocalcemia in patients with primary hypoparathyroidism and pseudohypoparathyroidism; it can be combined with a calcium supplement (1 to 2 g/day of elemental calcium). When hypomagnesemia occurs with calcium, potassium, and phosphate deficiencies, correcting the hypomagnesemia makes treating the other deficiencies easier.

A thiazide diuretic or chlorthalidone can be used in some patients to increase phosphate excretion and decrease calcium excretion. Hypocalcemia from phosphate excess can be avoided by decreasing phosphate intake or by using aluminum hydroxide gel or large doses of calcium carbonate, which bind phosphate in the intestine and reduce its absorption.

An IV infusion of calcium is rarely needed but is used for the immediate treatment of tetany. Usually, 10% calcium gluconate is given IV over 5 to 10 minutes; subsequently, more may be added to a continuous IV drip. A large amount may be needed if much unmineralized osteoid is present, as often occurs in postoperative patients with primary or secondary hyperparathyroidism or hyperthyroidism and high-bone turnover (hungry bone syndrome); several grams of calcium may be needed during repletion. The dose is determined by closely monitoring the serum calcium concentration.

HYPERCALCEMIA

A corrected serum calcium concentration > 10.4 mg/dL (> 2.6 mmol/L) or an ionized calcium concentration > 5.2 mg/dL (> 1.3 mmol/L).

Hypercalcemia is common and dangerous in the elderly.

Etiology and Pathogenesis

Causes of hypercalcemia are listed in TABLE 58–2. In the elderly, hypercalcemia most often results from malignancy (eg, metastatic breast cancer, multiple myeloma). It can also result from primary hyperparathyroidism. Occasionally, patients with mild primary hyperparathyroidism develop severe hypercalcemia because of an intercurrent illness that causes dehydration. Immobilization can produce hypercalcemia in persons with rapid bone turnover; however, such rapid turnover is rare in the elderly, except in Paget's disease.

Familial benign hypocalciuric hypercalcemia is a hereditary form of hypercalcemia.

Symptoms and Signs

Mild hypercalcemia due to mild primary hyperparathyroidism is usually asymptomatic and is usually detected by the routine measurement of serum calcium. Affected patients may have related abnormalities, including hypertension, muscular weakness and irritability, mild GI disturbances, renal colic, bone cysts, impaired renal function (polyuria), and decreased bone mass.

Hypercalciuria and nephrolithiasis may occur and may be asymptomatic. Despite reversal of hypercalciuria and hypercalcemia, moderate or severe renal impairment may progress. The development of nephrocalcinosis produces irreversible damage.

Although symptomatic cystic bone lesions are rare, mild degrees of osteitis fibrosa cystica with subperiosteal bone resorption of the hands and a salt-and-pepper–like appearance of the skull can be observed radiologically. Patients with primary hyperparathyroidism usually lose cortical bone mass in the appendicular skeleton. Trabecular bone mass in the spine may be relatively well preserved, but elderly patients often lose trabecular bone, perhaps because they also have osteoporosis. With hyperparathyroidism, the risk of fracture (especially in the extremities) is probably increased, but data are limited.

In severe hypercalcemia, progressive dehydration may occur because of increased urinary output resulting from direct inhibition of renal tubular reabsorption of sodium and water and decreased fluid intake

TABLE 58-2.   CAUSES OF HYPERCALCEMIA IN THE ELDERLY

Increased bone resorption
Primary hyperparathyroidism
Persistent secondary (or tertiary)
hyperparathyroidism
Metastatic malignancy
Hematologic malignancy
Humoral hypercalcemia of malignancy
Immobilization
Hyperthyroidism
Increased intestinal absorption
Vitamin D toxicity
Milk-alkali syndrome
Sarcoidosis and other granulomas

Miscellaneous
Familial benign hypocalciuric
hypercalcemia
Addison's disease
Acute renal failure (recovery
phase)

False hypercalcemia
Hemoconcentration
Increased calcium-binding
proteins or anions

resulting from anorexia, nausea, and vomiting. Hypercalcemia can cause potassium loss, which may be aggravated by saline loading. When the serum calcium concentration is > 12 mg/dL (> 3 mmol/L), mental confusion can occur. As the patient becomes increasingly dehydrated, the calcium concentration may increase, resulting in coma and death. *Calcium concentrations > 16 mg/dL (> 4 mmol/L) are life threatening and constitute a medical emergency.*

Laboratory Findings and Diagnosis

In primary hyperparathyroidism, the serum calcium concentration is elevated and the phosphate concentration is decreased. Tubular reabsorption of calcium is increased, and tubular reabsorption of phosphate is decreased. Because the filtered load of calcium is also increased, calcium excretion may be high, although it rarely exceeds 500 mg/24 hours (12.5 mmol/24 hours). Many elderly patients with mild chronic primary hyperparathyroidism and minimal serum calcium elevation have a normal or low rate of urinary calcium excretion. Urine and serum calcium and phosphate concentrations may be the same in primary hyperparathyroidism and hypercalcemia of malignancy; therefore, these measurements are not useful in differential diagnosis.

Sustained mild hypercalcemia over several years strongly indicates primary hyperparathyroidism, although occasionally sarcoidosis may be the cause. Mild hyperchloremic acidosis can occur in patients with hyperparathyroidism but is less likely to occur with other forms of hypercalcemia.

A rapid onset of hypercalcemia, especially with anemia, weight loss, and hypoalbuminemia, suggests malignancy. Serum protein electrophoresis, thyroid function tests, and a chest x-ray should be obtained in all cases. Additional tests for specific malignant disorders should be performed when appropriate.

In vitamin D toxicity, milk-alkali syndrome, and hyperthyroidism, the serum phosphate concentration is usually normal or elevated. Vitamin D toxicity can be detected by measuring the serum 25-hydroxycholecalciferol concentration. 1,25-Dihydroxycholecalciferol is elevated in primary hyperparathyroidism, in sarcoidosis, and occasionally in hematopoietic malignancies.

Measuring intact circulating immunoreactive PTH is critical in the differential diagnosis of hypercalcemia. Most patients with primary hyperparathyroidism have elevated PTH concentrations (although PTH may be in the normal range), and most patients with malignancy have suppressed PTH concentrations. Patients with vitamin D intoxication, milk-alkali syndrome, and sarcoidosis also have low PTH concentrations. However, in the elderly, interpretation of PTH assays is complicated because concentrations normally increase slightly with age. Therefore, high, normal, or slightly elevated levels with normal serum calcium concentration do not indicate primary hyperparathyroidism.

Because coexisting hyperparathyroidism and malignancy are not rare in elderly patients, signs of malignancy (eg, hypoalbuminemia, anemia, weight loss) may occur. Patients with known malignancy and nonsuppressed PTH concentrations are likely to have primary hyperparathyroidism and may benefit from parathyroidectomy.

Localization of a parathyroid adenoma, although not strictly diagnostic, may help to avoid prolonged surgical exploration and permit the use of local anesthesia. The combined technetium-sestamibi and radioiodine scan is the most useful test for this purpose. However, false-negative test results are common and false-positive results can occur with a multinodular goiter, which is common in older patients.

In familial benign hypocalciuric hypercalcemia, PTH concentrations may be only modestly elevated, and urinary calcium excretion is low (which can also occur with primary hyperparathyroidism). Serum calcium concentrations of family members may be needed to confirm the diagnosis. Familial benign hypocalciuric hypercalcemia may be confused with primary hyperparathyroidism, possibly leading to inappropriate parathyroidectomy.

Treatment

Treatment depends on the serum calcium concentration, the rapidity of onset of hypercalcemia, the severity of associated symptoms, and the underlying cause. In patients with serum calcium concentrations > 12 mg/dL (> 3 mmol/L), especially if onset is recent, immediate efforts should be made to reduce concentrations while diagnostic studies are undertaken.

Because dehydration and impaired renal function often contribute to hypercalcemia, the first step is rehydration. Extracellular fluid volume should be expanded with IV 0.9% sodium chloride solution. Because elderly patients may have difficulty handling large fluid loads, furosemide may also be needed; this diuretic increases urinary calcium and sodium excretion but should be given only if necessary to prevent or treat fluid overload. Effective reduction of serum calcium with furosemide requires large doses (80 to 100 mg IV q 2 h), which can produce recurrent dehydration or hypotension in the elderly. Rarely, hemodialysis is used to treat severe hypercalcemia unresponsive to other therapy.

Serum potassium concentrations should be monitored and potassium replaced as necessary. Hypophosphatemia is usually not a problem, but when the serum inorganic phosphate concentration is < 1 mg/dL (< 0.3 mmol/L), IV phosphate replacement may be appropriate. (CAUTION: *Except under these circumstances, IV phosphate therapy should be avoided, particularly in the presence of hypercalcemia.*) IV phosphate therapy should be closely monitored and should be discontinued when serum phosphate concentrations become normal or when renal function decreases, because irreversible tissue damage can occur if calcium phosphate salts become deposited in the tissues of the kidneys, blood vessels, and lungs.∎

Calcitonin rapidly lowers serum calcium, although usually not to normal concentrations. However, despite continued administration of calcitonin, tachyphylaxis usually develops in 48 to 72 hours. Tachyphylaxis may be caused by down-regulation of calcitonin receptors or postreceptor desensitization. Nevertheless, calcitonin acts rapidly, is safe, and is often used in the initial treatment of hypercalcemia, together with other more effective drugs. Prednisone 20 to 40 mg/day po (which may be divided into bid or tid dosing) reduces hypercalcemia in patients with vitamin D intoxication and sarcoidosis. Rarely, patients with prostaglandin-dependent hypercalcemia respond to nonsteroidal anti-inflammatory drugs (eg, indomethacin). However, because these drugs can further impair renal function, particularly in patients who are dehydrated or who have renal damage, they should probably be avoided.

Patients with hypercalcemia of metastatic malignancy, humoral hypercalcemia of malignancy, or any type of hypercalcemia in which the serum calcium concentration remains markedly elevated after hydration require additional therapy. The best way to reduce the serum calcium concentration in such patients is to inhibit bone resorption with a bisphosphonate. The most potent bisphosphonate available for IV use is pamidronate. When given in a single IV infusion of 60 mg in 500 to 1000 mL of 0.9% sodium chloride or 5% dextrose in water over 4 hours, pamidronate can reduce serum calcium concentrations in most patients in 2 to 3 days; repeated infusions may be required. Often, the reduction in serum calcium is long-lasting. Pamidronate is relatively safe, although transient fever often occurs on the day after the infusion,

∎ see page 581

and large doses may inhibit bone resorption so much that hypocalcemia develops.

Etidronate, which is also available for IV infusion, must be given in larger doses (7.5 mg/kg in 250 mL of 0.9% sodium chloride solution daily for 3 to 6 days) and is less effective. Oral bisphosphonates such as alendronate can be used to maintain the inhibition of bone resorption.

Treatment for primary hyperparathyroidism is surgical, and exploration of the neck should be considered as soon as the diagnosis is made. Age alone is not a contraindication to surgery. When performed by a skilled head and neck surgeon, the operation is well tolerated even in patients > 80 years and often produces a substantial improvement in health. However, patients may develop transient hypocalcemia after adenoma removal, probably from a combination of suppression of the remaining parathyroid glands and the hungry bone syndrome (as a result of calcium returning to bone after the PTH stimulus is removed). Vigorous treatment with calcitriol and IV and oral calcium should be instituted early to avoid tetany. Surgery is curative in 80 to 90% of patients. In patients with single adenomas, recurrences are extremely rare. In patients with multiple gland hyperplasia in whom most of the parathyroid tissue is removed, disease may recur, although usually not for several years. Adenoma removal can reverse some of the symptoms and signs due to hypercalcemia; however, hypertension, renal impairment, and CNS symptoms may persist after surgery.

Because mild primary hyperparathyroidism is rarely progressive or life threatening, many patients may elect to be monitored without surgery. These patients must be monitored at 6-month intervals for an increase in serum calcium concentration, hypercalciuria, bone loss, or impaired renal function. In patients with low bone mass in whom surgery is contraindicated or refused, estrogens or bisphosphonates can prevent further loss. Patients should be warned to avoid dehydration and to contact a physician if vomiting or diarrhea occurs because the renal effects of hypercalcemia may begin a vicious cycle of increased serum calcium concentration and further dehydration.

In familial benign hypocalciuric hypercalcemia, treatment other than the occasional need for calcium-lowering measures is rarely needed.

PHOSPHATE METABOLISM

Serum phosphate concentrations vary much more than serum calcium concentrations. The normal range is 2.5 to 4.5 mg/dL (0.8 to 1.5 mmol/L) of phosphorus as inorganic phosphate. Eighty percent of the body's phosphate is stored in bone as hydroxyapatite; the remaining 20% is largely organic. Phosphate-containing nucleic acids, nucleotides, phospholipids, and phosphoproteins are vital to energy metabolism, membrane function, and cell replication.

HYPOPHOSPHATEMIA

A serum concentration of inorganic phosphorus < 2.5 mg/dL (< 0.8 mmol/L).

Etiology

Mild hypophosphatemia is common in the elderly and probably results from decreased intake and impaired intestinal absorption of phosphate. The age-related increase in parathyroid function might also lower the renal threshold for tubular reabsorption of phosphate. Severe hypophosphatemia (serum concentrations < 1.5 mg/dL [< 0.5 mmol/L]) usually results from prolonged, severe decreased dietary intake and impaired absorption or from renal tubular dysfunction. Vomiting, acidosis, and alcoholic ketoacidosis may also contribute to hypophosphatemia. Aluminum hydroxide antacids, renal dialysis, and a rapid recovery of renal function after acute renal failure or transplantation are other causes of phosphate loss. Serum phosphate concentrations may also be extremely low with relatively mild degrees of intracellular phosphate depletion when extracellular phosphate rapidly shifts into the cells. This shift usually occurs when insulin and glucose are administered together in the treatment of diabetes.

Symptoms and Signs

Hypophosphatemia is usually asymptomatic. However, chronic severe hypophosphatemia can cause anorexia, muscle weakness, and osteomalacia. Rhabdomyolysis, hemolytic anemia, and impaired leukocyte and platelet function may occur, as may progressive encephalopathy, coma, and death.

Treatment

Because IV phosphate therapy can cause hypocalcemia and soft tissue calcification and because many elderly patients have impaired renal function and do not handle phosphate loads well, IV phosphate must be administered cautiously, even when serum concentrations are extremely low. Patients with severe phosphate depletion often have depleted concentrations of other ions, particularly potassium and magnesium; determining which abnormality is causing the symptoms can be difficult. However, patients with extremely low phosphate concentrations and evidence of impaired central nervous system (CNS) function and muscular weakness should receive IV sodium phosphate; those who also have a potassium depletion should also receive IV potassium phosphate. Serum calcium, inorganic phosphate, potassium, and magnesium concentrations should be monitored.

Oral phosphate supplements are usually unnecessary in patients with adequate diets. However, in hypophosphatemic patients who also have hypercalcemia, these supplements may lower the serum calcium concentration. Elderly patients have difficulty taking > 1 to 2 g/day of oral phosphate, even when administered in divided doses, because of diarrhea.

HYPERPHOSPHATEMIA

A serum concentration of inorganic phosphorus > 4.5 mg/dL (> 1.5 mmol/L).

Hyperphosphatemia occurs most commonly in patients with chronic renal failure.∎ In rare cases, severe hyperphosphatemia occurs in patients who undergo rapid cell lysis with release of phosphate. This condition can occur in patients with leukemia or other tumors who receive chemotherapy. Excessive intake of phosphate rarely causes hyperphosphatemia, partly because a high phosphate concentration leads to diarrhea and partly because renal excretion is efficient. Hyperphosphatemia caused by large volumes of phosphate-containing enemas has been reported. If the serum phosphate concentration is extremely high, calcium phosphate salts are deposited in bone and soft tissue, and the serum calcium concentration may fall, producing tetany. Most patients are asymptomatic.

Treatment

When renal function is normal and hydration is maintained, hyperphosphatemia is usually transient. If tetany occurs, IV calcium may be needed. (CAUTION: *Excessive administration of IV calcium in the presence of a high phosphate concentration can cause deposition of calcium phosphate salts and lead to acute kidney, blood vessel, and lung damage.*)

In chronic renal failure, hyperphosphatemia can be controlled by a low phosphate intake and administration of calcium or aluminum salts, which bind phosphate.

MAGNESIUM METABOLISM

Maintaining normal serum magnesium concentration depends mainly on dietary intake, although renal and intestinal mechanisms usually conserve magnesium. Magnesium, a cation abundant in the body, is distributed almost equally between bone and soft tissue. Intracellular magnesium is needed for many enzyme activities, particularly those involving nucleotide phosphate metabolism, and plays a vital role in DNA, RNA, and protein synthesis. Unlike serum calcium concentration, serum magnesium concentration is not tightly regulated and can vary considerably depending on diet and changes in cellular uptake. The normal serum magnesium concentration is 1.7 to 2.2 mg/dL (1.4 to

∎ see page 962

1.8 mEq, 0.7 to 0.9 mmol/L). About 20 to 30% of serum magnesium is bound to plasma proteins; magnesium may compete with calcium for protein binding.

Evidence of primary regulation of serum magnesium is scant, but high concentrations can inhibit parathyroid hormone (PTH) secretion, presumably acting at the same sites as extracellular calcium. Although low magnesium concentrations may stimulate PTH secretion transiently, marked depletion (< 0.9 mg/dL [< 0.4 mmol/L]) can impair PTH secretion, possibly leading to hypocalcemia.

HYPOMAGNESEMIA

Serum magnesium concentration < 1.7 mg/dL (< 1.4 mEq, < 0.7 mmol/L).

Common in elderly patients, mild to moderate hypomagnesemia is probably not an accurate reflection of intracellular or bone stores, which can be maintained long after serum concentrations begin to decrease. Nevertheless, hypomagnesemia is a warning sign that depletion may develop. Conversely, tissue depletion of magnesium may occur with normal serum concentrations.

Etiology

Causes of magnesium depletion include dietary deprivation, renal loss, and GI disorders, including vomiting, diarrhea, and malabsorption syndrome. Renal loss can occur in many conditions, including aldosterone excess, diuretic therapy, and diabetes mellitus. A few patients develop severe magnesium depletion because of a primary defect in renal tubular reabsorption of magnesium. Alcoholism often causes magnesium depletion. Serum magnesium concentrations fall rapidly in some patients after parathyroid adenomas are removed, presumably because of a rapid uptake in bone.

Symptoms and Signs

Symptoms and signs are nonspecific. Neuromuscular irritability and muscle weakness are common. Because hypomagnesemia is often associated with low serum concentrations of calcium, potassium, and phosphate, attributing particular symptoms or signs to magnesium depletion is difficult. Magnesium depletion may cause arrhythmias and increased sensitivity to cardiac glycosides and may contribute to hypertension and atherosclerosis.

Treatment

When possible, magnesium depletion should be avoided by maintaining adequate dietary intake. Mild hypomagnesemia can usually be reversed with a magnesium-rich diet. If hypomagnesemia has been prolonged or if parathyroid and cell functions are likely to be impaired,

50% magnesium sulfate (4 mEq/mL) 2.5 mL IM can be given. Patients at high risk of hypotension should receive a smaller dose. Magnesium sulfate can be given IV (1 mEq/kg) but only as a more dilute solution ($\leq$ 10%) over 24 hours with half the dose given in the first 3 hours and the remaining half over the rest of the day.

Replacement of magnesium by the oral route is difficult because magnesium salts are powerful laxatives and because magnesium depletion often occurs in persons with GI disorders. Small amounts of oral magnesium hydroxide or magnesium chloride can be used, but some patients require magnesium sulfate IM at regular intervals to prevent deficiency.

When hypomagnesemia occurs with calcium, potassium, or phosphate deficiencies, correcting the hypomagnesemia makes treating the other deficiencies easier.

HYPERMAGNESEMIA

Serum magnesium concentration > 2.5 mg/dL (> 2.0 mEq/L, > 1 mmol/L).

Hypermagnesemia is rare except in renal failure or after parenteral magnesium administration. It can depress central nervous system and cardiac functions. ECG changes include PR prolongation, QRS widening, and T-wave amplitude increase. Furosemide or ethacrynic acid, administered IV, increases magnesium excretion if hydration is maintained and renal function is adequate. Severe magnesium intoxication requires 10 to 20 mL of 10% calcium gluconate given IV, together with circulatory and respiratory support. Dialysis is required occasionally.

59 ▮ DISORDERS OF ACID-BASE METABOLISM

The normal pH of extracellular fluid (range, 7.35 to 7.45) is unaffected by age. However, age-related changes do occur in certain respiratory and renal regulatory processes involved in maintaining normal pH, and the ability to respond to a challenge may be limited. For example, the ability to hyperventilate in response to acute metabolic acidosis may be blunted, leading to a further decline in pH. The aging kidney is slower to respond to an acid load, and the blood pH may take longer to recover. Many disorders common in the elderly (eg, heart failure, anemia, sepsis, diabetes mellitus, renal and pulmonary disease) can overwhelm the regulatory systems and contribute to acid-base disturbances.

Also, many commonly used drugs (eg, salicylates, diuretics, laxatives) may precipitate acid-base disturbances. The combination of impaired homeostatic mechanisms and the high prevalence of drug use and disease in the elderly make acid-base disturbances common.

METABOLIC ACIDOSIS

A condition characterized by a primary decease in extracellular fluid bicarbonate; serum pH and carbon dioxide content are decreased.

The serum anion gap, which may help identify the cause of metabolic acidosis (see TABLE 59–1), is determined as follows: Serum sodium – (serum chloride + total CO_2) = ± 2. The urine anion gap is calculated as follows: (urine sodium + urine potassium) – urine chloride ≤ 0.

A non-anion gap metabolic acidosis (NAGMA) is due to a failure of bicarbonate homeostasis and is characterized by a compensatory retention of the other main body anions, which results in hyperchloremia. NAGMA results from renal tubular acidosis or from a loss of bicarbonate or organic acid anions in patients with diarrhea.

If there is a serum NAGMA and the urine anion gap is ≤ 0, gastrointestinal loss of bicarbonate (diarrhea) is the cause of the metabolic acidosis. A NAGMA with a urine anion gap ≥ 0 suggests type 1 (distal) or type 4 renal tubular acidosis. A urine pH > 5.5 with metabolic acidosis suggests distal tubular inability to acidify the urine and occurs with type 1 or type 4 renal tubular acidosis. In the elderly, type 1 renal tubular acidosis may be caused by amphotericin therapy or by tubular dysfunction

TABLE 59–1.   METABOLIC ACIDOSIS IN THE ELDERLY

Non-anion gap
  Urine anion gap < 0 → GI losses of bicarbonate
  Urine anion gap ≥ 0
    Urine pH < 5.5 → type 2 (proximal) RTA or carbonic anhydrase
    inhibitors
    Urine pH always > 5.5 + low or normal potassium → type 1
    (distal) RTA due to amphotericin or myeloma
    Urine pH always > 5.5 + hyperkalemia → type 4 RTA due to
    urinary tract obstruction, diabetes mellitus, or drugs that interfere
    with the prostaglandin-renin-aldosterone axis

Anion gap elevation
  Ketoacidosis
  Uremia
  Salicylate ingestion
  Methanol intoxication
  Alcohol ingestion
  Lactic acidosis

GI = gastrointestinal; RTA = renal tubular acidosis.

due to the myeloma protein in multiple myeloma. Type 2 (proximal) renal tubular acidosis is uncommon in the elderly as a primary defect of tubular function but can result from the bicarbonate diuresis caused by carbonic anhdrase inhibitors used to treat glaucoma. In this disorder, there is NAGMA, but after the bicarbonate diuresis, urine pH is < 5.5 during acidosis due to normal distal hydrogen ion urine acidification capability.

Type 4 renal tubular acidosis is caused by urinary tract obstruction, diabetes mellitus, or drugs that interfere with aldosterone (eg, distal angiotensin-converting enzyme inhibitors, angiotensin-receptor blockers). Acidosis with an increased anion gap (such as occurs with lactic acidosis, diabetic ketoacidosis, salicylate toxicity, toxic alcohol ingestion, and renal failure) is more common. Type 4 renal tubular acidosis is characterized by tubular dysfunction that is worse than that in type 1. The added tubular dysfunction is suggested by concomitant hyperkalemia.

Diagnosis is usually established by the history, physical examination findings (eg, hyperpnea), and laboratory findings (eg, blood gas determinations; urine pH; and blood urea nitrogen [BUN], creatinine, blood glucose, and ketone levels).

Initial treatment aims to correct the underlying disease process. When severe acidosis (pH < 7.2) is accompanied by anorexia, nausea, lethargy, hyperventilation, and decline in cardiac output, treatment should be started with IV sodium bicarbonate. Acute complete correction of arterial pH is not a goal of therapy, and caution must be used to avoid volume and sodium overload. Commonly, 2 to 3 ampules (44 mEq/L each) of sodium bicarbonate are dissolved in 5% dextrose in water and administered at a rate of 50 to 100 mL/h.

METABOLIC ALKALOSIS

A condition characterized by a primary increase in extracellular fluid bicarbonate; pH and carbon dioxide content are increased.

Metabolic alkalosis results from net acid loss or alkali gain in the extracellular fluid. Acid loss can result from vomiting, prolonged gastric suctioning, and diuretic use. The concomitant chloride deficiency requires that the high bicarbonate be reabsorbed with sodium and will not correct until adequate chloride ion is available (ie, treated with sodium chloride, potassium chloride, or hydrochloride). The chloride-resistant forms of metabolic alkalosis common in the elderly include an excessive mineralocorticoid effect of chronic prednisone administration, renin-angiotensin-aldosterone stimulation due to renal atherosclerosis, Cushing's disease, primary aldosteronism, and ectopic corticotropin (ACTH) production due to malignancy. In these cases, the mineralocorticoid excess dictates excessive renal generation of bicarbonate because of stimulated sodium/hydrogen exchange. Treatment is directed toward mineralocorticoid antagonism. Lethargy and stupor may occur from adverse effects on the cerebral circulation. Arrhythmias, especially due to digitalis toxicity, are common. Therapy depends on whether the metabolic alkalosis is sensitive or resistant to chloride. The chloride-sensitive forms respond to administration of chloride, such as in normal saline. Gastric acid and chloride losses can be reduced by giving a histamine-2 blocker or a proton pump inhibitor. Bicarbonate diuresis can also be accomplished using carbonic anhydrase inhibition; acetazolamide 250 mg IV can be given bid or qid in severe cases or when patients are unable to take drugs orally. Chloride-resistant forms require treatment of the underlying disorder or mineralocorticoid antagonism with spironolactone. A dose of 50 to 100 mg/day po in divided doses may help patients with chronic alkalosis.

RESPIRATORY ACIDOSIS

A primary increase in arterial carbon dioxide partial pressure; pH is decreased and total carbon dioxide content is increased if renal function is intact.

Respiratory acidosis is caused by carbon dioxide retention from alveolar hypoventilation, which may result from disorders that depress the central respiratory center, restrict chest wall mobility, reduce pulmonary alveolar surface area, or narrow the upper airway. The elderly are at risk because of their reduced vital capacity and ventilatory responses to hypoxia and hypercapnia. Common causes are drugs that can produce respiratory depression, neuromuscular disorders, and pulmonary disorders. Respiratory acidosis is often accompanied by hypoxia. Progressive respiratory failure often results in a metabolic encephalopathy with headache, drowsiness, and ultimately stupor and coma. Asterixis and myoclonus may develop.

Treatment aims to improve the underlying pulmonary disorder and may include intubation and assisted mechanical ventilation. Hypoxia must be corrected with the lowest possible oxygen concentration to avoid further depression of respiratory drive. Many patients also have concomitant metabolic alkalosis.

RESPIRATORY ALKALOSIS

A primary decrease in arterial carbon dioxide partial pressure; pH is increased and total carbon dioxide content is decreased.

The hyperventilation usually present leads to an excessive loss of carbon dioxide. Common causes include mechanical overventilation, hypoxemia, sepsis, pulmonary embolism, heart failure, hepatic failure, primary central nervous system disorders, and salicylate toxicity. Anxiety can cause a mild, acute respiratory alkalosis with a characteristic hyperventilation syndrome. Physiologic consequences of respiratory alkalosis include cerebral vasoconstriction, with resulting cerebral hypoxia and decreased ionized serum calcium concentrations leading to tetany and hypophosphatemia. Treatment consists of correcting the underlying disorder or, in the case of hyperventilation syndrome, supervised breathing into a paper bag.

60 ■ VITAMIN AND TRACE MINERAL DISORDERS

Mild vitamin deficiencies are very common among elderly persons (particularly frail and institutionalized elderly) and are associated with cognitive impairment, poor wound healing, anemia, and an increased propensity for developing infections. Trace mineral deficiencies are associated with immune system dysfunction and many other disorders.

Elderly persons who are at risk of or who are suspected of having protein-energy undernutrition■ should be presumed to also be at risk for multiple vitamin deficiencies. Undernutrition of < 1 year usually causes deficiencies in the B vitamins and in vitamin C (ie, the water-soluble vitamins). Undernutrition of longer duration usually also causes deficiencies in vitamins A, D, E, and K (ie, the fat-soluble vitamins) and in vitamin B_{12}, which have larger body stores. Deficiencies can also be associated with certain diseases, high-risk behaviors (eg, smoking, alcohol abuse), and medication use (see TABLE 60–1).

Tests to diagnose early vitamin deficiencies can be difficult and expensive; thus, supplementation with a multivitamin containing at least the recommended dietary allowances (RDAs) is recommended for elderly patients at risk. Because extreme vitamin deficiency can cause irreversible organ damage, supplementation should begin before signs appear.

The benefit of routine vitamin supplementation for healthy elderly persons is controversial. A diet that includes at least five or six daily servings of fruits and vegetables usually contains sufficient vitamins (as well as other healthful phytochemicals available only in food). However, a less healthful diet probably requires daily supplementation. There is also evidence that a multivitamin supplement improves immune status in healthy elderly persons. The new Dietary Reference Intakes (an expansion of the RDAs) issued by the Food and Nutrition

■ see page 595

TABLE 60-1.   SUBSTANCES THAT MAY AFFECT VITAMIN OR MINERAL FUNCTION

Substance	Vitamin or Mineral Affected
Alcohol	Thiamine (B_1), other B vitamins, folic acid, magnesium
Antacids	Vitamin B_{12}, calcium, iron
Anticonvulsants	Vitamin D, folic acid
Cholestyramine	Vitamin B_{12}
Fiber in diet	Calcium, iron, zinc
Hydralazine	Pyridoxine (vitamin B_6)
Iron	Vitamin C
Isoniazid	Pyridoxine (vitamin B_6)
Levodopa	Pyridoxine (vitamin B_6)
Methotrexate	Folic acid
Penicillamine	Pyridoxine (vitamin B_6)
Sulfasalazine	Folic acid
Tobacco	Vitamin C
Trimethoprim	Folic acid

Board at the Institute of Medicine lists the recommended daily requirements of vitamins and minerals for healthy persons, including tolerable upper intake levels.

VITAMINS

VITAMIN A

Vitamin A deficiency is uncommon except with prolonged starvation. Toxicity may occur with intake above the RDA of 800 to 1000 µg retinol equivalents (> 2700 to 3300 IU); the symptoms of toxicity (liver, skin, mucous membrane, and mental changes) are nonspecific and difficult to recognize.

A diet rich in fruits and vegetables, which contain carotenoids (including β-carotene), is highly recommended for everyone. β-Carotene is often called pro-vitamin A but does not have the toxicity of regular vitamin A. Supplementation with β-carotene alone, however, is not recommended, because high intake can turn the skin yellow-orange, and there is some concern that it may increase the risk of cancer.

VITAMIN D

For the elderly, daily vitamin D intake of up to 600 to 800 IU (RDA = 200 IU [5 µg]) may strengthen bones and protect against some cancers (eg, prostate cancer).**1** Higher intakes are not recommended because the resulting hypercalcemia rapidly increases the toxicity.**2**

1 see also page 657   **2** see page 576

Dietary sources of vitamin D include fortified dairy products (8 oz of fortified milk contains 100 IU). Vitamin D is also produced by exposure to moderate direct sunlight, although such exposure can have photoaging and carcinogenic effects on the skin. Synthetic forms of vitamin D are under study.

VITAMIN E

A low-fat diet may be deficient in vitamin E, which is found primarily in vegetable oils and the products made from these oils (eg, margarine, mayonnaise). Vitamin E is a common supplement. When taken in doses exceeding the RDA (ie, > 8 to 10 IU), the antioxidant effects of vitamin E may lower the risk of cardiovascular disease, peripheral vascular disease, and certain eye diseases. This high dose also acts as an anticoagulant, which may lower the risk of myocardial infarction. Whether the high dose increases the risk of bleeding remains unclear. Vitamin E improves cellular immune function, which potentially lowers the risk of infection. Its hypothetical protective effect against certain neurologic diseases (eg, Parkinson's disease, Alzheimer's disease) is under study.

The long-term consequences of high-dose supplementation are unknown. Vitamin E has very low toxicity at intakes < 800 IU, but vitamin E can affect coagulation in patients taking warfarin. Daily supplemental doses > 800 IU generally are not recommended. Vitamin E complex, which contains various subtypes of vitamin E, may be more beneficial than α-tocopherol alone.

THIAMINE

(Vitamin B$_1$)

Thiamine deficiency usually occurs with deficiency of the other B vitamins. Symptoms of deficiency, which are vague, include anorexia, weight loss, confusion, apathy, and weakness. Isolated thiamine deficiency can lead to beriberi, causing heart failure and peripheral nerve damage. Deficiency is very rare in developed countries but can occur with psychiatric eating disorders. Thiamine supplementation (100 mg daily) is recommended for persons with chronic alcoholism to prevent Wernicke's encephalopathy and psychosis (Korsakoff's syndrome).

RIBOFLAVIN

(Vitamin B$_2$)

Riboflavin deficiency generally occurs with other B-vitamin deficiencies and can manifest as inflammation of the mouth and tongue or cracking of the lips. The possible role of riboflavin in preventing migraine headaches is under study.

PYRIDOXINE

(Vitamin B$_6$)

Several drugs can affect pyridoxine function (see TABLE 60–1). Pyridoxine deficiency usually occurs with other water-soluble B-vitamin deficiencies. Pyridoxine may play a minor role, compared with folic acid, in causing an elevated homocysteine level in the blood and an increased risk of vascular disease. Supplementation does not lessen symptoms of carpal tunnel syndrome, contrary to some health food advertisers' claims. High intake of pyridoxine (ie, > 100 mg daily [RDA = 1.5 to 1.7 mg daily]) may increase toxicity or decrease efficacy of many drugs used to treat Parkinson's disease and seizures and can cause sensory neuropathy in the lower extremities.

VITAMIN B$_{12}$

In younger adults, vitamin B$_{12}$ deficiency is usually due to loss of intrinsic factor secretion needed to absorb the vitamin in the distal ileum. In the elderly, however, more common causes of vitamin B$_{12}$ deficiency are decreased gastric acid production (hypochlorhydria— occurring in up to 15% of persons > 65) and *Helicobacter pylori* infection of the stomach. Thus, the Schilling test, which is used to measure intrinsic factor in younger adults, usually is not used to detect vitamin B$_{12}$ deficiency in the elderly.

Vitamin B$_{12}$ deficiency causes hematologic and neurologic signs and symptoms. Hematologic signs include anemia with macrocytosis and megaloblastic changes noted as hypersegmented polymorphonuclear leukocytes.∎ Neurologic damage is independent of the hematologic changes and results in nonspecific paresthesias (eg, numbness) of the extremities, abnormal position and vibration sense, difficulty walking (ie, gait ataxia from degeneration of the posterolateral columns of the spinal cord), and mental confusion, each of which can occur in many other age-related diseases. However, vitamin B$_{12}$ deficiency only rarely causes symptoms similar to the slowly progressive mental changes typical of Alzheimer's disease. Although vitamin B$_{12}$ plays a role in homocysteine metabolism and arteriosclerosis, folic acid appears to play a much more significant role.

Vitamin B$_{12}$ deficiency has four hematologic stages: negative vitamin B$_{12}$ balance, vitamin B$_{12}$ depletion, vitamin B$_{12}$-deficient erythropoiesis,

∎ see page 685

and vitamin B_{12} deficiency anemia. The first two stages are characterized by a serum vitamin B_{12} level of < 350 picograms [pg]/mL (< 260 picomoles [pmol/L]) and a reduced holotranscobalamin II and transcobalamin II saturation. (The latter two tests are not commercially available.) In the third stage, hypersegmented neutrophils appear, the holotranscobalamin II and the transcobalamin II saturation fall further, and serum methylmalonic acid levels begin to increase slightly. The patient is still not anemic, and the mean corpuscular volume is often normal. By the fourth stage, all standard laboratory test results are abnormal, and the patient is anemic.∎

The stage at which neurologic damage occurs is not known but may predate macrocytosis and anemia. Irreversible neurologic damage and dementia can occur before hypersegmentation develops and before methylmalonic acid levels rise; therefore, screening frail elderly persons for low serum vitamin B_{12} levels is recommended. Persons who are vegans, who are infected with HIV, who are receiving prolonged antacid therapy, or who have had stomach or small-bowel surgery or disease should be monitored for early deficiency.

The serum vitamin B_{12} determination remains the most practical way to discover vitamin B_{12} depletion. Diagnosis is confirmed by a serum vitamin B_{12} level < 200 pg/mL (< 150 pmol/L). Low-normal levels—those between 200 and 350 pg/mL (150 and 260 pmol/L)—should be confirmed by demonstrating an elevated serum or urine methylmalonic acid level. Early (and reversible) vitamin B_{12} deficiency may elevate the methylmalonic acid level before the serum vitamin level falls. The Schilling test is not as useful in the elderly because decreased vitamin B_{12} absorption is usually not due to lack of intrinsic factor, and treatment of all vitamin B_{12} deficiency is similar.

Because it is not known which cases will progress to anemia or neurologic injury if untreated, treatment is recommended (see TABLE 60–2). Oral and nasal replacement forms of vitamin B_{12} are available, but elderly persons with symptoms or signs of deficiency should be given monthly IM injections of vitamin B_{12}. The RDA for vitamin B_{12} is only 2.4 μg, but supplemental doses as high as 1000 to 2000 μg (daily if given orally, monthly if given by injection) may be necessary when treating deficiency.

FOLIC ACID

(Folate)

Deficiency of folic acid, one of the water-soluble B-vitamins, is often seen with malnutrition, alcohol abuse, or use of certain substances (see TABLE 60–1). Folic acid plays a major role in lowering homocysteine

∎ see page 685

TABLE 60–2.   GUIDELINES FOR MANAGEMENT OF VITAMIN B$_{12}$ DEFICIENCY

1. Frail elderly patients should undergo routine screening of serum vitamin B$_{12}$ levels. A serum vitamin B$_{12}$ level of < 200 pg/mL (< 150 pmol/L) indicates vitamin B$_{12}$ deficiency. A serum vitamin B$_{12}$ level of 200–350 pg/mL (150–260 pmol/L) suggests vitamin B$_{12}$ depletion, and the test should be repeated in 1–3 mo or a methylmalonic acid level should be obtained.

2. For most elderly patients, a Schilling test is unnecessary unless the patient is otherwise known to be at risk of autoimmune pernicious anemia.

3. Even if the patient has no hematologic or neurologic abnormalities or the routine fasting Schilling test result is normal, a serum vitamin B$_{12}$ level of < 200 pg/mL requires treatment.

4. Vitamin B$_{12}$ 1000–2000 μg/day po should be given until serum vitamin B$_{12}$ levels increase to > 350 pg/mL.

5. A patient with any symptoms or signs of vitamin B$_{12}$ deficiency, an abnormal Schilling test result, or a vitamin B$_{12}$ serum level that does not increase to > 350 pg/mL with oral vitamin B$_{12}$ should be treated with parenteral vitamin B$_{12}$ (as if the patient has pernicious anemia).

levels. High homocysteine levels (> 10 to 15 μmol/L) are associated with a 2- to 40-fold increased risk of coronary artery disease, cerebrovascular disease, and peripheral vascular disease. The role of folic acid in preventing or treating these diseases is being studied. The RDA is 400 μg daily for adults. Intake should not exceed 1000 μg daily; a higher intake can mask hematologic signs of vitamin B$_{12}$ deficiency and perhaps delay its diagnosis.

Macrocytosis and anemia may develop with prolonged deficiency.∎ Folic acid deficiency may also play a role in depression but does not cause a slowly progressive dementia. Measurement of serum folic acid levels is a reasonable test for deficiency unless the patient's diet has changed recently, in which case red blood cell folic acid levels should be measured.

VITAMIN C

Vitamin C is found in many fresh or frozen fruits and vegetables; the RDA is 60 mg (100 mg for smokers), about the amount contained in one orange. Its antioxidant effects may be protective against certain eye diseases (eg, cataracts, macular degeneration). It also helps to reactivate vitamin E, another antioxidant. Whether vitamin C plays a role in protecting against or treating cancer or viral infections is controversial.

∎ see page 686

Persons with skin fragility, easy bruisability, or poor wound healing may benefit from increased vitamin C intake ($\leq$ 500 to 1000 mg daily). However, doses >1000 mg daily are not recommended for several reasons. First, vitamin C increases iron absorption; high levels of iron may be associated with an increased risk of cardiac disease. In addition, many people carry the hemochromatosis gene and are unaware that they do so.∎ These people accumulate toxic levels of iron and may be harmed by vitamin C supplementation. Another concern about consuming high doses of any antioxidant is that under certain conditions, antioxidants can have the opposite effect (ie, can become a pro-oxidant) and perhaps damage cells and DNA.

TRACE MINERALS

CHROMIUM

Chromium is involved in glucose metabolism. Studies suggest that it may play a role in insulin action and may improve blood glucose control in patients with diabetes mellitus. Recommendations regarding requirements and supplementation remain controversial because of difficulty in assessing chromium status and because there is no clearly defined chromium deficiency syndrome. Any role for chromium in changing muscle or fat distribution, in treating obesity, or in affecting lipid metabolism remains under investigation.

SELENIUM

Epidemiologic data suggest an inverse relationship between selenium levels and cancer incidence. In a recent study, decreased risk of total cancer incidence (excluding skin cancers) and mortality was found for middle-aged to older adults who took 200 μg of selenium (RDA = 55 to 70 μg) daily. Further studies are needed before selenium supplementation can be recommended, because high intake may cause vague gastrointestinal and skin symptoms (eg, upset stomach, fingernail changes, hair loss) and fatigue.

ZINC

Zinc is needed for adequate wound healing, immunity, and a healthy appetite (RDA = 12 to 15 mg). It may also slow progression of age-related macular degeneration. Zinc deficiency is common among mal-

∎ see page 1072

nourished elderly persons, particularly among those who also have cirrhosis or diabetes mellitus or who are taking diuretics. A high-fiber diet may interfere with zinc absorption.

Deficiency is difficult to diagnose: Serum zinc levels are a poor marker of zinc nutrition, and zinc status is difficult to accurately assess. Supplementation may be useful for patients at risk of deficiency, but high doses may cause stomach upset or interfere with copper metabolism and cause anemia. Supplementation for treatment of benign, self-limited viral upper respiratory infections is controversial; studies have had conflicting conclusions.

61 ■ PROTEIN-ENERGY UNDERNUTRITION

(Malnutrition)

A deficiency syndrome caused by inadequate intake or absorption of macronutrients.

Marasmus and kwashiorkor are two forms of protein-energy undernutrition. **Marasmus** is a condition of borderline nutritional compensation in which a patient has a marked depletion of muscle mass and fat stores but normal visceral protein and organ function. Because the patient has depleted nutritional reserves, any additional metabolic stress (eg, surgery, infection, burn) may rapidly lead to **kwashiorkor** (hypoalbuminemic protein-energy malnutrition). Kwashiorkor is characterized by a loss of visceral protein and is often associated with edema.

About 16% of elderly persons living in the community consume < 1000 kcal/day, an amount that does not maintain adequate nutrition. Undernutrition also affects 17 to 65% of those in acute care hospitals and 5 to 59% of those in long-term care institutions. Protein-energy undernutrition can lead to many acute and chronic conditions (see TABLE 61–1). Studies show that elderly persons who are underweight in middle age and later are at greater risk of death than those who are overweight.

Failure to thrive, a term borrowed from the pediatric literature to describe children with delayed physical growth, is applied to the elderly to indicate a deterioration in functional status disproportional to their disease burden. The causes of failure to thrive are multifactorial and include protein-energy undernutrition, loss of muscle mass (sarcopenia), problems with balance and endurance, declining cognition, and depression.

TABLE 61-1.   CONDITIONS RESULTING FROM PROTEIN-ENERGY
UNDERNUTRITION

Anemia	Fatigue
Anergy	Hip fracture
Cognitive dysfunction	Increased drug-drug interactions (due
Decreased CD4$^+$:CD8 ratio	to decreased albumin binding and fat
Decreased muscle strength (frailty)	depots)
Decreased natural killer cell activity	Infections
Decreased serum antibody response to	Orthostatic hypotension
antigen challenge	Pedal edema
Euthyroid sick syndrome	Pressure sores

Pathophysiology

The physiologic changes of aging place elderly persons at risk of undernutrition. For example, a physiologic decline in food intake occurs. The reasons for this decline are not known, but several factors may be involved.

Elderly persons appear to feel fuller with less food, which may be caused by a decrease in the opioid (dynorphin) feeding drive and an increase in the satiety effect of cholecystokinin. Recent studies suggest that early satiety in the elderly may be caused by a nitric oxide deficiency, which decreases the adaptive relaxation of the fundus of the stomach in response to food.

Leptin, a recently discovered protein hormone produced by fat cells, decreases food intake and increases energy metabolism. In normal younger adults, an increase in body fat triggers an increase in leptin levels, and vice versa. In contrast, abnormally elevated leptin levels are strongly correlated with decreased body fat, and leptin deficiency in children has been reported to result in massive obesity. In elderly women, leptin levels decline with the decline in body fat that occurs after age 70. In elderly men, however, leptin levels increase despite the decline in body fat. This increase is related to the decline in testosterone levels that occurs with age. The importance of leptin in decreasing food intake with age is unknown. Postmenopausal women with high leptin levels tend to eat somewhat less than those with low leptin levels.

A number of cytokines (eg, tumor necrosis factor, interleukin-2, interleukin-6) decrease food intake. Some elderly persons have elevated levels of these cytokines, which may contribute to anorexia. Stressors (eg, surgery, infection, burns) usually result in cytokine release, which inhibits the production of albumin and causes it to move from the blood into the extravascular space. This occurrence explains the often dramatic decrease in albumin (which has a relatively long half-life of 21 days) of newly hospitalized patients. Characteristically, elderly patients experience this reduction more rapidly than younger patients; even relatively minor stress may be the cause. Usually, susceptible elderly patients are underweight, but even those who appear to have ample fat and muscle mass are susceptible if they have a recent history of rapid weight loss.

Activin, a hormone produced by the testes and ovaries, has been associated with the wasting syndrome in transgenic mice. With age, activin levels increase in men, but not in women; this finding may explain the greater decrease in food intake seen in men compared with women.

Etiology

Except in a hypermetabolic or malabsorption state (eg, hyperthyroidism), malnutrition is generally caused by anorexia. Anorexia has been related to the physiologic changes that occur with age and with various pathologic conditions (see TABLE 61–2).

A diminished sense of smell and taste may decrease the pleasure of eating, but changes in taste appear to play a minor role in decreased food intake, even though many elderly persons complain that food does not taste as good as it used to. Changes in taste are variable and are often associated with lifelong cigarette smoking, poor dental hygiene, and disease.

Dysphagia due to a stroke, another neurologic disorder, or esophageal pain caused by candidiasis may lower food intake, as may dental problems and xerostomia.

Tremors and other physical problems that make eating difficult (eg, an inability to cut food after a stroke) can also be causative. Continuous

TABLE 61–2.   CAUSES OF PROTEIN-ENERGY UNDERNUTRITION IN THE ELDERLY

Addison's disease	Hyperthyroidism
Alcoholism	Late-life paranoia
Anorexia nervosa, anorexia tardive	Loneliness
Cancer	Malabsorption syndrome (eg, late-onset celiac disease, pancreatic insufficiency)
Cholelithiasis	
Chronic infection (eg, tuberculosis, *Clostridium difficile* diarrhea, *Helicobacter pylori* infection)	Mania
	Pheochromocytoma
Chronic obstructive pulmonary disease	Physical disability (eg, tremors)
Dementia	Poverty
Dental problems	Stroke
Depression	Therapeutic diets
Difficulty shopping for or preparing food	Use of drugs (eg, digoxin, theophylline)
Diminished sense of smell and taste	Withdrawal from drugs (eg, anxiolytics and other psychoactive drugs)
Dysphagia	Xerostomia
Hypercalcemia	

tremors from such conditions as Parkinson's disease may cause weight loss by markedly raising the metabolic rate.

The use of certain drugs can result in weight loss by causing anorexia (eg, digoxin, fluoxetine, quinidine, hydralazine, vitamin A, psychoactive drugs); by causing nausea (eg, antibiotics, theophylline, aspirin); by increasing energy metabolism (eg, thyroxine, theophylline); or by causing malabsorption (eg, the sorbitol vehicle in theophylline elixir, cholestyramine). Also, withdrawal from certain drugs (eg, from alcohol, anxiolytics, or psychoactives) may cause weight loss. Alcoholism in late life is often associated with weight loss, squalor syndrome (living in unhygienic conditions), and depression.

Depression is one of the most common reversible causes of weight loss in the elderly. Depressed elderly persons are more likely to lose weight than depressed younger persons. Some very old persons may stop eating because they have lost the joy of living but are not clinically depressed. Loneliness can diminish the desire to prepare meals.

Poverty can also cause low food intake. Problems with shopping and food preparation may result in insufficient food being available in the home.

Anorexia nervosa may recur in elderly persons who had an episode in their teens; this disorder is being increasingly recognized. Abnormal attitudes about food intake and body image are not rare among the underweight elderly. When these abnormal attitudes are associated with severe weight loss, the condition is called anorexia tardive.

Paranoia and mania may have a late-life onset and are also associated with weight loss.

Dementia usually results in weight loss because the person forgets to eat. In addition, persons who wander can use up large amounts of calories in a single day, but persons with Alzheimer's disease do not have increased metabolism. Persons with dementia may have pica, including coprophagy (the ingestion of feces). In advanced dementia, self-feeding and even assisted feeding may become impossible.

Other medical causes of weight loss include hyperthyroidism, Addison's disease, hypercalcemia, pheochromocytoma, cancer, and chronic infections (eg, tuberculosis, recurrent *Clostridium difficile* diarrhea). In some elderly persons, *Helicobacter pylori* infections have been associated with severe anorexia and weight loss. Malabsorption syndromes, particularly late onset of celiac disease and pancreatic insufficiency, should also be considered. Cholelithiasis can result in early satiation and weight loss.

Screening and Diagnosis

The Mini Nutritional Assessment is the best validated nutritional screening device for elderly persons (see FIGURE 61–1) and has been translated into numerous languages. The SCALES screening device has been cross-validated with the Mini Nutritional Assessment; it is easy to

Nestlé NESTLÉ NUTRITION SERVICES

Last name: _____   First name: _____   Sex: _____   Date: _____

Age: _____   Weight, kg: _____   Height, cm: _____   I.D. Number: _____

Complete the screen by filling in the boxes with the appropriate numbers.
Add the numbers for the screen. If score is 11 or less, continue with the assessment to gain a Malnutrition Indicator Score.

SCREENING

A   Has food intake declined over the past 3 months
due to loss of appetite, digestive problems,
chewing or swallowing difficulties?
0 = severe loss of appetite
1 = moderate loss of appetite
2 = no loss of appetite   ☐

B   Weight loss during last months
0 = weight loss greater than 3 kg (6.6 lbs)
1 = does not know
2 = weight loss between 1 and 3 kg (2.2 and
6 6 lbs)
3 = no weight loss   ☐

C   Mobility
0 = bed or chair bound
1 = able to get out of bed/chair but does not
go out
2 = goes out   ☐

D   Has suffered psychological stress or acute
disease in the past 3 months
0 = yes   2 = no   ☐

E   Neuropsychological problems
0 = severe dementia or depression
1 = mild dementia
2 = no psychological problems   ☐

F   Body Mass Index (BMI) (weight in kg) / (height in m)^2
0 = BMI less than 19
1 = BMI19 to less than 21
2 = BMI 21 to less than 23
3 = BMI 23 or greater   ☐

Screening Score (subtotal max. 14 points)   ☐☐

12 points or greater   Normal—not at risk—
no need to complete assessment

11 points or below   Possible malnutrition—
continue assessment

ASSESSMENT

G   Lives independently (not in a nursing home or
hospital)
0 = no   1 = yes   ☐

H   Takes more than 3 prescription drugs per day
0 = yes   1 = no   ☐

I   Pressure sores or skin ulcers
0 = yes   1 = no   ☐

J   How many full meals does the patient eat daily?
0 = 1 meal
1 = 2 meals
2 = 3 meals   ☐

K   Selected consumption markers for protein intake
• At least one serving of dairy products
(milk, cheese, yogurt) per day?   yes ☐ no ☐
• Two or more servings of legumes
or eggs per week?   yes ☐ no ☐
• Meat, fish or poultry every day   yes ☐ no ☐
0.0 = if 0 or 1 yes
0.5 = if 2 yes
1.0 = if 3 yes   ☐.☐

L   Consumes two or more servings of fruits or
vegetables per day?
0 = no   1 = yes   ☐

M   How much fluid (water, juice, coffee, tea, milk. . .)
is consumed per day?
0.0 = less than 3 cups
0.5 = 3 to 5 cups
1.0 = more than 5 cups   ☐.☐

N   Mode of feeding
0 = unable to eat without assistance
1 = self-fed with some difficulty
2 = self-fed without any problem   ☐

O   Self view of nutritional status
0 = views self as being malnourished
1 = is uncertain of nutritional state
2 = views self as having no nutritional problem   ☐

P   In comparison with other people of the same age,
how do they consider their health status?
0.0 = not as good
0.5 = does not know
1.0 = as good
2.0 = better   ☐.☐

Q   Mid-arm circumference (MAC) in cm
0.0 = MAC less than 21
0.5 = MAC 21 to 22
1.0 = MAC 22 or greater   ☐.☐

R   Calf circumference (CC) in cm
0 = CC less than 31   1 = CC 31 or greater   ☐

Assessment (max. 16 points)   ☐ ☐.☐

Screening score   ☐☐

Total Assessment (max. 30 points)   ☐ ☐.☐

Malnutrition Indicator Score

17 to 23.5 points   at risk of malnutrition   ☐

Less than 17 points   malnourished   ☐

® Société des Produits Nestlé S.A., Vevey, Switzerland,
Trademark Owners

FIGURE 61–1.   The Mini Nutritional Assessment. (From the Société des Produits Nestlé S.A., Vevey, Switzerland; reprinted with permission.)

TABLE 61–3. "SCALES" PROTOCOL FOR EVALUATING RISK OF MALNUTRITION IN THE ELDERLY*

Item Evaluated	Assign One Point	Assign Two Points
Sadness (as measured on the Geriatric Depression Scale—see TABLE 33–4)	10–14	≥ 15
Cholesterol level	< 160 mg/dL (< 4.15 mmol/L)	—
Albumin level	3.5–4 g/dL	< 3.5 g/dL
Loss of weight	1 kg (or 1/4 in. midarm circumference) in 1 mo	3 kg (or 1/2 in. midarm circumference) in 6 mo
Eating problems	Patient needs assistance	—
Shopping and food preparation problems	Patient needs assistance	—

*A total score ≥ 3 indicates that the patient is at risk of malnutrition.
Modified from Morley JE, Miller DK: "Malnutrition in the elderly." *Hospital Practice* 27(7):95–116, 1992; used with permission.

use in the outpatient setting (see TABLE 61–3). The Specific Global Assessment of nutritional status has been validated for use in hospitalized patients with gastrointestinal disorders but requires further validation for determining malnutrition among elderly persons. The Nutrition Screening Index was developed to identify elderly persons at risk of nutritional problems but has poor specificity and sensitivity.

Weight loss is the single best factor for predicting persons at risk of malnutrition. Adequate height and weight tables for optimum body mass for the elderly are not available, but a body mass index < 21 kg/m^2 (weight/height^2) suggests a problem. Midarm circumference or midarm muscle circumference (which corrects for triceps skinfold thickness by allowing for subtraction of fat mass) can help detect muscle mass changes in persons retaining fluid. Skinfold thickness measurements have little diagnostic value.

Albumin is an excellent measure of protein status. Healthy ambulatory elderly persons have serum albumin levels > 4 g/dL (3.5 g/dL because of fluid shifts when recumbent). Albumin levels < 3.2 g/dL in hospitalized elderly persons are highly predictive of subsequent mortality. Measurement of short-lived proteins (eg, prealbumin, retinol binding protein) has little diagnostic value but, in certain situations (eg, in intensive care units), may help evaluate the response to therapy.

Cholesterol levels < 160 mg/dL (< 4.15 mmol/L) in nursing home residents predict mortality, presumably because such levels reflect malnutrition. Acute illness associated with cytokine release can also lower cholesterol levels.

Anergy (failure to respond to common antigens, such as mumps, injected into the skin) can occur in healthy as well as in malnourished elderly persons. The combination of anergy and signs of malnutrition correlates more strongly with a poor outcome than does either one alone.

In persons with **marasmus,** edema is absent; serum albumin and hemoglobin levels, total iron-binding capacity, and test results of cell-mediated immune function (to detect anergy) are usually normal. In persons with **kwashiorkor,** anergy and edema are often present. The serum albumin level is < 3.5 g/dL, and anemia, lymphocytopenia, and hypotransferrinemia (evidenced by a total iron-binding capacity < 250 μg/dL [< 45 μmol/L]) are likely.

Treatment

Overall, undernutrition is poorly recognized and treated in elderly persons. Thorough examination for treatable causes of weight loss is essential. Appropriate use of short-term aggressive caloric supplementation can save lives (ethical concerns regarding the appropriate withdrawal of nutritional support are discussed elsewhere).◼

Two recent studies have suggested that at least half of elderly persons in hospitals receive insufficient calories to meet their basic needs. These patients have much worse outcomes than those who receive adequate calories. Also, recent studies show that elderly persons with hip fractures benefit from oral caloric supplements or, if their albumin level is < 3 g/dL, from short-term tube feeding. Total parenteral nutrition should be reserved for severely undernourished persons (those with an albumin level < 3 g/dL) and for those who cannot tolerate enteral feedings. Peripheral vein parenteral nutrition (see TABLE 61–4) appears to be underused in acutely ill elderly persons, in part because it has been poorly studied.

There are little data to guide the choice of nutrient supplements. High-protein supplements are generally used for persons with infections. High-fat, high-fiber diets may lessen the glycemic response in persons with diabetes. High-fiber diets may reduce tube feeding–induced diarrhea but may result in fecal impaction in immobile patients. In most cases, the choice of a supplement should be based on the patient's preference. For tube feeding, the most cost-effective supplement should be used.

Adverse effects (eg, electrolyte abnormalities, hyperglycemia, aspiration pneumonia) may result from the feeding of a malnourished elderly person. Food can cause a significant drop in blood pressure,

◼ see pages 123 and 139

TABLE 61–4.   COMPARISON OF NASOGASTRIC TUBE FEEDING AND PERIPHERAL PARENTERAL NUTRITION

Feature	Nasogastric Tube Feeding	Peripheral Parenteral Nutrition
Ease of initiation	Difficult	Easy
Side effects of placement	Multiple	Few
Patient comfort	Poor	Good
Ease of maintenance	Problematic	Relatively easy
Calories delivered per 24 hours	Variable	Prescribed amount
Interference with satiation	Yes	No
Aspiration risk	Increased	None
Allows for oral feeding	Possibly not, because of throat discomfort	Yes

which is associated with falls and syncope. The decrease in blood pressure results from carbohydrate, which releases the vasodilatory calcitonin gene-related peptide.

For long-term tube feedings, most patients prefer percutaneous enteral gastrostomy tubes to nasogastric tubes. Patients with dementia tend to pull out gastrostomy tubes less often than nasogastric tubes. All types of tube feedings carry the risk of aspiration. Recent studies have shown that long-term tube feeding is associated with multiple compli-

TABLE 61–5.   NURSING STRATEGIES FOR NURSING HOME RESIDENTS WITH PROTEIN-ENERGY UNDERNUTRITION

- Determine food preferences, including ethnic meal preferences
- Provide snacks between meals and at night
- Do not interrupt meals by dispensing medications at mealtimes
- Suggest family members visit at mealtimes and help feed the resident
- If caloric supplements are being used, give them between meals
- Encourage the resident to eat in the dining room so that the environment is conducive to the enjoyment of eating
- Ensure that the resident is given adequate time to eat
- Consider "med pass" supplement (a program in which caloric supplements are given with medications)
- Consider recommending an exercise program for appetite stimulation
- Consider the need for special feeding devices; if necessary, consult the occupational therapist
- Remind demented patients to swallow, because they may have apraxia of swallowing
- Use a feeder table for residents who require long feeding times

cations and that in many cases outcomes are no better than when tube feeding is not used. This finding suggests the need for more careful targeting of elderly persons who will benefit from tube feeding. Recombinant growth hormone has been used to retain nitrogen and increase weight in severely malnourished elderly persons. Some of the newer growth hormone secretagogues may be ideal for this purpose. Use of medroxyprogesterone has led to weight gain in elderly persons with lung cancer and in nursing home residents (in one study). Use of dronabinol has led to weight gain in nursing home residents with dementia (in one study). Use of oxoglutarate (not available in the USA) has had dramatic effects on weight gain in elderly persons in Europe.

For patients with tremors or other physical problems with eating (eg, an inability to cut food after a stroke), using adaptive utensils, such as a heavy-handled spoon or a rocker-bottom knife, can help.

Nursing Issues

Food intake of nursing home residents is often underestimated. Nurses need training in appropriate estimation of the amount of food eaten. A number of simple procedures can improve the food intake of nursing home residents (see TABLE 61–5).

62 ■ OBESITY

Excessive accumulation of body fat.

Total body fat (visceral and nonvisceral) increases until about age 40 in men and age 50 in women and then remains steady until age 70, after which it decreases. The decrease is due to loss of both lean and adipose tissue. Percentage of body fat peaks at middle age and may decline slightly in extreme old age. Intra-abdominal and intramuscular fat increases with age. Visceral body fat also tends to increase with age.

Fat acts as a storage organ for excess calories, providing protection during times of acute illness. Fat also protects vital organs from injury during falls and plays an important role in maintaining core body temperature. The excessive accumulation of body fat, however, may cause certain medical complications in the elderly (see TABLE 62–1). A low waist-to-hip ratio protects against some of these complications. An increased waist-to-hip ratio suggests an increase in visceral fat, which in turn is associated with increased risk of hypertension, diabetes mellitus, coronary artery disease, and premature death. Women have lower waist-to-hip ratios than men.

TABLE 62–1.   COMPLICATIONS OF OBESITY IN THE ELDERLY

Moderate Obesity	Morbid Obesity*
Colon and prostate cancer (in men)	Decreased longevity
Coronary artery disease	Diagnostic problems
Deep vein thrombosis	Immobility
Diabetes mellitus	Increased surgical risk
Gallbladder disease	Intertrigo
Gout	Pickwickian syndrome
Hypertension	
Impaired functional status	
Osteoarthritis	
Pressure sores	
Pulmonary embolism	
Sleep apnea	
Uterine, breast, cervical, and ovarian cancer (in women)	

*These complications are in addition to those that occur in the moderately obese.

Persons who weigh 120 to 130% of their desirable weight are considered moderately obese; those who weigh more than 130% of their desirable weight are considered morbidly obese. In the USA, the prevalence of obesity in men is highest during middle age, declining to 26% by age 65 to 74. The prevalence in women is highest between ages 65 and 74 (36% for whites and 60% for blacks). In nursing homes, only morbid obesity has been associated with increased mortality.

Animal studies, particularly in rodents, have shown that dietary restriction may improve longevity. Primate studies are beginning to suggest that dietary restriction produces some biochemical improvements associated with longevity. However, the ideal body mass for an elderly person has not been established, although it is probably higher than that for a younger person.

Etiology

In elderly men, obesity appears to result from a decrease in physical activity; in elderly women, from the loss of estrogen; and in both sexes, from decreased levels of growth hormone. Genotype appears to account for 25% of a person's visceral body fat, ie, about 25% of the visceral fat pool is attributable to genes.

Overeating coupled with a decrease in physical activity and resting metabolic rate is the most common cause of obesity. Compared with younger men, elderly men experience a 20% decrease in total energy expenditure. Elderly women, however, experience only a minimal change in total energy expenditure. The explanation for this is that men tend to markedly reduce their physical activity with retirement, whereas women continue doing the bulk of the housework throughout their life. Resting metabolic rate decreases by 20% in men and 13% in women. These age-related reductions in resting metabolic rate result from a small decrease in triiodothyronine levels, reduced responsiveness to norepinephrine, reduced muscle tone and strength of muscle contraction, and reduced Na^+,K^+-ATPase activity. However, the major factor affecting resting metabolic rate is decreased food intake with age. Nonsmoking women aged 55 to 74 consume 300 kcal/day less than women aged 19 to 29; for men, the decrease is 950 kcal/day. Elderly persons also have a decreased thermic response to food.

Other causes of obesity include hypothyroidism, Cushing's syndrome, tumors of the ventromedial hypothalamus, and therapy with glucocorticoids, monoamine oxidase inhibitors, and moderate doses of phenothiazines.

Treatment

Obesity generally is a less important problem in elderly persons than in younger persons. The risk/benefit ratio of any therapeutic intervention should be evaluated. Some evidence suggests that excessive weight loss in elderly persons is associated with increased mortality.

Because the major identifiable cause of weight gain in elderly persons is lack of physical activity, an exercise program is the most reasonable approach to weight reduction. Walking 1 mile burns about 100 kcal. Thus, a mall-walking program in which a person walks 2 to 3 miles four times a week may induce gradual weight loss, as long as caloric intake is restricted. For persons with osteoarthritis, an upper body exercise program is recommended.

The diet of elderly persons trying to lose weight should provide at least 800 kcal/day and should always be supplemented with vitamins and trace minerals. Elderly persons on a weight-reduction diet should drink at least 1 L of fluid daily. Any dietary program should be supplemented with a behavior modification program, because a change in lifetime habits is often needed. Because of the risk of developing protein deficiency, an elderly patient on a weight-reduction diet should have his albumin level monitored monthly. If the level falls below 3.5 g/dL (35 g/L), a high-protein diet should be prescribed or the current diet discontinued. Rarely is a weight-reduction diet indicated for long-term nursing home residents.

Weight-loss drugs such as sibutramine or fluoxetine are not recommended for the elderly, because the possible benefits do not outweigh the adverse effects. Orlistat (an inhibitor of fat absorption) may be useful for obese elderly persons, particularly those with diabetes mellitus or hypertension.

Any operation that decreases stomach size is contraindicated in the elderly unless obesity is associated with sleep apnea.

The most common lipoprotein disorders are hypercholesterolemia (type II hyperlipoproteinemia); hypertriglyceridemia (primarily types IV and V hyperlipoproteinemia); hypoalphalipoproteinemia; and high lipoprotein(a) (Lp[a]) levels. However, hypercholesterolemia and hypoalphalipoproteinemia may not be as prevalent among the elderly as among the general population because mortality risk is so high that patients with these disorders do not survive to old age.

The association between high serum cholesterol levels and coronary artery disease (CAD■), whose prevalence and mortality rate increase with age, is well established. High levels of low-density lipoprotein cholesterol (LDL-C) and Lp(a) and a low level ($<$ 35 mg/dL [$<$ 0.91 mmol/L]) of high-density lipoprotein cholesterol (HDL-C) are significant independent positive risk factors for CAD and carotid artery atherosclerosis. A high level ($\geq$ 60 mg/dL [$\geq$ 1.55 mmol/L]) of HDL-C is a significant independent negative risk factor. However, the total cholesterol (TC)/HDL-C ratio is a more valuable measure of CAD risk than TC or LDL-C levels alone; the risk is higher in men when the ratio is $>$ 6.4 and in women when the ratio is $>$ 5.6.

For the elderly, the predictive value of high cholesterol levels in determining the risk of CAD is unclear, and the value of lowering high cholesterol levels—in terms of quality of life, morbidity, and mortality—is disputed. Some studies suggest that high cholesterol levels are an important risk factor for CAD in the elderly, others suggest that the risk decreases with age, and still others suggest a U-shaped relationship in which both high and low cholesterol levels are associated with an increased risk of morbidity and mortality. Some studies suggest sex differences: the mortality rate was lowest at a TC level of 215 mg/dL (5.55 mmol/L) for elderly men and 270 to 280 mg/dL (7.00 to 7.25 mmol/L) for elderly women.

There may also be a U-shaped relationship between cholesterol levels and death due to stroke. High cholesterol levels have been associated with increased risk of death due to nonhemorrhagic stroke, whereas low cholesterol levels have been associated with increased risk of death due to hemorrhagic stroke.

Studies of lipid-lowering treatments in the elderly, particularly primary prevention studies, have not consistently shown a significant reduction in the overall mortality rate. However, most studies have shown that for patients who have had a myocardial infarction (MI) or who have hemodynamically significant CAD, lowering lipid levels can stop or reverse disease progression and reduce the incidence of CAD events, CAD mortality, and all-cause mortality.

■see page 853

Classification and Etiology

Lipoprotein disorders may be primary (usually familial and usually classified based on lipoprotein elevation patterns—see TABLE 63–1) or secondary. However, genetic and secondary factors, such as various disorders and drugs (see TABLE 63–2), diet, obesity, physical activity, alcohol use, and cigarette smoking, are often interrelated.

The most common cause of secondary hypercholesterolemia is probably a diet high in saturated fat or cholesterol, whether or not a polygenic tendency for hypercholesterolemia exists. Covert hypothyroidism (with normal thyroxine and high thyroid-stimulating hormone levels) is a relatively common cause of high TC and LDL-C levels and is associated with an increased risk of premature MI.

The most common causes of secondary hypertriglyceridemia among the elderly are excessive alcohol intake, exogenous estrogen supplementation, poorly controlled diabetes, uremia, corticosteroid use, and β-blocker use. Isolated low HDL-C levels with normal triglyceride (TG) levels may result from smoking, androgenic steroid use, severe restriction of physical activity, or morbid obesity.

Generalized obesity may cause an increase in TG levels but not in cholesterol levels and, in persons > 60, may not contribute to risk of CAD. However, abdominal/upper body (male-pattern) obesity appears to be correlated with increased risk.

Age and sex have a major influence on lipid levels. For persons living in most industrialized countries, cholesterol and TG levels increase through middle age. In men, mean levels of TC increase until about age 50, then plateau, and then decrease starting at about age 70. In women, they increase more gradually up to age 65 to 69, then decrease. Starting at about age 55 to 60, women have higher TC levels than men. The age-related increase in TC, particularly in women, results primarily from an increase in LDL-C levels and much less from a small increase in very-low-density lipoprotein cholesterol (VLDL-C) levels.

TG levels progressively increase from birth through adulthood. The rate of increase is greater in men than in women. TG levels increase until age 55 in men and until about age 70 in women, then decrease, gradually in men.

In men, mean levels of HDL-C decrease at puberty, increase at about age 45, and then level off at age 50 to 59. These changes may be an effect of testosterone; generally, levels of plasma testosterone and HDL-C are positively correlated in adult men. After puberty, women have higher HDL-C levels than men despite a decrease after age 65.

Premenopausal women have lower LDL-C and higher HDL-C levels than men, partly because of endogenous estrogens. This difference may contribute to the lower CAD rates in premenopausal women. At menopause (whether natural or surgical), women lose this protection against CAD: LDL-C and Lp(a) levels increase and HDL-C levels decrease.

TABLE 63-1. PRIMARY LIPOPROTEIN DISORDERS

Disorder	Principal Lipoprotein Abnormality	History and Clinical Findings*	Primary Mode of Inheritance; Estimated Prevalence
Type I hyperlipoproteinemia (exogenous or familial hypertriglyceridemia, hyperchylomicronemia)	High TG, primarily chylomicrons	Typically, presentation in childhood Recurrent abdominal pain Pancreatitis Eruptive xanthomas Hepatosplenomegaly Lipemia retinalis	Recessive; 1/1,000,000
Type IIA hyperlipoproteinemia	High TC and LDL-C	Severe premature atherosclerosis MI, angina†,‡ Tenosynovitis (Achilles, patellar) Periorbital xanthelasma§ Tendinous xanthomas‖ Tuberous xanthomas‖,¶ Arcus juvenilis corneae	Dominant; 1/200– 1/500
Type IIB hyperlipoproteinemia	High TC, TG, and LDL-C	Same as for type IIA	Same as for type IIA
Type III hyperlipoproteinemia (familial dysbetalipoproteinemia)	High TC, TG, and IDL (β-migrating VLDL)	Severe premature atherosclerosis MI, stroke, peripheral vascular disease, claudication, carotid obstruction†,‡ Glucose intolerance§ Hyperuricemia§ Essential hypertension Obesity Palmar-planar xanthomas‖ Tuberous xanthomas‖ Tendinous xanthomas‖,¶	Recessive; 1/1000 #
Type IV hyperlipoproteinemia (includes familial hyperprebetalipoproteinemia and familial combined hyperlipidemia)	High TC, TG, and VLDL-TG	Premature atherosclerosis MI, stroke†,‡ Glucose intolerance Hyperuricemia Obesity Essential hypertension Periorbital xanthelasma§	Dominant; 1/200

TABLE 63-1.   (*Continued*)

Disorder	Principal Lipoprotein Abnormality	History and Clinical Findings*	Primary Mode of Inheritance; Estimated Prevalence
Type V hyperlipoproteinemia (mixed hypertriglyceridemia)	High TG, VLDL-TG, and chylomicron TG	Premature atherosclerosis MI, stroke†,‡ Abdominal pain Pancreatitis Glucose intolerance Hyperuricemia Essential hypertension Obesity Eruptive xanthomas§ Hepatosplenomegaly Peripheral sensory neuropathy	Dominant; 1/1000
Hypoalphalipoproteinemia	Low HDL-C	Severe premature atherosclerosis MI, stroke†,‡ Hyperuricemia Glucose intolerance Essential hypertension Obesity	Dominant; 1/200
High Lp(a) levels	High Lp(a)	Severe premature atherosclerosis, stroke, peripheral vascular disease	Uncertain
Hyperalphalipoproteinemia	High HDL-C	Longevity	Uncertain
Hypobetalipoproteinemia	Low LDL-C	Longevity	Uncertain

*Findings are common unless otherwise noted.
†Common in the patient and in first-degree relatives.
‡Premature cardiovascular disease in the patient and, commonly, in first-degree relatives.
§Occasional.
‖Rare.
¶If present, almost always diagnostic of familial hyperlipidemia.
#Although the genes that cause type III are relatively common, the disorder probably develops in only about 1% of persons with the genes.
TG = triglycerides; TC = total cholesterol; LDL-C = low-density lipoprotein cholesterol; MI = myocardial infarction; IDL = intermediate-density lipoprotein; VLDL = very-low-density lipoprotein; HDL-C = high-density lipoprotein cholesterol; Lp (a) = lipoprotein (a).

TABLE 63–2.   SOME CAUSES OF SECONDARY LIPOPROTEIN DISORDERS

Category	High TC and High LDL-C Levels	High TG and/or Low HDL-C Levels
Disorder	Acute intermittent porphyria* Anorexia nervosa* Cushing's syndrome* Diabetes that is poorly controlled Dysproteinemias (eg, myeloma, Waldenström's macroglobulinemia)* Hypothyroidism Nephrotic syndrome† Obstructive liver disease† Orthostatic proteinuria Uremia†	Alcoholic hepatitis, alcoholism Chlorinated hydrocarbon exposure† Diabetes that is poorly controlled Dysproteinemias* Glycogen storage disease* Hypothyroidism Idiopathic hypercalcemia* Nephrotic syndrome† Obstructive liver disease, acute hepatitis† Severe metabolic stress (myocardial infarction, stroke) Systemic lupus erythematosus* Uremia (with or without dialysis)
Drugs	Androgenic steroids Corticosteroids Progestins Thiazide diuretics	Androgenic steroids (decrease HDL-C) β-Blockers Corticosteroids Estrogens, oral contraceptives Nicotine (decreases HDL-C) Synthetic vitamin A compounds (for acne) Zinc (decreases HDL-C)
Diet	Excess intake of saturated fat or cholesterol	Excess intake of alcohol (may increase TG and HDL-C)

*Rare.
†Occasional.
TC = total cholesterol; LDL-C = low-density lipoprotein cholesterol; TG = triglycerides; HDL-C = high-density lipoprotein cholesterol.

Diagnosis

Patients who have had an MI, a stroke, or other manifestations of significant atherosclerosis (eg, peripheral arterial disease, carotid artery stenosis) before age 60 should be screened for familial lipoprotein abnormalities. The Lp(a) level should be measured in patients who have had an MI or a stroke or who have CAD and in patients who have other major CAD risk factors, because a high Lp(a) level probably acts synergistically with other risk factors. If a lipoprotein abnormality is detected, the physician should try to determine whether the lipoprotein disorder is primary or secondary and assess the patient for other CAD risk factors (eg, smoking, hypertension, a high-fat diet, physical inactivity). If secondary causes can be ruled out, the disorder is usually one of the common familial hyperlipoproteinemias.

Screening and identification criteria for hypercholesterolemia are controversial. The National Cholesterol Education Program (NCEP) provides guidelines for identifying high TC and LDL-C levels (see TABLE 63–3) and low and high HDL-C levels.

According to NCEP guidelines, no single cholesterol value should be used to classify a patient clinically, because values may vary from day to day. If the first screening test detects an abnormality, two subsequent tests are recommended. The NCEP does not give guidelines by age group; its guidelines are based on data from middle-aged persons and do not consider the increase in serum lipids that occurs with age. (As a result, 60% of persons > 65 would be classified as candidates for treatment.)

In contrast, the American College of Physicians guidelines recommend a single measurement of TC alone to identify patients who would benefit from lipid-lowering therapy. These guidelines note that evidence is insufficient to recommend or discourage the screening of men and women aged 65 to 75 for primary prevention, and screening is not recommended for persons > 75.

If elderly persons are screened, a full lipid profile should be obtained. For many elderly persons, the predominant reason for a high TC level is a high HDL-C level, not a high LDL-C level; therefore, their risk of CAD is decreased, not increased. Some persons have normal TC and TG levels but an HDL-C level below the 10th percentile and thus have a very high risk of CAD.

TG levels can be accurately measured only after a fast. If the TG level is < 400 mg/dL (< 4.52 mmol/L), the LDL-C component of the lipid profile can be estimated using the Friedewald equation: LDL-C = TC – [HDL-C + (TG/5)].

Basal lipoprotein measurements usually cannot be determined in the following situations: during a fever or major infection; within 4 weeks of an acute MI, a stroke, or major surgery; immediately after acute excessive alcohol intake; in diabetes mellitus that is severely out of control (fasting blood glucose level > 250 mg/dL (> 13.9 mmol/L), glycosylated hemoglobin > 9%); or during rapid weight loss.

Certain characteristic findings (eg, tendinous, tuberous, or palmar-planar xanthomas; arcus juvenilis corneae) are diagnostically useful (see TABLE 63–1). Obesity (with or without essential hypertension), glucose intolerance, and hyperuricemia may indicate primary hypertriglyceridemia or hypoalphalipoproteinemia.

Secondary lipoprotein disorders are common, even among patients with a well-defined primary lipoprotein disorder, and may exacerbate

TABLE 63–3. TREATMENT DECISIONS BASED ON LDL CHOLESTEROL LEVEL

Patient Category	Initiation Level for Dietary Treatment	Initiation Level for Drug Treatment	Goal
Without CAD and with fewer than two risk factors	≥ 160 mg/dL (≥ 4.14 mmol/L)	≥ 190 mg/dL (≥ 4.92 mmol/L)	< 160 mg/dL (< 4.14 mmol/L)
Without CAD and with two or more risk factors	≥ 130 mg/dL (≥ 3.37 mmol/L)	≥ 160 mg/dL (≥ 4.14 mmol/L)	< 130 mg/dL (< 3.37 mmol/L)
With CAD	> 100 mg/dL (> 2.59 mmol/L)	≥ 130 mg/dL (≥ 3.37 mmol/L)	≤ 100 mg/dL (≤ 2.59 mmol/L)

LDL = low-density lipoprotein; CAD = coronary artery disease.
From Grundy SM, Bilheimer D, Chait A, et al: "Summary of the Second Report of the National Cholesterol Education Program (NCEP) Expert Panel on Detection, Evaluation, and Treatment of High Blood Cholesterol in Adults (Adult Treatment Panel II)." *Journal of the American Medical Association* 269(23):3015–3023, 1993.

the expression of the primary disorder, particularly severe hypertriglyceridemia. Thus, when a primary lipoprotein disorder is first diagnosed, a physical examination should be performed, and a drug, occupational, family, dietary, and alcohol-intake history should be obtained. Levels of thyroxine, thyroid-stimulating hormone, blood urea nitrogen or creatinine, and fasting blood glucose should be measured, and urinalysis and liver function tests should be performed.

Treatment

The NCEP guidelines recommend treatment of persons in the top quintile for TC levels (although in the elderly, use of TC levels alone can be misleading) and of persons with an LDL-C level ≥ 160 mg/dL (≥ 4.14 mmol/L) or lower depending on the number of CAD risk factors and the presence of CAD or other atheromatous disease. Patients are considered at high risk if they have two or more CAD risk factors (age > 45 for men or > 55 for women, premature menopause without estrogen replacement therapy, a family history of CAD, current cigarette smoking, hypertension, low HDL-C levels, and diabetes). One risk factor is subtracted if HDL-C levels are ≥ 60 mg/dL (≥ 1.55 mmol/L).

Therefore, NCEP recommendations for initiation of dietary or drug treatment are based on LDL-C levels (see TABLE 63–3). The goals of treatment are to lower TC and LDL-C levels to the recommended levels, to lower TG levels to < 500 mg/dL (< 5.65 mmol/L) and thus avoid pancreatitis, and to increase HDL-C levels to > 35 mg/dL (> 0.91

mmol/L), preferably to ≥ 40 mg/dL (≥ 1.03 mmol/L). For post-menopausal women, a high TG level is an important independent risk factor for CAD; thus, lowering the level to < 250 mg/dL (< 2.82 mmol/L) is probably valuable.

Because the NCEP guidelines are not based on data from nor designed specifically for the elderly, several factors should be considered when deciding whether elderly patients with a lipoprotein abnormality should be treated:

- Decisions should not be based primarily on the patient's age. Many elderly patients are physiologically and mentally much younger than their chronologic age.

- Some benefits of treatment may be realized almost immediately: Significant lowering of LDL-C levels can lead to increased endothelial cell production of nitrous oxide (a potent vasodilator) and can reduce platelet aggregation; significant lowering of TG levels sharply decreases plasminogen activator inhibitor activity and increases fibrinolysis. Often, treatment stops progression of atherosclerotic lesions or induces regression within 1 to 2 years.

- If patients have other life-limiting conditions, aggressive lipid-lowering treatment may be inappropriate or less useful.

- Elderly patients who take many drugs may be less likely to comply with drug regimens, and their risk of drug-drug interactions is increased. Although lipid-lowering treatment can reduce long-term costs for some patients, elderly patients with a fixed income may have difficulty affording the better tolerated and more effective drugs.

- Strict lipid-lowering diets may be effective in the elderly but may lead to or exacerbate malnutrition, as may voluntary dietary restriction. Unappetizing low-fat diets can cause anorexia and eventually lead to nutritional deficiencies. The potential morbidity of protein-energy malnutrition probably outweighs that of moderate hypercholesterolemia.

Dietary treatment: Because the elderly have difficulty maintaining adequate caloric and protein intake and are at risk of malnutrition, a moderate approach to diet is generally recommended (see TABLE 63–4). Patients can be advised to trim fat from meat; to increase intake of fish, soybean products, and beans; to avoid fried foods; and to use monounsaturated fats (eg, olive oil). Consumption of foods rich in soluble fiber (eg, oat bran) may also lower lipid levels. Phytosterols, present in soybean products, and stanol esters, available as a margarine product, decrease cholesterol absorption.

A strict diet may be preferred for some patients. Aerobic exercise should be included as part of treatment because the benefits of diet

TABLE 63–4. PRACTICAL APPROACH TO A LOW-CHOLESTEROL, LOW-SATURATED-FAT DIET

Food Category	Foods to Reduce	Foods to Choose	Substitutes
Meats and meat products	Fatty cuts of beef, lamb, and pork; spareribs; organ meats; regular cold cuts; sausage; hot dogs	Fish, chicken, and turkey (without the skin); lean cuts of beef, lamb, pork, and veal	Cold cuts prepared from processed turkey, except those containing organ meats
Dairy products	Whole milk (4% fat), evaporated or condensed whole milk, cream, half-and-half, most nondairy creamers, whipped toppings	Skim milk, 1% fat milk, buttermilk	Polyunsaturated fat–based cream substitutes
	Whole-milk yogurt, whole-milk cottage cheese, all natural cheeses (blue, Roquefort, Camembert, cheddar, Swiss), cream cheese, sour cream, ice cream	Nonfat (0% fat) or low-fat yogurt, low-fat cottage cheese (1%, 2%), low-fat cheeses (labeled ≤ 6 g fat/oz)	Sherbet, sorbet, frozen low-fat yogurt made from skim milk and without eggs
	Butter; butter-margarine mixture	Margarines made from liquid vegetable oils and packaged in a tub or squeeze bottle	Diet margarine made from liquid oils
	Eggs (to < 3/wk)	Egg whites (2 whole egg whites = 1 egg in recipes)	Egg substitutes; cholesterol-free egg substitutes
Commercial baked goods	Pies, cakes, doughnuts, croissants, pastries, muffins, biscuits, high-fat crackers, high-fat cookies, egg noodles, breads in which eggs are a major ingredient	Homemade bread goods made with unsaturated oils; angel food cake; low-fat cookies, crackers, and pretzels; rice; pasta; whole-grain (oatmeal, bran, rye, multigrain)* breads and cereals	Pastries made with polyunsaturated or monounsaturated oils and egg substitutes or egg whites
Saturated fats and oils, dressings	Chocolate	—	Cocoa powder, carob
	Coconut oil, palm oil, kernel oil, lard, bacon	Unsaturated vegetable oils: corn, olive, rapeseed, safflower, sesame, soybean, sunflower	—
	Dressings made with egg yolk	Low-fat mayonnaise, salad dressings made with liquid oils, as above	Low-fat diet dressings made with liquid oils
	Coconut	Seeds and nuts*	—
Fruits and vegetables	Fruits and vegetables prepared in butter, saturated fats, cream, or sauces with saturated fat	Fresh, frozen, canned, and dried fruits or vegetables*	—

* Fruits, vegetables, grains, seeds, and nuts contain no cholesterol, and most contain no saturated fat.

without exercise may be limited. A low-saturated-fat, low-cholesterol diet should be tried for 6 months before drug therapy is instituted. For patients with a **high LDL-C level,** the American Heart Association and NCEP recommend a two-step diet (see TABLE 63–5). High-risk patients should start with the step 1 diet. Patients who are already following the equivalent of a step 1 diet should start with the step 2 diet. Elderly persons may have difficulty consuming adequate calories and protein, so the diet must be modified cautiously. However, the step 1 and 2 dietary guidelines and the practical approach shown in TABLE 63–4 should be safe for most elderly persons. The full effects of dietary treatment at either step may not be achieved for 8 to 12 weeks; therefore, patients should advance to step 2 only if the therapeutic goal is not reached in 8 to 12 weeks. Weight loss helps lower TC, LDL-C, and TG levels but is at least as difficult for the elderly as for younger persons.

For patients with **hypertriglyceridemia,** a low HDL-C level, and an increased risk of CAD, dietary interventions are important. The major goal is to increase the HDL-C level, although lowering the TG level alone may be valuable for women > 50. When the TG level is > 1000 mg/dL (> 11.29 mmol/L), a sharp reduction in total fat intake (to < 30 g/day) helps prevent TG-induced pancreatitis. Other goals are to lose weight, because modest weight loss can markedly lower TG levels; to reduce alcohol intake to ≤ 3 drinks per week or, if TG levels are ≥ 500 mg/dL (≥ 5.65 mmol/L), to discontinue alcohol; and to reduce the intake of total fat, saturated fat, and cholesterol using the step 2 diet.

For patients who have a TG level ≥ 1000 mg/dL (≥ 11.29 mmol/L) with high levels of chylomicron and VLDL-TG or who have the much rarer primary hyperchylomicronemia, total fat intake should be restricted to 10 to 20% of total calories, primarily to prevent TG-induced pancreatitis. Also, the sharp decrease in VLDL-C levels and the increase in HDL-C levels that result may help prevent patients with high levels of chylomicron and VLDL-TG from developing severe premature CAD. Weight loss is crucial for obese patients. For patients with severe hypertriglyceridemia, estrogen is contraindicated.

For patients who have **type III hyperlipoproteinemia** and are overweight, the single most important strategy is weight loss. Patients should reduce intake not only of total fat, saturated fat, and cholesterol but also of dietary sugars.

For patients with **hypoalphalipoproteinemia,** the only consistently effective dietary strategy is weight loss, which may increase HDL-C levels. Other strategies to increase HDL-C levels include supplementation with fish oils rich in omega-3 fatty acids (4 to 12 g/day), smoking cessation (or at least reduction), and aerobic activity (three to five 30-minute periods per week). At least initially, exercise should be supervised by a physician.∎ Intake of moderate amounts of alcohol can

∎ see page 297

TABLE 63–5.   STEP DIET FOR TREATMENT OF HYPERCHOLESTEROLEMIA*

Nutrient	Step 1	Step 2
Total fat (% of total calories)	≤ 30%	≤ 30%
Saturated fatty acids (% of total calories)	8–10%	≤ 7%
Polyunsaturated fatty acids (% of total calories)	≤ 10%	≤ 10%
Monounsaturated fatty acids (% of total calories)	≤ 15%	≤ 15%
Carbohydrate (% of total calories)	≥ 55%	≥ 55%
Protein (% of total calories)	About 15%	About 15%
Cholesterol (mg/day)	< 300	< 200
Total calories	To achieve and maintain desirable weight	To achieve and maintain desirable weight

*Recommended by the American Heart Association and the National Cholesterol Education Program.

increase HDL-C levels, but only if hepatic synthetic function is normal.

Drug treatment: If hyperlipoproteinemia persists after secondary causes have been identified and treated when possible and after dietary treatment has been tried, drug treatment should be used (see TABLE 63–6). When a single drug is inadequate, two drugs may be required.

Bile acid–binding resins (eg, cholestyramine, colestipol) interrupt the normal enterohepatic circulation of bile acids and indirectly increase the liver's catabolism of LDL-C by stimulating hepatocytes to synthesize more LDL receptors. These drugs can reduce CAD risk.

Resins are effective and safe as first-line drugs to lower the LDL-C level in patients whose primary abnormality is a high LDL-C level and whose TG level is < 250 mg/dL (< 2.82 mmol/L). However, they may increase the TG level. If the TG level increases to > 300 mg/dL (> 3.38 mmol/L) during resin therapy, nicotinic acid or gemfibrozil (1200 mg/day) may be added, particularly if the patient has high LDL-C and TG levels; the resin and nicotinic acid act synergistically. Alternatively, an HMG-CoA reductase inhibitor (statin) can be used instead of the resin or resin combination therapy. ∎

Resins should be started in small doses (8 to 10 g/day), particularly for the elderly. Many patients respond to the lowest dose, but the dose should be adjusted according to effect on LDL-C levels. Constipation, the most common adverse effect, can usually be avoided by increasing dietary fiber or by using stool softeners. Because resins are not system-

∎see page 617

ically absorbed, they have essentially no systemic adverse effects (except for rare, mild, reversible changes in liver enzymes).

Resins can augment warfarin's effects; however, if a resin and warfarin are taken within a short time, the resin can also bind warfarin. Thus, resins should be used cautiously, if at all, with warfarin-like anticoagulants. Resins should not be given concurrently with exogenous thyroid hormones, sex hormones, prednisone, or digoxin, all of which may be bound in the intestine by resins. These drugs should be given at least 2 hours before the first resin dose of the day.

Resins are probably contraindicated as single-drug therapy in patients with a high LDL-C level and a TG level > 300 mg/dL and in those with severe hemorrhoids or a history of bowel resection or severe constipation; a statin may be used.

Nicotinic acid (niacin) inhibits secretion of VLDL from the liver, lowering VLDL-C and LDL-C levels. In patients with CAD, it reduces the incidence of recurrent MI and all-cause mortality. Nicotinic acid can be used as a first-line drug, but it is usually added to resin therapy if the resin does not lower LDL-C levels sufficiently. The initial dose is 100 mg bid or tid. The frequency of administration and total daily dose should be increased slowly at about weekly intervals, as necessary. Generally, an initial maintenance dosage of 1.5 to 2 g/day is required. Every 6 to 8 weeks, liver function tests and stool tests for occult blood should be performed, and blood glucose, uric acid, and LDL-C levels should be measured.

Adverse effects of nicotinic acid are common, bothersome, and often severe (see TABLE 63–6). Flushing may be ameliorated by taking aspirin 80 to 325 mg 30 to 60 minutes before taking nicotinic acid, but aspirin may cause gastrointestinal adverse effects in the elderly. Fast-release formulations of nicotinic acid are preferable because hepatotoxicity appears to be more common and more severe with slow-release formulations. If possible, nicotinic acid should not be used concurrently with a statin, because risk of myositis and hepatotoxicity is increased.

HMG-CoA reductase inhibitors (statins) block intracellular cholesterol biosynthesis and force cells to synthesize more LDL receptors, thus increasing the catabolism of LDL cholesterol. Statins include atorvastatin, cerivastatin, fluvastatin, lovastatin, pravastatin, and simvastatin. Statins are becoming the cholesterol-lowering drugs of choice because they are generally safe, have a relatively favorable adverse effect profile, and effectively lower TC levels (by 15 to 45%) and LDL-C levels (by 20 to 40%) and increase HDL-C levels (by 5 to 15%). Statins also effectively lower TG levels (by 10 to 35%). Lovastatin should be taken with food. The others do not have this restriction and are usually taken at bedtime.

Adverse effects are relatively rare and usually transient. Because liver enzyme (particularly transaminase) levels may increase, liver function tests should be performed before treatment, at 6 and 12 weeks

TABLE 63–6. LIPID-LOWERING DRUGS

Drug Category	Indications	Drug	Usual Maintenance Dosage	Adverse Effects
Bile acid–binding resins	High LDL-C Type II hyperlipoproteinemia	Cholestyramine*,†	8–24 g (2–4 packets or scoops) daily in 2–4 divided doses‡	Constipation (common) and other GI symptoms, increased VLDL and TG, binding of other drugs, augmentation of warfarin's effect (possible), elevated liver enzymes (rare and reversible)
		Colestipol†	10–30 g (2–6 packets or scoops) daily in 2–4 divided doses‡	
Nicotinic acid (niacin)†	High LDL-C with high TG (type IIB hyperlipoproteinemia) Isolated low HDL-C Types III, IV, and V hyperlipoproteinemia (if other therapies are ineffective)	—	2–6 g daily in 3 divided doses, taken with meals to minimize flushing§	Cutaneous flushing, pruritus, tachycardia, GI symptoms, ulcers, gastritis, liver function abnormality (common), impaired glucose tolerance, hyperuricemia, amblyopia (very rare)
3-Hydroxy-3-methylglutaryl coenzyme A reductase inhibitors (statins)	High LDL-C Type IIB hyperlipoproteinemia	Atorvastatin‖	10–80 mg/day	Liver function test abnormalities, myalgia or myopathy, headaches, skin rashes, fatigue, GI symptoms
		Cerivastatin‖	0.3 mg/day; 0.2 mg/day for patients with moderate to severe renal dysfunction (CrCl < 60 mL/min/1.73m²)	
		Fluvastatin‖	20–40 mg/day	
		Lovastatin *,†	20–80 mg/day (20–40 mg dose given in evening; 60–80 mg dose given in divided doses, AM and PM)	
		Pravastatin*	10–40 mg/day	
		Simvastatin*	5–80 mg/day	

Drug class	Indication	Drug	Dose	Adverse effects
Fibric acid derivatives	High TG Low HDL-C High LDL-C with high TG Types III, IV and V hyperlipoproteinemia Hypoalphalipoproteinemia	Gemfibrozil¶	600 mg bid; maximum dose 1200 mg/day	Minor GI symptoms, rash, eosinophilia, anemia, increased gallstones, muscle cramps and aches (myopathy, which is rare but is more common among patients who have uremia or who are taking a statin or cyclosporine)
Probucol‖	High LDL-C Type II hyperlipoproteinemia	—	500 mg bid	Minor GI symptoms, decreased HDL-C (as much as or more than LDL-C), foul-smelling sweat (rare), prolonged QT interval
Omega-3 fatty acids‖	High TG that does not respond optimally to gemfibrozil or nicotinic acid	—	4–15 g/day	Fishy taste after belching, diarrhea
Bile acid–binding resin plus nicotinic acid	LDL-C higher than target with single-drug therapy	A resin *plus* nicotinic acid	Recommended dose Recommended dose	Same as for individual drugs
Bile acid–binding resin plus a statin	LDL-C higher than target with single-drug therapy	A resin *plus* a statin	Recommended dose Recommended dose	Same as for individual drugs
Probucol plus a bile acid–binding resin	LDL-C higher than target and HDL-C lower than target with single-drug therapy	Probucol *plus* a resin	500 mg bid Recommended dose	Less constipation than with a resin alone; less diarrhea than with probucol alone; HDL-C higher than with probucol alone

Table continues on the following page.

TABLE 63–6. LIPID-LOWERING DRUGS (*Continued*)

Drug Category	Indications	Drug	Usual Maintenance Dosage	Adverse Effects
Gemfibrozil plus a bile acid—binding resin	LDL-C at target, TG > 250 mg/dL (> 2.82 mmol/L), and HDL-C < 35 mg/dL (< 0.91 mmol/L) after resin therapy; or TG and HDL-C at target and LDL-C higher than target after gemfibrozil therapy	Gemfibrozil *plus* a resin	600 mg bid Recommended dose	Same as for individual drugs
A statin plus gemfibrozil	LDL-C at target, TG > 250 mg/dL (> 2.82 mmol/L), and HDL-C < 35 mg/dL (< 0.91 mmol/L) after statin therapy; or TG and HDL-C at target and LDL-C higher than target after gemfibrozil therapy	A statin *plus* gemfibrozil#	Lowest effective dose 600 mg bid	Myopathy and increased creatine kinase much more common than with either drug alone

* Reduction in CAD event rate has been proved in controlled clinical studies.
† Cessation of CAD progression and/or CAD regression has been proved in controlled clinical studies.
‡ The initial dose should always be low (1 pack or 1 scoop per day); the dose is increased gradually as needed.
§ The initial dose should always be low (500 mg/day); the dose is increased gradually, by 500-mg increments.
‖ Reduction in CAD event rate has not been proved.
¶ The dose should be reduced if uremia is present.
# This combination should generally be avoided.

LDL-C = low-density lipoprotein cholesterol; GI = gastrointestinal; VLDL = very-low-density lipoprotein; TG = triglycerides; HDL-C = high-density lipoprotein cholesterol; CrCl = creatinine clearance; CAD = coronary artery disease.

after initiation of treatment or after elevation in dose, and at 6-month intervals thereafter. Increases in transaminase levels should be monitored until levels return to normal. Usually, a statin is not discontinued unless the liver enzyme elevations exceed three times the upper limit of normal.

A statin may be the drug of choice for patients with a high LDL-C level and a TG level > 300 mg/dL and for those with severe hemorrhoids or a history of bowel resection or severe constipation. Gemfibrozil may be added if the TG level remains > 300 mg/dL and the patient is at high risk of or has had an atherosclerotic event.

Statins can be used effectively with resins but probably should not be used with nicotinic acid because the risks of myopathy and hepatotoxicity are increased.

The concurrent use of a statin and cyclosporine commonly produces myopathy and may also produce rhabdomyolysis and myoglobinuria. This drug combination should thus be restricted to situations in which other lipid-lowering regimens are ineffective, and patients should be closely monitored.

Erythromycin and its derivatives should not be given concurrently with a statin because the risk of myopathy is increased.

Gemfibrozil, a fibric acid derivative, increases the hydrolysis of VLDL-TG and the synthesis of HDL-C and apolipoprotein A-I. Gemfibrozil lowers LDL-C and TG levels and reduces CAD morbidity and mortality rates in appropriate patients. It is the drug of choice for elderly patients with hypertriglyceridemia or hypoalphalipoproteinemia. Gemfibrozil should be considered for patients with a high TG level (> 300 mg/dL), a low HDL-C level (< 35 mg/dL [< 0.91 mmol/L]), and a moderately high LDL-C level (< 190 mg/dL [< 4.92 mmol/L]). Well tolerated by most patients, gemfibrozil rarely causes gastrointestinal upset or myopathy, although myopathy is more common when the drug is given to patients with impaired renal function. For such patients, especially if they are also receiving cyclosporine, the dose should be reduced.

Combined gemfibrozil–statin therapy may be necessary for patients at highest risk of CAD who have evidence of atherosclerosis. Such patients often have combined hyperlipidemia, usually with high TC, high TG, and low HDL-C levels, which are maintained despite significant dietary, weight, and exercise modification. When these patients are treated with gemfibrozil alone, TG levels can usually be normalized and HDL-C levels can often be increased to > 35 mg/dL (> 0.91 mmol/L), but TC and LDL-C levels may not be adequately lowered and often increase. Conversely, when these patients are treated with a statin alone, LDL-C levels can usually be normalized, but TG levels often remain high, and HDL-C levels often remain low (< 35 mg/dL).

Because myopathy, rhabdomyolysis, myoglobinuria, and renal injury have been reported in patients taking combined gemfibrozil–statin therapy, the following guidelines are recommended:

- It should be reserved for secondary prevention.
- It should not be used if patients have a very low creatinine clearance rate, because the risk of myopathy is increased.
- It should not be used concurrently with cyclosporine or nicotinic acid, because the risk of myopathy is increased.
- It can be used if patients are reliable and are well informed about the possibility of myopathy.
- Creatine kinase levels should be measured and liver function tests should be performed at baseline and every 6 to 8 weeks thereafter.
- Patients should take gemfibrozil 1.2 g/day po and the lowest starting dose of the statin. The statin dose should be adjusted to the lowest dose that will lower LDL-C levels to the target range.

Probucol appears to increase the rate of LDL-C catabolism, probably through pathways not mediated by LDL receptors. One hypothesis is that the antioxidant effect of probucol may reduce atherosclerosis by reducing the atherogenic effect of oxidized LDL-C. The effect of probucol on CAD risk has not been established.

Probucol is considered a second-line drug in the NCEP guidelines. Probucol usually lowers LDL-C levels by about 8 to 15%, but because it also lowers HDL-C levels by as much as 25%, its role in treating patients with a high LDL-C level is uncertain. Xanthoma regression has been reported as HDL-C levels decrease.

Generally, probucol is well tolerated; diarrhea is the most common adverse effect. Because the drug can prolong the QT interval, it is probably contraindicated in patients with ventricular irritability and an initially prolonged QT interval and in those taking other drugs that prolong the QT interval. The combination of probucol and a resin is effective; the reduction in the HDL-C level is less than that with probucol alone, and constipation is much less common than with a resin alone.

Fish oils containing omega-3 fatty acids are available over the counter but can also be obtained in reasonable amounts by eating a 3-oz (cooked) portion of oily fish (eg, herring, mackerel, salmon, shad, trout). Data about the long-term effectiveness and adverse effects of fish oil supplements are scarce; however, for short-term use, doses of ≤ 15 g/day appear to be safe and can lower TG levels, but they are not useful in lowering cholesterol levels. They may increase the hydrolysis of VLDL-TG. In patients with hypertriglyceridemia, fish oils may increase HDL-C levels by 10 to 15%. At much higher doses (usually > 50 g/day), they may be associated with thrombocytopenia and increased bleeding time; such doses are almost never used clinically. In rare cases when doses of > 20 g/day are used, platelet counts and bleeding time should be monitored. At such doses, fish oils may interfere with glucose control in patients with diabetes.

Estrogen replacement therapy: Postmenopausal women who receive unopposed estrogen replacement therapy have lower LDL-C levels (by 15 to 25%) and higher HDL-C levels (by 16 to 21%) than those who do not receive this therapy; as a result the LDL-C/HDL-C ratio is substantially decreased. Such therapy also lowers Lp(a) levels. Unopposed estrogen therapy appears to reduce the risk of cardiovascular death. The addition of a progestin to reduce the risk of endometrial hyperplasia and endometrial cancer probably does not have a significant adverse effect on lipoprotein levels.

Estrogen replacement therapy can be used alone or with other lipid-modifying treatments. Estrogen substantially elevates TG levels in women with preexisting hypertriglyceridemia, occasionally to levels that can cause lethal pancreatitis. Consequently, fasting TG levels should be measured before initiating estrogen replacement therapy (with or without a progestin). Estrogen replacement therapy is contraindicated in women with familial hypertriglyceridemia and a TG level > 300 mg/dL after modification of diet and alcohol intake.

Antioxidant therapy: The toxicity of LDL-C may be reduced by the use of antioxidants. According to one hypothesis, atherosclerosis progresses because "toxic LDL" triggers the development of fatty streaks. Toxic LDL is formed when the lipid component of the lipoprotein is oxidized by endothelial cells and smooth muscle cells. Oxidation occurs via a free radical mechanism involving superoxide anions and hydrogen peroxide. The oxidized LDL functions as a chemotactic agent for monocytes, transforming them to macrophages, which stimulate cholesterol esterification and the formation of foam cells.

α-Tocopherol (vitamin E) inhibits the oxidation of LDL in vitro. In several studies, vitamin E consumption appeared to be strongly and inversely correlated with CAD risk. Vitamin E supplementation for short periods produced no benefit, but supplementation for at least 2 years was associated with a lower risk of CAD in men and women.

Vitamin A, a β-carotenoid, may affect atherosclerosis by scavenging oxidizing free radicals. In observational studies, the CAD mortality rate appeared to be strongly and inversely correlated with dietary carotene intake.

Ascorbic acid (vitamin C) is considered a secondary antioxidant; it works synergistically with vitamin E, regenerating vitamin E from the vitamin E radical. Vitamin C may also enhance the transformation of cholesterol into bile acids.

Treatment of special conditions: Treating elderly patients with an **isolated low HDL-C level** (usually well below 35 mg/dL [0.91 mmol/L]), a TC level < 200 mg/dL (< 2.26 mmol/L), and a TG level < 250 mg/dL (< 2.82 mmol/L) is a challenge. If lifestyle changes (weight loss, increased aerobic exercise, cessation of cigarette smoking) do not increase the HDL-C level and particularly if the patient has had an atherosclerotic event or is at high risk because of primary hypoalphalipoproteinemia or other CAD risk factors, drug treatment is warranted. However, the best approach has not been established. Nicotinic acid 1.5 to 6.0 g/day or gemfibrozil 1.2 g/day may be effective, particularly if the Lp(a) level is also high. If these drugs are ineffective or cannot be tolerated, a statin may be given to lower the TC level to < 160 mg/dL (< 4.14 mmol/L) or the LDL-C level to < 100 mg/dL (< 2.59 mmol/L); the HDL-C level usually does not change, but the TC/HDL-C ratio is usually substantially decreased.

High Lp(a) levels cannot be lowered by diet and can be lowered only modestly by nicotinic acid. Most other drugs that lower LDL-C levels do not substantially alter Lp(a) levels. Therefore, aggressive modification of other CAD risk factors, if present, is important.

64 ▆▆▆ DISORDERS OF CARBOHYDRATE METABOLISM

DIABETES MELLITUS

A syndrome characterized by hyperglycemia with repeated fasting blood glucose levels > 125 mg/dL (> 6.9 mmol/L) or any postprandial level > 200 mg/dL (> 11.1 mmol/L) resulting from absolute or relative impairment of insulin secretion and/or insulin action.

Type II diabetes mellitus (DM) is much more common than type I in the elderly. Type I can usually be distinguished from type II by its early onset and dependency on insulin therapy. This chapter focuses primarily on type II DM.

The prevalence of type II DM increases with age (from about 3 to 5% in persons in the 4th to 5th decade of life to about 10 to 20% in persons in the 7th to 8th decade). Type II DM is often diagnosed during a routine medical examination.

Etiology and Pathogenesis

Type II DM encompasses a heterogeneous group of disorders in which hyperglycemia results from an impaired insulin secretory response to glucose and a decreased insulin effectiveness in stimulating glucose uptake by skeletal muscle and in restraining hepatic glucose production (insulin resistance). However, insulin resistance is common, and most patients with insulin resistance do not develop type II DM because the body compensates by adequately increasing insulin secretion. Although insulin resistance in type II DM is not the result of genetic alterations in the insulin receptor or glucose transporter, genetically determined postreceptor intracellular defects likely play a role. The resulting hyperinsulinemia may lead to the syndrome of insulin resistance, which is characterized by visceral/abdominal obesity, hypertension, hyperlipidemia, and coronary artery disease.

Type II DM is commonly associated with obesity, especially of the upper body (visceral/abdominal), and often presents after a period of weight gain. Although the patient's weight may be normal, the waist-to-hip ratio is increased (> 1). Type II DM patients with upper body obesity may have normal blood glucose levels after losing weight.

Genetic factors appear to be major determinants for the development of type II DM (the concordance rate for type II DM in monozygotic twins is > 90%), yet only a minor association between type II DM and specific human leukocyte antigen (HLA) phenotypes or islet cell cytoplasmic antibodies has been demonstrated. One exception is a subset of lean adults with detectable islet cell cytoplasmic antibodies who carry one of the HLA phenotypes and who may eventually develop type I DM. Another subset of lean elderly persons (who are not insulin-resistant) have a decreased ability to secrete adequate insulin, although they have neither anti-islet antibodies nor the relevant HLA.

In type II DM, the pancreatic islets retain β cells (insulin-secreting cells) in ratios to α cells (glucagon-secreting cells) that are not consistently altered, and normal β- and α-cell mass appears to be preserved in most patients. Pancreatic islet amyloid, resulting from a deposition of amylin, is found in many type II DM patients at autopsy, but its relationship to the pathogenesis of type II DM is unknown.

Before diabetes develops, patients generally lose the early insulin secretory response to glucose and may secrete relatively large amounts of proinsulin. In established diabetes, although fasting insulin levels may be normal or even increased in type II DM patients, glucose-stimulated insulin secretion is decreased. The decreased insulin levels reduce insulin-mediated glucose uptake and fail to restrain hepatic glucose production.

Hyperglycemia may not only be a consequence but also a cause of further impairment in glucose tolerance in the diabetic patient (glucose toxicity) because hyperglycemia decreases insulin sensitivity and increases hepatic glucose production. Once a patient's metabolic control improves, the insulin or hypoglycemic drug dose is usually lowered.

Brittle diabetes is characterized by frequent, rapid swings in blood glucose levels without apparent cause. It is most common in patients with low residual insulin secretory capacity and in those who have autonomic neuropathy with impaired gastric emptying. These patients may have sustained hyperglycemia, which further impairs gastric emptying.

Chronic pancreatitis, particularly in alcoholics, often leads to diabetes. Such patients lose insulin-secreting and glucagon-secreting islet cells. Therefore, they may be mildly hyperglycemic, are not prone to diabetic ketoacidosis (DKA), and are usually sensitive to low doses of insulin. Given the lack of effective counterregulation (exogenous insulin that is unopposed by glucagon), they often experience rapid onset of hypoglycemia. Diabetes can be caused by other endocrine diseases (eg, Cushing's syndrome, acromegaly, pheochromocytoma, glucagonoma, primary hyperaldosteronism, somatostatinoma). Most of these disorders are associated with peripheral or hepatic insulin resistance. Many patients become diabetic once insulin secretion also decreases. The prevalence of type I DM is increased in patients with certain autoimmune endocrine diseases (eg, Graves' disease, Hashimoto's disease, idiopathic Addison's disease).

Symptoms and Signs

DM has diverse initial presentations. Type I DM often presents with symptomatic hyperglycemia or DKA, whereas type II DM may present with symptomatic hyperglycemia, nonketotic hyperglycemic-hyperosmolar coma (NKHHC), or as a clinical manifestation of a late complication of diabetes.

Asymptomatic hyperglycemia is usually associated with elevated blood glucose levels ≤ 200 mg/dL (≤ 11.1 mmol/L). Such levels rarely result in significant glucosuria and catabolism and are much easier to treat than higher levels.

In symptomatic hyperglycemia (usually > 200 mg/dL [> 11.1 mmol/L]), polyuria followed by polydipsia and weight loss occurs when elevated blood glucose levels cause marked glucosuria and osmotic diuresis, resulting in dehydration. However, because the kidneys' ability to reabsorb filtrated glucose often increases with age, elderly patients may have significant hyperglycemia without polyuria. Hyperglycemia may also cause blurred vision, fatigue, and nausea and lead to fungal and bacterial infections. In type II DM, symptomatic hyperglycemia may persist for days or weeks before medical attention is sought; in women, type II DM with symptomatic hyperglycemia is often associated with perineal itching due to vaginal candidiasis.

Complications

Although hyperglycemia increases the risk of **macrovascular** disease (eg, atherosclerosis) ◘ fivefold, other factors (eg, hypertension, cigarette smoking) increase the risk 10- to 20-fold. Another contributing factor is dyslipidemia of type II DM, which is characterized by elevated triglyceride levels and decreased high-density lipoprotein (HDL) levels. Although low-density lipoprotein (LDL) levels are not strikingly differ-

◘ see page 849

ent from those of nondiabetic persons, they contain a preponderance of smaller, denser, more atherogenic LDL particles. Macrovascular disease may lead to stroke, symptomatic coronary artery disease, claudication, skin breakdown, and infections. Aspirin helps prevent macrovascular complications in diabetic patients. However, the positive effects may be achieved only with doses higher than those found to be effective in nondiabetics to prevent stroke and heart attack. Treatment of concomitant risk factors, such as hypertension (particularly with angiotensin-converting enzyme inhibitors) and/or dyslipidemia (particularly with statins) ▇ has been shown to further reduce morbidity and mortality in elderly diabetic patients. Amputation of a lower limb for severe peripheral vascular disease or gangrene remains common.

Microvascular complications (eg, retinopathy, nephropathy, peripheral and autonomic neuropathies) usually occur after several years of poorly controlled hyperglycemia. However, many type II DM patients have some of these complications at diagnosis. Most microvascular complications can be prevented, delayed, or even reversed by tight glycemic control.

Background **retinopathy** (the initial retinal changes seen on ophthalmoscopic examination or in retinal photographs) does not significantly alter vision, but it can progress to macular edema or proliferative retinopathy with retinal detachment or hemorrhage, which can cause blindness. ▇ About 85% of all diabetic patients eventually develop some degree of retinopathy, beginning at least 7 years before the diagnosis of type II DM is made. Some data support the use of oral pentoxifylline.

Diabetic nephropathy develops in about one third of type I DM patients and in a smaller percentage of type II DM patients. Glomerular filtration rate may be increased initially with hyperglycemia. Clinically detectable albuminuria ($\geq$ 300 mg/L), which is unexplained by other urinary tract disease, may develop after about 5 years of diabetes. Albuminuria is almost 2.5 times higher in diabetic patients with diastolic blood pressure (BP) > 90 mm Hg than in those with diastolic BP < 70 mm Hg. Thus, both hyperglycemia and hypertension accelerate the progression to end-stage renal disease. Diabetic nephropathy is usually asymptomatic until end-stage renal disease develops, but the nephrotic syndrome may result. Albuminuria and renal disease may be prevented or delayed with captopril, an angiotensin-converting enzyme inhibitor.

Diabetic neuropathy commonly occurs as a distal, symmetric, predominantly sensory polyneuropathy that causes sensory deficits, which begin with and are usually most marked by a stocking-glove distribution. Diabetic polyneuropathy may cause numbness, tingling, and paresthesias in the extremities and, less often, debilitating, severe, deepseated pain and hyperesthesias. Ankle jerks are usually decreased or absent. Acute, painful mononeuropathies affecting the 3rd, 4th, or 6th cranial nerve as well as other nerves, such as the femoral, may spontaneously improve over weeks to months, occur more often in elderly patients, and are attributed to nerve infarctions. Autonomic neuropathy occurs primarily in patients with polyneuropathy and can cause postural hypotension, disordered sweating, impotence and retrograde ejaculation in men, impaired bladder function, delayed gastric emptying (sometimes with dumping syndrome), esophageal dysfunction, constipation or diarrhea, and nocturnal diarrhea. A blunted decrease in heart rate in response to the Valsalva maneuver or standing and a blunted decrease in heart rate slowing with deep breathing are evidence of autonomic neuropathy.

Foot ulcers and joint problems are important causes of morbidity in diabetic patients. The major predisposing cause is diabetic polyneuropathy. The sensory denervation impairs the perception of trauma from such common causes as ill-fitting shoes or pebbles. Alterations in proprioception lead to an abnormal pattern of weight bearing and sometimes to the development of Charcot's joints.

Infection risk from fungi and bacteria is increased because of decreased cellular immunity caused by acute hyperglycemia and circulatory deficits caused by chronic hyperglycemia. Peripheral skin infections and oral and vaginal thrush occur most commonly. A fungal infection may lead to wet interdigital lesions, cracks, fissures, and ulcerations that favor secondary bacterial invasion. Patients with infected foot ulcers often feel no pain because of neuropathy and have no systemic symptoms until late in a neglected course. Early surgical debridement is essential, but amputation is sometimes necessary.

Elderly diabetic patients may be more at risk of **cognitive dysfunction and depression.** One retrospective study demonstrated that elderly diabetic patients had similar cognitive function as had nondiabetic patients but were twice as likely to exhibit symptoms of depression. Other studies suggest that good blood glucose control may reduce the likelihood and severity of cognitive dysfunction. Still other studies demonstrated that diabetes and functional decline were risk factors for increased mortality.

Diagnosis

In asymptomatic patients, **fasting blood glucose levels** ≥ 126 mg/dL (≥ 7.0 mmol/L) are considered diagnostic for types I and II DM (see TABLE 64–1). These criteria are based on evidence that complications occur at these levels and that, in most patients, more severe DM follows. Although hyperglycemia in the elderly is usually caused by type II DM, other causes (eg, diseases of the exocrine pancreas, endocrinopathies, drug- or chemical-induced causes) should be considered.

An **oral glucose tolerance test** (OGTT; with 75 g anhydrous glucose dissolved in water) is not routinely needed but may help diagnose type

TABLE 64-1.   CRITERIA FOR DIAGNOSIS OF DIABETES MELLITUS IN THE ELDERLY*

Symptoms of diabetes plus casual plasma glucose level $\geq$ 200 mg/dL ($\geq$ 11.1 mmol/L). Casual is defined as any time of day without regard to time since last meal. The classic symptoms of diabetes include polyuria, polydipsia, and unexplained weight loss.

or

Fasting plasma glucose level $\geq$ 126 mg/dL ($\geq$ 7.0 mmol/L). Fasting is defined as no caloric intake for at least 8 hours.

or

Two-hour plasma glucose level $\geq$ 200 mg/dL ($\geq$ 11.1 mmol/L) during an oral glucose tolerance test using a glucose load containing the equivalent of 75 g of anhydrous glucose dissolved in water.

*In the absence of unequivocal hyperglycemia with acute metabolic decompensation, these criteria should be confirmed by repeat testing on a different day. The oral glucose tolerance test is not routinely recommended.

Adapted from American Diabetic Association: "Report of the Expert Committee on the Diagnosis and Classification of Diabetes Mellitus (Committee Report)." *Diabetes Care* 22 (Suppl. 1):S5–S19, January 1999.

II DM in patients whose fasting blood glucose level is between 110 and 126 mg/dL (6.1 and 7.0 mmol/L). Such levels are common in lean elderly patients who develop hyperglycemia postprandially. Test results are positive if blood glucose levels are $\geq$ 200 mg/dL ($\geq$ 11.1 mmol/L) at 2 hours.

Glycosylated hemoglobin (Hb A$_{1c}$) is not specific for diagnosing diabetes; however, elevated Hb A$_{1c}$ often indicates existing diabetes. Hb A$_{1c}$ should be determined every 1 to 3 months to estimate blood glucose control. In poorly controlled diabetic patients, the level ranges from 9 to 12%; the goal is to maintain a level of $\leq$ 8%. Measuring the **fructosamine level** is another indirect test of glucose control. Fructosamine is formed by a chemical reaction of glucose with plasma protein and reflects glucose control in the previous 1 to 3 weeks. Therefore, this assay may show a change in control before Hb A$_{1c}$ does and is often helpful when the patient undergoes intensive treatment and in short-term clinical trials.

Prognosis and Treatment

On each physician visit, a diabetic patient should be assessed for symptoms or signs of complications, including a check of the feet and the pulses and sensation in the feet and legs, and be given a urine test for albumin. Laboratory evaluation every year includes lipid profile, blood urea nitrogen and serum creatinine levels, ECG, and a complete annual ophthalmologic examination. ∎

∎see also page 1303

The elderly should be treated as aggressively, in terms of glycemic control, as their general situation allows. Hyperglycemia is responsible for most of the long-term microvascular complications of diabetes. A linear relationship exists between Hb A_{1c} levels and the rate at which complications develop; Hb $A_{1c} < 8\%$ is a threshold below which most complications seem to be prevented. Thus, in type I DM, therapy should try to intensify metabolic control to lower Hb A_{1c} while avoiding hypoglycemic episodes. In type II DM, intensive treatment with oral hypoglycemic drugs or insulin is also beneficial. However, treatment in the elderly can be difficult (see TABLE 64–2).

Weight management is important. In the overweight diabetic patient, weight loss is usually the goal. Insulin sensitivity increases when obese patients are in negative caloric balance, which occurs within weeks of starting a weight-loss diet (long before much of the extra weight is lost). As hyperglycemia lessens, glucose toxicity may improve, leading to better metabolic control. Weight maintenance or even weight gain may be the goal for the significant percentage of the oldest old diabetics who are lean. Because these patients are relatively insulin-deficient, insulin therapy may increase appetite and help manage body weight.

Diet management is also important and is often best achieved by working with a dietitian; coordination with other caregivers is often required. In insulin-treated diabetics, diet management aims to restrict variations in the timing, size, or composition of meals, which could make the prescribed insulin regimen inappropriate and result in hypoglycemia or marked postprandial hyperglycemia. All insulin-treated patients require detailed diet management, including a prescription for

TABLE 64–2. FACTORS AFFECTING DIABETES TREATMENT IN THE ELDERLY

Altered sense	Neoplasia
Decreased vision	Decreased exercise and mobility
Decreased smell	Drugs
Altered taste perception	Medications (non–potassium-sparing
Decreased proprioception	diuretic, glucocorticoids, phenytoin)
Difficulties in food preparation and	Alcohol
consumption	Neuropsychiatric problems
Tremor	Bereavement
Arthritis	Depression
Poor dentition	Cognitive impairment and dementia
Alterations in gastrointestinal function	Social factors
and nutrient absorption	Inadequate education
Altered recognition of hunger and thirst	Poor dietary habits
Altered renal and hepatic function	Living alone
Acute infections	Poverty

Modified from Lipson LG: "Diabetes in the elderly: Diagnosis, pathogenesis and therapy." *American Journal of Medicine* 80 (Suppl 5A):10–21, 1986; used with permission.

their total daily caloric intake; guidelines for proportions of carbohydrate, fat, and protein in their diets; and instruction on distributing calories among meals and snacks. A dietitian can tailor the plan to meet the patient's needs. Patient motivation is enhanced when the plan is flexible.

Regular exercise is beneficial, especially in obese patients to burn calories. Exercise also increases insulin sensitivity (ie, patients respond better to insulin injection or endogenous insulin). However, for this effect to occur, exercise must be sufficient to lower the resting heart rate. Although some elderly patients cannot undertake a vigorous exercise program, all diabetic patients should be encouraged to exercise as much as they can, especially walking, swimming, and other aerobic activities. However, in patients receiving insulin, moderate to vigorous exercise can lead to hypoglycemia, primarily because absorption from the injection site increases.

Pharmacotherapy: Oral antidiabetic drugs (see TABLE 64–3) are used only for type II DM. Single or combination drug therapy with oral antidiabetic drugs is often successful in achieving good metabolic control for many years. Oral antidiabetic drugs include the antihyperglycemic drugs (biguanides, α-glucosidase inhibitors, and thiazolidinediones) and the oral hypoglycemic drugs (sulfonylureas and a meglitinide analog). In contrast with oral hypoglycemic drugs, oral antihyperglycemic drugs rarely cause hypoglycemia and should be used for patients diagnosed with diabetes early.

Metformin (a biguanide) decreases hepatic glucose production and may improve insulin sensitivity. Metformin should be considered the drug of choice for treating newly diagnosed, obese type II DM patients. However, metformin is contraindicated in patients with kidney disease (creatinine level $\geq$ 1.4 mg/dL [$\geq$ 120 μmol/L]), in patients $\geq$ 80 because their renal function is difficult to assess, and in patients with liver disease, alcoholism, or lactic acidosis; it should not be used in most patients during acute hospitalization. It is as effective as a sulfonylurea as monotherapy (although when used alone it rarely causes hypoglycemia) and is synergistic in combination with sulfonylurea therapy. It promotes weight loss and decreases lipid levels. Metformin reduces diabetes-related complications (eg, myocardial infarction) and diabetes-related deaths by about 30 to 40%. Gastrointestinal (GI) adverse effects are common but are often transient and may be prevented if the drug is taken with meals and if the dose is increased gradually (at weekly intervals by 500 to 850 mg/day up to 2.55 g/day).

Repaglinide, which activates signals downstream from the sulfonylurea receptor, has a short half-life and biologic action, so that insulin secretion tends to decrease postprandially. Repaglinide has a similar safety profile to that of the sulfonylureas.

Acarbose (an α-glucosidase inhibitor) may be ideal for elderly patients with mild hyperglycemia (fasting blood glucose levels between

TABLE 64–3. CHARACTERISTICS OF ORAL ANTIDIABETIC DRUGS

Generic Name	Daily Dosage Range (mg)	Duration of Action (h)	Comments
Antihyperglycemic drugs			
Biguanide			
Metformin	500–2550 divided with meals	6–10	Applied as monotherapy or combination therapy with sulfonylurea. Contraindicated with kidney and liver diseases, alcoholism, and lactic acidosis and in patients $\geq$ 80
α-Glucosidase inhibitors			
Acarbose, miglitol	25–300 divided with meals	2–6	Applied as monotherapy or combination therapy with sulfonylurea to decrease postprandial blood glucose levels. GI side effects are common
Thiazolidine-diones			
Rosiglitazone	2–8 once a day	24	Applied as monotherapy or combination therapy; rosiglitazone may have an adverse hepatic effect
Pioglitazone	15–45 once a day	24	
Oral hypoglycemic drugs			
Sulfonylureas			
First-generation			
Tolbutamide	500–3000	6–12	Rarely drug of choice in the elderly
Chlorpropamide	100–750	60	*Do not use in the elderly*
Acetohexamide	250–1500	12–24	
Tolazamide	100–1000	12–24	
Second-generation			
Glyburide	1.25–20	12–24	Applied as monotherapy or combination therapy with other oral agents and insulin; has risks for hypoglycemia
Micronized glyburide	0.75–12	12–24	
Glipizide	2.5–40	12–24	
Glipizide-GITS	5–20	24–36	
Glimepiride	1–8	24	
Meglitinide analog			
Repaglinide	0.25–16	1–3	

GI = gastrointestinal; GITS = gastrointestinal therapeutic system.

100 and 150 mg/dL [between 5.6 and 8.3 mmol/L]) or with postprandial hyperglycemia. Acarbose competitively inhibits hydrolysis of oligosaccharides and monosaccharides, which delays carbohydrate digestion in the small intestine and subsequent absorption, resulting in less postprandial elevation of blood glucose levels. Acarbose has a weaker antihyperglycemic effect as monotherapy than metformin or the sulfonylureas. GI adverse effects are common in the elderly but are often transient. The drug must be taken three times daily with each main meal (with the first bite), and the dosage should be gradually increased from 25 mg up to 50 to 100 mg with each meal.

Miglitol (another α-glucosidase inhibitor) has an efficacy and adverse effect profile similar to that of acarbose.

Thiazolidinediones (eg, pioglitazone, rosiglitazone, troglitazone [no longer available in the USA]) are recent additions to the available therapy for type II DM. These drugs improve insulin sensitivity in skeletal muscle and suppress hepatic glucose output. Thiazolidinediones have a weaker antihyperglycemic effect than metformin or the sulfonylureas and are most appropriate as reserve drugs to control blood glucose in patients taking other oral drugs or insulin. Rosiglitazone and pioglitazone are useful in elderly patients with impaired renal function, in whom metformin and sulfonylureas are contraindicated. These drugs increase body weight and may cause small changes in total, low-density lipoprotein (LDL), and high-density lipoprotein (HDL) cholesterol. Troglitazone is no longer marketed in the USA because a worrisome number of patients taking troglitazone developed idiosyncratic liver disease, and some developed hepatic failure, which led to liver transplantation or death. Rosiglitazone may cause hepatotoxicity also. Pioglitazone does not appear to do so.

The **sulfonylureas** lower blood glucose levels primarily by stimulating insulin secretion, but they also improve peripheral and hepatic insulin sensitivity. The sulfonylureas differ in potency and duration of action. Allergic reactions and other adverse effects of sulfonylureas (eg, cholestatic jaundice) are relatively uncommon. The 2nd-generation sulfonylureas (eg, glipizide, glyburide, glimepiride) are about 100 times more potent than the 1st-generation ones and are absorbed rapidly.

Among the 1st-generation sulfonylureas, acetohexamide may be used in patients who are allergic to other sulfonylureas. Chlorpropamide should not be used in elderly patients because it has a prolonged half-life and can potentiate the action of antidiuretic hormone, often leading to hyponatremia and impaired mental status.

For initial treatment, many authorities prefer the shorter-acting sulfonylureas, and most do not recommend using a combination of different sulfonylureas. Treatment is started with a low dose, which is adjusted after several days until a satisfactory response is obtained or the maximum recommended dose is reached. About 10 to 20% of patients fail to respond, and patients who fail to respond to one sulfonylurea often fail to respond to others. Of those who initially respond, 5 to 10% per year experience secondary failures. In such cases, insulin may be added to the sulfonylurea treatment.

Hypoglycemia, which is the most important complication of sulfonylurea treatment in the elderly, occurs most often with long-acting sulfonylureas (eg, glyburide, chlorpropamide). Sulfonylurea-induced hypoglycemia can be severe and last or recur for days after treatment is stopped. Therefore, all patients treated with sulfonylureas who develop hypoglycemia should be closely monitored in the hospital for 2 to 3 days.

Combination therapy is often useful when oral antidiabetic drugs with different mechanisms of action are used together. For example, the combination of metformin and glyburide is likely to decrease Hb A_{1c} by about 2% more than glyburide can alone. When combined with insulin, metformin and thiazolidinediones allow for decreased insulin dosage while improving metabolic control. Although the incidence of hypoglycemia is low when these drugs are combined with insulin, patients should be instructed to decrease their daily insulin dosage by 10 to 20% when blood glucose levels decline to 8 to 11 mmol/L.

Insulin therapy: Most type II DM patients do not need insulin. In general, oral drugs should be adequately tried first. Human insulin is often preferred because it is less antigenic than animal-derived varieties. However, detectable insulin antibody levels, usually very low, develop in most insulin-treated patients, including those receiving human insulin preparations.

Insulin is injected subcutaneously with disposable syringes. The 1/2-mL syringes are generally preferred by patients who routinely inject doses of 50 U or less, because these syringes facilitate the accurate measurement of smaller insulin doses. A multiple-dose insulin injection device (eg, NovolinPen), commonly referred to as an insulin pen, uses a cartridge containing several days' dosage. The accuracy and simplicity of this method may be beneficial to elderly patients. Insulin should be refrigerated *but never frozen;* however, most insulin preparations are stable at room temperature for months, which facilitates their use when working and traveling. Some elderly patients have difficulty accurately drawing insulin doses. Magnifying lenses and syringe guides may help; alternatively, a visiting nurse can prepare a week's worth of syringes.

Insulin preparations are rapid-acting (short-acting), intermediate-acting, or long-acting. The usual onset of action, time of peak action, and duration of action of the most commonly used preparations are listed in TABLE 64–4; these data should be used only as guidelines, because patients and different doses of the same preparation in the same patient vary considerably. Mixtures of insulin preparations with different onsets and durations of action are often given in a single injection by drawing measured doses of two preparations into the same syringe

TABLE 64–4.   TIME COURSE OF ACTION OF INSULIN PREPARATIONS*

Insulin Preparation	Onset of Action†	Peak Action (h)	Duration of Action (h)
Rapid-acting Lispro	0–15 min	$\frac{1}{2}$–1$\frac{1}{2}$	4
Rapid-acting regular	15–30 min	2–4	6–8
Rapid-acting Semilente (prompt insulin zinc suspension)	1–2 h	4–9	10–16
Intermediate-acting (NPH and Lente)	1–3 h	6–12	18–26
Long-acting (Ultralente and PZI)	4–8 h	14–24	28–36

*Extreme variability among patients accounts for the broad ranges indicated.
†Subcutaneous injection.
NPH = neutral protamine Hagedorn; PZI = protamine zinc insulin.

immediately before use. The critical determinant of the onset and duration of action is the rate of insulin absorption from the injection site.

Treatment should be started with bedtime neutral protamine Hagedorn (NPH) insulin. Type II DM patients, nearly all of whom have significant insulin resistance, usually require more insulin than type I DM patients. The initial total daily dose may be later divided so that half is administered before breakfast, one quarter before dinner, and one quarter at bedtime. Adjustments in the amounts, types, and timing are made based on blood glucose determinations. The insulin dose is adjusted to maintain the preprandial blood glucose level between 80 and 150 mg/dL (between 4.4 and 8.3 mmol/L). Increments in insulin dose are generally restricted to 10% at a time, and the effects are assessed over about 3 days before any further increment is made. More rapid adjustments of regular insulin are indicated if hypoglycemia threatens.

Many patients with **brittle diabetes** improve when switched to more intensive therapy or when their GI dysfunction is effectively managed, often with metoclopramide. The aim is not to achieve a near-normal blood glucose level but to stabilize the fluctuations within a range that prevents symptomatic hyperglycemia and hypoglycemia.

Complications of insulin treatment: Hypoglycemia may occur because of an error in insulin dosage, a small or missed meal, unplanned exercise (patients are usually instructed to reduce their insulin dose or to increase their carbohydrate intake before planned exercise), or without apparent cause. Patients should be taught to recognize symptoms of hypoglycemia. However, patients with good metabolic control should be aware that they may not experience adrenergic symptoms and may lose the ability to recognize hypoglycemia, although they still experience central nervous system (CNS) dysfunction and can deteriorate rapidly into a coma. All diabetic patients should carry candy, lumps of sugar, or glucose tablets. An identification card, bracelet, or necklace indicating that the patient is an insulin-treated diabetic aids in an emergency. Family members should be instructed to administer glucagon with an easy-to-use injection device.

The **dawn phenomenon** refers to the normal tendency of the blood glucose level to rise in the early morning hours before breakfast, which is frequently exaggerated in patients with type I DM and in some patients with type II DM. Fasting blood glucose levels rise because of an increase in hepatic glucose production, which may be secondary to the midnight surge of growth hormone. In some patients with diabetes, nocturnal hypoglycemia may be followed by a marked increase in fasting blood glucose with an increase in plasma ketones (**Somogyi phenomenon**).

Local allergic reactions at the site of insulin injections are less common with purified porcine and human insulins. These reactions can produce immediate pain and burning followed several hours later by local erythema, pruritus, and induration, the latter sometimes persisting for days. Most reactions spontaneously disappear after weeks of continued insulin injection and require no specific treatment, although antihistamines are sometimes used.

Local fat atrophy or hypertrophy at injection sites is relatively rare and usually lessens by switching to human insulin and injecting it directly into the affected area. No specific treatment of local fat hypertrophy is required, but injection sites should be rotated.

Generalized **insulin allergy** (usually to the insulin molecule) is rare but can occur when treatment is discontinued and restarted after a lapse of months or years. Symptoms usually develop shortly after an injection and may include urticaria, angioedema, pruritus, bronchospasm, and, in some cases, circulatory collapse. Treatment with antihistamines may help, but epinephrine and IV glucocorticoids may be required. If insulin treatment needs to be continued after the condition stabilizes, skin testing with a panel of purified insulin preparations and desensitization should be performed by an experienced physician.

Insulin resistance is an increase in insulin requirement to 200 U/day and is associated with marked increases in the plasma insulin-binding capacity. Most patients treated with insulin for 6 months develop antibodies to insulin. In patients with insulin resistance, switching to purified porcine or human insulin may lower the requirement. Remission may be spontaneous. Prednisone may decrease the insulin requirement within 2 weeks; treatment is usually initiated with about 30 mg po bid and is tapered as the requirement decreases.

Treatment of diabetic patients during concurrent illness: Diabetic patients commonly have coexisting illnesses that aggravate hyperglycemia (eg, an infection, coronary artery disease). Bed rest and a regular diet may also aggravate hyperglycemia. Conversely, if the patient is anorectic or vomits or if food intake is reduced, continuation of drugs may cause hypoglycemia. In hospitals, a sliding scale for insulin administration is commonly used; however, the scale should not be the only intervention because it is reactive rather than proactive. Hypoglycemic drugs may be discontinued during an acute condition associated with decreased food intake or one that has a tendency to cause hypoglycemia (eg, renal failure). Insulin may be added if blood glucose levels remain high. However, hospitalized type II DM patients often do well without any change in their antidiabetic drugs.

Because DM patients are at increased risk of acute renal failure, x-rays that require IV injection of contrast dyes should be performed only when absolutely necessary and only when the patient is well hydrated.

Treatment of diabetic patients during surgical procedures: The effects of surgical procedures (including the prior emotional stress, the effects of general anesthesia, and the trauma of the procedure) can markedly increase blood glucose levels in diabetics and induce DKA in type I DM patients. Sulfonylureas should be withheld 2 to 4 days before surgery, and blood glucose levels should be measured preoperatively and postoperatively and every 6 hours while patients receive IV fluids. Metformin should be withheld after the operation until cardiovascular and renal functions are confirmed to be normal. Insulin is not required for diabetic patients who maintain a satisfactory blood glucose level by diet alone or in combination therapy before surgery.

Patient and Caregiver Issues

Because of the evolving technology of diabetes treatment, the multifactorial drug regimen, and necessary lifestyle changes for the patient, the diabetic patient is often referred to a diabetes center. The first appointment should immediately follow the initial diagnosis, and other visits can be scheduled on an individual basis, depending on the success or failure of the therapy initiated by the primary care physician. When educating the elderly diabetic patient, one should recognize the patient's previous experiences and choose teaching materials and methods that will actively include the patient (eg, large-print materials, additional time for practicing skills).

Group classes can provide needed socialization and support for the elderly, are more cost-effective than one-on-one sessions, and often encourage participation from elderly patients. Factors that may influence learning include the aging process, the patient's emotional state, other medical conditions, and drug treatment. Many elderly diabetic patients are enthusiastic and motivated learners and are actively involved in all aspects of their treatment. When elderly patients are appropriately educated, they can self-monitor their blood glucose level as accurately as younger patients. Including family members in the assessment and education process is essential.

Appropriate aids should be provided to circumvent some of the patient's limitations (eg, poor vision, limited dexterity). Glucose meters should be easy to use, have large display screens and memory capabilities, and require no cleaning. Patients must recognize indications for seeking immediate medical attention and exercise appropriate foot care.∎ Clinical dietitians have an important role in teaching weight and food management. Insulin-treated patients should be taught to adjust their insulin doses based on self-monitoring of glucose, which can be tested with easy-to-use home analyzers using a drop of fingertip blood. A spring-powered lancet is recommended to obtain the fingertip blood sample. The frequency of testing is determined individually. Insulin-treated patients ideally should test their blood glucose level daily before meals, 2 to 3 hours after meals, and at bedtime. However, in practice, two to four measurements may be obtained each day at different times, so that an overall assessment can be made after a week or so of treatment.

NONKETOTIC HYPERGLYCEMIC-HYPEROSMOLAR COMA

A syndrome characterized by hyperglycemia, extreme dehydration, and hyperosmolar plasma, leading to impaired consciousness, sometimes accompanied by seizures.

Nonketotic hyperglycemic-hyperosmolar coma (NKHHC) is a complication of type II DM that has a high mortality rate. It usually develops after a period of symptomatic hyperglycemia during which fluid intake is inadequate to prevent extreme dehydration from the hyperglycemia-induced osmotic diuresis. It is more common in the elderly and is often accompanied or precipitated by acute infection, particularly gram-negative pneumonia or sepsis associated with a urinary tract infection. In some patients, NKHHC can occur when patients with undiagnosed or neglected type II DM receive drugs that impair glucose tolerance (eg, glucocorticoids) or increase fluid loss (eg, diuretics). Persons with severe dementia may be particularly insensitive to hunger or thirst—the former leading to weight loss, the latter to dehydration and, if uncorrected, to NKHHC.

Symptoms, Signs, and Diagnosis

NKHHC produces CNS dysfunction and symptoms and signs of dehydration. The state of consciousness at presentation varies from mental cloudiness to coma. Focal or generalized seizures may occur and are more common in the elderly. Transient hemiplegia may occur. Laboratory studies show extreme hyperglycemia, hyperosmolarity,

---

∎ see TABLE 56–2 on page 547

mild metabolic acidosis without marked hyperketonemia, and prerenal azotemia (or preexisting chronic renal failure). The blood glucose level is usually > 500 mg/dL (> 27.8 mmol/L—higher than in most cases of diabetic ketoacidosis). The calculated serum osmolality on admission is > 350 mOsm/kg, whereas the normal level is about 290 mOsm/kg. Initial plasma bicarbonate levels are often depressed, reflecting increased lactate levels from poor perfusion or associated sepsis. However, these patients are often positive for ketones, reflecting low insulin levels (glucose toxicity) and high glucagon levels. Serum Na and K levels are usually normal, but blood urea nitrogen and serum creatinine levels are markedly increased.

The average fluid deficit is 10 L, and acute circulatory collapse is a common terminal event in NKHHC. Widespread in situ thrombosis is a frequent finding on autopsy, and in some cases bleeding ascribed to disseminated intravascular coagulation or gangrenous-appearing digits has been found.

Treatment

The immediate aim of treatment is to rapidly expand the contracted intravascular volume to stabilize blood pressure (BP) and to improve circulation and urine flow.

Treatment is started by infusing 2 to 3 L of 0.9% sodium chloride solution over 1 to 2 hours. If BP and circulation stabilize and good urine flow is restored, then the IV infusion can be changed to 0.45% sodium chloride solution to provide additional free water. The rate of the 0.45% sodium chloride solution infusion must be adjusted in accordance with frequent assessments of BP, cardiovascular status, and the balance between fluid input and output. Potassium replacement is usually started by adding 20 mEq/L (20 mmol/L) potassium as a phosphate salt to the initial liter of the IV-infused 0.45% sodium chloride solution, provided urine flow is adequate and the resulting initial rate of potassium infusion does not exceed 10 to 20 mEq/hour.

Insulin treatment should not be aggressive and may be unnecessary, because adequate hydration usually decreases blood glucose levels. Patients with NKHHC are more sensitive to insulin than are patients with diabetic ketoacidosis, and large doses can decrease plasma glucose precipitously, leading to cerebral edema. If insulin is administered, 5% glucose should be added to the IV fluids when the blood glucose level reaches about 250 mg/dL (13.9 mmol/L) to avoid hypoglycemia.

DIABETIC AND ALCOHOLIC KETOACIDOSIS

Diabetic ketoacidosis: Metabolic acidosis from the accumulation of ketones due to severely depressed insulin levels. Alcoholic ketoacidosis: Ketoacidosis accompanied by mild hyperglycemia.

Diabetic ketoacidosis occurs mainly in type I DM and is accompanied by hyperglycemia as a result of low insulin and high glucagon levels. It is treated with insulin. Additional supportive treatment is similar to that used in NKHHC. Sometimes, patients with NKHHC (typically with blood glucose levels much higher than 500 mg/dL [27.8 mmol/L]) develop ketones and acidosis (often referred to as Flatbush diabetes). The ketones may be due to glucose toxicity and features of starvation. The acidosis is mainly the result of dehydration and decreased perfusion, combined with insulin deficiency. Many patients with NKHHC recover and do not need insulin or oral antidiabetic drugs.

In alcoholic ketoacidosis, blood alcohol levels may be elevated, but blood glucose levels are usually normal or low. Treatment is with glucose and thiamine.

HYPOGLYCEMIA

An abnormally low blood glucose level that leads to symptoms of sympathetic nervous system stimulation or of CNS dysfunction.

The causes of hypoglycemia are insulin, alcohol, sulfonylureas, and end-stage liver or renal disease. A non–insulin-secreting mesenchymal tumor may cause hypoglycemia because it secretes an insulin-like growth factor (IGF) molecule that mimics insulin. Prolonged starvation may rarely be a cause, but reactive (postprandial) hypoglycemia is very rare in the elderly.

Symptoms and Signs

The major symptoms and signs of hypoglycemia are listed in TABLE 64–5. Hypoglycemia has two distinct patterns: adrenergic symptoms

TABLE 64–5. SYMPTOMS AND SIGNS OF HYPOGLYCEMIA

Adrenergic	Central Nervous System
Weakness	Headache
Sweating	Hypothermia
Tachycardia	Visual disturbances
Palpitations	Mental dullness
Tremor	Confusion
Nervousness	Inappropriate behavior (can be mistaken for
Irritability	inebriation)
Tingling of mouth and fingers	Amnesia
Hunger	Seizures
Nausea (unusual)	Stupor
Vomiting (unusual)	Coma

attributed to increased sympathetic activity and epinephrine release (they can occur in adrenalectomized patients) and CNS manifestations. The blood levels at which symptoms of either type develop vary markedly among individual patients. Well-controlled diabetic patients often lose the ability to recognize hypoglycemia and tend not to have adrenergic symptoms but do have CNS symptoms.

Diagnosis

Whether the patient presents with unexplained CNS manifestations or unexplained adrenergic symptoms, diagnosis requires evidence that the symptoms occur in association with an abnormally low blood glucose level, which is usually defined as < 50 mg/dL (< 2.8 mmol/L) in men or < 45 mg/dL (< 2.5 mmol/L) in women (below the lower limits occurring in normal men and women after a 72-hour fast). A portion of the initial blood sample should be saved as frozen plasma to determine the initial plasma insulin, proinsulin, and C-peptide levels or to perform a drug scan when necessary. Blood lactate and pH should be determined and the plasma checked for ketones.

If the cause is not clear from the history, different causes may be distinguished by laboratory testing. Patients with insulin-secreting pancreatic tumors (insulinomas, islet cell carcinomas) usually have increased proinsulin and C-peptide levels that parallel the insulin levels. An increased C-peptide level would be expected in patients taking a sulfonylurea, but a high level of the drug should be detectable. Several imaging techniques have improved the localization of these tumors, and intraoperative ultrasound detects most.

Patients with hypoglycemia induced by exogenous insulin injections (commonly given by health care workers or the diabetic patient's family members) have normal proinsulin levels and suppressed C-peptide levels. In the rare cases of autoimmune hypoglycemia, the plasma-free insulin level during a hypoglycemic episode is usually markedly elevated, the plasma C-peptide level suppressed, and plasma insulin antibodies readily detectable.

Patients with non–insulin-secreting mesenchymal tumors may suffer from hypoglycemia due to production of a large IGF-II molecule, which cannot bind to plasma proteins and therefore exerts its hypoglycemic effect. In these patients, although the unbound IGF does not change measurable total IGF levels, a helpful test is to identify low levels of plasma growth hormone during hypoglycemia (because of inhibition by IGF).

Treatment

Oral ingestion of glucose or sucrose is usually adequate for relieving acute adrenergic and early CNS symptoms. Patients treated with insulin or a sulfonylurea are advised to drink a glass of fruit juice or water with 3 tablespoons of table sugar added and to teach family members to give such treatment if they suddenly exhibit confusion or inappropriate behavior. In patients treated with a sulfonylurea, especially the long-acting ones such as chlorpropamide, hypoglycemia may recur over many hours or even days if oral intake is inadequate. When oral glucose is unavailable or inadequate, IV glucose may be used (25 to 50 mL of 50% glucose followed by an infusion of 5% glucose [or even 10% glucose] in water).

Glucagon is used to treat severe hypoglycemic reactions when oral glucose is inadequate and IV glucose is unavailable. It is mainly useful for emergencies away from medical settings.

Surgical excision often resolves hypoglycemia due to a non–insulin-secreting mesenchymal tumor. When surgical removal of most of the tumor is not feasible, corticosteroid therapy may be tried. A gastrostomy may be needed for continuous feeding of the enormous amounts of carbohydrate required throughout the day.

An insulin-secreting islet cell tumor requires surgical treatment. Most often, a single insulinoma is found, and its enucleation is usually curative. If this fails, the surgeon usually performs a blind partial pancreatectomy. Before the operation, diazoxide and octreotide (a long-acting octapeptic analog of somatostatin) may be used to inhibit insulin secretion.

65 ▬ THYROID DISORDERS

The prevalence of hypothyroidism and thyroid nodules increases dramatically in elderly persons. Although the prevalence of hyperthyroidism is similar for younger and elderly patients, its presentation in elderly patients may be nonspecific and it may be difficult to diagnose.

Thyroid Function in Normal Aging

The thyroid gland produces thyroxine (T_4) and triiodothyronine (T_3). With age, the thyroid gland undergoes moderate atrophy and develops nonspecific histopathologic abnormalities: fibrosis, increasing numbers of colloid nodules, and some lymphocytic infiltration. Production of T_4 decreases by about 30% between young adulthood and advanced age. However, because serum T_4 levels remain unchanged with age, the decrease in T_4 is considered to be physiologic compensation for decreased use of the hormone by tissue and not a manifestation of primary thyroid failure.

The body's decrease in use of T_4 correlates with the age-related decline in lean body mass, suggesting that the mass of metabolically active, protein-rich tissue (ie, muscle, skin, bone, and viscera) decreases, which may lead to reduced use and catabolism of thyroid hormones. Thyroid hormone levels rise subtly, and thyroid-stimulating hormone (TSH) output decreases. T_3 and T_4 output decreases, and serum T_4 levels return to normal. When stimulated by increased TSH, the healthy aged thyroid gland can increase its hormone production normally.

Serum T_3 and free T_3 levels decrease moderately with age. This decline is thought to be due to a combination of decreased monodeiodination of the outer ring of T_4 and decreased pituitary secretion of TSH. In healthy centenarians, the decline in serum T_3 may be as much as 35%.

The average serum TSH level rises with age. Although this increase appears to contradict the explanation given for the constancy of serum T_4, it probably reflects the high prevalence of Hashimoto's disease leading to hypothyroidism in elderly patients. Hashimoto's disease (also called chronic autoimmune thyroiditis) is an autoimmune inflammatory disease of the thyroid gland. The increase in serum TSH level correlates with elevated antibody levels and disappears when patients with Hashimoto's disease are excluded from consideration.

HYPOTHYROIDISM

(Myxedema)

The clinical expression of thyroid hormone deficiency.

Epidemiology and Etiology

The prevalence of overt hypothyroidism is 2 to 5% in persons $\geq$ 65 years. Another 5 to 10% of those $\geq$ 65 have subclinical hypothyroidism (isolated elevation of TSH levels with normal T_4 and T_3, with or without symptoms). The prevalence rises with age, is much higher in women than in men at all ages, and is higher in elderly institutionalized patients than in elderly patients living in the community.

The causes of sustained overt and subclinical hypothyroidism in elderly persons are similar to those in younger persons. The most common causes are Hashimoto's disease, previous irradiation or surgical removal of the thyroid gland, and idiopathic hypothyroidism, which may be simply the result of nongoitrous Hashimoto's disease. Less common causes include pituitary and hypothalamic disorders causing TSH deficiency, iodine-induced hypothyroidism (from radiocontrast agents, amiodarone, or supplemental potassium iodide), and use of lithium or other antithyroid drugs. Transient hypothyroidism may occur after thyroid surgery, after treatment with radioactive sodium iodide (^{131}I), or during episodes of subacute thyroiditis when the thyroid gland has depleted its store of hormone and the follicular cells have not yet recovered sufficiently to replace it.

Pathogenesis and Pathophysiology

Thyroid glands of older persons are more susceptible to the destructive autoimmune effects of Hashimoto's disease than are those of younger persons. The pathogenesis of Hashimoto's disease appears to change little with age. Four types of thyroid-directed antibodies may appear in the serum of patients with the disease, but the inflammatory and cytotoxic lesion is probably cell-mediated.

Hypothyroidism after ^{131}I therapy for hyperthyroidism is common in elderly patients because the incidence of hypothyroidism continues to increase at an annual rate of 2 to 5% for 20 or 30 years after the initial treatment. Also, hypothyroidism after ^{131}I therapy is caused by a failure of DNA repair and replication, and these processes are less efficient with age. Thyroid antibodies and Hashimoto's disease also are much more common in patients with Graves' disease; therefore, organ failure may often be due to a combination of radiation and autoimmune destruction. Thus, cases of hypothyroidism accumulate as patients with treated Graves' disease age.

Symptoms, Signs, and Complications

Hypothyroidism in older persons is a great masquerader. Elderly patients have significantly fewer symptoms of hypothyroidism than do younger adults and complaints are often subtle and vague. Chilliness, weight gain, muscle cramps, and paresthesias are significantly less common in patients ≥ 70 than in those ≤ 55. Fatigue, weakness, depression, constipation, and dry, coarse skin may also be less common. Many elderly patients with hypothyroidism present with nonspecific geriatric syndromes—confusion, anorexia, weight loss, falling, incontinence, and decreased mobility. Musculoskeletal symptoms (especially arthralgias) occur often, but arthritis is rare. Muscular aches and weakness, often mimicking polymyalgia rheumatica or polymyositis, and an elevated creatine phosphokinase level may occur.

The term subclinical hypothyroidism implies that the patient has no symptoms attributable to hypothyroidism. However, patients with isolated elevations of serum TSH levels have more symptoms consistent with hypothyroidism than do patients with normal TSH levels.

Physical findings may be difficult to interpret. Puffiness around the eyes and myxedematous facies are difficult to distinguish from normal facial changes in elderly persons. The most reliable sign—prolonged relaxation time after muscular contraction—may not be detectable in older patients because of decreased amplitude or absent reflexes. Occasionally, noninflammatory effusions may occur in the joints and in pleural, pericardial, and peritoneal cavities. Basal body temperature may decrease.

Because elderly persons have more circulating antidiuretic hormone (vasopressin), they are susceptible to excessive water retention without proportionate sodium retention. Hypothyroidism accentuates these tendencies, often leading to hyponatremia. Complications of hypothyroidism include hypertension and hyperlipidemia. Hypothyroidism is also associated with elevation of lipoprotein(a), an independent risk factor for coronary artery disease. Myocardial infarction and heart failure are serious but uncommon complications of early disease. Untreated hypothyroidism may lead to myxedema coma, a life-threatening emergency. Mental confusion progresses to stupor and coma and is often accompanied by hyponatremia, hypoglycemia, or hypercapnia.

Diagnosis

Diagnosis is based on precise, reliable assays of serum TSH and T_4 levels. The most sensitive indication of hypothyroidism due to primary thyroid gland failure is a marked elevation of serum TSH. The most specific test finding is a subnormal serum free T_4 level, because it corrects for abnormalities in the T_4-binding proteins. The serum T_3 level has little value because it is normal in about one third of patients with hypothyroidism and because subnormal levels are often due to illness or inadequate caloric intake.

Because of its great sensitivity and adequate specificity, the serum TSH level alone should be measured in patients suspected of having hypothyroidism and in those in whom it needs to be excluded. If the serum TSH level is normal, hypothyroidism is essentially ruled out, and the serum free T_4 rarely needs to be measured. A serum TSH level above normal (usually > 4.5 mU/L) suggests a possible diagnosis of hypothyroidism. Serum free T_4 should be measured to differentiate overt hypothyroidism (subnormal free T_4) from subclinical hypothyroidism (normal free T_4).

Subclinical hypothyroidism is usually indicated by a serum TSH level between the upper limit of normal (about 5 mU/L) and 15 mU/L; occasionally the level may be higher. The serum free T_4 level is, by definition, within the normal range but tends to be below the mean of the euthyroid elderly population. The serum TSH measurement may need to be repeated in patients with concurrent illnesses because it may be subnormal during the illness and elevated during the recovery phase.

Measurement of thyroid antibodies is neither sensitive nor specific; only a minority of elderly patients with elevated antibody levels have hypothyroidism, and only 40 to 70% of patients with hypothyroidism have elevated antibody levels. However, this measurement is prognostically useful in patients with subclinical hypothyroidism, in whom the rate of progression to overt hypothyroidism is much higher in those with positive antibody titers.

Although serum cholesterol and creatine kinase levels are elevated in hypothyroidism, these measurements are rarely useful diagnostically.

However, obtaining serum TSH levels and thereby making a diagnosis of hypothyroidism may explain elevated cholesterol and creatine kinase levels.

Hypothyroidism must be differentiated from **euthyroid sick syndrome,** which is characterized by abnormal thyroid function test results in clinically euthyroid patients with severe nonthyroidal systemic illness. Findings may include low serum T_3 and free T_3 levels and high serum reverse T_3 levels, but the difficulty arises because of low serum T_4, free T_4 index, and free T_4 levels in the most seriously ill patients. A subnormal serum TSH level (0.02 to 0.4 mU/L) is generally but not always detectable by 3rd-generation TSH assay. Diagnosis of hypothyroidism in the critically ill patient can be made only if the serum TSH level is markedly elevated ($>$ 15 mU/L) or if the free T_4 levels are markedly subnormal ($<$ 0.6 ng/dL [$<$ 8 pmol/L]); hypothyroidism is more likely when both findings occur. Although pituitarigenic hypothyroidism may rarely be the cause of low serum TSH and free T_4 levels, these findings are almost always explained by the euthyroid sick syndrome.

Screening, Prognosis, and Treatment

Screening every 5 years by measuring serum TSH is recommended for all men $\geq$ 65 and for all women $\geq$ 35. For those with risk factors for thyroid disease, the serum TSH level should be checked more often. Screening for hypothyroidism is as cost-effective as screening for hypertension, hypercholesterolemia, and breast cancer. This single test is highly sensitive and specific in diagnosing or excluding two prevalent and serious disorders (hypothyroidism and hyperthyroidism), both of which can be treated effectively.

Proper treatment of hypothyroidism completely corrects the metabolic condition. Long-standing, untreated hypothyroidism is a risk factor for coronary artery disease. Therefore, cardiac stress testing is indicated, and the response of blood lipid levels to treatment should be monitored.

Treatment of choice is T_4 replacement with levothyroxine sodium. The average dose for patients $\geq$ 65 years is 0.075 to 0.1 mg/day po. If the patient has coronary artery disease, the initial dose of levothyroxine sodium should be only 0.0125 to 0.025 mg/day po. For patients with hypothyroidism short of myxedema coma, replacement therapy should be given cautiously, starting with a dose of 0.025 mg/day po and increasing at intervals of 2 to 4 weeks. The increases should be by 0.0125 mg/day if the interval is 2 weeks and by 0.025 mg/day if the interval is $\geq$ 4 weeks. About 1 to 2 months after reaching a dose of 0.075 mg/day po of levothyroxine sodium, the serum TSH level should be measured (always by a 2nd- or 3rd-generation TSH assay capable of detecting $\geq$ 0.01 mU/L). If the TSH level is still above normal, the dose may be increased to 0.1 mg/day. If the TSH is below normal ($<$ 0.4 mU/L), the dose should be lowered. Serum T_3 and T_4 measurements usually are not needed. If the serum TSH level is still high 1 to 2 months after reaching a dose of 0.1 mg/day of levothyroxine sodium, the dose should be maintained for another 2 months. If the TSH level is still elevated, the dose should be raised to 0.112 or 0.125 mg/day.

The physician should emphasize to the newly diagnosed patient with hypothyroidism that treatment with levothyroxine sodium must be maintained for life. This counsel should be repeated at follow-up visits at least once a year.

Treatment of myxedema coma involves large IV doses of thyroid hormones (eg, 0.2 to 0.5 mg levothyroxine sodium on the first day, then 0.1 to 0.3 mg IV on day 2, and 0.05 to 0.1 mg daily thereafter [until the patient is able to take oral levothyroxine]) supplemented by IV adrenal corticosteroids (eg, hydrocortisone sodium succinate 50 to 100 mg immediately and 50 to 100 mg q 6 h thereafter) and measures to treat hyponatremia, hypoglycemia, and respiratory failure, if present.

HYPERTHYROIDISM

(Thyrotoxicosis)

The clinical expression of excess thyroid hormone.

Some controversy continues over the terms hyperthyroidism and thyrotoxicosis. Some authorities refer to thyrotoxicosis as the clinical expression of excess thyroid hormone, whatever its source, and hyperthyroidism as a condition in which there is increased synthesis and secretion of thyroid hormones from the thyroid gland. In this chapter, hyperthyroidism is used synonymously with thyrotoxicosis.

Epidemiology, Etiology, and Pathophysiology

In elderly patients, the prevalence of overt hyperthyroidism is 0.2 to 2%, which is similar to that in the general population. The prevalence of subclinical hyperthyroidism (suppression of TSH levels with normal T_4 and T_3 levels and usually without symptoms) is unknown.

Hyperthyroidism in elderly patients is more often due to multinodular and uninodular toxic goiter than to Graves' disease, which is the most common cause in younger adults. Adenomas autonomously produce and secrete excessive thyroid hormone even though TSH production is fully suppressed. In Graves' disease, an autoimmune disorder, an antibody to the TSH receptor on thyroid follicular cells is produced that has TSH-like activity. In granulomatous or lymphocytic subacute thyroiditis, damaged follicles leak thyroglobulin, T_3, and T_4 into the circulation. In certain cases of Hashimoto's disease, a similar leakage may occur, usually of short duration.

A common cause of hyperthyroidism among elderly patients is iodine-induced hyperthyroidism, often from the use of amiodarone, a cardiac drug containing iodine that deposits in tissue and delivers iodine to the circulation over very long periods of time. Hyperthyroidism also may result from excessive ingestion of T_4 or T_3 (either therapeutic or patient-initiated).

Regardless of the cause of hyperthyroidism, the result is supranormal levels of thyroid hormones in T_3-responsive tissues. The various types of hyperthyroidism are characterized by overproduction of T_3 and, to a lesser extent, T_4. In T_3 hyperthyroidism, which accounts for $< 5\%$ of hyperthyroidism at all ages, the serum T_4 level is normal despite clinical evidence of hyperthyroidism.

In hyperthyroidism, extrathyroidal tissues convert the excess secreted T_4 to T_3. Thus, a supraphysiologic concentration of T_3 arrives at target tissues and is transported into the nucleus, where it binds to a receptor. The hormone-receptor complex then binds to the promoter region of T_3-responsive genes, leading to an overproduction of enzymes and other proteins that mediate the characteristic actions of T_3.

Symptoms, Signs, and Complications

Hyperthyroidism in elderly patients is even more of a masquerader than hypothyroidism. Older patients have fewer symptoms and signs and a different complex of symptoms than do younger patients. Only about 25% of hyperthyroid patients ≥ 65 present with typical symptoms and signs (see TABLE 65–1). Many of the age-related differences in symptoms are the result of the aging process and of concomitant disease that modifies the effects of excessive thyroid hormone. For example, the response to catecholamines decreases in elderly patients, possibly because of a decreased number or affinity of catecholamine receptors. Because catecholamines act synergistically with T_3 to produce the typical symptoms and signs of hyperthyroidism, reduced responsiveness to catecholamines may explain some atypical symptoms.

The classic triad in older patients is tachycardia, weight loss, and fatigue (or weakness or apathy), whereas in younger patients it is tachycardia, goiter, and exophthalmos. Ocular signs are usually absent. Decreased appetite is common; increased appetite is the exception. Because the baseline heart rate decreases with age, heart rates > 90 beats/minute (rather than the standard of 100) must be interpreted as tachycardia in elderly hyperthyroid patients. Regarding goiter, the thyroid gland is normal in size or impalpable in about 40% of cases, enlarged and nodular in 35%, and enlarged and diffuse in 25%. Diarrhea is uncommon, whereas constipation is present in $> 20\%$ of elderly patients. Sweating is also far less common in elderly hyperthyroid patients. A subjective sense of nervousness and anxiety is less commonly reported by elderly hyperthyroid patients, although observed tremor is almost as frequently seen as in younger patients. Hyperactive

TABLE 65–1.   CLINICAL FEATURES OF HYPERTHYROIDISM IN THE ELDERLY

Feature	Comment
More common	
Smaller thyroid gland	Normal or decreased in size in about 40% of patients
Multinodular gland	More common than Graves' disease
Tachycardia	Heart rates > 90 beats/min are regarded as tachycardia in elderly patients
Fatigue, weakness	—
Atrial fibrillation	Affects about 27% of elderly hyperthyroid patients
Arrhythmias	—
Angina, heart failure	Common because excess thyroid hormone stresses the aging or diseased heart
Constipation	Due to decreased GI motility
Changes in appetite	Decreased in 33% of elderly patients; increased in only 10%
Neuropsychiatric symptoms (eg, apathy, listlessness, anorexia, weight loss, mental confusion)	May be due to depression concomitant with hyperthyroidism
Myopathy	—
Less common	
Diarrhea	Due to decreased gastrointestinal motility
Nervousness and anxiety	—
Hyperkinesis	—
Sweating	Aging skin is less able to perspire in a hot environment
Hyperreflexia	—
Ocular signs (eg, exophthalmos)	—

reflexes with quick recoil are far less common in older than in younger patients.

Symptoms of heart failure and angina may dominate the clinical picture to the exclusion of the usual features of hyperthyroidism. Because cardiac disease is common in elderly persons, the possibility of underlying hyperthyroidism may not be suspected. Gastrointestinal (GI) symptoms may be confused with GI malignancy.

The most common complication in elderly patients is atrial fibrillation, which occurs in 27% of elderly hyperthyroid patients at presentation. Prognosis for heart failure and early death is increased if atrial fibrillation does not convert to normal sinus rhythm when euthyroidism is restored. Atrial fibrillation also carries a high risk of embolic stroke. Other important complications are depression (called apathetic thyroidism), myopathy, and osteoporosis.

Thyroid storm is a rare, life-threatening episode that may occur in the course of hyperthyroidism. It usually occurs when a stressful illness or event is superimposed on hyperthyroidism or occasionally when ^{131}I therapy leads to massive leakage of thyroid hormones into the circulation. The symptoms and signs of hyperthyroidism are present, but the following also occur: fever, extreme tachycardia, nausea, vomiting, heart failure, and changes in mental status or consciousness. Serum T_4 and T_3 levels are no higher than in patients with usual degrees of hyperthyroidism. Thus, thyroid storm is a clinical diagnosis.

Diagnosis

The best single test is the serum TSH measurement, whose sensitivity and specificity are ≥ 0.98. A subnormal value suggests hyperthyroidism, and an undetectable value by a 2nd- or 3rd-generation assay (< 0.01 mU/L) is almost pathognomonic.

Serum T_4, T_3, and thyroglobulin levels are on the average lower in older patients with hyperthyroidism than in younger patients.

Serum thyroid hormone levels should *not* be performed with the initial TSH test; they may be measured subsequently to confirm the diagnosis or to establish that the patient is not euthyroid when the serum TSH level is normal but clinical suspicion is strong. Starvation or serious disease (severe hyperthyroidism, thyroid-induced heart failure, or intercurrent disease) lowers the serum T_3 level, so a patient with hyperthyroidism may have a normal serum T_3 level. With more serious disease, the serum T_4 and free T_4 index may also decline into the normal range. If this occurs, the diagnosis is usually indicated by an elevated free T_4 level (measured by equilibrium dialysis), a supranormal radioiodine uptake test, or an undetectable serum TSH by 2nd- or 3rd-generation assay.

Hyperthyroidism must be differentiated from **euthyroid hyperthyroxinemia** in patients with acute systemic disease and in patients with acute psychiatric disorders. A serum TSH measurement and a repeat measurement of the serum T_4 level after 2 weeks (by which time the serum T_4 level has generally returned to normal) help establish the correct diagnosis.

Prognosis and Treatment

The prognosis for hyperthyroidism is excellent. Treatment usually leads to a euthyroid state. If hypothyroidism results, it is treated easily with levothyroxine sodium.

Treatment of choice for most elderly patients with **Graves' disease** or a **single autonomous nodule** is radioactive sodium iodide (^{131}I). It is preferred because it is easy to administer and it avoids any age-related postoperative complications of surgery.∎ Antithyroid drugs (eg, propylthiouracil, methimazole) are effective in the treatment of Graves' disease if the patient's adherence with the regimen is good. However, in patients with uninodular toxic goiter, antithyroid drugs are slow to work and almost never lead to permanent remission.

In **multinodular toxic goiter,** the response to ^{131}I therapy is often delayed and incomplete. Because many doses of ^{131}I may be needed, the patient remains hyperthyroid many months after the diagnosis. Thus, surgery may be preferred, at least for patients at low risk of postoperative complications. For patients at high risk, large and repeated doses of ^{131}I should be given.

When hyperthyroidism is due to **subacute thyroiditis, Hashimoto's disease,** or **acute radiation damage,** the only effective treatment is to give β-blockers and to closely observe the patient for complications. Antithyroid drugs and ^{131}I are not helpful because they do not decrease the uncontrolled output of hormone from damaged thyroid follicles.

The usual treatment of **iodine-induced hyperthyroidism** is high doses of antithyroid drugs and a β-blocker. Treatment may be difficult because the large store of thyroid hormone in the gland blunts the effect of antithyroid drugs, and the large pool of iodine throughout the body markedly decreases the uptake of ^{131}I.

^{131}I: No consensus exists on an appropriate dose of ^{131}I for hyperthyroidism. One option is a low dose calculated on the basis of thyroid size and ^{131}I uptake intended to produce a euthyroid state. Another option is a large, arbitrary dose (usually 10 mCi or more) intended to produce hypothyroidism (followed by levothyroxine sodium therapy when hypothyroidism occurs). Even with low-dose therapy, hypothyroidism develops in 50% of patients by 20 years, but this option cuts in half the probability that levothyroxine sodium will be needed later when patients are likely to be already taking multiple drugs. However, the large dose may be advantageous by providing the patient with more years of well-being because the relief of hyperthyroidism is faster and more reliable.

Antithyroid drugs: The indications for antithyroid drugs are similar for all ages: if ^{131}I is refused by the patient, before or after ^{131}I is administered to relieve hyperthyroidism faster, before surgical subtotal thyroidectomy is performed, and as primary, long-term therapy to try to keep the patient in a euthyroid state until remission of the underlying disease is achieved. The advantage of giving antithyroid drugs before ^{131}I administration is that not only does the patient become euthyroid but also the therapy depletes the thyroid gland of its stored hormone, thus minimizing the risk of hyperthyroidism due to "dumping" into the blood after ^{131}I therapy.

∎ see page 250

Long-term antithyroid drug treatment usually lasts 1 to 2 years. If the elderly patient follows instructions, antithyroid drug therapy is usually successful. Because mild hyperthyroidism and a small thyroid gland are characteristic in elderly patients, the chance of permanent remission is enhanced. If hyperthyroidism recurs after antithyroid drug treatment, ^{131}I should be given.

Antithyroid drugs as primary therapy in elderly persons are administered in the same way as in younger persons. **Propylthiouracil** is given initially at 150 to 300 mg/day po in divided doses q 8 h. Maintenance dosing is 100 to 150 mg/day in divided doses q 8 to 12 h. The dosage is lowered sequentially based on symptoms and signs and serum hormone levels, which are monitored every 2 months. Serum TSH levels are useful. If the therapeutic response is inadequate, the dosage may be increased to 300 mg q 8 h.

Methimazole can be given as a single daily dose; the initial dose is 15 to 40 mg/day. The dose needs to be adjusted every 1 or 2 months, depending on the response. If the patient's course is erratic with methimazole or propylthiouracil (eg, the patient slips quickly into hypothyroidism after small dose increases), the simplest solution is to add a small dose of levothyroxine sodium, usually 0.05 mg/day.

A pharmacologic dose of **inorganic iodide** (any dose > 6 mg/day) acts by inhibiting the release of thyroid hormone. The dose is generally effective for only 10 to 14 days. Iodide may be administered as Lugol's solution (5% iodine and 10% potassium iodide), 2 to 6 drops tid (50 to 150 mg/day) or as saturated solution of potassium iodide (1 g potassium iodide/mL); the recommended dose is 5 to 10 drops tid, although this dose provides far more than is needed (750 to 1500 mg/day).

Symptomatic treatment: Propranolol and other β-blockers can help manage symptoms of hyperthyroidism. Ipodate sodium and iopanoic acid (cholecystographic contrast materials) are extremely effective in lowering the serum T_3 level to the normal range within 48 to 72 hours (although they are not approved in the USA for treating hyperthyroidism). In patients with atrial fibrillation and high thyroid hormone levels, cardioversion should not be attempted until a euthyroid state is achieved. Once it is, the atrial rhythm spontaneously reverts to normal in about two thirds of patients. Psychiatric symptoms usually resolve when the patient becomes euthyroid but should be treated if necessary. Standard measures to prevent osteoporosis are indicated, particularly in elderly women. ∎

Thyroid storm: Thyroid storm is treated as an emergency. Treatment includes large doses of propylthiouracil (150 to 300 mg q 6 h) by nasogastric tube, if necessary; propranolol (1 mg by slow IV push q 5 min to decrease heart rate to between 90 and 110 beats/minute), and a glucocorticoid IV (eg, hydrocortisone sodium succinate 100 mg imme-

---

∎see page 472

diately and 50 mg q 6 h thereafter). Oral or IV sodium iodide (500 mg/day) can also be given, but ipodate sodium (3 mg in a single dose po or by nasogastric tube) is much more effective because it lowers the serum T_3 level to normal within 24 hours.

THYROID NODULES

The prevalence of thyroid nodules increases markedly with age. Even in iodine-sufficient regions (all of the USA), about 80% of persons >70 have one or more thyroid nodules based on gross pathologic examination, and during life 45% show nodules by ultrasonography and about 10% by palpation.

Radiation-induced cancer does not appear to occur after latent periods of > 50 years; therefore, a history of radiation to the face, neck, or thorax in childhood is probably not relevant in elderly patients.

Symptoms, Signs, and Diagnosis

Findings are similar in the elderly and in younger persons. A nodule may be merely an enlarged lobe, a lobule in a diffuse goiter, or a pyramidal lobe. Nodules may also be regenerating areas after subtotal resection of the thyroid, localized subacute or chronic thyroiditis, cysts, or hemorrhage and calcification in a colloid adenoma. Concern about malignancy may be lower if the dominant nodule is not the only one, if both lobes are abnormal on palpation, or if the history reveals a sudden appearance with pain and tenderness, suggesting hemorrhage in a degenerating colloid adenoma.

Hashimoto's disease causes the gland to feel very firm with multiple small nodules. Colloid adenomas may be softer than normal, although their consistency varies from patient to patient. Tenderness suggests hemorrhage into a colloid adenoma. Fluctuation suggests cystic changes, but these are more likely to result from hemorrhage or necrosis of a colloid adenoma than from a simple water-clear cyst.

Anaplastic carcinoma often has features that clearly suggest malignancy. The patient has a large, growing, stony hard thyroid mass that is irregular, immobile, and fixed to other tissues. Also, the patient may be hoarse.

Evaluation of thyroid nodules remains controversial, regardless of the patient's age. Most experts recommend at least a fine-needle aspiration, which has high sensitivity and specificity for a cancer diagnosis. Thyroid function tests are usually normal except with the relatively uncommon hyperfunctioning nodule, in which case serum T_4 and T_3 levels may be high and serum TSH may be subnormal or undetectable. When these findings are obtained, a radionuclide scan should be performed to prove that the nodule is functioning. When results of thyroid function tests are normal, a radionuclide scan is often performed to exclude a functioning lesion, which is almost always benign, and ultrasonography is performed to identify simple cysts, also usually benign. However, these expensive procedures have a low diagnostic yield because of their extremely poor specificity for malignancy. Serum thyroglobulin measurement has low specificity. X-rays of microcalcifications, representing psammoma bodies, have low sensitivity but high specificity for the diagnosis of papillary adenocarcinoma. Elevated antithyroid antibodies suggest Hashimoto's disease as the cause of nodularity but cannot rule out a coexisting carcinoma, so fine-needle aspiration is indicated for the dominant nodule.

Prognosis and Treatment

Most nodules are benign or behave benignly, even if they appear malignant on histologic examination. The 5-year survival rate for all patients with thyroid cancers is 93%, which is comparable with the average survival of the age-adjusted population. In elderly patients, nodules tend to be somewhat more invasive and malignant, but most are still papillary or papillofollicular and have excellent prognoses.

Surgery is indicated when fine-needle aspiration indicates cytologic evidence of or suspicion of malignancy unless concomitant medical conditions absolutely contraindicate it. If the physician doubts the cytologic impression (eg, the cytologist can diagnose a follicular neoplasm but usually cannot tell if it is benign or malignant), a better treatment choice is levothyroxine sodium to suppress TSH to subnormal (ie, 0.1 to 0.4 mU/L) but not to the point that the patient becomes hyperthyroid. Another fine-needle aspiration should be performed in 6 to 12 months. Overall, 6% of thyroid nodules are malignant, and 25% of those with suspicious cytologic results are malignant.

If thyroid cancer is discovered during surgery, the next step is controversial. Most physicians recommend a near-total thyroidectomy followed by ^{131}I therapy to ablate the remainder. Then a total body scan is performed to search for residual tissue capable of capturing [131]I. If the results are positive, a therapeutic dose of 50 to 150 mCi is administered. Although it has a logical rationale and is widely accepted, this approach has not proved to be superior to near-total thyroidectomy alone; its alleged advantage derives from nonrandomized studies with possible selection bias.

At all times, except when preparing for a radionuclide scan or a therapeutic dose of ^{131}I, the patient should receive long-term treatment with levothyroxine sodium as described above. Long-term TSH-suppressive therapy may cause accelerated osteoporosis and cardiac abnormalities if thyrotoxic doses are given.

Because levels of many hormones decrease with age (see TABLE 66–1), restoring low hormone levels might seem a logical way to help reverse some of the effects of aging. However, any resulting improvement in functional status might theoretically be gained at the expense of reduced longevity. For example, increased metabolism, which often results from hormone administration, can lead to tissue damage because of free radical generation. Therefore, indications for hormonal supplementation should be restricted to correcting documented low hormone levels or to ameliorating symptoms resulting from such low levels.

ESTROGEN

At menopause, ovarian follicles no longer respond to stimulation by gonadotropins; consequently, estrogen levels decrease despite an increase in gonadotropin levels.

The short-term benefit of estrogen replacement therapy[1] is amelioration of menopausal symptoms. The major long-term benefits are a reduced rate of postmenopausal bone loss, with consequent reduced risk of spine and hip fractures, and possibly reduced cardiovascular risk.

Long-term adverse effects of estrogen replacement therapy are increases in risk of breast and endometrial cancer; however, the increased risk of endometrial cancer can be opposed by concomitant progesterone administration.

Selective estrogen receptor modulators (eg, raloxifene) were developed to avoid the adverse effects of estrogen on the uterus and breast. However, these agents seem to be not as effective as estrogen at delaying bone loss and appear to have only minimal protective effects on the cardiovascular system.

TESTOSTERONE

Testosterone levels decrease with age because of a failure of the hypothalamic-pituitary axis to secrete gonadotropin (secondary hypogonadism). About 5% of men aged 50 and 70% of men aged 70 are hypogonadal,[2] resulting in a symptom complex of reduced muscle mass, strength, and cognitive function. Low testosterone levels are associated with an increased incidence of coronary artery disease in elderly men.

In elderly men, testosterone replacement therapy increases libido, muscle strength and mass, bone mineral density, and visuospatial cog-

---

[1] see also page 1211   [2] see also page 1171

TABLE 66-1.   COMPARISON BETWEEN THE EFFECTS OF AGING AND HORMONAL DEFICIENCY

	Aging	Hormonal Deficiency		
		Growth Hormone	Testosterone	Estrogen
Nitrogen balance	↓	↓	↓	—
Muscle mass	↓	↓	↓	↓
Muscle strength	↓	—	↓	↓
Bone density	↓	↓	↓	↓
Hematocrit	↓ (only in men)	—	↓	—
Renal blood flow	↓	↓	—	—
Libido	↓	—	↓	↓(?)
Facial hair	↓	—	↓	—
Cognition	↓	—	↓	—
Immunity	↓	↓	—	—

↓ = decrease; — = no effect.

nitive performance; it decreases leptin levels. Coronary artery vasodilation is increased through release of nitric oxide; cardiac electrophysiologic function may improve in elderly men with coronary artery disease. Testosterone replacement therapy appears to have no deleterious effects on lipid levels. Most studies used a dose of 200 mg IM q 10 to 14 days of testosterone enanthate or testosterone cypionate.

However, testosterone replacement therapy increases Hct, sometimes to levels > 55%, which increases the risk of stroke. Testosterone replacement therapy does not appear to increase prostate-specific antigen levels or increase the incidence of benign prostatic hypertrophy; however, it should not be administered to elderly men with prostate cancer.

The effects of testosterone replacement therapy on longevity are unknown.

PREGNENOLONE

Levels of pregnenolone, which is a hormone derived from cholesterol, decrease with age. In rodents, pregnenolone is the most potent memory enhancer known. In humans, it has been shown to improve sleep and to enhance productivity but not to affect mood, strength, cognition, or overall function. Currently, no evidence supports the use of pregnenolone in the elderly.

DEHYDROEPIANDROSTERONE

Dehydroepiandrosterone (DHEA) and its sulfate (DHEAS) are abundant in the body, but their physiologic role is not understood. Circulating DHEA and DHEAS levels decrease with age. Low DHEA levels are associated with osteoporosis and possibly with coronary artery disease, but whether these associations are causal or incidental is unknown.

In animal studies, DHEA has been shown to slow the rate of growth of pancreatic and colorectal cancer. DHEA is a potent memory-enhancing drug in mice and has various immunostimulant effects in rodents.

In humans, the effects of DHEA on mood are conflicting. At relatively high doses (100 mg/day), DHEA increases insulin-like growth factor I, lean body mass, and muscle strength in men but not in women. The effects on the immune system have been minor and inconsistent. In a study of nursing home residents, DHEA levels were directly related to function. However, DHEA supplementation had minimal or no effect on memory.

There is insufficient evidence to support the use of DHEA as an antiaging agent. Moreover, DHEA available in health food stores has variable bioavailability.

VITAMIN D

Vitamin D is a prohormone that is absorbed from milk products in the diet and is also synthesized in the skin by exposure to sunlight. With age, vitamin D levels decrease, but the effects are minimal except in elderly persons living in northern latitudes (because of reduced biosynthesis of vitamin D from sunlight), institutionalized or homebound elderly persons who have little sunlight exposure, and those who do not ingest enough milk products. Vitamin D deficiency tends to cause osteomalacia■, which may result in accelerated osteoporosis in the elderly; severe vitamin D deficiency can result in a painful myopathy.

Vitamin D supplementation may decrease the rate of osteoporosis and risk of hip fractures and increase survival. Vitamin D has various effects on immune function; whether vitamin D supplementation enhances immune function in healthy elderly persons is unknown. In epidemiologic studies, vitamin D supplementation was associated with impaired glucose tolerance.

Elderly persons at increased risk of vitamin D deficiency may benefit from ingestion of 600 to 800 IU of vitamin D daily, particularly during the winter.

■ see page 483

MELATONIN

Melatonin is a hormone produced by the pineal gland; production is suppressed by light. Levels can be measured in serum, saliva, or urine (as sulfatoxymelatonin). Melatonin levels peak during early childhood and then decrease throughout life until they become negligible in the elderly.

The major effect of melatonin is to promote sleep; it may also protect against free radical damage. Melatonin has been shown to increase cortisol in older but not in younger women. Insufficient evidence exists to support routine use of melatonin in the elderly.

GROWTH HORMONE

Levels of growth hormone (GH) decrease with age, as do levels of insulin-like growth factor I (IGF-I), which mediates many of the effects of GH in adults. Many of the symptoms and signs of GH deficiency (eg, decreased muscle mass, weakness, fatigue) are similar to those occurring during normal aging.

The causes of age-related decline in GH are multifactorial. Secretion of somatostatin, a neuropeptide that inhibits GH release, increases with age. Secretion of growth hormone–releasing hormone (GHRH) decreases with age, resulting not only in decreased circulating GH levels and fewer daily peaks of GH secretion, but also, possibly, in sleep fragmentation (because GHRH affects slow-wave sleep). Age-related declines in estrogen and testosterone (which converts to estrogen through aromatization) may also decrease GH secretion.

Unlike in younger adults, GH supplementation in the elderly produces only a slight increase in muscle mass, with no increase in muscle strength. It decreases adipose tissue stores and increases skin thickness but does not increase bone mineral density. GH supplementation has minor effects on the immune system (eg, increased natural killer T-cell activity). The effects of GH supplementation on cognitive function are unknown. The adverse effects of GH supplementation include carpal tunnel syndrome, arthralgias, headaches, lethargy, fluid retention, and gynecomastia. Whether the use of more physiologic doses of GH would result in positive effects with fewer adverse effects is unknown. However, long-term effects are unclear; middle-aged persons with high levels of GH and IGF-I have higher mortality than do those with lower levels of GH and IGF-I.

As an alternative to GH supplementation, IGF-I administration decreases adipose tissue stores and increases lean body mass in the elderly. However, its use is limited because the incidence of adverse effects (eg, carpal tunnel syndrome) is high. GHRH administration increases levels of GH and IGF-I in the elderly. Certain small peptide molecules, called growth hormone secretagogues, increase GH, IGF-I, and IGF-binding protein-3 levels when administered orally daily for 28 days. Treatment is well tolerated; however, some patients experience appetite stimulation. Overall, little evidence supports the routine use of GH supplementation in the elderly.

67   HYPERTHERMIA AND HYPOTHERMIA

HYPERTHERMIA

Abnormally high body temperature due to inadequate or inappropriate responses of heat-regulating mechanisms.

Physiologic changes resulting from normal aging and from diseases more common in the elderly combine to impair optimal heat regulation. Heat exacerbates chronic diseases, and heatstroke causes many pathophysiologic changes. The number of deaths resulting from most diseases increases during hot, humid weather, particularly among older persons. Of persons who die of heatstroke, about 80% are > 50 years. Deaths attributed to diabetes, lung disease, and hypertension increase by > 50% during heat waves; thus, the risk of hyperthermia-related death may depend more on severity of associated disease than on severity of heat stress.

AGING AND TEMPERATURE REGULATION

Under usual environmental conditions, convection and radiation account for 65% of heat loss; evaporation from skin and lungs contributes another 30%. The hypothalamus regulates heat loss through neuroendocrine and autonomic mechanisms. Heat causes blood vessels in the skin to dilate, and sweating increases as a result of cholinergic discharge. Vasodilation, in turn, reflexly increases heart rate and cardiac output.

When ambient temperature exceeds body surface temperature, heat is no longer lost through convection and radiation, but instead is absorbed. Evaporation of sweat becomes the last mechanism by which heat is lost, but increased humidity can prevent cooling by this mechanism.

Aging appears to reduce the effectiveness of sweating in cooling the body. Many eccrine glands become fibrotic, and the remainder may not function properly. Surrounding connective tissue becomes less vascular. Elderly persons begin to sweat at higher core temperatures and have less maximal sweat output per gland.

Heart disease increases the risk of heat stress. Under experimental conditions, increased ambient heat and humidity exacerbate heart failure. The greater the degree of cardiac impairment, the less a person is able to withstand high ambient temperatures.

DISORDERS CAUSED BY HEAT

HEAT CRAMPS

Heat cramps are muscle cramps that often occur during intense physical activity performed in hot, humid weather. Heat cramps are preceded by profuse sweating and polydipsia without an elevation in body temperature and result when fluids and electrolytes lost through sweating are replaced mainly with water. Oral replacement with electrolyte-rich beverages such as Gatorade is likely to prevent heat cramps.

HEAT EXHAUSTION

Heat exhaustion is characterized by anorexia, nausea, vomiting, disorientation, and postural hypotension. Cramping may occur, and body temperature may be normal or elevated. Patients may be thirsty and weak and generally display some central nervous system signs—usually light-headedness, dizziness, or loss of consciousness. The two major forms of heat exhaustion are **water depletion,** which produces hypertonic dehydration, and **salt depletion,** which results when fluid and sodium chloride lost through sweating are replaced with electrolyte-free water, as occurs in heat cramps. Because elderly patients tend to present late with advanced symptoms, treatment is usually IV replacement of fluids and electrolytes, based on abnormal laboratory values. Oral therapy with electrolyte-rich beverages may be tried when symptoms are mild and patients are physiologically vigorous. Death and major complications are rare.

HEATSTROKE

The inadequacy or failure of heat loss mechanisms resulting in dangerously elevated body temperature accompanied by an absence of sweating and severe central nervous system disturbance.

Risk Factors

Heatstroke occurs 12 to 13 times more commonly in persons ≥ 65 years than in younger persons. Risk factors for heatstroke in the elderly include low socioeconomic status, impaired self-care ability, alcoholism, mental illness, unavailability of air-conditioning, and concomitant medical disorders (eg, cardiovascular or cerebrovascular disease, diabetes, chronic obstructive pulmonary disease).

TABLE 67-1.   TYPES OF DRUGS THAT IMPAIR RESPONSE TO HEAT

Drugs that can cause hypohidrosis
Anticholinergics
Antihistamines
Antiparkinsonian drugs
Antipsychotics
  Butyrophenones
  Phenothiazines
  Thioxanthenes
Antidepressants
  Monoamine oxidase inhibitors
  Tricyclic antidepressants
Drugs that can cause hypovolemia
Diuretics

Many drugs, particularly psychoactive ones, can predispose the patient to heatstroke (see TABLE 67–1). Anticholinergics (eg, synthetic and belladonna alkaloids), phenothiazines, tricyclic antidepressants, and antihistamines impair hypothalamic function centrally and sweat output peripherally. In addition, these drugs, as well as opioids, sedative-hypnotics, and alcohol, alter a person's awareness of heat and diminish the ability to respond to heat stress. Amphetamines can raise body temperature by acting directly on the hypothalamus. Diuretics (by causing additional fluid loss) and β-blockers (by impairing cardiovascular responsiveness) can also increase the risk of heatstroke. Therefore, a thorough drug history can be helpful in preventing heatstroke or in elucidating its cause.

Symptoms and Signs

Heatstroke is characterized by a high fever (generally > 41° C [>106° F], although the temperature may be lower if other criteria are met), absence of sweating, and severe central nervous system disturbance. Prodromal light-headedness, dizziness, headache, weakness, dyspnea, and nausea may occur transiently, but loss of consciousness is usually the first manifestation. Heatstroke has a bimodal population distribution, occurring in younger persons who overexert themselves at high ambient temperatures and in older persons, in whom it develops insidiously as the ability to dissipate heat declines.

Two common patterns of **cardiovascular response** have been identified. In the hyperdynamic response, generally seen in younger persons, pulse is typically very rapid (160 to 180 beats/minute), cardiac output is normal or increased, blood pressure (BP) is usually normal, and central venous pressure is commonly elevated. In the hypodynamic response, more typical in the elderly, pulse is usually slow and thready, BP may be low or imperceptible, hypovolemia is often present, and capillary wedge pressure is normal. The hypodynamic response may be due to an inability to respond to heat stress with a sufficient rise in heart rate or appropriate change in peripheral vascular resistance. In addition, the more protracted development and later diagnosis of heatstroke in older patients may result in greater fluid loss. Other cardiovascular manifestations include ECG changes in ST segments and T waves, premature ventricular contractions, supraventricular tachycardias, and conduction abnormalities.

Signs of CNS involvement may include lethargy, stupor, or coma. The electroencephalogram is usually normal initially, in the absence of seizures, and cerebrospinal fluid is unremarkable. Neurologic deficits may be permanent in < 5% of patients who recover. At autopsy, edema, patchy congestion, and diffuse petechial hemorrhages are found in the brain.

Renal manifestations range from mild proteinuria to acute tubular necrosis in 10 to 30% of cases. Rhabdomyolysis, which causes acute renal failure, may occur in both exercise-induced heatstroke and heatstroke from other causes. Generally, heatstroke is accompanied by metabolic acidosis and an elevated lactate level, with compensatory respiratory alkalosis. **Severe hypokalemia** is common and is thought to be secondary to increased aldosterone secretion.

Hepatic damage is unusual, although transient elevations of transaminases are common, and jaundice may be seen.

Coagulation defects include elevated prothrombin and partial thromboplastin times and a decreased fibrinogen level; the full-blown syndrome of disseminated intravascular coagulation is rare.

Specific prognostic signs remain undefined, but in the absence of comorbidity, elderly patients with the highest fever, the most severe hypotension, or the greatest neurologic impairment have the highest mortality rate.

Prevention

Heatstroke is both a public and an individual health problem; morbidity and mortality rates can be reduced by increased awareness and action. Caregivers should be alert to the symptoms of heatstroke in elderly persons at high risk and, in very hot weather, should try to move them to an air-conditioned environment, even if only for brief periods. If this is not possible, providing fans may be helpful. At times of greatest risk, they may need to move to temporary shelters. Elderly persons should wear light clothing and should keep their windows open at night and shaded during the day. Adequate fluid intake and avoidance of exercise are also important. Drugs that predispose one to heatstroke should be avoided or given in reduced doses whenever possible. Physicians should be aware of the nonspecific presentation of heatstroke.

Treatment

Heatstroke is a medical emergency requiring hospitalization and continuous monitoring. Normal body temperature must be restored as quickly as possible, because many metabolic and cardiovascular problems are temperature-dependent. Core temperature should be continuously monitored with a thermocouple while the patient is immersed in cool water. It is best to remove the patient from the bath when body temperature reaches 38.8° C (102° F) to avoid overcooling and hypothermia. The cooling process can then continue with wet sponging.

Because heatstroke may be either hyperdynamic, often associated with pulmonary edema, or hypodynamic, with major fluid loss, central venous pressure or pulmonary capillary wedge pressure monitoring to guide fluid replacement is advisable. Close monitoring of hematologic and renal parameters during the acute event is essential, as is a search for predisposing factors, including infection.

HYPOTHERMIA

(Accidental Hypothermia)

The unintentional decrease in body temperature to ≤ 34.4° C (≤ 94° F).

Prevalence, incidence, and mortality data for hypothermia are scanty, particularly in the USA. In a study conducted in two London hospitals, hypothermia was found in 3.6% of patients ≥ 65 years admitted during the winter. In a large community study conducted in Great Britain during an average winter, 10% of the elderly population had early morning core temperatures of ≤ 35.5° C (≤ 96° F). No correlation was found between low body temperature and living alone, being housebound, or being without central heating or indoor plumbing.

Estimates of deaths due to hypothermia are difficult to calculate because no definitive clinical or pathologic findings are available. Most corpses are already cold when discovered, making it difficult to attribute death to hypothermia. Accordingly, figures indicating that only a few hundred deaths each year in the USA are caused by hypothermia are probably an underestimation.

In the USA, about 75,000 "excess winter deaths" occur among the elderly, including deaths from hypothermia and deaths associated with many other winter risks, such as influenza and pneumonia. Among identified cases of hypothermia, the mortality rate is 50%. Of persons with hypothermia, those >75 years are five times more likely to die than those < 75 years. Mortality correlates more closely with the presence and severity of associated illness than with the degree of hypothermia.

Elderly patients with diabetes have a sixfold greater risk of hypothermia, probably due to vascular disease, which alters thermoregulatory mechanisms.

Etiology and Pathophysiology

The factors usually implicated in the genesis of hypothermia are a cold environment, age-related physiologic changes in thermoregulation, certain drugs (see TABLE 67–2), and diseases that decrease heat production, increase heat loss, impair thermoregulation, or diminish activity (see TABLE 67–3).

An ambient temperature only a few degrees cooler than body temperature can cause hypothermia in severely debilitated elderly persons. Most episodes of hypothermia are initiated by ambient temperatures $\leq$ 15.5° C ($\leq$ 60° F), but frail elderly persons may become hypothermic while at home at temperatures as warm as 22 to 24° C (70 to 75° F). Also, many age-related physiologic changes predispose elderly persons to hypothermia, including a diminished perception of cold. Changes in response to endogenous catecholamines reduce the vasoconstrictor and shivering responses to cold. A decrease in lean body mass reduces the efficiency of shivering for producing heat. Less physical activity and reduced caloric intake also affect the ability to produce heat.

Symptoms and Signs

The symptoms and signs of hypothermia are insidious and may be transient. Although elderly persons with body temperatures between 35° and 36.1° C (95° and 97° F) often report feeling cold, patients with established hypothermia usually do not, although they feel cool to the touch. Clinical findings are nonspecific; they can suggest other conditions (eg, stroke, a metabolic disorder).

Although shivering may occur normally at body temperatures > 35° C (> 95° F), it is absent in most hypothermic elderly patients. Instead, marked rigidity accompanied by a generalized increase in muscle tone and, occasionally, a fine tremor may be present.

Although many people have cold hands or feet in winter, hypothermic patients also have cold abdomens and backs. Their skin has a

**TABLE 67–2.   DRUGS THAT CAN PREDISPOSE PATIENTS
TO HYPOTHERMIA**

Alcohol
Antidepressants
Barbiturates
Benzodiazepines
Opioids
Phenothiazines
Reserpine

TABLE 67–3.   RISK FACTORS FOR HYPOTHERMIA

Mechanism of Action	Disorder
Decreased heat production	Diabetic ketoacidosis Hypoglycemia Hypopituitarism Malnutrition or starvation Myxedema Hypothyroidism
Impaired thermoregulation	Neuropathy: alcoholism, diabetes Primary CNS disease: head trauma, polio, stroke, subarachnoid hemorrhage, subdural hematoma, tumor, Wernicke's encephalopathy Systemic disease influencing hypothalamus Carbon monoxide poisoning, uremia
Increased heat loss	Arteriovenous shunt Inflammatory dermatitis: exfoliation, ichthyosis, psoriasis Paget's disease Alcohol-induced vasodilation Cold exposure Reduction in subcutaneous fat, malnutrition
Diminished activity	Parkinson's disease, parkinsonism Arthritis Dementia A fall or other injury Paralysis or stroke

CNS = central nervous system.

cadaveric pallor and chill, and pressure points have erythematous, bullous, or purpuric patches. Subcutaneous tissues are firm, probably from edema, which also causes puffiness, especially of the face.

Neurologic findings include thick, slow speech; ataxic gait; and depressed deep tendon reflexes. Sleepiness and confusion may progress to coma. Pathologic reflexes and plantar responses may be present, and pupils may be dilated and sluggishly reactive. Focal signs, seizures, paralysis, and sensory loss may also occur.

The **cardiovascular system** is initially stimulated by cold, resulting in peripheral vasoconstriction, tachycardia, and elevated BP. As hypothermia progresses, the myocardium is depressed, causing hypotension and progressive sinus bradycardia. Severe hypothermia can lower BP and heart rate to barely detectable levels, which in rare cases leads to an erroneous pronouncement of death. Various cardiac arrhythmias may be precipitated by cold temperatures, including atrial fibrillation and flutter, premature ventricular beats, and idioventricular rhythm. Cardiac arrest, from either ventricular fibrillation or asystole, is increasingly likely as body temperature falls below 30° C (86° F).

Renal responses occur early in hypothermia, when increased heart rate, cardiac output, and renal blood flow cause diuresis. In addition, cold suppresses antidiuretic hormone secretion and diminishes tubular responsiveness to its action, further increasing diuresis. As volume depletion reduces glomerular filtration and renal blood flow, oliguria and tubular necrosis follow.

Pulmonary findings include depression of respiration and cough reflex. Atelectasis is almost universal, and pneumonia is common. Pulmonary edema during recovery may be related to increased vascular permeability as well as to heart failure.

The gastrointestinal response includes decreased peristalsis or even ileus, producing abdominal distention and diminished or absent bowel sounds. Less often, acute gastric dilation occurs with vomiting. Pancreatitis may also occur but is usually not apparent until after warming. Because hepatic metabolism is depressed, drug metabolism may be sharply reduced.

Diagnosis

Hypothermia is often missed; the usual clinical practice is to search for and exclude fever, not to search for and exclude hypothermia. Hypothermia should be suspected if the history or physical examination is suggestive.

The diagnosis of hypothermia depends on the ability to measure body temperature < 34.4° C (< 94° F). A low-reading thermometer or more expensive thermistors or thermocouples can be used. Rectal thermometers, which are calibrated from 28.9 to 42.2° C (84 to 108° F), are available from most hospital suppliers, although they are not commonly used. Standard clinical thermometers, which are calibrated from 34.4 to 42.2° C (94 to 108° F), probably will not detect hypothermia.

Clinical laboratory data generally are not specific for hypothermia. Hemoconcentration, leukocytosis, lactic acidosis, and thrombocytopenia are common findings. Laboratory evaluation should include CBC; platelet count; clotting studies; measurements of blood urea nitrogen, creatinine, electrolytes, blood glucose, and serum and urine amylase levels; thyroid and liver function tests; arterial blood gas studies; ECG with constant monitoring; chest and abdominal x-rays; and constant monitoring and recording of core temperature.

Blood glucose findings in patients with hypothermia can be confusing. Usually, hyperglycemia is found. In most cases, hypothermia triggers hyperglycemia through corticosteroid- and catecholamine-induced gluconeogenesis. Although insulin secretion is also stimulated, cold interferes with its action, further raising blood glucose levels. When hypoglycemia occurs in a hypothermic patient, it is usually drug-induced; ie, the drug-induced hypoglycemia is the cause of the hypothermia.

ECG findings can provide a major diagnostic clue. A junctional (J), or Osborne, wave, although present in only about one third of hypothermic patients, is specific for hypothermia. This wave appears as a small deflection early in the ST segment: it is positive in the left ventricular leads and negative in the right ones. An ECG finding frequently seen in the nonshivering patient is a fine regular oscillation of the baseline produced by increased muscle tone with an imperceptible tremor.

Prevention

Elderly persons with identifiable predisposing problems should keep ambient temperatures ≥ 18.3° C (≥ 65° F) and should keep a reliable thermometer available (separate from the thermostat) for determining room temperature. The thermometer should be checked daily, especially during very cold weather. Extra clothing, particularly for hands, feet, and head, should be worn indoors. Adequate caloric intake is important. In addition, frequent periods of exercise can increase heat production. Drugs that may alter thermoregulatory mechanisms should be discontinued whenever possible.

For elderly patients undergoing surgery, special care must be taken to regulate body temperature and thus reduce the risk of hypothermia. The shivering that sometimes accompanies hypothermia increases oxygen consumption; if oxygen demand exceeds supply, hypoxemia, acidosis, and circulatory changes occur, and the elderly patient may be unable to compensate. Warming the operating room, inspired gases, IV solutions, and antibacterial solutions used to prepare the surgical site can minimize the risk of hypothermia and its sequelae. Forced-air warming blankets should be used.

Treatment

An elderly patient with hypothermia usually is treated initially for some other disorder, either because a cause or complication of hypothermia is the exclusive focus, or because the symptoms and signs of hypothermia are erroneously attributed to one of the diseases that commonly affects the elderly. In either case, therapy is too often delayed.

Once the body temperature falls into the hypothermic range, thermoregulation quickly fails and the patient reacts like a poikilotherm. Accordingly, *even mild hypothermia should be considered a medical emergency, and patients should be monitored under hospital conditions* (usually in an intensive care unit) until recovery is complete. However, movement or excessive stimulation of hypothermic patients may provoke arrhythmias and should be performed cautiously.

Therapy can be divided into two foci: (1) primary treatment by warming and (2) secondary treatment of the direct effects and complications of hypothermia. General medical care demands comprehensive evaluation, close monitoring, and anticipation of likely complications.

Primary measures aim to restore normal body temperature and to abort the pathophysiologic consequences of hypothermia. In younger patients, rapid active warming is performed. In elderly patients, however, *rapid active warming can lead to a syndrome characterized by profound hypotension, new cardiac arrhythmias, and deteriorating metabolic abnormalities, culminating in death.* Therefore, slow spontaneous warming is recommended for elderly patients. By preventing further heat loss and conserving the heat still being produced by the patient, slow spontaneous warming allows the body temperature to rise slowly, at a rate of about 0.6° C (1° F)/hour. A more rapid rise in core temperature, even when slow spontaneous warming is used, is associated with warming hypotension. The ambient temperature is kept above 21.1° C (70° F), and blankets or more sophisticated insulating materials are used to retain body heat.

If slow spontaneous warming does not raise body temperature, rapid active warming of the core is necessary. Techniques for core warming include the use of heated, moist inspired air; IV fluids warmed to 37° C (98.6° F); and heated peritoneal dialysis. *Rapid active warming in elderly patients requires scrupulous, comprehensive intensive care.* When ventricular fibrillation or cardiac standstill occurs at temperatures < 29.4° C (< 85° F), warming must be accomplished as quickly as possible, because the heart is unresponsive to electrical defibrillation at temperatures below this level. Bradycardia resulting from myocardial depression is not influenced by atropine. The need for ventilatory assistance, intracardiac monitoring and pacing, and full circulatory support should be anticipated, because collapse and profound hypotension associated with warming are common under such conditions.

Ventricular arrhythmias, if not rapidly responsive to warming, are suppressed with lidocaine. Countershock and pacing are less effective at low temperatures; if critical arrhythmias occur, appropriate treatment is given while the patient is warmed. If cardiac arrest or ventricular fibrillation is unresponsive to usual measures, CPR is continued until warming has been accomplished; treatment is then repeated. All IV fluids are warmed to normal or slightly above normal body temperature.

Although some studies have recommended the routine use of drugs such as corticosteroids, thyroid hormone, anticoagulants, antibiotics, and digoxin, none of these agents has proved effective unless specifically indicated. Myxedema is a well-known cause of hypothermia; when hypothermia and hypothyroidism occur together, they result in a very high mortality rate.

Although hyperglycemia is common in hypothermic patients, insulin is rarely given unless blood glucose levels are very high (> 400 mg/dL

[> 22.2 mmol/L]), because insulin is ineffective at low temperatures. Any previously administered insulin can produce severe hypoglycemia during warming. Even without exogenous insulin, hypoglycemia may occur during warming due to production of endogeous insulin. In general, most drugs are less active during hypothermia but have exaggerated pharmacologic effects as body temperature rises. When death occurs, cardiac arrest or ventricular fibrillation is usually the cause. The body temperature at which each cardiac event appears varies, but at temperatures < 29.4° C (< 85° F), risk of death is high, particularly in patients with underlying heart disease. *Resuscitation during warming should be aggressive and prolonged in patients who are profoundly hypothermic;* unexpected recoveries have been reported in such cases. Most authorities agree that patients should not be pronounced dead until CPR is shown to be ineffective after body temperature has been raised to at least 35.8° C (96.5° F).

SECTION 9

HEMATOLOGIC DISORDERS AND CANCER

HEM/
ONC

68 ▌ AGING AND THE BLOOD

Age-related hematologic changes derive mostly from changes in the bone marrow, which are rarely clinically significant. However, the reduced capacity to make new blood cells quickly when disease has occurred is a feature of aging and can be a problem in the elderly.

CHANGES IN BONE MARROW

The percentage of marrow space occupied by hematopoietic tissue declines progressively from birth until about age 30, when it levels off. After about age 70, it again declines progressively, starting with the long bones, especially the femur; the flat bones are relatively spared. Whether the second decline results from an intrinsic reduction in blood-forming elements or from an increase in bone marrow fat displacing hematologic tissue is not known.

Several age-related changes occur in marrow function. The number of stem cells in marrow decreases significantly with age, although the length of time that marrow can be maintained in tissue culture by serial transplantation is the same for elderly and younger adults. The rate of incorporation of iron in marrow culture is comparable in elderly and younger adults, but in the elderly, the rate increases less with erythropoietin stimulation. Iron uptake from the intestines is normal in the elderly, but slowed erythropoiesis reduces incorporation of iron into red blood cells (RBCs). Clonal hematopoiesis, resulting from oncogene mutations, has been observed in healthy elderly persons without morphologic or functional hematologic abnormalities.

In animal studies, healthy older subjects are unable to produce reticulocytes in response to hemorrhage or hypoxemia as efficiently as younger subjects. Whether this defect is due to ineffective erythropoiesis, to changes in the hematopoietic elements, to a decrease in growth factors, or to age-related architectural changes in the marrow is unclear. In elderly patients, such findings (slow recovery of peripheral hematologic values after hemorrhage or severe infection) are termed decreased marrow reserve. However, some studies suggest that the response to hemorrhage in the elderly is just as effective as that in younger adults and that hematopoietic response to administered growth factors (eg, erythropoietin, granulocyte colony-stimulating factor, granulocyte-macrophage colony-stimulating factor, interleukin-3) is well maintained in the elderly.

These changes in marrow function are not secondary to nutritional deficiencies, because total body iron and bone marrow iron increase with age, and folate and vitamin B_{12} levels in healthy elderly persons remain within the normal range.

CHANGES IN PERIPHERAL BLOOD

With age, average values of hemoglobin and hematocrit decrease slightly but remain within the normal adult range. Mean corpuscular volume increases slightly, but RBC morphologic characteristics do not change significantly. RBC content of 2,3-diphosphoglycerate decreases, and RBC osmotic fragility increases. ESR increases significantly. Levels of fibrinogen and coagulation factors V, VII, and IX increase.

RBC life span, total blood volume, RBC volume, and platelet morphologic characteristics do not change with age. Platelet counts have been reported as either normal or slightly decreased, and platelet function has been reported as normal, decreased, or increased.

CHANGES IN THE LYMPHOID SYSTEM

Age-related changes in the lymphoid system (immune senescence) affect cellular and humoral immunity.∎ They include a significant decrease in humoral antibody response (especially the primary response), a decrease in T-cell function, production of antibodies that have less affinity for antigen, and increased production of autoidiotype antibody (which has an inhibitory effect on immune response). The resulting reduction in immunity may contribute to the increased susceptibility of the elderly to infections and malignancy.

In the healthy elderly, total lymphocyte and granulocyte counts have been reported as either normal or slightly decreased.

∎ see also page 1351

69 ANEMIAS

Decreases in red blood cell (RBC) or hemoglobin resulting from blood loss, impaired production of RBCs, or RBC destruction.

The prevalence of anemia varies greatly in outpatients, depending on the population examined. Although anemia is common in the elderly, it is never normal. Normal values for Hct and RBC volume are not altered with aging. Because anemia is a sign, not a diagnosis, an evaluation is almost always warranted to identify the underlying cause. At the very least, enough testing should be performed to determine the type of anemia. With that information, the need for further evaluation can better be determined. Often anemia is caused by benign disease and, indeed, may simply be a marker of chronic illness. However, it may be the presenting sign of serious disease, including cancer.

The most diagnostically useful way to classify anemias is by mean corpuscular volume (MCV). This method groups anemias into three categories: microcytic, normocytic, and macrocytic (see TABLE 69–1). However, some anemias fall into more than one category.

Symptoms and signs generally are similar across age groups, although some may be more common or prominent in the elderly because of underlying, possibly unrelated, diseases. For example, fatigue, shortness of breath, worsening angina, and peripheral edema

TABLE 69–1. ANEMIAS CLASSIFIED BY MEAN CORPUSCULAR VOLUME

Microcytic anemia (MCV < 80 fL)	Iron deficiency anemia (can be normocytic)
	Thalassemia minor
	Myelodysplastic syndromes (can be normocytic or macrocytic)
Normocytic anemia (MCV 80–100 fL)	Anemia of chronic disease (can be microcytic)—eg, chronic liver disease, endocrine disorders, malnutrition
	Anemia of primary autonomic failure
	Hemolytic anemias (can be macrocytic)
	Aplastic anemia
	Anemia caused by malignancy (bone marrow replacement by metastases, multiple myeloma, myeloid metaplasia, leukemia)
	Sideroblastic anemia (can be microcytic or macrocytic)
	Unexplained anemia (can be microcytic or macrocytic)
Macrocytic anemia (MCV > 100 fL)	Vitamin B_{12} deficiency anemia
	Folate deficiency anemia

MCV = mean corpuscular volume; fL = femtoliters.

are more common with anemia when elderly patients also have preexisting atherosclerotic heart disease or heart failure. Mental status changes, including confusion, depression, agitation, and apathy, may occur as presenting symptoms of anemia, even in previously unimpaired elderly persons. Dizziness is also common. Pallor may be less noticeable in the elderly, although it can usually be noticed on the oral mucosa and the conjunctiva.

MICROCYTIC ANEMIAS
Anemias in which the MCV is < 80 femtoliters.

In the elderly, common microcytic anemias include iron deficiency anemia and thalassemia minor. Anemia of chronic disease may be microcytic but is more commonly normocytic. Myelodysplastic syndromes ◘ may also be microcytic or normocytic or even macrocytic.

IRON DEFICIENCY ANEMIA

Normally, total body and bone marrow iron stores increase with age, because the body cannot eliminate excessive iron. Therefore, iron deficiency is never normal in elderly persons, although iron deficiency anemia is common in persons > 65.

Dietary iron deficiency in adults is virtually unknown in the USA, and iron malabsorption occurs only after total gastrectomy or with severe, generalized malabsorption. ◙ If these conditions do not exist, iron deficiency implies blood loss, most commonly from the gastrointestinal (GI) ▣ or genitourinary tract, and evaluation is necessary. Common sources of chronic occult or other bleeding in the elderly include carcinoma, ulcer, atrophic gastritis, gastritis from drug ingestion, postmenopausal vaginal bleeding, bleeding hemorrhoids, recurrent hemoptysis, and angiodysplasia of the colon.

Symptoms and Signs

The principal symptoms are those of anemia, although mild disease may be asymptomatic. Symptoms related to the cause, such as melanotic stools, acid reflux, and weight loss, may also occur and give clues to the etiology. Atrophy of the tongue and buccal mucosa as well as angular stomatitis may occur. Abnormalities of the gastric mucosa, especially superficial gastritis, frequently develop. Iron deficiency may lead to central nervous system dysfunction. Fatigue, irritability, and decreased cognitive function have been reported in children, but whether they occur in the elderly is unknown.

◘see page 739   ◙see page 1095   ▣see page 1105

Diagnosis

Iron deficiency anemia is characterized by small, pale RBCs and depleted iron stores. The peripheral blood smear is populated with microcytic hypochromic cells, and the MCV, the mean corpuscular Hb, and the mean corpuscular Hb concentration are usually reduced. In early iron deficiency, however, these values may still be normal. Many elderly persons with iron deficiency anemia and chronic disease have normal RBC indices and distribution width.

A transferrin saturation ratio (serum iron to total iron-binding capacity [TIBC]) of < 16% may indicate iron deficiency. However, this ratio frequently is not useful because serum iron and TIBC decrease with age and in cases of chronic disease.

Serum ferritin levels usually accurately reflect bone marrow iron stores. However, infection, inflammation, liver disease, and states of increased RBC turnover (eg, ineffective erythropoiesis and hemolysis) can falsely elevate these levels. Serum ferritin levels < 10 μg/L are diagnostic of iron deficiency.

If a conclusive diagnosis of iron deficiency still cannot be made, a bone marrow aspirate stained for iron may be performed. In iron deficiency, iron is either present in trace amounts or is absent. Another option is to give a 1-month trial of oral iron in the form of ferrous salts. If the anemia results from iron deficiency, both Hb and Hct will increase. If no increase occurs, either the patient is not iron deficient, blood loss is exceeding new blood formation, an inflammatory or malignant process is contributing to the anemia, or the patient has protein-energy malnutrition.

For all patients, stools should be screened for occult blood. When iron deficiency is discovered, additional GI tract evaluation (ie, barium studies or endoscopy) may be necessary but depends on the individual patient.

Treatment

Treatment involves finding and eliminating the source of bleeding and correcting the iron deficiency. Oral iron therapy is inexpensive, safe, and convenient. Only ferrous iron salts should be used; enteric-coated and sustained-release preparations are not well absorbed because they are transported past the duodenum, where most iron absorption occurs. One 300-mg tablet of ferrous sulfate contains 60 mg of elemental iron. A single daily dose generally provides enough iron and reduces the likelihood of constipation and gastric irritation; increasing the dose increases iron absorption only minimally. Liquid preparations are available for patients unable to swallow tablets. Many frail elderly patients are unable to tolerate ferrous sulfate because of GI symptoms (including constipation), but they may be able to tolerate a polysaccharide-iron complex, 1 tablet/day, which provides 150 mg of elemental iron. Therapeutic response is monitored by serially measuring serum Hb, Hct, and ferritin levels. Reticulocyte response should begin within 1 to 2 weeks; however, $\geq$ 6 months (often up to 1 year) of therapy usually is needed after bleeding has stopped to fully replenish iron stores.

Parenteral iron may be used for patients who have severe malabsorption, who cannot tolerate oral iron, or when iron losses exceed what can be replaced orally (eg, during continued bleeding). Parenteral iron is available as iron dextran and may be given IV or by deep IM injection into the buttocks using the Z-track technique to avoid tissue staining. A test dose of 0.5 mL IV or IM should be given before treatment begins, because this therapy has been associated with anaphylactic shock. Other adverse effects include pain at the injection site, fever, and arthralgias. The maximum recommended dosage is 2 mL/day, which delivers 100 mg of elemental iron. A daily IV infusion should be given at a rate of $\leq$ 1 mL/minute for about 2 minutes (2 mL/day) until iron is replenished.

The most expensive and potentially hazardous way to replace iron is by transfusion. Each milliliter of transfused RBCs delivers 1 mg iron.

THALASSEMIA MINOR

Thalassemia minor occurs in persons who are heterozygous for genes that produce few or no α- or β-globin chains. Because thalassemia minor is asymptomatic, the microcytosis throughout life may have been overlooked or misdiagnosed as iron deficiency; thus it is not unusual to have thalassemia minor diagnosed in old age. Other anemias caused by abnormal Hbs are usually diagnosed in younger persons, because they are symptomatic or the patient has a more pronounced anemia.

Thalassemia minor produces microcytosis with or without mild anemia. The reticulocyte count is usually normal, and serum iron, TIBC, and serum ferritin are normal. Hb electrophoresis may reveal an increase in the minor Hbs, particularly fetal Hb or Hb A_2 in β-thalassemia; Hb electrophoresis may be normal in α-thalassemia. No treatment is required for thalassemia minor, and iron therapy is contraindicated because it may cause iron overload.

NORMOCYTIC ANEMIAS

Anemias in which the MCV is 80 to 100 femtoliters.

Normocytic anemia is often worrisome in the elderly. Although it may be caused by obvious concurrent illness (anemia of chronic disease), this type of anemia can also indicate life-threatening conditions, such as multiple myeloma, hemolysis, and myelofibrosis (see TABLE 69–1).

ANEMIA OF CHRONIC DISEASE

Anemia of chronic disease is the most common normocytic anemia in the elderly, accounting for up to 10% of anemias in this population. The most common and most important causes are chronic infection or inflammation, cancer, renal insufficiency, chronic liver disease, endocrine disorders, and malnutrition. The diagnosis is made by excluding other causes of anemia and by finding a chronic disease process.

Chronic infection or inflammation commonly produces anemia, usually after 4 to 8 weeks of illness. The anemia is usually mild and normochromic-normocytic but may be slightly microcytic and hypochromic. It probably results from slightly decreased erythropoietin production, decreased RBC survival, and impaired delivery of iron from the reticuloendothelial system to the bone marrow. The reticulocyte count is low, serum iron and TIBC are normal or reduced, and serum ferritin is normal or elevated. When the underlying disorder is treated, the anemia disappears.

Renal insufficiency produces anemia resulting from decreased erythropoiesis and decreased RBC survival, which are caused by decreased erythropoietin production. Serum iron stores are normal. The anemia occurs independent of nutritional deficiencies common in renal disease (eg, iron or folate deficiency). In hemodialysis patients, injections of erythropoietin correct the anemia. In nondialysis patients, erythropoietin may not completely reverse the anemia, because erythropoietic inhibitors can accumulate. Erythropoietin is given IV to hemodialysis patients and subcutaneously or IV to nondialysis patients with renal failure. The starting dosage is 50 to 100 U/kg 3 times/week, although single weekly doses are now commonly prescribed. The target Hct is 30 to 33%. The maximum recommended dosage is 300 U/kg 3 times/week. Newer studies show that subcutaneous doses are often preferred because, although peak levels are lower, the kinetics are different, leading to more prolonged bone marrow stimulation even with lower doses. This can be an important cost-saving approach, especially in patients who require long-term use of erythropoietin.

Chronic liver disease results in decreased RBC production and survival and produces a normochromic-normocytic or a normochromic-macrocytic anemia. Large quantities of alcohol are toxic to the bone marrow as well as to the liver. Unless liver disease is complicated by bleeding, TIBC is decreased and serum iron is increased, resulting in an increased transferrin saturation. Serum ferritin is also increased and often reflects total body iron overload. Treatment must be directed toward the underlying liver disorder.

Endocrine disorders (eg, pituitary insufficiency, adrenal insufficiency, hypothyroidism) commonly produce a normochromic-normocytic anemia. Unless a specific deficiency of iron, vitamin B_{12}, or folate is identified, treatment focuses on the underlying disorder. **Malnutrition** results in an anemia due to deficiency of essential nutrients, such as folic acid, vitamin C, trace minerals (eg, copper), and essential amino acids. In malnutrition, Hb synthesis and RBC production decrease, as does all other protein synthesis (eg, prealbumin and albumin in the liver) and cell (lymphocyte) and fibroblast production.

ANEMIA CAUSED BY MALIGNANCY

Cancer in its later stages is almost always accompanied by anemia of chronic disease. Frequently, there is no correlation between the degree of anemia and the extent of the tumor. Poor nutrition can lead to calorie, protein, and vitamin deficiency.

Cancer can also cause other types of anemia; eg, bleeding from GI or genitourinary tract tumors or from vascular lesions of the skin can cause iron deficiency anemia. In some cancers there is a microangiopathic hemolytic anemia; in others, splenomegaly leads to increased RBC destruction. Replacement of normal marrow by a neoplasm is a relatively uncommon cause of normochromic-normocytic anemia.

Bone marrow invasion by cancer is often associated with the release of immature leukocytes and nucleated erythrocytes, but the extent of bone marrow metastases correlates poorly with the degree of anemia. Serum iron, vitamin B_{12}, and folate values are normal or elevated, and the ESR is usually elevated.

HEMOLYTIC ANEMIAS

Acquired hemolytic anemia (ie, hemolysis not resulting from a congenital abnormality of the RBCs) increases in incidence with age.

Etiology

Idiopathic autoimmune hemolysis may result from warm-reactive antibodies of the IgG class; from cold agglutinins that are usually of the IgM class but that may be of the IgG class; or from a nonagglutinating cold-activated hemolysin of the IgG class. Idiopathic cold-agglutinin disease occurs primarily in old age.

Secondary immune hemolysis occurs in a wide variety of illnesses. About 30% of secondary immune hemolytic anemias are caused by lymphoproliferative diseases, including chronic lymphocytic leukemia, non-Hodgkin's lymphoma, Hodgkin's disease, and multiple myeloma. Agnogenic myeloid metaplasia, systemic lupus erythematosus, viral infections, *Mycoplasma pneumoniae* infection, syphilis, and various nonhematologic malignancies are also associated with immune hemolytic anemia.

Drug-induced hemolysis is another major cause of hemolytic anemia. The elderly are prone to this problem because they generally take more drugs than younger persons. Three types of drug-induced hemolysis have been described (see TABLE 69–2).

Some drugs cause autoantibody formation with antibodies directed against normal RBC antigens. Methyldopa creates these antibodies in 10 to 40% of persons taking it. These antibodies attach to the RBC, resulting in a positive direct Coombs' test result against IgG; however, < 1% of those taking methyldopa actually develop hemolysis. Other drugs that commonly produce autoantibodies but rarely produce autoimmune hemolysis include L-dopa and procainamide. Discontinuing the drug usually corrects the anemia, but autoantibodies may persist for months to years.

Other drugs bind to the surface of the RBC, acting as a hapten. Antibodies, usually IgG, are produced against the drug-RBC complex. The direct Coombs' test result is positive, and if the drug is added to test RBCs, the indirect Coombs' test result is also positive. The anemia clears quickly when the drug is discontinued.

Still other drugs stimulate the production of antibodies to the drug. Drug-antibody immune complexes form in the circulation and bind briefly to the RBC. Hemolysis occurs because the complex activates complement on the RBC surface. The Coombs' test result is positive for complement but not for IgG. Hemolysis ceases quickly when the drug is withdrawn.

Microangiopathic hemolytic anemia (traumatic hemolytic anemia) is commonly caused by obstruction of the microvasculature. Chronic forms may be due to diabetes mellitus, atherosclerosis, or collagen-vascular diseases. A similar anemia occurs in persons with mechanical heart valves, particularly if the valves are malfunctioning. The peripheral blood smear shows fragmented cells (schistocytes).

TABLE 69–2. SELECTED DRUGS CAUSING HEMOLYTIC ANEMIA

Autoimmune response	Immune complex response	
L-Dopa	*p*-Aminosalicylic acid	Quinine
Methyldopa	Cephalosporins	Rifampin
Procainamide	Chlorpromazine	Streptomycin
	Doxepin	Sulfonamides
Hapten-type response	Insecticides	Sulfonylureas
Cephalosporins	Isoniazid	Tetracyclines
Penicillins	Phenacetin	Thiazides
Tetracyclines	Quinidine	

Acute forms of microangiopathic hemolytic anemia occur in persons with malignant hypertension, vasculitis, disseminated intravascular coagulation, and thrombotic thrombocytopenic purpura.

Diagnosis

Increased peripheral destruction of RBCs results in increased production of immature RBCs by the bone marrow, producing an elevated reticulocyte count and polychromatophilia on the peripheral blood smear. If the reticulocytosis is marked, the RBC indices may become macrocytic, because reticulocytes are larger than mature RBCs. Destruction of RBCs results in increased serum levels of unconjugated bilirubin, aspartate transaminase, and lactic dehydrogenase; decreased serum haptoglobin; and increased urine urobilinogen. If hemolysis is intravascular, urine hemosiderin increases. The direct antiglobulin (Coombs') test is used to detect antibody or complement on the RBC and can also identify the antigen to which the antibody is reacting.

Treatment

All hemolytic anemias require folic acid treatment, because this vitamin is used up with the increased bone marrow production of erythrocytes.

Idiopathic autoimmune hemolysis secondary to warm-reactive antibodies of the IgG class responds, in about 75% of cases, to corticosteroid therapy. Prednisone 60 mg/day in divided doses is given initially, although occasionally 100 mg/day is needed. A rise in Hb and Hct and a drop in the reticulocyte count usually occur within 3 to 14 days, but the response may be delayed up to 8 weeks. After remission, the dosage may be tapered by 5 mg/week. A relapse requires increasing the dosage by 15 to 20 mg/day, followed by a more gradual tapering. Some patients continue to need a small daily dose or alternate-day therapy for months or even years.

If after 4 to 8 weeks, prednisone produces no response, higher doses may be tried or 200 mg bid to qid of danazol (an androgen) may be added. If this fails, the next step is usually splenectomy, which achieves long-term remission in 50 to 75% of cases. In patients who do not respond to these measures or who are poor surgical candidates, immunosuppressants (cyclophosphamide 150 mg/day or azathioprine 200 mg/day) may be useful.

Transfusion is rarely used to treat warm-antibody autoimmune hemolysis except in those patients with severe symptoms of anemia. Blood compatibility testing is problematic, and the autoantibodies reduce the survival of the transfused RBCs. Plasmapheresis is usually not successful, because IgG has a large volume of distribution in the body.

Idiopathic cold-agglutinin disease is treated by avoiding exposure to cold. If transfusion is necessary, it should be performed with warmed, washed RBCs. Plasmapheresis may lead to temporary improvement, because IgM is confined to the intravascular space. Corticosteroids and splenectomy are seldom helpful. **Secondary immune hemolysis** usually improves only with treatment of the underlying illness. If this approach is not possible, treatment may be tried as described above for idiopathic disease, but success is less likely.

Drug-induced hemolysis is usually treated by simply discontinuing the responsible drug. In rare cases, methyldopa-induced autoimmune hemolysis continues long enough to require corticosteroid therapy, as described above for idiopathic autoimmune hemolysis.

Microangiopathic hemolytic anemia is treated by correcting the underlying disease process. Management includes treatment with iron to replace the loss in the urine, which occurs only with intravascular hemolysis. In the extravascular hemolytic anemias, iron is conserved and recycled via the reticuloendothelial system.

APLASTIC ANEMIA

This normochromic-normocytic anemia results from decreased bone marrow production of RBCs alone (pure RBC aplasia) or of all cell lines. Aplastic anemia is not very common, but its incidence increases with age. In this disorder, the reticulocyte count is low; serum levels of iron, vitamin B_{12}, and folate are normal; and the bone marrow is hypoplastic. If thrombocytopenia occurs, bleeding may become a problem. The overall mortality rate is > 50%.

Idiopathic aplastic anemia is usually a disease of adolescents and young adults but can occur in old age. The most common pathogenesis involves T-cell–mediated suppression of the hematopoietic stem cell. **Secondary aplastic anemia** can be caused by chemicals, radiation, or drugs, especially chemotherapeutic drugs, chloramphenicol, gold, and anticonvulsants (see TABLE 69–3). Thymoma and chronic lymphocytic leukemia sometimes cause pure RBC aplasia.

Treatment

All potentially causative drugs must be discontinued. An oral androgen (eg, oxymetholone 1 to 2 mg/kg/day) may be given but is rarely successful. Bone marrow transplantation, the only curative therapy, usually is not an option in patients > 65, who can rarely tolerate it. Ongoing supportive treatment with transfusions is, therefore, required. Pure RBC aplasia may respond to prednisone or cyclophosphamide; if it is associated with thymoma, tumor resection may be helpful. Usually, attempts are made to suppress cellular immunity with cyclosporine or high doses of antithymocyte immunoglobulins. The use of corticosteroids is controversial. Recombinant human granulocyte-macrophage

TABLE 69-3. DRUGS THAT CAN CAUSE APLASTIC ANEMIA

Analgesics (phenylbutazone)
Antibiotics (daunorubicin, doxorubicin) and antimicrobials (chloramphenicol, organic arsenicals, quinacrine)
Anticonvulsants (mephenytoin, trimethadione)
Antimetabolites (cytarabine, mercaptopurine, thioguanine)
Antimitotics (colchicine, vinblastine, vincristine)
Benzene
Gold compounds
Inorganic arsenic
Ionizing radiation
Sulfur or nitrogen mustard and congeners (busulfan, cyclophosphamide, melphalan)

colony-stimulating factor, granulocyte colony-stimulating factor, interleukin-3, erythropoietin, and thrombopoietin may be useful.

ANEMIA OF PRIMARY AUTONOMIC FAILURE

This rare normochromic-normocytic anemia occurs in 38% of elderly patients with primary autonomic dysfunction (Shy-Drager syndrome) and appears to be caused by reduced erythropoietin secretion. A dilutional effect on Hb concentration from fluid overload may also be a factor. Erythropoietin levels are low in the absence of renal disease, and no other cause of anemia is present. In about 80% of these cases, the anemia is corrected with low-dose erythropoietin treatment (50 U/kg 3 times/week).

SIDEROBLASTIC ANEMIAS

Sideroblastic anemias are a heterogeneous group of disorders characterized by impaired heme synthesis. Iron continues to go into the mitochondria of the bone marrow erythroblasts, but since heme is not being synthesized, the iron accumulates and ultimately damages the mitochondria and the cell, resulting in ineffective erythropoiesis. Ringed sideroblasts can be seen in bone marrow stain for iron; they represent iron in the mitochondria that encircle the nucleus of the erythroblast. Eventually, this iron accumulation leads to an iron overload in the body.

Sideroblastic anemias may be primary or secondary to other conditions. The primary genetic form usually is diagnosed in younger people. The primary acquired form is often a myelodysplastic syndrome ∎

∎see page 739

in elderly people. Chronic alcohol use is probably the most common cause of a secondary sideroblastic anemia. Sideroblastic anemias also occur secondary to hematologic malignancies (eg, multiple myeloma, acute leukemias); vitamin B_{12} and/or folate deficiencies; rheumatic disorders; use of drugs that inhibit heme synthesis (eg, phenytoin, isoniazid, chloramphenicol); and exposure to toxins, especially lead.

In sideroblastic anemias, the MCV may be low, normal, or high, but the reticulocyte count is always low. Serum iron, transferrin saturation, and ferritin levels are high. A hypochromic anemia in an elderly person without iron deficiency is usually a sideroblastic anemia. In bone marrow examination, there is usually erythroid hyperplasia, and 15% of erythroid cells are ringed sideroblasts.

Any possibly offending drug should be stopped, and any underlying disorders should be treated. Any nutritional disorder should also be treated. If there is no response, pyridoxine 200 mg/day should be given for 1 to 2 months. If there is still no response, transfusions may be required if the anemia is severe (Hb < 8 g/dL) or if the patient is symptomatic from the anemia.

OTHER CAUSES OF ANEMIA

A mild normochromic-normocytic anemia without any underlying disease or deficiency (Hb usually between 11 and 12 g/dL) has been reported in people > 70, accounting for up to 30% of the normochromic-normocytic anemias in this age group. The bone marrow does not contain ringed sideroblasts. Unexplained anemia may be associated with low neutrophil, lymphocyte, and platelet counts and with increased RBC 2,3-diphosphoglycerate levels, implying that this condition is not merely a normal age-related variant. Its significance is unknown, but it is probably a myelodysplastic syndrome,∎ even though there are no ringed sideroblasts in the bone marrow.

MACROCYTIC ANEMIAS

Anemias in which the MCV is > 100 femtoliters.

With age, the MCV increases slightly, but rarely enough to produce significant macrocytosis. Macrocytic anemia in the elderly is often megaloblastic because of vitamin B_{12} or folate deficiency. Macrocytic anemia may also be caused by hypothyroidism, chronic liver disease, or hemolytic anemia as well as by certain drugs (ie, chemotherapeutic drugs and anticonvulsants).

∎ see page 739

VITAMIN B$_{12}$ DEFICIENCY ANEMIA

Vitamin B$_{12}$ deficiency anemia accounts for up to 9% of all anemias in the elderly, and 3 to 12% of all elderly persons have low serum vitamin B$_{12}$ levels. Neurologic damage and dementia may occur before anemia or any hematologic changes are found.◻

Etiology

In the elderly, the most common cause of low serum vitamin B$_{12}$ is an inability to split vitamin B$_{12}$ from the R (rapid electrophoretic) proteins in food, to which it is bound. This inability probably results from a deficiency of hydrochloric acid or pancreatic enzymes. Low stomach acidity is present in 15% of elderly persons and is the major known cause of vitamin B$_{12}$ deficiency in this population.

Vitamin B$_{12}$ deficiency anemia may also result from a lack of intrinsic factor, which prevents vitamin B$_{12}$ absorption (**pernicious anemia**). In this autoimmune disease, antibodies are produced against parietal cells in which intrinsic factor is synthesized or against intrinsic factor itself. Pernicious anemia occurs in about 1% of persons > 60 and is often associated with other autoimmune disorders.

Other causes of vitamin B$_{12}$ deficiency anemia include gastrectomy, small-bowel disease or surgery, *Helicobacter pylori* infection, prolonged use of antacids, intestinal bacterial overgrowth, and a strict vegan diet.

Symptoms, Signs, and Diagnosis

Vitamin B$_{12}$ deficiency takes years to develop, and its symptoms are subtle. Neurologic changes may or may not occur but may predate the anemia. Various neuropsychiatric syndromes, including dementia, depression, and mania, may occur with or without anemia and often remain after the deficiency is treated. The neuropsychiatric problems may be related to the elevated homocysteine level and to microvascular disease in the brain. The anemia is usually reversible, but the neurologic changes are often irreversible.

Vitamin B$_{12}$ deficiency has four stages: negative vitamin B$_{12}$ balance, vitamin B$_{12}$ depletion, vitamin B$_{12}$–deficient erythropoiesis, and vitamin B$_{12}$ deficiency anemia. The standard laboratory test results (eg, deoxyuridine suppression test, serum methylmalonic acid levels, serum homocysteine levels) may not be abnormal until the patient becomes anemic.

Besides macrocytic anemia, laboratory abnormalities include the presence of hypersegmented polymorphonuclear leukocytes on peripheral blood smear. The platelets are large. The MCV and RBC distribution width are typically elevated. Leukopenia and thrombocytopenia

◻ see page 591

may occur. Serum levels of bilirubin, ferritin, and lactic dehydrogenase may be elevated because of ineffective erythropoiesis. When anemia is present, bone marrow examination will show megaloblastic changes. Use of the Schilling test in the elderly is rarely needed because the cause is almost always gastric hypoacidity, and the treatment is the same. If bacterial overgrowth is suspected, the full stages of the Schilling test should be performed.

Treatment

Treatment of vitamin B_{12} deficiency in pernicious anemia or hypochlorhydria consists of lifelong vitamin B_{12} administration. A common regimen is 1000 μg/day for the first week, then 1000 μg/week for 4 weeks or until the Hct is normal, and then 1000 μg/month for life. Sublingual (500 μg/day) or nasal vitamin B_{12} is also effective, but at a higher cost. If the vitamin B_{12} deficiency results from an inability to split vitamin B_{12} from food proteins, as is the case in most elderly patients, vitamin B_{12} may be given orally as 1000 μg/day on an empty stomach. Even in patients with pernicious anemia, this amount of vitamin B_{12} usually corrects the deficiency by mass action absorption even in the absence of intrinsic factor, but patients should be monitored closely for improvement.

Reticulocytosis usually begins within 1 week. Anemia is usually corrected within 1 month, although abnormalities in the peripheral blood smear may persist for 1 year. Transfusion is rarely necessary. Treatment with folic acid alone may improve the hematologic disorder; however, it will not prevent or improve the neurologic changes associated with vitamin B_{12} deficiency.

FOLATE DEFICIENCY ANEMIA

Folate deficiency produces changes in the peripheral blood smear and bone marrow that are indistinguishable from those caused by vitamin B_{12} deficiency. Folate deficiency∎ is probably uncommon in the ambulatory elderly who are well nourished, but the actual incidence is unknown, partly because of varying definitions of the lower limits of the normal range and differences in radioimmunoassay and microbiologic methods used to measure serum and RBC folate levels.

Normal body stores of folate can be depleted in 3 to 6 months. Rapid folate deficiency can be caused by malabsorption, poor nutrition, alcoholism, and states of increased folate utilization, such as hemolytic anemia and neoplasia. Drugs (eg, anticonvulsants, nitrofurantoin, triamterene, trimethoprim) also can cause folate deficiency.

∎ see also page 592

Symptoms, Signs, and Diagnosis

Pure folate deficiency may result in neurologic changes that are virtually indistinguishable from those caused by vitamin B_{12} deficiency. This may be due, in part, to elevated serum levels of homocysteine in folate, vitamin B_{12}, and vitamin B_6 deficiencies.

A diagnosis of folate deficiency anemia is confirmed by the presence of macrocytic RBCs and hypersegmented neutrophils in the peripheral blood smear, a normal serum vitamin B_{12} level (unless B_{12} deficiency coexists), and a low serum folate level (< 2 ng/mL [< 5 nmol/L]) or a low RBC folate level (< 100 ng/mL [< 227 nmol/L]). However, serum folate levels fluctuate rapidly and do not necessarily reflect body stores; RBC folate levels are more stable and, therefore, are more clinically reliable. Serum homocysteine is elevated, but methylmalonic acid levels are normal. Bone marrow is histologically indistinguishable from that seen in vitamin B_{12} deficiency, but bone marrow aspiration or biopsy is rarely needed.

Treatment

Therapy consists of folic acid 1 mg/day po. Higher doses are sometimes needed for resistant cases. A parenteral form is available for patients with severe malabsorption. In patients with megaloblastic anemia secondary to vitamin B_{12} deficiency, treatment with folic acid alone may correct the anemia but will not reverse neurologic damage.

70 ▪ HYPERCOAGULABILITY AND ANTICOAGULATION

The incidence of venous thromboembolism, including deep vein thrombosis (DVT) and pulmonary embolism, and arterial thromboembolism, which can lead to myocardial infarction (MI) and stroke, increases with age, particularly after age 55. The comparatively low incidence of thrombotic events in women up to age 60 decreases over time; by age 60, incidence rates among men and women are essentially equal.

The predisposition to intravascular thrombosis among the elderly is difficult to explain but most likely reflects a multifactorial process with variable clinical expression. The predominant risk factors for arterial thrombosis may, in fact, originate within the vasculature itself in the form of atherosclerosis. However, the venous circulatory system is also affected, suggesting that one or more systemic factors are also involved.

Pathophysiology

Virchow's triad organizes the understanding of intravascular thrombosis and provides a platform for a comprehensive approach to its differential diagnosis. The three components of Virchow's triad are (1) abnormalities in the vessel wall, (2) abnormalities within the circulating blood, and (3) stasis of blood flow. Although many prothrombotic states are characterized by more than one defect, profound isolated defects may be sufficient to provoke thrombosis.

Vessel walls: The vascular (luminal) surface that is continuously exposed to circulating blood must be nonthrombogenic to avoid hypercoagulability. Yet, it must have prothrombotic capabilities in case protective clotting is needed. Profound structural abnormalities may be sufficient to stimulate thrombosis; however, usually an abnormality of clotting also exists.

Atherosclerosis plays an important role in stimulating unwanted clotting. It is considered the most common acquired hypercoagulable state. The atherosclerotic process may be influenced directly by abnormalities in platelet activation, coagulation, and fibrinolysis, each contributing to fibrin deposition and, ultimately, plaque growth. Rupture of plaque may stimulate abnormal clotting.

Atherosclerosis has an inflammatory aspect that represents a chronic inflammatory disease of the vasculature. Inflammation, in addition to producing a thrombogenic surface, is responsible for the release of mediators (eg, cytokines, chemokines) that may contribute to thrombosis directly or indirectly.

Vasculitis may also affect vessel walls and lead to abnormal clotting. It is characterized by various stages of inflammation, involving small-, medium-, or large-caliber vessels (depending on the disorder). Inflammation with accompanying structural and functional endothelial abnormalities and shear stress—increasing as a result of changes in luminal dimension—foster platelet adherence, activation, and fibrin deposition. Although some vasculitides may be associated with circulating procoagulant factors (eg, antiphospholipid antibodies), most increase thrombotic tendency primarily by creating focal abnormalities involving the vessel wall. Locally, active vasculitis can cause arterial thrombosis, including MI. In addition, healed vasculitis of the coronary arteries can accelerate atherosclerosis, itself a procoagulant state. Overall, the vasculitides most commonly associated with arterial thrombosis are polyarteritis nodosa[1] and giant cell arteritis.[2]

Circulating blood abnormalities: Under normal circumstances, blood circulates freely, and the plasma coagulation factors exist in a nonactivated state. Upon activation, intrinsic regulatory mechanisms prevent excess clotting (ie, more than is required for hemostasis).

[1] see page 509   [2] see page 506

Abnormalities in either activation of the clotting cascade or deactivation once it has started can lead to hypercoagulability. Those abnormalities may develop as a result of abnormalities in clotting levels, intrinsic abnormalities of their protein structure, or circulating antibodies that abnormally activate the cascade.

Fibrinogen levels increase with age, with the greatest proportional increase occurring between ages 65 and 85. There is little difference between men and women. The relationship between fibrinogen level and cardiovascular risk appears to be independent of age. Whether factor VII activity and factor XII activity are independent risk factors for thrombotic events among the elderly remains open to debate. They may represent epiphenomena of disease activity (eg, atherosclerosis) rather than true prothrombotic risk factors.

Stasis of blood flow: Venous stasis occurs during prolonged periods of immobilization, such as following trauma, major surgery, or serious medical illnesses. Comparatively long periods of recovery and convalescence are common among the elderly, increasing their risk of stasis and venous thromboembolism.

HYPERCOAGULABLE STATES

The hypercoagulable (thrombophilic) states, which involve excess clotting factors and/or defective intrinsic regulatory (thromboresistance) mechanisms, can be inherited or acquired (see TABLE 70–1). Although inherited thrombophilias can manifest for the first time at an advanced age, most elderly people who experience a thrombotic event should be evaluated for an acquired thrombophilia.

TABLE 70–1.   HYPERCOAGULABLE STATES

Acquired	Inherited (Congenital)
Anticardiolipin syndrome	Activated protein C resistance
Antiphospholipid antibodies	Antithrombin deficiency
Cancer and chemotherapy	Dysfibrinogenemia
Disseminated intravascular coagulation	Heparin cofactor II deficiency
Elevated factor VIII, VII, I (fibrinogen), and von Willebrand factor	Hyperhomocysteinemia
	Plasminogen activator inhibitor 1 excess
Heparin-induced thrombocytopenia	Plasminogen deficiency
Hormone replacement therapy use	Protein C deficiency
Lupus anticoagulant	Protein S deficiency
	Prothrombin G20210A defect
	Thrombomodulin defect
	Tissue plasminogen activator deficiency

INHERITED THROMBOPHILIAS

With most inherited thrombophilias, venous thromboembolism is more common than arterial thromboembolism. However, MI and stroke have been reported (in some cases the result of paradoxical embolism or cerebral sinus thrombosis).

ACTIVATED PROTEIN C RESISTANCE

Nearly 30% of patients with spontaneous venous thrombosis have a defect in factor V that renders it resistant to activated protein C neutralization. The specific gene mutation, referred to as factor V Leiden defect, is present in nearly 5% of the general population, making activated protein C resistance by far the most common inherited thrombophilia. Activated protein C resistance increases the risk of venous thromboembolism approximately fivefold, with 30 to 40% of persons with this disorder experiencing a thrombotic event by age 60. Therefore, a relatively large proportion of affected persons either remain event-free or experience their first event later in life. Nearly 30% of men with their first venous thromboembolism after age 60 have the factor V Leiden mutation. The risk of recurrent idiopathic venous thromboembolism among these persons is increased fourfold to fivefold.

Activated protein C resistance is an important defect to be aware of when hormone therapy is being considered. Among women who experience venous thromboembolism during oral contraceptive use, 60% have the defect. The risk for women receiving postmenopausal estrogen replacement therapy has not been established. An association between protein C resistance and MI has been described in women who smoke.

HYPERHOMOCYSTEINEMIA

Several inherited defects in methionine metabolism can lead to either mild, moderate, or marked increases in plasma homocysteine levels. Acquired hyperhomocysteinemia is observed in persons with vitamin B_6 (pyridoxine), B_{12} (cobalamin), and folate deficiency as well as in those with chronic renal failure and drug-induced abnormalities in folic acid (methotrexate, anticonvulsants), cobalamin (nitrous oxide), or pyridoxine (theophylline) metabolism.

Several epidemiologic studies have identified a relationship between hyperhomocysteinemia and venous thromboembolism. An association with arterial thrombosis (MI, stroke) has also been reported.∎ If confirmed, hyperhomocysteinemia may represent one of the most common hypercoagulable states, given its worldwide prevalence and ability to manifest in both inherited and acquired forms.

∎ see also page 852

OTHER INHERITED THROMBOPHILIAS

Antithrombin deficiency, previously referred to as antithrombin III deficiency, may affect the elderly. Antithrombin is a glycoprotein that binds and inactivates thrombin and other coagulation proteins. The inhibitory effect of antithrombin is markedly accelerated by heparin administered exogenously (for therapeutic reasons) and by endogenous heparin sulfate found on the vascular endothelial surface.

Protein C deficiency (prevalence, about 1/100) occurs either because the quantity (type I protein C deficiency) of the protein is low or its quality (type II protein C deficiency) is abnormal. Up to 50% of persons with this disorder experience venous thromboembolism by age 50, and 75% experience it by age 60. Variable expression of disease and concomitant risk factors are responsible for first thromboembolism in later years.

Protein S deficiency usually produces a first venous thromboembolism by age 40. Protein S is a vitamin K–dependent glycoprotein synthesized in the liver that serves a pivotal supporting role for protein C activity.

There are no detailed data on the elderly. The prevalence of disease for inherited abnormalities would not change over time unless the events are fatal. Most people with deficiency of antithrombin, protein C, or protein S experience their first venous thromboembolism by age 40. However, in some cases, patients have not sought medical attention or been tested thoroughly for an inherited thrombophilia.

ACQUIRED THROMBOPHILIAS

ANTIPHOSPHOLIPID ANTIBODY SYNDROME

Antiphospholipid antibodies are a heterogeneous group of circulating polyclonal (IgG, IgM, IgA) or mixed immunoglobulins directed against negatively charged or neutral phospholipids. Within this group, the lupus anticoagulant and anticardiolipin antibodies are the most commonly acquired. They predispose to both arterial and venous thrombosis. Antiphospholipid antibodies occur in a variety of autoimmune disorders, malignancies, lymphoproliferative disorders, and systemic viral infections; however, most persons experiencing thromboembolism have no identifiable clinical condition. These persons are considered to have primary antiphospholipid antibody syndrome.

MALIGNANCY

A strong association exists between malignancy and venous thromboembolism. The overall incidence of venous thromboembolism among cancer patients ranges from 1 to 15% in clinical series and up to 30% in autopsy-based reports. Malignancies with the highest rates of thromboembolism include mucin-producing adenocarcinomas of the gastrointestinal tract followed by tumors of the lung, breast, and ovary. Myeloproliferative disorders and leukemias are also associated with an increased incidence of thromboembolism. In elderly patients, it is not uncommon for DVT or pulmonary embolism to be the initial manifestation of malignancy. Therefore, careful screening should be carried out in all patients > 60 who experience idiopathic (spontaneous) venous thromboembolism.

DISSEMINATED INTRAVASCULAR COAGULATION

Abnormal generation of fibrin in the circulating blood.

Disseminated intravascular coagulation (DIC) can accompany a wide variety of conditions, including sepsis, metabolic acidosis, acute and chronic leukemias, malignancy, and hemolytic transfusion reactions. The initial event is often mediated by tissue factor that is released by vascular endothelial cells, monocytes, or amnionic cells. The trigger itself varies from endotoxins to amnionic fluid and procoagulant factors released by tumor cells.

DIC begins with a stimulus for intravascular thrombosis followed by a consumption of coagulation factors and stimulation of fibrinolysis. The clinical expression of DIC is a combination of thrombosis, characteristically affecting the microcirculation, and hemorrhage. Acute DIC is a fulminant process that causes both tissue necrosis and life-threatening hemorrhage. When chronic DIC accompanies malignant conditions, thrombosis often predominates.

Diagnosis

The prothrombin time (PT), activated partial thromboplastin time (aPTT), and thrombin time are typically prolonged, and the fibrinogen level and platelet count are decreased. Schistocytes (evidence of intravascular hemolysis) are present in about 50% of patients, a finding shared by other conditions that cause microangiopathic hemolytic anemia. Fibrinogen (fibrin) degradation products (FDP) are elevated in 85 to 100% of patients with DIC; however, they too are nonspecific even when quantitated using a latex agglutination assay. Nonetheless, because enhanced fibrinolysis is a feature of DIC, many clinicians still use the FDP as an initial screening test.

In contrast to FDP, D-dimers are specific for factor X activation and fibrin formation. Although D-dimers may also be elevated in patients with DVT and pulmonary embolism (without DIC), the assay is considered the most reliable method for diagnosing DIC. Results are elevated in nearly 95% of cases.

Antithrombin levels and quantitative thrombin-antithrombin complexes represent important means for diagnosing and monitoring DIC. Antithrombin is consumed in DIC as antithrombin-thrombin complexes are generated. Determination of fibrinogen levels does not add additional diagnostic information, but levels should be measured in patients with uncontrolled hemorrhage, because patients with low fibrinogen levels and DIC accompanied by life-threatening hemorrhage may benefit from cryoprecipitate transfusion.

Once the diagnosis of DIC is confirmed by finding high D-dimer and FDP titers (in combination with low antithrombin levels), subsequent monitoring (and assessment of DIC status) can be carried out as needed with serial D-dimer assays.

Treatment

The keys to managing DIC center on the diagnosis and treatment of the underlying disorder. The specific treatment of DIC is limited but can be broken down into three categories: (1) restoration of hemostasis, (2) prevention of thrombosis, and (3) removal of thrombus. Transfusion of packed RBCs and fresh frozen plasma may be required to restore intravascular volume and to replace consumed coagulation factors. Cryoprecipitate and platelet transfusions can be used in patients with severe bleeding, although there is a theoretical risk that this will worsen clotting. Low-dose heparin (300 to 400 U/hour) can prevent microthrombosis in patients in whom the risk of bleeding is relatively minor compared with the probability of thrombosis. Low-dose heparin is most useful in patients with septic shock and DIC. It also should be considered when a thrombotic event (eg, pulmonary embolism) is the precipitating cause of DIC. In this case, standard heparin doses may be used if bleeding is not evident. When bleeding occurs, thrombectomy (surgical, extraction catheter) and filter placement should be considered.

PROPHYLAXIS OF VENOUS AND ARTERIAL THROMBOEMBOLISM

Venous thromboembolism remains a major cause of death and disability among hospitalized patients. Recent estimates suggest that > 250,000 cases are diagnosed yearly in acute care hospitals, with as many, if not more, cases going unrecognized. Some believe that the incidence of venous thromboembolism may be higher, perhaps twice as high, in rehabilitation centers and nursing homes.

DVT and pulmonary embolism are particularly common in elderly patients; the incidence of both of these conditions increases with age, with no particular predilection for sex or race. Additional risk factors for surgical and medical patients are listed in TABLE 70–2.

The rationale for venous thromboembolism prophylaxis is based on the clinically silent nature of the disease. In fact, most events cause few specific symptoms, and the clinical diagnosis is notoriously unreliable. Beyond the immediate complications of pulmonary embolism, which can lead to death within 30 minutes, unrecognized and untreated DVT

TABLE 70-2.   RISK FACTORS FOR VENOUS THROMBOEMBOLISM

Acute myocardial infarction
Age > 40 years
Heart failure
Hypercoagulable state
Immobilization > 3 days
Malignancy
Paralytic stroke
Previous venous thromboembolism
Trauma

can cause long-term morbidity from chronic venous stasis (post-phlebitic syndrome) and predispose patients to recurrent venous thromboembolism (see TABLE 70–3).

The postphlebitic syndrome is characterized by varying degrees of chronic venous stasis and its accompanying manifestations of peripheral edema, stasis dermatitis, and, in the most severe cases, venous ulcers that are difficult to treat. Patients at risk for the postphlebitic syndrome include those with extensive proximal and recurrent DVT, in whom damage and, ultimately, incompetence of the venous valves ensue. The key to prevention is early treatment. Long-term therapy includes fitted support stockings, avoidance of stasis (eg, sedentary life style), leg elevation during periods of inactivity to minimize peripheral edema, and meticulous skin care.

The risk of venous thromboembolism is greatest in the early postoperative or postevent period but varies according to the overall risk profile. After orthopedic procedures, prophylaxis should be continued for 10 to 14 days (or longer if the patient has experienced postoperative complications that delay rehabilitative efforts and ambulation). For patients undergoing general surgery, 5 to 7 days of prophylaxis is probably adequate, with the exception of patients with underlying malignancy (or prior venous thromboembolism in whom a longer period of prevention may be beneficial).

The approach in patients with medical conditions must be individualized. In general, prophylaxis should be continued until full ambulation is resumed. As with venous thromboembolism, strategies for prophylaxis have been developed to prevent arterial thromboembolism in patients at risk. Specific conditions warranting prophylaxis are outlined below.

Orthopedic procedures: The risk of DVT after an orthopedic procedure has been performed is high, particularly when surgery is performed semi-electively or urgently after traumatic fracture.

For **total hip replacement,** the incidence of proximal DVT (in the absence of prophylaxis) approaches 25%, with an alarming 3 to 4%

TABLE 70-3.   RISK STRATIFICATION AND PREVENTIVE STRATEGIES
FOR VENOUS THROMBOEMBOLISM

Risk	Patient Profile	Incidence of Events	Prophylactic Regimens
Low	Uncomplicated surgery Patient ≤ 40 years No other risk factors	Proximal DVT 0.4% PE 0.2% Fatal PE 0.002%	No specific prophylaxis Early ambulation
Moderate	Major surgery Patient > 40 years No other risk factors	Proximal DVT 2–4% PE 1–2% Fatal PE 0.1–0.4%	Heparin 5000 U sc bid *or* IPC boots *or* Elastic stockings
High	Major surgery Patient > 40 years One or more of the following: myocardial infarction, heart failure, neurosurgery, immobilization > 3 days	Proximal DVT 4–8% PE 2–4% Fatal PE 0.4–1.0%	Heparin 5000 U sc tid *or* LMWH *or* IPC boots
Very high	Major surgery Patient > 40 years One or more of the following: malignancy, previous venous thromboembolism, orthopedic surgery, hip fracture, stroke, spinal cord injury	Proximal DVT 10–20% PE 4–10% Fatal PE 3–5%	LMWH *or* Warfarin *or* Adjusted-dose heparin *plus* IPC boots

DVT = deep vein thrombosis; IPC = intermittent pneumatic compression; LMWH = low-molecular-weight heparin; PE = pulmonary embolism.

incidence of fatal pulmonary embolism. Prophylaxis reduces the occurrence of venous thromboembolism by 30 to 50%. The most effective regimens include low-molecular-weight heparin (eg, enoxaparin 30 mg sc q 12 h or 40 mg sc q 24 h), oral anticoagulants (warfarin to target the international normalized ratio [INR] between 2.0 and 2.5), and adjusted-dose IV heparin (titrated to aPTT in the upper range of normal).

For **traumatic hip fracture,** the approach to DVT prophylaxis remains a substantial challenge because of the concomitant risk of bleeding in these typically elderly patients. The incidence of venous thromboembolism (in the absence of prophylaxis) is about 50%. Either warfarin or low-molecular-weight heparin is the anticoagulant of choice and should be instituted preoperatively whenever possible. Although intermittent pneumatic compression boots are used frequently in clinical practice, there are limited data on their effectiveness. **Total knee replacement** is associated with an incidence of DVT approaching 60%. Low-dose subcutaneous heparin and oral warfarin provide marginal benefit. The greatest benefit has been achieved with low-molecular-weight heparin and intermittent pneumatic compression boots; however, the incidence of proximal DVT remains 5 to 10% even with this prophylaxis.

Atrial fibrillation: The formation of thrombi within the atria and atrial appendices (the left far more often than the right) is a well-recognized phenomenon among all patients with atrial fibrillation. Anticoagulation reduces thromboembolism and the most feared and devastating manifestation—stroke. Anticoagulation is recommended for at least 3 weeks before and 4 weeks after successful cardioversion. Transesophageal echocardiography may have a role in identifying patients at low and high risk for thromboembolism.

Atrial flutter: Patients with atrial flutter/fibrillation and atrial flutter with concomitant valvular diseases or a reduced left ventricular function probably warrant treatment with warfarin or, at the very least, further evaluation in the form of transesophageal echocardiography. In the absence of valvular heart disease or compromised left ventricular performance, atrial flutter most likely represents a very low risk condition. Guidelines for managing anticoagulation for patients with atrial flutter have not yet been established; however, some clinicians choose to treat patients with warfarin as they would those with atrial fibrillation.

Acute myocardial infarction: The overall incidence of venous thromboembolism is about 20%; elderly patients and those with infarctions complicated by heart failure, recurrent angina, or ventricular arrhythmias are at greatest risk. Prophylaxis is recommended in the form of low-dose heparin, low-molecular-weight heparin, or intermittent pneumatic compression boots. Comparative trials of low-dose heparin and low-molecular-weight heparin in high-risk medical patients are in progress.

Patients with large infarctions (ejection fraction < 35%), particularly those involving the anterior and apical walls of the myocardium, are at risk for mural thromboses and cardioembolic events. Serial echocardiograms may be a useful diagnostic strategy. Prophylactic therapy includes unfractionated heparin or low-molecular-weight heparin. Warfarin (target INR 2.0 to 3.0) is an effective outpatient therapy and is typically continued for 2 to 3 months after an MI. Patients experiencing a cardioembolic event should receive warfarin therapy for ≥ 1 year if their ventricular performance remains poor.

Ischemic stroke: In patients with stroke and a paralyzed lower extremity, the incidence of DVT is about 30 to 40%. Both low-dose heparin and low-molecular-weight heparin reduce the occurrence of

DVT by at least 50%. Intermittent pneumatic compression boots are likely to be beneficial.

SPECIFIC ANTICOAGULANTS

There are many different anticoagulants available, many of which have distinct uses, especially as prophylaxis for venous thromboembolism (see TABLE 70–3). In general, drugs given intravenously, such as heparin or the fibrinolytic agents, are used short-term for hospitalized patients, and oral drugs, such as warfarin and antiplatelet drugs, are used long-term for outpatients. Low-molecular-weight heparins, administered subcutaneously, can be used in almost any setting.

UNFRACTIONATED HEPARIN

Heparin, the most widely used anticoagulant, accelerates the inhibitory interaction between antithrombin and several hemostatic proteins, most notably thrombin and factor X. After IV administration, about one third of circulating heparin molecules bind to antithrombin; the remaining two thirds have minimal anticoagulant activity. Heparin is cleared from the circulation through a combination of a rapid saturable mechanism (binding) and a much slower first-order mechanism (renal).

Unfractionated heparin is indicated in elderly patients at risk of venous or arterial thromboembolism. The prevention of venous thromboembolism is achieved with doses of 5000 U given sc 2 or 3 times/day. Treatment of DVT or pulmonary embolism requires a larger dose, typically initiated as a bolus (60 U/kg) followed by a continuous IV infusion (15 U/kg/hour) to a target aPTT of 1.5 to 2.5 times control. Dose requirements are influenced by body weight and acute-phase responses. The latter is particularly important in clinical practice because acute vascular thrombosis is associated with both inflammation and platelet activation, neutralizing heparin in the circulation (through direct binding) and increasing initial dose requirements. Age and renal function also affect heparin dosing, but minimally.

After its IV administration, heparin binds to vascular endothelial cells, macrophages, and plasma proteins. Because of these complex kinetics, the anticoagulant effect of heparin at therapeutic doses is not linear, although usually both intensity and duration increase as the dose increases. Therefore, the biologic half-life of heparin increases from 30 minutes after an IV dose of 25 U/kg, to 60 minutes after a dose of 100 U/kg, to 150 minutes with a dose of 400 U/kg.

The anticoagulant effects of heparin are usually monitored with the aPTT, a test sensitive to the inhibitory effects of heparin on thrombin and factor X. A therapeutic state of systemic anticoagulation (1.5 to 2.5 times control) is a prerequisite when heparin is used in the treatment of venous and arterial thromboembolic disorders. Because the pharmaco-kinetics and pharmacodynamics of heparin are complex, frequent monitoring during the course of treatment is required.

The most common adverse effect of heparin is hemorrhage. Other complications include thrombocytopenia (with or without thrombosis), skin necrosis, alopecia, hypersensitivity reactions, and hypoaldosteronism. The risk of bleeding increases with heparin dose (and anticoagulant effect), age, decreasing body weight, trauma, recent surgery, invasive procedures, and the concomitant use of aspirin.

Mild to moderate bleeding should initially be addressed by reducing the heparin dose (particularly if the aPTT is excessively prolonged) or by discontinuing the infusion for 30 minutes. More severe bleeding often requires discontinuation of heparin or, with life-threatening hemorrhage, neutralization with protamine sulfate (1 mg for each 100 U of heparin administered in the preceding 4 hours). However, it may be in the patient's best interest to continue systemic anticoagulation, particularly if the bleeding is not life-threatening and can be adequately controlled with local measures (eg, manual pressure over a site of vascular trauma).

LOW-MOLECULAR-WEIGHT HEPARIN

Low-molecular-weight heparins (LMWHs) are used for DVT prophylaxis and in the treatment of DVT and acute coronary syndromes (unstable angina, MI without ST-segment elevation).

LMWH can be given IV or subcutaneously. Dosing strategies (eg, prophylactic dose: enoxaparin 30 mg sc bid or 40 mg sc daily; treatment of DVT or acute coronary syndromes: enoxaparin 1 mg/kg sc bid) have been established that, because of predictable bioavailability and pharmacokinetics, yield a safe and effective plasma concentration (peak anti-Xa level of about 1.5 U/mL and steady state level of about 0.5 U/mL). Because of their short chain length and unique anticoagulant properties (factor Xa inhibition), LMWHs do not prolong the aPTT and are not fully neutralized (about 60%) by protamine sulfate.

The bleeding risk associated with LMWH administration is similar to or slightly lower than the risk observed with unfractionated heparin and is related to dose and molecular weight (higher molecular weight fractions cause a greater risk of bleeding).

WARFARIN

Like heparin, warfarin is a frequently used anticoagulant in clinical practice. Warfarin is indicated for elderly patients at risk of thromboembolism (venous or arterial) as well as for those with established thromboembolism.

Warfarin is rapidly absorbed from the gastrointestinal tract after oral administration, reaches maximal plasma concentration in 90 minutes,

TABLE 70-4.   DISORDERS AND SUBSTANCES THAT INFLUENCE THE ACTION OF WARFARIN

Decreased effect of warfarin	Increases response (direct pharmacodynamic effect)
Impairs absorption of warfarin	2nd- and 3rd-generation cephalosporins
Cholestyramine	Clofibrate
Increases metabolic clearance of warfarin	Heparin
Barbiturates	Potentiates effect of warfarin
Carbamazepine	Hyperthyroidism
Ethanol	Liver disease
Hypothyroidism	Low vitamin K intake
Rifampin	Malnutrition (decreased serum albumin)
Increases vitamin K intake	Reduced vitamin K absorption
Leafy green vegetables	Unknown mechanisms
Nutritional supplements	Anabolic steroids
Increased effect of warfarin	Fluconazole
Inhibits metabolic clearance of warfarin	Isoniazid
Amiodarone	Ketoconazole
Cimetidine	Phenytoin
Disulfiram	Propafenone
Metronidazole	Quinidine
Sulfa derivatives	Tamoxifen

and has a circulating half-life of 36 to 42 hours. It circulates bound to plasma proteins, particularly albumin. The dose-response profile of warfarin differs among individuals and is influenced by pharmacokinetic and pharmacodynamic factors. Conditions that affect the availability of vitamin K also influence warfarin response (see TABLE 70-4).

The hepatic clearance (metabolism) of warfarin declines with age. Thus, it is considered safe to initiate warfarin therapy at lower doses ($\leq$ 5 mg/day) in the elderly. Some studies have suggested that the elderly are more prone to hemorrhagic complications with warfarin use. Nonetheless, most elderly patients in need of prolonged anticoagulation can be treated safely and effectively with warfarin if treatment includes education, meticulous attention to comorbid illnesses and concomitant drugs, and dose monitoring through a coordinated anticoagulant program.

Bleeding is the most common complication of long-term warfarin therapy. Other complications include skin necrosis and thrombosis in protein C–deficient patients. The risk of bleeding is directly influenced by the intensity of anticoagulant therapy, age, renal insufficiency, and occult disease of the gastrointestinal and genitourinary tracts.

The anticoagulation effect of warfarin can be reduced or entirely reversed by lowering the dose, discontinuing treatment, administering vitamin K, or replacing the defective coagulation factors with fresh frozen plasma. The amount of green leafy vegetables in the diet substantially alters warfarin response.

The prothrombin time (PT) is the method most commonly used for monitoring warfarin therapy. The PT increases in response to depression of three of the four vitamin K–dependent coagulation proteins—factors II, VII, and X. In the initial stages of warfarin administration, prolongation of the PT primarily reflects factor VII depression (shortest half-life). The desired level for the PT (and its corresponding INR) varies according to the disease being treated. For example, an INR of 1.5 to 2.0 may be adequate for DVT, but an INR of 3.0 may be required to treat thromboembolism associated with the cardiolipin syndromes.

The prevention of venous thromboembolism following orthopedic surgical procedures is achieved with a target INR of 2.0 to 2.5, while treatment requires an INR of 2.0 to 3.0. The prevention of arterial thromboembolism in patients with atrial flutter, atrial fibrillation, and mural thrombosis is effectively achieved with an INR of 2.0 to 3.0. The target INR for patients with mechanical heart valves is 2.5 to 3.5.

DIRECT THROMBIN ANTICOAGULANTS

Direct thrombin anticoagulants, including hirudin, bivalirudin, and argatroban, have yielded mixed results in clinical trials; hemorrhagic events are a major concern. Although use in arterial thrombotic disorders may be limited, hirudin (lepirudin-recombinant hirudin) has shown promise in the management of heparin-induced thrombocytopenia and for DVT prophylaxis. Investigation of factor Xa antagonists (oral, intravenous), tissue factor pathway inhibitor, and other unique anticoagulant compounds is ongoing.

FIBRINOLYTIC AGENTS

The available fibrinolytic agents, including tissue plasminogen activator (t-PA), streptokinase (SK), anisoylated plasminogen-streptokinase activator complex (APSAC), urokinase, and 3rd-generation agents recombinant plasminogen activator (r-PA), novel plasminogen activator (n-PA), and TNK-tPA convert the inactive proenzyme plasminogen to the active enzyme plasmin, which then is responsible for dissolution of fibrin.

Evidence suggests that elderly patients with acute MI derive significant benefit from fibrinolytic-based reperfusion; however, their risk of serious hemorrhage, including intracranial bleeding, is increased. Fibrinolytic agents have also been used in the treatment of elderly patients with ischemic stroke. The most encouraging results have been achieved with t-PA when administered within 3 hours of symptom onset. Before fibrinolytic agents are administered for ischemic stroke, careful screen-

TABLE 70-5. RISK FACTORS FOR SEVERE HEMORRHAGE FOLLOWING FIBRINOLYTIC THERAPY

Active bleeding (current or within previous 2 months)
Age > 70 years
Bleeding diathesis (congenital or acquired)
History of stroke, intracranial neoplasm, arteriovenous malformation, or aneurysm
Hypertension (> 180/110 mm Hg), acute or poorly controlled
Recent major surgery (within previous 4 weeks)
Recent puncture or noncompressible vessel or organ biopsy (within previous 7 days)
Significant trauma (within previous 2 months)

ing, including a scan of the brain, must be undertaken to exclude hemorrhagic stroke.

Fibrinolytic agents may also be considered for patients with massive pulmonary embolism. As with other indications, careful screening must be undertaken to exclude those at risk for hemorrhagic complications.

Severe bleeding occurs in about 5% of patients treated with fibrinolytic agents (see TABLE 70-5). However, most patients also receive adjuvant treatment with antiplatelet agents (aspirin) and anticoagulants (heparin). This practice probably increases the risk of bleeding, particularly if careful coagulation monitoring is not carried out in the first 24 to 48 hours.

To counter the effects of fibrinolytic agents when bleeding occurs, fresh frozen plasma provides factors V and VIII, α2-antiplasmin, and plasminogen activator inhibitor. Cryoprecipitate (1 U/10 kg) is the preferred source of fibrinogen (200 to 250 mg/10 to 15 mL) and factor VIII (80 U/10 to 15 mL). If the platelet count is low (< 80,000/μL), platelets (6 to 10 U random donor) should be given. Desmopressin (0.3 mg/kg IV over 20 minutes) can be used to correct *qualitative* platelet abnormalities. Persistent and potentially life-threatening hemorrhage unresponsive to standard measures (as outlined above) may require antifibrinolytic therapy with aminocaproic acid or tranexamic acid. This intervention should be used with caution because it may precipitate serious thrombotic complications.

PLATELET ANTAGONISTS

Platelets participate in the thrombotic process by adhering to an abnormal surface, aggregating to form an initial platelet plug, stimulating further aggregation, and triggering the coagulation cascade.

Aspirin irreversibly acetylates cyclooxygenase, impairing prostaglandin metabolism and thromboxane A_2 synthesis, thereby inhibiting platelet aggregation in response to collagen, adenosine diphosphate, and thrombin. Adherence and platelet release, however, are not affected. Aspirin's inhibitory effect persists for the life span of the platelet (7 ± 2 days), because platelets lack the synthetic capacity to regenerate cyclooxygenase. The antithrombotic effect of aspirin can be achieved with doses ranging from 160 to 325 mg/day (and possibly lower); maintenance of 80 to 160 mg/day is probably adequate in most clinical settings. Although nonsteroidal anti-inflammatory drugs also inhibit cyclooxygenase, they do so in a reversible manner. These compounds have not been adequately tested in large randomized clinical trials for this purpose.

Aspirin is indicated for primary and secondary prevention of MI and stroke and is also used in combination with clopidogrel or ticlopidine after intracoronary stent procedures. The addition of low-dose aspirin to warfarin may be beneficial for patients with mechanical heart valves; such is particularly indicated in patients who have experienced thrombotic events while taking appropriately adjusted warfarin doses.

Platelet glycoprotein IIb/IIIa antagonists—abciximab, tirofiban, and eptifibatide—are indicated for patients with acute coronary syndromes and those undergoing high-risk percutaneous coronary interventions. They completely block in vitro platelet aggregation induced by agonists thought to function in vivo.

Ticlopidine is structurally distinct from all other antiplatelet agents. It is a potent inhibitor of platelet aggregation induced by adenosine diphosphate and variably inhibits aggregation provoked by collagen, epinephrine, arachidonic acid, thrombin, and platelet-activating factor. Ticlopidine also inhibits the platelet release action and may impair platelet adhesion as well.

Ticlopidine has been used in the treatment of transient ischemic attacks, strokes (particularly those occurring while aspirin is already being taken), and unstable angina and after placement of an intracoronary stent (probably the most common indication). Neutropenia and thrombotic thrombocytopenic purpura are infrequent but potentially life-threatening complications.

Clopidogrel reduces the risk of MI (and recurrent MI) among patients with atherosclerotic vascular disease. Its adverse effect profile, based on experience to date, is superior to that of ticlopidine, and its relatively long half-life permits once-daily dosing.

71 ■ CHRONIC MYELOID DISORDERS

The chronic myeloid disorders, which become more prevalent with age, can be categorized as either *bcr/abl*-positive (ie, positive for the Philadelphia chromosome, which is characteristic of chronic myelocytic leukemia)◧ or *bcr/abl*-negative. The *bcr/abl*-negative chronic myeloid disorders can be subdivided into the chronic myeloproliferative disorders (see TABLE 71–1 and FIGURE 71–1) and the myelodysplastic syndromes. The classic myelodysplastic syndromes◨ include refractory anemia and chronic myelomonocytic leukemia.

However, not all myeloid processes can be categorized as myelodysplastic syndromes or chronic myeloproliferative disorders, and certain variants may show features of both (see FIGURE 71–1). In the chronic myeloproliferative disorders, patients present with erythrocytosis, thrombocytosis, or leukocytosis (or some combination). In contrast, in myelodysplastic syndromes, patients present with significant dyshematopoiesis and intramedullary apoptosis, resulting in ineffective hematopoiesis and peripheral pancytopenia (see TABLE 71–1).

CHRONIC MYELOPROLIFERATIVE DISORDERS

A group of disorders characterized by abnormal proliferation of one or more hematopoietic cell lines or connective tissue elements.

The classic chronic myeloproliferative disorders are primary thrombocythemia, polycythemia vera, and myelofibrosis; the atypical ones are atypical chronic myelocytic leukemia (which is *bcr/abl*-negative), chronic neutrophilic leukemia, hypereosinophilic syndrome (chronic eosinophilic leukemia), and mast cell disease.

PRIMARY THROMBOCYTHEMIA

(Essential Thrombocythemia; Essential Thrombocytosis; Thrombocythemia Vera)

A disease characterized by an increased platelet count, megakaryocytic hyperplasia, and a tendency toward hemorrhage or thrombosis.

Primary thrombocythemia is the most common of the chronic myeloproliferative disorders, with an approximate incidence of 2.5/100,000 per year. The median age at presentation is 60 years (female:male ratio = 1.6:1); only 20% of patients present before age 40. Primary thrombocythemia is usually discovered incidentally during routine blood testing.

◧ see page 728   ◨ see page 739

TABLE 71–1. COMPARISON OF LABORATORY AND CLINICAL FEATURES OF MYELODYSPLASTIC SYNDROME AND THE CHRONIC MYELOPROLIFERATIVE DISORDERS

Examination	Myelodysplastic Syndrome	Chronic Myeloproliferative Disorders
History	Exposure to chemotherapy	History of thrombosis
Clinical presentation	Vasculitic-like syndrome in about 15% of cases Symptoms of cytopenia (anemia symptoms, hemorrhage, infections)	Vasomotor symptoms (PV, primary thrombocythemia) Thrombosis, hemorrhage (PV, primary thrombocythemia) Pruritus (PV) Hypercatabolic symptoms (myelofibrosis) Extramedullary hematopoiesis resulting in spinal cord compression, ascites, etc.
Physical examination	Pallor, cutaneous signs of infection	Splenomegaly (myelofibrosis > PV > primary thrombocythemia)
Peripheral blood smear	Anemia with or without other cytopenias Dimorphic red blood cells Pelger-Huët anomaly	Erythrocytosis Thrombocytosis (always in primary thrombocythemia; sometimes in PV or myelofibrosis) Leukocytosis (may occur in PV, primary thrombocythemia, or myelofibrosis)
Bone marrow	Mostly hypercellular but can be hypocellular Trilineage dysplasia Fibrosis (occasional)	Hypercellular Atypical megakaryocytes Fibrosis (myelofibrosis)
Cytogenetics	−7, 5q−, +8, −5, del(20)	del(13) (myelofibrosis, PV) del(20) (PV, myelofibrosis) del(5), del(20), del(12), +8, +9, +21, −7

PV = polycythemia vera.
From Tefferi A: "The Philadelphia chromosome negative chronic myeloproliferative disorders: A practical overview." *Mayo Clinic Proceedings* 73:1177–1184, 1998. By permission of Mayo Foundation for Medical Education and Research.

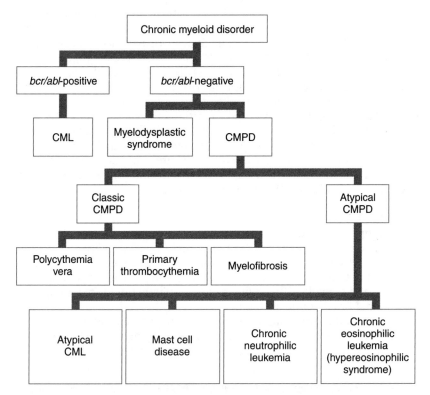

FIGURE 71–1. **Classification of chronic myeloid disorders.** *bcr/abl* is a fusion gene resulting from a chromosomal translocation between chromosomes 9 and 22 (the Philadelphia chromosome). CML = chronic myelocytic leukemia; CMPD = chronic myeloproliferative disease. (From Tefferi A: "The Philadelphia chromosome negative chronic myeloproliferative disorders: A practical overview." *Mayo Clinic Proceedings* 73:1177–1184, 1998. By permission of Mayo Foundation for Medical Education and Research.)

The pathogenetic basis of vasomotor symptoms is believed to be platelet-mediated endothelial injury of small vessels. However, the risk of thrombosis and hemorrhage has not been correlated with quantitative or qualitative platelet abnormalities.

Symptoms, Signs, and Complications

Most patients are asymptomatic. Vasomotor symptoms occur in one third of patients and include headache, erythromelalgia (burning pain and erythema of the hands or feet), paresthesias, and visual disturbances.

Major hemorrhagic complications are infrequent (5%) and usually result from the use of nonsteroidal anti-inflammatory drugs (NSAIDs). Thrombotic complications occur in 15% of patients at presentation and in 11% during follow-up. They can be life threatening, although they occur less frequently and are less likely to be fatal than in polycythemia vera. They can be arterial or venous and include ischemic stroke, transient ischemic attacks, myocardial infarction, deep vein thrombosis, digital ischemia, and superficial thrombophlebitis. Characteristic thrombotic syndromes include Budd-Chiari syndrome, portal vein thrombosis, superior sagittal vein thrombosis, and skin necrosis. Acquired von Willebrand's disease is a rare complication associated with extreme thrombocytosis and is related to abnormal platelet adsorption of circulating von Willebrand's multimers.

Diagnosis

The first step in diagnosis is to rule out secondary (reactive) thrombocythemia (see TABLE 71–2). Shorter duration of thrombocytosis, low levels of serum ferritin (which is diagnostic of iron depletion), and an increase in C-reactive protein suggest secondary thrombocythemia. The presence of Howell-Jolly bodies in the peripheral blood smear indicates functional or anatomic asplenia.

If the initial evaluation does not suggest secondary thrombocythemia, a bone marrow examination with cytogenetic studies and a reticulin stain is recommended. Bone marrow examination in primary

TABLE 71–2.   CAUSES OF SECONDARY (REACTIVE) THROMBOCYTHEMIA

Acute conditions
  Immediate postsurgical period
  Acute hemorrhage
  Acute hemolysis
  Infections
  Tissue damage (eg, acute pancreatitis, myocardial infarction, trauma,
    burns)
  Coronary artery bypass graft
  Rebound effect from chemotherapy or immune thrombocytopenia

Chronic conditions
  Iron deficiency anemia
  Surgical or functional asplenia
  Metastatic cancer, lymphoma
  Inflammation (rheumatoid arthritis, vasculitis, allergies)
  Renal failure, nephrotic syndrome

From Tefferi A: "The Philadelphia chromosome negative chronic myeloproliferative disorders: A practical overview." *Mayo Clinic Proceedings* 73:1177–1184, 1998. By permission of Mayo Foundation for Medical Education and Research.

thrombocythemia shows megakaryocyte clusters in most cases, mild reticulin fibrosis in about 15% of cases, and cytogenetic abnormalities in < 5% of cases.

The following disorders associated with thrombocytosis can be distinguished from primary thrombocythemia by their diagnostic features:

* Chronic myelocytic leukemia is diagnosed through karyotypic analysis revealing the Philadelphia chromosome [t(9;22)]. Cases undetectable by karyotypic analysis may be diagnosed by a fluorescence in situ hybridization study of peripheral blood.

* Polycythemia vera is diagnosed by demonstrating an increase in red blood cell (RBC) mass, although this finding does not always indicate polycythemia vera.

* Myelodysplastic syndrome is diagnosed by demonstrating dyserythropoiesis and other bone marrow morphologic and cytogenetic features.

Prognosis

Elderly persons with primary thrombocythemia are at significantly increased risk of thrombosis compared with younger persons (1.7 thrombotic events/100 person-years in patients < 40; 15.1 thrombotic events/100 person-years in patients > 60). A history of thrombosis raises the risk even further, to almost 20% per year. Primary thrombocythemia may transform into leukemia (≤ 5%); postthrombocythemic myeloid metaplasia (< 5%), which is a fibrotic stage; or polycythemia vera (< 5%).

Treatment

Hydroxyurea (starting dose, 500 mg po bid) decreases the significant risk of thrombotic complications in high-risk patients and may be given to most elderly patients with primary thrombocythemia. The goal of therapy is to keep the platelet count below 400,000/µL. Because of concern about potential leukemogenicity that may be associated with long-term use of hydroxyurea, alternative agents, including anagrelide and interferon-α, may be considered for patients < 60 and for some elderly patients.

The starting dose of anagrelide is 0.5 mg po qid. Adverse effects, occurring in one third of patients, include headache, fluid retention, dizziness, palpitations, tachycardia, diarrhea, and, rarely, heart failure. The response rate is > 90%, and response occurs at a median of 3 weeks. Anagrelide does not affect the leukocyte count or the Hb level.

Interferon-α controls thrombocytosis, splenomegaly, and disease-associated symptoms in about 80% of patients. The starting dose is 3 to 5 million U sc daily, and the average response time is 12 weeks. Short-term adverse effects include a transient influenza-like syndrome of fever and chills, myalgias, headache, and arthralgias. Long-term adverse effects include fatigue, nausea, anorexia, weight loss, diarrhea, increased liver transaminase, altered mental status, and depression.

For patients with vasomotor symptoms, a low dose of aspirin (81 mg daily) is effective, presumably by reducing thromboxane production. For high-risk patients > 60, hydroxyurea plus a low dose of aspirin is usually appropriate.

POLYCYTHEMIA VERA

An idiopathic chronic myeloproliferative disorder characterized by an increase in Hb concentration and RBC mass (erythrocytosis).

Polycythemia vera (PV) is almost as common as primary thrombocythemia, with an incidence of 2.3/100,000 per year. The median age at presentation is 60 years (male:female = 1.2:1), with only 7% of patients presenting before age 40.

Symptoms, Signs, and Complications

Presenting symptoms may include headache, dizziness, visual disturbances, paresthesias, fatigue, abdominal discomfort, weight loss, and night sweats. Postbathing pruritus is a poorly understood, common complaint. Clinical examination may reveal plethora (facial fullness and erythema), retinal vein distention, and palpable splenomegaly. Erythromelalgia may occur.

Three major complications of PV are early thrombotic events, development of myelofibrosis, and leukemic conversion (transformation into acute leukemia), the latter two occurring after 10 to 20 years of disease.

Thrombotic events are common (20% of cases) and include ischemic stroke, transient ischemic attacks, retinal vein thrombosis, central retinal artery occlusion, myocardial infarction, angina, pulmonary embolism, hepatic and portal vein thrombosis, deep vein thrombosis, and peripheral arterial occlusion. The risk of fatal or debilitating thrombotic events is much greater than with primary thrombocythemia. Patients receiving high doses of NSAIDs may have severe gastrointestinal (GI) hemorrhage. The risk of bleeding and thrombosis is significantly increased during periods of stress, including trauma and surgery.

The risk of thrombotic complications during the first 3 years in patients who have received adequate phlebotomy treatment (Hct ≤ 45% in men, ≤ 42% in women) ranges from 3% in low-risk patients to 15% in high-risk patients. Risk factors for thrombosis in PV include age > 60, history of thrombosis, and a need for phlebotomy more than 4 times/year. About 20% of all patients with PV present with thrombosis, and ≤ 25% subsequently develop thrombosis. The rate is higher in the elderly.

The cumulative risk of transformation to myelofibrosis increases with time and is estimated to be about 10% in the first 10 years and 20% in the first 20 years. Risk of leukemic conversion depends on the type of treatment. Studies have shown risks of 1.5% for phlebotomy alone, 9.6% for phlebotomy plus chlorambucil, and 13.2% for phlebotomy plus radiophosphorus. The risk of transformation into a fibrotic state ("spent phase," or postpolycythemic myeloid metaplasia) is 10% over 10 years and 20% over 25 years and does not appear to be influenced by treatment.

Diagnosis

Unlike all other causes of erythrocytosis, the erythroid proliferation in PV is erythropoietin-independent and down-regulates erythropoietin production. Consequently, serum levels of erythropoietin are usually low, occasionally normal, but never increased. Similarly, endogenous erythroid colony growth is suggestive of PV rather than of secondary erythrocytosis.

Diagnostic criteria according to the Polycythemia Vera Study Group are shown in TABLE 71–3. These criteria require increased RBC mass as a diagnostic prerequisite. However, increased RBC mass does not always indicate PV and may be due to an erythropoietin-mediated secondary erythrocytosis (see TABLE 71–4).

Leukocytosis or thrombocytosis occurs in > 50% of patients. Microcytosis is common and indicates iron deficiency, usually from repeated phlebotomy for treatment or occult GI blood loss. Nonspecific additional laboratory abnormalities include increases in leukocyte alkaline phosphatase score, serum level of vitamin B_{12}, and uric acid.

TABLE 71–3.   DIAGNOSTIC CRITERIA FOR POLYCYTHEMIA VERA*

Major Criteria	Minor Criteria

1. Increased red blood cell mass
    Males: ≥ 36 mL/kg
    Females: ≥ 32 mL/kg
	1. Platelets > 400,000/μL

	2. Leukocytes > 12,000/μL

2. Normal arterial oxygen saturation
    ≥ 92%
	3. Leukocyte alkaline phosphatase
	    score > 100
	    or vitamin B_{12} > 900 pg/mL

3. Splenomegaly	(> 664 pmol/L)
	    or unbound vitamin B_{12} binding
	    capacity > 2200 pg/mL
	    (> 1623 pmol/L)

*Diagnosis of polycythemia vera requires the presence of all three major criteria *or* the presence of the first two major criteria and any two minor criteria.
NOTE: Diagnostic criteria are from the Polycythemia Vera Study Group.

TABLE 71–4.   CAUSES OF SECONDARY ERYTHROCYTOSIS

Congenital
  Low P_{50}
    High oxygen-affinity Hb
    2,3-Diphosphoglycerate deficiency
  Normal P_{50}
    Autosomal dominant (benign) familial erythrocytosis
    Autosomal recessive familial erythrocytosis

Acquired
  Appropriate erythropoietin response
    Chronic lung disease
    Arteriovenous or intracardiac shunts
    High-altitude habitat
    Chronic carbon monoxide exposure (smoking)
  Pathologic erythropoietin production
    Tumors (liver, kidney, cerebellum)
    Uterine fibroids
    After renal transplantation

P_{50} = the partial pressure of oxygen at which Hb becomes 50% saturated.

Prognosis and Treatment

Median survival without therapy is < 2 years and is about 12 years for patients treated with phlebotomy alone.

Phlebotomy significantly reduces the risk of thrombosis. Therefore, all patients should undergo regular phlebotomy. About 500 mL of blood may be removed daily (in symptomatic patients) or weekly (in asymptomatic patients) until the Hct is < 45% in men and < 42% in women. Thereafter, the frequency is adjusted to maintain the Hct at this level.

Hydroxyurea has been shown to decrease the risk of early thrombosis without significantly increasing the risk of leukemic conversion. Thus, hydroxyurea (starting dose, 500 mg po bid) is recommended as a supplement to phlebotomy in elderly patients, particularly those who have a history of thrombosis.

Interferon-α (3 million U sc 3 times weekly) may be used for patients who cannot tolerate hydroxyurea because of adverse effects or neutropenia.

Radiophosphorus (2.3 mCi/m^2 given IV q 3 months) may be considered if the life expectancy of the patient is < 10 years and when compliance with drug treatment is poor.

A low dose of aspirin (81 mg daily) alleviates vasomotor symptoms and should be used if there are other reasons for giving aspirin. Whether aspirin is safe and effective for preventing early thrombosis associated with PV is being evaluated.

Pruritus associated with PV is often difficult to alleviate. In patients with adequate phlebotomy treatment, the addition of hydroxyurea or the alternative use of interferon-α may control refractory pruritus. Some patients may benefit from starch baths and the avoidance of brisk rubbing with a towel and showering. Although some medications, including cimetidine (900 mg daily), cyproheptadine (12 mg daily), and aspirin (81 mg daily) may be used, they have not shown consistent effectiveness and have major adverse effects in the elderly. Low doses of antidepressants (doxepin, 50 mg daily; paroxetine, 20 mg daily) are sometimes beneficial. In refractory cases, phototherapy or cholestyramine (20 g daily) may be tried.

MYELOFIBROSIS
(Agnogenic Myeloid Metaplasia)

A chronic, usually idiopathic disease characterized by bone marrow fibrosis, splenomegaly, and leukoerythroblastic anemia with teardrop-shaped RBCs.

Myelofibrosis is the least common of the chronic myeloproliferative diseases, with an incidence of 1.3/100,000 per year. The median age at presentation is 60 years (male:female = 1.2:1). Only about 5% of patients present with myelofibrosis before age 40.

The cause is unknown. Myelofibrosis may complicate the course of chronic myelocytic leukemia, primary thrombocythemia, and polycythemia vera. Fewer than 5% of patients with primary thrombocythemia and about 20% of those with polycythemia vera develop myelofibrosis after 10 to 20 years of disease. Such transformations are called postthrombocythemic myeloid metaplasia and postpolycythemic myeloid metaplasia, respectively, and their clinical course is similar to that of myelofibrosis. Together, all three are called myelofibrosis with myeloid metaplasia.

The spleen and liver are sites of extramedullary hematopoiesis, which is largely responsible for the enlargement of these organs.

Symptoms, Signs, and Complications

Most patients present with anemia and marked splenomegaly, the latter usually causing early satiety. Progressive anemia and massive hepatosplenomegaly usually develop during the course of the disease. Hypercatabolic symptoms include severe fatigue, low-grade fever, night sweats, and weight loss. Occasionally, severe left upper quadrant pain results from splenic infarction. Thrombotic complications are less common than in polycythemia vera.

Hemorrhagic complications are usually due to thrombocytopenia, esophageal varices, the use of NSAIDs, or acquired deficiency of factor V. Marked splenomegaly or intrahepatic obstruction may lead to portal hypertension. In some patients, extramedullary hematopoiesis develops in the spinal cord (causing cord compression), in the pleural or peritoneal cavity (causing pleural effusion or ascites), in the lymph nodes (causing lymphadenopathy), or in other organs.

Diagnosis

Diagnosis is suggested by examination of the peripheral blood smear and confirmed by bone marrow biopsy. In addition to normocytic (sometimes microcytic) anemia, laboratory findings often include an increased or decreased number of granulocytes and platelets. The peripheral blood smear demonstrates characteristic features of myelophthisis (bone marrow infiltration), including teardrop-shaped RBCs (dacryocytes), and of leukoerythroblastosis (the presence of nucleated RBCs and granulocyte precursors). In addition, the peripheral blood smear may show giant platelets and polychromasia (indicative of reticulocytosis). The latter finding is consistent with a component of hemolytic anemia that may occur in a small proportion of patients.

Nonspecific laboratory findings include increased blood levels of vitamin B_{12}, uric acid, and liver enzymes, including markedly increased levels of alkaline phosphatase. The bone marrow is often difficult to aspirate, and a bone marrow biopsy reveals extensive collagen fibrosis that is best seen with reticulin stain. Fibrosis often is associated with atypical megakaryocytic hyperplasia and thickening and distortion of the bony trabeculae (osteosclerosis). Cytogenetic studies of the bone marrow reveal clonal abnormalities in about 30% of patients.

The differential diagnosis of diseases associated with myelofibrosis is summarized in TABLE 71–5. Thorough morphologic and cytogenetic examinations are required for a diagnosis of myelofibrosis.

Prognosis

Median survival is estimated to be between 3 and 5 years. Risk factors for decreased survival are age > 60, hepatomegaly, weight loss, anemia (Hb < 10 g/dL), leukocytosis (white blood cell [WBC] count > 30,000/μL), leukopenia (WBC count < 4000/μL), circulating blasts ≥ 2%, male sex, thrombocytopenia (platelet count < 150,000/μL), and abnormal karyotype. Anemic patients with leukocytosis or leukopenia have a median survival of about 1 year. Patients with either anemia or leukocytosis/leukopenia have a median survival of about 2 years. Causes of death include leukemic conversion in about 10% of patients, heart failure, and infection. Splenomegaly and the degree of bone marrow fibrosis do not affect survival. Conversely, factors for longer survival include Hb ≥ 10 g/dL and a WBC count between 4,000 and 30,000/μL, forming the basis of a prognostic scoring system (Dupriez score).

TABLE 71-5.   DISORDERS ASSOCIATED WITH MYELOFIBROSIS

Myeloid disorders	Nonhematologic disorders
Chronic myeloproliferative diseases	Metastatic cancer
Myelodysplastic syndrome	Systemic lupus erythematosus
Acute myelofibrosis	Connective tissue disease
Acute myeloid leukemia	Infections
Mast cell disease	Vitamin D deficiency (rickets)
Malignant histiocytosis	Renal osteodystrophy
Lymphoid disorders	Gray platelet syndrome
Lymphomas	
Hairy cell leukemia	
Multiple myeloma	

Treatment

Allogeneic bone marrow transplantation (ABMT) may offer a possible "cure" to some patients. Five years after receiving ABMT, 50% of patients are alive and about 25% are disease-free. Generally, patients with a low Dupriez score fare better than those with a higher score.

Patients who are not candidates for ABMT receive palliative treatment. The combination of an androgen (fluoxymesterone, 10 mg po bid) and a corticosteroid (prednisone, 30 mg po daily) reduces anemia in one third of patients. If the patient responds after 1 month of treatment, fluoxymesterone is continued and the corticosteroid dosage is tapered. Before starting androgen therapy, men should be screened for prostate cancer (by digital rectal examination and measurement of prostate-specific antigen), because men with prostate cancer cannot receive androgen. All patients should have periodic monitoring of liver function. Women should be warned about virilizing adverse effects.

Erythropoietin does not usually alleviate anemia resulting from myelofibrosis. Patients who do not respond to androgen therapy receive supportive treatment with periodic RBC transfusions. Secondary hemosiderosis from long-term blood transfusion may be managed with desferoxamine (2 g daily by sc infusion pump), which may prevent complications of iron overload.

Hydroxyurea (starting at 500 mg po bid) may reduce spleen size and control thrombocytosis and leukocytosis in some patients but may worsen anemia.

Splenectomy is considered for patients who have symptomatic splenomegaly (mechanical discomfort, hypercatabolic symptoms, portal hypertension). Laboratory evidence of disseminated intravascular coagulation before splenectomy may increase the risk of perioperative hemorrhage; splenectomy should therefore be postponed until the abnormalities are corrected. At experienced centers, the mortality rate for splenectomy is generally < 10%. Postsurgical complications include intra-abdominal hemorrhage, subphrenic abscess, sepsis, large vessel thrombosis, extreme thrombocytosis, and accelerated hepatomegaly. The thrombocytosis and hepatomegaly may be controlled transiently with hydroxyurea (starting dosage, 500 mg po tid) or 2-chlorodeoxyadenosine (0.14 mg/kg given over 2 hours IV daily for 5 days).

After splenectomy, hypercatabolic symptoms and portal hypertension subside in almost all patients, and refractory anemia subsides in about 25% of the patients.

For patients unable to tolerate splenectomy, splenic irradiation (50 to 200 cGy delivered in 10 to 15 daily fractions) usually provides a transient (3 to 6 months) benefit. Irradiation is also useful in reducing extramedullary hematopoiesis at other sites, eg, spinal cord or pleural cavity.

As the factors that indicate a worsening prognosis increase, treatment is increasingly directed to end-of-life palliative care.∎

▇ 72 ▇ CANCER

Although cancer occurs in persons of every age, it is fundamentally a disease of aging. Sixty percent of new cancer cases and two thirds of cancer deaths occur in persons > 65 years (see FIGURE 72–1). The incidence of common cancers (eg, breast, colorectal, prostate, lung) increases with age. However, incidence of many cancers levels off after age 80, suggesting the possibility of intrinsic resistance to the development of cancer in late life or some selection bias.

The age-related increase in cancer incidence predicts that as the U.S. population ages, cancer incidence will continue to increase. There are several theoretical reasons why cancer incidence increases in the elderly (see TABLE 72–1): age-related alterations in the immune system (decreased immune surveillance); accumulation of random genetic mutations leading to oncogene activation or amplification or decreased tumor-suppressor gene activity; lifetime carcinogen exposure (especially for colorectal and lung cancers); hormonal alterations or exposure; and long latency periods. There may be increased susceptibility to carcinogens, possibly caused by decreased DNA repair. Multiple genetic changes are necessary for the development of cancer, most clearly exemplified by the stepwise genetic changes shown by many colon polyps

∎ see page 115

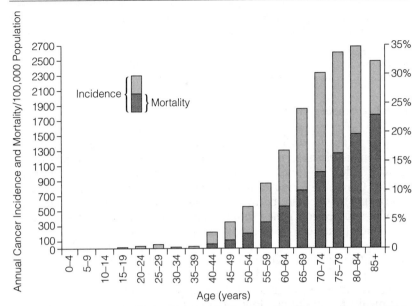

FIGURE 72–1. **Age-specific incidence and mortality for all types of cancer.** (Data from *SEER Cancer Statistics Review: 1973–1994*, Bethesda, MD, National Cancer Institute, 1997.)

progressing to cancer. The exponential rise in many cancers with age fits with an increased susceptibility to the late stages of carcinogenesis by environmental exposures. Lifetime exposure to estrogen may lead to breast or uterine cancer; exposure to testosterone, to prostate cancer. The decline in cellular immunity may lead to certain types of cancer that are highly immunogenic (eg, lymphomas, melanoma).

Controversy continues over whether cancer is less aggressive in the elderly. Growth and metastasis of several types of cancer (breast, colon,

TABLE 72–1.   THEORIES FOR WHY CANCER INCIDENCE INCREASES WITH AGE

Lifetime carcinogenic exposure
Increased susceptibility of cells to carcinogens
Decreased ability to repair DNA
Oncogene activation or amplification (accumulation)
Decreased tumor-suppressor gene activity
Microenvironment alterations, including hormonal alterations or exposure
Decreased immune surveillance due to immune senescence

lung, prostate) appear to be slower in the elderly. Yet, death occurs with smaller tumor burdens. Reasons for the difference in mortality appear to be complex: Diagnosis is often made later, treatment tends to be less aggressive, and competing causes of death are more likely; all of these factors result in shorter survival in older patients.

Risk Factors and Prevention

The part of cancer prevention we know the most about is the avoidance of toxins that induce or promote cancer. Induction refers to the earliest genetic change induced by a carcinogen. Promotion refers to cell growth induction that fixes and then further alters the genetic abnormality. Carcinogens may alter normal growth-promoting genes (protooncogenes), which are permanently turned on. They may also damage growth-suppression genes (tumor suppressors) such that they become permanently turned off. Both may be necessary to create a cancer. Since prolonged exposure is one of the necessary ingredients to both induction and promotion, prevention of cancer in the elderly must begin before people become old. The best evidence strongly recommends avoiding smoking, overuse of alcohol, and exposure to known toxic chemicals. Maintaining a low-fat, high-fiber diet may be helpful.

Hormonal exposure is implicated in the development of breast, prostate, and uterine cancers. Studies have been inconsistent as to whether exogenous estrogen exposure increases breast cancer risk, but the relative risk is probably in the range of 1.3. Early menarche, late menopause, and late or no pregnancies are confirmed risk factors. Estrogenic stimulation of the endometrium, when allowed to go unchecked, increases the risk of uterine cancer 2- to 2.5-fold.

Drugs may also reduce the risk of some cancers. Tamoxifen has recently been approved for breast cancer prevention. Aspirin and other nonsteroidal anti-inflammatory drugs (NSAIDs) appear to reduce the risk of colon cancer. Retinoids may be helpful in reducing the risk of new primary squamous cell cancers in persons with previous such cancers related to tobacco use. The role of antioxidants in preventing cancers remains unclear. Inhibiting the conversion of testosterone to 5-α-dihydroxytestosterone may prevent prostate cancer.

Screening

Because cancer is more common in the elderly than in younger populations, screening is more likely to detect cancer in older populations. Cancers for which screening has proved beneficial in reducing mortality include breast, cervical, and colon cancer. It is unclear whether immune surveillance of early cancers is effective. Most cancers are poorly immunogenic and are unlikely to raise an immune response with low tumor volumes. With prostate-specific antigen (PSA) testing, prostate cancer is detected at an earlier stage, but most studies have not shown that screening with PSA reduces mortality. ▉ Screening for ovarian cancer, even in high-risk women, has proved disappointing. Most published recommendations for cancer screening focus on populations younger than considered here. Thus, the main concern regarding the elderly is when to discontinue routine screening. No studies show benefit of screening past age 75 for any cancers. Despite the lack of data, recommendations on cancer screening in the elderly have been published (see TABLE 72–2).

Treatment

Research that focuses on cancer in younger populations may not be applicable to the elderly, the segment of the population at highest risk for cancer, leaving us with a paucity of knowledge on how best to manage cancer in the age group that experiences it most.

Treatment goals must be individualized based not only on treatability of the cancer, but also on comorbid conditions, functional status (one of the best predictors of response and tolerance ▉), social situation (which may preclude treatments involving travel or expense), and willingness of the patient to tolerate side effects of treatment. Surgery, chemotherapy, radiation therapy, and hormonal therapy are the mainstays of treatment. However, symptomatic and supportive therapy with analgesics, antidepressants, anxiolytics, and antiemetics, as well as support groups and individual and family counseling, must be integrated into treatment programs. Access to support services and to trained health care practitioners varies depending on the patient's geographic location, financial resources, mobility, and support of family and friends. Referral to major cancer centers may prolong survival but may not be the most humane course of action for debilitated and relatively immobile patients.

Age per se is not usually the deciding factor as to whether aggressive treatment is warranted: that decision must assess the likelihood that the cancer will respond to treatment, the extent of spread, comorbid conditions that could limit therapy, and the patient's wishes. Chemotherapy or radiation therapy should be strongly considered in clinical situations in which cure, prolonged survival, or definable palliation can be achieved with these modalities.

Chemotherapy: A variety of older chemotherapeutic drugs remain effective and useful. In addition, newer antineoplastics are becoming more commonly used in the treatment of cancer in the elderly (see TABLE 72–3). Chemotherapy may be less well tolerated by elderly patients because of kinetic and dynamic changes that occur with age, decreased

---

▉ see page 1183   ▉ see TABLES 81–3 and 81–4 on pages 803 and 804

TABLE 72–2. RECOMMENDATIONS FOR CANCER SCREENING IN ELDERLY PATIENTS

Cancer	Test	ACS Guideline	USPSTF Guideline
Breast	Breast self-examination	Monthly	No recommendation
	Breast physical examination	Annually	Every 1–2 yr until age 69
	Mammography	Annually	Age ≥ 70, individual discretion
Cervix	Papanicolaou test	Annually until three or more smears normal, then physician's discretion	Every 1–3 yr until age 65; stop if normal
Colon	Digital rectal examination	Every 5 yr	No recommendation
	Fecal occult blood test	Annually	Annually
	Sigmoidoscopy	Every 5 yr	Periodically
	or colonoscopy	Every 10 yr	No recommendation
	or double-contrast barium enema	Every 5–10 yr	No recommendation
Prostate	Digital rectal examination	Should be discussed annually	Not recommended
	PSA	Annually*	Not recommended
Ovary	Ultrasound	Not recommended	Not recommended
	Serum markers	Not recommended	Not recommended
	Pelvic examination	Not recommended	Not recommended
Lung	Chest radiography	Not recommended	Not recommended
	Sputum cytology	Not recommended	Not recommended
Skin	Skin inspection	Annually	No recommendation
Oral	Mouth inspection and palpation	Annually	No recommendation

*With life expectancy ≥ 10 yr.
ACS = American Cancer Society; USPSTF = U.S. Preventive Services Task Force; PSA = prostate-specific antigen.
NOTE: *No recommendation* indicates insufficient evidence exists to recommend for or against. *Not recommended* is a specific recommendation against testing.

organ reserve, and poorer wound healing. Comorbid conditions such as diabetic neuropathies, renal insufficiency, heart failure, and decubitus ulcers may contraindicate specific treatments. However, nausea and vomiting from chemotherapy tend to be less intense in the elderly.

Age-related decreases in liver size, blood flow, and metabolic reserve and use of drugs that inhibit cytochromes may inhibit drug metabolism. The neurotoxicity of drugs such as vincristine, cisplatin, and paclitaxel is especially troublesome in the elderly, and severe neuropathies or constipation may result. Hematopoietic toxicity of most drugs and of radiation therapy is increased to some degree. Gastrointestinal toxicities of 5-fluorouracil and doxorubicin may be increased, and frail patients are less able to tolerate short episodes of diarrhea or decreased oral intake from mucositis. Reduced cardiac reserve makes it more difficult for the elderly to tolerate anthracyclines, and decreased renal reserve decreases tolerance to platinum drugs and methotrexate, requiring adjustments in dose or choice of drug. With curable malignancies, great care must be taken not to reduce doses without documented need.

Advancements in hematologic manipulation have made the use of chemotherapy safer in the elderly. For example, granulocyte colony-stimulating factor (G-CSF) and granulocyte-macrophage colony-stimulating factor (GM-CSF) diminish duration of chemotherapy-induced neutropenia. Erythropoietin is often effective in treating chemotherapy-induced anemia and is well tolerated. Oprelvekin, a nonspecific growth factor for megakaryocytes, has been approved for preventing and treating severe thrombocytopenia associated with chemotherapy. However, oprelvekin prevents, at most, 30% of needed platelet transfusions and often causes significant adverse effects (edema, dyspnea, tachycardia). It should be used with caution in patients at risk of heart failure or with central nervous system tumors. Pamidronate is effective treatment of tumor-induced hypercalcemia. Other bisphosphonates may be as effective.

Antiserotonin antiemetics (ondansetron, granisetron, dolasetron) are more effective than older drugs and have few side effects. Dolasetron may cause a prolonged QT interval and therefore must be used with caution in patients at risk of ventricular arrhythmias. Expense is a major deterrent to the use of the antiserotonin antiemetics, and they lose effectiveness 48 to 72 hours after chemotherapy. Phenothiazines, benzodiazepines, and dexamethasone are more effective for delayed nausea.

Amifostine is a chemoprotectant that is beneficial in treating neurotoxicity and nephrotoxicity caused by cisplatin. Dexrazoxane is a cardioprotectant used with anthracyclines. The clinical usefulness of amifostine and dexrazoxane has not been fully defined.

Radiation therapy: This modality has become more tolerable and safer with newer technologies and improved techniques, such as high-energy linear accelerators, better control of target areas, three-dimensional CT planning, and improved dosimetry. Patients who have conditions such as arthritis, kyphoscoliosis, parkinsonism, or dementia may require special positioning or immobilization. The elderly appear to be at increased risk of radiation lung damage, coronary artery injury, esophagitis, and enteritis, necessitating precise planning and dosimetry. Mucositis, esophagitis, or enteritis may lead to more rapid dehydration in the elderly. Despite these problems, some seemingly frail elderly patients can tolerate radiation therapy.

TABLE 72–3. NEWER ANTINEOPLASTIC DRUGS FOR TREATMENT OF CANCER IN THE ELDERLY

Drug	Commonly Responsive Tumors	Toxicity	Comments
Taxanes (docetaxel, paclitaxel)	Breast, lung, ovarian, head and neck, upper GI tract cancers	Myelosuppression, fluid retention (docetaxel), neurotoxicity (paclitaxel)	Premedication with dexamethasone is required with either drug
Fludarabine	Chronic lymphocytic leukemia, low-grade lymphomas	Myelosuppression, profound cellular immune suppression, neurologic toxicity	Has highest response rate for tumors mentioned Prophylactic TMP/SMX may be used on weekends to prevent *Pneumocystis* pneumonia
Cladribine	Hairy cell leukemia	Leukopenia (may be profound and prolonged)	Most active drug for tumor mentioned; may be curative; generally well tolerated
Gemcitabine	Pancreatic, lung, ovarian cancers	Leukopenia	Provides palliation for pancreatic cancer; relatively good response rates in lung and ovarian cancers
Capecitabine	Breast cancer (and probably other cancers for which 5-FU is effective)	Inflammation and desquamation of the skin of the hands and feet (hand-foot syndrome [palmar-plantar dysesthesia])	Capecitabine is an oral 5-FU analog
Doxorubicin (liposomal encapsulated)	Kaposi's sarcoma, ovarian cancer, breast cancer	Palmar-plantar dysesthesia	Fewer cardiac and myelosuppressive side effects than other drugs
Tamoxifen	Breast cancer, including prevention	Endometrial cancer (rare), hot flashes, hypercoagulability	A SERM with both estrogen agonist and antagonist activity. It has been most commonly used to treat postmenopausal breast cancer in the case of metas-

Raloxifene	Breast cancer	Endometrial cancer (?), hot flashes, hypercoagulability	Raloxifene, a new SERM, may be superior to tamoxifen in retaining bone density and may not cause endometrial cancer, but long-term safety data are not available, and extensive testing for prevention and treatment has not been performed
Toremifene	Breast cancer (advanced)	Hot flashes	A SERM with mainly anti-estrogenic properties. Occasional responses among patients who relapse after initial tamoxifen use
Astemizole; letrozole	Breast cancer	Hot flashes	Astemizole and letrozole block the production of adrenal estrogens by blocking aromatase enzyme activity. They are useful in second-line hormonal therapy of breast cancer with better efficacy and fewer side effects than megestrol

tases or as postsurgical adjuvant therapy, but new data indicate usefulness in treating premenopausal women and in preventing breast cancer. It is ineffective against cancers that are both estrogen- and progesterone-receptor negative, but as a preventive agent, it reduces the risk of second primary tumors. The reduction in risk of death from breast cancer far outweighs the small increase in risk of death from endometrial cancer

5-FU = 5-fluorouracil; GI = gastrointestinal; SERM = selective estrogen receptor modulator; TMP/SMX = trimethoprim-sulfamethoxazole.

Pain control: Pain control is especially important in the care of elderly cancer patients.◘ Although pain control is often considered part of end-of-life care, persons with cancer may have chronic pain or intermittently painful complications of cancer during any stage of their disease and it may continue over the course of many years. The goal is to achieve an acceptable level of pain control with tolerable adverse effects. Comfort must be emphasized and the patient reassured that pain will be aggressively managed. Treating the source of pain is important. Radiation therapy to painful bony or other lesions should be considered. Chemotherapy may be of palliative benefit.

Opioids are used to treat severe pain not relieved by NSAIDs. Addiction should not be an issue for prescribers, and patients should be reassured that fear of addiction should not affect their use of the drug. Timed-release morphine and oxycodone as well as transdermal fentanyl relieve baseline pain. Fast-acting drugs, such as hydrocodone, oxycodone, morphine, hydromorphone, and transmucosal fentanyl lollipops, relieve intermittent or breakthrough pain. Fentanyl clearance is decreased in the elderly. Methadone, meperidine, pentazocine, and propoxyphene should not be used in the elderly. Stimulant laxatives are essential for an elderly patient receiving opioid therapy.

Elderly patients may become somnolent while being treated with opioids. Methylphenidate, taken periodically at a dose of 5 to 10 mg, is often useful, especially for those patients desiring more social interaction when taking opioids.

Pain not relieved by opioids requires adjunctive treatment. Antidepressants, anticonvulsants, or antiarrhythmics may be used for neuropathic pain. Epidural or intrathecal opioids or clonidine infusion may be extremely effective without causing side effects. Nerve blocks may be helpful for intra-abdominal or dermatomal distribution pain.

Pamidronate given intravenously monthly is effective at reducing bone pain in metastatic breast cancer, multiple myeloma, and probably prostate cancer. Radioactive strontium or samarium localizes in blastic bone metastases and reduces bone pain, but results have been less promising than first expected.

Nursing Issues

Oncology nursing is now a specialization of nursing. Oncology nurses educate and counsel patients and their families as well as administer chemotherapy, interpret and manage treatment-related side effects, coordinate community and medical services, and provide palliative care. Triage and initial management of problems in elderly cancer patients are often handled by nursing personnel with the use of standard protocols. The nurse must be able to recognize the altered presentations

◘ see also pages 116 and 387

of illness and side effects in the elderly as well as pharmacologic differences in the use of commonly prescribed drugs. Examples of enhanced side effects of drugs used in the elderly include increased risk of disorientation, light-headedness or falls from the use of antiemetics or opioids, and increased risk of dehydration from drugs that cause vomiting and diarrhea in elderly patients with decreased thirst response. The oncology nurse is a key provider in assessing and managing pain because of the prolonged contact with patients in a variety of settings. The oncology nurse is also on the front lines of managing nutritional support and other symptoms.

Social Issues

Many social issues arise in the care of elderly cancer patients. These issues often become complex and require the expertise of a social worker or an interdisciplinary team. Services may have to be coordinated to help with home care, travel, meal preparation, and drug adherence. Counseling may be warranted to help patients and their families cope with the seriousness of the illness. Efforts to overcome these difficulties frequently require alterations in treatment plans and interdisciplinary approaches. [1]

Finances may pose problems as well. Oral chemotherapy drugs are covered 80% by Medicare if there is also an approved IV form of the drug. Other drugs taken orally, including pain medications (especially timed-release formulations), can be very expensive and are not covered by Medicare. Most pharmaceutical companies have indigent patient programs.

End-of-Life Issues

It must not be forgotten that cancer is often fatal. [2] Sometimes treatment becomes futile, exposing an elderly patient to suffering that outweighs any potential benefit. Even at the time of initial diagnosis, treatment is not always warranted. An honest discussion of what is likely to be gained and what the side effects of treatment are likely to be is the best course of action. Most patients understand when it is time to make a transition to more palliative goals of care (palliative care is defined by the World Health Organization as the active total care of patients whose disease is not responsive to treatment). This understanding can be fostered by direct and forthright discussions regarding prognosis and benefits and risks of therapy and is enhanced by a trusting physician-patient relationship.

Involvement of hospice services early in the course of palliative care can be helpful. [3] The financial benefits alone of switching to the Medicare hospice benefit may be substantial. Hospice personnel have

[1] see page 74   [2] see page 115   [3] see page 90

expertise in preparing patients and families spiritually, financially, and legally for the end of life. Most patients wish to remain at home. Every effort should be made to accommodate this wish, but attention needs to be paid to caregiver burden. Short stays in a hospital or nursing home, which are covered by Medicare, may be necessary for respite to caregivers. Interventions and clinic visits should be kept to the minimum necessary for palliation. Although Medicare reimburses physicians for time spent on hospice issues, the reimbursement is rarely adequate and does not compensate for the amount of documentation required. ◨

73 ■ HEMATOLOGIC MALIGNANCIES

ACUTE LEUKEMIAS

Accumulation of neoplastic, immature lymphoid or immature myeloid cells in the bone marrow and peripheral blood; tissue invasion by these cells; and associated bone marrow failure.

Acute leukemias are categorized as acute lymphoblastic (lymphocytic) leukemia (ALL) or acute myelogenous (myelocytic, myeloblastic) leukemia (AML), according to the morphologic characteristics of leukemic cells in peripheral blood and bone marrow smears and to the cells' histochemical staining and immunologic markers. The French-American-British (FAB) Cooperative Group classification, the system most widely used to facilitate clinical studies, allows some degree of prognostication.

Acute leukemia is primarily a disease of children and the elderly. In the USA, acute leukemia has an incidence of about 15/100,000 across all age groups. However, the incidence begins rising at age 40 and by age 80 is about 160/100,000. About 80% of adults with acute leukemia have AML.

Etiology and Pathophysiology

In most cases of acute leukemia, the etiology is unknown. Radiation exposure has been causally implicated in some cases. Atomic bomb survivors from Hiroshima and Nagasaki have a 10 to 20% increase in the incidence of AML. Likewise, the risk of developing AML is 2.5 times

◨ see also page 166

greater in diagnostic radiologists and 14 times greater in patients who received radiation therapy for ankylosing spondylitis earlier this century. High-level benzene exposure in the workplace has been strongly implicated as a risk factor for AML. Also, long-term low-dose therapy with virtually any chemotherapeutic alkylating agent can cause acute leukemia, usually the myelogenous type. Combining a chemotherapeutic agent with radiation therapy increases the risk.

Chronic bone marrow disorders (eg, myelodysplasia, polycythemia vera, aplastic anemia) are sometimes followed by a rapidly progressive leukemic phase in patients of all ages.

Viruses have long been suspected as the cause of some acute leukemias, particularly the lymphocytic varieties. Oncogenes appear to have a role in inducing and maintaining malignancy. In some cases, specific oncogenes are involved in particular chromosome translocations or in chromosome deletion or reduplication.

In acute promyelocytic leukemia (FAB M3 classification), the t(15;17) translocation, which involves the retinoic acid receptor gene on chromosome 17, is present as a unique feature in virtually all cases, which may explain the response to treatment with all-*trans*-retinoic acid.

In acute leukemia, primitive lymphoblasts and myeloblasts accumulate rapidly in the bone marrow and invade many tissues, including the liver, spleen, lymph nodes, and central nervous system (CNS). Normal bone marrow and normal leukocytes are replaced by these blasts, resulting in severe anemia, thrombocytopenia with marked bleeding, and great susceptibility to infection.

Symptoms and Signs

Acute leukemia frequently presents as an apparent infection with an acute onset of malaise and high fever. An associated thrombocytopenia usually produces petechiae, ecchymoses, and bleeding from the nose, mouth, and gastrointestinal and genitourinary tracts. Often, the liver, spleen, and lymph nodes are enlarged. In the elderly, the disease can present insidiously with progressive weakness, pallor, an altered sense of well-being, and delirium.

Diagnosis

The total peripheral white blood cell (WBC) count may be low, normal, or elevated. Blasts are usually present in the peripheral blood smear, but a bone marrow aspiration should be performed to confirm the diagnosis. The bone marrow in acute leukemia contains excessive blast cells and an absence or decreased number of normal erythrocytic, granulocytic, and megakaryocytic cells. Histochemical stains, immunophenotype, and chromosome abnormalities help identify the type of acute leukemia.

Elderly patients with ALL often have one or more of the following: a WBC count > 20,000/μL, mediastinal mass, L2 to L3 morphologic changes, T-cell or B-cell leukemia, and meningitis.

Prognosis

Without treatment, death usually occurs within 4 to 6 months of clinical onset.**1** Some patients die within days. Indicators of a poor prognosis include advanced age, infection, bleeding, high blast counts, and chromosomal abnormalities (the elderly have more complex karyotypic abnormalities than do younger patients). Auer rods (in AML) have been reported to be an indicator of a good prognosis. A prior bone marrow disorder (eg, polycythemia vera, myelodysplasia) or leukemia secondary to previous therapy with an alkylating agent seems to indicate a poor prognosis. However, data regarding all prognostic signs are contradictory.

Advanced age has typically been considered an unfavorable prognostic factor. The major problem in treating the elderly is their relative inability to tolerate the prolonged pancytopenia that accompanies aggressive chemotherapy. Of patients with ALL, the elderly have a much worse prognosis than do children, who have an excellent prognosis. T-cell leukemia has a slightly better prognosis than does B-cell leukemia.

Treatment

Acute lymphoblastic leukemia: Therapy traditionally consists of a combination of drugs, including vincristine, prednisone, an anthracycline, and asparaginase (which is tolerated poorly by elderly patients). Most elderly patients experience relapse within the first year of treatment, and no accepted standard salvage therapy exists. Bone marrow transplantation is rarely used for patients > 65. Patients with true B-cell ALL (FAB L3 classification) are treated with regimens for small noncleaved cell non-Hodgkin's lymphoma (high-grade non-Hodgkin's lymphoma).**2**

Acute myelogenous leukemia: The initial aim is to induce a complete remission, ie, to reduce leukemic blasts to an undetectable level (in practice, < 5% marrow blasts). In the induction phase of treatment, comprehensive care is critical, because the patient is often infected and bleeding and has a large tumor burden with little normal hematopoiesis. Many induction regimens are being used; the standard combination is cytarabine 100 to 200 mg/m²/day as a continuous IV infusion for 5 to 7 days and daunorubicin 45 mg/m²/day IV for the first 3 days. A low-dose cytarabine regimen of 50 to 100 mg/m²/day lowers the mortality rate

1 see also page 115   **2** see page 751

during induction but does not improve the complete remission rate. With the use of fresh, frozen, and packed red blood cells (RBCs), platelets, antibiotics, and growth factors, the complete remission rate in patients > 60 ranges from 40 to 76%. Median survival is 1 to 2 years. The value of maintenance and consolidation chemotherapeutic regimens is under study. As in ALL, bone marrow transplantation is rarely used for patients > 65.

In acute promyelocytic leukemia, oral administration of all-*trans*-retinoic acid can induce differentiation of the leukemic cells and produce a histologic and cytogenetic remission; however, this regimen has not been studied specifically in the elderly. Moreover, the remissions are temporary, and standard chemotherapy is also required.

Complications of treatment: Infections are the major cause of morbidity and mortality in patients with acute leukemia. Infections result from the severe leukopenia (with polymorphonuclear leukocytes often < 500 to 1000/µL) and destruction of normal cutaneous and mucosal barriers. In many patients, endogenous bowel flora is the source of infection, but the pharynx, lungs, perirectal area, and skin are also common sources. The genitourinary tract and CNS are rare sources. Because the source of infection is usually internal, isolation has limited value. Viruses, protozoa, and anaerobic bacteria are uncommon pathogens early in therapy. Fungal infections usually occur after 7 to 14 days of antibiotic therapy in neutropenic patients.

The initial choice of antibiotics depends on the predominant organisms causing infection in a given hospital. In most hospitals the most common organisms are *Pseudomonas* and *Escherichia coli*; therefore, an aminoglycoside plus a semisynthetic penicillin or a cephalosporin is usually the combination of choice. Trimethoprim-sulfamethoxazole has been suggested as prophylaxis, particularly in patients who have been admitted frequently with fever and neutropenia.

Metabolic problems are common during induction therapy. Hyperuricemia should be treated prophylactically with allopurinol 300 mg/day. Oliguric renal failure will develop from uric acid nephropathy unless the patient is vigorously hydrated, is treated with allopurinol, and undergoes urine alkalinization. Natriuresis and hyponatremia often develop from increased osmolar clearance as a result of electrolytes, water, and urea released from dead blasts. Hypokalemia can occur from natriuresis, the syndrome of inappropriate antidiuretic hormone secretion (SIADH), physiologic hypervasopressinemia, or proximal renal tubular dysfunction. A renal tubular acidosis–like syndrome, with hypokalemia, aminoaciduria, and hyperphosphaturia, occurs but is probably not related to lysozyme, because it occurs when the leukemic cells are not releasing large amounts of this enzyme, and the serum and urinary lysozyme levels are not elevated. Metabolic alkalosis, metabolic acidosis, hypocalcemia, and hyperphosphatemia are also common complications.

Aggregates of blasts and thrombi may occlude small blood vessels throughout the body, particularly in the brain and lungs. Therapy consists of hydration and rapid reduction of the blast count by promptly initiating chemotherapy. Leukapheresis may be palliative.

The CNS is the most common site of extramedullary relapse in acute leukemia; patients present with headache, vomiting, and irritability. The need for prophylactic meningeal therapy with cranial irradiation and intrathecal methotrexate and/or cytarabine has not been formally addressed in the elderly. Therefore, these treatments must be used with extreme caution, if at all. Spinal cord compression with resulting motor and sensory deficits may occur; it usually responds to local radiation. The acute T-cell lymphocytic leukemias are most likely to cause either CNS or gonadal invasion. However, the role of prophylactic testicular irradiation in the elderly is unclear.

Disseminated intravascular coagulation (DIC)**◻** is an uncommon complication occurring mainly in promyeloblastic leukemia. The patient presents either with massive sudden bleeding (acute DIC) or, more commonly, with slow bleeding (chronic DIC). Generally, DIC is self-limited and is most problematic during the rapid cell lysis of induction chemotherapy. Use of prophylactic heparin to treat this condition is controversial.

End-of-Life Issues

Acute leukemia in elderly patients is most often fatal within 1 to 2 years. Patients and family members should understand that, even with aggressive treatment, the best that can usually be hoped for is a short prolongation of life. The patient must weigh this prognosis against the unpleasant side effects of chemotherapy. Often, older patients decide not to undergo chemotherapy. Hospice care, palliative care (including pain relief), and patient comfort are the goals.**◻**

CHRONIC LEUKEMIAS

Accumulation of neoplastic, mature lymphoid or mature myeloid cells in the blood, which usually progresses far more slowly than that in acute leukemia.

If the neoplastic cells are of the lymphoid type, the disease is called chronic lymphocytic leukemia (CLL); if they are of the myeloid type, it is called chronic myelocytic (myeloid, myelogenous) leukemia (CML). In > 95% of cases, CLL involves the neoplastic proliferation of B cells.

CLL, primarily a disease of the elderly, is the most common leukemia in Western society, accounting for 25 to 40% of all leukemias.

◻ see page 692   ◻ see page 115

The incidence is about 4/100,000 for all ages and about 80/100,000 for persons > 80. About 90% of all patients are > 50, with the majority > 60. Men are affected twice as often as women. CML usually occurs in persons in their 30s and 40s and is rare in the elderly.

Etiology and Pathophysiology

A genetic component seems to be involved in CLL, because the illness is more common in certain families. Some of these families have immunologic abnormalities. Chronic viral infections (eg, with Epstein-Barr virus) have also been suggested as a possible cause. Ionizing radiation plays no part in the etiology of CLL.

In > 95% of CLL cases, the neoplastic proliferation involves lymphocytes of B-cell origin; in the remaining cases, the proliferation involves lymphocytes of T-cell origin. Cells appear morphologically mature but have receptors for mouse erythrocytes, human leukocyte antigen (HLA)-DR, and small amounts of surface immunoglobulin, suggesting some degree of immaturity. Trisomy 12 has been identified in about 25% of cases. Monoclonal lymphocytes accumulate in the peripheral blood, bone marrow, lymphoid tissues, and sometimes other organs. Infiltration of the bone marrow may eventually result in pancytopenia. Deficiency of normal B cells often leads to bacterial infection. Transformation to a diffuse large cell lymphoma (Richter's syndrome) or to acute prolymphocytic leukemia may occur as a terminal event.

In CLL, the anemia and thrombocytopenia may result from marrow replacement, hypersplenism, or suppressor mechanisms such as antiplatelet antibodies.

Symptoms and Signs

Presentation varies greatly. More than 25% of patients are asymptomatic; the disease is diagnosed during routine physical examination or by blood count. The most common initial symptoms are fatigue, malaise, and decreased exercise tolerance. In many elderly patients, an exacerbation of coronary artery disease or cerebrovascular disease is the initial manifestation.

Splenomegaly is clinically detectable in 50% of patients at presentation; it can cause abdominal pain or early satiety. Lymphadenopathy commonly occurs in the cervical, axillary, and supraclavicular areas. Inguinal adenopathy is rare. Hepatomegaly may develop as the disease progresses. Jaundice usually suggests hemolysis, although biliary obstruction can result from periportal lymph node enlargement. Lymphocytic infiltration can occur in any organ. In the late stages, ecchymoses and petechiae may result from thrombocytopenia.

Fever is usually secondary to bacterial infection, which is the most common complication of CLL, particularly affecting the lungs and urinary tract. Gram-positive cocci, gram-negative bacilli, fungi, *Listeria,* and *Pneumocystis carinii* are the most common causative organisms.

Fever, in the late stages, may indicate the development of acute prolymphocytic leukemia or aggressive lymphoma. Clinically significant hyperviscosity∎ (which may result in skin and mucosal bleeding, visual disturbances, headache, and other changing neurologic manifestations) is rare, occurring only when the WBC count is ≥ 800,000/μL.

T-cell CLL usually is a more aggressive disorder than B-cell CLL, with massive splenomegaly, marked neutropenia, skin infiltration, modest bone marrow infiltration, and a rapid clinical course leading to death in about 50% of these patients. However, some cases have an indolent course. There is a high concurrence with rheumatoid arthritis.

Diagnosis

The diagnosis of CLL requires demonstration of sustained lymphocytosis and bone marrow lymphocyte infiltration in the absence of other causes. The absolute lymphocyte count is generally > 4800/μL, commonly > 15,000/μL. The cells appear mature and tend to smudge when the blood smear is prepared.

In **B-cell CLL,** the number of T cells and B cells increases, but the malignant B cells increase preferentially, accounting for 40 to 90% of all lymphocytes. They are of monoclonal origin and express the surface immunoglobulins of one light chain class. The usual surface immunoglobulin is IgM; less commonly, it is IgD. The ratio of helper (CD4) to suppressor (CD8) T cells is reversed because of an increased number of suppressor cells. This reversal may account for the development of pure RBC aplasia, which occurs in a few patients.

In **T-cell CLL,** CD4 or CD8 cells predominate over B cells. T-cell CLL is characterized by lymphocytes that form rosettes with sheep RBCs. The lymphocytes often exhibit cytoplasmic azurophilic granules. The malignant cell may have a more convoluted nucleus and is usually of CD4 immunophenotype. CD8 T-cell CLL is rare and usually presents with marked anemia and neutropenia disproportionate to the extent of bone marrow and organ involvement.

In **either type,** the RBC morphologic characteristics are usually normal. Anemia occurs in 10 to 20% of patients and is usually normochromic and normocytic. The Coombs' test reveals IgG coating of RBCs in about 20% of patients; however, an autoimmune hemolytic anemia occurs only 8% of the time. Thrombocytopenia occurs in 10 to 20% of patients. Bone marrow morphologic examination shows interstitial or nodular infiltration in the early stages of disease and diffuse infiltration in the advanced stages.

In about 5% of patients, the immunoglobulin found on the cell surface is also found in the serum as a monoclonal protein. Hypogammaglobulinemia or agammaglobulinemia is found in 50 to 75% of patients.

∎ see page 735

Prognosis

The 5-year survival rate is only about 50%; however, 25 to 30% of patients with CLL live 10 years or more. Patients with CLL have at least a fourfold risk of developing a second malignancy.

Two common approaches to staging are the Rai, which is primarily based on hematologic changes, and the Binet, based on extent of disease (see TABLE 73–1). Using the Binet classification, patients in stage A, with ≤ 2 involved sites, usually survive > 7 years. Patients in stage B, with 3 to 5 involved sites (possibly including the cervical, axillary, supraclavicular, and inguinal lymph nodes as well as the liver and spleen), usually survive < 5 years. Patients in stage C have anemia (Hb < 10 g/dL) or thrombocytopenia (platelets < 100,000/μL) and usually survive < 2 years. Generally, the disease progresses in a stepwise pattern from less severe to more severe.

Other unfavorable prognostic signs include diffuse replacement of bone marrow, trisomy 12 plus other abnormal chromosomes, and surface IgM rather than IgD.

Treatment

Treatment is outlined for the Binet stages.

Stage A patients and **stage B** patients usually do not require treatment, because the complications of chemotherapy (eg, infection, development of acute nonlymphocytic leukemia) may be more deleterious than the disease itself. However, stage B patients are treated as de-

TABLE 73–1.   CLINICAL STAGING OF CHRONIC LYMPHOCYTIC LEUKEMIA

Classification and Stage	Description
Rai	
Stage 0	Absolute lymphocytosis of > 10,000/μL in blood and ≥ 30% lymphocytes in bone marrow
Stage I	Stage 0 plus enlarged lymph nodes
Stage II	Stage I plus hepatomegaly or splenomegaly
Stage III	Stage II plus anemia with Hb < 11 g/dL
Stage IV	Stage III plus thrombocytopenia with platelet counts < 100,000/μL
Binet	
Stage A	Absolute lymphocytosis of > 10,000/μL in blood and ≤ 30% lymphocytes in bone marrow; Hb ≥ 10 g/dL, platelets > 100,000/μL, ≤ 2 involved sites*
Stage B	As for stage A, but 3–5 involved sites
Stage C	As for stage A or B, but Hb < 10 g/dL or platelets < 100,000/μL

*Sites considered: cervical, axillary, inguinal, hepatic, splenic, lymphatic.

scribed for stage C patients if they are troubled by progressive, disabling constitutional symptoms clearly attributable to the leukemia.

For **stage C patients,** chlorambucil is the most commonly used agent. It induces responses in 50 to 80% of patients and complete remission in 10 to 20%. Chlorambucil may be given orally at a daily dosage of 0.08 to 0.2 mg/kg or for 1 day every 4 weeks at 0.4 mg/kg as a single dose. The dosage is tapered as the WBC count falls and is discontinued when the lymphocyte count falls below 20,000/μL. Prednisone 0.8 mg/kg/day is often used concomitantly and may improve the response rate. Corticosteroids alone are used only in patients with autoimmune hemolytic anemia or thrombocytopenia. Some patients may benefit from the newer agents fludarabine or pentostatin. Certain combination chemotherapy regimens, such as cyclophosphamide, doxorubicin, vincristine, and prednisone, may be useful in advanced stages.

Radiation therapy is used to reduce locally bulky disease, vital organ compromise, or painful bone lesions. Patients with refractory CLL may benefit from repeated leukapheresis, which lowers the WBC count, reduces organomegaly, and reduces cytopenia.

When transformation to either an acute prolymphocytic leukemia or an aggressive lymphoma occurs, response to chemotherapy or radiation is generally poor.

End-of-Life Issues

Although elderly patients often live with chronic leukemia for years or decades, it is still likely to cause death. As the disease advances, patients should be helped through preparations for death, and their wishes regarding terminal care should be documented.❚

MULTIPLE MYELOMA

A neoplastic disorder resulting from the proliferation and accumulation of neoplastic immature plasma cells in the bone marrow.

In the USA, the annual incidence is about 3/100,000 persons. Multiple myeloma usually occurs in people > 50, and incidence increases with age. The disease is more common in blacks than in whites. It occurs equally in men and women.

Etiology

An increased occurrence of myeloma in first-degree relatives and in blacks and the higher frequency of the 4C complex of HLA antigens in multiple myeloma patients suggest that genetic factors play a role. However, the risk of developing multiple myeloma seems to increase after high radiation exposure, as demonstrated in Hiroshima and Naga-

❚ see pages 115 and 134

saki atomic bomb survivors. Other possible causes include chronic antigenic stimulation from factors such as cholecystitis, osteomyelitis, repeated allergen injections, rheumatoid arthritis, hereditary spherocytosis, and Gaucher's disease. Asbestos exposure and viral illnesses (eg, human herpesvirus 6) have also been suggested as possible etiologic factors.

The age-related decrease in cell-mediated immunity may play a role. As T-cell numbers decrease, B-cell clones may proliferate excessively. Then, because of this monoclonal expansion, spontaneous or externally induced genetic alteration of the B-cell clone may occur, allowing it to proliferate and produce large amounts of its immunoglobulin. The clone would remain under some control of the immune system and thus would be a benign monoclonal gammopathy.◻ A second external oncogenic event might then result in uncontrolled proliferation of these cells (ie, multiple myeloma).

Pathophysiology

The consequences of abnormal plasma cell growth are plasma cell tumors, osteolytic lesions, bone marrow functional impairment, hypogammaglobulinemia, paraproteinemia, paraproteinuria, and renal disease. Neoplastic plasma cells almost always synthesize abnormal amounts of monoclonal immunoglobulin (IgG, IgA, IgD, or IgE) or κ or λ light chains. Therefore, they are usually classified according to their immunoglobulin class as determined by immunoelectrophoresis. In rare cases, there is no detectable immunoglobulin production.

Plasma cell tumors usually develop in areas of hematopoietically active bone marrow. They occur in virtually any bone but rarely in extraskeletal sites. Even plasma cell tumors that seem solitary eventually become widespread.

Osteolytic lesions, which are very common, are thought to result from the release of osteoclast-activating factor (interleukin-6) by the neoplastic plasma cells. Interleukin-6 stimulates osteoclasts to resorb bone, which can result in osteolytic lesions or diffuse osteoporosis.

Bone marrow functional impairment occurs in direct proportion to the number of plasma cells in the bone marrow. Anemia is most common, but neutropenia and thrombocytopenia may also occur.

An actual or functional hypogammaglobulinemia occurs, due to a single clone of abnormal plasma cells producing an excess of a single type of immunoglobulin or a portion of the immunoglobulin molecule, thereby suppressing the other normal classes of immunoglobulins. In > 50% of patients with monoclonal gammopathies, the monoclonal protein is IgG; in 20%, IgA; in 12%, IgM (Waldenström's macroglobulinemia); and in 2%, IgD. An IgE monoclonal protein is rare. About

---

◻ see page 737

10% of patients produce only light chains, and < 1% produce only heavy chains. About 1% of patients have no monoclonal protein in serum or urine. Rarely, patients produce two or more monoclonal proteins. Renal disease occurs in about 50% of patients. Glomerular amyloid deposits, urinary tract infections, calcium or uric acid calculi, and plasma cell infiltration of the kidney may occur. However, the major cause of renal failure is the tubular damage associated with the excretion of light chains, called Bence Jones proteins. All light chain proteins are not nephrotoxic, and some patients may excrete large amounts of light chains for years without developing renal failure.

Symptoms and Signs

Multiple myeloma is usually progressive. The abnormal plasma cells are estimated to double in 3 to 10 months. In rare cases, however, the preclinical stage may last for years. The major manifestations of multiple myeloma result from the direct effect of neoplastic cells, the characteristic proteins they produce, and their secondary effects on other organ systems.

Bone pain is the most common symptom of multiple myeloma, occurring in about 70% of patients. Pain often occurs in the lower back or ribs and gradually increases in intensity. A sudden onset may mean that a vertebra has collapsed or that a spontaneous pathologic fracture has occurred (eg, in the shaft of a long bone, the pelvis, a rib, or a clavicle).

Systemic symptoms and signs include pallor, weakness, fatigue, dyspnea on exertion, and palpitations—all due to normochromic-normocytic anemia, which is present in about 70% of patients at diagnosis. Signs of thrombocytopenia (eg, ecchymoses, purpura, epistaxis, excessive bleeding from trauma) are common. Infection also occurs frequently because of neutropenia and immunoglobulin deficiency, and the patient may present with pneumonia, pyoderma, or pyelonephritis. Cold sensitivity and urticaria may result from cryoglobulinemia. Rarely, patients present with nephrotic syndrome.

Hypercalcemia, common in patients with destructive bone lesions, may result in anorexia, nausea, vomiting, polyuria, polydipsia, constipation, and dehydration. Particularly in the elderly, hypercalcemia may produce drowsiness, confusion, and coma.

Renal disease may be acute or chronic. Acute disease is usually accompanied by azotemia and may be caused by hypercalcemia, hyperuricemia, hypotension, dehydration, infections, or treatment with nephrotoxic drugs. Dehydration often results from fluid deprivation or IV use of hypertonic contrast media during a diagnostic procedure. Procedures such as IV or retrograde urograms or open bone biopsies should *not* be performed unless urine production is ample and hypercalcemia and hyperuricemia have been corrected.

Hyperviscosity syndrome occurs in about 50% of cases in which the monoclonal immunoglobulin is IgM (Waldenström's macroglobulinemia). The syndrome is uncommon in multiple myeloma with other immunoglobulin classes. Purpura, ecchymoses, epistaxis, gastrointestinal bleeding, blurred vision (resulting from venous congestion, intraocular hemorrhages, and exudates), and ischemic neurologic symptoms are common. Neurologic symptoms and signs in multiple myeloma include mental confusion from hypercalcemia, spinal cord and nerve root compression, myelomatous meningitis, carpal tunnel syndrome from amyloid deposits, and sensorimotor polyneuropathy not due to amyloid or plasma cell infiltration. Less commonly, CNS symptoms may result from intracerebral plasmacytomas, herpes zoster, and multifocal leukoencephalopathy.

Diagnosis

Virtually all patients have normochromic-normocytic anemia. Elderly patients with unexplained normochromic-normocytic anemia should be evaluated for multiple myeloma. Many also have thrombocytopenia in the range of 80,000 to 130,000/μL and leukopenia in the range of 3000 to 4000/μL.

Multiple myeloma is diagnosed by the presence of osteolytic bone lesions or osteoporosis, monoclonal proteins in serum, and > 10% mature and immature plasma cells in the bone marrow. Daily excretion of light chains (Bence Jones protein) into the urine of > 60 mg/24 hours and serum levels of monoclonal protein > 2 g/dL are highly suggestive of multiple myeloma. If bone marrow plasmacytosis is not demonstrated along with these findings, repeated bone marrow aspirations and a search for an extraskeletal plasma cell tumor should be undertaken. Idiopathic monoclonal components may occur with other cancers.

Prognosis and Treatment

Once a diagnosis of multiple myeloma is made, the patient may be classified as a good or a poor risk. Good-risk patients have laboratory values of Hb $\geq$ 9.0 g/dL, serum creatinine < 2 mg/dL (< 177 μmol/L), and calcium $\leq$ 12 mg/dL ($\leq$ 3 mmol/L) after hydration. With therapy, the good-risk group has a median survival of 42 months; the poor-risk group, only 21 months. The groups respond equally well to initial therapy. In some good-risk elderly patients, the disease progresses slowly (smoldering myeloma). If the patient is asymptomatic or only mildly symptomatic, the disease can be followed over time to determine its pace. Occasionally, elderly patients with advanced-stage multiple myeloma do well.

Because multiple myeloma is a disseminated neoplastic disorder, the mainstay of treatment is chemotherapy. Many chemotherapeutic regimens are used for multiple myeloma. In elderly persons, the two most common regimens are intermittent melphalan with prednisone and low-dose continuous melphalan. In the intermittent regimen, the dosage of melphalan is 0.25 mg/kg/day po for 4 days, and the dosage of prednisone is 2 mg/kg/day for 4 days. This dosage is repeated every 4 to 6 weeks, depending on the degree of bone marrow suppression. In the continuous regimen, the patient is generally first given melphalan 8 to 10 mg/day for about 1 week (loading dose). The dosage is then reduced to 2 mg/day but must be adjusted frequently, depending on bone marrow sensitivity. In the very old, the loading dose is usually reduced to 4 mg/day for 1 week.

Radiation is useful for localized tumor burden and is widely used to relieve back pain from osteolytic lesions. Large osteolytic lesions should be irradiated before fractures occur. A fracture through a lytic lesion requires placement of an intramedullary pin and radiation therapy. However, if back pain results from extensive demineralization of bone, radiation usually will not relieve it, and chemotherapy should be begun promptly.

A variety of experimental therapies are available. In severe cases, mini-autologous bone marrow transplantation is being attempted up to age 75, depending on the patient's functional status. High-dose chemotherapy and bone marrow transplantation have been successful in younger patients, even though the malignant clone of plasma cells is rarely eliminated. The use of high-dose pulse dexamethasone seems to be as effective as more toxic combination chemotherapy regimens. Cyclosporine may reverse drug-resistance. Maintenance therapy with interferon can be used for the patient who has achieved a stable tumor level (as measured by M protein).

All patients should be encouraged to stay active to prevent further bone demineralization. Lumbar corsets and braces may help relieve pain and reduce the risk of pathologic fractures. All infections must be treated promptly. Patients must drink sufficient fluid (2 to 3 L/day) to increase urine output and increase the excretion of light chains, calcium, uric acid, and other metabolites. Hydration with saline or saline plus furosemide IV may also be used temporarily. Hyperuricemia should be treated with allopurinol 300 mg/day. For hyperviscosity, treatment with plasmapheresis may be effective in the short term.

Hypercalcemia is usually treated with pamidronate (90 mg diluted in 500 mL of sterile 0.45% or 0.9% sodium chloride or 5% dextrose administered over a 4-hour period on a monthly basis) and corticosteroids (40 to 100 mg for 4 to 5 days). This combination of drugs is also used in patients with osteolytic lesions, even without hypercalcemia. Vigorous saline hydration is an integral part of treatment. The patient's blood volume must be adequate prior to therapy, particularly if there is Bence Jones proteinuria. *Pamidronate should never be mixed with a calcium-containing solution (eg, Ringer's lactate) and should be given in its own separate IV line.* An alternative—calcitonin 4 to 8

IU/kg sc q 12 h, often with corticosteroids—can be used, but it is very expensive. Plicamycin 25 μg/kg IV over 4 to 6 hours may be used if pamidronate and calcitonin fail. Sodium or potassium phosphate 2 g/day may also be useful in some patients with mild or moderate hypercalcemia.

End-of-Life Issues

Multiple myeloma involves a great deal of pain and is ultimately fatal. Because this disease occurs mainly in the elderly, treatment protocols were devised with this age group in mind. Treatment, therefore, is not a harder burden for the elderly to bear compared with younger patients. However, treatment eventually fails, and death is inevitable. It is essential to prepare the patient for dying and to discuss such issues as advance directives, resuscitation, feeding tubes, and pain relief.∎

MONOCLONAL GAMMOPATHY OF UNDETERMINED SIGNIFICANCE

The presence of M protein in the serum or urine of asymptomatic, apparently healthy persons.

Monoclonal gammopathy of undetermined significance—usually a benign disorder—is a likely diagnosis in a patient with elevated serum levels of monoclonal protein but with no other symptoms and neither osteolytic lesions nor plasma cell infiltration. Confirming findings for this diagnosis include no significant amounts (ie, < 60 mg/24 hours) of a single type of light chain (ie, Bence Jones protein) in the urine and serum levels of monoclonal protein < 2 g/dL.

Only time will determine if a diagnosis of monoclonal gammopathy of undetermined significance is really early multiple myeloma. Over 20 years, about 25% of patients initially diagnosed with monoclonal gammopathy develop overt multiple myeloma or other lymphoproliferative lesions. No evidence indicates that not treating these patients is harmful.

WALDENSTRÖM'S MACROGLOBULINEMIA

(Primary Macroglobulinemia)

A neoplastic disorder in which there is a proliferation of B cells that produce an M protein of the IgM class.

Waldenström's macroglobulinemia is an uncommon disease with an incidence of about one tenth that of multiple myeloma.

∎see pages 115 and 134

Etiology and Pathophysiology

The etiology is unknown, but the etiologic associations are similar to those of multiple myeloma.
Lymphocytic infiltration of the bone marrow crowds out the normal hematologic elements, producing cytopenic complications, such as anemia. Abnormal B cells produce large amounts of IgM proteins. The manifestations of the illness frequently result from high plasma viscosity resulting from increased levels of these IgM proteins in the plasma.

Symptoms and Signs

Plasma hyperviscosity leads to visual changes, CNS symptoms, heart failure, acute myocardial infarction, and strokes. Infections, bleeding, and anemia (eg, with resulting pallor, weakness, vertigo) are a consequence of lymphocytic infiltration of the bone marrow. Bone pain and lytic lesions are not common. Lymphadenopathy and hepatosplenomegaly are common. Retinal hemorrhages and vascular segmentation in the retinal vessels (sausage links) are characteristic. A history of cold sensitivity or Raynaud's phenomenon may be associated with a cryoglobulin or a cold agglutinin. The course of the illness is similar to that of a low-grade B-cell lymphoma with bone marrow involvement.

Diagnosis

Waldenström's macroglobulinemia is diagnosed when there is both a B-cell lymphocyte proliferation and an overproduction of a monoclonal IgM. In contrast to multiple myeloma, there is no plasma cell proliferation and no bone destruction.

The serum protein electrophoresis shows a sharp protein peak, with gamma motility. Serum immunoelectrophoresis demonstrates that the M protein is an IgM. Urine immunoelectrophoresis frequently reveals a monoclonal light chain (usually κ), but gross Bence Jones proteinuria is rare. Osteolytic lesions are not usually found. The bone marrow shows a variable increase in lymphocytes and plasmacytoid lymphocytes. Lymph node biopsy usually resembles a diffuse well-differentiated B-cell lymphoma. Serum viscosity commonly is elevated and must be treated.

Other laboratory findings include moderate anemia, high ESR, and rouleaux formation of RBCs on peripheral blood smear. Leukopenia, relative lymphocytosis, and thrombocytopenia occasionally occur. Cryoglobulins, rheumatoid factor, and cold agglutinins may be present. A variety of platelet and coagulation abnormalities may be found.

Prognosis and Treatment

The prognosis is variable, but the course tends to be much more benign than in multiple myeloma. When hyperviscosity is controlled, the course seems to be similar to that of CLL. Hyperviscosity is treated by plasmapheresis. Daily plasma exchanges of 3 to 4 L are recommended until the patient is asymptomatic. Chemotherapy is reserved for patients who have symptoms due to lymphomatous spread. Chlorambucil is the mainstay of chemotherapy; the regimens are identical to those used in CLL.⬛ Fludarabine is sometimes effective for patients refractory to chlorambucil. Regimens identical to those used to treat multiple myeloma have also been used.⬛

MYELODYSPLASTIC SYNDROMES

A heterogeneous group of syndromes in which the hematopoietic precursors are abundant but morphologically abnormal.

The actual incidence of the myelodysplastic syndromes is not known, but they are fairly common in the elderly. Ineffective erythropoiesis, which is a key feature of these syndromes, increases with age, and in some studies, up to 20% of people > 65 have unexplained refractory anemia. The syndromes are twice as common in men and are rare in persons < 40.

Etiology and Pathophysiology

In most patients, the cause is unknown, but prior treatment with alkylating agents increases the risk of developing a myelodysplastic syndrome—the longer a patient is treated, the greater the risk. Myelodysplastic syndrome tends to progress into acute myelogenous leukemia (AML); a protracted myelodysplastic syndrome lasting up to 20 years precedes 5 to 10% of cases of AML. The AML that develops in 2 to 7% of patients treated with alkylating agents is invariably fatal. This progression, a long-term complication of successful chemotherapy, may become more prevalent as more patients survive. Chemotherapeutic drugs that are not alkylating agents (eg, methotrexate, hydroxyurea) do not seem to produce this complication.

Other possible causes of myelodysplastic syndromes include RNA viruses, somatic mutations, radiation, environmental toxins, and autoimmune mechanisms. Yet, the ability of any of these factors to induce myelodysplasia may be enhanced by aging. Accumulated genetic mutations from various causes, including aging, are more likely to result in dysplastic and malignant change than are single genetic insults, a concept sometimes called the multihit theory. Familial instances of myelodysplastic syndromes are rare.

Myelodysplastic syndromes are thought to arise from an undefined cytopathologic alteration of the pluripotential hematopoietic stem cell

⬛ see page 728   ⬛ see page 732

pool, evolving from the clonal expansion of a single stem cell (or a very small number of stem cells). The major pathophysiologic consequence is ineffective hematopoiesis caused by defective maturation of marrow precursor cells. Proliferation of progenitor and early precursor cells is usually normal or enhanced (creating a hypercellular marrow). However, circulating mature cells are deficient; they also have a slightly shorter life span, which contributes to cytopenia.

Classification

Exact characterization is difficult; refractory anemia often progresses to a refractory dysmyelopoietic anemia involving the red cell, white cell, and megakaryocytic lines.

The syndromes are classified by morphologic criteria. In refractory anemia and refractory anemia with ringed sideroblasts,◧ platelets and WBCs are usually normal. In refractory anemia with excess blasts, chronic myelomonocytic leukemia, and refractory anemia with excess blasts in transformation, all three cell lines are often abnormal. These terms have generally replaced the term preleukemia, because only about 10 to 30% of patients with a myelodysplastic syndrome develop an acute leukemia.

Symptoms and Signs

Because cytopenia develops slowly, many patients are asymptomatic, and the diagnosis is made incidentally or the anemia is falsely attributed to aging. Symptomatic patients generally seek medical care for symptoms of anemia, thrombocytopenia, or leukopenia, such as fatigue, decreased exercise tolerance, purpura, fever, or infections. Hepatomegaly occurs in about 5% of patients, splenomegaly in about 10%, and pallor in about 50%. Often the patient complains of arthralgias.

Most patients have increased iron stores, and many have clinical hemochromatosis with diabetes, cirrhosis, infiltrative heart disease, and pituitary dysfunction.

Diagnosis

The hallmark of myelodysplastic syndromes is anemia with reticulocytopenia. The RBC morphologic appearance is usually abnormal. The RBCs are usually dimorphic; some cells are microcytic and hypochromic, and others are normochromic and normocytic or macrocytic. At first analysis, laboratory values may result in the anemia being classified as normochromic-normocytic, but the red cell distribution width will likely be elevated. Basophilic stippling, target cells, schistocytes, siderocytes, and nucleated RBCs often appear.

◧ see page 683

Leukopenia is moderate; the WBC count ranges from 1000 to 4000/μL. Neutropenia is more pronounced than lymphopenia. The neutrophils are often sparsely granulated, and the acquired Pelger-Huët nuclear anomaly (hypolobulation of the nuclei of mature neutrophils) may be present. Neutrophil alkaline phosphatase activity may be low. Granulocytes often function abnormally, which further impairs resistance to infection. Monocytosis occurs in 30% of patients, which may elevate serum and urinary lysozyme levels. Thrombocytopenia is common, although occasionally, patients have thrombocytosis. The platelets may have functional defects. Immature myeloid cells may be present in the peripheral blood smear.

Diagnosis is made by histologic examination of a bone marrow aspirate and biopsy. Erythroblasts may have double or fragmented nuclei or intranuclear bridging; budding, ringed sideroblasts may be prominent. These are usually found in patients with abnormalities in the RBC precursors. With primarily erythroid dysplasia, the ratio of myeloid to erythroid precursors (M:E ratio) is between 1:1 and 1:10 (normal is 3:1). Dyserythropoiesis results in moderately elevated levels of serum lactic dehydrogenase and indirect bilirubin.

Marrow myeloid cells may show immature to mature neutrophils, may have the acquired Pelger-Huët nuclear anomaly, and are often sparsely granulated. Eosinophils and basophils may also be dysplastic. In patients with primarily myeloid dysplasia, the M:E ratio is between 3:1 and 20:1. Megakaryocytes may be immature and dysplastic as well.

Reticuloendothelial iron is increased, as are the serum iron and ferritin levels. Iron stores are increased in most patients. Iron turnover rate is increased, but incorporation of iron into circulating erythrocytes is decreased, indicating ineffective erythropoiesis.

Prognosis

Prognosis is highly variable, with survival ranging from a few months to 15 years. The median survival is about 3 years. Although about 10 to 30% of patients die as a result of acute blastic transformation (AML), individual prognosis cannot be predicted. Patients with primarily erythroid dysplasia are at lower risk than those with involvement of the other cell lines.

Treatment

Transfusion of blood products is the mainstay of treatment but should be limited and given only if the patient is symptomatic from the anemia or is in danger of cardiac compromise. Transfusing packed RBCs risks iron overload; alloimmunization to RBC, WBC, and platelet antigens; and transmission of various infections. Washed RBCs may slow the development of alloimmunization. Platelets should be transfused only if the patient is bleeding or if surgery is needed. Granulocyte colony-stimulating factor is used in neutropenic patients. Granulocyte transfusions should be given only to neutropenic patients with documented gram-negative infections that are unresponsive to antibiotics alone.

Occasionally, patients with ringed sideroblasts**1** respond to pyridoxine 100 to 200 mg/day po. However, the response is only partial, and an abnormal RBC morphologic appearance usually persists. Androgens and corticosteroids have benefited a small number of patients. Recombinant hematopoietic growth factors including erythropoietin have been tried, but no consistent improvement has been shown in those whose serum erythropoietin level is lower than expected for the measured Hct. Continuous overnight (12-hour) IV or subcutaneous administration of deferoxamine by portable pump should be considered when the patient is receiving blood transfusions monthly or more often. A convenient regimen is 2 g of deferoxamine given sc over 12 h by portable infusion pump for 5 days/week.

Chemotherapy as early treatment of myelodysplasia with excessive blasts has not increased survival. Administering low-dose cytarabine to induce differentiation of blasts is controversial. For patients who develop AML, the remission rate is even lower than for patients with leukemia who did not previously have myelodysplasia. Patients with this secondary form of AML have prolonged marrow aplasia after chemotherapy. One approach in the elderly consists of giving supportive care with blood products and attempting to keep the WBC count < 50,000/μL by giving hydroxyurea 10 to 80 mg/kg/day po.

End-of-Life Issues

Seventy to ninety percent of patients with myelodysplasia will not die of the illness. However, in the patients with an increasing percentage of blasts and decreasing RBCs, WBCs, and platelets, the likelihood of AML transformation is great. The AML that develops is usually totally refractory to treatment. These patients and their families will need help in preparing for a rapid death.**2**

74 ■ LYMPHOMAS

Primary malignancies of the lymph nodes.

The major types of lymphoma—Hodgkin's disease and non-Hodgkin's lymphoma—are distinct entities characterized by different cells of origin, patterns of spread, and clinical manifestations. Hodgkin's disease usually has a predictable pattern of spread to contiguous lymph node areas; non-Hodgkin's lymphoma is usually widespread at diagnosis and is more likely to involve extranodal areas. Both

---

1 see page 683   **2** see page 115

can be subdivided into types based on the histologic appearance of the lymph nodes.

Patient and End-of-Life Issues

Some lymphomas are curable with radiation and/or intensive combination chemotherapy. Age alone is not a consideration for whether or not to recommend therapy; however, comorbidity is often a consideration. Patients and their families should be informed that treatment is usually long and uncomfortable and should weigh potential benefits against risks. To ease care, elderly patients who live alone usually need help at home as they undergo therapy. Therapy often weakens the patient for at least 6 months, and some degree of independence must be suspended.

If treatment is unsuccessful or if the disease relapses, the prognosis is poor and the hope for a cure dwindles. A continuing dialogue with the physician and a support system of family and friends are helpful. Supportive and palliative measures are often the goals of treatment. ∎

HODGKIN'S DISEASE

Localized or disseminated malignant proliferation of tumor cells arising from the lymphoreticular system, primarily involving lymph node tissue and the bone marrow.

The annual incidence of Hodgkin's disease is 2/100,000 in the USA. There is a bimodal age distribution, with an initial peak between ages 15 and 35 and a second peak between ages 50 and 80. At age 75, incidence is 7/100,000 annually, slightly higher in men. Hodgkin's disease is more common in people at higher socioeconomic levels. Geographic, occupational (woodworkers), and family clusters of Hodgkin's disease have been noted.

Etiology and Pathophysiology

The cause of Hodgkin's disease is unknown. However, seroepidemiologic studies suggest that the Epstein-Barr virus may be involved. Patients with immunodeficiencies and autoimmune disease are at increased risk (suggesting that the immune system plays a role), as are those taking hydantoin drugs, such as phenytoin.

Histologically, Hodgkin's disease is subdivided into four major types: lymphocyte-predominant (mainly lymphocytes with few Reed-Sternberg cells); mixed cellularity (a cellular response of mature lymphoid cells, plasma cells, eosinophils, and Reed-Sternberg cells); lymphocyte-depleted (few lymphoid cells with a majority of histiocytes,

∎ see page 115

fibrotic reaction, and Reed-Sternberg cells); and nodular sclerosis (effacement of lymphoid structure by nodular aggregates of mature lymphoid cells and lacunar variants of Reed-Sternberg cells separated by bands of birefringent collagen).

In all types, normal lymphoid tissue is replaced by the malignant lymphoma, resulting in immunodeficiency and infections. The bone marrow may be replaced, resulting in pancytopenia and subsequent bleeding and infection. Tumor bulk may obstruct or invade vital organs, ultimately causing death.

Symptoms and Signs

Patients with Hodgkin's disease usually present with enlarged lymph nodes in the neck. The lymph nodes may be painful or tender, and drinking alcohol may make them more so. Although any nodal group can be involved, the central or axial lymph nodes are most commonly affected. The patient may be asymptomatic (when the disease is clinically staged as A) or may have fever, night sweats, or loss of ≥ 10% of body weight (stage B). These systemic symptoms are often associated with extensive disease. Patients with extensive disease may also present with diffuse adenopathy and involvement of the spleen, liver, bone marrow, or lungs.

Diagnosis

The diagnosis is made when biopsy of a lymph node reveals the histologic picture of Hodgkin's disease. Fundamental to the diagnosis is the histologic finding in the lymph node of the giant Reed-Sternberg cell, which usually has twin nuclei and nucleoli that give it the appearance of owl's eyes. The Reed-Sternberg cell is probably the malignant cell, and the surrounding cells probably represent tissue reaction.

Clinical staging in Hodgkin's disease is extremely important in determining treatment. The currently accepted stages are listed in TABLE 74–1. Clinical staging is based on a complete physical examination with special attention to all lymph node areas. Laboratory studies include a routine blood chemistry profile and CBC count and CT scans of the abdomen, pelvis, and, in some cases, the chest. Lymphangiograms via the pedal lymphatics to outline the femoral, inguinal, pelvic, and paraaortic nodes are being replaced by positron emission tomography, spiral CT scans, and MRI. In cases in which the clinical stage may change the treatment modality, laparotomy including splenectomy, liver biopsies, and biopsies of grossly suspicious lymph nodes are performed as needed. A bone marrow biopsy is required only if the findings will affect treatment. A staging laparotomy, by providing additional findings, results in a change in clinical and pathologic stages in up to 30% of patients. In the elderly, Hodgkin's disease is more likely to present as advanced disease (stage III or IV). Some authorities

TABLE 74–1.   CLINICAL STAGING OF HODGKIN'S DISEASE*

Stage	Definition
I	Disease limited to one anatomic region
II	Disease in two or more anatomic regions on the same side of the diaphragm†
III	Disease on both sides of the diaphragm but limited to lymph nodes, spleen, and Waldeyer's tonsillar ring‡
IV	Extranodal disease not contiguous to a nodal area, ie, bone marrow, lung, pleura, liver, plus disease above the diaphragm

*All stages are subclassified as A if the patient is asymptomatic or B if the patient has unexplained fever, night sweats, or loss of ≥ 10% of body weight.

† In stage II disease, the number of lymph node regions involved may be indicated by a subscript.

‡ Stage III disease may be subdivided by anatomic distribution of abdominal involvement. Stage III₁ indicates involvement that is limited to the upper abdomen above the renal vein. Stage III₂ indicates involvement of pelvic and/or para-aortic nodes.

believe that patients > 40, particularly those with mixed cellularity or lymphocyte depletion, may not benefit from the findings gained by laparotomy.

Prognosis

Hodgkin's disease is often curable, even though older age is an unfavorable prognostic factor because the elderly cannot tolerate as much chemotherapy and have more concomitant illnesses. The 5-year survival rate for patients < 40 is about 80%; for those 40 to 60, 60%; and for those > 60, about 30%. Other unfavorable prognostic signs are bulky disease, high serum lactic dehydrogenase (LDH) levels, and extranodal involvement. However, the stage at the time of treatment is by far the most predictive of outcome. Hodgkin's disease in the elderly may have a different etiology than that occurring in the young, since elderly patients often present with stage IV disease and a greater number of unfavorable prognostic signs. Alternatively, aging might alter the presentation.

Before the introduction of potentially curative treatment, the lymphocyte-predominant and nodular sclerosis types carried better prognoses than the other types.

Treatment

Elderly persons in advanced stages do not do as well as younger persons because they are usually unable to tolerate maximum doses of radiation and chemotherapy.

Recommendations for treatment depend on stage (see TABLE 74–2). However, the regeneration of bone marrow after radiation therapy or

TABLE 74-2.   TREATMENT RECOMMENDATIONS FOR PATIENTS WITH HODGKIN'S DISEASE

Stage	Therapy	Disease-Free Survival (%) for All Ages
IA, IIA, and II₁A*	Mantle and para-aortic irradiation†	90
III₁A	Total nodal irradiation	50
	Chemotherapy and extended field irradiation†	85
IB and IIB	Similar to IA and IIA therapy‡	80–90
III₂A and IIIB	Chemotherapy and involved field irradiation§	80–85
IVA and IVB	Chemotherapy with or without irradiation of bulk disease	25–40

*Local extension into an organ from a lymph node but otherwise meeting criteria for IIA.
†If the mediastinal mass is > 1/3 the diameter of the chest, combined modality therapy consisting of chemotherapy and mantle irradiation is preferable to radiation alone.
‡Some authorities now use chemotherapy for stage IIB disease.
§Some authorities reserve chemotherapy for stage IV disease and use only radiation therapy for stages I to III. The overall disease-free intervals are similar.

chemotherapy is markedly diminished in patients > 40, and the gastrointestinal (GI) side effects are much more severe. Thus, consideration should be given to limiting the usual field of radiation in elderly patients with early-stage disease. Similarly, administering the optimum dose of chemotherapy may be impossible in elderly patients, even though the benefit of aggressive therapy generally outweighs the risk. Many elderly patients can tolerate only 30 to 50% of the optimum doses of chemotherapy, although the survival rate of patients given less than the optimum doses is dramatically lower.

The most frequently used regimens in the elderly are MOPP, British MOPP, and ABVD, each of which consists of four drugs (see TABLE 74–3). The duration of chemotherapy is 6 to 8 months or for at least 2 months after complete remission. The incidence of a second malignancy (usually acute leukemia or non-Hodgkin's lymphoma) increases in patients who have Hodgkin's disease and who are receiving or have received chemotherapy, especially when combined with total nodal irradiation.

Hemolymphopoietic growth factors can sometimes be used to help overcome loss of normal lymphatic cells, which occurs through destruction of lymphoid tissue by lymphoma. Fifteen of these factors have been characterized; three of them—erythropoietin, granulocyte colony-stimulating factor (G-CSF), and granulocyte-macrophage colony-stimulating factor (GM-CSF)—are commercially available.

TABLE 74-3.   CHEMOTHERAPY FOR HODGKIN'S DISEASE

Regimen*	Dosage
MOPP	
Mechlorethamine (nitrogen mustard)	6 mg/m² IV on days 1 and 8
Oncovin (vincristine)	1.4 mg/m² IV on days 1 and 8†
Prednisone	40 mg/m²/day po on days 1 to 14 (cycles 1 and 4 only)
Procarbazine	100 mg/m²/day po on days 1 to 14
British MOPP (ChlVPP)	
Chlorambucil	6 mg/m²/day po on days 1 to 14
Vinblastine	6 mg/m² IV on days 1 and 8
Prednisone	40 mg/m²/day po on days 1 to 14
Procarbazine	50 mg/m²/day po on days 1 to 14
ABVD	
Adriamycin (doxorubicin)	25 mg/m² IV on days 1 and 15 (do not exceed 550 mg/m² total—450 mg/m² if patient received radiation therapy)
Bleomycin	10 mg/m² IV on days 1 and 15 (do not exceed 200 mg/m² total)
Vinblastine	6 mg/m² IV on days 1 and 15
Dacarbazine	375 mg/m² IV on days 1 and 15

*Each regimen is given every 28 days until there is complete response, after which 2 additional cycles are given for a minimum of 6 and a maximum of 8 cycles.
† Maximum dose, 2.5 mg.

Human G-CSF is also used in patients who are receiving myelosuppressive anticancer drugs, which can cause severe neutropenia. The recommended starting dose is 5 µg/kg/day sc or IV. The use of G-CSF varies with different chemotherapeutic regimens. Human GM-CSF has been used mainly after bone marrow transplantation and, therefore, no data exist in the elderly. The use of other growth factors (including all the interleukins) is still experimental.

NON-HODGKIN'S LYMPHOMA

Malignant monoclonal proliferation of lymphoid cells in sites of the immune system, including lymph nodes, bone marrow, spleen, liver, and GI tract.

In the USA, the annual age-adjusted incidence of non-Hodgkin's lymphomas (NHLs) ranges from 2.6 to 5.8/100,000. Increasing incidence with age is similar to that of acute leukemia. At age 80, the annual incidence is about 40/100,000.

The NHLs are a heterogeneous group of lymphoid malignancies that share certain features. Classification of NHLs is controversial and has undergone many revisions. Currently, there are two complementary approaches: one based on descriptions of lymph node architecture and histologic features (see TABLE 74–4) and the other based on the use of immunologic markers. A new classification based on immunologic markers and histologic features is shown in TABLE 74–5.

Etiology and Pathophysiology

The cause of most NHLs is unknown. However, immunosuppressed patients (eg, renal transplant patients) and patients with abnormally high immune function (eg, those with collagen-vascular disease) are at greater risk, as are those taking hydantoin drugs (eg, phenytoin), suggesting that the immune system plays a role. A virus is involved in at least some cases. Burkitt's lymphoma, endemic in Central Africa, is

TABLE 74–4. HISTOLOGIC CLASSIFICATION OF NON-HODGKIN'S LYMPHOMAS

Classification	Working Formulation	Rappaport Classification
Low-grade	Small lymphocytic	Well-differentiated lymphocytic lymphoma or chronic lymphocytic leukemia
	Plasmacytoid lymphocytic	Waldenström's macroglobulinemia
	Follicular small cleaved lymphocytic	Nodular poorly differentiated lymphocytic lymphoma
	Mixed follicular small cleaved cell and large cell lymphocytic	Nodular mixed lymphoma
Intermediate-grade	Follicular, predominantly large cell	Nodular histiocytic lymphoma
	Diffuse small cleaved cell	Diffuse poorly differentiated lymphocytic lymphoma
	Diffuse large cells (cleaved or noncleaved)	Diffuse histiocytic lymphoma
High-grade	Diffuse large cell immunoblasts (B cell, T cell, polymorphous, epithelial cell component)	Diffuse histiocytic lymphoma
	Lymphoblastic, convoluted or nonconvoluted	Lymphoblastic lymphoma
	Small noncleaved, Burkitt's or non-Burkitt's	Diffuse undifferentiated lymphoma

TABLE 74-5.   REVISED CLASSIFICATION OF NON-HODGKIN'S LYMPHOMAS

B Cell

1. Precursor B-cell neoplasms (pre–B-cell lymphoblastic leukemia/lymphoma)
2. Peripheral B-cell neoplasms
   a. B-cell CLL/small lymphocytic lymphoma
   b. Lymphoplasmacytoid lymphoma/immunocytoma
   c. Mantle cell lymphoma
   d. Follicle center lymphoma, follicular
      Small cell
      Mixed small and large cell
      Large cell
      Diffuse, predominantly small cell
   e. Marginal zone B-cell lymphoma
      Extranodal (MALT ± monocytoid)
      Nodal (± monocytoid)
      Splenic (± villous)
   f. Hairy cell leukemia
   g. Plasmacytoma/myeloma
   h. Diffuse large B cell
   i. Primary mediastinal B-cell subtype
   j. Burkitt's lymphoma

T Cell

1. Precursor T-cell neoplasms
   a. T-cell lymphoblastic lymphoma/leukemia
2. Peripheral T-cell and NK-cell neoplasms
   a. T-cell CLL/prolymphocytic
   b. Large granular lymphocyte leukemia
      T cell
      NK cell
   c. Mycosis fungoides/Sézary syndrome
   d. Peripheral T-cell lymphoma
      Mixed medium and large cell, lymphoepithelioid
   e. Angioimmunoblastic T-cell lymphoma
   f. Angiocentric lymphoma
   g. Intestinal T-cell lymphoma (± enteropathy)
   h. Adult T-cell lymphoma/leukemia (HTLV-I)
   i. Anaplastic large cell lymphoma
      CD30+ cell
      T cell
      Null cell

CLL = chronic lymphocytic leukemia; HTLV-I = human T-cell lymphotropic virus type I; MALT = mucosa-associated lymphoid tissue; NK = natural killer.

associated with Epstein-Barr virus infection. An aggressive T-cell leukemia-lymphoma is associated with human T-cell lymphotropic virus type I (HTLV-I) infection in Japan and the Caribbean. Patients with HIV often develop aggressive NHL.

In the pathophysiology of NHL, normal lymphoid tissue is replaced by the malignant lymphoma, resulting in immunodeficiency and infections. The bone marrow may be replaced, resulting in pancytopenia and subsequent bleeding and infection. Tumor bulk may obstruct or invade organs, ultimately causing death.

Symptoms and Signs

NHL appears to be multicentric in origin and is often widespread at presentation. A leukemic phase, detectable by peripheral blood testing, may occur. Most patients initially seek medical care because of cervical or inguinal lymph node enlargement. However, the skin, GI tract, bone, liver, and central nervous system constitute up to 10 to 20% of the primary sites of lymphoma at presentation. Occasionally, splenomegaly, bone marrow failure, autoimmune hemolytic anemia, and autoimmune thrombocytopenia are presenting features. Systemic symptoms (fever, night sweats, loss of weight, pruritus) are not as common as in Hodgkin's disease. Waldeyer's tonsillar lymphatic ring is commonly involved in patients with GI lesions. Hypercalcemia is prominent in HTLV-I–related NHL but is rare in other types. Hypogammaglobulinemia may occur. However, occasionally a monoclonal serum M spike is found on serum protein electrophoresis and on immunoelectrophoresis.

Diagnosis

The diagnosis is made by a biopsy of a lymphatic site revealing the histologic features of malignant lymphoma. Clinical staging of NHL is similar to that of Hodgkin's disease, although a staging laparotomy is rarely required because the illness is usually disseminated when discovered. After a complete physical examination, CBC, blood chemistry profile, bone marrow aspirate, lymph node biopsy, chest x-ray, and abdominal CT scan, about 90% of patients are found to have stage III or IV disease. Other studies (eg, serum protein electrophoresis, skeletal x-rays, IV urography) are sometimes useful.

Prognosis and Treatment

In NHL, indicators of a good prognosis are nodular histologic pattern, limited stage, low number of extranodal sites, and younger age. Marrow involvement is a poor prognostic sign for high-grade lymphomas but not for low- or intermediate-grade lymphomas. Other poor prognostic signs are poor performance status, bulky abdominal disease, Hb < 12 g/dL, and serum LDH > 250 U/L. The rapidity of response to chemotherapy also predicts survival.

Chemotherapy has the potential to cure only patients with intermediate- and high-grade lymphomas. Paradoxically, aggressive therapy does not even prolong survival of patients with low-grade lymphomas, even though these tumors are extremely sensitive to chemotherapy. Therefore, therapy should be minimal with low-grade tumors and aggressive with intermediate- and high-grade tumors. Hemolymphopoietic growth factors may also be used.**1**

Low-grade lymphomas: In stage I or II disease, often no therapy is indicated. The disease at these stages usually is asymptomatic, except in patients with lymphadenopathy. The clinical course of low-grade NHL is identical to that of chronic lymphocytic leukemia.**2** Particularly in the elderly, a practical approach is to withhold treatment and to monitor closely until problems of progressive disabling constitutional symptoms clearly due to the NHL develop (ie, progression to stages III and IV). Regional radiation can be used in stage I or II disease to reduce the local bulky nodes and any resulting compromise of vital organs. Since most of these patients relapse despite regional radiotherapy, chemotherapy may be indicated to prevent relapses and to reduce disabling constitutional symptoms. However, even without chemotherapy, the disease is usually so indolent that it does not recur for 5 to 10 years.

In stages III and IV, most patients experience only lymphadenopathy. Although most patients respond to chemotherapy, the relapse rate is 10 to 20% annually. Even though 80 to 90% of patients with favorable prognostic histologic findings achieve a complete remission, only 10 to 20% are without disease after 10 years. Thus, it seems wise to avoid both the serious systemic toxicity inherent in aggressive combination chemotherapy and the risk of acute nonlymphocytic leukemia caused by chronic low-dose alkylating agents. Chemotherapeutic treatment is reserved for patients with progressive disabling constitutional symptoms. Most oncologists use a single alkylating agent (eg, chlorambucil 0.4 mg/kg as a single dose for 1 day every 28 days). This so-called pulse therapy has less myelotoxicity and, perhaps, less leukemogenic potential. Some physicians use relatively mild combination chemotherapy regimens (see Table 74–6). Local radiation can be used to reduce bulky nodes.

Intermediate- and high-grade lymphomas: These aggressive NHLs are rapidly growing tumors with a short natural history. In elderly patients with intermediate- and high-grade lymphomas who have good functional status and normal organ function, curative combination chemotherapy is generally feasible. In those elderly patients with poor functional status and cardiopulmonary, renal, or central nervous system impairment, chemotherapy is poorly tolerated and rarely successful. Clearly, the physician must weigh all of these factors before recommending chemotherapy.

Regimens developed specifically for the elderly are available. One such regimen, as shown in Table 74–6, uses cyclophosphamide, doxorubicin, procarbazine, bleomycin, vincristine, and prednisone

TABLE 74-6. CHEMOTHERAPY FOR NON-HODGKIN'S LYMPHOMAS

Regimen	Dosage
Low-grade lymphomas*	
CVP (COP)	
Cyclophosphamide	750 mg/m² IV on day 1
Vincristine (Oncovin)	1.4 mg/m² IV on day 1†
Prednisone	100 mg/m²/day po on days 1 to 5 (CVP)
	60 mg/m²/day po on days 1 to 5 (COP)
C-MOPP	
Cyclophosphamide	650 mg/m² IV on days 1 and 8
Vincristine (Oncovin)	1.4 mg/m² IV on days 1 and 8†
Prednisone	40 mg/m²/day po on days 1 to 14
Procarbazine	100 mg/m²/day po on days 1 to 14
Intermediate and high-grade lymphomas‡	
CAP/BOP§	
Cyclophosphamide	650 mg/m² IV on day 1
Doxorubicin (Adriamycin)	50 mg/m² IV on day 1
Procarbazine	100 mg/m² po on days 1 to 7
Bleomycin	10 mg/m² sc on day 15
Vincristine (Oncovin)	1.4 mg/m² IV on day 15†
Prednisone	100 mg/day po on days 15 to 21

* Cycles are repeated every 21 to 28 days.
† Maximum dose, 2 mg.
‡ One-third reduction of myelosuppressive drugs for patients > 70.
§ Regimen is repeated every 21 to 28 days or when absolute granulocyte count is > 2.0 × 10⁸/L. The patients are restaged after 3 cycles and if in complete remission, 2 more cycles are given. If only in partial remission, another 2 cycles are given and the patient is restaged, always continuing to 2 cycles past complete remission or to a maximum of 9 cycles.

(CAP/BOP). However, doxorubicin is not well tolerated by the elderly (nor is methotrexate because it causes renal complications). Nearly identical complete remission rates were found for patients > 60 and those < 60 treated with this regimen. The toxicity was the same in both age groups, as was the duration of remission. Overall survival was 62% for those < 60 but only 35% for those > 60. However, most of the excess morbidity was related to factors other than lymphoma.

SECTION 10

PULMONARY DISORDERS

75   AGING AND THE LUNGS

The effects of aging on the lungs are physiologically and anatomically similar to those that occur during the development of mild emphysema.∎ Although aging affects ventilation, gas exchange, compliance, and other parameters of lung function as well as the defense mechanisms of the lungs, pure age-related changes do not lead to clinically significant airway obstruction or dyspnea in the nonsmoker. However, in smokers and ex-smokers with emphysema, dyspnea worsens with age.

Pulmonary Compliance

Pulmonary compliance is the change in lung volume per unit change in elastic recoil pressure. Age-related changes in ventilation and gas

∎ see page 779

distribution result primarily from changes in compliance of the lungs and the chest wall.

At about age 55, the respiratory muscles begin to weaken. In addition, the chest wall gradually becomes stiffer, probably as a result of age-associated kyphoscoliosis, calcification of intercostal cartilage, and arthritis of the costovertebral joints. Weakened outward muscular force combined with increased stiffness of the chest wall (decreased compliance) is counterbalanced by a loss of elastic recoil of the lungs (increased compliance), which probably results from a decrease in the number of parenchymal elastic fibers. Airway size decreases with age, and the proportion of collapsible small airways increases.

The increased outward pull of the stiffer chest wall combined with the reduced ability of the lung to pull inward results in a small increase in functional residual capacity (the volume at which the lung comes to rest at the end of a quiet expiration) and residual volume (the volume that remains in the lung after a maximal expiration). Total lung capacity remains fairly constant.

With age, the diaphragm may weaken by up to 25%. Without concurrent disease, this weakening is not usually relevant. However, in the presence of disease that requires high minute ventilation, such as pneumonia, this weakening predisposes the elderly to serious respiratory problems.

Rates of Airflow

Airway collapse is prevented by intra-alveolar pressure generated by the elastic recoil of the lung. Age-related loss of this elastic recoil results in early collapse of poorly supported peripheral airways, which in turn may result in decreased flow at low lung volumes, similar to the small airway obstruction produced by long-term cigarette smoking (see FIGURE 75–1).

The forced expiratory volume in 1 second (FEV_1) decreases by about 30 mL/year in men and 23 mL/year in women after about age 20. The annual decline in FEV_1 is small at first but accelerates with age. The forced vital capacity (FVC) decreases as well, by about 14 to 30 mL/year in men and 15 to 24 mL/year in women.

The decreases in FEV_1 and FVC that occur until age 40 are thought to result from changes in body weight and strength rather than from loss of tissue. With age, airway obstruction may also be partially due to an accumulation of inflammatory injuries. It is not certain whether the decreases in FEV_1 and FVC that occur after age 40 are due to aging itself or to the cumulative effects of respiratory illness, smoking, or exposure to environmental toxins. For example, cigarette smoking repeatedly disrupts inflammatory mediators, humoral protection (elastase and antielastase, oxidant and antioxidant), neutrophil recruitment, and tissue repair, culminating in inflammatory lung destruction and air-

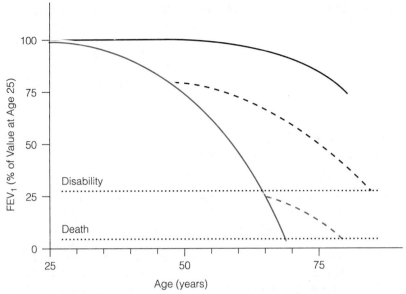

FIGURE 75–1.   Smoking cessation and risk of chronic obstructive pulmonary disease (COPD). Solid black line indicates the expected decline in the forced expiratory volume in 1 second (FEV_1) that occurs with age in patients who have never smoked or are not susceptible to smoke. Solid red line indicates the expected decline in FEV_1 that occurs with age in patients who smoked regularly and are susceptible to the effects of smoke. Dotted black line indicates the expected decline in FEV_1 that occurs with age in patients who stopped smoking at age 45 (these patients are at risk of mild COPD). Dotted red line indicates the expected decline in FEV_1 that occurs with age in patients who stopped smoking at age 65 (these patients are at risk of severe COPD). (Adapted from Fletcher C, Peto R: "The natural history of chronic airflow obstruction." *British Medical Journal* 1:1646, 1977.)

way obstruction. Accumulated environmental oxidant injuries could produce the same type of damage.

In most pulmonary conditions, survival parallels preservation of ventilatory function. In the elderly with diseases that cause airway obstruction (except chronic bronchitis), there is a higher mortality from concurrent diseases (eg, cardiovascular disease) as compared with younger adults. Airway obstruction increases the risk of death from chronic obstructive pulmonary disease (COPD) and heart disease and increases the risk of lung cancer.

Diffusing Capacity

Diffusing capacity (the ability of the lung to transfer gases between the lung and the blood) peaks in persons in their early 20s and then declines; from middle age onward, it declines at a rate of about 2.03

mL/minute/mm Hg per decade in men and at a rate of about 1.47 mL/minute/mm Hg in women. This decline results from decreased surface area caused by destruction of alveoli, increased alveolar wall thickness, and small-airways closure; these changes lead to ventilation and perfusion inequality. Estrogen may slow this decline in women aged 25 to 46, presumably because of preserved vascular integrity; the effects of estrogen replacement therapy on this decline in postmenopausal women is unknown.

Partial Pressure of Oxygen

The linear deterioration of the partial pressure of oxygen (Pa_{O_2}) that occurs with aging (about 0.3%/year) is estimated by the equation $Pa_{O_2} = 109 - (0.43 \times age)$. However, after age 75, the Pa_{O_2} level of healthy nonsmokers remains stable at about 83 mm Hg.

The gradual decline in Pa_{O_2} that occurs with age parallels the decrease in elastic recoil and the increase in physiologic dead space. These changes may lead to the collapse of peripheral airways, which decreases ventilation to distal gas exchange units but with much less effect on perfusion. This ventilation/perfusion imbalance accounts for most of the reduction in Pa_{O_2}. Also, lower cardiac output in the elderly results in increased tissue oxygen uptake, decreased mixed venous oxygenation, and, consequently, decreased Pa_{O_2}.

Control of Breathing

Heart rate and ventilatory responses to hypoxia and hypercapnia diminish with age because of diminished responsiveness of peripheral and central chemoreceptor function and integration of central nervous system pathways with age. Age also decreases neural output to respiratory muscles and lowers chest wall and lung mechanical efficiency. As a result, the ventilatory response to hypoxia is reduced by 51% in healthy men aged 64 to 73 compared with healthy men aged 22 to 30; the ventilatory response to hypercapnia is reduced by 41%. These reductions increase the risk of developing diseases that produce low oxygen levels (eg, pneumonia, COPD, obstructive sleep apnea). Effects are even greater in persons who are deconditioned.

Exercise Capacity

Maximal oxygen consumption ($\dot{V}_{O_2}max$) is the body's ability to maximally deliver oxygen to the tissues. It is the standard measurement of physical work (exercise) capacity. Work capacity increases during childhood, peaks in the late teens, plateaus until the mid-20s, then gradually declines. The gradual decline in oxygen delivery is 32 mL/minute/year in men and 14 mL/minute/year in women. The increase in work capacity that occurs during childhood results from the growth of muscle, heart, and lungs, and the decline results in part from gradual reductions in maximal heart rate and muscle mass that occur with age. The reduced $\dot{V}O_2$max in elderly persons may be due in part to cardiovascular deconditioning associated with lower levels of habitual physical activity or from changes in cardiovascular function. Although pulmonary function measurements such as FEV_1 decline with age, reduced ventilation seldom limits exercise in healthy persons. The ventilatory response to exercise (ie, breathing rate or minute ventilation at maximal exercise) is actually increased in the elderly and may compensate for inefficient gas exchange. Regular aerobic training can substantially slow the decline in $\dot{V}O_2$max.

The age-related decrease in aerobic exercise capacity is due only in part to pulmonary changes. It is predominantly due to altered cardiovascular responses,[1] which may result from a sedentary lifestyle, a decreased left ventricular ejection fraction, a lower maximum heart rate, decreased myocardial contraction, and a decreased response to β-adrenergic stimulation.

Defense Mechanisms

Clearance mechanisms: With age, the rate of mucociliary transport declines, although the effect of decreased clearance on clinical infection has not been proved. More significantly, loss of an effective cough reflex occurs in $> 70\%$ of elderly patients with community-acquired pneumonia (compared with only 10% of age-matched controls). Loss of cough reflex is likely due to the prevalence in the elderly of conditions associated with reduced consciousness, such as sedative use and neurologic diseases. Dysphagia or impaired esophageal motility, conditions that occur more often in old age, may exacerbate the tendency to aspirate.

Cellular detoxification: Cumulative oxidant exposure may lead to an age-related decline in lung function. Multiple enzymes and antioxidants have been the subject of much recent research because of their effect on lung injury and repair. For example, preliminary results show that intake of vitamin E (an antioxidant) may be associated with a significantly higher FEV_1 and FVC.

Immunity: The acute antibody response to extrinsic antigens, such as pneumococcal and influenza vaccines, is considerably reduced with age.[2] The age-related decline in cellular immunity correlates with an increasing incidence of secondary tuberculosis (reactivation tuberculosis).

[1] see page 815   [2] see page 1358

PNEUMONIA

An inflammatory reaction to microbes or to microbial products involving the pulmonary parenchyma.

Pneumonia is one of the most common and significant health problems in the elderly. It is the 4th leading cause of death and the leading infectious cause of death in this age group. Pneumonia is often the terminal event after prolonged serious illness; it has been called the "old man's friend."

The annual incidence in the elderly varies from 20 to 40/1000 for community-acquired pneumonia to 100 to 250/1000 for pneumonia acquired in long-term care facilities. At any given time, an estimated 2.1% of elderly residents of long-term care facilities have pneumonia. Nosocomial pneumonia is common among hospitalized elderly patients who have undergone thoracic or abdominal surgery, mechanical ventilation, or tube feeding.

The major risk factor for developing pneumonia in the elderly is the presence of other serious illness. Additionally, the likelihood of a serious outcome with pneumonia, including death, is directly related to the number of comorbid illnesses; the mortality rate increases from 9/100,000 without comorbidity to 217/100,000 with one high-risk condition and 979/100,000 with two or more high-risk conditions. Elderly patients are likely to experience more complications from pneumonia, such as bacteremia, empyema, and meningitis.

Etiology

The most common identifiable organisms causing pneumonia in the elderly are discussed below. In 30 to 50% of cases, no specific pathogen is detected. Colonization of the respiratory tract with potentially pathogenic gram-negative and gram-positive bacteria occurs more often in the elderly than in younger persons, owing in part to such factors as repeated antibiotic therapy, endotracheal intubation, smoking, malnutrition, surgery, and therapy that lowers gastric acidity, thereby raising pH.

Streptococcus pneumoniae: *S. pneumoniae* (causing pneumococcal pneumonia) is the most common bacterial cause of community-acquired pneumonia in the elderly. It accounts for 15 to 50% of all culture-diagnosed pneumonias in adults. The attack rate of pneumococcal pneumonia is estimated to be 46/1000 in persons > 65. Patients > 65 years are 3 to 5 times more likely to die of pneumococcal pneumonia than their younger counterparts.

Gram-negative bacilli: These pathogens are more common in institutional settings, where *Klebsiella, Pseudomonas aeruginosa, Enterobacter* sp, *Proteus* sp, *Escherichia coli,* and other gram-negative bacilli account for about 40 to 60% of all culture-diagnosed pneumonias. Gram-negative bacilli may colonize the posterior pharynx in debilitated and seriously ill patients.

Anaerobic bacteria: Anaerobes cause 20% of community-acquired and 31% of nosocomial cases of pneumonia in the elderly. Pneumonia caused by anaerobes usually results from aspiration. Elderly patients tend to aspirate because of conditions associated with aging that alter consciousness, such as sedative use and medical conditions (eg, neurologic disorders, weakness). Anaerobes frequently implicated include *Fusobacterium nucleatum,* black-pigmented anaerobes (formerly called *Bacteroides melaninogenicus*), peptostreptococci, peptococci, and, occasionally, *B. fragilis.*

Haemophilus influenzae: Strains of *H. influenzae* account for 8 to 20% of pneumonias in the elderly. These organisms are more frequent causes of pneumonia in patients with chronic bronchitis.

Legionella sp: Susceptibility to *Legionella* infections (5% of all culture-diagnosed pneumonias) increases with age. *L. pneumophila* accounts for about 85% of all *Legionella* pneumonias among the elderly, and *L. micdadei* for about 15%. Although legionnaires' disease occurs sporadically, outbreaks have been reported in hotels and hospitals.

Viruses: Viral causes of pneumonia in elderly patients include influenza and parainfluenza viruses, respiratory syncytial virus, and possibly adenoviruses. Parainfluenza viruses infrequently invade healthy adults; their relatively frequent occurrence among the elderly may reflect waning immunity.

Influenza is the most important cause of pneumonia in the elderly. Its incidence in persons ≥ 70 is about 4 times that in persons < 40. About 90% of influenza-associated deaths in the USA occur in persons ≥ 65. Secondary bacterial pneumonia may complicate a course of influenza.

Pathogenesis

Two major factors predisposing the elderly to pneumonia are oropharyngeal colonization and silent aspiration. Colonization of the oropharynx with various gram-negative bacilli is especially common among hospitalized and critically ill patients. Predisposing factors include poor oral hygiene; abnormal swallowing; increased adherence of gram-negative bacilli to mucosal cells; debility from cardiac, respiratory, or neoplastic diseases; decreased ambulation; and exposure to broad-spectrum antibiotics. Silent aspiration of oropharyngeal secretions is often related to alcoholism, use of sedatives or narcotics, cerebrovascular disease, esophageal disorders, and nasogastric intubation.

Microorganisms reach the tracheobronchial tree via four routes: inhalation, aspiration, direct inoculation from contiguous sites, and hematogenous spread. Inhalation and aspiration are the most common routes.

Inhalation pneumonia: Aerosolized pathogens inhaled into the lower airways as microparticles include *Mycobacterium tuberculosis, Legionella* sp, and the influenza virus. *M. tuberculosis* and the influenza virus are transmitted via aerosolized secretions produced by coughing. Although most cases of pneumococcal pneumonia are acquired by aspiration, in rare cases, especially in an epidemic, the organism is inhaled. *Legionella* infection is not transmitted from person to person, but rather, is acquired by inhaling infected aerosols from a waterborne source (eg, from air conditioners or shower heads). Waterborne organisms may also be introduced into the lower airways by instrumentation or delivered by small-particle aerosols from a contaminated reservoir nebulizer used with ventilation equipment.

Aspiration pneumonia: In community-acquired aspiration pneumonia, the usual pathogens are the anaerobic bacteria that normally reside in the gingival crevices (eg, peptostreptococci, fusobacteria, black-pigmented anaerobes). In nosocomial aspiration pneumonia, the usual pathogens are gram-negative bacilli, sometimes in association with anaerobes. Most cases of pneumococcal and gram-negative bacillary pneumonia presumably follow microaspiration, in which a fairly small inoculum of bacteria travels from the posterior pharynx into the lungs. Large-volume aspiration results in a relatively large inoculum of oropharyngeal bacteria into the lower airways and occurs with conditions that compromise consciousness or that cause dysphagia.

Symptoms, Signs, and Diagnosis

The characteristic clinical features of pneumonia—fever, cough, and sputum production—are often subtle and incompletely expressed in elderly patients. Only 33 to 60% of elderly patients present with a high fever. Instead, elderly patients with pneumonia commonly present with acute confusion or delirium and deterioration of baseline function. Tachypnea and tachycardia may be presenting signs.

Chest x-ray is usually diagnostic but does not indicate cause. Progression and multilobe involvement are seen more often in elderly patients. Leukocytosis with immature white blood cells develops less often in elderly patients. Blood cultures should routinely be performed.

The diagnosis should not be made based on expectorated sputum, because expectorated sputum does not distinguish colonization from true pulmonary infection. However, expectorated sputum is useful for culturing *M. tuberculosis,* pathogenic fungi (*Histoplasma, Blastomyces,* and *Coccidioides*), and *Legionella* sp. A gram stain of expectorated specimens may be useful if a predominance of one organism is seen along with a large number of neutrophils. Transtracheal aspiration (sputum sample removal through a cannula passed to the lower airways through a percutaneous puncture at the cricothyroid membrane), transthoracic aspiration, and fiberoptic bronchoscopy using a protected brush may produce reliable results but are rarely used in elderly patients for routine diagnostic evaluation. Obtaining a specimen for anaerobic culture and etiologic identification is often problematic because of contamination of the expectorated sputum specimens by the normal flora of the upper airways.

Prevention

Two types of pneumonia can be prevented—influenza and pneumococcal. A yearly influenza vaccine█ is highly protective. Even when the vaccine fails to prevent infection, the severity of disease and the frequency of complications are reduced. Pneumococcal vaccine█ is recommended for all persons ≥ 65. There is a 60% protection rate in immunocompetent adults. In healthy elderly persons, protection is presumed to be lifelong; thus, reimmunization is unnecessary. In high-risk elderly patients, however, including those with chronic renal failure, diabetes mellitus, heart failure, chronic obstructive pulmonary disease (COPD), or an underlying malignancy, reimmunization with pneumococcal vaccine is recommended every 6 to 10 years.

Treatment

Treatment includes antimicrobial drug therapy, respiratory and other forms of supportive care, and drainage of empyemas and large pleural collections.

Recommendations for antimicrobial drug use depend on the specific organism (see TABLE 76–1). They are similar across age groups, although the elderly require closer therapeutic monitoring. Potentially nephrotoxic drugs, primarily aminoglycosides, require close serum monitoring and frequent measurements of renal function and should be avoided unless a non-nephrotoxic drug cannot be used. Because elderly persons have reduced cardiac reserve, IV fluids and electrolytes and other forms of osmotic loading must be given cautiously. With age, the risk of antibiotic-associated diarrhea or colitis increases with ampicillin, cephalosporin, or clindamycin use. Antimicrobials may interact with other drugs (eg, warfarin) commonly used to treat the elderly. Sedatives that decrease deep inspiration and cough should be avoided.

Chest percussion and pulmonary hygiene measures are often useful in frail elderly patients with a diminished cough reflex. Such measures aid in clearing thick, inspissated secretions, thereby reducing the risk of mucous plugs, which often lead to lung collapse.

Patient and Caregiver Issues

Stable elderly patients with pneumonia who have no comorbid diseases can often be treated as outpatients. The caregiver's role is to

---

█ see page 1364   █ see page 1365

TABLE 76-1.   ANTIMICROBIAL DRUGS RECOMMENDED FOR SPECIFIC PNEUMONIAS

Causative Organism	Antimicrobial Drug
Streptococcus pneumoniae	Penicillin, 1st-generation cephalosporins, a macrolide, a fluoroquinolone (eg, levofloxacin)
Haemophilus influenzae	Cefuroxime, 3rd-generation cephalosporins, trimethoprim-sulfamethoxazole, levofloxacin
Pseudomonas aeruginosa	An antipseudomonal penicillin or ceftazidime plus an aminoglycoside (tobramycin or amikacin); sensitivity tests are required
Legionella sp	Erythromycin with or without rifampin, a newer macrolide, or a fluoroquinolone
Staphylococcus aureus	An antistaphylococcal penicillin (nafcillin or oxacillin), cephalothin, cefamandole, or vancomycin; vancomycin is preferred for methicillin-resistant strains
Gram-negative bacilli	3rd-generation cephalosporins, imipenem, or aztreonam; an aminoglycoside is often added; sensitivity tests are required
Anaerobic bacilli	Penicillin or clindamycin
Influenza A virus	Amantadine or rimantadine and an antibiotic if superimposed bacterial infection is suspected

ensure compliance with and completion of the treatment regimen. Frail and bedridden elderly patients for whom outpatient treatment is being considered may require home health care services.◧ Elderly persons often have an increased risk of delirium associated with infection, poor adherence with drugs, and polypharmacy, which can result in drug-drug interactions. Regular communication between the physician and the patient and caregiver should be emphasized.

End-of-Life Issues

Pneumonia in the elderly is often the terminal event of comorbid diseases such as diabetes mellitus, COPD, heart failure, malignancy, and dementia. Elderly patients with comorbidity are more likely to develop complications, eg, adult respiratory distress syndrome, empyema, and septic shock. In some cases, comfort measures may be more appropriate than antibiotics. Advance directives in such severe cases can often assist the physician in making appropriate decisions regarding resuscitative measures.◨ When palliative care is the goal, opioids often help patients with dyspnea.

◧see page 87   ◨see page 134

TUBERCULOSIS

An infectious disease caused by Mycobacterium tuberculosis.

In the USA, the number of reported cases of tuberculosis (TB) has declined since 1992. However, the number of cases among foreign-born persons residing in the USA is steadily rising, particularly in adults > 45. The elderly are especially at risk of infection; 20 to 30% of newly diagnosed cases of TB occur in persons ≥ 65. Elderly residents of long-term care facilities are at increased risk of reactivation of latent infection and are susceptible to new infection. About 90% of TB cases in the elderly are due to reactivation of a primary infection.

About 75% of all cases of TB in the elderly occur in the respiratory tract. Common extrapulmonary sites include the bones and joints, particularly the spine, and the genitourinary tract. Miliary TB, a form of disseminated TB, is also relatively common in the elderly.

Pathogenesis

Primary TB infection (ie, no previous exposure to *M. tuberculosis*) is acquired by inhaling droplet nuclei of viable organisms. Tubercle bacilli may evade the host immune mechanisms in the upper lung zones, brain and meninges, bone, and kidneys, often remaining dormant as long as the host immune system remains intact. Factors such as poor nutrition, homelessness, imprisonment, alcoholism or drug addiction, and immune dysfunction caused by disease, drugs, or aging can reactivate dormant bacilli. In the elderly, reactivation is often caused by diseases common to this age group (eg, diabetes mellitus, malignancies, chronic renal failure), poor nutrition, and the use of immunosuppressants, especially corticosteroids. The major component of the immune system affected by aging is T-lymphocyte–mediated responses,◻ although this component may not be entirely responsible for the increased susceptibility of the elderly to TB.

Some infected persons eventually eliminate the viable tubercle bacilli and revert to negative tuberculin reactor status. These persons have no lasting immunity and are thus susceptible to reinfection.

Persons who have contained the primary infection and who remain asymptomatic with a positive tuberculin skin test are described as having TB infection; those who have symptoms of infection are said to have TB disease. Persistent TB infection without disease occurs in 30 to 50% of cases. Some elderly persons who were previously infected with *M. tuberculosis* lose their cellular immune reactivity (as indicated by a negative tuberculin skin test) to the organism. Consequently, they are at risk of reinfection with *M. tuberculosis.*

◻ see page 1354

Symptoms and Signs

Pulmonary TB typically produces respiratory and systemic symptoms of cough, excessive sputum production, hemoptysis, fever, anorexia, weight loss, night sweats, and fatigue, although these symptoms are less common in the elderly.

Miliary TB may occur in elderly patients in either of two forms. The elderly are more likely to present with the nonreactive form, which is an overwhelming tuberculous infection consisting of numerous small caseous lesions with large numbers of replicating bacilli, sparse neutrophil infiltrate, and no granulomatous reaction. Clinical features include acute onset of fever, weight loss, hepatosplenomegaly, and, occasionally, fever of undetermined origin. The chronic hematogenous form consists of repeated episodes of low-grade *M. tuberculosis* bacillemia, with a slowly progressive protracted illness associated with low-grade fever without localizing symptoms or signs. Radiographic changes of miliary mottling may not be present.

Tuberculous meningitis in the elderly produces clinical features similar to those seen in younger persons, ie, headache, fever, weakness, and confusion. In addition, elderly patients may present with unexplained dementia or obtundation.

Tuberculous spinal infection may cause paravertebral abscesses. Presenting symptoms are pain over the involved vertebrae, fever, weight loss, and constitutional symptoms; in advanced cases, neurologic deficits or sinus tracts may develop.

Tuberculous arthritis can involve large weight-bearing joints, such as the hips, but in the elderly, other peripheral joints, such as the knees, wrists, ankles, and metatarsophalangeal joints, may be involved as well. Degenerative joint disease, common in the elderly, may make the diagnosis more difficult.

Genitourinary TB may involve any part of the genitourinary tract, including the kidneys, ureters, bladder, prostate, epididymis, and seminal vesicles. About 20 to 33% of patients with kidney involvement are asymptomatic. Symptoms, when present, include flank pain, dysuria, and gross hematuria. Abnormal urinary sediment, especially sterile pyuria and hematuria, is a common finding. Rarely, genitourinary TB involves the genitals, and the patient may present with a scrotal or pelvic mass or draining sinus and no systemic symptoms.

Other sites that may be affected by TB include the lymph nodes, pleura, liver, gallbladder, small intestine, large intestine, pericardium, middle ear, and carpal tunnel, although virtually any organ may be infected with *M. tuberculosis.*

Diagnosis

TB in the elderly often is difficult to diagnose because of nonspecific symptoms and clinical presentations that are often remote from the disease site. TB should be considered in the differential diagnosis in elderly persons who present with the clinical manifestations described above that involve specific organ systems, as well as in elderly persons with a mild decline in their health status, functional capacity, or state of well-being. Because chest x-rays may be atypical, some authorities recommend that any elderly person who requires hospitalization for pneumonia have at least one sputum culture for TB.

Tuberculin skin test: The Mantoux method of skin testing with polysorbate-stabilized purified protein derivative (PPD) antigen is the standard screening procedure for TB infection and reflects the delayed-type hypersensitivity response to *M. tuberculosis* antigen. A positive test result indicates that the person harbors viable organisms, although the test does not distinguish TB infection from TB disease. The dose of 5 tuberculin units is biologically standardized and routinely used for skin testing. The skin is examined 48 to 72 hours after intradermal PPD injection, at which time the diameter of induration is measured. The size of the induration reaction correlates to some extent with the probability of TB; induration of ≥ 10 mm is significant. A smaller reaction (5 to 10 mm of induration) is suspect in high-risk populations. The bacille Calmette-Guérin vaccine, which may have been administered to some foreign-born elderly persons in childhood, has an unpredictable effect on PPD skin test reactivity, but reactivity to the vaccine often wanes after 10 years.

Because skin-test reactivity to tuberculin wanes with time, a test that produces a negative result in the elderly should be repeated (using the same dose) a week later to detect the booster phenomenon. Most elderly patients with TB disease have positive test results. The higher-strength (250 tuberculin units) PPD test generally should be avoided, and patients with a history of having positive test results should not be retested.

Chest x-ray: Primary TB can involve any lung segment but usually involves the middle or lower lobes as well as the mediastinal or hilar lymph nodes. The usual sites of lung involvement for reactivated TB are the apical and posterior segments of the upper lobes and the superior segments of the lower lobes. However, the lower lung fields and anterior segment of the upper lobes may also be involved. Infiltrates in the elderly may be interstitial, lobar, patchy or cavitary, and bilateral.

Laboratory findings: Clinical specimens taken from suspected sites of TB are initially examined by smear to detect acid-fast bacilli and are subsequently cultured for *M. tuberculosis*. In the case of possible pulmonary or genitourinary involvement, three consecutive early morning sputum or urine specimens, respectively, are recommended for routine mycobacteriologic studies. Induced-sputum or bronchoscopic specimens may be needed for patients who cannot expectorate sputum. Sterile body fluids and tissues can be inoculated into a liquid medium, which allows growth and detection of *M. tuberculosis* 7 to 10 days earlier than the solid medium techniques.

On histologic examination, tissue that shows caseous necrosis with granuloma formation with or without acid-fast bacilli also strongly supports the diagnosis.

Polymerase chain reaction testing detects very small numbers of TB, may help increase the sensitivity of diagnosis, and may be used to predict drug resistance before standard results are available. The nucleic acid amplification test uses transcription-mediated amplification to detect *M. tuberculosis*–complex ribosomal RNA. Serologic tests for detecting antibodies against mycobacterial antigens have not been refined sufficiently for routine clinical use.

Prevention and Treatment

The Centers for Disease Control and Prevention (CDC) has established recommendations for surveillance, control, and reporting of TB in long-term care facilities and acute-care institutions. All new employees and new residents in long-term care facilities should undergo an initial skin test and then annual testing. The two-step PPD screening is recommended as part of the initial comprehensive assessment of all elderly patients. Chest x-rays are recommended for all persons who test tuberculin positive on admission to a long-term care facility to ensure that they do not have pulmonary infiltrates consistent with TB. In addition, the CDC recommends that all persons suspected of having TB have a chest x-ray, regardless of the primary site of infection.

TB infection: High-risk persons of any age who do not have active disease should undergo treatment of TB infection with isoniazid 300 mg/day po for 6 to 12 months. Persons considered to be at high risk are household members and other close contacts of potentially infectious persons; newly infected persons (those who have had a tuberculin skin test conversion within the previous 2 years); persons with positive skin tests and abnormal chest x-rays compatible with previous TB; and persons with positive skin tests and clinical situations favorable to infection, such as silicosis, diabetes, immunosuppression (including that resulting from corticosteroid administration and cancer chemotherapy), HIV-positive serologic findings, hematologic and reticuloendothelial malignancies, end-stage renal disease, and associated conditions characterized by rapid weight loss or chronic malnutrition.

TB disease: Patients with active TB require four antituberculous drugs, usually isoniazid, rifampin, pyrazinamide, and ethambutol. Treatment is given for 2 months, until sensitivity test results are available. All *M. tuberculosis* isolates should undergo sensitivity testing for resistance. Patients with strains of TB sensitive to isoniazid and rifampin should receive these drugs for an additional 4 months. Isoniazid and rifampin are usually effective because most elderly patients acquired their original strains many decades before, when most TB strains were susceptible to these drugs. A 9-month course of isoniazid and rifampin is also acceptable as an alternative therapy for most elderly patients. Pyridoxine 25 to 50 mg/day po is given to prevent peripheral neuropathy caused by isoniazid use. These recommendations are modified if in vitro sensitivity tests indicate infection with resistant strains.

All patients with TB should remain under observation until adherence with their treatment regimen is established. **Treatment monitoring** includes obtaining baseline measurements of liver enzyme, bilirubin, and serum creatinine levels; a CBC; and a platelet count or estimate. Serum uric acid concentration should be measured when pyrazinamide is used. Patients should be monitored at least monthly for symptoms suggesting hepatitis (eg, jaundice, fever, anorexia, dark urine), which is more common in the elderly and is a common adverse effect of isoniazid use. Testing liver function with aspartate transaminase is recommended, especially during the first 6 months of treatment, when hepatitis is most likely to occur. If transaminase levels increase $\geq$ 5 times higher than the upper limit of normal values, isoniazid should be discontinued. For patients with active disease, sputum should be examined at least monthly until cultures convert to negative. In about 90% of patients, cultures convert within 3 months of initiating the recommended regimens.

INFLUENZA

Infection with influenza A or B virus, which causes an acute febrile illness of the respiratory tract.

Infections with influenza viruses occur every year, either sporadically as local outbreaks or as a widespread epidemic. In the Northern Hemisphere, epidemics occur almost exclusively during December through April; in the Southern Hemisphere, during May through September. Attack rates during such outbreaks may be as high as 10 to 40% over 5 to 6 weeks. The overall annual risk of dying of influenza is about 1/5,000 to 1/10,000; death rates are higher among the elderly and among those with chronic diseases. Elderly persons, especially those with chronic medical conditions, account for at least 50% of all hospitalizations and for > 80% of all deaths attributed to influenza.

Influenza is transmitted via aerosol droplets expelled during coughing or sneezing. Low relative humidity and low environmental temperature foster the survival of airborne virus.

Symptoms and Signs

The clinical manifestations of influenza A and B viruses are similar. Influenza A is generally more severe and requires hospitalization much more frequently.

The classic syndrome is characterized by the abrupt onset of fever, chills, rigors, headache, myalgias, malaise, anorexia, sore throat, and a nonproductive cough. Early in the course of illness, the patient appears to be in a toxic condition: the face is flushed, and the skin is hot and moist. Prostration may occur in severe cases.

Fever is a consistent feature of influenza infection. Among elderly persons, fever is common, although the temperature may not rise as high as it does in children and young adults. The temperature usually rises rapidly within 12 hours on the first day of illness, concurrent with the onset of systemic symptoms. Myalgias may involve the extremities or the long muscles of the back. Lateral gaze may elicit pain in the eye muscles; photophobia and other ocular symptoms (including injected, watery, and burning eyes) occur in up to 20% of patients. Diarrhea occurs in < 5% of patients. Respiratory symptoms (ie, dry cough, a clear nasal discharge) are usually present at the onset of illness but are overshadowed by nonrespiratory symptoms. Nasal obstruction, hoarseness, and a dry or sore throat may also occur. Hyperemia of the mucous membranes of the nose and throat develops, but exudate generally does not. Most persons with influenza develop bronchitis without other involvement of the lower respiratory tract. Small, tender cervical lymph nodes develop in about 25% of patients.

On the 2nd and 3rd days of illness, as systemic symptoms and signs decline, respiratory symptoms and signs, especially cough, become more apparent. Scattered wheezes or localized crackles are observed in < 20% of patients. Elderly patients are often left extremely weak even after other symptoms resolve. Full recovery can take ≥ 2 weeks.

Complications

Pneumonia and severe bronchitis commonly accompany influenza in the elderly; the rate increases progressively in persons > 50 and is high in persons > 70. Pneumonia may be due to primary influenza viral infection or to secondary bacterial infection. ◼

Primary influenza pneumonia most often affects persons with cardiovascular disease, especially rheumatic heart disease with mitral stenosis. Other chronic illnesses may increase risk as well. Fever, cough, dyspnea, cyanosis, and hemoptysis may occur. Auscultation reveals fine inspiratory crackles and inspiratory and expiratory wheezes. Chest x-rays usually show diffuse perihilar infiltrates. The mortality rate associated with primary influenza pneumonia is high.

Patients at risk of **secondary bacterial pneumonia** include those with chronic pulmonary, cardiac, metabolic, or other chronic diseases. A classic influenza illness is followed by a period of improvement (4 to 14 days) before the clinical course worsens and symptoms and signs of

◼see page 758

bacterial pneumonia appear. The syndrome consists of fever, productive cough, and an area of decreased breath sounds and dullness to percussion. Chest x-rays show lobar or lobular infiltrates. Bacterial causes of pneumonia include pneumococcus, *Staphylococcus aureus*, *H. influenzae*, and other gram-positive and gram-negative organisms.

Many **nonpulmonary complications** have been described in patients with influenza, including myositis (sometimes with myoglobinuria and renal failure), myocarditis and pericarditis, toxic shock syndrome (probably from colonization of the trachea with *S. aureus*), Goodpasture's syndrome, and central nervous system complications, such as Guillain-Barré syndrome, transverse myelitis, and encephalitis. Anosmia and ageusia (loss of smell and taste) can develop and, although usually temporary, may last for months.

Diagnosis

The local or state health department or the CDC often can confirm that influenza virus is affecting a region or community. In such cases, most persons with fever, muscle aches, and cough are likely to have influenza.

Although rarely indicated, specific diagnostic procedures can be used to detect virus or viral antigens in respiratory secretions. Early in the course of illness, the virus can be isolated from nasal or throat swab specimens, nasal washes, or sputum; bronchoalveolar lavage and lung tissue specimens can also be used to isolate the virus. Positive results appear in about two thirds of cases within 3 days of testing and in the remainder of cases in 5 to 7 days. Virus can also be cultured by the inoculation of embryonated hens' eggs.

Serologic tests, although sensitive and specific, do not yield data within a clinically relevant time because sera must be obtained from convalescing patients at least 10 days after the onset of illness.

Prevention

Vaccination: Prevention of influenza is best accomplished by using inactivated virus vaccines.▪ All persons ≥ 65 and the medical personnel who care for them should receive the influenza vaccine annually. In addition, annual vaccination may be advisable for all persons who have extensive contact with elderly persons. Vaccination should be given several weeks before the start of the influenza season. In the USA, vaccination should be given in October, although it can be given throughout the influenza season until the late winter.

Efficacy rates for preventing influenza illness in the frail elderly are 30 to 70%; however, the vaccine is 50 to 60% effective in preventing hospitalization and pneumonia and about 75% effective in reducing

▪see also page 1364

deaths from influenza in hospitalized high-risk elderly patients. Diminished responses to the vaccine may occur in very elderly persons and in those who have renal failure or who are immunocompromised. The only contraindication to vaccination is hypersensitivity to hens' eggs. About 25 to 50% of patients have some discomfort at the vaccine site 8 to 24 hours after vaccination. About 1 to 2% of patients have fever or other systemic reactions. The vaccine cannot cause influenza or other respiratory infection.

Antiviral drugs: The new neuraminidase inhibitors oseltamivir and zanamivir appear effective in the prevention of influenza A and B. Amantadine and rimantadine provide prophylaxis against influenza A; their efficacy is about 75 to 90%. Rimantadine is as effective as amantadine in preventing clinical influenza and has a lower incidence of adverse effects. It is recommended for short-term (5 to 7 weeks) prophylaxis during a presumed outbreak of influenza A for unvaccinated persons and for vaccinated persons (especially those in a long-term care facility) who are becoming ill at a high rate. Prophylaxis may be particularly useful for unvaccinated residents of long-term care facilities. In addition, amantadine and rimantadine may be used to supplement protection in patients expected to have a poor antibody response to vaccination. Household contacts of a person infected with the virus may also be given prophylaxis, as may staff members and patients in hospitals or institutions, to prevent an outbreak. Use of these drugs should not exceed 2 weeks if vaccine is given simultaneously. The suggested dose for rimantadine for elderly persons without renal failure is 100 mg po once daily.

Treatment

Oseltamivir and zanamivir are effective for influenza A and B. These drugs must be given within 48 hours of symptom onset. They reduce symptom duration, including fever, by about 1 to 1.5 days, and substantially decrease viral shedding. These drugs lack CNS toxicity; however, oseltamivir may have GI adverse effects.

Amantadine and rimantadine can reduce the symptoms and signs of influenza A infection and shorten its course by 1 or 2 days if given within 48 hours of symptom onset. Neither drug inhibits influenza B virus. For healthy elderly persons with normal renal function, the usual dose of rimantadine is 100 mg/day po. When the index of suspicion is high (ie, during the winter months and when influenza has been reported in or near the community), patients who have an influenza-like illness and temperature > 37.8° C (> 100° F) are given rimantadine for 3 to 5 days even if they have been vaccinated.

Rimantadine is generally better tolerated than amantadine. Amantadine is associated with minor reversible CNS adverse effects, such as nervousness, insomnia, dizziness, and difficulty concentrating; such effects are common in the elderly, although they can occur with rimantadine as well. In patients with a known seizure disorder, seizures occur more often even when anticonvulsant therapy is maintained. In elderly persons with severe liver dysfunction, the apparent clearance of rimantadine is reduced by 50% compared with that of elderly patients with normal liver function; thus, this drug must be administered cautiously. In influenza viral pneumonia, these drugs may reduce peripheral airway resistance.

Adjunctive therapy for influenza includes measures to provide symptomatic relief. Patients should remain on bed rest and receive additional fluids. Aspirin or acetaminophen is effective in reducing fever.

Patient and Caregiver Issues

Elderly patients without comorbidity can be treated as outpatients, because the treatment of influenza is largely supportive. However, frail and bedridden elderly patients must be closely monitored for evidence of superimposed bacterial pneumonia. Caregivers should maintain communication with the physician in such cases.

In cases of poor family support, home health care **1** is generally an effective alternative to institutionalized care. Because severe influenza can be a terminal disease, issues regarding advance directives must be addressed. **2**

77 ■ PULMONARY EMBOLISM

An obstruction of the pulmonary arteries caused by a blood clot (embolus) or other material carried to the pulmonary vasculature by the circulatory system.

In the USA, pulmonary emboli and its primary cause, deep vein thrombosis, **3** are estimated to lead to 110,000 hospitalizations annually in patients > 65 years. Annual incidence rates per 1000 persons aged 65 to 69 are 1.3 and 1.8 for pulmonary emboli and deep vein thrombi, respectively. Both rates increase with age.

Because the symptoms and signs are nonspecific, pulmonary embolism may be overdiagnosed or underdiagnosed, especially in the elderly. Patients with cardiac and respiratory disorders are especially at risk of misdiagnosis.

Etiology

Although a blood clot is the most common cause of pulmonary embolism, air, fat, bone marrow, foreign bodies, arthroplasty cement, and tumor cells also can obstruct the pulmonary vessels.

---

1 see page 87   **2** see page 134   **3** see page 923

Bed rest and inactivity pose the greatest risk for developing deep vein thrombosis. Certain medical conditions common among the elderly (eg, trauma to leg vessels, obesity, heart failure, malignancy, hip fracture, myeloproliferative disorders) predispose them to venous thrombosis, as do smoking, estrogen use, tamoxifen therapy, the presence of a femoral venous catheter, surgery, and immobility. Risk factors for venous thrombosis are vessel wall injury, stasis, and conditions that increase the tendency of the blood to clot, including rare deficiencies of antithrombin III, protein C, and protein S as well as disseminated intravascular coagulation, polycythemia vera, or the presence of a lupus anticoagulant or antiphospholipid antibodies.∎ Aging is also associated with increased coagulation and products of fibrinolysis, resulting in an overall prethrombotic state.

About 90% of blood clots that cause pulmonary embolism originate in the legs. The risk that a clot will embolize and lodge in the lungs is greater if the clot is in the popliteal or iliofemoral vein (about 50%) than if it is confined to the calf veins ($< 5\%$). Less common sites of thrombosis that may lead to pulmonary embolism are the right atrium, the right ventricle, and the pelvic, renal, hepatic, subclavian, and jugular veins.

Symptoms and Signs

In elderly patients, the most common symptoms are tachypnea (respiratory rate > 16 breaths/minute), shortness of breath, chest pain that may be pleuritic, anxiety, leg pain or swelling, hemoptysis, and syncope. Patients who have small thromboemboli may be asymptomatic or have atypical symptoms. Nonspecific symptoms suggestive of pulmonary emboli in the elderly include persistent low-grade fever, change in mental status, or a clinical picture that mimics airway infection.

Patients with pulmonary embolism usually present with one of the following symptom patterns: (1) diagnostically confusing syndromes (confusion, unexplained fever, wheezing, resistant heart failure, unexplained arrhythmias); (2) transient shortness of breath and tachypnea; (3) pulmonary infarction (pleuritic pain, cough, hemoptysis, pleural effusion, pulmonary infiltrate); (4) right-sided heart failure along with shortness of breath and tachypnea secondary to pulmonary embolism; or (5) cardiovascular collapse with hypotension and syncope. Fewer than 20% of elderly patients have the classic triad of dyspnea, chest pain, and hemoptysis. If tachypnea is absent, pulmonary embolism is unlikely.

The most common physical findings are tachypnea, tachycardia, fever, leg edema or tenderness, cyanosis, and a pleural friction rub. Although most elderly patients with pulmonary embolism have deep

___

∎ see also pages 690–692

vein thrombosis ▯ as the initial source of the embolus, only 33% have clinical signs of leg thrombosis—eg, leg swelling, tenderness, increased warmth, and Homans' sign. About 33% of elderly patients with pulmonary embolism have pleural effusions, which are usually unilateral. About 67% of these effusions are bloody (red blood cell count > 100,000/mL) and must be distinguished from cancer and trauma. Patients with pulmonary embolism and a bloody pleural effusion generally have a pulmonary infiltrate on chest x-ray that suggests hemorrhagic consolidation of the lung parenchyma. The infiltrate usually resolves over several days. About 10% of patients with pulmonary emboli, especially those with severe heart failure, develop pulmonary infarction. The remainder of nonbloody effusions due to pulmonary embolism are exudates with elevated white blood cell counts (up to 75,000/mL) that mimic infected pleural effusions.

Syncope, a systolic blood pressure < 100 mm Hg, or a markedly decreased systolic blood pressure in a hypertensive patient suggests the possibility of a massive pulmonary embolism or, in a patient with marginal cardiopulmonary function, a significant embolus. Hypotension is ominous, because decreased aortic diastolic pressure may significantly reduce coronary artery blood flow to the overworked right ventricle, establishing a vicious circle.

A patient who is hypotensive because of pulmonary embolism has elevated right atrial and ventricular pressures (as measured by a pulmonary arterial catheter). Thus, a normal right atrial or ventricular pressure in a patient with hypotension argues against pulmonary embolism as the cause. An echocardiogram can help distinguish pulmonary embolism from right ventricular pressure overload, dissection of the aorta, pericardial tamponade, and myocardial infarction.

Diagnosis

The most important consideration for determining the extent of testing is the clinical assessment of pretest probability. The clinical pretest probability of pulmonary embolism places patients into low-, moderate-, or high-probability groups. This grouping is combined with the results of ventilation-perfusion scans or of spiral chest CT scans (see Laboratory Findings, below) to determine whether further testing is needed.

Patients with a normal ventilation-perfusion scan do not have pulmonary emboli, although about 1% have deep vein thrombosis, as determined by ultrasonography. Patients with a high-probability ventilation-perfusion scan and either a moderate or high pretest probability (about 10% of patients) almost certainly have pulmonary emboli and need treatment. Patients with a high-probability ventilation-perfusion

---

scan but a low pretest clinical probability (about 2% of patients) need to undergo bilateral venous ultrasonography. If the results are positive (about 20% of patients), the patient should receive treatment; if they are negative (about 80% of patients), pulmonary angiography is usually necessary.

If patients with indeterminate ventilation-perfusion scans have a high pretest clinical probability (about 3% of patients), they should undergo venous ultrasonography. If the ultrasonography results are positive (about 30% of patients), anticoagulation therapy is indicated. If results are negative (about 70% of patients), pulmonary angiography is indicated.

Patients with indeterminate ventilation-perfusion scans who have either a low or moderate pretest clinical probability should undergo ultrasonography. If the results are positive, treatment is indicated. If the initial ultrasonography results are negative and there is adequate cardiopulmonary reserve, then anticoagulation therapy is unnecessary. However, serial ultrasonography should be performed on day 3 and possibly on day 7. During a 3-month follow-up, these patients have a rate of venous thromboembolic events of about 1%, which is similar to the rate in patients with normal ventilation-perfusion scans and normal initial ultrasonograms.

Pulmonary angiography should be strongly considered if there is great discordance between clinical suspicion and the ventilation-perfusion scan. In general, the greater the risk of not treating the patient for pulmonary embolism or the greater the risk of therapy, the greater the need for definitive angiographic diagnosis. Of patients with a low pretest clinical probability, a high-probability ventilation-perfusion scan, and a negative ultrasonogram, 33% have an embolus. Of patients with a high pretest probability, an indeterminate ventilation-perfusion scan, and a normal venous ultrasonogram, 50% have an embolus, as detected by pulmonary angiography.

Laboratory Findings

A chest x-ray, an ECG, and arterial blood gas values should be obtained. If pulmonary embolism is still considered likely, the next step is usually to obtain a ventilation-perfusion lung scan. If the lung scan is likely to be indeterminate (because of underlying lung disease), spiral chest CT scans may be useful. Finding deep vein thrombosis with ultrasonography indicates the need for anticoagulation and usually eliminates the need for further testing for pulmonary emboli. The gold standard for diagnosing pulmonary embolism is pulmonary angiography.

Lung scan: Ventilation-perfusion scans are usually the first test done to confirm pulmonary embolism. They are interpreted as normal, high probability, or indeterminate probability. A normal scan shows no perfusion defect and excludes pulmonary embolism. A high-probability scan shows one or more segmental or greater perfusion defects with normal ventilation or two or more large subsegmental perfusion defects (> 75% of a segment) with normal ventilation. High-probability scans indicate a 90% probability of pulmonary embolism. Many scans are, however, indeterminate and thus neither confirm nor rule out pulmonary embolism.

Pulmonary angiography: This test is not needed in everyone. It is invasive, and the dye load can cause severe renal complications. It should be used only when its outcome will definitively change treatment. In patients with renal failure, gadolinium-enhanced magnetic resonance pulmonary angiography is a better alternative because it determines the anatomy without the risk of contrast nephrotoxicity.

Two findings are pathognomonic: a constant intraluminal filling defect and a sharp cutoff of a vessel > 2.5 mm in diameter. A single small embolus may be missed, but multiple emboli are rarely missed. Because most patients with pulmonary embolism have many emboli, the incidence of false-negative pulmonary angiograms is low.

Spiral chest CT scan: Spiral chest CT scans are excellent for detecting pulmonary emboli in the central pulmonary arteries (sensitivity, 94%; specificity, 94%; positive predictive value, 93%; negative predictive value, 95%). Spiral chest CT scans, however, do not detect emboli in subsegmental vessels (which occur in about 6 to 16% of patients). In patients with known cardiopulmonary abnormalities or abnormal chest x-rays, spiral chest CT scans may be preferred to ventilation-perfusion lung scans.

Chest x-rays: Results of chest x-rays may be normal or may show nonspecific abnormalities, eg, atelectasis, an elevated hemidiaphragm, pleural effusion, or an infiltrate. An enlarged pulmonary artery on one side, hyperlucency of one lung because of reduced pulmonary vascular markings, or a pleural-based pyramidal infiltrate that points toward the hilus (Hampton's hump) is uncommon. A chest x-ray cannot establish or exclude a diagnosis of pulmonary embolism but can help diagnose other conditions with similar symptoms (eg, pneumothorax, pneumonia, rib fracture, heart failure).

ECG: ECG findings are usually nonspecific; 33% of patients with pulmonary embolism have a normal ECG. The most common abnormal findings are sinus tachycardia and nonspecific ST-segment and T-wave changes. Uncommon changes that strongly suggest pulmonary embolism indicate strain on the right side of the heart; these changes include T-wave inversion in precordial leads V_1 through V_4, transient right bundle branch block, new right or left deviation of the QRS axis, sudden onset of atrial fibrillation or other atrial arrhythmia, and ECG signs of right ventricular hypertrophy or right atrial enlargement. The $S_1Q_3T_3$ pattern (prominence of S wave in lead I, Q wave in lead III, and T-wave inversion in lead III) also suggests pulmonary embolism. This pattern of right-sided heart strain is usually accompanied by T-wave inversion in the precordial leads.

Arterial blood gas studies: Pulmonary embolism often results in arterial hypoxemia because a low ventilation/perfusion ratio develops secondary to airway closure and bronchoconstriction in lung segments adjacent to the emboli. Intrapulmonary shunting of blood and a reduced mixed venous oxygen tension also contribute. Rarely, right-to-left shunting of blood occurs through a patent foramen ovale due to right atrial hypertension from massive pulmonary embolism.

An elevated alveolar-arterial gradient is nonspecific in the elderly population and is of minimal use in the diagnosis of acute pulmonary embolism. Conversely, a normal alveolar-arterial oxygen gradient does not exclude the diagnosis. However, a sudden decrease in partial pressure of arterial O_2 (Pa_{O_2}) that cannot be easily explained by another diagnosis is significant. If tachypnea is present, arterial blood gas values typically show a decrease in partial pressure of arterial CO_2 (Pa_{CO_2}).

D-Dimer: Levels of D-dimer, a fibrin-specific product, are increased in patients with acute thrombosis. About 60% of patients < 50 who are suspected of having a pulmonary embolus have an abnormal D-dimer result. In contrast, 92% of patients > 70 have abnormal D-dimer levels, probably due to comorbid conditions. Therefore, if D-dimer test results are negative, deep vein thrombosis or pulmonary embolism is unlikely, but positive test results are not useful in patients > 70.

Venous ultrasonography and venography: For patients with an indeterminate ventilation-perfusion scan, serial ultrasonography performed at 3, 7, and 14 days may help exclude extension of a calf vein clot.∎

Digital subtraction angiography, MRI, and fiberoptic angioscopy: These tests are under study and are not yet routinely used. Digital subtraction angiography and MRI are less invasive and use less dye than pulmonary angiography.

Prognosis

The mortality rate for hospitalized patients > 65 with pulmonary embolism is 21%. If pulmonary embolism is the primary diagnosis, the mortality rate is 13%; if it is a secondary diagnosis, the rate is 31%. Thus, many diseases and medical conditions—including heart failure, chronic obstructive pulmonary disease, cancer, myocardial infarction, stroke, and hip fracture—greatly increase the risk of death among hospitalized patients > 65 with pulmonary embolism. Prognosis is poorest for patients with severe underlying cardiac or pulmonary disease.

Pulmonary embolism is believed to recur in 5 to 10% of patients despite ongoing heparin therapy. The likelihood of recurrent emboli is greatest in patients who have massive pulmonary embolization or for

∎ see page 925

whom anticoagulant therapy is inadequate. If recurrence develops in the first few days of heparin or thrombolytic therapy, this treatment is usually continued.

In patients > 65 with a pulmonary embolus, the recurrence rate in the first year is 8%, and the 1-year mortality rate is 39% (21% inpatient mortality and an additional 18% mortality during the first year). Elderly patients with deep vein thrombosis but without pulmonary emboli have a 21% mortality rate in the first year. Recurrent pulmonary embolism leading to chronic pulmonary hypertension and cor pulmonale is uncommon.

Right ventricular hypokinesis, as identified by echocardiography, is present in about 60% of elderly patients with pulmonary emboli and a normal systemic arterial pressure. These patients have a twofold to threefold increase in mortality at 2 weeks, 3 months, and 1 year compared with patients with normal right ventricular function. The high incidence of right ventricular dysfunction in elderly patients may contribute to the high mortality rate.

Treatment

Supportive therapy includes providing supplemental O_2 to achieve a Pa_{O_2} of 60 to 70 mm Hg, providing adequate intravascular fluid to maintain cardiac output, monitoring the patient for evidence of bleeding due to anticoagulant therapy, and avoiding drugs that adversely affect platelet function (eg, aspirin, other cyclooxygenase blockers).

If the patient is hypotensive, treatment includes volume expanders, thrombolytics, and an infusion of norepinephrine to increase aortic diastolic pressure and maintain coronary artery blood flow. In patients for whom thrombolysis is contraindicated or unsuccessful, transvenous catheter embolectomy to fragment the clot should be considered. Rarely, immediate surgery to remove a large clot from a major vessel may be attempted, but the survival rate among elderly patients is low.

Heparin prevents clot formation and extension. ◘ Because the risk of death from pulmonary embolism is greatest in the first few hours of development of a clot and because diagnostic test results often are not available for 8 to 12 hours, heparin should be given to patients with a moderate to high clinical probability of pulmonary embolism or deep vein thrombosis until all diagnostic results are available. Low-molecular-weight heparin (LMWH) is preferred to unfractionated heparin. LMWH can be given subcutaneously once or twice a day, and laboratory monitoring may not be necessary.

Long-term anticoagulation is begun in the hospital with heparin and is continued after discharge, usually with **warfarin.** ◙

◘ see pages 697 and 926   ◙ see pages 698 and 928

Thrombolytic (fibrinolytic) therapy∎ should be considered for patients with deep vein thrombosis involving the iliofemoral system. It is also useful for patients with massive pulmonary embolism who have significant pulmonary hypertension, obstruction of multiple segments of the pulmonary circulation, right ventricular dysfunction, or systemic hypotension.

Clot lysis may reduce the incidence of recurrent thrombi and post-phlebitic syndrome and returns pulmonary arterial pressure to normal more quickly than does heparin therapy. Thrombolytic therapy also relieves strain on the right side of the heart more quickly than heparin does. However, thrombolytic therapy does not improve survival. Risks include hemorrhage, including an approximate 1 to 2% risk of intracranial bleeding. The hemodynamic response and the rate of bleeding are similar across age groups.

Contraindications to thrombolytic therapy include eye or central nervous system surgery within the preceding 2 weeks, intracranial neoplasms or vascular abnormalities, stroke within the preceding 2 months, active bleeding, severe hypertension, and allergy to thrombolytic agents. Age is not a consideration.

Interruption of the inferior vena cava∎—usually with a Greenfield filter—may be required in patients who have a contraindication to anticoagulation; who do not respond to anticoagulant therapy, as demonstrated by recurrent emboli; who have pulmonary emboli from septic thrombophlebitis; or who have massive embolization from a clot in the legs.

Endarterectomy may be helpful in patients who have chronic pulmonary hypertension due to a clot occluding the main or lobar pulmonary arteries.

Prophylaxis decreases the incidence of fatal pulmonary emboli by two thirds in hospitalized patients at risk of developing venous clots. LMWH (eg, enoxaparin 40 mg sc once daily) is as effective and safe as prophylaxis with subcutaneous heparin (5000 IU sc bid or tid) and may reduce drug-induced adverse effects. Postoperative prophylaxis with LMWH (eg, enoxaparin 30 mg sc q 12 h for up to 14 days) also dramatically reduces the incidence of venous thrombosis after knee or hip replacement. For total hip replacement, some investigators find that 4 to 6 weeks of LMWH postoperatively may be more effective.

End-of-Life Issues

In some clinical situations, a decision is made not to attempt prevention, diagnosis, or treatment of deep vein thrombosis or pulmonary embolism. Such a decision should be based on a thorough understanding of the patient's wishes and quality of life. Palliative care at the end of life is discussed in Ch. 13.

∎ see pages 700 and 929   ∎ see page 929

CHRONIC OBSTRUCTIVE PULMONARY DISEASE

A group of diseases, usually defined as including chronic bronchitis and emphysema, characterized by chronic airflow obstruction with reversible or irreversible components or both.

Chronic bronchitis is a clinical diagnosis and is characterized by a productive cough occurring most days of the month for at least 3 months of the year for 2 consecutive years. **Emphysema** is a pathologic diagnosis and is characterized by enlarged alveolar spaces and destructive changes in the alveolar walls that reduce the surface area for gas exchange.

Epidemiology and Etiology

The prevalence of chronic obstructive pulmonary disease (COPD) in North America may be as high as 10% in persons aged 55 to 85. Over the past 15 years, the incidence of COPD has risen more rapidly than that of any of the other nine leading causes of death. COPD ranks second to coronary artery disease as a Social Security–compensated disability.

About 3% of the U.S. population have chronic bronchitis, whereas 4 to 7% of elderly persons have it. About 1% of the U.S. population have emphysema. However, only 5% of persons with chronic bronchitis and about 40% of persons with emphysema have clinically significant airway obstruction.

A combination of genetic predisposition and environmental exposure leads to COPD. Cigarette smoking, the most common environmental risk factor, is believed to contribute to COPD in > 80% of cases. Pollution, occupational contacts, and other environmental exposures are less important contributors. Other risk factors for COPD include age, male sex, low socioeconomic status, and a history of significant childhood respiratory illnesses.

Pathophysiology

Cigarette smoking contributes to airway obstruction by causing an inflammatory reaction with or without mucus production in the airways; by promoting the influx of polymorphonuclear leukocytes, which release inflammatory mediators and elastases that break down lung elastin, leading to emphysema; and by inhibiting the body's endogenous elastase inhibitors.

Patients with chronic bronchitis have an increased number of mucous glands, smooth muscle hyperplasia, and reduced structural support of the airways. Pathologic changes of chronic bronchitis include increased peribronchial muscle, fibrosis, goblet cell metaplasia, and increased intraluminal mucus. Patients with severe emphysema may have large bullous lesions scattered throughout the lungs. The severity of emphysema correlates with airway obstruction.

Symptoms and Signs

The most common symptoms of COPD are cough, increased sputum production, dyspnea, and wheezing. Disabling symptoms worsen rapidly in elderly patients and are more common among men than women.

A productive cough usually begins several years after a person starts to smoke. The sputum is usually opalescent and varies in volume from < 1 teaspoon to several tablespoons. Larger quantities or color variations (eg, green, yellow) suggest infection or, less commonly, bronchiectasis. Especially in persons with osteoporosis, coughing can cause painful rib fractures.

Dyspnea, the most disabling symptom, usually begins after age 50 and worsens progressively. Large day-to-day variation in the degree of dyspnea may indicate bronchospasm. Dyspnea is more severe and more common among men. Wheezing, when present, is usually first noted when the patient is supine. Later, it may occur in any position and is usually associated with bronchospasm.

If hypoxemia develops, subtle signs of mental dysfunction, such as an inability to concentrate and reduced short-term memory, may occur. Hypercapnia may develop later and slowly lead to brain swelling and further dysfunction, resulting in confusion, lethargy, and increasing somnolence.

Signs of severe obstruction include pursed-lip breathing, which delays airway closure so that a large tidal volume can be maintained and respiratory muscles can function more efficiently; breathing in the sitting position with elbows resting on the thighs or a table, which may fixate the upper thorax and increase the curvature of the diaphragm, making breathing more efficient; and use of extrathoracic muscles (eg, the sternocleidomastoid).

Exacerbations of obstructive bronchitis in COPD patients usually result from infection with viruses, *Haemophilus influenzae,* or *Streptococcus pneumoniae.* Fever and leukocytosis may not appear. Worsening airway obstruction often leads to increasing dyspnea. Hypoxemia or hypercapnia accompanying a respiratory infection may lead to confusion and restlessness, which may be misinterpreted as an age-related change.

In severe COPD, two stereotypes—the pink puffer and the blue bloater—help define the extremes of the disease. Most patients have features of both stereotypes. The pink puffer is typically an asthenic, barrel-chested emphysematous patient who exhibits pursed-lip breathing and has no cyanosis or edema. Usually, such a patient uses extrathoracic muscles to breathe, produces minimal sputum, and experiences little fluctuation in the day-to-day level of dyspnea. Diaphragmatic excursions are reduced, and breath and heart sounds are distant. The barrel-shaped chest is nonspecific because elderly persons commonly have increased lung compliance and larger resting lung volumes. The blue bloater is typically overweight, cyanotic, and edematous and has a chronic productive cough. Elderly blue bloaters are uncommon because blue bloaters often have cor pulmonale, which rapidly leads to death if not treated appropriately.

Diagnosis

Chest x-rays are not sensitive in early or moderate COPD. Patients with chronic bronchitis may have normal chest x-rays or increased interstitial markings and enlarged pulmonary arteries. Patients with severe emphysema typically have a flattened diaphragm, a narrow heart, enlarged lungs, decreased peripheral vascular markings, and an increased retrosternal air space.

Spirometry (measured before and after an aerosolized bronchodilator treatment) documents the obstructive component of the disease. In early or moderate COPD, prolonged forced expiration (> 4 seconds) is the first clinically measurable change. Normal aging results in a gradual reduction (25 to 30 mL/year) of the forced expiratory volume in 1 second (FEV_1) and a slight increase in functional residual capacity (FRC) and residual volume (RV). Obstruction is present when the FEV_1 is $< 80\%$ of the forced vital capacity (FVC). Patients are usually not dyspneic until the FEV_1 approaches 1.5 to 1.75 L. With emphysema, a determination of lung volume by the helium dilution technique or body plethysmography shows an increased FRC and RV; with chronic bronchitis, FRC and RV may be near normal. The diffusing capacity is low in emphysema but is near normal in chronic bronchitis. An increased dead space is common in patients with emphysema.

Arterial blood gas levels are typically abnormal in moderate and severe COPD. Hypoxemia, when present, results from ventilation/perfusion mismatching because of bronchospasm, intrabronchial mucus, premature airway collapse, and destruction of alveoli. Hypoxemia may also result from reduced alveolar oxygen pressure with hypoventilation. When hypoventilation is present, hypercapnia also occurs. Chronic hypercapnia is confirmed by a near-normal blood pH and an elevated serum bicarbonate level. Care must be taken in diagnosing hypoxemia in elderly persons because the normal partial pressure of oxygen (Po_2) of a 75-year-old is about 75 mm Hg, compared with 100 mm Hg in younger persons.

Prognosis

COPD is the fourth leading cause of death in the USA. The mortality rate appears to be leveling off among white men but increasing among the elderly, women, and blacks. Mortality rates at age 55 are similar for both sexes but by age 85 are 3.5 times higher among men. Continuing to smoke worsens the prognosis. In smokers, FEV_1 decreases at a rate of 50 to 100 mL/year, and FEV_1 correlates with survival rate. An $FEV_1 > 1.5$ L is usually associated with a normal age-adjusted life span; an $FEV_1 \leq 1$ L is associated with an average survival of ≤ 5 years. Other conditions associated with a poor prognosis include resting tachycardia, ventricular arrhythmias, and hypercapnia.

Hospitalization for a COPD exacerbation in elderly patients is associated with an average survival time of 5 years, with women having a more favorable prognosis. Aging is associated with longer hospitalizations in COPD patients and a greater likelihood of discharge to institutional care. Therefore, assessment of likelihood of return to independent living and discharge planning should begin early in the hospitalization.

Longevity probably cannot be significantly improved with any treatment except for those with hypoxemia, who can benefit from supplemental O_2 therapy. However, close monitoring and intensive rehabilitation programs,█ including drug therapy and reconditioning through exercise, can improve quality of life and reduce the number of hospitalizations for elderly COPD patients as effectively as for younger patients.

Treatment

Treatment for chronic bronchitis and emphysema is palliative, not curative. It is considered successful when it produces a favorable balance between symptomatic relief and drug-related adverse effects. Clear written directions are important, because the COPD patient's cognitive skills may be impaired by hypoxemia and hypercapnia.

The primary goal is to maximize functional independence and avoid repeated hospitalizations. Respiratory compromise eventually leads to functional impairment and loss of independence, often accompanied by anxiety, lowered self-esteem, depression, role reversal, and sexual dysfunction. Education about exercise, nutrition, and avoidance of infections can help improve the patient's quality of life.

Cough and sputum: When coughing and sputum production are not caused by infection, avoiding irritants is the most important and effective therapy. Because cough is a natural protective mechanism, it should not be completely suppressed pharmacologically; however, forceful or frequent coughing can cause rib fractures or syncope. Over-the-counter drugs containing dextromethorphan often provide moderate cough suppression. When necessary, stronger narcotic derivatives may be used for short periods.

█ see page 806

TABLE 78–1.   REDUCING DYSPNEA IN ELDERLY PATIENTS WITH CHRONIC OBSTRUCTIVE PULMONARY DISEASE

Goal	Therapy
Strengthen respiratory muscles	Diaphragm-strengthening exercises: Patient lies supine with one hand on the abdomen and the other on the chest, then inhales deeply through the nose while concentrating on making the hand on the abdomen move upward, using the diaphragm. The patient breathes out through pursed lips. Placing a 5- to 8-lb book on the abdomen facilitates diaphragm movement during expiration and forces the diaphragm to work harder on inspiration. This exercise is performed for 10 to 15 min several times a day Adequate nutrition Use of theophylline preparations
Reduce the amount of respiratory muscle work	Dilation of the narrowed airways using bronchodilators, corticosteroids, and a regimen of pulmonary care, including mucus-thinning agents when indicated Low-carbohydrate, high-fat diet, which decreases CO_2 production, thereby decreasing ventilation
Reduce oxygen requirements	Aerobic conditioning exercises (simultaneous supplemental oxygen may be required for the patient to exercise long enough to benefit from the program)
Ensure adequate oxygen delivery	Instruction in pursed-lip breathing

Liquefaction and expectoration of sputum may be aided by adequate hydration and, occasionally, by potassium iodine solutions. The elderly tend to become dehydrated because of altered renal function and loss of the sensation of thirst, so they must be told to drink adequate amounts of fluids daily. Mucolytic drugs have not been proved effective when inhaled by patients with bronchitis, nor have expectorants been proved effective in removing secretions. Postural drainage after bronchodilator inhalation is effective only in patients with bronchiectasis.

Dyspnea: Dyspnea[1] is thought to result from respiratory muscle fatigue caused by an inappropriate amount of work for a given level of ventilation or hypoxemia. Therefore, attempts are made to strengthen respiratory muscles, reduce the amount of respiratory muscle work, reduce oxygen requirements, and ensure adequate oxygen delivery (see TABLE 78–1). Pursed-lip breathing may reduce dyspnea by allowing for

[1] see also page 116

more complete emptying of the lungs, which in turn allows the diaphragm to achieve a more efficient length. There is some evidence that blowing cool air with a fan on the cheeks of patients with COPD reduces the sensation of dyspnea.

Bronchospasm: A reversible component of bronchospasm is documented when spirometry shows a 15% improvement in FEV_1 after bronchodilator use. However, a lack of improvement in FEV_1 on a single test does not mean that a bronchodilator offers no therapeutic benefit.

Theophylline, besides being a bronchodilator, may also be a mild respiratory stimulant. In elderly patients, the half-life of theophylline preparations is prolonged; the proper dosage may be half the usual amount. Plasma levels should be checked at least every 6 months. Multiple drug interactions (eg, with warfarin) may occur.

Ipratropium bromide, an atropine derivative, is considered the inhaled drug of choice for patients with COPD and bronchospasm because it reverses bronchospasm and has few cardiovascular adverse effects. Rarely, patients with glaucoma or prostatic hypertrophy experience adverse effects and must stop taking the drug.

Inhaled β_2-sympathomimetics also are often effective. Long-acting ones may be preferable to short-acting inhaled or oral ones in the elderly because they are less likely to produce cardiovascular adverse effects. The disadvantage of hand-held, metered-dose, aerosolized delivery systems is that up to one third of persons > 65 cannot synchronize drug aerosolization with inspiration. Administration is helped by use of either a spacer, which is attached to the metered-dose inhaler, or a compressor nebulizer, which does not require patient coordination. A compressor nebulizer delivers a continuous fine mist of sterile saline mixed with a bronchodilator. However, it is more expensive and has not proved to be more effective. Breath-activated devices deliver a dry-powder medication.

Corticosteroids are beneficial during acute exacerbations of bronchospasm in elderly patients with severe COPD and may reduce the length of stay in the intensive care unit and in the hospital. Long-term systemic corticosteroid therapy (prednisone 10 to 20 mg/day or its equivalent) is also beneficial in selected patients with end-stage COPD in whom all other forms of therapy are ineffective. Prolonged use of high-dose corticosteroids should be avoided if possible because of the risk of osteopenia, cataracts, subcutaneous hemorrhage, hyperglycemia, cutaneous fragility, and cardiovascular disease. High doses should be supplemented with calcium 1 to 1.5 g/day. Inhaled corticosteroids have not yet been demonstrated to be effective in elderly patients with COPD, although they are often prescribed.

Infection: Preventive measures include receiving annual influenza vaccinations and a polyvalent pneumococcal vaccination. Although most elderly persons need only one pneumococcal vaccination in their lifetime, high-risk patients (such as those with COPD) may need revaccination every 6 to 10 years. Other preventive measures include washing hands after contact with persons who have viral syndromes and avoiding crowds in poorly ventilated spaces during influenza epidemics.

At the first sign of purulent sputum in a patient with significant obstruction, an oral antibiotic such as tetracycline 500 mg qid for 10 days, amoxicillin 250 to 500 mg tid for 10 days, erythromycin 500 mg qid for 10 days, clarithromycin 500 mg bid for 10 days, azithromycin 500 mg on day 1 followed by 250 mg/day on days 2 to 5, trimethoprim-sulfamethoxazole 160 mg to 800 mg (one double-strength tablet) bid, or one of the quinolones should be given, even though the efficacy of such therapy is uncertain. Higher doses of bronchodilators and oral corticosteroids may also be necessary during acute infections.

Heart failure: Right-sided heart failure and biventricular failure are the two most common forms of cardiac decompensation in elderly patients with COPD. Right-sided heart failure usually results from alveolar hypoxia–induced pulmonary hypertension. Pulmonary vasodilators (eg, nifedipine, hydralazine) may be helpful for selected patients with severe pulmonary and systemic hypertension.

Hypercapnia: Hypercapnia commonly accompanies severe airway obstruction, but it is generally not dangerous when blood pH is near normal. A rapid rise in the partial pressure of CO_2 (PCO_2) with a drop in pH suggests that the patient has fatigued respiratory muscles and needs more intensive therapy, perhaps including ventilatory support.

Acute respiratory failure: Acute respiratory failure ◘ may result when a viral infection or other cause of exacerbation decreases respiratory reserve, and adequate ventilation is not possible. Mechanical ventilation may also cause complications (eg, pneumothorax), and successful weaning is often difficult.

Hypoxemia: The physician should determine if and when hypoxemia (PO_2 < 55 mm Hg; arterial saturation < 90%) occurs. If hypoxemia occurs at rest, oxygen should be administered continuously. If hypoxemia does not occur at rest, oximetry measurements during exercise and sleep are often indicated. If hypoxemia is documented, supplemental oxygen should be given to raise the PO_2 to about 65 mm Hg or > 90% arterial saturation. A 5 to 10 mm Hg rise in PCO_2 is acceptable, provided no significant mental status changes occur.

Supplemental oxygen devices vary in price and convenience. An oxygen concentrator allows the patient to move throughout one floor of a home, but the machine is not portable and uses a lot of electricity. Compressed oxygen tanks are relatively inexpensive but are heavy and difficult to move. Liquid oxygen systems come with a large reserve tank

◘ see page 787

for in-home use and a small portable tank. This small tank, which can be refilled by the patient, can be carried in a shoulder bag or backpack or wheeled on a metal carrier. It provides oxygen for 3 to 8 hours, depending on its size, the flow rate, and the method of delivery (oxygen may be delivered continuously or through a valve that opens only when the patient inhales). It is ideal for use with vigorous activities, including exercise. A demand valve system is best for most patients with COPD because they use less oxygen, thus they can go longer between refills of the small tank.

Exercise should be continued year-round. Walking is an excellent form of exercise and can be done outdoors in good weather or indoors (eg, in a mall, on a treadmill) in inclement weather. Stair climbing and bike riding are other alternatives.

Patient and Caregiver Issues

Although many activities must be curtailed or modified, many others can be continued. COPD patients need education and encouragement to remain active.

Sexual activity is often still possible. However, the patient should be rested, schedule sexual activity for the "best-breathing" time of day, use a bronchodilator 20 to 30 minutes beforehand, avoid consuming large amounts of food or alcohol beforehand, and assume a position that does not put pressure on the chest or abdomen or require arm support.

Caregivers must guard against "caregiver fatigue." They need periods of time when they are relieved of the burden of caring for the terminally ill patient.

End-of-Life Issues

Patients should be encouraged to discuss end-of-life care with their family and physician, including issues of resuscitation and intubation. An advance directive in the form of a living will or durable power of attorney∎ is the best way for patients to document their wishes.

Signs of a near-terminal state are progressive weight loss not explained by other diseases; progressively less activity leading to severe dyspnea; rising resting P_{CO_2} over time; and a chronically fatigued state. If patients truly have no respiratory reserve and are nearing the end of life, exercise is unwarranted and activities of daily living should be decreased to minimize dyspnea. The physician may suggest that patients live on a single level of their home, not wear shoes that require tying, avoid tight belts, and eat five or six small meals a day rather than three larger ones.

Ideally, end-of-life care is discussed in the outpatient setting before either a life-threatening pulmonary infection develops or a comorbid ill-

∎ see page 134

ness is exacerbated. Patients with end-stage COPD who need assisted ventilation often have difficulty being weaned from the machine. In some cases, it is more appropriate (with the patient's and family's consent) to forgo artificial ventilation and instead use morphine and supportive measures to keep the patient comfortable. ◻

◼79◼ RESPIRATORY FAILURE

Impairment of gas exchange between ambient air and circulating blood, occurring in intrapulmonary gas exchange or in the movement of gases in and out of the lungs.

Respiratory failure can be defined with numeric constants, such as a partial pressure of oxygen (Pao_2) < 60 mm Hg (hypoxemia) or a partial pressure of carbon dioxide ($Paco_2$) > 45 mm Hg(hypercapnia). However, many patients function quite well with hypoxemia and chronic hypercapnia. Therefore, understanding and treating the continuum of the causative disease and the limited reserves and endurance of a patient are usually more valuable than relying on specific laboratory test values.

Etiology and Pathophysiology

The respiratory system can fail to eliminate CO_2 (ventilatory failure), to bring in O_2 (hypoxemia), or to defend the lung against damage and disease. It is rare for only one aspect to fail.

Ventilatory failure: Normal changes of aging, including decreased elastic recoil of the lung, loss of some of the supporting structure around the airways, stiffening of the rib cage, and decreased muscle mass, ◻ can predispose the elderly to ventilatory failure

Ventilatory failure is synonymous with an inappropriate elevation in $Paco_2$; the absolute level is less important. For example, a patient with a previous $Paco_2$ of 30 mm Hg because of compensation for metabolic acidosis may be in respiratory failure when the $Paco_2$ rises to 39 mm Hg because of respiratory muscle fatigue.

The most common cause of ventilatory failure in the elderly is probably the increased work of breathing associated with chronic obstructive pulmonary disease (COPD). Recognizing impending ventilatory respiratory failure can be difficult in such patients. A history of labile bronchospasm or of gradual worsening of symptoms (suggesting that the patient's pulmonary reserve is depleted), inherent in COPD, puts these patients at high risk of respiratory failure.

◻see pages 115 and 139   ◻see page 753

Other common causes of ventilatory failure include decreased respiratory muscle strength and impairment of the central drive to breathe, which can be caused by drug toxicity. Increased CO_2 production as a result of fever or agitation or changes in metabolism based on dietary intake can induce respiratory failure in a patient with concomitant respiratory disease and limited pulmonary reserve.

Hypoxemia: Hypoxemia (decreased oxygen content of the arterial blood) may lead to hypoxia (decreased oxygen at the tissue level). The predicted Po_2 for age can be estimated by subtracting one third of the patient's age from 105. Forms of hypoxia include hypoxemic hypoxia (reduced arterial oxygen content), anemic hypoxia (low Hb, which reduces oxygen-carrying capacity), circulatory hypoxia (inadequate cardiac output, leading to inadequate oxygenation of the tissues), and cytotoxic hypoxia (interference with intracellular oxygen transport, which can be caused by a poison such as cyanide). The most common cause of hypoxemia is ventilation/perfusion ($\dot{V}/\dot{Q}$) mismatch. Other causes include a decrease in the inspired oxygen concentration (as occurs at high altitude) and hypoventilation.

A common cause of hypoxic respiratory failure is capillary leak pulmonary edema as a result of adult respiratory distress syndrome (ARDS). ARDS represents a common pathway of lung injury, the cause of which may include aspiration of gastric contents, sepsis, hypotension, shock, and inhalation of toxic gas. Pulmonary edema is caused by a leaking at the alveolar capillary interface so that high-protein fluid moves from the vascular space into the interstitium and alveoli. Unlike cardiac edema, the mechanism is not hydrostatic pressure. Rather, it is a diffuse inflammatory process, a potent cause of shunt and refractory hypoxemia. In addition, the lung becomes stiff, and lung compliance decreases.

Inadequate lung defense: In elderly patients, the defense functions of the airway are altered,∎ so that pneumonia is more common and often more serious than in younger patients. Pneumonia can lead to ventilatory or hypoxemic respiratory failure.

Diagnosis

Ventilatory failure is confirmed by the inability to eliminate CO_2, resulting in elevation of $Paco_2$. A pulsus paradoxicus (a greater-than-normal decrease in systolic blood pressure with inspiration) suggests that the work of breathing is increased. Measurement of peak flow can be helpful in difficult cases and in patients who minimize their symptoms. The response of flow rate to bronchodilator therapy is very important: peak flow that remains < 70% of predicted after bronchodilator therapy indicates serious disease that necessitates inpatient

---

∎ see page 757

care; a flow rate remaining $< 50\%$ of predicted indicates critical disease that requires observation in an intensive care unit.

Hypoxemic respiratory failure may be difficult to diagnose in the elderly. Heart rate during hypoxemia may not increase because of blunted autonomic drive. Cyanosis may occur late in patients with anemia (because at least 5 g of unsaturated Hb is needed), although cyanosis may occur early in patients with chronic lung disease and polycythemia.

Arterial blood gases can help determine the severity of the process but not the cause. Patients in acute distress should not have their supplemental oxygen removed to obtain a room air blood gas for a baseline $Paco_2$ measurement or because of concern about possible CO_2 retention. Pulse oximeters, although useful, may give inaccurate readings in patients with poor perfusion. Heavy smokers or patients exposed to exogenous carbon monoxide may register falsely elevated Pao_2 levels.

Chest x-rays and ECGs can identify causes of dyspnea, such as flash pulmonary edema or an unsuspected pneumothorax. ARDS often manifests as tachypnea and diffuse whitening of the lungs (due to increased lung water). It usually begins diffusely, although areas with prior emphysematous change are sometimes spared.

When **inadequate lung defenses** produce respiratory failure, pneumonia is almost always present. It can usually be diagnosed on the basis of typical symptoms and laboratory findings.■

Treatment

Ventilatory failure: The usual therapy is assisted ventilation; other therapy is directed at the underlying problem that increases the work of breathing.

A nasal bilevel continuous positive airway pressure (BiPAP) mask (in which gas flow is delivered at a higher pressure during inspiration than during expiration) allows noninvasive ventilation. This method can temporarily assume some of the work of breathing while treatment is directed at the underlying disease. BiPAP is difficult to maintain with a patient who is uncooperative or whose mental status is altered. The patient must be closely monitored for persistent elevation of $Paco_2$ or failure to tolerate the mask or pressure. Some patients need assisted ventilation at night only. Temporary ventilation with heliox, a mixture of helium (80%) and oxygen (20%), may increase mid–vital capacity flow rates by as much as 50%, substantially reducing the work of breathing.

More severe respiratory failure may require acute intervention with airway adjuncts, such as bag-and-mask ventilation. Ventilation with a bag may be easier when dentures are left in place, allowing a tighter seal. However, mechanical ventilation is usually started as quickly as

■ see page 760

possible using intubation. Special care must be taken to avoid unnecessary neck extension and damage to the jaw and teeth during efforts to place an endotracheal tube.

Hypoxemia: The primary goal is to restore proper delivery of oxygen to the tissues. The lowest concentration of oxygen that prevents hypoxia should be used. Oxygen concentrations $> 60\%$ can cause alveolar injury within 48 to 72 hours (through the generation of free oxygen radicals) and within 12 hours at 100% inspired oxygen fraction (Fi_{O_2}). A 100% Fi_{O_2} can produce absorptive atelectasis, which can be avoided by using $\leq 90\%$ Fi_{O_2}. Bronchociliary function is impaired at oxygen concentrations as low as 30%.

Treatment with oxygen may require the use of a high-flow device (eg, ventimask), which provides a blended oxygen concentration, or a low-flow device (eg, nasal cannula) set at a particular flow rate (L/minute). High-flow devices provide more consistently delivered Fi_{O_2}, but low-flow devices may be more comfortable. A close-fitting mask equipped with a reservoir bag and nonrebreathing valves over exhalation ports in the mask body provide the highest Fi_{O_2} (about 90%) without requiring intubation. Nebulizer masks with 100% oxygen delivered through a nebulizer bottle with water can provide the same high Fi_{O_2} with humidity, which can increase patient comfort.

The specific therapy for ARDS depends on the underlying cause. In most cases, therapies are mainly supportive, maintaining oxygen delivery to the tissues until the inflammatory process resolves, the capillary leak is reversed, and the alveolar fluid is cleared. Corticosteroids are not useful in the treatment of acute ARDS.

Inadequate lung defense: Therapy is directed at the underlying disorder and any subsequent infection. Defense may be further impaired by the presence of an endotracheal tube, which bypasses a number of respiratory defenses and eliminates the possibility of glottic closure and the initiation of an effective cough.

Intubation

Intubation should be considered early in the course of a respiratory illness, because if delayed, it may need to be performed as an emergency procedure. Oral endotracheal tubes generally allow better suctioning and produce less resistance but may be occluded by a patient who is biting or may be moved by the patient's tongue, resulting in malposition or additional trauma to the trachea. In addition, endotracheal tubes are often more difficult to secure in edentulous patients.

Intubation of some patients, particularly those in marked distress, is often followed by hypotension. This complication may be due to the loss of sympathetic tone when the work of breathing is quickly reduced, to sedative use, to alkalosis due to overventilation, or to increased positive intrathoracic pressures leading to diminished venous return and lower cardiac output. Elderly patients who are hypovolemic as a result of an underlying disease are particularly at risk of hypotension and its sequelae.

The endotracheal tube reduces the normal protective mechanisms that defend the airway from aspiration and colonization with bacteria. About 20% of patients with endotracheal tubes aspirate; elderly patients aspirate at a rate that may be as high as 70%. Other complications of prolonged endotracheal intubation include pressure necrosis on the tracheal mucosa from overinflated cuffs or from movement of cuffs with movement of the tube. The cuff pressure should not exceed 25 mm Hg because blood flow to the mucosa is decreased and necrosis may occur. The "minimal leak" approach, in which the cuff is inflated until there is no leak and then very slowly deflated, usually maintains pressure within the safe limit, but direct measurement of pressures in the cuff provides greater assurance.

When prolonged intubation ($>$ 2 weeks) is necessary, a tracheostomy should be considered. Many patients feel more comfortable with a tracheostomy.

Mechanical Ventilation

Initially, most patients are best treated by a mode of mechanical ventilation that completely assumes the work of breathing and minimizes the patient's efforts. Minimizing airway pressure and providing the most uniform ventilation possible is an important goal, especially when stiff lungs limit maximum volume.

Most ventilators are volume-cycled: they provide inspiratory flow until a set volume is delivered. The frequency of breaths and the inspiratory flow are also programmed, leaving the inspiratory/expiratory ratio and the pressure in the airways as the resulting dependent variables. A ventilator in control mode delivers its set volume at a specific frequency and will not respond to the patient's efforts to take more frequent breaths. In assist-control mode, the ventilator provides a preset number of breaths at a given volume per minute, but in between these breaths, the patient can trigger the ventilator by making an inspiratory effort; the ventilator then resets its clock to wait for the next appropriate interval until another breath is given. A ventilator in pressure-support mode provides specific airway pressure during inspiration only. Pressure may be set high to do most or all of the inspiratory work of breathing or low to provide partial support. Pressure-support mode may be helpful during weaning efforts and when patients need only a minimal level of support and have an adequate respiratory drive.

Ventilator settings: Tidal volumes between 5 and 8 mL/kg and respiratory rates around 20 breaths/minute are usually recommended. Positive end-expiratory pressure (PEEP) allows airway pressure during expiration to remain at a small positive value; PEEP recruits and stabilizes damaged alveoli (as in ARDS), brings them to larger volume, and helps prevent complete alveolar collapse. However, PEEP increases the risk of barotrauma, diminishes venous return, may increase intracranial pressure, and may increase fluid retention through changes in antidiuretic hormone and atrial natriuretic factor.

Pharmacotherapy: Many patients placed on mechanical ventilation require sedation to be comfortable. Opioids decrease breathlessness but may cause hypotension and ileus. Benzodiazepines are effective and are commonly used. Patients must always receive adequate sedation when receiving neuromuscular blockade, which may be needed when patients have difficulty matching their respiratory pattern to the ventilator. Neuromuscular blockade may reduce airway pressures and risk of barotrauma.

Nutrition: Adequate nutrition during assisted ventilation is very important. Elderly patients with nutritional problems may have less muscle mass, especially the fast twitch fibers that may be related to inspiratory work. Nutritional deficiency may worsen host defenses. However, because carbohydrates produce more CO_2 per calorie than fat, feedings with large proportions of carbohydrates require greater ventilation.

Complications: Complications from mechanical ventilation are often abrupt and dramatic. Problems include inadvertent disconnection of the patient from the ventilator; barotrauma-related events, such as pneumothorax or pneumomediastinum; and ventilator malfunction. When adequate ventilation is in doubt, the patient should be removed from the ventilator and immediately supported with bag ventilation at 100% O_2. If bag ventilation is not successful and the examination does not suggest a pneumothorax, a quick attempt at endotracheal tube suctioning can be made to determine whether a large mucous plug is the problem. Larger mucous plugs that cannot be removed effectively by positioning or unguided suctioning may require bronchoscopy.

Weaning: The underlying disease that caused the respiratory failure should be under control, hemodynamics should be stable, mental status and neurologic function should be good, secretions should be minimal, nutritional support should be adequate, and sedating drugs should be stopped.

Determinants of a patient's readiness to be weaned from a ventilator include a negative inspiratory pressure more negative than -20, tidal volumes > 5 to 10 mL, vital capacities twice the associated tidal volume, and minute volumes < 10 L/minute. The patient should also be on minimal PEEP (5 cm) and on $\leq 50\%$ $F_{I_{O_2}}$. However, about one third of patients who meet these criteria cannot be weaned successfully. A "rapid-shallow" breathing index (calculated by dividing the respiratory rate by the tidal volume in liters) < 105 may predict successful weaning.

The patient should be well rested and positioned for maximal chest bellows effectiveness (eg, sitting partially upright). Weaning techniques include spontaneous breathing through a T-piece, synchronized intermittent mandatory ventilation with reduced machine-assisted breaths, and pressure support. Spontaneous breathing while intubated can be permitted by providing continuous gas flow through large-bore tubing and attaching the tubing to the end of the patient's endotracheal tube (T-piece ventilation). When performed with a ventilator, this spontaneous breathing is called CPAP (continuous positive airway pressure). A patient breathing spontaneously when the ventilator is set not to deliver any additional pressure other than what the patient generates is on a CPAP of zero.

Patients who do not wean successfully may be considered for transfer to a long-term care facility that accepts ventilated patients.

End-of-Life Issues

Some patients choose not to spend their last days in the hospital and prefer to die at home or in a nursing home. Supportive care can be arranged in both settings. Hospice care is an option in either setting.[1] Families and caregivers should be taught how to treat worsening distress and what to do when death comes.[2]

When a patient has made a decision to have mechanical ventilation withdrawn, the physician should ensure the patient's comfort during this process. Comfort measures may include the use of drugs to relieve pain or dyspnea, even though such use may hasten death.

80 ■ INTERSTITIAL LUNG DISEASES

A heterogeneous group of disorders that diffusely affect the lung parenchyma.

The interstitial lung diseases (ILDs) are classified together because of their similar clinical, physiologic, pathologic, and radiologic manifestations (see TABLE 80–1). ILD is usually related to occupational or environmental exposure, especially to inorganic or organic dusts. Sarcoidosis, idiopathic pulmonary fibrosis (IPF), and pulmonary fibrosis associated with connective tissue diseases have an unknown etiology. Limited information exists regarding the incidence and outcomes of these diseases in the elderly.

Deterioration of patients with ILD may be secondary to disease progression, to disease-related complications, or to therapy-associated complications. This latter phenomenon may be especially problematic

[1] see page 90   [2] see page 115

TABLE 80–1. SELECTED INTERSTITIAL LUNG DISEASES

Disease	Etiology	Symptoms and Signs	Treatment	Special Considerations in the Elderly
Idiopathic pulmonary fibrosis (IPF)	Unknown	Gradually worsening dyspnea; cough with dry inspiratory rales; digital clubbing; reticular opacities in the mid and lower lung zones; resting hypoxemia; steady progression	Immunosuppressants (cyclophosphamide or azathioprine with prednisone)	IPF is the most common ILD among the elderly
Idiopathic bronchiolitis obliterans with organizing pneumonia (BOOP)	Unknown	Flu-like symptoms (fever, cough, malaise, weight loss); leukocytosis; restrictive pulmonary function; excessive proliferation of granulation tissue within small airways and alveolar ducts	Corticosteroids	BOOP is common among the elderly (mean age at presentation, 58 yr); mortality is higher among the elderly than among patients < 50
Drug-induced ILD	Direct toxic injury to pulmonary parenchyma and/or indirect immune-mediated mechanisms	Manifestations ranging from acute fulminant deterioration to an insidious, progressive process mimicking IPF	Discontinuation of offending drug (eg, nitrofurantoin, amiodarone); corticosteroids	The disease is more severe in the elderly than in younger patients
Occupational/ environmental ILD				
Silicosis	Silica exposure (≥ 5 yr)	Dyspnea and cough from chronic bronchitis; low titers of ANA	None	The latency period between exposure and disease manifestation is long

Asbestosis	Asbestos exposure	Dyspnea; nonproductive cough; inspiratory rales; bilateral digital clubbing	None	The latency period between exposure and disease manifestation is long; death from respiratory failure or malignancy is common
Hypersensitivity pneumonitis	Inhalation of finely dispersed organic dusts, simple chemicals, or fungal spores	Granulomatous inflammatory responses; fever, chills, dyspnea, cough; normal or fleeting reticular or alveolar opacities on chest x-ray; steady, progressive deterioration in function associated with irreversible pulmonary fibrosis	Avoidance of antigen exposure; corticosteroids (efficacy is debatable)	Elderly patients may be more prone to a chronic progressive course because of insidious disease secondary to prolonged, low level exposure (eg, to domestic caged birds); the lack of acute episodes, failure to identify serum precipitins to a suspected antigen, and atypical x-ray appearance may result in misdiagnosis (especially IPF)
ILD associated with connective tissue diseases (eg, scleroderma, systemic lupus erythematosus, dermatomyositis or polymyositis, Sjögren's syndrome, rheumatoid arthritis)	Unknown	Lung involvement (occasionally the first manifestation), including an interstitial inflammatory pattern that is histopathologically indistinguishable from idiopathic pulmonary fibrosis	Immunosuppressants (cyclophosphamide or azathioprine with prednisone)	Prevalence peaks between 25 and 55 yr; rheumatoid arthritis–associated ILD is the most prevalent form in the elderly

Table continues on the following page.

TABLE 80–1. SELECTED INTERSTITIAL LUNG DISEASES (*Continued*)

Disease	Etiology	Symptoms and Signs	Treatment	Special Considerations in the Elderly
Sarcoidosis	Unknown	Dyspnea, cough, chest pain; hypercalcemia, hypergamma-globulinemia, liver function test abnormalities; symmetric bilateral hilar adenopathy	Corticosteroids	Sarcoidosis is most common in persons aged 20 to 40 but can occur in persons in their 70s
Eosinophilic pneumonia (acute and chronic)	Drug toxicity, parasitic infections	Acute form: dyspnea, nonproductive cough, low-grade fever. Chronic form: subacute onset with cough and dyspnea; increased serum IgE level common	Corticosteroids; maintenance with prednisone, 5 to 20 mg for chronic form	Acute form tends to affect younger patients who require short-term (≤ 3 months) treatment; chronic form is more common in elderly patients
Chronic, recurrent aspiration pneumonitis	Gastroesophageal disorders, GERD, neurologic disease, sedative use	Proximal dysphagia, swallowing dysfunction; reticular and/or alveolar opacities, commonly migratory, in dependent lung zones; GERD; fat-containing macrophages in sputum or bronchoalveolar fluid (using Sudan or oil red O stains)	Discontinuation of the offending agent (eg, mineral oil); corticosteroids; gastric tube feedings	Bedtime use of mineral oil to prevent constipation or of petroleum-based products (eg, Vaseline) to lubricate nasal passages increases risk in the elderly
Pulmonary lymphangitic carcinomatosis	Adenocarcinoma from the breast, lung, stomach, prostate, or pancreas (80% of cases)	Septal Kerley B lines on chest x-ray	Chemotherapy may be indicated	

ILD = interstitial lung disease; ANA = antinuclear antibody; GERD = gastroesophageal reflux disease.

in elderly patients, whose tolerance of the drugs used to treat ILDs is 2 to 3 times less than that of younger patients.

Symptoms, Signs, and Diagnosis

Although ILDs do not present differently in the elderly, concurrent disease may confuse the diagnosis. The insidious onset of breathlessness or cough is common, as are other nonspecific findings such as fatigue, arthralgias, and myalgias. Frank arthritis, myositis (muscle tenderness, weakness), photosensitivity, visual problems, or Raynaud's phenomenon suggests a systemic process, such as collagen vascular disease, vasculitis, or sarcoidosis.

A detailed drug history is needed to exclude the possibility of drug-induced disease. An occupational/environmental history is needed to evaluate exposure in the workplace (eg, to asbestos or silica) and in the home (eg, to pets [particularly birds], humidifiers, evaporative coolers, or materials used for hobbies).

The physical examination usually reveals resting tachypnea and bibasilar rales. Cardiac test results may be normal, but a thorough search for signs of left ventricular dysfunction and mitral valve disease (both common in the elderly) should be made. Signs of pulmonary hypertension (right-sided gallops or heaves, accentuated pulmonary component of the second heart sound) may occur late in any of the ILDs. Digital clubbing is common in IPF, collagen vascular disease–related ILD, and asbestosis but is uncommon in hypersensitivity pneumonitis, silicosis, sarcoidosis, and idiopathic bronchiolitis obliterans with organizing pneumonia (BOOP). A thorough inspection of mucosal surfaces, skin, and joints may give clues to systemic processes.

The chest x-ray may provide the earliest evidence of ILD by showing reticular or nodular opacities with reduced lung volume. Other abnormalities indicative of ILD include alveolar or ground-glass opacities, septal Kerley B lines, pleural involvement, and mediastinal or hilar adenopathy. High-resolution CT (HRCT) of the chest may show distinctive patterns of various ILDs. HRCT is significantly more sensitive and specific than chest x-ray for diagnosing and assessing the extent of ILD.

Pulmonary function tests often reveal a restrictive pattern of lung dysfunction. The ratio of forced expiratory volume in 1 second to forced vital capacity (FEV_1/FVC) is normal or increased because of increased elastic recoil of the stiff lung parenchyma. Several ILDs (eg, chronic sarcoidosis, chronic hypersensitivity pneumonitis, advanced pulmonary histiocytosis X) cause airway obstruction and normal or increased volumes secondary to air trapping and hyperinflation. Lung compliance is increased in ILD. The diffusing capacity for carbon monoxide (DL_{CO}) is generally reduced, even when corrected for alveolar volume and Hb. Arterial blood gases obtained at rest may be normal early in ILD; hypoxemia and mild hypocarbia are common as the disease progresses.

Multistage and steady-state exercise testing are considered the most sensitive methods for assessing severity. They reveal the patient's functional limitations. In mild to moderate disease, the ratio of dead space volume to tidal volume (VD/VT) ventilation is often normal at rest but usually remains stable or decreases with exercise. In advanced disease, the VD/VT ratio commonly increases with exercise; if this occurs in milder cases of ILD, however, pulmonary vascular involvement should be suspected.

Routine blood and serologic tests are often unremarkable. Abnormal results of hepatocellular injury tests and high serum calcium levels are clues to the diagnosis of sarcoidosis or metastatic malignancy with pulmonary lymphangitic spread. Renal insufficiency or microscopic hematuria raises the possibility of Wegener's granulomatosis, Goodpasture's syndrome, systemic lupus erythematosus, or systematic necrotizing vasculitis. However, these conditions rarely present in the elderly. Low titers of antinuclear antibodies and rheumatoid factor are nonspecific findings in a number of ILDs, especially IPF. High titers of antinuclear antibodies suggest collagen vascular disease.

Specialized procedures for obtaining lung cells or tissue are often required to confirm a specific diagnosis. These include fiberoptic bronchoscopy with bronchoalveolar lavage (BAL) of subsegmental regions of the lung with or without biopsy. BAL is considered safe for use in elderly patients, although caution should be used when anesthetizing and premedicating patients with sedatives (eg, midazolam). Transbronchial lung biopsy, the least invasive way to obtain lung tissue for diagnosis, is of limited value in diagnosing ILD, because only small pieces of tissue can be obtained. Surgical lung biopsy by means of video-assisted thoracic surgery is the procedure most often used to obtain a definitive diagnosis of ILD. Elderly patients tolerate thoracoscopic biopsy well, incurring much less pain and fewer complications than with traditional open thoracotomy. Complications include postoperative atelectasis with hypoxemia, pneumonia, and persistent bronchopleural fistulas.

Treatment

Diagnosing and treating the disease early helps delay or prevent functional limitation and disability. End-stage fibrosis is irreversible and untreatable, regardless of etiology.

In general, any possible offending agent should be identified and removed before other medical treatment is started. The mainstay of treatment, especially for IPF, sarcoidosis, and pulmonary fibrosis associated with connective tissue diseases, is suppression of inflammatory and cellular immune responses with corticosteroids and immunosuppressants. Supportive care, including physical and pulmonary rehabilitation, psychosocial therapy, and supplemental oxygen therapy, seems to greatly improve quality of life for many patients.

Corticosteroids: Corticosteroids, which are used to suppress active ongoing alveolar and interstitial inflammation and injury, have long been the drug of choice for treating patients with ILD. Unfortunately, only 15 to 20% show improvement by objective measures.

The dosage and duration of corticosteroid therapy depend on the specific disorder. Patients with fibrosing alveolitis (IPF or collagen vascular disease—related ILD) often require up to 6 months to respond. Patients with sarcoidosis or idiopathic BOOP may respond more quickly to lower doses. Some conditions, such as IPF, commonly require therapy for ≥ 12 months.

Immunosuppressants: Variable success has been achieved with use of immunosuppressants, such as cyclophosphamide or azathioprine (at 1 mg/kg/day lean body weight for 6 to 8 weeks to a maximum dose of 2 mg/kg/day po). Dosing should begin at 50 to 100 mg/day and after the initial dosing period be increased gradually at 4-week intervals in 25-mg increments until the maximum dose is reached. Therapy is usually combined with corticosteroids (prednisone 0.25 mg/kg/day). Immunosuppressants are associated with substantial toxicity and adverse effects, including hemorrhagic cystitis; leukopenia; anorexia, nausea, and vomiting; infection; and development of hematologic malignancies. Therefore, the decision to use immunosuppressants in elderly patients should not be taken lightly.

Patient and End-of-Life Issues

Patients with ILD, especially those with IPF, may stop exercising regularly and may even stop performing normal daily activities because of dyspnea caused by physical exertion. Education in energy management techniques may provide these patients with the means to perform more of their daily activities and improve their quality of life. Patients with severe disease may benefit from a comprehensive pulmonary rehabilitation program.[1]

ILD is often chronic, progressive, and irreversible. Endotracheal intubation and mechanical ventilation for respiratory failure in patients with end-stage ILD should be avoided, because these patients rarely recover adequately to be extubated or discharged from intensive care. Consequently, patients with progressive ILD should be encouraged to issue advance directives indicating their wishes with respect to life-sustaining therapies.[2] There comes a time when symptomatic relief and supportive care are often preferred over aggressive and uncomfortable treatment.[3]

---

[1] see page 806   [2] see page 134   [3] see page 115

Lung cancer is the most common cause of cancer-related deaths among both men and women in the USA. It is predominantly a disease of the elderly: incidence increases with age, reaching 482/100,000 men > 65 years, and peaks at age 75, reaching about 502/100,000 men. A man aged 65 has a 50 times greater risk of developing lung cancer than a man aged 25, and a 3 to 4 times greater risk than men aged 45 to 64.

Etiology and Pathology

About 90% of lung cancer cases in men and 80% in women are attributable to cigarette smoking. The risk of lung cancer is related to the total years of smoking, which exposes smokers to carcinogens and promoting agents. Risk also increases in the elderly because of the age-related decline in cellular DNA repair. From initial exposure to cigarette smoke to clinical presentation, lung cancer probably has a 15- to 20-year natural history.

The four major histologic patterns of lung cancer are squamous cell carcinoma, adenocarcinoma, large cell carcinoma, and small cell carcinoma. Often, two or more of these patterns occur simultaneously.

Squamous cell carcinoma is the most common lung cancer among the elderly, accounting for 40 to 50% of lung cancers among patients > 65. These tumors often grow slowly and usually arise in central airways.

Adenocarcinoma is the second most common lung cancer, accounting for 30 to 35% of lung cancers among the elderly. These tumors probably arise from bronchial and mucosal glands. Except for stage I lesions (see TABLE 81-1), adenocarcinoma generally has a worse prognosis than squamous cell carcinoma.

Large cell carcinoma accounts for 15% of all lung cancers. Usually, it is distinguished by the absence of the distinctive characteristics of the other types. Newer staining techniques allow some tumors once classified as large cell to be reclassified as poorly differentiated squamous cell carcinoma or adenocarcinoma. The site of origin of large cell carcinoma is similar to that of adenocarcinoma.

Small cell (oat cell) carcinoma accounts for 15 to 20% of all lung cancers and is somewhat more common in patients > 65, accounting for slightly more than 25% of all lung cancers in this population. Small cell tumors invade the submucosa early in their growth, and patients usually present with regional or distant metastases at diagnosis. Small cell carcinoma is the most rapidly growing and most chemoresponsive of all lung cancers.

Symptoms, Signs, and Diagnosis

The symptoms and signs that commonly accompany local and regional lung cancer are listed in TABLE 81-2. Patients ≥ 50 who are

TABLE 81–1.   LUNG CANCER TNM STAGING SYSTEM

Stage	Description	5-Yr Survival*
0	Carcinoma in situ, no involvement of nodes, no distant metastases (TisN0M0)	90%
IA	Tumor 3 cm, no involvement of nodes, no distant metastases (T1N0M0)	67%
IB	Tumor > 3 cm or any size tumor either invading visceral pleura or causing obstructive pneumonitis and atelectasis to hilum and ≥ 2 cm distal to the carina at bronchoscopy, no involvement of nodes, no distant metastases (T2N0M0)	57%
IIA	Tumor 3 cm, node involvement limited to peribronchial or ipsilateral hilum, no distant metastases (T1N1M0)	55%
IIB	Tumor > 3 cm or any size tumor invading visceral pleura or causing obstructive pneumonitis and atelectasis to hilum and ≥ 2 cm distal to the carina at bronchoscopy, node involvement limited to peribronchial or ipsilateral hilum, no distant metastases (T2N1M0)	39%
IIIA	Tumor extending beyond visceral pleura, ie, into chest wall, diaphragm, pericardium, or < 2 cm distal to the carina at bronchoscopy; no involvement of nodes; no distant metastases (T3N0M0)	38%
	Tumor extending beyond visceral pleura, ie, into chest wall, diaphragm, pericardium, or < 2 cm distal to the carina at bronchoscopy; node involvement limited to peribronchial or ipsilateral hilum; no distant metastases (T3N1M0)	25%
	Tumor of any size with involvement of subcarinal or ipsilateral mediastinal nodes, no distant metastases (T1–3N2M0)	23%
IIIB	Tumor invasion of mediastinal structures or malignant pleural effusion, involvement of any nodes (Any T4)	7%
	Tumor of any size with involvement of contralateral intrathoracic or any scalene or supraclavicular nodes, no distant metastases (Any N3M0)	< 5%
IV	Tumor of any size with distant metastases, eg, brain, bone, liver (Any M1)	< 5%

* 5-yr survival refers only to non–small cell lung cancer.
T = tumor; N = node; M = metastases.
Modified from Mountain CF: "Revisions in the International System for Staging Lung Cancer." *Chest* 111:1710–1717, 1997; used with permission.

current or former smokers and who present with community-acquired pneumonia should raise particular concern. The routine practice of waiting up to 3 months for community-acquired pneumonia in an elderly smoker to clear may delay early detection of lung cancer. An

TABLE 81–2.   SYMPTOMS AND SIGNS OF LOCAL AND REGIONAL LUNG CANCER

Type of Growth	Description	Symptoms and Signs
Local	Endobronchial growth	Cough Dyspnea (secondary to endobronchial obstruction) Chest pain Hemoptysis Wheeze or stridor Pneumonic symptoms (fever, productive cough)
	Peripheral growth	Pain (pleural or chest wall) Cough Dyspnea (secondary to restriction, effusion)
Regional	Nerve entrapment	Hoarseness (recurrent laryngeal nerve) Hemidiaphragm elevation with dyspnea (phrenic nerve)
	Vascular obstruction	Superior vena cava syndrome
	Pericardial or cardiac extension	Tamponade Arrhythmia Heart failure
	Pleural involvement	Pleural effusion
	Mediastinal extension	Esophageal compression with dysphagia Bronchoesophageal fistula Lymphatic obstruction with pleural effusion

Modified from Cohen MH: "Signs and symptoms of bronchogenic carcinoma," in *Lung Cancer: Clinical Diagnosis and Treatment,* ed. 2, edited by MJ Straus. New York, Grune & Stratton, 1983, pp. 97–111; used with permission.

elderly current or former smoker with a cough and an infiltrate without fever and purulent sputum should be assumed to have lung cancer until tests prove otherwise.

Cytologic screening may be useful in detecting squamous cell carcinoma in elderly cigarette smokers. Overall, however, routine cytologic screening fails to detect lung cancer cells at a stage early enough to perform surgical resection or to lengthen survival.

Chest x-ray is usually the initial diagnostic tool, although it is not useful as a screening tool. CT scans are a valuable addition to chest x-rays for determining mediastinal tumor extension. However, CT scans yielded false-negative results in 5 to 9% of cases, in which they indicated only local involvement.

Mediastinoscopy is often used to stage lung cancer and as a prelude to surgical resection of the involved lung to confirm the clinical staging.

Prevention and Treatment

Smoking cessation reduces the risk of lung cancer mortality at any age, and the earlier a smoker quits, the better. The approach to smoking cessation is no different for the elderly than it is for younger patients.

In the elderly, lung cancer usually manifests at a less advanced stage, and treatment, therefore, is usually more successful. However, the diagnostic and therapeutic options offered to the elderly are often substantially less aggressive. Treatment decisions should be based not on age, but rather on cancer type and stage, functional status (see TABLES 81–3 and 81–4), organ function, pulmonary function, cardiopulmonary test results, and comorbidities. For some elderly patients with severe disease, such as advanced dementia or renal, cardiac, or pulmonary disease, treatment may be best aimed at relieving symptoms rather than at attempting cure.

Treatment for non–small cell lung cancer depends on tumor stage, as categorized by the international TNM staging system (see TABLE 81–1). Small cell lung cancer is usually metastatic; thus, treatment is based on whether cancer is limited or extensive rather than on whether it is localized or metastatic.

Surgery: Age alone is not a contraindication to potentially curative surgery. For patients with adequate pulmonary reserve and no evidence of extrathoracic (bone, brain, or liver) metastases, the extent of mediastinal and thoracic lymph node involvement determines whether curative resection is possible. Tissue (surgical) staging must be performed in patients who are otherwise acceptable candidates for surgical resection but who have enlarged mediastinal lymph nodes. Staging is sometimes

TABLE 81–3.   EASTERN COOPERATIVE ONCOLOGY GROUP PERFORMANCE SCALE

Grade	Definition
0	Fully active, able to carry out all pre-disease activities without restrictions
1	Restricted in physically strenuous activity but ambulatory and able to carry out work of a light or sedentary nature
2	Ambulatory and capable of all self-care but unable to carry out any work activities. Up and about > 50% of waking hours
3	Capable of only limited self-care, confined to bed or chair > 50% of waking hours
4	Completely disabled. Cannot carry out any self-care. Totally confined to bed or chair

TABLE 81-4.   KARNOFSKY PERFORMANCE SCALE

Grade	Definition
100	Normal, no complaints, no evidence of disease
90	Able to carry out normal activity, minor symptoms or signs of disease
80	Able to carry out normal activity with effort, some symptoms or signs of disease
70	Able to care for self; unable to carry out normal activity or do active work
60	Requires occasional assistance but is able to care for most of his/her needs
50	Requires considerable assistance and frequent medical care
40	Disabled; requires special care and assistance
30	Severely disabled, hospitalization indicated; death is not imminent
20	Very sick, hospitalization necessary, active and supportive treatment necessary
10	Moribund, fatal processes (eg, intracranial metastasis, massive hemoptysis) progressing rapidly

accomplished through mediastinoscopic or needle transtracheal lymph node sampling. If the tumor is found to extend to the mediastinum, the disease is considered incurable and surgery is not beneficial. Surgery is not recommended for most patients with advanced (stage IIIB, stage IV) non–small cell lung cancer.

Curative surgical treatment for non–small cell lung cancer may be considered for patients with stage I or II disease. However, only 20 to 25% of all patients with lung cancer meet the criteria even before clinical staging is completed. The success of lung cancer resection, the choice of adjuvant therapy, and prognosis for resected non–small cell lung cancer depend on the extent of metastases.

A predicted postoperative forced expiratory volume in 1 second (FEV_1) of > 800 mL is usually considered a minimum for consideration of surgery, because hypercapnia often occurs below this level. Hypoxia (partial pressure of arterial O_2 [Pa_{O_2}] < 50 mm Hg) and hypercapnia (partial pressure of arterial CO_2 [Pa_{CO_2}] > 45 mm Hg) are also risk factors for increased perioperative mortality.

Perioperative pulmonary complications in the elderly can be minimized by preoperative smoking cessation, intensive pulmonary physical therapy, antibiotic therapy (for existing bronchitis), bronchodilator therapy, and postoperative pulmonary rehabilitation.■ Perioperative complications correlate with preoperative physiologic measurements (eg, FEV_1, maximum minute ventilation, maximal oxygen consumption).

■see page 806

Postoperative mortality is 1.3% for patients < 60, 4.1% for patients 60 to 69, and 7.1% for patients ≥ 70. Mortality is at least partially dependent on the operation performed. Expected postoperative mortality rates for lung cancer surgery are 11.6% for pneumonectomy, 4.2% for lobectomy, and 3.7% for segmentectomy. Pneumonectomy is associated with a two to seven times greater risk of mortality for the elderly than for patients < 65. Respiratory complications occur twice as often in patients ≥ 75. Elderly cigarette smokers, who are most likely to develop lung cancer, commonly have coronary artery disease and ventilatory obstruction as well, thus increasing the risk of surgery. When patients also have chronic obstructive pulmonary disease and emphysema (frequently due to cigarette smoking), the risk of postoperative pneumonia and atelectasis increases.

Chemotherapy: Cure with chemotherapy is rare. Length of survival may be improved with chemotherapy, but quality of life may be compromised by significant adverse effects of treatment. How well chemotherapy is tolerated depends more on functional status than on age (see TABLES 81–3 and 81–4), even in patients with extensive disease. Thus elderly patients must weigh the same considerations as must younger patients. Response rates to treatment for advanced lung cancer are similar across age groups. In the case of advanced-stage small cell lung cancer, the response rate approaches 80% and the 2-year survival rate is up to 10%, so that chemotherapy is often appropriate.

Radiation therapy: Radiation can be used as primary therapy or for palliation and pain control in advanced disease. Local control of unresectable disease often can be achieved with radiation therapy, although control of metastases and cure are uncommon. Patients with locally (T3, T4) or regionally (N2, N3) advanced non–small cell cancer often receive radiation therapy alone or combined with chemotherapy as primary treatment. Patients with distant metastases (M1) receive radiation therapy for palliation and pain control. When staging studies confirm that small cell cancer is limited, reported median survival is 10 to 16 months with radiation therapy. However, radiation may not prolong survival.

In general, elderly patients tolerate palliative radiation therapy as well as younger patients. However, radiation pneumonitis is more clinically severe among the elderly. Newer radiation modalities and computer-assisted or computer-directed treatment may lessen the severity of pneumonitis.

Nursing and Caregiver Issues

Nursing care must be tailored to the patient's prognosis as determined by the type and stage of cancer as well as any comorbidities. For patients who require surgical intervention, pain management and pulmonary function are likely to be key nursing issues. Early in the postoperative period, pain is usually acute at the incisional site and later tapers off. The use of drugs for pain management must be appropriate to the degree and extent of pain expressed by the patient.[1] Deep-breathing and coughing exercises help maintain adequate ventilation in the postoperative phase. For patients receiving radiation therapy or chemotherapy, any adverse effects must be assessed and treated appropriately. For patients who have previously smoked or have been exposed to lung irritants, chest physical therapy and regular auscultation to detect early symptoms and signs of adverse events such as pneumonia, atelectasis, and pneumothorax are essential.

For patients whose disease has been newly diagnosed, support groups and patient education may be helpful. Family and friends should be included to the greatest degree possible to ensure adequate support and educational impact.

End-of-Life Issues

Although lung cancer may be curable if detected early, most cases are ultimately fatal. The realistic chances that treatment will prolong life or improve the quality of life must be discussed with the patient. The patient should also be informed of the likely adverse effects of treatment. The patient's wishes regarding terminal care should be discussed and documented early.[2]

In the late stages of lung cancer, patients are likely to experience pain, shortness of breath, anorexia, and weight loss and may become depressed. Such symptoms should be fully treated.[3] In the terminal stages, full doses of opioids may be needed for patients distressed by hypoxia.

82 ▬▬ PULMONARY REHABILITATION

A multidimensional continuum of services directed to persons with pulmonary disease and their families, usually by an interdisciplinary team of specialists, with the goal of achieving and maintaining the person's maximum level of independence and functioning in the community.

For many patients with chronic respiratory disease, medical therapy only partially allays the symptoms and complications of their illness. A comprehensive program of pulmonary rehabilitation may lead to significant clinical improvement by reducing shortness of breath, increasing

---

[1] see page 387   [2] see page 134   [3] see page 115

exercise tolerance, improving overall quality of life, and, to a lesser extent, decreasing the number of hospitalizations. However, these programs do not improve survival. Because chronic obstructive pulmonary disease (COPD) is the most common chronic respiratory disease among the elderly, ◼ most research in pulmonary rehabilitation has addressed COPD patients. Furthermore, although most studies have involved patients aged 50 to 70 years, patients > 70 have also been shown to benefit from pulmonary rehabilitation programs.

Dyspnea is the most common symptom of COPD and often produces a vicious circle of inactivity, anxiety, and depression. The inactivity leads to deconditioning and reduction in muscle strength and cardiac function, which exacerbate activity-provoked dyspnea. Anticipatory dyspnea is another component of the vicious circle; the patient experiences anxiety when anticipating an activity that the patient thinks will lead to shortness of breath. This anxiety leads to an increased heart and respiratory rate, which in turn increases dyspnea. Anxiety and limitations on activity commonly lead to depression. Pulmonary rehabilitation programs are designed to break the vicious circle of dyspnea by lessening each symptom in the circle.

Patient Selection

Comprehensive pulmonary rehabilitation programs are effective for patients with significant impairment despite maximal medical therapy. Problems that must be addressed include severe dyspnea, which impairs quality of life; impaired exercise capacity, which may affect daily activities; and multiple hospitalizations or emergency room visits because of pulmonary disease. Other significant impairments may be attributable to anxiety and depression or to suboptimal adherence to drug regimens (especially with oxygen therapy). Education is a key component. Pulmonary rehabilitation programs may also help coordinate complex medical services (eg, by arranging transportation, home services, medical equipment, and physician visits).

The Pulmonary Rehabilitation Team

Although some elements of pulmonary rehabilitation may be successfully carried out by a single health care professional, the wide range of services needed often requires the skills of a variety of health care professionals. ◪ For example, patients may need exercise training, education, pharmacotherapy, psychosocial counseling, and nutritional guidance, which often require the expertise of a respiratory or physical therapist, a nurse, a physician, a psychologist or social worker, and a dietitian. Communication among team members and with the patient is

◼ see page 779   ◪ see also page 74

paramount, and one team member is usually designated as the leader to ensure effective communication and coordination of services.

Patient Evaluation and Goal Setting

The first step in pulmonary rehabilitation is to clarify the patient's reasons for enrolling in rehabilitation and the desired long-term goals so as to develop realistic, achievable short-term goals. For example, an elderly patient may desire to travel by air to visit a grandchild. If the person can walk only 300 feet (91.4 meters) because of shortness of breath but must be able to walk 1000 feet (304.8 meters) to board the airplane, the initial short-term goal may be to walk 500 feet (152.4 meters). Achieving that goal motivates the patient to try for the next goal of 1000 feet (304.8 meters). Continued encouragement by staff is essential. Periodic reevaluation is important to ensure that goals are being met. An ongoing maintenance program is also essential. Identifying factors that may limit the program's effectiveness is also important. These include problems with financial resources, transportation, cognition, and family dynamics.

Exercise Training

Exercise training■ is probably the most important component of pulmonary rehabilitation. It reduces the effects of inactivity and deconditioning. An intensive conditioning program can result in lower lactate levels during exercise and thus reduce the ventilatory demands associated with activity. In patients who have limited ventilatory reserve because of intrinsic pulmonary disease, lower ventilatory needs during activity lessen dyspnea and increase exercise capacity. However, physical limitations may limit the types of exercise training to be used.

Most elderly patients, particularly those with limited functional capacity due to pulmonary disease and the effects of aging, are not motivated to initiate or maintain an exercise program. The rehabilitation team provides motivation and psychologic support to patients during exercise, helps patients better understand their physical limitations and gain a sense of control over shortness of breath, and ensures patient safety during exercise.

Lower extremity exercise is the cornerstone of pulmonary rehabilitation. Because walking is necessary for most activities of daily living, many programs use walking as the preferred mode of training. Walking may be initiated on a treadmill, which provides an objective measure and control of distance and speed. Many patients continue to use a treadmill, although some prefer walking outdoors or in an enclosed shopping mall. A stationary bicycle may be preferred by some patients. Choosing exercise that is comfortable and satisfying for the patient enhances long-term adherence.

■ see page 298

Psychosocial Counseling

Because strong emotions may worsen dyspnea, patients may not express their emotions and thus may be caught in an emotional straitjacket. Yet, anxiety and depression are common. Dyspnea, along with anxiety and depression, may interfere with sexual activity, which need not be given up. Patients may be unable to manage stress and relax. Pulmonary rehabilitation programs use counseling, group therapy, and, when needed, drugs to treat psychosocial problems.

Nutritional Evaluation and Counseling

Patients with severe COPD may experience weight loss. Weight loss may be due to pulmonary cachexia or to the patient's inability to buy food because of insufficient funds or lack of transportation. Through nutritional counseling and supplementation, pulmonary rehabilitation programs help patients avoid loss of muscle mass. Loss of muscle mass impairs the ability of the patient to fully participate in an exercise program and limits the benefits of pulmonary rehabilitation. Rehabilitation programs help pulmonary patients maintain adequate caloric intake while avoiding satiety that can interfere with respiration.

Weight gain may occur from a reduced level of activity associated with dyspnea on exertion and may further exacerbate dyspnea. In such cases, the goal becomes weight loss using a weight loss diet. ∎

Drugs

Patients with advanced pulmonary disease usually take multiple drugs on complex schedules requiring precise dosing. Patients are educated about the appropriate timing and doses of regularly scheduled and prn drugs prescribed by the physician. The proper technique for use of inhaled drugs is emphasized. Because nonadherence is a serious complicating factor in management, programs closely monitor and educate patients and families about the importance of appropriate drug use.

The goal of education is to improve the patient's long-term adherence to the prescribed drug regimen. Education often includes information about the nature of the pulmonary condition and the role of drug therapy, including expected benefits and potential adverse effects. Other important goals include teaching patients to recognize changes in their pulmonary condition and to recognize when the medical program needs to be modified in response to changes in symptoms, so that they will contact their physician promptly. The patient's physicians should emphasize and reinforce the education and training provided by the rehabilitation staff and communicate frequently with them.

∎see page 605

SECTION 11

CARDIOVASCULAR DISORDERS

83 AGING AND THE CARDIOVASCULAR SYSTEM

Differences between cardiovascular function in older and younger persons have been extensively quantified. However, interactions between age, disease, and lifestyle are often overlooked. Whether the high prevalence of cardiovascular disorders such as hypertension, coronary artery disease, and heart failure is due to an aging process, or these disorders merely occur more frequently in elderly persons because of a longer exposure to risk is not yet established (see TABLE 83–1).

CARDIOVASCULAR STRUCTURE

The Heart

With age, the heart can atrophy, remain unchanged, or develop moderate or marked hypertrophy. Atrophy usually coincides with various wasting diseases and is not observed during aging in healthy persons. A modest increase in left ventricular wall thickness is normal with age; an exaggerated increase occurs in persons with hypertension.█ Other normal age-associated changes may include enlargement of the left atrium and slight enlargement of the left ventricular cavity and of the cardiac silhouette, seen on chest x-ray.

The amount of fibrous tissue within the myocardium increases with age but does not contribute appreciably to cardiac mass. Rather, myocardial wall thickening occurs largely because cardiac myocytes increase in size. Some myocytes are replaced by fibrous tissue, so that the number of myocytes probably decreases with age. However, cardiac myocytes are probably able to reenter the cell cycle and proliferate, thereby partly offsetting cell loss due to necrosis or apoptosis.

In nearly half of persons > 70 years, amyloid can be detected in the heart, and the incidence increases sharply with age. About half of these persons have only small amounts of amyloid confined to the atria.

█ see page 833

TABLE 83–1. RELATIONSHIP OF AGE-ASSOCIATED CHANGES TO CARDIOVASCULAR DISEASE

Category	Age-Associated Change	Likely Mechanisms	Possible Disease Outcomes
Cardiovascular structure	Increased vascular intimal thickness	Increase in migration of and in matrix production by vascular smooth muscle cells Possible derivation of intimal cells from other sources	Early stages of atherosclerosis
	Increased vascular stiffness	Elastin fragmentation Increased elastase activity Increased collagen production by vascular smooth muscle cells and increased cross-linking of collagen Altered growth factor regulation and tissue repair mechanisms	Systolic hypertension Stroke Atherosclerosis
	Increased left ventricular wall thickness	Decreased number of myocytes (due to necrosis and apoptosis) but increased left ventricular myocyte size Altered growth factor regulation Focal collagen deposition	Slowed early diastolic cardiac filling Increased cardiac filling pressure Lower threshold for dyspnea
	Increased left atrial size	Increased left atrial pressure and volume	Lone atrial fibrillation
Cardiovascular function	Altered regulation of vascular tone	Decreased nitric oxide regulation and effects Decreased β-adrenergic receptor responses	Vascular stiffening Hypertension
	Decreased cardiovascular reserve	Increased vascular load Decreased intrinsic myocardial contractility Decreased β-adrenergic modulation of heart rate, myocardial contractility, and vascular tone	Lower threshold for and increased severity of heart failure

TABLE 83-1.   (*Continued*)

Category	Age-Associated Change	Likely Mechanisms	Possible Disease Outcomes
Lifestyle	Reduced physical activity	Learned lifestyle	Exaggeration of some age-associated changes in cardiovascular structure and function Increased risk of vascular disease, hypertension, and heart failure

Whether cardiac amyloidosis is part of normal aging is debatable; it is not present in all elderly persons, not even in centenarians.

The Vasculature

With age, the walls of large distributing arteries (eg, the aorta) thicken, and the arteries become dilated and elongated. The thickening results mainly from an increase in intimal thickness due to cellular accumulation and to matrix deposition; fragmentation of the internal elastic membrane also occurs. These changes may partly explain the elderly's increased likelihood of developing atherosclerosis. With age, increases in collagen and changes in the cross-linking of collagen within the vascular media may make the media less elastic. Glycoprotein eventually disappears from elastin fibrils, and elastin becomes frayed. An age-associated increase in elastase activity and in Ca^{++} and cholesterol deposition on elastin may contribute to elastin fragmentation or to a reduction in elastin content. The total mucopolysaccharide content (ground substance) of the interstitial matrix is unaltered with age, but the amount of dermatan and heparan sulfate contained in the matrix increases and that of hyaluronate and chondroitin sulfate decreases.

CARDIOVASCULAR FUNCTION

Cardiovascular function is determined by the interaction of several variables, which may be affected by age (see TABLE 83–2). However, aging does not alter overall systolic cardiac pump function at rest in normotensive elderly persons.

Compliance, Cardiac Filling, and Preload

An age-associated reduction in ventricular compliance remains unproved, because proof would require the simultaneous measurement

TABLE 83–2.   AGE-ASSOCIATED CHANGES IN CARDIAC FUNCTION*

Variable	Seated Rest	Upright Cycle Exercise
Cardiac index	In men, no change In women, ↓	↓ (25%)
Heart rate	↓ (10%)	↓ (25%)
Stroke volume	In men, ↑ (10%) In women, no change	No change
Preload		
End-diastolic volume	In men, ↑ (12%) In women, no change	↑ (30%)
Early filling	↓	†
Late filling	↑	
Afterload		
Compliance	↓	N/A
Pulse wave reflection	↑	N/A
Inertance	↑	N/A
Peripheral vascular resistance	Modest ↑	↑ (30%)
End-systolic volume	In men, ↑ In women, no change	↑ (275%)
Contractility	No change	↓ (60%)
Ejection fraction	No change	↓ (15%)
Oxygen consumption		↓ (50%)
A-Vo$_2$		↓ (25%)
Plasma catecholamine (norepinephrine, epinephrine) levels	↑ or no change (variable)	↓
Cardiac and vascular responses to β-adrenergic stimulation	↓	↓

*Change between ages 20 and 80 in healthy persons.
†Early and late filling cannot be separated during exercise.
↓ = decreased; ↑ = increased; A-Vo$_2$ = arteriovenous oxygen difference; N/A = not applicable.

of pressure and volume; such invasive measurements are not usually attempted in healthy persons.

The early diastolic left ventricular filling rate progressively slows after age 20, so that by age 80, the rate is reduced by up to 50% (see FIGURE 83–1). This reduction is attributed to structural (fibrous) changes in the left ventricular myocardium or to residual myofilament Ca^{++} activation from the preceding systole, resulting in prolonged isovolumic relaxation.

Although left ventricular filling in early diastole is less in older than in younger persons, filling in later diastole is greater, because the atrial contraction is augmented. Thus, end-diastolic volume in the supine or seated position is not usually decreased in healthy older women and increases slightly with age in men as long as the atrial contraction is normal. The augmented atrial contraction is accompanied by atrial enlargement and is manifested on auscultation as a fourth heart sound (atrial gallop). Lack of an augmented atrial contraction in elderly patients with acute atrial fibrillation or with a pacemaker that does not stimulate atrial contraction can be clinically significant if ventricular function is compromised for other reasons. The result may be heart failure, particularly if the ventricular rate is rapid.

Afterload

The extent to which aging affects afterload (which depends on peripheral vascular resistance, aortic impedance, and aortic pulse wave velocity) varies dramatically from person to person. Some studies have reported that peripheral vascular resistance at rest increases with age. An age-associated increase has been measured in aortic impedance, which is usually < 10% of total vascular impedance.

Aortic pulse wave velocity increases with age. As a result, pressure waves from peripheral sites are returned to the heart more quickly in elderly persons. In healthy elderly men and women, pressure in the aortic root continues to rise and peaks later in systole, thereby altering the pressure pulse contour (see FIGURE 83–2) and causing a late augmentation of systolic blood pressure. Arterial stiffening, the resulting increase in pulse wave velocity, and late augmentation of systolic blood pressure may explain the overall increase in systolic blood pressure with age. The increase in systolic blood pressure may reflect a resetting of the baroreceptor reflex to a higher level in the elderly. The same structural changes that make the aorta stiffer and cause pulse wave velocity to increase may explain the decreased baroreceptor stimulation required

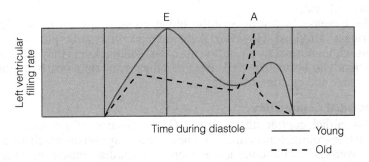

FIGURE 83–1.   **Age-associated changes in left ventricular diastolic filling.** The first wave (E wave) occurs during early filling; the second (A wave) is due to atrial contraction. Modified from Schulman SP, Lakatta EG, Fleg JL, et al: "Age-related decline in left ventricular filling at rest and exercise." *American Journal of Physiology* 263(6 Pt 2):H1932–1938, 1992.

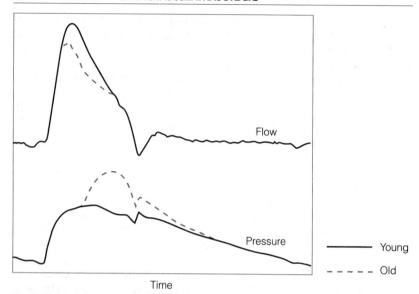

Time

FIGURE 83–2. **Age-associated differences in ascending aortic blood flow velocity and pressure wave forms.** Peak pressure and flow occur simultaneously in younger persons. Peak pressure occurs later during the cardiac cycle in older persons and increases with age. From Nichols WW, O'Rourke MF, Avolio AP et al: "Effects of age on ventricular-vascular coupling." *American Journal of Cardiology* 55:1179–1184, 1985.

for a given change in aortic pressure. Alternatively, the baroreceptor response may be blunted because of age-associated changes in afferent nerve impulses from the baroreceptors or in efferent nerve impulses to the arterial system.

The increase in resting systolic blood pressure affects resting left ventricular afterload. However, if the increase in systolic pressure remains within normal limits, left ventricular wall thickness may increase sufficiently to normalize wall stress and thus maintain a nearly normal cavity size and ejection fraction.

Myocardial Contractility

Myocardial contractility involves Ca^{++} activation of myofilaments (excitation-contraction coupling). The effects of age on the mechanisms that govern excitation-contraction coupling in cardiac muscle have been studied in animal models. Some of the age-associated changes are partly related to alterations in gene expression. In rats, contractile force production, at least at low stimulation rates, is preserved in old age. Although passive stiffness in isolated cardiac muscle has not been shown to increase with age, stiffness during contraction increases. The increase in myoplasmic Ca^{++} after excitation at low rates and the affinity of myofibrils for Ca^{++} do not change with age. At higher rates of excitation, the amplitude of the Ca^{++} transient (a brief increase in the cytosolic concentration of calcium) is not well characterized with respect to aging.

Relaxation is prolonged in senescent cardiac muscle, probably because Ca^{++} is removed more slowly from the myoplasm during diastole. This slow removal probably occurs because the sarcoplasmic reticulum sequesters less calcium. The action potential lasts longer in senescent cardiac muscle, but the role of this change in prolonging contraction is unclear. Action-potential changes may reflect age-associated changes in sarcolemmal ionic conductances or may result from the prolonged myoplasmic Ca^{++} transient elicited by excitation.

In isolated senescent cardiac muscle, myosin isoenzymes shift to slower forms, and adenosine triphosphatase activity decreases. These changes may explain why shortening velocity decreases during isotonic contraction.

A reduction in the myocardial relaxation rate results in less complete myocardial relaxation when the mitral valve opens and in a reduction in the early diastolic left ventricular filling rate.

Ejection Fraction and Stroke Volume

The resting ejection fraction is not reduced in healthy older men and women. Resting stroke volume increases slightly in older men (commensurately with the slightly larger end-diastolic volume) and remains constant in older women.

Heart Rate

With age, the supine resting heart rate does not change in healthy men; the heart rate while seated decreases slightly in men and women. Spontaneous variations in heart rate during a 24-hour period decrease in men without coronary artery disease, as do variations in the sinus rate with respiration. The intrinsic sinus rate (ie, measured after sympathetic and parasympathetic blockade) decreases significantly with age. For example, the average intrinsic sinus rate is 104 beats/minute at age 20 compared with 92 beats/minute at age 45 to 55. Data from persons > 55 are lacking.

Cardiac Output

The resting cardiac index (cardiac output per unit of time [L/minute], measured while seated and divided by body surface area [m^2]) is not reduced in healthy older men who have been rigorously screened to exclude occult heart disease and who live independently in the community. However, in older women, resting cardiac output decreases slightly because neither end-diastolic volume nor stroke volume increases to compensate for the modest reduction in heart rate. These sex-related differences appear to be due in part to differences in fitness, even between sedentary men and women.

AEROBIC CAPACITY AND CARDIOVASCULAR FUNCTION DURING EXERCISE

Aging affects aerobic capacity and cardiovascular performance during exercise (see TABLE 83–2). Peak exercise capacity and peak oxygen (O_2) consumption decrease with age, but interindividual variation is substantial. Aerobic capacity decreases by 50% between ages 20 and 80, because maximum cardiac output decreases by 25% and peripheral O_2 utilization decreases (ie, the arteriovenous O_2 difference decreases by 25%) as a result of age-associated reductions in muscle mass and strength. Other possible mechanisms include inefficient redistribution of blood flow to working muscles and reduced O_2 extraction and utilization per unit of muscle. With age, heart rate during exhaustive exercise decreases, but heart volume at end-diastole and throughout the cardiac cycle (including end-systole) is larger during exercise in older than in younger persons. Thus, in older persons, the early diastolic left ventricular filling volume increases during exercise. As a result, the end-diastolic volume, even at peak exercise, is not compromised because of a "stiff heart," and stroke volume during exercise is maintained in older persons. The 25% reduction in maximum cardiac index that occurs between ages 25 and 85 is completely due to the age-associated reduction in maximum heart rate.

During all levels of exercise, the older heart, on average, pumps blood from a larger filling volume. However, stroke volume in older persons does not exceed that in younger persons, because the end-systolic volume in older persons remains larger than it does in younger persons. Consequently, the ejection fraction does not increase as much in response to an increase in end-diastolic volume. Thus, although the stroke volume during exercise is maintained at the same level in older persons as in younger persons, the Frank-Starling mechanism is blunted with age. These changes result from a combination of age-associated factors, including augmented vascular and cardiac components of afterload, reduced maximal intrinsic myocardial contractility, and reduced augmentation of contractility by β-adrenergic stimulation.

β-Adrenergic Modulation

The activity of the sympathetic nervous system seems to increase with age, as suggested by higher blood levels of norepinephrine and epinephrine in older than in younger persons during any effort. Because levels of norepinephrine and epinephrine are higher, more β-adrenergic receptors on cardiac and vascular cell surfaces are occupied. The result is a desensitization of β-adrenergic receptors, thereby causing a down-regulation of associated intracellular signaling pathways. Such desensitization may account for all or a substantial portion of the age-associated postsynaptic reduction in responsiveness to β-adrenergic stimulation.

β-Adrenergic stimulation of pacemaker cells partially accounts for an increased heart rate during exercise. When a rapid intra-arterial infusion of a β-adrenergic agonist (eg, isoproterenol) is used to mimic exercise, the increase in heart rate and in ejection fraction is smaller and forearm vascular dilation and venorelaxation are less in older than in younger men. (In isolated human cardiac muscle and in myocytes, response to β-adrenergic stimulation is also reduced with age.) However, α-adrenergic–mediated venoconstriction during exercise is not impaired with age and is a major factor in facilitating the return of blood to the heart.

β-Adrenergic blockade during exercise abolishes age-associated differences in heart rate, in early diastolic left ventricular filling rate, and in end-diastolic volume. Thus, the cardiovascular response to exercise is similar in younger persons during acute β-blockade and in older persons.

Animal studies confirm the age-associated reduction in contractile response of cardiac myocytes to β-adrenergic stimulation. The contractile response is reduced because with age, β-adrenergic stimulation is less able to increase L-type sarcolemmal Ca^{++} channel availability and thus to augment the brief increase in cytosolic calcium concentration (Ca^{++} transient). The age-associated reduction in the postsynaptic response of myocytes to β-adrenergic stimulation appears to be due to multiple changes in coupling of $β_1$- and $β_2$-adrenergic receptors to postreceptor intracellular machinery. The major age-associated change that limits this signaling pathway appears to involve the coupling of the β-adrenergic receptor to adenylyl cyclase via the stimulatory G (G_S) protein. Because of this change, not enough intracellular cyclic adenosine monophosphate (cAMP) is produced to adequately activate protein kinase A, which phosphorylates key proteins, leading to altered protein function and augmented cardiac function. The reduced response to β-adrenergic stimulation in healthy older persons resembles that in patients with chronic heart failure. However, unlike the case in chronic heart failure, neither β-adrenergic kinase activity nor inhibitory G (G_i) protein activity (G_i inhibits intracellular adenylyl cyclase) appears to be involved in the age-associated blunting of β-adrenergic effects.

CARDIOVASCULAR FUNCTION IN HYPERTENSION

The same vascular and cardiac (hemodynamic) changes that are observed in normotensive persons as they age also occur in hypertensive persons but at a younger age, and in some, the changes are exaggerated. However, with age, hypertensive persons undergo some changes that do not occur in normotensive persons. In hypertensive persons, peripheral vascular resistance increases substantially with age. The increase in peripheral vascular resistance elevates diastolic and mean arterial pressures and plays a greater role in the vascular afterload of the heart than it does in normotensive persons. Also, resting stroke volume and cardiac output are lower in hypertensive persons than in normotensive persons.

EFFECTS OF LIFESTYLE

Diet, exercise habits, and smoking may affect the heart and blood vessels of older persons, as suggested by cross-cultural studies. For instance, a difference in dietary sodium may account for some of the differences in age-associated blood pressure changes that occur among persons of different countries. However, some changes occur because the sodium sensitivity of arterial pressure regulation increases with age.

Physical conditioning appears to lessen the vascular stiffening associated with aging.■ Late augmentation of resting systolic blood pressure, which is an index of arterial stiffness, is increased by only about half as much in endurance-trained elderly persons as it is in sedentary ones.

Physical conditioning can also improve the aerobic capacity of older persons by increasing cardiac output and O_2 utilization. Older persons in good physical condition can match or exceed the aerobic capacity of unconditioned younger persons.

Effects of exercise in older animals are consistent with those in older persons: Some of the age-associated changes in cardiac function (eg, prolonged myocardial relaxation, reduced sarcoplasmic reticulum function) are reversed. However, conditioning does not affect the prolonged action potential or the myosin isoenzyme shift to slower forms.

84 ■ DIAGNOSTIC EVALUATION

The patient's overall health and level of functioning help determine diagnostic approach and therapeutic goals. A clinician must consider both the quality and the quantity of remaining years, along with risks from significant comorbid disorders, while weighing the potential benefits of tests against their risk. Some tests pose risks directly; others do so because they lead to further tests and treatments.

HISTORY AND PHYSICAL EXAMINATION

When taking the history, a physician should remember that age-related changes in lifestyle may mask important symptoms; for example, exertional angina pectoris and dyspnea may not occur if a patient no longer walks far or fast enough to experience them. Other symptoms may be atypical; for example, the age-related decrease in left ventricular compliance may produce exertional dyspnea rather than angina in patients with myocardial ischemia. Memory or attention deficits may prevent a patient from accurately recalling or describing a cardiac symptom. Drugs commonly used by the elderly may affect cardiac function. For example, a nonsteroidal anti-inflammatory drug may cause sodium retention, which may exacerbate heart failure.

Elderly patients should be asked about cardiovascular risk factors, including smoking, hypertension, hyperlipidemia, and diabetes mellitus. In the elderly, aggressive risk factor modification is well tolerated and is accompanied by a reduction in risk of coronary events. Whether arterial pulse wave velocity and carotid artery intimal-medial thickness are useful markers of cardiovascular risk is unclear; therefore, tests to determine these parameters should not be routinely performed.

Blood pressure measurement is essential because hypertension (systolic blood pressure $\geq$ 140 mm Hg or diastolic pressure $\geq$ 90 mm Hg, regardless of age) is the most common treatable cardiovascular risk factor in the elderly. Blood pressure is measured with the patient supine, sitting, and standing (after 2 minutes). In about 20% of persons > 65 years, standing causes blood pressure to decrease by > 20 mm Hg.◨ Absence of compensatory tachycardia suggests autonomic insufficiency, sinus node dysfunction, or a drug adverse effect.

Arterial blood pressure is measured in both arms to exclude significant stenosis distal to the origin of the subclavian artery. Systolic blood pressure is first estimated by palpation, because an auscultatory gap (disappearance and later reappearance of the Korotkoff sounds) is more prevalent among the elderly than among younger patients and may lead to systolic blood pressure's being greatly underestimated. Measurements of systolic blood pressure in the peripheral arteries cannot be used to accurately estimate central systolic blood pressure because such measurements do not consider the exaggeration of late systolic peak pressure in central arteries that occurs with age. A sclerotic noncompressible brachial or radial arterial wall that remains palpable at suprasystolic cuff pressure suggests generalized arteriosclerosis. Generalized arteriosclerosis may result in falsely high systolic blood pressure—a condition called pseudohypertension. Pseudohypertension is suspected when cuff pressure is very high but no target-organ damage is apparent. The diagnosis can be confirmed by measuring intra-arterial pressure. (Osler's sign—the ability to palpate the radial artery when the sphygmomanometric cuff is inflated to suprasystolic pressure—was thought to suggest pseudohypertension, but this sign is neither sensitive nor specific for pseudohypertension.)

◨ see page 845

Central venous pressure is best estimated by observing the right internal jugular vein because the left brachiocephalic (innominate) vein is often compressed by the aortic arch and the left external jugular vein.

Heart sounds are usually softer in the elderly, probably because the distance between the heart and the chest wall increases with age. Splitting of the second heart sound (S_2) can be heard in only about 30 to 40% of elderly patients. Wide splitting that increases with inspiration suggests right bundle branch block. In the elderly, the heart relies on atrial contraction to compensate for diminished early left ventricular filling. Consequently, a fourth heart sound (S_4) is normal, but a third heart sound (S_3) is always abnormal. In younger persons, the reverse is true. Kyphoscoliosis and other deformities of the chest wall complicate interpretation of the apical impulse and other precordial movements.

Systolic ejection murmurs (most often aortic) are detected in about half of elderly patients. These benign murmurs are distinguished from murmurs due to significant aortic valve stenosis or hypertrophic obstructive cardiomyopathy by their short duration, low intensity (usually grade 1 or 2), and failure to radiate. Age-related stiffening of the arterial tree may result in an apparently normal, brisk upstroke of the carotid artery pulse tracing, even in patients with severe aortic stenosis. Pulmonary valve murmurs are much less common among the elderly.

A **bruit** in the neck, abdomen, or groin strongly suggests carotid, aortorenal, or peripheral vascular disease, respectively. A prominent midline abdominal pulse with bruit suggests an abdominal aortic aneurysm.

Pulmonary rales are more likely to represent atelectasis, pulmonary fibrosis, or an acute inflammatory process (and not pulmonary edema) in elderly patients than in younger ones. Emphysematous lungs can produce factitious hepatomegaly by displacing the liver inferiorly.

Peripheral edema may be secondary to right-sided heart failure or to venous varicosities, lymphatic obstruction, or low serum albumin.

DIAGNOSTIC PROCEDURES

Noninvasive procedures provide important information in addition to that provided by the history and physical examination. Invasive procedures may also be needed (see TABLE 84–1).

ELECTROCARDIOGRAPHY

Although left ventricular wall thickness and mass tend to increase with age, ■ no age-specific criteria for ECG diagnosis of left ventricular hypertrophy have been developed. Limb lead and precordial

---

■see page 813

TABLE 84–1.   PROCEDURES COMMONLY USED FOR DIAGNOSING CORONARY ARTERY DISEASE

Procedure	Sensitivity	Specificity	Technical Difficulty	Complications
Resting ECG	ND	↓	↔	None
Exercise ECG	↑	Mild ↓	↑	↔
Pharmacologic stress testing*	↔	Mild ↓	↑ or ↔	↔
Echocardiography	ND	ND	↑	None
Transesophageal echocardiography	ND	ND	↔	↔
Rest and exercise radionuclide ventriculography	↔	↓	↔†	↔
Exercise thallium scintigraphy	↔	↔	↔†	↔
Electron-beam CT	↑	↓	↔	↔
Cardiac catheterization	NM	NM	↑	↑

*Pharmacologic stress testing is usually performed with echocardiography or thallium scintigraphy.

†Radionuclide ventriculography and thallium scintigraphy are not more difficult to perform in the elderly, but they are often combined with exercise testing, which can be hampered by age-related difficulties in performing maximal aerobic exercise.

ND = no data available; NM = not meaningful.

NOTE: Arrows denote whether there is an increase (↑), a decrease (↓), or no difference (↔) in elderly persons compared with younger persons.

QRS voltages decrease with age. Age-related increases in the frequency of ectopic beats, in PR and QT intervals, in left axis deviation, and in the frequency of right bundle branch block have no prognostic significance for elderly persons without clinical evidence of heart disease.

The most common ECG abnormality in the elderly is nonspecific changes in ST segments or T waves, which are often due to use of digoxin, a diuretic, an antiarrhythmic, or a psychoactive drug; such changes have little independent prognostic significance. However, if the patient is not using any of these drugs and if voltage criteria for left ventricular hypertrophy are met, these changes predict an increased risk of cardiovascular morbidity and mortality.

In the elderly, an ECG pattern of poor R-wave progression in leads V_1 to V_4 has low specificity and predictive value for anterior myocardial infarction (MI), probably because of age-related increases in resting lung volume and anteroposterior chest diameter. Thus, ECG may not be as useful in detecting silent MI in the elderly as in younger persons.

Ambulatory ECG monitoring, usually for 24 hours, is useful for elderly patients with unexplained syncope, palpitations, or other evidence suggesting major arrhythmias or conduction disorders. Patients with known organic heart disease, especially those who have had an MI, are appropriate candidates because they are the most likely to have a major arrhythmia during monitoring. However, because complex arrhythmias during ambulatory ECG monitoring are relatively common among healthy elderly persons, patients should record symptoms in a diary so that symptoms can be correlated with ECG rhythm disturbances. Ambulatory ECG monitoring is also useful for detecting asymptomatic episodes of myocardial ischemia.

When symptoms are infrequent and nondisabling, an ECG event recorder is a better choice because it is economical and can provide up to 6 weeks of intermittent monitoring. Loop event recorders can capture up to 4 minutes of retrospective ECG data before patient activation and can transmit the ECG via telephone to a central recording facility when symptoms occur.

ELECTROPHYSIOLOGIC TESTING

Electrophysiologic testing includes recording of His bundle activity, atrial pacing, programmed atrial or ventricular stimulation, and mapping of tachyarrhythmias. However, in elderly patients, it is used mainly for programmed ventricular stimulation when coronary artery disease (CAD) or a life-threatening ventricular arrhythmia is present. Electrophysiologic testing in the elderly has a low morbidity rate and helps determine the need for antiarrhythmic drugs or for an implantable cardioverter-defibrillator. ▪

TILT TABLE TESTING

Tilt table testing is usually recommended for patients who have unexplained syncope but do not have structural heart disease. Patients are typically tilted at a 60 to 80° angle on a motorized table for 15 to 20 minutes while their blood pressure and heart rate are continuously monitored. If hypotension (with or without bradycardia) does not occur, patients are given an infusion of isoproterenol sufficient to accelerate the heart rate by 20 beats/minute, and the test is repeated. The procedure produces many false-positive results and must be used only for patients with definite syncope and negative ambulatory ECG results.

▪ see page 894

TABLE 84-2.   TYPES OF STRESS TESTS

Type	Stress	Advantages	Disadvantages
Exercise	Treadmill	Is inexpensive; has a large diagnostic and prognostic database	Requires exercise, which many elderly patients cannot perform because of conditions unrelated to the heart; is often nondiagnostic
	Bicycle	Is inexpensive; has a large database; does not require gait stability	Same as for treadmill
	Arm ergometry	Does not require use of legs	May be insufficient to achieve target heart rate
Pharmacologic	Dipyridamole or adenosine	Is short in duration; is well tolerated by the elderly	Has lower sensitivity than dobutamine; has high incidence of minor adverse effects; is contraindicated in patients with COPD
	Dobutamine	Simulates exercise physiology; can be titrated by operator to patient's response; is well tolerated by the elderly	Requires close monitoring and dose titration; is time-consuming
Electrical	Atrial pacing	Avoids use of a drug	Is invasive; has not been used extensively

COPD = chronic obstructive pulmonary disease.

Diagnostic sensitivity tends to be lower but specificity tends to be higher in elderly patients with syncope than in younger patients.

EXERCISE TESTING

Exercise testing is generally safe for the elderly (see TABLE 84–2). Treadmill or bicycle exercise testing with continuous ECG monitoring is an efficient, inexpensive procedure for diagnosing CAD and determining the prognosis for patients with known CAD, especially those who have had an MI.■ Test sensitivity increases with patient age, from 56% in patients < 40 to 85% in those > 60. This correlation is consistent with the higher prevalence and greater severity of CAD in the

■ see also page 854

elderly. Test specificity decreases modestly with patient age, from 84% in patients < 40 to 70% in those > 60, probably because left ventricular hypertrophy, nonspecific resting ST-segment abnormalities, and valvular heart disease are more common among elderly patients.

Exercise-induced ST-segment depression has diagnostic and prognostic significance for elderly patients with chest pain. A reduced exercise capacity, a blunted increase in the heart rate–blood pressure product, and the occurrence of major ventricular arrhythmias during exercise indicate high risk of cardiac death for elderly patients who have had an MI.

The following age-related changes should be considered when exercise testing is performed in elderly patients:

- The elderly have a lower maximal aerobic capacity, so testing should begin at a level requiring low energy expenditure.

- Maximal heart rate decreases progressively by about 1 beat/minute yearly until at least about age 90.

- Systolic blood pressure at rest and at any given submaximal external workload is higher in the elderly, although age-related differences are less prominent at maximal effort.

- The ability to exercise is often limited by conditions unrelated to the heart (eg, arthritis, neurologic disorders, peripheral vascular disease).

- Elderly persons may not exercise maximally because of psychologic factors (eg, unfamiliarity with vigorous exercise, fear, insufficient motivation).

Alternatives to treadmill exercise testing include bicycle ergometry, arm ergometry, atrial or esophageal pacing, and pharmacologic stress testing with IV dipyridamole, adenosine, or graded IV infusions of dobutamine. If dobutamine increases the heart rate to < 85% of predicted maximum, atropine may be added. These pharmacologic stress tests are safe and effective for elderly patients and are preferred when patients cannot perform treadmill or bicycle exercise—eg, because of musculoskeletal or pulmonary disorders.

Thallium-201 myocardial perfusion scintigraphy during exercise or pharmacologic stress testing is considered the most accurate noninvasive test for detecting CAD in all age groups. Perfusion defects detected at rest generally indicate a previous MI. Segmental defects that are detected during exercise (or pharmacologic stress testing) and that resolve or improve within 3 to 4 hours indicate exercise-induced ischemia. This imaging procedure can be used to screen for CAD in the many elderly patients who have left ventricular hypertrophy or bundle branch block or who are receiving digoxin or other antiarrhythmic drugs.

The procedure's sensitivity and specificity for CAD is nearly 90% for patients of all ages. The extent of the exercise-induced defect is a useful prognostic indicator for elderly patients with known or suspected CAD. Adding tomographic imaging increases sensitivity but may decrease specificity for mild disease. In patients ≥ 70, IV dipyridamole-thallium imaging has a sensitivity of 86% and a specificity of 75%. Use of IV adenosine instead of dipyridamole results in a higher incidence of adverse effects, such as conduction system disturbances or arrhythmias caused by impulse formation.

Technetium-99m sestamibi produces better images than thallium and is useful for elderly patients with chronic obstructive pulmonary disease or marked obesity.

CHEST X-RAY

When rales are detected, a chest x-ray may be indicated to document left-sided heart failure. When pulmonary hypertension is suspected, a chest x-ray can confirm the diagnosis by showing large central pulmonary arteries with oligemic lung fields.

Aortic knob calcification is detected in about 30% of the elderly but has no pathologic significance. In contrast, intracardiac calcification, most commonly on the aortic valve and the mitral annulus, is almost always pathologic; it signifies valvular stenosis. In the elderly, coronary artery calcification, best seen with fluoroscopy, does not necessarily signify major stenosis, as it does in younger patients. Calcification of the pericardium (due to constrictive pericarditis) or the left ventricular wall (due to an old MI) is occasionally also seen.

ECHOCARDIOGRAPHY

In the elderly, echocardiography is useful for assessing left ventricular chamber size and function after diagnosis of heart failure or after acute MI; for assisting in the differential diagnosis of systolic murmurs, especially those grade 3/6 or higher in loudness; for measuring left atrial size and assessing left ventricular function in patients with new atrial fibrillation; for determining pulmonary artery pressures in patients with heart failure; for confirming the presence of pericardial effusion or tamponade; and for detecting a left ventricular aneurysm. Echocardiography can detect thickened aortic or mitral valve leaflets or a calcified mitral annulus, which are the most common sources of systolic murmurs in the elderly. Atrial myxomas, left ventricular thrombi, and valvular vegetations are best detected by echocardiography.

Echocardiography performed immediately after treadmill or pharmacologic stress testing may be used instead of radionuclide perfusion imaging to detect myocardial ischemia (which is indicated by wall motion abnormalities) and to determine prognosis. For patients $\geq$ 70, dobutamine stress echocardiography, which is the preferred noninvasive test for the elderly by many clinicians, has a sensitivity of 87%, a specificity of 84%, and an accuracy of 86% for the diagnosis of CAD. Adenosine stress echocardiography has a sensitivity of 66%, a specificity of 90%, and an accuracy of 73%. Exercise echocardiography has a sensitivity of 85% and a specificity of 77%.

M-mode echocardiography can detect age-related changes such as small increases in aortic root and left atrial dimensions, an increase in left ventricular wall thickness with no change in cavity size, and a decrease in mitral valve E-F closure slope (the rate of mitral valve closure in early diastole). Despite these changes, values for elderly persons usually remain within the limits of what is considered normal for younger persons.

Doppler echocardiography is used to quantify aortic valve stenosis. It is also used to assess diastolic dysfunction, particularly in patients with heart failure of unclear etiology. ◨ Doppler echocardiography can be used to predict length of survival for elderly patients with heart failure on the basis of E- and A-wave velocity measurements. Color Doppler echocardiography, with flow mapping, is useful for detecting and estimating the severity of valvular regurgitation. Mild multivalvular regurgitation is common among otherwise healthy elderly persons, so regurgitation is significant only if it is moderate or severe.

Transesophageal echocardiography is safe for elderly patients and should be considered for those with suspected heart disease if transthoracic echocardiography is not diagnostic. Transesophageal echocardiography is particularly useful for detecting aortic dissection, valvular vegetations, thrombi in the left atrium or left atrial appendage, and prosthetic valve dysfunction in patients who have the appropriate clinical presentation. Elderly patients with intra-aortic atherosclerotic debris detected by transesophageal echocardiography are at increased risk of thromboembolic events during cardiac surgery.

Intravascular ultrasonography allows detailed morphologic assessment of CAD but is expensive and invasive. This procedure may be useful for determining the suitability of a specific intervention (eg, balloon angioplasty, laser therapy, stent placement) for patients with CAD.

RADIONUCLIDE VENTRICULOGRAPHY

Radionuclide ventriculography is the most accurate procedure for assessing global left and right ventricular function. It is especially useful for patients with chest wall abnormalities or pulmonary hyperinflation (about 25% of elderly patients), because technically adequate echocardiograms cannot be obtained in them. Two techniques are used:

◨ see page 900

With the first-pass technique, the initial passage of technetium 99m through the cardiac chambers is recorded. With the more commonly used gated blood pool (equilibrium) technique, technetium 99m is allowed to equilibrate in the blood, and then ECG-gated (synchronized) images are recorded during many cardiac cycles. Both techniques can accurately measure global and regional left ventricular systolic performance as well as changes in left ventricular volume.

In elderly patients with suspected CAD, the first-pass or gated technique can be used to measure the left ventricular ejection fraction during bicycle exercise. Radionuclide ventriculography (as well as myocardial perfusion imaging) is particularly useful when ST-segment changes cannot be reliably interpreted because of left bundle branch block, left ventricular hypertrophy, or treatment with digoxin. An abnormal exercise response in elderly persons is best defined as any decrease in ejection fraction from the resting value. A regional wall motion abnormality that occurs during exercise is considered a specific indicator of CAD.

POSITRON EMISSION TOMOGRAPHY

Positron emission tomography is used to assess myocardial blood flow and metabolism. The procedure is very sensitive, but its diagnostic usefulness in the elderly is unknown. It is costly and requires an on-site cyclotron to generate radioisotopes.

COMPUTED TOMOGRAPHY

CT of the heart is useful for diagnosing cardiac masses and pericardial effusions and may help detect pericardial thickening and distinguish pericardial fat from effusion. Echo-free pericardial spaces, indicating fat or effusion, increase in prevalence with age and occur in about 10% of women > 80.

Electron-beam CT detects CAD by determining the density of calcifications in the arterial wall; a calcium score above a predetermined threshold suggests significant luminal narrowing. The presence of calcium in coronary arteries is highly specific for CAD in younger patients; however, with age, this specificity decreases, from 74% in patients < 40 to 34% in those > 50. Because of the low specificity, this procedure is not recommended for diagnosing CAD in the elderly. The patency of coronary artery bypass grafts can be assessed using this procedure. It may be used instead of cardiac catheterization after bypass surgery, but IV injection of iodinated contrast media is required.

MAGNETIC RESONANCE IMAGING

MRI can characterize cardiac anatomy and metabolism without use of ionizing radiation. It can assess myocardial viability in patients who

TABLE 84-3.   COMPLICATIONS OF CORONARY ANGIOGRAPHY

	Incidence*	
Complication	Age ≤ 60 yr	Age > 60 yr
Arrhythmia	4.3	5.1
Contrast reaction	2.7	2.0
Death	0.7	1.2
Hemorrhage	0.5	1.0
Myocardial infarction	0.7	0.6
Stroke	0.5	0.9
Vascular events	4.2	4.9

*Per 1000 cases.
Data from Johnson LW, Lozner EC, Johnson S, et al: "Coronary arteriography 1984–1987: A report of the Registry of the Society for Cardiac Angiography and Interventions. I. Results and complications." *Catheterization and Cardiovascular Diagnosis* 17:5–10, 1989.

have had an infarction and in those who have chronic heart failure or many other disorders. It is an alternative to echocardiography for measuring chamber size and thickness. ECG-gated imaging allows ventricular function assessment; however, it is expensive, restricting its use in primary diagnosis.

CARDIAC CATHETERIZATION AND CORONARY ANGIOGRAPHY

Cardiac catheterization with coronary angiography remains the gold standard for diagnosis and quantitation of CAD. It is the only procedure that directly measures intracardiac pressures and defines coronary artery anatomy. The risks of cardiac catheterization, including cerebral and peripheral embolization, renal failure, and death, are increased for the elderly. Risks may be increased because elderly patients are more likely to have preexisting coronary and peripheral vascular disease, renal insufficiency, and left ventricular dysfunction.

The incidence of death and major complications associated with coronary angiography in patients ≥ 60 is low but is still significantly higher than that in younger patients (see TABLE 84-3). The incidence is higher in the elderly partly because cardiomegaly and left ventricular dysfunction are more common and because obtaining vascular access is more difficult. Nonetheless, coronary angiography is appropriate for elderly patients with CAD when revascularization is being considered.

Digital subtraction angiography, a computer-enhanced imaging technique, may be safer because the amount of contrast media can be reduced by 75%.

A persistent elevation of systolic and/or diastolic arterial pressure.

Hypertension is usually defined as a systolic blood pressure of ≥ 140 mm Hg or a diastolic pressure of ≥ 90 mm Hg, regardless of age. Isolated systolic hypertension is defined as a systolic pressure of ≥ 140 mm Hg and a diastolic pressure of < 90 mm Hg.

For persons living in industrialized countries, systolic and diastolic blood pressures tend to increase until about age 60. After that, systolic pressure may continue to increase, but diastolic pressure tends to stabilize or decrease. More than 50% of Americans ≥ 65 have high systolic or diastolic pressure. However, for persons living in some developing countries, neither systolic nor diastolic pressure increases with age, and hypertension is practically nonexistent, possibly because of low intake of sodium (< 1.4 g/day [< 60 mEq/day]) and greater physical activity.

The high prevalence of hypertension in the USA might suggest that an age-related increase in arterial pressure is normal and innocuous. However, the higher the systolic or diastolic pressure, the higher the cardiovascular and total morbidity and mortality rates. High systolic pressure is a more accurate predictor of cardiovascular complications than is high diastolic pressure. Elevation of systolic blood pressure higher than 160 mm Hg increases cardiovascular mortality risk by 2 to 5 times, risk of stroke by 2½ times, and overall mortality risk by 1½ times.

In general, hypertension predisposes elderly persons to heart failure, stroke, renal failure, coronary artery disease, and peripheral vascular disease. Antihypertensive therapy reduces the risk of developing many of these catastrophic complications. For instance, treatment of hypertension reduces the incidence of fatal myocardial infarction (by 60% in one study), nonfatal myocardial infarction, and fatal and nonfatal stroke.

Etiology

The causes of arterial hypertension appear to be no different for elderly and younger patients. **Essential (primary) hypertension,** affecting at least 90% of the 50 million hypertensive persons in the USA, may result from changes in any of the pressor and depressor mechanisms that maintain normal arterial pressure. **Secondary hypertension** is less common than essential hypertension and may be caused by various conditions, which may also exacerbate existing essential hypertension. The most common of these conditions are renal disorders, including renal artery stenosis due to atherosclerosis, which is common among the elderly; renal parenchymal disease (eg, chronic glomerulonephritis or pyelonephritis, polycystic renal disease, collagen disease of the kidneys, obstructive uropathy); and renal neoplasms.

Endocrine disorders (eg, thyroid disorders, Cushing's syndrome, primary aldosteronism, pheochromocytoma, hypercalcemic diseases, release of humoral agents from malignant tumors) can cause hypertension and may account for recent onset of hypertension in elderly patients.

Drugs (eg, cyclosporine, tricyclic antidepressants, monoamine oxidase inhibitors, phenylpropanolamine or other vasoconstrictors in over-the-counter cold preparations, corticosteroids, estrogen preparations) may precipitate hypertension. Drugs may also aggravate or complicate existing hypertension. For example, use of nonsteroidal anti-inflammatory drugs can elevate blood pressure or make preexisting hypertension harder to control. Secondary hypertension may also be caused by use of cocaine, licorice, or excess alcohol or by coarctation of the aorta.

Atherosclerotic disease may lead to isolated systolic hypertension by reducing large artery compliance: The left ventricle ejects its stroke volume into a less compliant aorta, increasing systolic pressure afterload. Other conditions that can contribute to systolic hypertension in the elderly are hyperthyroidism, aortic insufficiency, malnutrition (with clinical or subclinical beriberi), arteriovenous fistulas, and fever.

Pathogenesis

The hemodynamic characteristics of elderly and younger hypertensive patients are similar.■ However, in the elderly, calculated total peripheral resistance may be higher and compliance of the large arteries may be reduced.

In most elderly patients with essential hypertension, intravascular volume contracts as arterial pressure and total peripheral resistance increase. Plasma renin activity and angiotensin II levels are reduced, suggesting an attenuated relationship between intravascular volume and the renin-angiotensin system. This attenuated relationship may explain why the responsiveness to diuretics and calcium channel blockers is enhanced in many elderly hypertensive patients, particularly in those with isolated systolic hypertension. However, calcium channel blockers have not been shown to reduce cardiovascular morbidity and mortality risk better than other drugs.

A tissue-based renin-angiotensin system probably exists within the vascular myocyte and may contribute to the tone of vascular smooth muscle and to arterial remodeling, including increased vascular mass and fibrosis. Such a system may explain the effectiveness of angiotensin-converting enzyme (ACE) inhibitors in the elderly, who usually have low plasma renin activity.

Hypertension and aging act synergistically to produce nephrosclerosis. Renal blood flow decreases, intrarenal vascular resistance increases, and the glomerular filtration rate and the ability to concentrate

■see page 821

urine decrease. Among elderly patients with untreated essential hypertension, the incidence of hyperuricemia is high, because the lower the renal blood flow, the higher the serum uric acid concentration.

Several factors may predispose elderly persons with hypertension to heart failure. As vascular resistance increases, so do systolic and diastolic pressures. The heart adapts to this increasing afterload by developing concentric left ventricular hypertrophy. Because of the frequent coexistence of myocardial ischemia, blood supply to the myocardium may be insufficient—even if arterial pressure is not dramatically elevated. Age-related changes independent of blood pressure (eg, reduced β-adrenergic responsiveness; focal deposition of collagen, amyloid, and other substances in the myocardium) contribute to the risk of developing heart failure by reducing myocardial contractility. Obesity may lead to expansion of intravascular volume, increased venous return to the heart, and increased cardiac output. This volume overload provides an eccentric component (increased septal hypertrophy) to the left ventricular hypertrophy.

Symptoms and Signs

Patients with uncomplicated essential hypertension (ie, without target organ damage) are usually asymptomatic. Headaches, epistaxis, and tinnitus are often attributed to hypertension, but these symptoms are as common among persons without hypertension. Symptoms and signs are more common among patients with secondary hypertension.

In patients with essential hypertension, the presence of symptoms or signs suggests target organ damage. Early manifestations of cardiac involvement include easy fatigability, palpitations, and atrial or ventricular ectopia. Chest pain in patients without occlusive coronary artery disease may result from increased myocardial oxygen demand with persistently high blood pressure and left ventricular hypertrophy. More extensive cardiac involvement is marked by symptoms and signs of heart failure: exertional dyspnea, orthopnea, peripheral edema, and increased ventricular irritability. A third heart sound may develop, usually in association with a fourth heart sound, which reflects the reduced compliance of the hypertrophic left ventricle. Sudden onset of back pain and hypertension suggests aortic dissection.

Sensory or motor deficits indicate brain involvement. Transient speech impediments, numbness of fingers and extremities, and unusual weakness suggest a transient ischemic attack; these symptoms are subtle. ◨ Sudden onset of a vertiginous headache and hypertension suggests a subarachnoid hemorrhage.

All patients should be examined for hypertensive retinopathy, which, in elderly patients, should be distinguished from the changes of arteriosclerosis (increased arteriolar light striping, arteriovenous nicking,

◨ see page 401

and tortuosity). Ophthalmoscopy may detect arteriolar and venular constriction, hemorrhages, exudates, and papilledema, suggesting advanced hypertensive vascular disease. Retinal changes due to hypertension can be classified (according to the Keith-Wagener-Barker classification) into groups with increasingly worse prognostic implications: 1—constriction of retinal arterioles only; 2—constriction and sclerosis of retinal arterioles; 3—hemorrhages and exudates in addition to vascular changes; and 4—papilledema (malignant hypertension).

The physician should listen for renal, carotid, aortic, brachial, and femoral artery bruits. A carotid artery bruit with symptoms of a transient ischemic attack suggests an embolus originating from that artery.

Diagnosis

Hypertension is diagnosed when systolic blood pressure is ≥ 140 mm Hg and/or diastolic pressure is ≥ 90 mm Hg. The high pressure should be documented on at least three separate occasions, with at least two separate measurements on each occasion.

Proper measurement technique is especially important in elderly patients. Blood pressure should be measured in both arms (during the initial examination and periodically thereafter), because occlusive atherosclerotic disease of the subclavian or brachial artery often reduces systolic pressure in one arm. Measurements should be made while the patient is sitting (after a 5-minute rest), then immediately after the patient stands, because orthostatic (postural) hypotension is common among elderly patients, particularly after meals.

Pseudohypertension may occur in elderly patients with very stiff arteries. In such patients, sphygmomanometry may detect spurious blood pressure elevations because the cuff cannot completely occlude the sclerotic brachial artery. (Osler's sign—the ability to palpate the radial artery when the sphygmomanometric cuff is inflated to suprasystolic pressure—was thought to suggest pseudohypertension, but this sign is neither sensitive nor specific for pseudohypertension.) Pseudohypertension is rarely diagnosed on the basis of physical examination before treatment. It may be diagnosed when elderly patients treated for hypertension develop excessive fatigue or severe orthostasis.

In patients with **secondary hypertension,** the cause may be suspected on the basis of symptoms. Pheochromocytoma may produce headaches, flushing, and dramatic blood pressure lability. Occlusive renal artery disease may produce headaches and renal artery bruits. Occlusive renal artery disease is more likely when a renal artery bruit has a diastolic component than when it has only a systolic component. Renal parenchymal disease may produce recurrent urinary tract infections, urinary frequency, nocturia, an impaired ability to concentrate urine, or microscopic or gross hematuria; anemia may develop with advanced disease. The coexistence of hypertension and anemia may indicate renal parenchymal disease in younger patients (if hemoglobinopathy is excluded) but may indicate a neoplasm in the elderly.

For patients with hypertension of recent onset and without renal artery disease or another evident cause, thyroid disorders must be ruled out, because elderly patients with thyroid disease may not have the characteristic symptoms of hyperthyroidism**◨** or hypothyroidism.**◩** Patients with primary aldosteronism have muscle weakness, nocturia, isosthenuria, altered carbohydrate metabolism, and hypokalemic alkalosis. Cushing's syndrome is suggested by hypokalemic alkalosis, the typical facies, hirsutism, purplish abdominal striae, buffalo hump, and new appearance of acneiform lesions.

Laboratory tests: A CBC count, an ECG (to detect left ventricular hypertrophy, left atrial abnormality, and arrhythmias), selected blood tests (eg, serum measurements of fasting glucose, creatinine, electrolytes, uric acid, potassium, thyroid-stimulating hormone, and lipids, including high-density and low-density cholesterol), and a urinalysis should be performed.

Proteinuria occurs late in the course of uncomplicated essential hypertension. If daily urinary protein excretion exceeds 400 mg, nephrosclerosis due to essential hypertension is not likely to be the cause; instead, other causes of renal parenchymal disease should be considered. An alkaline pH in a fresh urine sample suggests hypokalemia or primary aldosteronism.

The chest x-ray is less specific than the ECG for detecting cardiac enlargement. An enlarged left atrium does not indicate atrial disease per se but is probably secondary to reduced left ventricular compliance resulting from left ventricular hypertrophy.

An echocardiogram can show ventricular hypertrophy. Moreover, the echocardiogram can distinguish primarily systolic dysfunction from primarily diastolic dysfunction.

Treatment

Treatment is similar for elderly and younger patients in many ways. For both, blood pressure level and the presence of risk factors, target organ damage, and cardiovascular disease must be considered (see TABLES 85–1 and 85–2). However, for elderly patients, the greater potential for troublesome adverse effects from treatment must also be considered.

Usually, patients whose systolic blood pressure increases with age but remains within the normal limits are not treated. However, without treatment, such patients are at higher risk of cardiovascular events: the greater the increase in systolic blood pressure, the higher the risk.

◨ see page 648   ◩ see page 644

TABLE 85–1.   COMPONENTS OF RISK STRATIFICATION FOR PATIENTS WITH HYPERTENSION

Risk Factor	Target Organ Damage or Cardiovascular Disease
Age > 60 Diabetes mellitus Dyslipidemia Family history of cardiovascular disease (in female relatives < 65 and in male relatives < 55) Male sex Postmenopausal status Smoking	Heart disease (eg, left ventricular hypertrophy, angina, myocardial infarction, heart failure) Nephropathy Peripheral artery disease Retinopathy Stroke or transient ischemic attack

Modified from "The Sixth Report of the Joint National Committee on Prevention, Detection, Evaluation, and Treatment of High Blood Pressure." *Archives of Internal Medicine* 157(21): 2413–2446, 1997.

Lifestyle modifications to lower blood pressure are recommended for all patients with hypertension. They include maintaining a desirable body weight, moderating alcohol intake ($\leq$ 1 oz of ethanol equivalent per day), controlling dietary sodium ($\leq$ 2.3 g [$\leq$ 100 mEq]/day), exercising regularly, and stopping smoking. These measures may not con-

TABLE 85–2.   TREATMENT BASED ON RISK STRATIFICATION*

Blood Pressure Stage (mm Hg)	Risk Group A†	Risk Group B‡	Risk Group C§
High-normal (130–139/85–89)	Lifestyle modification	Lifestyle modification	Drug therapy‖
Stage 1 (140–159/90–99)	Lifestyle modification (up to 12 mo)	Lifestyle modification¶ (up to 6 mo)	Drug therapy
Stage 2 (160–179/100–109)	Drug therapy	Drug therapy	Drug therapy
Stage 3 ($\geq$ 180/$\geq$ 110)	Drug therapy	Drug therapy	Drug therapy

*Lifestyle modification is recommended for all patients with hypertension.

† No risk factors, no target organ disease, no clinical cardiovascular disease (see TABLE 85–1).

‡ At least 1 risk factor, excluding diabetes; no target organ disease; no clinical cardiovascular disease.

§ Target organ disease or clinical cardiovascular disease, with or without other risk factors.

‖ For patients with heart failure, renal insufficiency, or diabetes.

¶ For patients with multiple risk factors, physicians should consider drugs for initial therapy.

Modified from "The Sixth Report of the Joint National Committee on Prevention, Detection, Evaluation, and Treatment of High Blood Pressure." *Archives of Internal Medicine* 157(21): 2413–2446, 1997.

TABLE 85-3.   ORAL ANTIHYPERTENSIVE DRUGS

Class	Examples	Usual Total Daily Dose (mg)*	Selected Adverse Effects and Comments†
Diuretics‡			
Thiazide and thiazide-like diuretics	Chlorthalidone	12.5–50 once daily	Short-term increased cholesterol, triglyceride, and glucose levels (with indapamide, less or no hypercholesterolemia); decreased potassium, sodium, and magnesium levels; increased uric acid and calcium levels; rarely, blood dyscrasias, photosensitivity, pancreatitis, rashes, other allergic reactions, sexual dysfunction
	Hydrochlorothiazide	12.5–25 once daily	
	Indapamide	1.25–5 once daily	
	Metolazone (rapidly available form)	0.5–1 once daily	
	Metolazone	1.25–5 once daily	
Potassium-sparing diuretics			Hyperkalemia, gastrointestinal disturbances
	Amiloride	5–10 once daily	
	Spironolactone	12.5–100 once daily or in 2 divided doses	(Gynecomastia)
	Triamterene	50–100 once daily or in 2 divided doses	
Adrenergic blockers			
Peripherally acting adrenergic inhibitors	Guanadrel§	10–75 in 2 divided doses	(Orthostatic hypotension, diarrhea)
	Guanethidine§	10–50 once daily	(Orthostatic hypotension, bradycardia, diarrhea)
	Reserpine§,‖	0.05–0.1 once daily	(Nasal congestion, sedation, depression, activation of peptic ulcer)
Centrally acting α-agonists			Sedation, dry mouth, bradycardia, rebound hypertension when drug is withdrawn
	Clonidine	0.1–0.6 in 2 or 3 divided doses	(Rebound hypertension with sudden withdrawal)
	Clonidine (transdermal)	One patch weekly (0.1–0.3 mg/day)	(Rash)

Table continues on the following page.

TABLE 85-3.   ORAL ANTIHYPERTENSIVE DRUGS (Continued)

Class	Examples	Usual Total Daily Dose (mg)*	Selected Adverse Effects and Comments†
Centrally acting α-agonists (cont'd)	Guanabenz§	4–32 in 2 divided doses	
	Guanfacine§	1–3 once daily	(Less severe rebound hypertension than with clonidine)
	Methyldopa§	250–2000 in 2 divided doses	(Depression, heart block, orthostatic hypotension, hepatic and autoimmune disorders; no rebound hypertension)
α₁-Blockers			Syncope with first dose, palpitations, fluid retention, anticholinergic effects, orthostatic hypotension, urinary frequency, priapism
	Doxazosin	1–16 once daily	
	Prazosin	1–20 in 2–3 divided doses	
	Terazosin	1–20 once daily	
β-Blockers			Bronchospasm, bradycardia, heart failure, possible masking of insulin-induced hypoglycemia, impaired peripheral circulation, insomnia, fatigue, decreased exercise tolerance, hypertriglyceridemia (unless the drug has intrinsic sympathomimetic activity), depression, Raynaud's phenomenon, vivid dreams, hallucinations, erectile dysfunction
	Acebutolol ¶,#	200–1200 once daily or in 2 divided doses	(Positive antinuclear antibody test results; very rarely, drug-induced systemic lupus erythematosus)
	Atenolol ¶	25–100 once daily or in 2 divided doses	
	Betaxolol ¶	5–40 once daily	
	Bisoprolol ¶	5–20 once daily	
	Carteolol#	2.5–10 once daily	

TABLE 85-3.   (*Continued*)

Class	Examples	Usual Total Daily Dose (mg)*	Selected Adverse Effects and Comments†
β-Blockers (*cont'd*)	Metoprolol succinate ¶ (extended-release)	50–400 once daily	
	Metoprolol tartrate	50–200 once daily or in 2 divided doses	
	Nadolol	20–240 once daily	
	Penbutolol	10–20 once daily	
	Pindolol	10–60 in 2 divided doses	
	Propranolol	40–240 in 2 divided doses	
	Propranolol (extended-release)	60–240 once daily	
	Timolol	10–40 in 2 divided doses	
α-β-Blockers			Orthostatic hypotension, bronchospasm
	Carvedilol	12.5–50 in 2 divided doses	
	Labetalol	200–1200 in 2 divided doses	
Direct vasodilators			Headache, fluid retention, tachycardia
	Hydralazine hydro-chloride	40–200 in 2 to 4 divided doses	(Lupus-like syndrome, hepatitis)
	Minoxidil	2.5–40 once daily or in 2 divided doses	(Hirsutism, pericardial effusion)
Calcium channel blockers Nondihydro-pyridines			Atrioventricular block, bradycardia, heart failure, conduction defects, worsening of systolic dysfunction, gingival hyperplasia
	Diltiazem	120–360 in 2 divided doses	(Nausea, headache)
	Diltiazem (extended-release)	120–360 or 480 once daily, depending on formulation	
	Verapamil	120–480 in 2 or 3 divided doses**	(Constipation)

Table continues on the following page.

TABLE 85-3.   ORAL ANTIHYPERTENSIVE DRUGS (*Continued*)

Class	Examples	Usual Total Daily Dose (mg)*	Selected Adverse Effects and Comments†
	Verapamil (extended-release)	120–480 once daily	
Dihydropyri-dines			Dizziness, edema of the ankle, flushing, headache, gingival hypertrophy
	Amlodipine	2.5–10 once daily	
	Felodipine	2.5–10 once daily	
	Isradipine	5–10 in 2 divided doses	
	Isradipine (extended-release)	5–10 once daily	
	Nicardipine (extended-release)	60–120 in 2 divided doses	
	Nifedipine (extended-release)	30–90 once daily	
	Nisoldipine	10–60 once daily	
Angiotensin-converting enzyme inhibitors			Commonly, cough; rarely, angioedema, hyper-kalemia, rash, loss of taste, leukopenia, acute renal failure with unilat-eral or bilateral renal artery stenosis
	Benazepril	10–40 once daily or in 2 divided doses	
	Captopril	12.5–150 in 2 or 3 divided doses	
	Enalapril	2.5–40 once daily or in 2 divided doses	
	Fosinopril	10–40 once daily or in 2 divided doses	
	Lisinopril	5–40 once daily	
	Moexipril	7.5–30 once daily or in 2 divided doses	
	Quinapril	5–80 once daily or in 2 divided doses	
	Ramipril	1.25–20 once daily or in 2 divided doses	
	Trandolapril	1–4 once daily	

TABLE 85–3.   (*Continued*)

Class	Examples	Usual Total Daily Dose (mg)*	Selected Adverse Effects and Comments†
Angiotensin II receptor blockers			Hyperkalemia; very rarely, angioedema
	Irbesartan	150–300 once daily	
	Losartan	25–100 once daily or in 2 divided doses	
	Valsartan	80–320 once daily	

*Dosages may vary from those listed in the *Physicians' Desk Reference* (53rd edition), which may be consulted for additional information.

† Selected adverse effects are listed for the class of drugs; exceptions for individual drugs are noted in parentheses. The package insert includes a more detailed listing.

‡ Loop diuretics are not the diuretic of choice for elderly patients.

§ The drug is generally considered a poor choice for the elderly and is best avoided.

‖ The drug also acts centrally.

¶ The drug is cardioselective in low doses.

The drug has intrinsic sympathomimetic activity.

** Dosage varies depending on the formulation.

Modified from "The Sixth Report of the Joint National Committee on Prevention, Detection, Evaluation, and Treatment of High Blood Pressure." *Archives of Internal Medicine* 157(21): 2413–2446, 1997.

trol arterial pressure completely but may control it adequately or enable the drug dosage to be reduced.

When lifestyle modifications do not control hypertension, monotherapy with a diuretic, a β-blocker, an ACE inhibitor, a calcium channel blocker, an α-β-blocker, or an $α_1$-blocker in submaximal doses may be used (see TABLE 85–3). Thiazide diuretics (eg, hydrochlorothiazide 12.5 to 25 mg) or β-blockers are often recommended as initial therapy, because some controlled studies have shown that these drugs reduce cardiovascular and total mortality rates and cardiovascular morbidity rates in all age groups. However, recent data suggest that β-blockers may not be a good choice for the elderly except after a myocardial infarction. The issue remains controversial.

If the initial dose of an antihypertensive does not control blood pressure, the stepped-care approach may be used. The dose of the current drug may be increased, or a second drug may be added, thus avoiding dose-related adverse effects caused by increasing the dose of the first drug. Alternatively, a different antihypertensive may be tried.

Treatment based on special needs: Selecting drugs based on special needs, such as the pressor mechanism causing hypertension, may be useful. For example, black or obese patients, who are more volume-dependent and have low plasma renin activity, may respond well to a diuretic or calcium channel blocker. Patients with unilateral renal stenosis but two kidneys may respond better to an ACE inhibitor. For patients who have had a myocardial infarction or who have angina pectoris, migraine headaches, or glaucoma, a β-blocker may be appropriate. For hypertensive patients with heart failure, ACE inhibitors may be particularly valuable. For men with benign prostatic hyperplasia, $α_1$-blockers or α-β-blockers are particularly appropriate for lowering blood pressure; however, in the other elderly patients, $α_1$-blockers may cause urinary incontinence.

In smokers, certain antihypertensives, such as β-blockers (eg, propranolol), may cause more hypertensive complications (eg, stroke, myocardial infarction) than other drugs, such as thiazide diuretics. Generally, β-blockers are contraindicated in patients with peripheral vascular disease, lung disease, or heart block.

Adverse effects: Although elderly patients with hypertension have no more adverse effects from prolonged treatment than do younger patients, they are more likely to have orthostatic hypotension due to use of peripherally acting adrenergic inhibitors. Also, hypotension may occur when the first few doses of an ACE inhibitor are taken. Centrally acting drugs are more likely to cause depression, forgetfulness, vivid dreams, hallucinations, and sleep problems. Diuretics, peripherally acting adrenergic inhibitors, and β-blockers may cause impotence.

Long-term therapy: All hypertensive patients should continue therapy after blood pressure is controlled, because blood pressure is likely to increase if therapy is discontinued. Stepping down therapy can be tried slowly. If blood pressure increases, therapy must be stepped up again.

86 ■ HYPOTENSION

Subnormal arterial blood pressure.

Baroreflex mechanisms regulate systemic blood pressure by increasing or decreasing heart rate and vascular resistance in response to transient decreases or increases in arterial pressure. With age, the baroreflex response to hypertensive and hypotensive stimuli progressively declines, and the risk of hypotension increases. Baroreflex function is most impaired in elderly patients with hypertension. Signs of impairment include increased blood pressure lability in response to daily activities and hypotension in response to stimuli that lower arterial pressure, particularly drugs.

The diminished baroreflex response may be caused partly by arterial stiffening due to atherosclerosis, which results in dampening of baroreceptor stretch and relaxation during changes in arterial pressure. Reduced adrenergic responsiveness by the aged heart and vasculature may diminish baroreflex-mediated cardioacceleration and vasoconstriction in response to hypotensive stimuli. These changes become clinically significant when common hypotensive stresses, such as postural changes, can no longer be rapidly or completely offset by compensatory increases in heart rate or in vascular resistance. With age, cerebral blood flow decreases. Cerebral autoregulatory mechanisms usually compensate for acute reductions in blood pressure. Autoregulation of cerebral blood flow is generally maintained with age, except in persons who have symptomatic orthostatic hypotension. However, chronic hypertension raises the lowest blood pressure at which autoregulation can maintain cerebral blood flow. Below this level, blood flow may decrease, increasing the risk of cerebral ischemia. Hypertension, heart disease, diabetes mellitus, and hyperlipidemia further decrease cerebral blood flow. Because of age- and disease-related decreases in cerebral blood flow, elderly patients are vulnerable to cerebral ischemia and syncope if blood pressure decreases.

ORTHOSTATIC HYPOTENSION

A reduction of ≥ 20 mm Hg in systolic blood pressure or of ≥ 10 mm Hg in diastolic blood pressure on standing upright.

Orthostatic hypotension occurs in 15 to 20% of community-dwelling and in about 50% of institutionalized elderly persons. Its prevalence increases with age and with basal blood pressure elevation and is higher among patients with cardiovascular disease. Many elderly persons have wide variations in postural blood pressure, which is closely associated with basal supine systolic blood pressure; ie, when basal supine systolic blood pressure is highest, the decline in postural systolic blood pressure is greatest. Among elderly nursing home residents, orthostatic hypotension is most prevalent in the morning when residents first arise, after basal supine systolic blood pressure has been highest.

Orthostatic hypotension is a significant risk factor for syncope,[1] falls,[2] and all causes of mortality in the elderly, even for those without other evidence of autonomic nervous system dysfunction.

Etiology

Orthostatic hypotension in the elderly may be due to age-related physiologic changes in blood pressure regulation, to certain disorders, or to use of certain drugs (see TABLE 86–1).

When due to aging, orthostatic hypotension varies dramatically from day to day and is associated with the exaggerated plasma norepinephrine response to postural change that is characteristic of aging. Orthostatic hypotension is often provoked by common hypotensive stresses

---

[1] see page 173   [2] see page 195

TABLE 86-1.   CAUSES OF ORTHOSTATIC HYPOTENSION

Cause	Examples
Systemic disorders	Adrenocortical insufficiency Dehydration Inactivity
Central nervous system disorders	Brain stem lesions Multiple cerebral infarcts Multiple system atrophy (eg, Shy-Drager syndrome) Myelopathy Parkinson's disease
Peripheral and autonomic neuropathies	Alcoholic and nutritional diseases (eg, vitamin deficiencies) Amyloidosis Diabetes mellitus (insulin-dependent) Paraneoplastic syndromes Tabes dorsalis
Drugs	Anticholinergics (eg, most antihistamines, gastrointestinal antispasmotics, some antiemetics) Antihypertensives (eg, methyldopa, clonidine, α-blockers, β-blockers, calcium channel blockers, angiotensin-converting enzyme inhibitors, hydralazine, guanethidine, vasodilators) Diuretics Levodopa and other antiparkinsonian drugs Monoamine oxidase inhibitors Nitrates Phenothiazines and other antipsychotics Tricyclic antidepressants

such as dehydration, use of hypotensive drugs, or the Valsalva maneuver during voiding. Although generally asymptomatic, orthostatic hypotension in otherwise healthy elderly persons may be sufficient to compromise cerebral blood flow and cause dizziness or syncope. Prolonged bed rest may further compromise blood pressure homeostasis, resulting in severe orthostatic hypotension.

The most common cause of acute orthostatic hypotension is dehydration during an acute illness. Excessive cardioacceleration on standing (which suggests dehydration as the cause of orthostatic hypotension in younger patients) may not occur in elderly patients because cardioacceleration is often blunted with age. A much less common cause of acute orthostatic hypotension is adrenocortical insufficiency accompanied by hyponatremia and hyperkalemia.

Chronic orthostatic hypotension is usually due to disorders of the autonomic nervous system and is associated with symptoms of autonomic nervous system dysfunction (eg, a fixed heart rate, incontinence, constipation, inability to sweat, heat intolerance, impotence, fatigability). Drugs—even when given in therapeutic doses—are a common cause of orthostatic hypotension (see TABLE 86–1). Drugs that reduce venous return, particularly nitrates and diuretics, commonly produce orthostatic hypotension in the elderly. The elderly depend on adequate venous return to generate a normal cardiac output because of age-related impairments in ventricular diastolic filling.◼ Drugs that slow heart rate can also precipitate orthostatic hypotension.

If no cause is identified, orthostatic hypotension is usually due to pure autonomic failure (previously called idiopathic orthostatic hypotension). Compared with other causes of orthostatic hypotension, pure autonomic failure produces lower basal plasma norepinephrine levels in the supine position, no increase in norepinephrine levels on standing, a lower threshold for the pressor response to infused norepinephrine, and an increased pressor response to tyramine despite the release of less norepinephrine at sympathetic nerve endings.

Diagnosis

A clinician should not assume that an elderly patient who reports postural dizziness and light-headedness has orthostatic hypotension. Blood pressure and pulse rate should be measured after the patient has been recumbent for at least 5 minutes and after the patient has been standing quietly for 1 minute and then for 3 minutes. A hypotensive response may be immediate or delayed. Measurements after a longer period of standing or a tilt test may be needed to detect a delayed hypotensive response.

Treatment

Symptoms can usually be reduced or eliminated, even without completely correcting orthostatic hypotension. Regardless of the cause, orthostatic hypotension should be managed in the following stepwise fashion:

Nonpharmacologic therapy: Patients with acute orthostatic hypotension due to dehydration should be treated with fluid replacement therapy. Patients with chronic orthostatic hypotension should be instructed to rise slowly after lying in bed or sitting in a chair for a long time. Dorsiflexing the feet before standing often promotes venous return to the heart, accelerates the pulse, and increases blood pressure. Crossing the legs while upright may also help increase blood pressure. A high-salt diet aimed at producing a modest weight gain blunts the symptoms of orthostatic hypotension in many patients. Elastic compression stockings that cover the calf and thigh may be effective;

◼see page 816

abdominal binders help some patients. Elevating the head of the bed 5 to 20° prevents the diuresis and supine hypertension caused by nocturnal shifts of interstitial fluid from the legs to the rest of the circulation.

Pharmacotherapy: Patients who remain symptomatic may require drug therapy. Fludrocortisone, a mineralocorticoid, appears to be effective for mild to moderately severe orthostatic hypotension due to most conditions. The dose is increased gradually from 0.1 mg/day po up to 1.0 mg/day until orthostatic hypotension resolves or trace pedal edema develops. Fludrocortisone increases extracellular fluid and plasma volume and sensitizes blood vessels to the vasoconstrictive effect of norepinephrine. Complications include supine hypertension, heart failure, and hypokalemia. Supine blood pressure and serum potassium should be measured every few months during therapy. If a patient has supine systolic blood pressure > 180 mm Hg, the dose may have to be reduced. Fludrocortisone should not be given in the evening before bed.

If patients taking fludrocortisone remain symptomatic, midodrine, a direct α_1-agonist, often helps. The starting dose is 2.5 mg po tid; the dose is increased 2.5 mg each week up to a total dose of 10 mg tid. Because the drug can cause supine hypertension, the evening dose should be given before the evening meal and at least 3 hours before bedtime. Other adverse effects include paresthesias, pruritus, and urinary retention.

Other drugs that may be helpful include nonsteroidal anti-inflammatory drugs, the central α_2-antagonist yohimbine, the α_2-agonist clonidine, and β-blockers that block β_2-vasodilator receptors or have intrinsic sympathomimetic activity (eg, pindolol). Yohimbine can increase central sympathetic nervous system outflow. When such outflow is reduced (as in patients with multiple system atrophy), α_2-agonists, which inhibit central sympathetic outflow in healthy persons, can act on peripheral α_2-receptors in the veins. This action promotes venoconstriction, thereby increasing venous return.

Caffeine 200 to 250 mg each morning as two cups of brewed coffee or a 200-mg tablet can be effective and can be used safely by the elderly. Ergot alkaloids, including oral ergotamine tartrate and dihydroergotamine given subcutaneously with oral caffeine, help some patients. Sympathomimetics such as ephedrine and phenylephrine are not consistently useful. For severe, unresponsive cases, erythropoietin may be useful.

POSTPRANDIAL HYPOTENSION

A decline in arterial blood pressure that occurs after a meal.

In clinically stable, unmedicated elderly persons, blood pressure decreases significantly after morning and noon meals; such decreases do not occur in younger persons. In up to one third of elderly persons, blood pressure decreases ≥ 20 mm Hg within 75 minutes of eating a meal. The incidence of postprandial hypotension is greatest among elderly persons with hypertension or autonomic nervous system dysfunction. In one study of institutionalized elderly persons, postprandial hypotension accounted for 8% of syncopal episodes.

Postprandial hypotension is thought to be due to impaired baroreflex compensation for splanchnic blood pooling during digestion. Alterations in autonomic control of heart rate and vascular resistance are probably underlying causes of this syndrome. Patients with postprandial hypotension and autonomic dysfunction have impaired forearm vasoconstriction, reduced systemic vascular resistance, and abnormal sympathetic nervous system control of heart rate after a meal.

Blood pressure should be measured once before meals and again at 30 and 60 minutes after meals in elderly patients who have postprandial dizziness, falls, syncope, or other cerebral or cardiac ischemic symptoms.

Treatment

Symptomatic patients should not take hypotensive drugs before meals and should lie down after meals. Reducing the dose of hypotensive drugs and eating small, frequent meals may also help. Walking after a meal helps restore normal circulation in some patients; however, hypotension may recur when the activity is stopped.

Low doses of a nonsteroidal anti-inflammatory drug, caffeine 200 to 250 mg with or without dihydroergotamine 6 to 10 μg/kg sc, or octreotide 12 to 16 μg sc before a meal may help. Caffeine should be taken only in the morning so that the effect wears off by evening, allowing sleep and preventing drug tolerance.

87   ATHEROSCLEROSIS

A disorder affecting medium and large arteries in which patchy subintimal deposits of lipids and connective tissue (atherosclerotic plaques) reduce or obstruct blood flow.

Atherosclerosis (collectively termed atherosclerotic cardiovascular disease) includes coronary artery disease (CAD), [1] cerebrovascular disease, [2] and peripheral vascular disease. [3] Although atherosclerosis contributes significantly to disability and death in all age groups, its toll is heaviest among the elderly.

---

[1] see page 853   [2] see page 397   [3] see pages 915 and 923

Epidemiology

The incidence of all forms of atherosclerosis increases with age, even among the elderly. However, during the last 30 years, the mortality rate for atherosclerosis has markedly and progressively decreased in the USA and in several other industrialized countries. The decreasing mortality rate is probably primarily due to the widespread use of preventive strategies, resulting in decreased prevalence of such risk factors as untreated hypertension, abnormal lipid levels, and cigarette smoking. Improvements in diagnosis and treatment of established atherosclerosis probably have contributed less.

Risk Factors

Many major risk factors increase in prevalence and severity with age. Often, several risk factors coexist, especially in the elderly. Nonmodifiable risk factors include age ($\geq$ 45 for men; $\geq$ 55 for women), premature menopause without estrogen replacement therapy, male sex, and a family history of premature atherosclerosis (in male relatives before age 55 or in female relatives before age 65). Increased carotid intimal-medial thickness and large vessel stiffness also increase risk.

The following risk factors are modifiable:

Hypertension is strongly correlated with risk of atherosclerosis, particularly for the elderly. For men and women of all ages, the overall risk of atherosclerosis is 2 to 3 times higher in persons with moderate to severe hypertension than in those with normal blood pressure; risk is intermediate for those with mild hypertension. Risk at any given level of blood pressure is 2 to 3 times higher in elderly men and women than in younger ones, and the risk is nearly always higher in men than in women, regardless of age. High diastolic blood pressure is an important risk factor for elderly men but is less important for elderly women.

Abnormal blood lipid levels[1]—ie, a high level of total or low-density lipoprotein (LDL) cholesterol and a low level of high-density lipoprotein (HDL) cholesterol—are strongly correlated with risk of CAD in younger men and women; however, whether the correlation is as strong in the elderly is controversial. A high triglyceride level is a marker for obesity, glucose intolerance, and a low HDL level, all of which are risk factors for CAD.

Cigarette smoking increases the risk of CAD, stroke, peripheral vascular disease, and death. The prevalence of cigarette smoking appears to decrease with age, primarily because smokers tend to die before reaching old age.

High blood glucose level, when chronic, is strongly associated with risk of atherosclerosis[2].

---

[1] see page 606   [2] see page 626

Obesity, even at an advanced age, is a significant risk factor for atherosclerosis. Progressive increases in body weight correlate with several other risk factors for atherosclerosis: increases in blood pressure and in cholesterol, triglyceride, and blood glucose levels and a decrease in HDL cholesterol level.

Infection and inflammation may be involved in the atherosclerotic process. Several microorganisms, such as herpesviruses (eg, cytomegalovirus), *Chlamydia pneumoniae,* and *Helicobacter pylori,* have been identified in atherosclerotic plaques in coronary arteries and other tissues. Elevated titers of antibodies to these microorganisms have been used to predict the recurrence of coronary events after an acute myocardial infarction. Despite these findings, there is no direct evidence that these microorganisms can cause atherosclerotic plaques. However, according to one theory, chronic subclinical infection with these and other microorganisms (eg, those related to chronic periodontal disease) may contribute to an extended but highly variable inflammatory process that could promote atherogenesis and its complications. The observation that C-reactive protein and other nonspecific inflammatory markers are strong predictors of initial and recurrent coronary events supports this theory.

Exacerbating Factors

Several lifestyle choices and conditions can precipitate or exacerbate a cardiovascular event (eg, myocardial infarction, stroke) in persons with atherosclerosis.

Cigarette smoking can exacerbate ischemia because the carbon monoxide derived from cigarette smoke reduces the oxygen-carrying capacity of hemoglobin. Nicotine and other substances derived from cigarette smoke affect vascular smooth muscle and platelets, possibly initiating thrombotic events in persons whose circulation has been compromised by atherosclerosis. Smoking may trigger ventricular arrhythmias, causing sudden cardiac death in vulnerable persons, presumably by enhancing sympathetic tone and reducing the threshold for ventricular fibrillation.

Exercise reduces the overall risk of cardiovascular events; however, risk is increased during and immediately after strenuous exercise, especially for persons who do not exercise regularly. The primary mechanism is temporary elevation of catecholamine levels.

Blood abnormalities may contribute to risk. For elderly men but not for elderly women, a high plasma fibrinogen level increases the likelihood of atherosclerosis-related events. A high white blood cell count, a high Hct, and low vital capacity (which are correlated with the number of cigarettes smoked per day) are markers for increased risk of cardiovascular events and CAD in elderly men whether they smoke or not, but only in women who smoke.

Hyperhomocysteinemia[1] appears to be an independent risk factor for premature atherosclerotic disease and to increase the likelihood of myocardial infarction and stroke, especially for persons with abnormal lipid levels. Homocysteine may accelerate atherosclerosis by affecting blood coagulation and by increasing the atherogenic properties of LDL particles and the proliferation of vascular smooth muscle cells. It is considered to be toxic to vascular endothelium and thereby thrombogenic. Factors that may increase homocysteine levels include advancing age, heavy smoking, renal insufficiency, psoriasis, acute lymphoblastic leukemia, breast cancer, and drugs that interact with vitamin B_6, vitamin B_{12}, and folic acid (eg, methotrexate, carbamazepine, phenytoin) or that interfere with the absorption of homocysteine (eg, colestipol, niacin) or with its metabolism (eg, isoniazid). Homocysteine levels are moderately high in many elderly persons whose diets are high in protein and/or deficient in vitamin B_6, vitamin B_{12}, or folic acid. Atropic gastritis, which occurs in about 35% of women > 80, interferes with B_{12} absorption and thereby can increase homocysteine levels. Many experts advocate the treatment of hyperhomocysteinemia in patients with CAD and homocysteine levels > 90th percentile of the specific assay used. Supplementation with folic acid, pyridoxine (vitamin B_6), and/or cyanocobalamin (vitamin B_{12}) is effective in decreasing homocysteine levels as well as safe and inexpensive;[2] however, supplementation has not been shown to reduce mortality and morbidity rates.

Left ventricular hypertrophy detected by ECG or echocardiography increases the likelihood of atherosclerosis-related events in elderly persons.

Symptoms and Signs

Patients are asymptomatic until obstruction of the affected artery produces symptoms of ischemia (eg, angina, claudication, transient ischemic attack, stroke) or until a complication (eg, thrombus, embolus, aneurysm) occurs. Typically, onset of symptoms is gradual, as the artery gradually narrows, and acute exacerbation of symptoms occurs during periods of increased demand (eg, during exercise). However, onset may be dramatic, as when an artery is acutely occluded. CAD,[3] cerebrovascular disease,[4] and peripheral vascular disease[5] produce specific symptoms and signs.

Diagnosis and Treatment

The diagnosis is typically based on symptoms and signs. Arterial narrowing may be confirmed by arteriography or Doppler ultrasonography.

---

[1] see also page 690   [2] see also page 592   [3] see page 853
[4] see page 397   [5] see pages 915 and 923

Modifiable risk factors should be managed, preferably early in life but also in old age. Treatment of established atherosclerosis depends on the specific type of atherosclerotic disease and the presence of complications. Such treatment includes dietary restriction of fats, weight control, exercise, and lipid-lowering drug therapy. ∎

88 ▬ CORONARY ARTERY DISEASE

A disorder in which one or more coronary arteries are narrowed by atherosclerotic plaque or vascular spasm.

Of persons ≥ 65, 30% have clinical manifestations of coronary artery disease (CAD). In autopsy studies, 70% of persons > 70 have CAD with ≥ 50% atherosclerotic obstruction of one or more coronary arteries. The prevalence of CAD and the incidence of new coronary events are higher among men than among women < 75 but are similar among men and women ≥ 75. CAD is the most common cause of death in persons ≥ 65, and 80% of deaths due to CAD occur in persons ≥ 65. The incidence of sudden cardiac death as the initial manifestation of CAD increases with age.

During the last 30 years in the USA, the CAD mortality rate has decreased for all geographic regions, most major sex-race groups, and all age groups > 35. Between 1968 and 1978, the CAD mortality rate decreased by 28% for persons aged 65 to 74 and by 19% for those aged 75 to 84. Between 1987 and 1994, the CAD mortality rate decreased by 5.1% per year, the incidence of recurrent myocardial infarction (MI) decreased, and post-MI survival rates increased. Furthermore, persons appear to be reaching old age with less severe atherosclerotic disease, according to recent autopsy studies. Factors contributing to the decreased severity of atherosclerosis and CAD mortality rate include reductions in cholesterol levels and in smoking prevalence as well as improved medical care for persons with acute CAD and better control of hypertension.

Risk Factors

Risk factors for CAD in elderly men and women include cigarette smoking, systolic and/or diastolic hypertension, increased pulse pressure, increased serum total and low-density lipoprotein (LDL) cholesterol levels, decreased serum high-density lipoprotein (HDL) cholesterol levels, diabetes mellitus, obesity, physical inactivity,

∎ see page 612

advancing age, increased carotid intimal-medial thickness, and hyper-homocysteinemia. **1** Hypertriglyceridemia is a risk factor for women.

Diagnosis

The diagnosis of CAD is usually based on symptoms and signs and is confirmed by angiographic evidence of significant coronary artery obstruction or by a previously documented MI. Coronary angiography is the gold standard for detecting the presence of CAD and determining its severity; noninvasive procedures (ECG, exercise testing, and echocardiography) can be used to detect myocardial ischemia. **2**

Results of diagnostic procedures may help predict which patients are more likely to have new coronary events. Such patients include those with evidence of left ventricular hypertrophy on an ECG or an ischemic ST-segment depression of ≥ 0.5 mm on a resting ECG; those with electronic pacemaker rhythm, atrial fibrillation, left bundle branch block, intraventricular conduction defect, type II second-degree atrioventricular block, or complex ventricular arrhythmias; and those who, in response to exercise testing, have exercise-induced hypotension, an inadequate blood pressure response to exercise, a marked ST-segment depression (≥ 2.0 mm) or an ST-segment depression in both anterior and inferior leads during exercise testing, short exercise duration (< 6 minutes using a standard Bruce treadmill protocol), an ST-segment depression that begins within 6 minutes of starting exercise, or persistence of ST-segment depression for > 8 minutes during recovery after exercise. The incidence of new coronary events is higher in elderly patients with CAD and complex ventricular arrhythmias or silent myocardial ischemia detected by 24-hour ambulatory ECG monitoring. Patients with left ventricular hypertrophy or with an abnormal left ventricular ejection fraction detected by echocardiography are at particular risk of new coronary events.

Primary Prevention

Modifiable risk factors for CAD should be controlled. Cessation of cigarette smoking, treatment of hypertension **3** and hyperlipidemia, **4** maintenance of a normal body weight, and regular physical activity lower the risk of CAD and new coronary events. A diet low in saturated fat and cholesterol is recommended. For obese persons, regular aerobic exercise and a healthy diet are recommended. **5** Moderate exercise programs suitable for the elderly include walking, climbing stairs, swimming, and bicycling.

Because the incidence of coronary events is higher in the elderly than in younger persons, risk factor modification causes a greater reduction in the absolute number of coronary events in the elderly.

---

1 see page 852   **2** see page 824   **3** see page 837   **4** see page 612
5 see page 605

ANGINA PECTORIS

A clinical syndrome of CAD caused by myocardial ischemia and characterized by dyspnea, precordial discomfort, pressure, or pain, typically precipitated by exertion and relieved by rest or sublingual nitroglycerin.

Symptoms, Signs, and Diagnosis

Among the elderly, dyspnea on exertion is a more common manifestation of myocardial ischemia than is chest pain. Exertional dyspnea results from a transient increase in left ventricular end-diastolic pressure caused by ischemia superimposed on reduced ventricular compliance.

Typically, chest pain occurs as tightness, heaviness, or constricting, pressing, squeezing, strangling, or burning discomfort in the substernal or adjacent area of the chest. The discomfort may be confined to the chest, or associated aching may be felt in one or both shoulders and arms (especially the ulnar aspect of the left upper arm) and in the fingers (particularly on the left side). Aching may also be felt in the neck, jaws, teeth, or left interscapular region. A choking sensation in the throat may be felt.

Anginal pain is less likely to be retrosternal in elderly than in younger patients and thus is more likely to be misinterpreted. Anginal pain in the back and shoulders may be misinterpreted as due to degenerative joint disease, and burning postprandial epigastric pain may be misinterpreted as due to peptic ulcer disease or a hiatus hernia. Some elderly patients underreport anginal pain because of confusion or dementia.

Anginal symptoms may be precipitated by exertion, emotional stress, heavy meals, or exposure to cold weather, wind, or tobacco smoke. For the elderly, exertion is a less common precipitant because their physical activity tends to be limited. The pain, which lasts 1 to 15 minutes, can usually be relieved within 3 minutes by use of sublingual nitroglycerin, by rest, or by resolution of emotional stress.

Anginal attacks vary in frequency from several a day to occasional attacks separated by symptom-free intervals of weeks or months. Attacks may increase in frequency (a phenomenon called crescendo angina), often leading to death, or they may gradually decrease or disappear if adequate collateral circulation develops, if the ischemic area becomes infarcted, or if heart failure supervenes and limits activity.

In stable angina, the characteristics of angina are usually constant. Unstable angina refers to any worsening in the pattern of symptoms—increased frequency, intensity, or duration of episodes; reduced threshold of stimulus; or occurrence when the patient is sedentary or awakening from sleep. Such changes may be prodromal to acute MI. In the elderly, acute pulmonary edema not due to acute MI may be a manifestation of unstable angina.

Treatment

Stable angina: The physician should identify and correct reversible factors that can aggravate myocardial ischemia and angina, such as anemia, infection, obesity, hyperthyroidism, hyperlipidemia, uncontrolled hypertension, arrhythmias (eg, atrial fibrillation with a rapid ventricular rate), and severe valvular aortic stenosis. Smokers should be advised to stop smoking. An exercise program can improve exercise tolerance. Aspirin 160 to 325 mg daily reduces the incidence of MI, stroke, and cardiovascular death.

Nitrates prevent and relieve angina. Nitroglycerin as a sublingual tablet (0.3 to 0.6 mg) or as a sublingual spray (0.4 mg) is the drug most commonly used to relieve an acute anginal attack. Onset of action is 2 to 5 minutes, and duration of action is 10 to 30 minutes. Initiating nitrate therapy at a low dose and increasing the dose slowly are important.

Long-acting nitrates help prevent recurrent episodes of angina. Isosorbide dinitrate 5 to 40 mg po bid or tid is commonly used. Onset of action is 15 to 30 minutes, and duration of action is 3 to 6 hours. Other commonly used long-acting nitrates include isosorbide mononitrate 5 to 60 mg po bid and transdermal nitroglycerin 5 to 15 mg as 2% ointment applied directly to the skin or in a skin patch. When long-acting nitrates are used, a 12- to 14-hour nitrate-free interval every 24 hours is necessary to prevent tolerance.

Hypovolemia, use of concomitant vasodilator therapy, impaired venous valves, and an impaired baroreceptor reflex make the elderly more susceptible to the hypotensive effects of nitrates. Episodes of hypotension may cause symptoms ranging from light-headedness to syncope and are commonly precipitated by standing. Patients should be instructed to sit or lie down when they take the drug sublingually.

β-Blockers are effective in preventing myocardial ischemia. Propranolol 10 to 40 mg qid, extended-release propranolol 40 to 240 mg once daily, timolol 10 to 20 mg bid, metoprolol 25 to 100 mg bid, extended-release metoprolol 50 to 200 mg once daily, atenolol 25 to 100 mg once daily, and labetalol 100 to 600 mg bid are commonly used. Because metoprolol and atenolol are relatively more cardioselective than propranolol, they are less likely to induce bronchospasm and peripheral arterial vasoconstriction when given in low doses. These two drugs also cause less sedation. When sedation or depression is a concern, nadolol may be preferable because it has the least central nervous system penetration. Patients with both heart failure and angina may be treated with carvedilol 3.125 to 25 mg bid.

A nondihydropyridine calcium channel blocker (eg, verapamil 40 to 120 mg tid, extended-release verapamil 120 to 240 mg daily, diltiazem 30 to 90 mg tid, extended-release diltiazem 120 to 300 mg daily) should be used if nitrates and β-blockers are contraindicated in, are poorly tolerated by, or do not control anginal symptoms in patients who have a normal left ventricular ejection fraction. If patients with persistent angina have heart failure or an abnormal left ventricular ejection fraction, amlodipine 2.5 to 10 mg daily or felodipine 2.5 to 20 mg daily should be used.

Revascularization is recommended if angina persists and interferes with quality of life or if noninvasive studies or the clinical picture indicates that the patient is at high risk (despite optimal therapy with nitrates, β-blockers, and calcium channel blockers). Cardiac catheterization, which has greater risks for the elderly,▌ is used to evaluate the need for coronary revascularization by percutaneous transluminal coronary angioplasty (PTCA) or coronary artery bypass grafting (CABG).▌

Unstable angina: About 90% of elderly patients can be stabilized with medical management. Care of elderly patients does not differ substantially from that of younger patients. After initiation of treatment in the emergency department, patients should be admitted to a coronary care unit. Reversible factors causing unstable angina (eg, anemia, hyperthyroidism) should be identified and corrected. When hospitalized, the elderly are prone to certain problems (eg, intensive care unit psychosis), and care should be taken to prevent these problems.▌ Oxygen therapy should be guided by arterial saturation; it is unlikely to help if oxygen saturation exceeds 94%.

Unless contraindicated, aspirin 160 to 325 mg should be given at admission and a daily dose continued indefinitely to reduce the risk of MI and death. The first dose should be chewed to facilitate the rapid antiplatelet effect of aspirin. Ticlopidine 250 mg bid or clopidogrel 75 mg daily may be used if aspirin is contraindicated. Use of tirofiban or abciximab (given with aspirin and heparin) may also reduce the incidence of coronary events.

For patients with pain at rest, ST-T wave changes of myocardial ischemia, and no contraindications for anticoagulation, continuous IV heparin should be started and maintained for at least 48 hours.▌

Patients whose symptoms are not fully relieved with three sublingual nitroglycerin tablets should be given continuous IV nitroglycerin for at least 24 hours. After patients have been angina-free for 24 hours, they can be switched to oral or transdermal long-acting nitrates.

β-Blockers, unless contraindicated, should be started in the emergency department. They are given IV initially, then orally.

Revascularization should be considered for patients who continue to have angina 30 minutes after initiation of therapy, who have angina that recurs during hospitalization, or who have unstable angina plus major ischemic complications (eg, pulmonary edema, complex ventricular arrhythmias, cardiogenic shock). Such patients are at increased risk of MI

▌see page 832   ▌see page 942   ▌see page 251   ▌see page 697

or cardiac death, and emergency coronary angiography should be performed to determine if PTCA or CABG is needed.◨ Insertion of an intra-aortic balloon pump is necessary for some patients.

MYOCARDIAL INFARCTION

Ischemic myocardial necrosis usually resulting from abrupt reduction in coronary blood flow to a segment of myocardium.

Clinically recognized or unrecognized MI occurs in 35% of elderly persons; 60% of hospitalizations due to acute MI occur in persons ≥ 65.

Symptoms and Signs

Of elderly patients with documented acute MI, 19 to 66% present with chest pain, 20 to 59% with dyspnea, 15 to 33% with neurologic symptoms, and 0 to 19% with gastrointestinal symptoms (eg, epigastric distress, vomiting, nausea, heartburn, indigestion). Other symptoms and signs include peripheral gangrene, increased claudication, palpitations, renal failure, weakness, pulmonary embolism, restlessness, sweating, and sudden cardiac death. Elderly patients with acute MI tend to delay longer than younger patients in seeking medical assistance after the onset of chest pain or other presenting symptoms of MI.

Elderly patients with acute MI are more likely than younger ones to die of MI and to have pulmonary edema, heart failure, left ventricular dysfunction, cardiogenic shock, conduction disturbances requiring insertion of a pacemaker, and atrial fibrillation or atrial flutter. In such patients, rupture of the left ventricular free wall, of a papillary muscle (which results in severe mitral regurgitation), or of the interventricular septum is also more likely. These ruptures are more common among women and among patients with persistent peri-infarctional hypertension. The rupture usually occurs without warning, most commonly 1 to 4 days after MI.

Diagnosis

Non–Q-wave MI, which is more common among elderly patients with acute MI than among younger ones, may be diagnosed in a symptomatic elderly patient when the plasma level of the MB-isoenzyme of creatine kinase is increased ≥ 5% or when serial ECGs show

- a new ST-segment elevation of ≥ 0.1 millivolt (measured 0.02 second after the J point),
- a new ST-segment depression of ≥ 0.1 millivolt (measured 0.08 second after the J point), or

- a new T-wave inversion of at least 0.1 millivolt in leads II, III, and aVF, in at least two precordial leads, or in leads I and aVL plus an increase of ≥ 5% in the plasma level of the MB-isoenzyme of creatine kinase

The total creatine kinase level is not necessarily increased after MI.

Q-wave MI may be diagnosed in a symptomatic elderly patient when serial ECGs show pathologic Q waves with a depth of ≥ 0.2 millivolt and a duration of ≥ 0.04 seconds. If pathologic Q waves occur on a resting ECG in a patient with no history of MI, the diagnosis is unrecognized Q-wave MI, which is common among elderly patients with documented MI (prevalence, 31 to 68%; incidence, 21 to 43%). The incidence of new coronary events among elderly patients with Q-wave MI is similar whether the MI is clinically recognized or unrecognized and whether the patients are men or women.

Treatment

Unless contraindicated, aspirin (or if contraindicated, ticlopidine or clopidogrel) should be given.[1] The role of glycoprotein IIb/IIIa inhibitors (eg, tirofiban, abciximab) in the treatment of elderly patients with acute MI is under study.

For chest pain associated with acute MI, morphine sulfate 2 to 4 mg IV is the drug of choice, but nitrates and β-blockers may also be used. Oxygen may be given but is unlikely to help if the oxygen saturation exceeds 94%. For heart failure, oxygen therapy, furosemide 20 to 80 mg IV, and nitrates may be used. For hypotension, IV fluids or dobutamine may be needed.

Subcutaneous heparin 7500 U q 12 h should be given to reduce the incidence of venous thromboembolism after treatment of acute MI.[2] The role of IV heparin in treatment of these patients is controversial, and that of low-molecular-weight heparin is under study.

Unless contraindicated, a β-blocker should be given to patients at admission. It is given IV initially, then orally. Such therapy can reduce the mortality rate by 23% in elderly patients who have had an MI (but it has not been shown to significantly reduce the mortality rate in younger patients). Risk of recurrent MI is also reduced. Early IV β-blocker therapy may be given with or without thrombolytic therapy.

Nitrates probably do not reduce mortality in patients with acute MI but may be used for treatment of chest pain and heart failure.

Early and continued use of an angiotensin-converting enzyme (ACE) inhibitor is recommended for patients with acute MI who are hemodynamically stable (systolic blood pressure ≥ 100 mm Hg) and who have heart failure, a large anterior MI, or a left ventricular ejection fraction of ≤ 40%. Such therapy can reduce the risk of death, severe heart failure,

[1] see page 857   [2] see page 697

and severe left ventricular systolic dysfunction. The reduction in risk of death and severe heart failure is greater among elderly than among younger patients. When ACE inhibitor therapy is initiated during acute MI, the patient's blood pressure, renal function, and serum potassium should be closely monitored.

Use of calcium channel blockers during acute MI is not recommended, because these drugs do not benefit and may harm patients with acute MI. Switching elderly patients who have been taking calcium channel blockers to β-blockers may be advisable.

The use of IV magnesium during acute MI is controversial. Magnesium should not be routinely used in the treatment of elderly patients with acute MI.

The prophylactic use of antiarrhythmic drugs other than β-blockers does not improve the clinical outcome in patients with acute MI. In a meta-analysis, prophylactic lidocaine, once commonly used, did not improve survival and was associated with an increased incidence of asystolic cardiac arrest. Also, the elderly are at increased risk of lidocaine toxicity. Therefore, the use of lidocaine during acute MI should be limited to treatment of patients with life-threatening ventricular arrhythmias. Patients with supraventricular tachyarrhythmias ▯ may be treated with β-blockers or direct-current cardioversion.

The need for a pacemaker may be temporary (during acute MI by transvenous pacing) or permanent (after acute MI).

Reperfusion therapy (thrombolytics or PTCA) during acute MI can reduce the absolute and percent mortality rate more among elderly patients than among younger patients. In patients > 80 who had had an MI, the mortality rate was 41% lower for patients given streptokinase than for those given placebo, and 14.1 lives per 100 treated patients were saved. Medical therapy alone is preferred for most elderly patients who have had an MI, but if revascularization is indicated, PTCA is generally preferred to CABG. ▯

Unless contraindicated, reperfusion therapy should be considered for elderly patients who have ischemic symptoms that last ≥ 30 minutes and that occur within 6 to 12 hours of clinical presentation and who have an ST-segment elevation of at least 1 to 2 mm in ≥ 2 ECG leads or who have left bundle branch block. Elderly patients with persistent myocardial ischemia, hypotension, or cardiogenic shock occurring > 12 hours after the onset of symptoms may still benefit from PTCA. Intracoronary stent placement decreases the risk of restenosis after PTCA. The potential benefit of reperfusion therapy is higher for elderly patients with a large anterior acute MI.

Streptokinase (1.5 million U IV over 1 hour) may be preferable to recombinant human tissue plasminogen activator (rt-PA) for the elderly

▯ see page 889   ▯ see page 944

because it causes fewer episodes of stroke and cerebral hemorrhage; it is also less expensive. However, the choice of thrombolytic drug is controversial. Minimization of delays in treatment is more important than drug choice.

Long-term management (see TABLE 88–1):   Modifiable risk factors should be controlled. Long-term drug therapy may include antiplatelet drugs, anticoagulants, β-blockers, nitrates, and ACE inhibitors. Calcium channel blockers are generally avoided; use of a calcium channel blocker instead of a β-blocker after MI doubled the risk of mortality in one study. Automatic implantable cardioverter-defibrillators and surgical treatment (revascularization with PTCA or CABG)◨ are appropriate for some patients.

Long-term use of the β-blockers propranolol, timolol, and metoprolol reduces rates of recurrent MI and sudden cardiac death more in elderly patients than in younger ones, regardless of whether the initial MI was non–Q-wave or Q-wave.

Class I antiarrhythmic drugs and D-sotalol (not clinically available) increase mortality rates after MI and should not be used in elderly patients after MI. Amiodarone and D,L-sotalol (which is available) do not significantly affect mortality rates after MI. β-Blockers are the only antiarrhythmic drugs that reduce mortality rates in elderly patients with nonsustained ventricular tachycardia or complex ventricular arrhythmias after MI; unless specifically contraindicated, β-blockers should be used to treat these patients after MI.

Because estrogen replacement therapy does not appear to improve outcome after MI and may increase the incidence of venous thromboembolic events and of gallbladder disease, it is not recommended for postmenopausal women who have had an MI.

Complications: When the left ventricular free wall, papillary muscle, or interventricular septum ruptures after acute MI, mortality risk is very high unless surgical repair is promptly performed.

When the left ventricular free wall ruptures suddenly, emergency surgery is not feasible. If the rupture is subacute, emergency cardiac surgery, perhaps after rapid stabilization with pericardiocentesis, volume expansion, intra-aortic balloon pump placement, and other medical therapy, offers hope of survival.

For patients with rupture of the papillary muscle, an overall operative mortality rate of 27% has been reported. The short-term and long-term mortality rates were slightly higher for those with ejection fractions < 45%; age did not predict survival. Patients with papillary muscle rupture and severe mitral regurgitation require prompt surgery because they may deteriorate rapidly, and surgery generally has good results. Age should not be a major consideration in the decision to perform surgery.

◨see pages 942–947

TABLE 88–1.   LONG-TERM MANAGEMENT AFTER MYOCARDIAL INFARCTION

Therapy	Indications	Specific Treatment
Risk factor modification	All patients as appropriate	Cessation of cigarette smoking Management of obesity with regular exercise and a healthy diet Management of hypertension Management of hyperlipidemia Management of diabetes
Antiplatelet drugs	All patients, unless use is contraindicated	Aspirin 160–325 mg daily, continued indefinitely
Anticoagulant drugs	Patients who cannot tolerate daily aspirin, who have atrial fibrillation, or who have a left ventricular thrombus	For elderly patients, oral warfarin in a dose that produces an INR of 2.0–3.0, continued indefinitely
β-Blockers*	All patients, especially patients with silent ischemia, angina, nonsustained ventricular tachycardia, complex ventricular arrhythmias, heart failure associated with an abnormal or a normal LVEF, diabetes mellitus, or a decreased LVEF (even without symptoms), unless use is contraindicated	Initiated during acute MI or within a few days of MI and continued indefinitely
Nitrates	Patients with angina	Requirement of a nitrate-free interval of 12–14 h each day to avoid nitrate tolerance, with β-blockers used during the interval to prevent angina and rebound myocardial ischemia
Angiotensin-converting enzyme inhibitors	Patients with clinical evidence of heart failure, an anterior MI, or an LVEF ≤ 40%, unless use is contraindicated	Instituted within 24 h of acute MI if the patient is hemodynamically stable or within a few days of MI and continued indefinitely
Calcium channel blockers	Contraindicated except for patients who have angina that persists despite use of β-blockers and nitrates or hypertension inadequately controlled by other drugs	Verapamil or diltiazem if LVEF is normal; amlodipine or felodipine if LVEF is abnormal

TABLE 88–1. (*Continued*)

Therapy	Indications	Specific Treatment
AICD	Patients with life-threatening ventricular tachycardia or ventricular fibrillation after MI; possibly other patients at very high risk of sudden cardiac death (eg, those who, after MI, have an LVEF of ≤ 35%, asymptomatic ventricular tachycardia, and inducible ventricular tachycardia)	—
Revascularization	Patients whose life would be prolonged or whose symptoms are unacceptable despite optimal medical therapy; patients > 80 whose quality of life would be improved	PTCA or, if necessary to achieve revascularization goals, CABG; aggressive medical therapy must be continued

*β-Blockers with intrinsic sympathomimetic activity should not be given.
INR = international normalized ratio; LVEF = left ventricular ejection fraction; MI = myocardial infarction; AICD = automatic implantable cardioverter-defibrillator; PTCA = percutaneous transluminal coronary angioplasty; CABG = coronary artery bypass grafting.

The results of surgery for rupture of the interventricular septum are somewhat less encouraging. Among one group of patients with cardiogenic shock, the only survivors were those who underwent prompt surgical repair, with a mortality rate of 62%. Age appears to be an independent predictor of survival. Operative mortality rates of 27 to 47% for early repair of septal rupture have been reported. Patients who survive the operation seem to have a favorable prognosis. Prompt surgery is therefore advised for most patients with postinfarction rupture of the interventricular septum.

89 ■ VALVULAR HEART DISEASE

With age, fibrotic thickening and increased opacity occur in the mitral and aortic valves. The aorta becomes stiffer (increasing systolic blood pressure and stress on the mitral valve), and afterload on the left ventricle increases (increasing myocardial oxygen demand and thus the requirement for myocardial blood flow). These age-related effects influence the development of symptoms and complications in elderly patients with valvular heart disease.

In elderly patients, the predominant causes of valvular heart disease are degenerative calcification, myxomatous degeneration, papillary muscle dysfunction, and infective endocarditis; valvular damage from rheumatic and syphilitic diseases is uncommon. Most often, valvular heart disease is suspected when murmurs are detected during the physical examination. Noninvasive imaging techniques help identify the etiology, establish the diagnosis, and assess disease severity.

Medical management is appropriate for many elderly patients; surgery **1** is indicated when symptoms interfere with daily activities or when hemodynamically significant valvular heart disease cannot be controlled medically. Although age per se is not a contraindication to surgery, comorbid disorders and the overall clinical condition may make surgery inappropriate. Generally, for patients > 75 years, the goal of surgery is to improve the quality of life rather than to prolong life.

Antibiotic prophylaxis for infective endocarditis is recommended before dental, gastrointestinal, gynecologic, and genitourinary procedures. **2**

AORTIC VALVE STENOSIS

Abnormal narrowing of the aortic valve orifice.

The prevalence of aortic valve stenosis, the most clinically significant valvular lesion in the elderly, increases with age. The severity of the stenosis is often underestimated because its progression is so gradual and because symptoms may be attributed to normal aging.

In the elderly, common causes of aortic valve stenosis are calcification of a congenital bicuspid aortic valve and degenerative aortic stenosis. Rheumatic heart disease is the cause in 20%; mitral valve disease often coexists. Regardless of the cause, calcification occurs in patients with aortic valve stenosis by age 65. A congenital bicuspid valve, if present, tends to become calcified in patients aged 45 to 60, and typically, the aortic aspect of the tricuspid semilunar aortic valve is calcified in patients > 75.

Pathophysiology

In aortic valve stenosis, the systolic gradient across the aortic valve during systole produces turbulence, which results in a systolic ejection murmur. The increased left ventricular systolic pressure leads to concentric left ventricular hypertrophy, and these two changes lead to an increase in myocardial oxygen demand. As the aortic valve narrows to < 0.8 cm², aortic pressure takes longer to reach its peak, and systolic pressure may decrease. During systole, tissue pressure on the coronary microvasculature increases coronary vascular resistance and decreases blood flow into the midmyocardium and epicardium. These factors decrease myocardial blood flow, especially to the subendocardium, and result in myocardial ischemia, subendocardial fibrosis, angina pectoris, and ventricular arrhythmias. Significant coronary artery disease (CAD) develops in almost 50% of elderly patients.

During exercise, systemic vascular resistance decreases normally. If stroke volume cannot increase, systolic blood pressure can decrease. This drop in blood pressure plus transient and rapid ventricular arrhythmias can result in exertional syncope.

Symptoms and Signs

Most patients with aortic valve stenosis are asymptomatic. Those with symptoms have an extremely poor prognosis without valve replacement. Chest discomfort, which is usually characteristic of angina pectoris, is an early symptom. During exertion, presyncope (transient alteration of consciousness) or syncope occurs in about one third of symptomatic patients. Exertional dyspnea may progress to pulmonary edema, or pulmonary edema may occur suddenly without previous symptoms. If aortic valve stenosis is severe, the left ventricle becomes stiff, and the left atrium may become dilated, resulting in atrial fibrillation. Absence of an atrial contraction markedly decreases the late filling of the noncompliant left ventricle, and stroke volume may decrease, resulting in a marked worsening of symptoms and in heart failure. Heart failure develops in about one half of elderly patients with severe aortic valve stenosis. Because of vascular stiffening, systolic hypertension may coexist with severe aortic stenosis in elderly patients. About one fourth of deaths due to aortic stenosis occur suddenly.

Physical findings may include a narrow pulse pressure, especially when stroke volume decreases, and a slow-rising, small-volume carotid pulse. However, the poorly compliant arterial wall may mask these abnormalities, so that the carotid pulse appears relatively normal. The cardiac apex impulse is forceful and sustained, but this finding may be masked by kyphosis (in which the anteroposterior diameter of the chest is increased). The first heart sound is soft. The aortic component of the second heart sound is also soft; it may be inaudible when stenosis is severe and the valve is heavily calcified. Reverse splitting of the second heart sound may occur in patients with left ventricular failure. A fourth heart sound is common but disappears in the one fourth of elderly patients who develop atrial fibrillation. Ejection sounds are rare because the valve cusps are immobile.

A harsh, loud crescendo-decrescendo systolic murmur, often associated with a thrill, is maximal at the upper right sternal border. The murmur peaks in mid to late systole and often radiates throughout the precordium and into the neck. This late peaking is often the best clue to severe aortic stenosis. The murmur's high-frequency components are often transmitted to the lower left sternal border and the cardiac apex during most of systole and may resemble the murmur of mitral regurgitation. In patients with heavily calcified aortic valves, the murmur sometimes has a musical high-pitched quality (termed seagull murmur). The murmur's intensity does not correlate with the severity of the obstruction. Basal diastolic murmurs of aortic regurgitation are heard in more than one half of patients with aortic valve stenosis.

The ECG shows evidence of left ventricular hypertrophy, but hyperinflated lungs may mask increased left ventricular voltage. Even when left ventricular hypertrophy is severe, heart size often remains normal until heart failure develops; the heart then enlarges. Poststenotic aortic dilation is common.

Diagnosis

Dense calcification of the aortic valve, best seen on a lateral chest x-ray, suggests hemodynamically significant aortic stenosis. If calcification is not seen on the chest x-ray or echocardiogram, the diagnosis of critical (very severe) aortic valve stenosis is virtually excluded.

Two-dimensional echocardiography is used to assess cardiac chamber size, wall thickness, wall motion, valve leaflet motion, valve orifice size, and valvular calcification. Doppler echocardiography is used to measure intracardiac blood velocity, from which the severity of valvular regurgitation or obstruction can be calculated. Serial measurements can determine progression of the disorder. If the anteroposterior diameter of the chest is increased, the echocardiographic views of the heart may be limited, and the technician may have to spend a long time getting the maximum jet velocity to reflect the maximum aortic systolic gradient. For this reason, the severity of aortic stenosis can be underestimated in the elderly.

Frequently, the severity of aortic stenosis can be determined on the basis of Doppler-echocardiographic findings. However, if surgery is being considered for an elderly patient, catheterization is usually performed to determine whether CAD is present and, if present, how severe it is. Stress testing to the level of the patient's ordinary activity with ECG monitoring may be used to check for ischemic changes and arrhythmias, especially in patients with moderate aortic stenosis.∎ However, if severe aortic stenosis is suspected, exercise testing is contraindicated because exercise-related syncope and death are risks.

Two-dimensional echocardiography and Doppler studies help differentiate aortic valve stenosis from benign aortic sclerosis, which occurs in one third to one half of elderly persons. Benign aortic sclerosis typically produces no symptoms and is not hemodynamically significant;

∎ see page 827

the basal systolic murmur is short and peaks early, and the carotid pulse is normal.

Because the chest discomfort of aortic valve stenosis is due to myocardial ischemia, aortic valve stenosis cannot be distinguished from angina pectoris due to CAD on the basis of symptoms. Syncope due to aortic valve stenosis must be distinguished from that due to atrioventricular block or tachyarrhythmias, both common among elderly patients. Ventricular tachyarrhythmias may be due to CAD or to ischemia produced by severe aortic valve stenosis. Severe aortic valve stenosis should be suspected and ruled out in all elderly patients with heart failure and a systolic ejection murmur, especially if they have unexplained left ventricular hypertrophy.

Prognosis and Treatment

Elderly patients with noncritical aortic valve stenosis require serial surveillance because stenosis often progresses at an unpredictable pace.

Asymptomatic elderly patients with severe aortic stenosis can usually be managed medically; surgery is justified only if the risk of perioperative mortality is less than that of sudden death. However, a detailed history is very important for verifying that the patient is active and asymptomatic before concluding that the patient can be safely managed medically.

Aortic valve replacement is indicated for symptomatic patients with hemodynamically significant aortic valve stenosis, **1** because their expected life span is reduced. The 3-year mortality rate for untreated symptomatic patients is about 50%; life span is shorter for such patients if they have heart failure and longer if they have angina pectoris. Elderly patients with severe aortic stenosis may have a worse prognosis. In one series, the mortality rate was 50% at 1 year and 65% at 2 years.

Percutaneous balloon valvuloplasty is used only for symptomatic palliation of severely ill patients who are not candidates for surgery, because valvuloplasty has high rates of restenosis and mortality after hospital discharge. **2** Ultrasonic debridement of calcium is no longer performed.

ACUTE AORTIC REGURGITATION

Sudden development of retrograde blood flow through an incompetent aortic valve into the left ventricle during ventricular diastole.

Trauma, infective endocarditis, or aortic dissection may cause acute aortic regurgitation.

---

1 see page 947   **2** see page 949

Symptoms and Signs

Frequently, patients present with acute severe pulmonary edema and tachycardia; often, hypotension also occurs. Heart failure is precipitated by abrupt ventricular volume overload within a noncompliant left ventricle and pericardial sac; compensatory hypertrophy or dilation does not have time to occur. Because myocardial oxygen demand increases and subendocardial coronary blood flow decreases, myocardial ischemia and its complications, including sudden death, may occur early in the course of the disorder.

The carotid pulse has a collapsing quality, like that of the left ventricle pressure curve, because of rapid runoff back into the left ventricle. In acute aortic regurgitation compared with the chronic form, the collapsing quality is less pronounced, aortic diastolic pressure cannot decrease as low (because of the rapid elevation of left ventricular filling pressure), and systolic pressure does not increase as much (because of the smaller stroke volume). Therefore, pulse pressure is not as wide, and many of the peripheral signs of severe chronic aortic regurgitation are absent.

The rapid increase in left ventricular filling pressure causes the mitral valve to close late in diastole, making the first heart sound soft. Because pressure in the aorta and left ventricle equilibrates early in diastole, the diastolic murmur along the left sternal border can be harsh and short. In patients with tachycardia and a short diastole, the diastolic murmur can be so short that it is difficult to hear, or it may be absent.

Diagnosis and Treatment

Acute aortic regurgitation should be considered in patients with acute heart failure or pulmonary edema. Echocardiography helps confirm the diagnosis. The ECG may be normal initially. Echocardiography often shows early mitral valve closure.

Acute aortic regurgitation must be differentiated from other causes of acute severe heart failure (eg, myocardial infarction with papillary muscle, chordal, or septal rupture). Pulmonary edema may be erroneously attributed to myocardial infarction because the heart is not enlarged, the wide pulse pressure may be absent, and the murmur may not be detected. Doppler echocardiography and ECG are the most helpful procedures in differential diagnosis.

If the cause is aortic dissection involving the ascending aorta, **1** urgent aortic valve replacement **2** or resuspension of the valve is indicated. For all patients who have signs of acute aortic regurgitation due to other etiologies, even those who do not have obvious pulmonary edema, urgent aortic valve replacement should be performed because clinical deterioration of these patients is rapid and sudden death is pos-

1 see page 938   **2** see page 947

sible. If the cause is infective endocarditis, appropriate antibiotics should be given for 12 to 24 hours before aortic valve replacement. ∎

CHRONIC AORTIC REGURGITATION

Long-standing retrograde blood flow through an incompetent aortic valve into the left ventricle during ventricular diastole.

Chronic aortic regurgitation may be caused by disease of the aortic valve leaflets (due to congenital or rheumatic heart disease, myxomatous degeneration, or infective endocarditis) or by aortic annular root dilation or ascending aortic disease (eg, as occurs in syphilis, rheumatoid spondylitis, Marfan's syndrome, ascending aortic aneurysm, aortic dissection, and various types of aortitis).

Pathophysiology

The regurgitant volume increases the left ventricular end-diastolic volume. If the left ventricular end-diastolic volume increases gradually, eccentric hypertrophy (hypertrophy with dilation) of the left ventricle results; ie, the ventricle enlarges so that it can accommodate the increased left ventricular end-diastolic volume without an increase in left ventricular filling pressure. Left ventricular stroke volume increases sufficiently to maintain a normal aortic forward effective stroke volume and to accommodate the regurgitant volume. With the increased stroke volume, systolic aortic pressure and runoff into the left ventricle are increased, and diastolic pressure is decreased, increasing pulse pressure.

The enlarged ventricle and increased left ventricular systolic pressure increases myocardial oxygen demand, and the low diastolic aortic pressure limits subendocardial blood flow. Consequently, myocardial ischemia and its complications occur, usually late in the course of the disorder.

Symptoms, Signs, and Diagnosis

Most often, mild to moderate aortic regurgitation produces no symptoms for many years, and exercise tolerance is preserved.

Rheumatic aortic regurgitation, which occurs predominantly in men, often produces no symptoms, even in old age. A short, soft basal diastolic murmur is characteristic and may be accentuated by hypertension. Syphilitic aortic regurgitation is more severe, and the prognosis is worse, often because of an associated aortic aneurysm or coronary ostial involvement. A long, loud decrescendo basal diastolic murmur, often with a short basal systolic ejection murmur, is characteristic of hemodynamically severe aortic regurgitation. Because left ventricular stroke volume is increased, the systolic ejection murmur can be loud and long, sounding like that of aortic valve stenosis. The peripheral signs of severe aortic regurgitation distinguish predominant aortic regurgitation from predominant aortic valve stenosis.

Effort intolerance and dyspnea may develop and may progress to heart failure. Chest pain is often due to associated coronary atherosclerosis but can be due to myocardial ischemia. Usually, palpitations are not due to arrhythmias but to the forceful ejection of blood.

The findings of severe regurgitation include bounding peripheral arterial pulses, a wide pulse pressure, and a hyperactive precordium with a rocking motion. Occasionally, a bisferious pulse (pulsus bisferiens) is present. The high-pitched diastolic murmur is best heard at the cardiac base. It is louder at the upper right sternal border in aortic root disease and is more prominent along the left sternal border in aortic valve leaflet disease. An associated diastolic thrill and a systolic murmur of increased aortic outflow may be heard. Third and fourth heart sounds and an apical diastolic rumble (Austin Flint murmur) are common. If the femoral artery is compressed over the groin with the bell of a stethoscope, a to-and-fro diastolic bruit (Duroziez's murmur) can be heard because there is retrograde flow of blood across the compressed artery during diastole.

Chest x-ray shows characteristic cardiac enlargement with a dilated aorta. Occasionally, an ascending aortic aneurysm is seen. Linear calcification of the ascending aorta is typical in syphilitic aortic regurgitation; in contrast, calcification in aortic atherosclerosis is patchy and frequently denser and thicker. The ECG shows left ventricular hypertrophy. The echocardiogram shows an enlarged left ventricular cavity, often with early diastolic fluttering of the anterior mitral valve leaflet. Doppler echocardiography can be used to estimate the severity of aortic regurgitation.

Treatment

Patients with left ventricular failure and severe chronic aortic regurgitation should be stabilized medically even if the valve is to be replaced. ∎ Patients with heart failure are treated with a diuretic, an angiotensin-converting enzyme (ACE) inhibitor, and digoxin before valve replacement. Asymptomatic patients with moderate to severe aortic regurgitation and good left ventricular function should receive an ACE inhibitor, a vasodilating calcium channel blocker, or hydralazine to reduce afterload. Afterload reduction can slow progression of left ventricular dilation and even postpone the onset of symptoms that

∎see page 947

warrant valve replacement. Drugs that cause bradycardia should be avoided, because relative diastolic prolongation can increase regurgitation and accentuate symptoms.

Patients who have left ventricular failure, even if they become asymptomatic with medical management, and patients who remain symptomatic after receiving optimal medical therapy should be considered for aortic valve replacement, preferably with bioprosthetic valves. However, because these patients commonly have severe underlying ventricular dysfunction, the results are less satisfactory than those for patients with aortic valve stenosis. Because decreasing myocardial contractility is manifested by a decreasing ability to eject a large stroke volume, a progressive increase in left ventricular end-diastolic and end-systolic dimensions with a decreasing left ventricular ejection fraction (detected by echocardiography or radionuclide angiography) is an indication for aortic valve replacement. Most patients become symptomatic before these changes occur.

MITRAL STENOSIS

Abnormal narrowing of the mitral valve orifice.

Mitral stenosis is usually identified before patients reach old age. Most patients with severe mitral stenosis have surgery or die before reaching the age of 65; thus, elderly patients with mitral stenosis have a mild to moderate form of disease that has become severe because the valve has become heavily calcified in late life.

Mitral stenosis is due almost exclusively to rheumatic heart disease. Rheumatic fever, although its incidence has markedly decreased in the USA, was still prevalent when the elderly were children or adolescents. Also, in developing countries, the incidence of rheumatic heart disease is still high. A much less common cause of mitral stenosis is progressive extension of mitral annular calcification, which results in moderate mitral stenosis. One third of patients > 70 have calcium deposits in the mitral or aortic valve.

Pathophysiology

Acute rheumatic fever results in commissural fusion and fibrosis. Later, the chordae tendineae fuse and the valve calcifies. Some degree of mitral regurgitation often coexists.

As the mitral orifice narrows to < 2 cm^2 during diastole, blood flow through the valve is progressively obstructed, resulting in an increase in left atrial pressure and a diastolic gradient across the mitral valve. As left atrial pressure increases, pulmonary capillary pressure increases and right ventricular and pulmonary artery systolic pressures passively increase, leading to pulmonary hypertension. In 10 to 15% of patients, pulmonary arteriolar vasoconstriction is marked, pulmonary vascular resistance is greatly increased, and pulmonary hypertension is severe. Because afterload on the right ventricle is increased, right ventricular hypertrophy, dilation, and failure develop.

Increased pulmonary venous pressure results in collateral runoff to the bronchial veins; if they rupture, hemoptysis results. Dilation of the left atrium results in early atrial fibrillation and stasis of blood. Atrial fibrillation results in thromboembolic events and may cause heart failure.

Symptoms, Signs, and Diagnosis

Most elderly patients with mild to moderate mitral stenosis have few or no symptoms and are in sinus rhythm. If mitral stenosis is moderate (especially if atrial fibrillation develops) or is severe, exertional dyspnea, orthopnea, paroxysmal nocturnal dyspnea, and pulmonary edema can occur. Later, with the development of pulmonary hypertension, right ventricular failure supervenes.

Clinical features, comparable to those in younger patients, include a loud first heart sound, an apical diastolic rumble with presystolic accentuation, and an opening snap. The first heart sound and opening snap may soften or disappear if valvular calcification is present. The diastolic murmur may become softer, especially when stroke volume is decreased (as in heart failure) and when dilation of the right ventricle pushes the left ventricle away from the chest wall. A right ventricular parasternal impulse is often palpable, and venous pressure may be elevated. Atrial fibrillation and arterial embolism are more common among elderly patients. Atrial fibrillation often precipitates clinical deterioration; it sometimes causes pulmonary edema, peripheral arterial embolism, and stroke.

Left atrial enlargement is often seen on chest x-ray. ECG evidence of right ventricular hypertrophy is common when the stenosis is severe. Doppler echocardiography can document mitral stenosis and help estimate its severity. Left atrial myxoma, which may mimic mitral stenosis, can be differentiated by echocardiography.

Treatment

Most elderly patients with mild to moderate mitral stenosis respond well to medical therapy. If atrial fibrillation develops, digoxin, verapamil, or a β-blocker can slow the ventricular response rate and reduce symptoms. Pharmacologic or electrical cardioversion to sinus rhythm may relieve symptoms, especially if the patient can be maintained in sinus rhythm by antiarrhythmic drugs.

Although elderly patients are at increased risk of bleeding, anticoagulants are recommended. The risk of peripheral arterial embolism and of embolic stroke is much higher than the risk of complications from anticoagulant therapy. ◻ Prolongation of the international normalized ratio (INR) to 2 to 3 is optimal.

Valve replacement ◻ is warranted for symptomatic patients with progressively severe mitral stenosis, because the calcified valve is rarely amenable to commissurotomy. Embolization without symptomatic hemodynamically severe mitral stenosis is not an indication for valve replacement. For the few patients who have uncalcified or minimally calcified valves, flexible valve leaflets, and mild mitral regurgitation, percutaneous balloon valvuloplasty is the procedure of choice.

ACUTE MITRAL REGURGITATION

Sudden development of retrograde blood flow from the left ventricle into the left atrium through an incompetent mitral valve during systole.

Acute, often massive mitral regurgitation in elderly patients is commonly due to chordal rupture or development of a flail mitral valve. The underlying disorder may be myocardial infarction, papillary muscle rupture, infective endocarditis, trauma, or mucoid degeneration of the valve cusps. Chordal rupture, common among the elderly, may be idiopathic and often results in life-threatening heart failure.

Pathophysiology

With sudden valvular incompetence, a large regurgitant volume enters the left atrium, suddenly increasing the volume of the left atrium during systole. During diastole, this increased volume enters and suddenly dilates the left ventricle; left ventricular filling pressure increases sharply because the normal pericardial sac is relatively noncompliant. Left ventricular dilation produces compression of the right ventricle during diastole, increasing right ventricular filling pressure and leading to right-sided heart failure.

Symptoms and Signs

Typically, patients have symptoms of pulmonary edema or acute pulmonary congestion, both of which often develop rapidly. Sinus tachycardia and a harsh, early systolic apical murmur, often with a thrill, are characteristic. The murmur ends early, when the noncompliant left atrium can no longer accept additional volume. The first heart sound is soft, and the accentuated pulmonic component of the second heart

---

◻ see pages 697–700   ◻ see page 947

sound reflects acute pulmonary hypertension. An early diastolic sound (S_3) is characteristic, and an atrial gallop (S_4) may be present. Severe acute mitral regurgitation often leads to right ventricular failure. The ECG and chest x-ray may be normal initially but soon show pulmonary venous congestion.

Diagnosis and Treatment

Echocardiography confirms the diagnosis and often suggests the etiology. It can differentiate acute mitral regurgitation due to papillary muscle dysfunction or rupture from interventricular septal rupture and can detect the valvular vegetations of infective endocarditis. Transesophageal echocardiography, a safe procedure, allows the valve to be evaluated in greater detail, thus helping to determine whether the valve can be repaired or must be replaced.

Acute pulmonary edema due to acute mitral regurgitation is managed in the same way as that due to other cardiac disorders. Patients with hemodynamic instability, characterized by hypotension with pulmonary edema, require intra-aortic balloon counterpulsation to allow cardiac catheterization and the subsequent induction of anesthesia for surgery. Patients with infective endocarditis require treatment with appropriate antibiotics. **1**

Patients with acute massive mitral regurgitation and clinical deterioration typically require urgent valve surgery. **2**

CHRONIC MITRAL REGURGITATION

Long-standing retrograde blood flow from the left ventricle into the left atrium through an incompetent mitral valve during ventricular systole, with eccentric left ventricular hypertrophy.

Chronic rather than acute mitral regurgitation is the most common type of mitral valve disease in the elderly. About half of patients with rheumatic mitral regurgitation have associated aortic valve disease, usually aortic regurgitation.

In the elderly, isolated chronic mitral regurgitation often results from papillary muscle dysfunction after myocardial infarction. Chronic mitral regurgitation may also be due to mitral annular calcification, myxomatous valve degeneration (with mitral valve prolapse), chordal rupture, or rheumatic heart disease. Mitral annular calcification occurs in about 6% of persons > 60, predominantly women. The incidence of myxomatous valvular degeneration increases with age.

1 see page 882   **2** see page 947

Pathophysiology

In chronic mitral regurgitation, the regurgitant volume gradually increases, increasing the volume of the left atrium during systole and that of the left ventricle during diastole. Enlargement of the left ventricle results in eccentric hypertrophy. Eventually, stretching of the left atrium results in atrial fibrillation, and the left ventricle can no longer maintain a normal effective forward stroke volume because of decreased myocardial contractility. Left ventricular failure develops, leading to increased pulmonary artery and right ventricular systolic pressure. Thus, right ventricular failure develops very late in the course of the disorder.

Mitral regurgitation due to mitral annular calcification prevents annular systolic contraction and may limit valve leaflet closure. It is rarely hemodynamically significant; however, calcification may involve the conduction system, causing various degrees of atrioventricular block, and may double the risk of stroke.

Symptoms, Signs, and Diagnosis

Patients may be asymptomatic or present with only a pansystolic apical murmur or a decrease in exercise tolerance with easy fatigability. Atrial fibrillation may occur later than it does in patients with mitral stenosis. Atrial fibrillation may precipitate hemodynamic deterioration, with an apical holosystolic murmur engulfing the first heart sound, and symptoms and signs of left-sided heart failure. Systemic embolism occurs predominantly when atrial fibrillation or heart failure is present but is less common among patients with chronic mitral regurgitation than among those with mitral stenosis.

If the cause is mitral valve prolapse, presenting symptoms and signs may include atypical chest pain, palpitations or syncope due to arrhythmia, and heart failure (more common among men). A midsystolic click or clicks and a late systolic or holosystolic murmur may be heard. The mitral regurgitant murmur predominates in elderly patients, whereas clicks and late crescendo systolic murmurs predominate in younger patients. An ECG often shows ST-T wave changes, but when mitral regurgitation is severe, it may show left ventricular hypertrophy. Ventricular arrhythmias are common, even in patients with normal ventricular function. With severe mitral regurgitation, the onset of atrial fibrillation may accentuate mitral and tricuspid valve prolapse and often precipitates hemodynamic deterioration. Systemic embolism and sudden death may occur.

Doppler echocardiography can be used to determine the magnitude of the mitral regurgitation and to assess overall ventricular size and function. It can sometimes determine the etiology of the mitral insufficiency. For example, vegetations suggest infective endocarditis; prolapse and thickening of the leaflets suggest myxomatous degeneration;

flail mitral valve suggests chordal rupture; and thickened retracted leaflets and chordal fusion suggest rheumatic heart disease. Doppler echocardiography can differentiate mitral valve prolapse from other causes of mitral regurgitation. A ringlike calcification in the area of the mitral valve on a chest x-ray and dense horseshoe-shaped calcifications on an echocardiogram indicate mitral annular calcification.

Coronary arteriography may be needed to differentiate the chest pain due to mitral valve prolapse from that due to coronary atherosclerosis.

Treatment

Atrial fibrillation and heart failure are managed with standard therapy.[1] Anticoagulants are given to prevent systemic embolism. Most symptomatic elderly patients with chronic mitral regurgitation respond readily to medical therapy.

Surgery[2] is indicated when medical therapy does not control symptoms and/or when ventricular function deteriorates, as indicated by a progressive increase in left ventricular end-diastolic and end-systolic volumes and a decrease in ejection fraction. The ejection fraction should not be allowed to decrease below 55%. Elderly men with mitral valve prolapse are more likely to require surgery than are elderly women. If high-degree atrioventricular block occurs, a pacemaker should be placed.[3]

For patients with papillary muscle dysfunction due to CAD, an annuloplasty ring placed during coronary artery bypass grafting can reduce the degree of regurgitation.

TRICUSPID REGURGITATION

Retrograde blood flow from the right ventricle into the right atrium caused by inadequate closure of the tricuspid valve orifice during ventricular systole.

In the elderly, tricuspid regurgitation is most often caused by a dilated valve ring secondary to right ventricular failure, which usually results from left-sided heart failure or pulmonary hypertension related to primary pulmonary disease. Infective endocarditis is a less common cause. Tricuspid regurgitation may be silent, or a short ejection or holosystolic murmur may be present.

The diagnosis is made by finding the characteristic systolic murmur, usually heard in the third or fourth intercostal space at the left sternal border. The murmur increases in intensity with inspiration (Carvallo's

[1] see pages 890 and 904   [2] see page 947   [3] see page 899

sign) in about 50% of patients. If tricuspid regurgitation is severe, a prominent large V wave may be seen in the jugular venous pulse. The diagnosis is confirmed by Doppler echocardiography.

Medical treatment of heart failure ameliorates tricuspid regurgitation. Surgery is rarely necessary.

TRICUSPID STENOSIS

Abnormal narrowing of the tricuspid valve orifice.

Tricuspid stenosis is rare and is most often due to multivalvular rheumatic heart disease or the carcinoid syndrome. Patients with isolated tricuspid stenosis have signs of right-sided heart failure with elevated cervical venous pressure, hepatomegaly, edema, and ascites; dyspnea and orthopnea are often absent. Commonly, exercise tolerance decreases because of low cardiac output. Hepatomegaly is present without other signs of left-sided heart failure.

The lower left sternal border diastolic rumble increases during inspiration. A low-pitched murmur is heard in the third or fourth intercostal space at the left sternal border; it frequently becomes louder with inspiration. A prominent A wave with poor or absent Y descent is seen in the jugular venous pulse. The diagnosis is made by finding the characteristic murmur and jugular venous pulse.

Medical therapy is indicated for mild disease. Although surgical repair is rarely required, balloon valvotomy is the treatment of choice for patients with signs of right-sided heart failure or with markedly decreased exercise tolerance due to inability to increase cardiac output. If the valve is calcified (a rare finding), valve replacement is necessary.

PULMONIC VALVE REGURGITATION

Retrograde blood flow from the pulmonary artery into the right ventricle through an incompetent pulmonary valve.

Among the elderly, pulmonic valve regurgitation is rarely due to primary pulmonic valve disease. It is almost always a sequela of pulmonary hypertension, usually due to left-sided heart failure or to primary pulmonary disease. It is characterized by a high-pitched, blowing decrescendo diastolic murmur in the second and third intercostal space to the left of the sternum. Often, this murmur cannot be distinguished from the murmur of aortic regurgitation. Doppler echocardiography can help distinguish the two disorders.

Treatment is aimed at managing the underlying disorder and attempting to lower pulmonary artery pressure.

Infection of the heart valves or mural endocardial myo-cardium, resulting in the formation of endocardial vegeta-tions.

Infective endocarditis has become more prevalent among the elderly. More than one fourth of all cases occur in persons > 60 years. Prevalence has increased because the number of elderly persons and of persons with prosthetic valves has increased, hospital-acquired bacteremia has become more prevalent, and persons with valvular heart disease survive longer. Infective endocarditis affects eight times as many elderly men as elderly women.

Etiology and Pathophysiology

The underlying cardiac lesions that predispose the elderly to endocarditis tend to differ from those in younger patients. Calcification of the mitral or aortic annulus with insufficiency is more common among the elderly, whereas congenital heart defects are more common among younger persons. The increased incidence of atherosclerosis in the elderly may be a factor, because atheromatous deposits in valves can cause turbulence, resulting in endothelial damage and thrombus formation. About 30% of elderly patients with endocarditis have rheumatic lesions, about 25% have calcified valves, and about 5% have mitral valve prolapse; however, about 40% have unidentified or no valvular lesions. All forms of valvular heart disease◼ increase the risk of endocarditis.

The aortic valve is involved in 20 to 40% of elderly patients with infective endocarditis, probably reflecting the high prevalence of aortic stenosis with calcification. Aortic stenosis with calcification is most commonly caused by rheumatic heart disease in persons < 50, by a calcified congenital bicuspid valve in those aged 50 to 65, and by degeneration of a normal valve in those > 65. Infective endocarditis involves the mitral valve in 25 to 70% of patients and both the aortic and mitral valves in about 10 to 25%. Endocarditis involving congenital heart defects other than those of the bicuspid valve occur infrequently in the elderly.

The development of infective endocarditis requires two conditions: The first is an alteration in the endocardial surface, allowing the deposition of platelet and fibrin. The resulting thrombus or vegetation usually develops in areas of jet impingement and increased turbulence and acts as a site for bacterial attachment. The second condition is

---

◼ see page 863

bacteremia, which results in colonization of the lesion. The source of bacteremia is usually unknown. Sites of primary infection include the mouth, the genitourinary (GU) tract (particularly after procedures involving instrumentation), the gastrointestinal (GI) tract, the skin, decubitus ulcers, surgical wounds, and IV catheters.

Some bacteria have certain properties (eg, certain streptococcal and staphylococcal species have increased adherence) that make them more likely to cause infective endocarditis. *Streptococcus* sp account for 25 to 70% of cases; viridans streptococci are less prevalent among elderly than among younger patients. Enterococci, which often inhabit the GU and lower GI tracts, account for up to 25% of cases in elderly patients. The prevalence of enterococcal bacteremia and endocarditis is high because urinary tract infections are common among the elderly and procedures involving instrumentation are frequently performed, especially in men with prostate disorders. *S. bovis,* a nonenterococcal group D streptococcus, is isolated in up to 25% of patients > 55 who have endocarditis. Many cases involving *S. bovis* are associated with underlying, often asymptomatic malignant or premalignant GI lesions, especially colon cancer.

Staphylococci account for 20 to 30% of all cases of endocarditis in the elderly. The predominant species, *Staphylococcus aureus,* often causes nosocomial endocarditis. *S. epidermidis* is isolated in < 5% of patients with native valve endocarditis, but it is the most common cause of cases that involve prosthetic valves occurring early after surgery in elderly and in younger patients. Gram-negative aerobic bacilli and fungi cause 2 to 3% of all cases of endocarditis. Infections due to *Bacteroides* sp and mixed infections are rare among the elderly.

Culture-negative endocarditis accounts for 5 to 20% of all cases of endocarditis; culture results may be negative because of prior antibiotic administration, fastidious pathogens, or inadequate laboratory techniques. Uremia is associated with an increased incidence of culture-negative endocarditis.

The pathophysiology of infective endocarditis is due to the body's reaction to the infection: the development of antibodies to the foreign protein of the organism, with resultant immune complex disease; systemic emboli; and valvular disruption and regurgitation. The hemodynamic clinical picture depends on how rapidly valvular regurgitation develops and how severe it is.

Symptoms and Signs

Clinical manifestations are diverse and may involve almost any organ system. Symptoms and signs usually occur within 2 weeks of the bacteremia. Fever is the most common sign. Anorexia, fatigue, confusion, back pain, weight loss, and night sweats are also common. Elderly patients may present atypically, with no fever, unexplained anemia, large systemic emboli, renal failure, and central nervous system syndromes (eg, rapid-onset dementia, stroke).

During physical examination, cardiac murmurs, due to a preexisting valvular abnormality or to the infection itself, are heard in > 90% of patients. New or changing cardiac murmurs occur in 36 to 52% of all patients with infective endocarditis diagnosed by strict clinical criteria but occur less frequently in the elderly. Signs of heart failure may also be present. Splenic enlargement occurs in 25 to 60% of patients; the increasing incidence is associated with a longer duration of endocarditis. About 40% of patients have cutaneous or peripheral manifestations. Petechiae are the most common, occurring in crops on the conjunctivae, palate, buccal mucosa, extremities, and skin above the clavicles. Splinter hemorrhages (linear, dark streaks) occur beneath the fingernails or toenails but are also common among elderly persons who do not have infective endocarditis. Osler nodes (small, raised, tender subcutaneous nodules in the pads of the digits or on thenar eminences) and Janeway lesions (small, nontender hemorrhagic or erythematous macules on the palms or soles) may occur. Roth's spots (pale-centered oval hemorrhages in the retina) suggest infective endocarditis but also occur in patients with collagen vascular disease or hematologic disorders.

Other clinical manifestations may result from thromboemboli. Emboli to the spleen may cause left upper quadrant abdominal pain radiating to the shoulder, a splenic friction rub, or signs of a left pleural effusion. Emboli to the kidneys may cause flank or back pain, suggesting renal infarction. Large emboli obstructing large arteries, such as the external iliac, superficial femoral, and brachial arteries, are characteristic of endocarditis caused by fungi or HACEK organisms *(Haemophilus parainfluenzae, H. aphrophilus, Actinobacillus actinomycetemcomitans, Cardiobacterium hominis, Eikenella corrodens, Kingella kingae).*

Cerebral embolism and rupture of an intracranial mycotic aneurysm (which may be presaged only by persistent headache) are devastating complications. The patient may present with signs of a stroke (eg, hemiparesis, cranial nerve palsies, cortical sensory loss, aphasia, ataxia, alteration in mental status), which may distract the clinician from identifying the infectious cause of the disease. Infective endocarditis should be considered in any patient with a fever and a stroke syndrome. Most cerebral emboli involve the distribution of the middle cerebral artery or one of its branches.◨

Diagnosis

Often, endocarditis, especially culture-negative endocarditis, is missed in the elderly because the diagnosis is not considered. When

◨see page 407

TABLE 90-1.   ANTIMICROBIAL PROPHYLAXIS FOR INFECTIVE ENDOCARDITIS

Procedure	Patient Status	Drug Dosage
Dental, oral, respiratory tract, or esophageal procedures	Requiring general prophylaxis	Amoxicillin 2 g po 1 h before the procedure
	Requiring general prophylaxis parenterally	Ampicillin 2 g IM or IV within 30 min of the procedure
	Requiring general prophylaxis and allergic to penicillin	Clindamycin 600 mg po 1 h before the procedure *or* Azithromycin or clarithromycin 500 mg po 1 h before the procedure *or* Cephalexin* or cefadroxil* 2 g po 1 h before the procedure
	Requiring general prophylaxis parenterally and allergic to penicillin	Clindamycin 600 mg IV within 30 min of the procedure *or* Cefazolin* 1 g IM or IV within 30 min of the procedure
Genitourinary or gastrointestinal (excluding esophageal) procedures	At high risk (eg, with prosthetic valves or previous endocarditis)	Ampicillin 2 g and gentamicin 1.5 mg/kg (not to exceed 120 mg) IM or IV 30 min before the procedure; 6 h later, ampicillin 1 g IM or IV or amoxicillin 1 g po
	At high risk and allergic to ampicillin or amoxicillin	Vancomycin 1 g IV slowly over 1 h, beginning 1 h before the procedure, together with gentamicin 1.5 mg/kg IV or IM (not to exceed 120 mg)
	At moderate risk (eg, with acquired valve dysfunction, hypertrophic cardiomyopathy, or mitral valve prolapse with valvular regurgitation)	Amoxicillin 2 g po 1 h before the procedure *or* Ampicillin 2 g IM or IV 30 min before the procedure
	At moderate risk and allergic to penicillin	Vancomycin 1 g IV slowly over 1 h, beginning 1 h before the procedure

*Cephalosporins are contraindicated in patients with immediate-type hypersensitivity reaction (urticaria, angioedema, anaphylaxis) to penicillin.

Adapted from Dajani AS, Taubert KA, Wilson W, Bolger AF: "Prevention of bacterial endocarditis—Recommendations by the American Heart Association." *Circulation* 96:358–366, 1997.

patients present atypically, infective endocarditis may not be recognized and treated until it has progressed to a late stage. Such patients have an extremely poor prognosis.

The most important laboratory finding is a positive blood culture result, which is found in about 90% of patients. Because bacteremia is continuous in infective endocarditis, the timing of the culture in relation to occurrence of fever is usually unimportant. Laboratory tests may detect anemia (in 70 to 90%), elevated ESR (in 90 to 100%), proteinuria (in 50 to 65%), and microscopic hematuria (in 30 to 50%). Rheumatoid factor is commonly detected in patients who have been infected for > 6 weeks but is also present in 5 to 10% of healthy elderly persons.

Doppler echocardiography is very valuable. It can detect valvular vegetations, valvular destruction, extravalvular infection (annular abscesses), and the hemodynamic sequelae of regurgitation. In the elderly, valvular masses are not synonymous with vegetations and may result from valvular sclerosis or myxomatous degeneration of the valve. Transesophageal echocardiography is helpful when the standard transthoracic approach to imaging is too difficult technically or is not diagnostic. It can detect multiple vegetations, satellite lesions, fistulas, annular abscesses, valvular perforations, and aneurysms when transthoracic echocardiography shows only a vegetation.

Prophylaxis and Treatment

Antibiotic prophylaxis is indicated in elderly patients with valvular heart disease, particularly in patients with calcified or prosthetic heart valves and particularly before certain procedures (see TABLE 90–1).

Optimal treatment requires use of microbicidal drugs. For acutely ill patients, empiric therapy should be started immediately after obtaining blood for culture, so that valvular damage can be limited.

Initially, selection of antimicrobial therapy is based on which microorganism is most likely in the specific clinical setting. If onset is subacute in a patient who does not use IV drugs and who has native valve endocarditis, infection with streptococci or enterococci is likely. The standard empiric regimen consists of high-dose IV penicillin G (or ampicillin) with an aminoglycoside such as gentamicin. If onset is acute or if the patient uses IV drugs, therapy should target *S. aureus*. If onset is acute in a patient who does not use IV drugs and who has native valve endocarditis, a penicillinase-resistant penicillin (eg, nafcillin) or a cephalosporin (eg, cefazolin) is appropriate initial therapy. If the patient has a prosthetic valve, vancomycin can be used to target resistant strains of *S. aureus* and *S. epidermidis*.

After the infecting microorganism is identified, antimicrobial therapy is altered accordingly, to the most effective, least toxic, and least costly regimen (see TABLE 90–2). Therapy is continued at least 2 weeks longer if patients have prosthetic valves.

TABLE 90–2.   ANTIMICROBIAL THERAPY FOR INFECTIVE ENDOCARDITIS

Organism	Regimen*
Streptococci (penicillin MIC ≤ 0.1 µg/mL), including *Streptococcus bovis*	Aqueous penicillin G 12–18 mU/day IV for 4 wk† given continuously or in 6 equally divided doses *or* Aqueous penicillin G 12–18 mU/day IV plus gentamicin‡,§ 1 mg/kg (maximum, 80 mg) IM or IV q 8 h for 2 wk *or* Ceftriaxone 2 g/day IV or IM‖ for 4 wk†, ¶ *or* Vancomycin# 30 mg/kg/24 h IV in 2 equally divided doses (not to exceed 2 g/24 h unless serum levels are monitored) for 4 wk**
Streptococci (penicillin MIC > 0.1 and < 0.5 µg/mL)	Aqueous penicillin G†† 18 mU/day IV for 4 wk plus gentamicin 1 mg/kg (maximum, 80 mg) IM or IV q 8 h for first 2 wk *or* Vancomycin# 30 mg/kg/24 h IV in 2 equally divided doses (not to exceed 2 g/24 h unless serum levels are monitored) for 4 wk
Enterococci or streptococci (penicillin MIC ≥ 0.5 µg/mL)	Aqueous penicillin G 18–30 mU/day IV or ampicillin 2 g q 4 h IV plus gentamicin§ 1 mg/kg IM or IV (maximum, 80 mg) q 8 h for 4–6 wk *or* Vancomycin# 30 mg/kg/24 h IV in 2 equally divided doses (not to exceed 2 g/24 h unless serum levels are monitored) plus gentamicin 1 mg/kg IM or IV q 8 h for 4–6 wk
Staphylococci (methicillin-susceptible) on a native valve	Nafcillin 2 g IV q 4 h or oxacillin 2 g IV q 4 h for 4–6 wk with or without gentamicin§ 1 mg/kg (maximum, 80 mg) IM or IV q 8 h for first 3–5 days *or* Cefazolin (or another 1st-generation cephalosporin in an equivalent dose)‡‡ 2 g IV q 8 h for 4–6 wk with or without gentamicin 1 mg/kg IM or IV q 8 h for first 3–5 days¶ *or* Vancomycin#,** 30 mg/kg/24 h IV in 2 equally divided doses (not to exceed 2 g/24 h unless serum levels are monitored) for 4–6 wk
Staphylococci (methicillin-resistant) on a native valve	Vancomycin** 30 mg/kg/24 h (maximum, 2 g in 24 h) IV in 2 equally divided doses for 4–6 wk
Staphylococci (methicillin-susceptible) on a prosthetic valve	Nafcillin or oxacillin§§ 2 g IV q 4 h plus rifampin 300 mg po q 8 h for ≥ 6 wk and gentamicin 1 mg/kg IM or IV q 8 h for first 2 wk

Table continues on the following page.

TABLE 90-2.   ANTIMICROBIAL THERAPY FOR INFECTIVE ENDOCARDITIS *(Continued)*

Organism	Regimen*
Staphylococci (methicillin-resistant) on a prosthetic valve	Vancomycin** 30 mg/kg/24 h (maximum, 2 g in 24 h) IV divided q 6 or 12 h plus rifampin‖‖ 300 mg po q 8 h for ≥ 6 wk and gentamicin § 1 mg/kg IM or IV q 8 h for first 2 wk
HACEK organisms	Ceftriaxone 2 g once daily IV or IM‖ for 4 wk
	or
	Ampicillin 12 g/24 h IV continuously or q 4 h plus gentamicin 1 mg/kg IV or IM q 8 h for 4 wk
Enterobacteriaceae	Cefotaxime 2 g IV q 4 h or imipenem 0.5–1 g IV q 6 h or aztreonam 2 g IV q 6 h plus gentamicin 1.7 mg/kg IV or IM q 8 h for 4–6 wk
Pseudomonas aeruginosa	Piperacillin 3 g IV q 4 h or ceftazidime 2 g IV q 8 h or imipenem 0.5–1 g IV q 6 h or aztreonam 2 g IV or IM q 6 h plus gentamicin 8 mg/kg IV q 8 h
Fungi	Amphotericin B 0.5–1 mg/kg/day IV plus flucytosine ¶¶ 100 mg/kg/day po in 4 divided doses

* Used for patients with normal renal and hepatic function. Regimen should be continued for at least 2 wk longer in patients with a prosthetic valve.

† Preferred in the elderly because aminoglycosides are likely to result in toxicity.

‡ Age > 65 is a relative contraindication to use of gentamicin.

§ After a 20–30 min IV infusion or an IM injection, a serum concentration of about 3 µg/mL is desirable; trough concentration should be < 1 µg/mL.

‖ IM injection of ceftriaxone may be painful.

¶ Cephalosporins are not acceptable alternatives for patients with immediate-type hypersensitivity to penicillin.

Vancomycin is recommended for patients who are allergic to β-lactam antibiotics.

** Peak serum concentrations should be maintained at 30–45 µg/mL if drug is given q 12 h.

†† For patients with penicillin hypersensitivity that is not the immediate type, cefazolin or another 1st-generation cephalosporin may be substituted for penicillin.

‡‡ Regimen is appropriate for patients who are allergic to β-lactam antibiotics but should not be used for those with immediate-type hypersensitivity to penicillin.

§§ For patients who are allergic to β-lactam antibiotics, 1st-generation cephalosporins or vancomycin should be used. However, cephalosporins should not be used for patients with immediate-type hypersensitivity to penicillin or with methicillin-resistant staphylococci.

‖‖ Used for coagulase-negative staphylococci; value for coagulase-positive staphylococci is controversial.

¶¶ Serum concentrations should be maintained at 50–100 µg/mL. Some experts recommend that flucytosine be started at 75 mg/kg/day when it is used with amphotericin B, because nephrotoxicity is a risk.

MIC = minimal inhibitory concentration; HACEK = *Haemophilus parainfluenzae, H. aphrophilus, Actinobacillus actinomycetemcomitans, Cardiobacterium hominis, Eikenella corrodens, Kingella kingae.*

Adapted from Baldassarre JS, Kaye D: "Principles and overview of antibiotic therapy," in *Infective Endocarditis*, ed. 2, edited by D Kaye. New York, Raven Press, 1992, pp. 169–190; as based on material appearing in Bisno AL, Dismukes WE, Durack DT, et al: "Antimicrobial treatment of infective endocarditis due to viridans streptococci, enterococci, and staphylococci." *JAMA* 261:1471–1477, 1989.

Some patients with infective endocarditis need valve replacement. ∎ Indications for valve replacement are hemodynamic deterioration due to valve dysfunction, fungal endocarditis, persistent infection despite appropriate antimicrobial therapy, repeated relapses after completion of therapy, early postoperative or complicated endocarditis involving a prosthetic valve, extravalvular extension of the infection, and recurrent emboli.

91 ■ ARRHYTHMIAS AND CONDUCTION DISTURBANCES

In the elderly, changes in cardiac structure ∎ and the increased incidence of cardiovascular disease contribute to the striking increase in the incidence of arrhythmias and conduction disturbances. Diagnostic and therapeutic data about specific arrhythmias in the elderly are scarce.

ECTOPIC BEATS AND TACHYARRHYTHMIAS

The presence of supraventricular or ventricular ectopic beats, even if frequent or complex, is not an accurate marker for organic heart disease or for increased risk of cardiac mortality in the elderly (see Table 91–1). Supraventricular and ventricular arrhythmias appear to be benign in healthy elderly persons but may not be benign in patients with heart disease. Regardless of patient age, the nature and severity of underlying heart disease have much greater prognostic significance than does the arrhythmia.

Epidemiology and Pathogenesis

The incidence of supraventricular and ventricular ectopic beats and tachyarrhythmias is increased in the elderly for reasons that are not fully understood. The increased incidence may be partially accounted for by age-related increases in left atrial size and pressure, in left ventricular mass, and in catecholamine levels. Supraventricular and ventricular ectopic beats are more common and more complex among patients with structural heart disease, which dramatically increases in incidence with age.

∎ see page 947   ∎ see page 813

TABLE 91–1.   TACHYARRHYTHMIAS AND ECTOPIC BEATS

Disorder	Prevalence With Age	Effect on Mortality*	Usual Treatment
Supraventricular ectopic beats	Increased	None	None
Paroxysmal supraventricular tachycardia	Increased	Probably none	Digoxin, a β-blocker, or a calcium channel blocker
Atrial fibrillation (chronic)	Increased	Increased	Digoxin, a β-blocker, or a calcium channel blocker; attempt at cardioversion; possibly anticoagulants
Ventricular ectopic beats	Increased	Probably none	None for healthy patients; probably none for patients with heart disease, unless needed to control symptoms
Ventricular tachycardia	Increased	Probably none unless sustained	Possibly antiarrhythmic drugs for healthy patients; antiarrhythmic drugs, AICD, or endocardial resection for patients with coronary artery disease

*In otherwise healthy elderly patients.
AICD = automatic implantable cardioverter-defibrillator.

An overload of ionized calcium (Ca^{++}) in senescent myocardium may play an important role in arrhythmogenesis. Under conditions that enhance cell Ca^{++} loading, senescent myocardium is more likely to spontaneously release Ca^{++} from the sarcoplasmic reticulum (ie, to undergo diastolic afterdepolarization). This greater likelihood for Ca^{++} overload may make the senescent heart more susceptible to arrhythmias when calcium homeostasis is disturbed (eg, by use of inotropic drugs or during postischemic reflow). Furthermore, the threshold for Ca^{++}–dependent ventricular fibrillation is lower in the senescent heart.

Symptoms, Signs, and Diagnosis

Tachyarrhythmias may produce palpitations or, occasionally, symptoms of hemodynamic upset (eg, dizziness, syncope, heart failure). Patients often notice the onset and offset of intermittent tachyarrhythmias.

The diagnosis is suggested by characteristic symptoms and by a rapid, possibly irregular peripheral arterial pulse, which reflects ventricular activity. Examination of the jugular venous pulse, which reflects atrial and ventricular activity, may help differentiate atrial from ventricular arrhythmias. Standard 12-lead ECG confirms the diagnosis.

Treatment

Antiarrhythmics (see TABLE 91–2) are more likely to cause adverse effects in the elderly than in younger patients. ∎

Serum digoxin levels for the same dose are higher in the elderly than in younger patients because of reduced renal clearance. Digitalis toxicity is relatively common among the elderly. Concurrent use of quinidine (class I) increases serum digoxin levels by about 100%; concurrent use of verapamil (class IV) or amiodarone (class III) can also increase serum digoxin levels.

Clearance of quinidine is reduced by 34% and elimination half-life is prolonged from 7.3 to 9.7 hours in persons aged 60 to 69 compared with those aged 23 to 29. Clearance of procainamide and disopyramide (class I) is also reduced with age; disopyramide should not be used in the elderly because it has anticholinergic effects on bladder and bowel function.

Because hepatic flow decreases with age, the infusion rate of lidocaine (class Ib) should be reduced to avoid central nervous system toxicity, which is common among the elderly. Similar dosage reduction is advised for most β-blockers (class II) and for the calcium channel blockers (class IV) verapamil and diltiazem, partly because these drugs undergo first-pass hepatic metabolism.

How aging affects the clinical pharmacology of newer antiarrhythmic drugs (eg, class Ic drugs flecainide, encainide, and propafenone; class III drugs amiodarone and sotalol) is not well characterized. However, clearance of encainide but not flecainide is reduced in the elderly.

SUPRAVENTRICULAR ECTOPIC BEATS

Premature beats resulting from an abnormal electrical focus or from reentry in the atria or other supraventricular tissue.

The incidence of supraventricular ectopic beats—whether simple or complex or whether detected during rest, routine activity, or exercise—increases with age, even among persons carefully screened to exclude latent coronary artery disease (CAD). Isolated supraventricular ectopic beats have been detected by exercise ECG in 8% of apparently healthy persons aged 20 to 29 but in 76% of those aged 80 to 89. Frequent (> 100 in 24 hours) supraventricular ectopic beats have been detected during 24-hour ambulatory ECG monitoring in 26% of healthy persons aged 60 to 85 with no evidence of CAD.

Patients with supraventricular ectopic beats, even when frequent, are usually asymptomatic and rarely require treatment. However, they may have a propensity for sustained supraventricular tachyarrhythmia.

∎ see also page 70

TABLE 91–2. VAUGHAN WILLIAMS CLASSIFICATION OF ANTIARRHYTHMIC DRUGS

Class	Pharmacologic Effect	Representative Drugs	A–H Interval	H–V Interval	QRS Complex	QT Interval	Accessory Pathway Conduction Time	Atrial ERP	Main Clinical Indications
Ia	Sodium channel blocker	Quinidine, procainamide, disopyramide	↑↓	↑	↑	↑	↑	↑	Ventricular arrhythmias, supraventricular tachycardias, atrial fibrillation
Ib	Sodium channel blocker	Lidocaine, mexiletine, tocainide, moricizine, phenytoin	0	0	0	0	↑ or 0	0	Ventricular arrhythmias
Ic	Sodium channel blocker	Flecainide, propafenone	↑	↑↑	↑↑	↑	↑	↑ or 0	Ventricular arrhythmias, supraventricular tachycardias, atrial fibrillation
II	β-Blocker	Atenolol, propranolol, metoprolol	↑*	0	0	0	0	0	Ventricular arrhythmias, atrial fibrillation
III	Potassium channel blocker	Amiodarone, sotalol, bretylium	↑	↑	0	↑↑	↑	↑	Ventricular arrhythmias, supraventricular tachycardias, atrial fibrillation
IV	Calcium channel blocker	Verapamil, diltiazem	↑	0	0	0	0	0	Supraventricular tachycardias

*Rate related rather than a separate effect.
ERP = effective refractory period; ↓ = shortened; 0 = no effect; ↑ = prolonged; ↑↑ = markedly prolonged; ↑↓ = variable effects.

Supraventricular ectopic beats do not appear to be associated with an increased risk of coronary events, including sudden cardiac death.

ATRIAL (SUPRAVENTRICULAR) TACHYCARDIAS

(Narrow QRS Tachycardias)

Incidence increases with age. Nonsustained supraventricular tachycardia has been detected by exercise ECG in < 1% of apparently healthy persons aged 20 to 29 but in 10% of those aged 80 to 89. Risk of developing a spontaneous supraventricular tachyarrhythmia was 2% in the younger group and 10% in the older group; however, the tachycardia was not associated with an increased risk of coronary events.

Paroxysmal supraventricular tachycardia: A regular narrow QRS complex at 150 to 200 beats/minute is characteristic. Short asymptomatic episodes of paroxysmal supraventricular tachycardia have been reported in 13% of elderly patients with no evidence of heart disease.

This tachycardia is usually due to a reentrant mechanism. It can often be terminated by vagal maneuvers (eg, Valsalva's maneuver, gagging, carotid sinus massage). NOTE: *Because an arterial embolus can be precipitated, carotid sinus massage should not be performed on elderly patients until significant carotid stenosis (defined by a readily audible bruit) has been excluded by physical examination.*

If vagal maneuvers are unsuccessful and the patient does not have hypotension, verapamil 5 to 10 mg IV should be given slowly over a period of 2.5 to 5 minutes. Alternatively, adenosine IV, which has a rapid onset of action and low risk of hypotension, can be used. Adenosine is very effective and has the same low incidence of adverse effects in patients > 70 as in those < 70. If paroxysmal supraventricular tachycardia precipitates hypotension, cerebral ischemic symptoms, angina pectoris, or heart failure, immediate cardioversion is indicated, starting at 25 to 50 joules.

Digoxin, β-blockers, or calcium channel blockers, given once daily, are similarly effective in preventing recurrences of this tachycardia.

Atrial tachycardia with block: A rapid atrial rate with a slower ventricular rate due to atrioventricular (AV) block is characteristic. Digitalis toxicity is the most common cause. Treatment consists of withholding digoxin and correcting hypokalemia.

Multifocal atrial tachycardia: P-wave morphology, the PR interval, and cycle length vary from beat to beat. This tachycardia is common among elderly patients with chronic obstructive pulmonary disease. Treatment is directed at correcting the underlying pulmonary disorder; verapamil is usually effective as short-term therapy.

Accelerated junctional rhythm: A heart rate of 70 to 130 beats/minute is characteristic; the P wave is usually inverted and may precede, follow, or fall within the QRS complex. Among the elderly, digitalis toxicity and acute inferior myocardial infarction (MI) are the most common causes. Although this tachycardia is not usually a cause of hemodynamic impairment, it can cause heart failure. Sudden regularization of the ventricular rate in an elderly patient receiving digoxin for chronic atrial fibrillation suggests this diagnosis. Treatment is directed at the underlying disorder.

Atrial flutter: Rapid, regular atrial activity between 250 and 350 beats/minute with sawtooth flutter waves (best seen in leads II, III, and aVF) is characteristic. Ventricular response is often regular at 75 beats/minute (4:1 AV block), 150 beats/minute (2:1 AV block), or, less commonly, 100 beats/minute (3:1 AV block). Atrial flutter usually indicates the presence of organic heart disease. Among the elderly, common causes are CAD and chronic obstructive pulmonary disease. Palpitations usually occur when the ventricular rate is > 120 beats/minute; patients may be asymptomatic when the rate is slower. Diagnosis is suggested by a regular tachycardia at a ventricular rate close to 150 beats/minute. The diagnosis is confirmed if carotid sinus massage (and probably other vagal maneuvers as well; see warning, above) abruptly slows the ventricular response and causes the emergence of sawtooth flutter waves at about 300/minute on an ECG. Digoxin is the drug of choice for hemodynamically stable patients. For unstable patients, low-level DC cardioversion (25 to 50 joules) almost always·converts flutter to sinus rhythm.

For patients with pure atrial flutter, the risk of thromboembolism is probably low. However, patients who have mixed atrial flutter and fibrillation or who also have valvular heart disease or reduced left ventricular function should be evaluated with transesophageal echocardiography because their risk of thromboembolism may be increased. Treatment with warfarin may be warranted. ∎

Atrial fibrillation: A lack of organized atrial activity and totally irregular timing of the QRS complexes are characteristic. Atrial fibrillation, unlike other supraventricular tachyarrhythmias, is much more likely to be chronic than acute. Atrial fibrillation occurs in 1 to 2% of elderly persons with no evidence of heart disease, accounting for about 12% of atrial fibrillation cases. Risk doubles with each decade of age. In one study, the biennial incidence of atrial fibrillation was 6.2 per 1000 men and 3.8 per 1000 women aged 55 to 64 and 75.9 per 1000 men and 62.8 per 1000 women aged 85 to 94. Hypertension, CAD, mitral valve disease, and heart failure are the most common predisposing disorders for elderly as well as middle-aged patients. Less common causes include thyrotoxicosis, sick sinus syndrome, and amyloidosis.

Atrial fibrillation usually indicates the presence of organic heart disease, but the risk of cardiovascular morbidity and mortality is substan-

---

∎see pages 696 and 698

tially increased for elderly persons with atrial fibrillation even if they do not have organic heart disease. After adjustment for coexisting cardiovascular disorders, mortality risk is increased by 1.5 to 1.9. Risk is increased primarily because atrial fibrillation increases the risk of thromboembolic stroke by 4 or 5 times. In patients with atrial fibrillation, thrombi form in the atria or atrial appendages. Stroke attributable to atrial fibrillation has been reported in 1.5% of patients in their 50s but in 23.5% of those in their 80s.

Acute or paroxysmal atrial fibrillation usually produces disagreeable palpitations or chest discomfort because of the dramatic increase in heart rate and the irregular rhythm. Heart failure may result. However, chronic atrial fibrillation is often well tolerated, especially if the ventricular response is < 100 beats/minute.

About one third of elderly patients with atrial fibrillation have a controlled ventricular response (because of associated AV nodal disease) and require no specific therapy. For other patients, initial therapy is the same as that for younger patients: Digoxin, diltiazem, verapamil, or propranolol is given IV to slow the ventricular response to 60 to 100 beats/minute. These drugs, given orally and sometimes in combination, are also used for long-term control of the ventricular rate. Digoxin and verapamil are contraindicated in patients with the Wolff-Parkinson-White syndrome, which is rare among the elderly.

Before electrical cardioversion is performed in patients with chronic atrial fibrillation, the cause and duration of atrial fibrillation, atrial size, and the risks of anticoagulants should be considered. Because elderly persons with chronic (including lone) atrial fibrillation have a high risk of thromboembolic events, use of anticoagulants before conversion should be strongly considered.∎ For most elderly patients, an early attempt at cardioversion (generally after a few weeks of warfarin) is probably warranted; warfarin should be continued for 4 weeks after successful cardioversion. A proposed alternative is use of transesophageal echocardiography to rule out preexisting left atrial thrombi; if no thrombi are present, cardioversion can be performed immediately, without anticoagulant prophylaxis. Immediate cardioversion may also be considered if atrial fibrillation has been present for ≤ 48 hours. However, these approaches are controversial, because atrial dysfunction occurs for several days after cardioversion, increasing the risk of de novo atrial thrombi.

In elderly patients with nonrheumatic atrial fibrillation, warfarin has been reported to reduce stroke risk by 68%, with virtually no increase in major bleeding. Aspirin 325 mg daily has reduced stroke risk by 36%, although only in patients ≤ 75. Nevertheless, because the risk of major bleeding from anticoagulant use is higher for elderly than for younger

∎ see page 696

patients, the decision to use anticoagulants should be made case by case, considering factors such as patient compliance, risk of falling, and coexistence of other major disorders.

Chemical cardioversion using quinidine or other class I drugs may be considered for elderly patients with atrial fibrillation, although some analyses suggest that patients receiving long-term quinidine therapy have an increased mortality rate, presumably due to proarrhythmia. Alternatively, sotalol or amiodarone (class III), which may have a lower risk of proarrhythmia, can be used.

Whether restoration with attempted maintenance of sinus rhythm reduces long-term morbidity and mortality rates in the elderly more effectively than simple rate control of atrial fibrillation plus anticoagulation is under study.

VENTRICULAR ECTOPIC BEATS

Premature beats resulting from abnormal electrical foci in the ventricles.

Incidence of ventricular ectopic beats—whether simple or complex or detected during rest, routine activity, or exercise—increases with age, even among persons carefully screened to exclude latent CAD. Isolated ventricular ectopic beats have been detected by exercise ECG in 11% of apparently healthy persons aged 20 to 29 but in 57% of those aged 80 to 89. With 24-hour ambulatory ECG monitoring, isolated ventricular ectopic beats have been detected in 80% of healthy persons aged 60 to 85 who had no evidence of CAD; frequent ($>$ 100 in 24 hours) ventricular ectopic beats have been detected in 17%. Ventricular ectopic beats were detected by resting ECG in 8% of randomly selected patients $>$ 70.

Unless extremely frequent, isolated ventricular ectopic beats usually produce no symptoms. Symptomatic ventricular ectopic beats commonly are perceived as missed beats. This perception is probably related to the augmented stroke volume of the following sinus beats rather than to the ventricular ectopic beats themselves.

The presence of ventricular ectopic beats, whether isolated or frequent and complex, does not appear to increase the long-term risk of cardiovascular mortality in healthy elderly persons. In contrast, even isolated ventricular ectopic beats increase the risk in patients with documented CAD. However, treating patients with CAD and isolated ventricular ectopic beats has not been shown to reduce the long-term risk of mortality.

The risk of adverse reactions to antiarrhythmic drugs is generally higher in the elderly. These drugs should be used only when the ventricular ectopic beats cause ventricular tachycardia or intractable palpitations. The drugs should be started in low doses, which are gradually increased until the density of ventricular ectopic beats is reduced by 75% and ventricular tachycardia is eliminated.

Flecainide and encainide (class Ic) have been shown to increase the mortality rate for patients with asymptomatic or mildly symptomatic frequent ventricular ectopic beats after acute MI. Because of the increased mortality risk observed with class Ic drugs, they should not be given to elderly patients with heart disease unless other drugs are ineffective. β-Blockers are probably the initial drugs of choice, especially for elderly patients with CAD. If patients are unresponsive to or intolerant of β-blockers, amiodarone or sotalol (a β-blocker with class III effects) may be used. Using low-dose combination therapy with various drugs may minimize the risks of adverse effects from a single drug. Treatment should also be directed at controlling underlying or exacerbating factors (eg, electrolyte disturbances, hypoxia, heart failure).

VENTRICULAR TACHYCARDIA

Usually, a regular tachycardia with broad QRS complexes and a ventricular rate of 100 to 200 beats/minute.

With 24-hour ambulatory ECG monitoring, ventricular tachycardia has been detected in 4% of women and 10% of men aged 65 to 100. Asymptomatic runs of exercise-induced ventricular tachycardia (≤ 6 beats) have been reported in nearly 4% of apparently healthy persons ≥ 65—25 times the prevalence in younger persons.

In the elderly, severe myocardial ischemia, acute MI, digitalis toxicity, and heart failure are common precipitating disorders.

Ventricular tachycardia is associated with increased left ventricular mass and a higher incidence of left ventricular dysfunction and heart failure. Even when patients with known CAD are excluded, the incidence of abnormal left ventricular function is higher in patients with ventricular tachycardia. Some data suggest that unsustained exercise-induced ventricular tachycardia is not associated with angina, MI, syncope, or cardiac death in apparently healthy elderly persons.

Ventricular tachycardia may produce no symptoms, especially in persons without organic heart disease and with short runs (< 10 beats). More commonly, palpitations occur. Among patients with organic heart disease, significant hemodynamic upset, including hypotension and syncope, is common, particularly when the arrhythmia is sustained for > 30 seconds.

Ventricular tachycardia is strongly suggested by the presence of AV dissociation, fusion beats, and QRS duration of > 0.14 seconds or a QRS axis between − 90 and − 180°. However, it is often difficult to distinguish from paroxysmal supraventricular tachycardia when the QRS complex is widened.

Regardless of age, patients with ventricular tachycardia that is sustained or that produces hypotension or syncope must be treated immediately. If ventricular tachycardia is well tolerated hemodynamically, a rapid IV infusion (bolus) of lidocaine 50 to 75 mg (eg, 1 mg/kg) may be given initially, followed by 50 mg 2 minutes later. If the arrhythmia recurs, a full loading dose of 5 mg/kg may be required, followed by an infusion at 1 to 4 mg/minute. Patients who have recurrent ventricular tachycardia or who do not respond to lidocaine may be treated with IV procainamide or β-blockers. Data, largely from studies of younger patients, suggest that bretylium is the most effective drug for acute therapy in patients who do not respond to lidocaine.

One approach to symptomatic patients with primary recurrent ventricular tachycardia is intracardiac programmed electrophysiologic stimulation: The tachycardia is induced and the prophylactic efficacy of various antiarrhythmic drugs is then assessed in a specialized catheterization laboratory. Using this procedure to select antiarrhythmic therapy may result in a lower rate of symptomatic ventricular tachyarrhythmia than does an empiric approach and may markedly reduce the 1- to 2-year mortality rate. A less invasive and less expensive approach is ambulatory ECG monitoring, with or without exercise testing. In one study, this approach predicted antiarrhythmic drug efficacy more frequently than intracardiac programmed electrophysiologic stimulation and had a similar success rate for preventing recurrences of arrhythmia.

If therapy chosen by programmed electrophysiologic stimulation or ECG monitoring is ineffective, an automatic implantable cardioverter-defibrillator (AICD) or endocardial resection guided by intraoperative mapping may be appropriate. Almost two thirds of the patients who receive an AICD are > 65. Although age alone should not determine whether an AICD is used, the devices are not indicated for patients who have a life expectancy of < 6 months with treatment. The life expectancy of candidates for AICD implantation is determined primarily by the extent of heart disease and the severity of left ventricular dysfunction. The prevention of sudden cardiac death by AICD implantation appears to be unaffected by patient age. The use of a transvenous rather than an epicardial technique for AICD implantation has markedly reduced morbidity and mortality rates.

The benefits of AICDs compared with those of antiarrhythmic drugs (particularly amiodarone) for certain patients are unclear. Some data suggest that for elderly patients with life-threatening ventricular tachyarrhythmias, the mortality rate is lower with AICDs than with amiodarone or sotalol. For patients with heart disease and asymptomatic high-density ventricular ectopic activity, whether amiodarone reduces the mortality rate relative to conventional therapy for the underlying heart disease (without antiarrhythmics) is unclear, and the role of AICDs is controversial. Most studies have excluded patients > 75, although age has not been shown to affect study results.

Long-term prophylaxis is not required for ventricular tachycardia that was precipitated by an acute event (eg, MI, digitalis toxicity), because the tachycardia rarely recurs. However, aggressive prophylaxis is required for primary sustained ventricular tachycardia (without an obvious precipitant), because the tachycardia recurs within 1 year in about 35% of patients and mortality risk is increased. A 1-year mortality rate of 29% has been reported for patients (mean age, 68.5) who had an out-of-hospital cardiac arrest caused by a primary arrhythmia.

BRADYARRHYTHMIAS AND CONDUCTION DISTURBANCES

Intrinsic conduction system disease and acute disorders affecting the conduction system (eg, MI, digitalis toxicity) are more common among the elderly than among younger persons. Therefore, most bradyarrhythmias and conduction disturbances (see TABLE 91–3) are common among the elderly. However, sinus bradycardia with < 40 beats/minute, sinus pauses of > 1.6 seconds, and high-degree AV block are rare among healthy persons > 60 and are often associated with ischemic, hypertensive, or amyloid heart disease.

TABLE 91–3.   BRADYARRHYTHMIAS AND CONDUCTION DISTURBANCES

Disorder	Prevalence With Age	Effect on Mortality*	Usual Treatment
Sinus bradycardia	Probably not increased	None	None
First-degree atrioventricular block	Increased	None	None
Second-degree atrioventricular block			
Mobitz type I	Probably not increased	Probably none	None†
Mobitz type II	Increased	Increased	Pacemaker
High-grade	Increased	Increased	Pacemaker
Third-degree (complete) atrioventricular block	Increased	Increased	Pacemaker
Sick sinus syndrome	Increased	None	Pacemaker only for symptomatic patients with bradycardia
Left bundle branch block	Increased	Increased	None known
Right bundle branch block	Increased	None	None

*In otherwise healthy elderly patients.
†Digoxin, a β-blocker, or a calcium channel blocker, if being used, should be withdrawn.

Pathogenesis

Widespread age-related histologic changes in the conduction system may contribute to the striking age-related increase in the incidence of bradyarrhythmias and conduction disturbances. The number of pacemaker cells in the sinoatrial node begins to decline progressively by age 60; only about 10% of the cells are still present at age 75. The sinoatrial node becomes enveloped by fat, which may partially or completely separate the node from the atrial musculature.

Age-related changes in the His bundle include loss of cells, an increase in fibrous and adipose tissue, and amyloid infiltration. Some degree of idiopathic fibrosis may affect the left side of the cardiac skeleton (central fibrous body, mitral and aortic annuli, and proximal interventricular septum). The fibrosis may also affect the AV node, His bundle, and proximal left and right bundle branches because of their proximity. If extensive, the fibrosis may cause AV block. This fibrosis is the most common cause of chronic AV block in the elderly.

Some age-related histologic changes in the conduction system are apparent on the standard 12-lead ECG. Although resting heart rate does not change with age, respiratory variation in resting sinus rate (known as sinus arrhythmia) decreases. Heart rate variability is reduced, and PR and QT intervals are somewhat prolonged; however, QRS duration is unchanged. The increase in PR interval is due to a delay that is proximal to the His bundle; conduction time from the His bundle to the ventricle appears to be unrelated to age.

The QRS frontal plane axis shifts left with age, probably reflecting the combined effects of fibrosis in the anterior fascicle of the left bundle branch and a mild age-related increase in left ventricular wall thickness. This left axis deviation is the most common ECG abnormality among the elderly, occurring in about half. For elderly patients without organic heart disease, neither first-degree AV block nor a left axis deviation of $-30°$ is associated with increased cardiac morbidity or mortality rates.

Symptoms, Signs, and Diagnosis

Bradycardias may produce no symptoms, mild fatigue or faintness, or significant hemodynamic upset (eg, hypotension, angina, heart failure). The diagnosis may be suspected on the basis of symptoms and signs but is confirmed by ECG.

Treatment

Patients with a bradyarrhythmia must be treated immediately if they also have hypotension, cerebral or cardiac ischemia, heart failure, and/or, in acute MI, frequent ventricular ectopic beats. Placing the patient in the supine position with the legs elevated often ameliorates hypotensive sequelae. Atropine 0.5 to 1 mg is given rapidly IV; it may be repeated at 3- to 5-minute intervals up to a total dose of 0.04 mg/kg (total, 2 to 3 mg). If atropine is ineffective or causes intolerable adverse effects, an isoproterenol infusion can be started at 1 to 4 μg/minute, then adjusted to produce a ventricular rate of 60 beats/minute. If neither drug is successful or if isoproterenol is contraindicated because of ischemia or infarction, temporary transvenous pacing should be used.

Cardiac pacemakers: More than 85% of patients who receive a pacemaker are > 64; about half of these patients are treated for high-degree AV block and half for sick sinus syndrome. Use of a permanent ventricular pacemaker has reduced the high mortality rate formerly associated with complete heart block in patients aged 65 to 79 who do not have structural heart disease; the survival rate may be lower in patients > 80 who have a pacemaker than in patients of the same age who do not.

Pacemakers that improve maximal exercise cardiac output and work capacity (eg, dual-chamber AV synchronous pacemakers as opposed to traditional fixed-rate ventricular pacemakers) may especially benefit active elderly patients. The elderly's greater dependence on the atrial contribution to ventricular filling suggests that AV synchronous pacemakers should be particularly beneficial for them. In addition, the incidence of atrial fibrillation and the mortality rate are higher for patients who have ventricular pacemakers than for patients who have atrial or dual-chamber AV synchronous pacemakers. Atrial fibrillation has been reported in 47% of patients > 70 with sick sinus syndrome who received a ventricular pacemaker and in 9% of those who received a dual-chamber pacemaker after 7 years; the mortality rates were 72% and 51%, respectively. Thus, otherwise healthy elderly patients who are in sinus rhythm and require a pacemaker for sick sinus syndrome should probably receive an AV synchronous pacemaker.

Complications with permanent pacemakers are rare but significant. Abrupt loss of pacing (due to battery failure, fibrosis around the catheter site, myocardial perforation, lead fracture, or electrode dislodgment) may result in marked bradycardia or asystole. The catheter may perforate the right ventricle, causing a pericardial friction rub or, rarely, tamponade. In patients with little overlying subcutaneous tissue, the pulse generator may extrude or the pacing wire may erode through the skin. Some patients have difficulty adjusting psychologically to pacemaker implantation. All patients with a pacemaker should have regular follow-up physical and ECG examinations.

SINUS BRADYCARDIA

A sinus rate of < 60 beats/minute.

Sinus bradycardia may indicate excellent physical conditioning; however, in the elderly, it often indicates intrinsic sinus node disease.

Inferior MI, hypothermia, myxedema, or increased intracranial pressure may cause this arrhythmia. For apparently healthy persons aged 40 to 80 with sinus rates < 50 beats/minute, 5-year cardiovascular morbidity and mortality rates do not appear to be increased. Treatment is not needed unless symptoms of cerebral hypoperfusion are present. If such symptoms are chronic, pacemaker implantation is the definitive treatment.

SINOATRIAL BLOCK

Inability of sinus node impulses to depolarize the atria.

Sinoatrial block is often 2:1, resulting in atrial and ventricular rates that are exactly one half the sinus rate. In the elderly, common causes are intrinsic conduction system disease, ischemia, digitalis toxicity, and toxicity from class Ia antiarrhythmics. The diagnosis is made when an ECG shows a pause in the sinus rhythm equal to a multiple of the underlying PR interval. Treatment is similar to that for sinus bradycardia.

ATRIOVENTRICULAR BLOCK

Partial or complete interruption of electrical conduction from the atria or sinus node to the AV node and ventricles.

First-degree atrioventricular block: The PR interval is prolonged (≥ 0.22 seconds). First-degree block may occur in healthy persons with high vagal tone, or it may be caused by intrinsic conduction system disease or by various drugs (eg, digoxin, β-blockers, calcium channel blockers, class Ia antiarrhythmic drugs). Because cardiac morbidity and mortality rates are not increased in patients with this disorder, no treatment is required.

Second-degree atrioventricular block: There are three patterns. In Mobitz type I (Wenckebach) block, the PR interval is progressively prolonged until a ventricular complex is dropped. Because this block is usually proximal to the His-Purkinje system, the QRS complex typically appears normal. Digitalis toxicity and acute inferior MI are common precipitating factors. Mobitz type I block is usually transient and rarely requires specific treatment.

In Mobitz type II block, the PR interval is fixed, but QRS complexes are dropped. Because the block occurs at or below the His bundle, the QRS complex is often wide. Mobitz type II block is most often associated with acute anterior MI, myocarditis, or advanced sclerodegenerative conduction system disease. Patients with this block are usually symptomatic and often present with syncope due to inadequate cerebral perfusion (Stokes-Adams attack). Because of the symptomatic presentation and frequent progression to complete heart block, patients usually receive a permanent pacemaker.

In high-grade block, there is a mathematical relationship between the P waves and QRS complexes (eg, 2:1, 3:1). High-grade block may progress to complete heart block. Patients are often symptomatic and usually receive a permanent pacemaker.

Third-degree (complete) atrioventricular block: Atrial depolarizations cannot activate the ventricle. Block within the AV node is usually associated with normal QRS complexes and an escape rate of almost 60 beats/minute. Common causes are acute inferior MI and digitalis toxicity. This block is usually transient, and no specific treatment is required. If digitalis toxicity is the cause, the drug is withdrawn. Pacemakers may be used when hypotension or symptoms of cerebral hypoperfusion are present.

Block within the ventricles is accompanied by wide QRS complexes and a slow escape rate, often < 40 beats/minute. Such block may occur in patients with severe sclerodegenerative conduction system disease or extensive acute anterior MI. Because these patients usually respond poorly to atropine and isoproterenol, pacemaker implantation is necessary.

SICK SINUS SYNDROME

A variety of rhythm disturbances that reflect sinoatrial node dysfunction and are often associated with dysfunction elsewhere in the conduction system.

CAD and a primary sclerodegenerative process are the most common precipitating disorders, although many heart diseases may precipitate the syndrome. Patients may present with bradyarrhythmias (sinus bradycardia, sinus pauses or arrest, sinoatrial exit block, or atrial fibrillation with a slow ventricular response) or with the bradycardia-tachycardia syndrome, in which a supraventricular tachycardia terminates in a long period of asystole. Therefore, symptoms may consist of palpitations or chest pain during tachycardia and dizziness or syncope during bradycardia.

The long-term prognosis for patients with sick sinus syndrome depends primarily on the presence and severity of the underlying heart disease.

For tachycardia (paroxysmal supraventricular tachycardia, atrial flutter, or atrial fibrillation), digoxin, other antiarrhythmic drugs, or cardioversion is used. For bradycardia associated with syncope, a permanent pacemaker is needed.

BUNDLE BRANCH BLOCK

Partial or complete interruption of electrical conduction in the bundle branches.

Left bundle branch block is usually associated with ischemic or hypertensive heart disease in elderly men and women. In contrast, complete right bundle branch block often occurs in apparently healthy elderly men and appears to be benign, although it is highly predictive of underlying heart disease in elderly women.

Pacemakers are not warranted for asymptomatic elderly patients with chronic bifascicular block (either left or right bundle branch block plus left anterior-superior or left posterior-inferior division block), with or without a prolonged PR interval, because complete heart block rarely occurs (see TABLE 91–3).

92 ■ HEART FAILURE AND CARDIOMYOPATHY

HEART FAILURE

A condition in which cardiac output is insufficient to meet physiologic demands.

Heart failure is common among persons $\geq$ 65 years. Its prevalence increases exponentially after age 70 and, unlike that of other cardiac disorders, has been increasing over the past two decades. Heart failure is now the most common diagnosis among hospitalized elderly patients.

Etiology and Pathogenesis

The principal mechanisms of heart failure involve impediments to forward ejection, myocardial failure, impaired cardiac filling, and volume overload (see TABLE 92–1). In the elderly, heart failure usually results from systemic arterial hypertension, which impedes forward ejection and eventually results in myocardial failure, or from coronary artery disease, which leads directly to myocardial failure. Hypertension and coronary artery disease also impair cardiac filling. Valvular heart disease may lead to heart failure by impeding forward ejection, thereby causing impaired cardiac filling and chronic volume overload, which results in secondary myocardial failure. Heart failure due to idiopathic dilated cardiomyopathy and high-output heart failure due to disorders such as thyrotoxicosis, anemia, arteriovenous fistulas, fever, and thiamine deficiency are less common among the elderly than among younger patients.

Heart failure may result from reduced function of the left and/or right ventricle (reduced stroke volume); combined left- and right-sided heart failure is more common than isolated left- or right-sided heart failure.

TABLE 92-1.   PRINCIPAL CAUSES OF HEART FAILURE

Mechanism	Condition
Impediments to forward ejection	Systemic arterial hypertension Elevated systemic vascular resistance Aortic valve stenosis Supravalvular stenosis (coarctation) Subaortic stenosis Obstructive hypertrophic cardiomyopathy Pulmonary hypertension
Myocardial failure	Loss of functioning cardiac muscle (due to myocardial infarction or myocardial ischemia) Cardiomyopathy Myocarditis Drugs (eg, doxorubicin) Systemic disease (eg, hypothyroidism) Chronic overload
Impaired cardiac filling	Ventricular hypertrophy (symmetric or asymmetric) Myocardial diastolic dysfunction Pericardial disease (causing constriction or tamponade) Restrictive heart disease (endocardial or myocardial) Ventricular aneurysm
Volume overload	Valvular regurgitation Increased intravascular volume Increased metabolic demands (eg, due to thyrotoxicosis, anemia, or certain skin disorders) Arteriovenous shunts or fistulas

Reduced ventricular function can result from systolic dysfunction (involving abnormal contractility), from diastolic dysfunction (involving abnormal filling), or from both; combined systolic and diastolic heart failure is more common than isolated systolic or diastolic heart failure.

Diastolic dysfunction, which is relatively uncommon among younger patients, accounts for about 50% of heart failure cases among elderly patients and appears to be particularly common among elderly women. In diastolic dysfunction, prolonged myocardial relaxation and increased myocardial stiffness (which decrease filling rate and volume) increase left ventricular diastolic pressure and reduce stroke volume at rest and during exercise. As a result, heart failure develops, even if systolic function (as indicated by the ejection fraction) is normal or nearly normal.

Age-related changes in the heart and cardiovascular system **1** lower the threshold for expression of heart failure. Interstitial collagen within the myocardium increases, the myocardium stiffens, and myocardial relaxation is prolonged. These changes lead to a significant reduction in diastolic left ventricular function, even in healthy elderly persons. Modest decrements in systolic function also occur with age. An age-related decrease in myocardial and vascular responsiveness to β-adrenergic stimulation further impairs the ability of the cardiovascular system to respond to increased work demands.

As a result of these changes, peak exercise capacity decreases significantly (about 8% per decade after age 30), and cardiac output at peak exercise decreases more modestly. Thus, elderly patients are more prone than are younger ones to develop heart failure symptoms in response to the stress of systemic disorders or relatively modest cardiovascular insults. Stressors include infections (particularly pneumonia), hypothyroidism, hyperthyroidism, anemia, myocardial ischemia, hypoxia, hypothermia, hyperthermia, renal failure, nonadherence with drug or diet regimens, and use of certain drugs (including nonsteroidal antiinflammatory drugs, β-blockers, and certain calcium channel blockers).

Symptoms, Signs, and Diagnosis

The cardinal symptoms and signs of heart failure include dyspnea and fatigue (particularly with exertion), orthopnea, and dependent edema. They are common among young and elderly patients. Peripheral edema is less specific as a sign of heart failure in the elderly than in the young. Also, in bedridden patients, edema may occur in the sacral area rather than in the lower extremities. Jugular venous distention and hepatojugular reflux are also common. In patients with advanced, uncompensated heart failure, mild tachycardia occurs. However, elderly patients may also present with nonspecific symptoms and signs (eg, somnolence, confusion, disorientation, weakness, fatigue, failure to thrive).

In elderly persons, a fourth heart sound (S_4 gallop), particularly if soft, does not necessarily indicate clinically significant heart disease. However, a third heart sound (S_3 or early diastolic gallop) usually does. Coarse, wet inspiratory rales can be heard, particularly in the lower lung fields.

Classifying symptom severity according to the New York Heart Association (NYHA) classification **2** aids in selecting therapy, following progress, and determining the prognosis.

No test can provide a diagnosis of heart failure. Rather, the diagnosis is based on clinical findings. Diagnosis is complicated because patients often do not perceive substantial, progressive declines or they attribute such declines to old age. Consequently, patients should be encouraged

---

1 see page 813   **2** see TABLE 29–1 on page 280

to give concrete examples of their functional abilities, to compare them with those of their peers, and to recall tasks that have become difficult or that are now avoided.

Differentiating systolic heart failure from diastolic heart failure, which is often underdiagnosed, is important because therapy differs. Patients with diastolic heart failure are more often women and tend to be obese. Onset of symptoms may be acute, and clinical deterioration abrupt. This rapid deterioration, commonly known as flash pulmonary edema, is usually related to severe hypertension or acute ischemia. Atrial fibrillation with rapid ventricular response is also a common precipitant. Diastolic dysfunction is typically accompanied by a forceful, minimally displaced apical impulse and a fourth heart sound.

Systolic dysfunction of the left ventricle produces secondary signs of right-sided heart failure (jugular venous distention, pedal edema) more frequently than does diastolic dysfunction of the left ventricle. Systolic dysfunction is typically accompanied by a dilated left ventricle (with a laterally displaced or diffuse point of maximal impulse) and a third heart sound. Onset of symptoms can be rapid but is more often gradual (eg, when due to cardiomyopathy).

Despite these differences, systolic dysfunction and diastolic dysfunction usually cannot be reliably distinguished at bedside. Therefore, evaluation of new-onset heart failure should include an imaging test, usually echocardiography. Echocardiography can evaluate left ventricular systolic function (eg, ejection fraction), help determine the primary etiology of heart failure (eg, cardiac tamponade, aortic stenosis, severe valvular regurgitation), and exclude specific complications (eg, left ventricular aneurysms, mural thrombi).

Typically, patients with primarily diastolic heart failure have a normal (usually 50 to 65%) or high ($\geq$ 70%) ejection fraction (stroke volume divided by end-diastolic volume), a normal or small left ventricle, thickened ventricular walls with concentric hypertrophy, and no segmental wall motion abnormalities. Typically, patients with primarily systolic heart failure have a significantly reduced left ventricular ejection fraction (usually $\leq$ 40%), a dilated left ventricle, and multiple regional wall motion abnormalities. Patients who have combined systolic and diastolic dysfunction with an ejection fraction of 40 to 50% have mixed heart failure.

Ejection fraction, which can be measured with various imaging tests, provides a relatively reliable measure of systolic function. However, no comparable measure is available for diastolic function. Left ventricular diastolic filling indexes, including early/atrial (E/A) ratio and early deceleration time, can be assessed noninvasively (eg, with Doppler echocardiography). However, because these indexes are affected by factors other than abnormal diastolic function (eg, blood pressure, drugs, aging), they cannot be used to definitively diagnose diastolic dysfunction.

Two relatively inexpensive tests provide important supplemental information: A chest x-ray provides unique information about cardiomegaly, pulmonary vascular congestion, and pleural effusions; and a resting ECG provides information about cardiac rhythm and rate, hypertrophy, and infarction. Measurement of serum electrolytes and creatinine, albumin, and thyroid-stimulating hormone levels; liver function tests; and urinalysis are useful when heart failure is first diagnosed. Because patients with active myocardial ischemia can present with heart failure, a stress test or, if severe or unstable angina coexists, coronary angiography is often indicated.

Prognosis

Prognosis is determined largely by the primary cause and its severity, the presence of comorbid conditions, and the patient's age. Preliminary data suggest that among community-dwelling elderly persons with a mean age of 70, the annual mortality rate is 9% for diastolic heart failure and 18% for systolic heart failure. However, among hospitalized and very elderly patients, mortality rates for diastolic and systolic heart failure may be similar. Recent hospitalization for heart failure indicates a poor prognosis, whether the heart failure is systolic or diastolic. Other prognostic data regarding diastolic heart failure are scarce.

For systolic heart failure, prognostic data are relatively plentiful, although few studies have focused on elderly patients. A high NYHA class, low exercise capacity (which can be objectively measured with cardiopulmonary exercise testing), a very low ejection fraction, and ischemic etiology are important indicators of a poor prognosis. Renal failure is a particularly ominous comorbid condition and greatly complicates management. Other indicators of a poor prognosis include hyponatremia, even when mild; conduction abnormalities (eg, left bundle branch block); ventricular ectopy, identifiable on a resting ECG; abnormal liver function test results; and a severely dilated (> 60 mm) left ventricle and circumferential myocardial thinning, both identifiable on an echocardiogram. Shortened deceleration time of the early component of the Doppler mitral filling pattern is an important negative prognostic indicator for patients with dilated cardiomyopathy, who constitute a substantial portion of those with systolic dysfunction. When this filling pattern is accompanied by a restrictive diastolic filling pattern, the 2-year mortality rate appears to be about 50%.

Treatment

Treatment should be aimed at reducing symptoms, improving quality of life, and preventing acute exacerbations and hospitalization. A physician- or nurse-directed interdisciplinary team can help achieve these goals and thereby substantially reduce total health care costs. The team may include a social worker, dietitian, nurse case-manager, and physical therapist. Such a team can provide extensive education for the patient, family members, and other caregivers and can arrange appropriate posthospital support and access to follow-up care.

General measures: Measures include attempts to identify and manage exacerbating factors or disorders; common exacerbating factors include dietary (eg, sodium) indiscretion, drug nonadherence, and inadequate blood pressure control. Management of such factors can frequently prevent acute episodes. Other measures include smoking and alcohol cessation and control of hyperlipidemia and diabetes. Pneumococcal and influenza vaccinations are recommended. Selected elderly patients with heart failure may benefit from cardiovascular rehabilitation.◻ Most patients should be encouraged to engage in light to moderate physical activity regularly so that they can maintain function.

Pharmacotherapy: For the elderly, drugs are generally initiated at a low dose, which is increased gradually to the target maintenance dose. Usually, target maintenance doses are the doses used in clinical studies, but such doses are not always feasible for elderly patients. Therapy should be individualized, because elderly patients, especially those with systolic heart failure, often have limited physiologic reserves and multiple concomitant medical problems.

For patients who have **systolic heart failure** without significant edema and with only mild symptoms, usual therapy begins with an angiotensin-converting (ACE) inhibitor, which may be the only drug required for some time. If volume overload and edema are present, therapy begins with a diuretic; the dose is adjusted to the lowest dose that maintains euvolemia. Digoxin is added when more severe symptoms or atrial fibrillation develops.

Therapy for patients with **diastolic heart failure** is largely empiric; data from clinical studies are lacking. Because severe or inadequately controlled hypertension is so common among patients with diastolic heart failure and because increased afterload adversely affects diastolic function, blood pressure control should be a primary goal. ACE inhibitors, angiotensin II receptor blockers, β-blockers, and calcium channel blockers are often favored on theoretical grounds. However, no drug has been shown to directly enhance diastolic function in elderly patients with heart failure and a normal left ventricular ejection fraction.

Diuretics are not necessary for all patients or at all stages of the disease. However, most patients with moderate to severe heart failure have symptoms and signs of sodium and volume overload, which warrant cautious use of diuretics. Loop diuretics are most commonly used. For patients with acute pulmonary edema and normal or increased systemic pressure, IV loop diuretics (furosemide, bumetanide) often result in dramatic and rapid reduction of symptoms. Once the acute episode resolves, the dose should be decreased to the lowest dose that maintains

◻ see page 278

the patient in a relatively asymptomatic and euvolemic state; the patient's weight should be noted. Thiazide diuretics are sometimes adequate, particularly for patients with mild heart failure. The potassium-sparing diuretic spironolactone may reduce the mortality rate for patients with systolic heart failure when it is added in low doses to usual therapy, most often consisting of an ACE inhibitor and a loop diuretic, with or without digoxin.

Many patients with heart failure have an intrinsic diuretic dose threshold; doses below this threshold produce minimal diuresis, even when doses are repeated. Usually, a single morning oral dose slightly higher than the threshold can provide effective maintenance diuresis. Multiple daily doses are usually unnecessary, are inconvenient for patients, and can exacerbate urinary incontinence. Dosing can be timed to fit a patient's lifestyle so that incontinence is not precipitated when access to a bathroom is inconvenient. The need to increase the diuretic dose in a previously stable outpatient suggests disease progression, worsening renal dysfunction, poor absorption due to bowel edema, other systemic complications, or nonadherence.

For patients with end-stage disease, consultation with a specialist may help optimize diuretic therapy. Use of IV loop diuretics in high, pulsed, and/or intermittent doses can be effective. Oral metolazone 2.5 or 5.0 mg given 30 minutes before the loop diuretic can significantly enhance the diuretic effect. Adjuvant short-term therapy with low-dose dopamine or dobutamine may help promote diuresis by increasing renal flow. Nonsteroidal anti-inflammatory drugs can cause relative diuretic resistance and should be discontinued if possible. During active diuresis, the patient should be closely monitored, and electrolytes, particularly potassium and magnesium, should be replaced; fluid restriction may be needed to prevent or alleviate hyponatremia.

Vasodilators include ACE inhibitors, angiotensin II receptor blockers, hydralazine, and isosorbide dinitrate. Vasodilators can increase stroke volume by reducing impedance to ejection. Nearly all of them can produce short-term improvement in hemodynamics and can reduce symptoms. However, with long-term use, most have minimal benefit. Notable exceptions are ACE inhibitors and angiotensin II receptor blockers, which have multiple therapeutic mechanisms in addition to vasodilation.

ACE inhibitors substantially reduce symptoms, improve exercise tolerance, slow disease progression, and reduce hospitalization and long-term mortality rates for patients with left ventricular ejection fractions of $\leq$ 35 to 40%. These benefits occur even if patients have no overt heart failure symptoms and if symptom relief appears to be minimal. Benefits are so compelling that ACE inhibitor therapy, unless contraindicated, should be withheld only from patients who cannot tolerate it despite reasonably aggressive efforts to enable them to do so. With careful management, most patients can start and continue to take an

ACE inhibitor. Little information comparing the benefits of different ACE inhibitors is available. Selection is often based on half-life (dose frequency) and cost. Initially, a low dose (eg, enalapril 2.5 to 5.0 mg po bid, captopril 6.25 mg po tid) is given to avoid hypotension. The dose is slowly increased over several weeks to reach the doses that were shown to be optimally effective in large studies (eg, enalapril 10 to 20 mg bid, captopril 50 mg tid). Although adherence is usually better with once- or twice-daily regimens, dose frequency for captopril should not be reduced to twice daily for patients with heart failure.

Common adverse effects of ACE inhibitors include hypotension, rash, chronic dry cough, and increased serum creatinine and potassium levels. Except for angioedema, which is rare, adverse effects can be minimized by starting with a low dose. When adverse effects occur, they can often be minimized by decreasing the dose or by using a different ACE inhibitor. Patients can often tolerate persistent mild dry cough, particularly when they understand the significant reduction in mortality rate associated with the drug.

Hypotension is common but usually mild and asymptomatic; it is usually most prominent after the first one or two doses. Unless hypotension is unusually severe, the drug should not be discontinued. Patients who are very old and patients who have volume depletion due to excessive diuresis, severe left ventricular dysfunction, a baseline systolic blood pressure of < 100 mm Hg, or hyponatremia are at highest risk of severe first-dose hypotension. Volume depletion should be corrected before ACE inhibitor therapy is initiated.

Angiotensin II receptor blockers directly inhibit angiotensin II at the end-organ receptor level. These drugs have some theoretical advantages and possibly some disadvantages compared with ACE inhibitors. The angiotensin II receptor blocker losartan appears to have no advantage over the ACE inhibitor captopril in terms of mortality rate reduction for patients with systolic heart failure. The incidence of cough seems to be substantially lower with losartan than with captopril, but the incidence of renal dysfunction does not seem to differ. However, until the relative roles of ACE inhibitors and angiotensin II receptor blockers are determined, an ACE inhibitor should probably remain the initial therapy of choice, even for elderly patients with systolic heart failure. An angiotensin II receptor blocker is a rational alternative for patients who cannot tolerate ACE inhibitors, particularly because of cough.

Neither ACE inhibitors nor angiotensin II receptor blockers have been extensively studied in patients with diastolic heart failure. However, both drug classes decrease blood pressure, left ventricular hypertrophy, and interstitial myocardial collagen; all of these effects are theoretically beneficial for patients with diastolic heart failure. In animal models of heart failure, diastolic dysfunction is ameliorated after antagonism of angiotensin II. In one small study of elderly patients with heart failure and a normal left ventricular ejection fraction, enalapril, an ACE inhibitor, improved exercise tolerance. In another study, losartan, an angiotensin II receptor blocker, improved exercise tolerance and quality of life and reduced exercise blood pressure in elderly patients with mild diastolic dysfunction.

Compared with ACE inhibitors, the combination of **hydralazine and isosorbide dinitrate**—the first vasodilator regimen shown to reduce the mortality rate in patients with systolic heart failure—has a more cumbersome dosing regimen, is less well tolerated, and reduces the mortality rate less. However, this combination is useful for patients who cannot tolerate ACE inhibitors or angiotensin II receptor blockers, usually because of renal dysfunction or allergy, and has been used in patients with advanced systolic heart failure.

Calcium channel blockers have little, if any, role in primary therapy for patients with systolic left ventricular dysfunction. In some analyses, use of these drugs has been associated with an increased mortality rate for such patients. Calcium channel blockers with negative inotropic properties, including verapamil and diltiazem, can precipitate or exacerbate heart failure symptoms. A possible exception is the dihydropyridine calcium channel blocker amlodipine. Among patients with severe systolic left ventricular dysfunction, the addition of amlodipine to usual therapy seems to decrease the mortality rate for those without known coronary artery disease and not to increase the mortality rate for those with coronary artery disease.

In patients with diastolic heart failure, verapamil may reduce symptoms and improve exercise tolerance. In addition, verapamil can reduce symptoms in patients with hypertrophic cardiomyopathy, which is present in a subset of patients with diastolic heart failure.

β-Blockers have intrinsic negative inotropic properties that can precipitate or exacerbate heart failure symptoms in patients with significant systolic left ventricular dysfunction. However, these drugs, when added cautiously to usual therapy, may significantly reduce symptoms as well as hospitalization and mortality rates for selected patients with systolic left ventricular dysfunction and mild to moderate symptoms of heart failure. The greatest effect on mortality reduction appears to be in patients with heart failure after acute myocardial infarction. β-Blockers are important in the treatment of coronary artery disease (including myocardial infarction) and of ventricular arrhythmia, which are common concomitant disorders in patients with systolic heart failure. Carvedilol, bisoprolol, and metoprolol have been studied the most extensively. Carvedilol, a nonselective β-blocker, is approved for the treatment of systolic heart failure.

β-Blockers may be considered additive therapy for selected patients who have symptomatic systolic heart failure and have been stabilized with diuretics, ACE inhibitors, and possibly digoxin. β-Blockers should not be used in patients who are acutely symptomatic, who have severe

(NYHA class IIIS or IV) heart failure, or who have contraindications to β-blockers (eg, bronchospastic chronic obstructive pulmonary disease, significant conduction abnormalities).

β-Blockers should be initiated in very low doses (typically, carvedilol 3.125 mg bid, bisoprolol 1.25 mg once daily, or sustained-release metoprolol 12.5 mg once daily). The patient should be directly observed for at least 1 to 2 hours after administration of the first dose, or longer depending on the patient's condition. If tolerated, the initial dose should be continued at least 2 weeks before the dose is gradually increased. Generally, target maintenance doses are similar to the doses used in studies (eg, carvedilol 25 mg bid, bisoprolol 10 mg once daily, sustained-release metoprolol 50 to 100 mg once daily). Patients must be closely monitored during therapy.

β-Blockers can have substantial adverse effects; most occur early in therapy. Experience with β-blocker therapy in very elderly or debilitated patients with heart failure is relatively limited.

β-Blockers have been recommended as therapy for diastolic heart failure, because they have the theoretical benefits of heart rate reduction and negative inotropism. However, supportive data from clinical studies are lacking.

Digoxin therapy for symptomatic heart failure remains important. Regardless of whether sinus rhythm is normal, a third heart sound is present, or left ventricular ejection fraction is reduced, digoxin can improve exercise tolerance, alleviate symptoms, and reduce the incidence of heart failure exacerbations and the risk and duration of hospitalization.

For elderly patients with a wide range of left ventricular ejection fractions, digoxin seems to have a neutral effect on the overall mortality rate: A slight reduction in the number of deaths related to heart failure is balanced by a similar increase in the number of deaths due to other conditions, particularly sudden cardiac death. Thus, digoxin is indicated for relief of heart failure symptoms that persist despite ACE inhibitor and diuretic therapy, usually in patients with NYHA class III or IV heart failure.

For most patients > 70, digoxin should be initiated and maintained at 0.125 mg daily. For large patients with normal renal function (especially if they are < 70), the dose may be 0.25 mg/day. For elderly patients with renal dysfunction, 0.125 mg every other day or twice a week may be adequate. One assay may be performed shortly after initiation of therapy (ie, after at least 5 doses or half-lives), but thereafter, patients can usually be monitored clinically without routine assays.

Inotropic drugs such as IV dopamine and milrinone may help markedly symptomatic hospitalized patients who do not respond adequately to usual measures. These drugs can reduce symptoms and improve quality of life. For highly selected patients with severe, refractory end-stage systolic heart failure, IV dobutamine is appropriate as compassionate-use therapy or can be used as a bridge to surgical treatment. Oral inotropic drugs that initially showed promise, sometimes with dramatic reduction in symptoms, have been shown to increase mortality rates and have been abandoned in the USA.

Antiarrhythmic therapy, including drugs and electrical cardioversion, is often warranted to restore and maintain sinus rhythm in patients with atrial fibrillation. Elderly persons, in particular, depend on atrial contraction for adequate ventricular filling.

Use of amiodarone and/or an automatic implantable defibrillator can reduce the risk of sudden cardiac death, which is common among patients with systolic heart failure. High-risk patients who may benefit from such therapy include those with a history of sustained ventricular tachycardia, ventricular fibrillation, or resuscitated sudden cardiac death. β-Blockers may also provide protection. Type I antiarrhythmic drugs should generally be avoided in patients with heart failure and an ejection fraction ≤ 40% unless they have an automatic implantable defibrillator, because mortality risk is increased.

Warfarin is indicated for patients with systolic heart failure and atrial fibrillation or prior embolism. Its use in other patients with systolic heart failure is controversial. Warfarin has also been used in patients who have a markedly dilated left ventricle, who have an unstable cardiac thrombus or a ventricular aneurysm at high risk of rupture, who are at increased risk of thrombophlebitis, or who require prolonged bed rest. During bed rest, mechanical devices and leg and toe exercises can also help prevent venous thrombosis. **1** The elderly are at increased risk of adverse effects from warfarin and other anticoagulants. **2**

Surgical treatment: Coronary revascularization should be considered if patients have severe coronary artery disease and manifest myocardial ischemia. Valve replacement surgery is warranted for many patients with heart failure due to primary valvular disease. **3**

Survival rates after heart transplantation have improved steadily because of improved medical supportive posttransplant care and immunotherapy. However, because the availability of donor organs is limited, transplantation is rarely performed in elderly patients. Ventricular assist devices are generally appropriate only as a bridge to transplantation. New ventricular remodeling surgeries are considered experimental and should be performed only in highly selected patients.

Patient and Caregiver Issues

The patient, family members, and other caregivers must thoroughly understand the drug regimen, diet (including moderate sodium restriction), and need for regular moderate physical activity. Patients with heart failure should have a scale, weigh themselves regularly, and know what

1 see page 926   **2** see pages 697–702   **3** see page 947

steps to take if weight unexpectedly increases more than a specified amount, usually 3 to 5 pounds (1.4 to 2.2 kg). Nurses can communicate diuretic dose adjustments to patients by telephone, or patients may be able to adjust the dose themselves, using individualized algorithms.

End-of-Life Issues

When heart failure reaches a terminal stage, quality of life may be poor and therapeutic options may become limited; comfort issues and home services are important.∎ There should be timely discussion of advance directives∎ with patients.

CARDIOMYOPATHY

A functional abnormality of the ventricular myocardium.

Cardiomyopathy generally refers to a diffuse or generalized myocardial disorder, often without a known underlying cause; involvement of the myocardium is primary (idiopathic). However, valvular heart disease, hypertension, or coronary artery disease may coexist with primary cardiomyopathy. The main types of cardiomyopathy, which may overlap, are dilated (congestive), hypertrophic, and restrictive (infiltrative).

DILATED CARDIOMYOPATHY

Myocardial disorders characterized by systolic dysfunction with dilation of chambers and an increase in muscle mass without full compensatory increase in wall thickness.

About 10% of patients with dilated cardiomyopathy are > 65. Dilated cardiomyopathy is usually chronic, and patients present with effort dyspnea and fatigability because of elevated left ventricular diastolic pressure and low cardiac output. Less commonly, when an infective agent is the cause, onset is acute and is associated with fever; this syndrome is called acute myocarditis, which is rare among the elderly. Usually, no specific cause of myocarditis can be identified, although the disorder has been attributed to viruses (especially coxsackievirus) and rickettsiae. Acute myocarditis may be difficult to diagnose clinically.

The diagnosis of dilated cardiomyopathy is made by excluding other causes of diffuse myocardial dysfunction (eg, doxorubicin toxicity, radiation damage, chronic alcoholism) and is confirmed by echocardiographic evidence of four-chamber dilation with depressed systolic ventricular function. Dilated cardiomyopathy may be misdiagnosed as heart failure caused by coronary artery disease.

∎see page 115   ∎see page 134

Treatment should be aimed at managing heart failure due to systolic dysfunction.∎ Immunosuppressive therapy has not been shown to be effective as treatment for myocarditis.

HYPERTROPHIC CARDIOMYOPATHY

A disease of the myocardium characterized by marked ventricular hypertrophy and a nondilated left ventricle without other known cardiovascular disease.

Hypertrophic cardiomyopathy is relatively common among the elderly (4% in one series) and more common among women than among men. Causes of hypertrophic cardiomyopathy in the elderly are not well defined. Most cases are associated with severe, poorly controlled systemic hypertension and may be acquired. However, some cases appear similar to those in younger patients and are probably congenital.

Hypertrophic cardiomyopathy is characterized by normal or small chamber size, increased wall thickness, hyperdynamic systolic ejection, and impaired diastolic filling. Ventricular hypertrophy may be substantial and is usually concentric, especially in elderly patients with a history of hypertension, but it may be asymmetric, as in patients with congenital hypertrophic cardiomyopathy.

In some patients, septal thickening narrows the left ventricular outflow tract. During left ventricular ejection, the anterior leaflet of the mitral valve is drawn toward the septum, further narrowing the outflow tract and causing a systolic gradient. In other patients, a systolic gradient results from obstruction at the level of the mid left ventricular cavity, mitral annulus, or, rarely, the apex.

Symptoms and Signs

Elderly and younger patients commonly present with chest pain, dyspnea, dizziness, palpitations, and syncope (due to tachyarrhythmias or decreased cardiac output resulting from outflow obstruction). Although CAD may be present, chest pain does not necessarily indicate CAD. Ischemic infarction occasionally occurs, even in patients with normal coronary arteries. Ventricular tachycardia, which increases the likelihood of sudden death, may be present but appears to be less common in elderly than in younger patients. Supraventricular tachyarrhythmias are also common as the left atrium enlarges. Atrial fibrillation may cause rapid hemodynamic deterioration.

A late systolic murmur that is heard from the lower left sternal border to the apex and terminates before the second heart sound is charac-

∎ see page 905

teristic. Other signs include a rapid bisferious carotid pulse and a prominent fourth heart sound. Provocative maneuvers (eg, Valsalva maneuver, standing after squatting) accentuate the systolic murmur, which decreases or disappears when the patient squats; however, many elderly patients cannot adequately perform these maneuvers. With the patient supine, passive lifting of the legs to 90° increases venous return, enlarges the left ventricular outflow tract, and decreases the murmur. The murmur may also disappear as systolic function deteriorates and the cavity dilates.

Diagnosis

Hypertrophic cardiomyopathy should be considered in patients with a systolic murmur and anginal chest discomfort or syncope. Often, the disorder is not suspected because prominent carotid pulses, basal systolic murmurs, and fourth heart sounds are common among elderly persons without heart disease.

Echocardiography is diagnostic and characterizes the pattern of left ventricular hypertrophy, the site and severity of dynamic outflow obstruction, systolic and diastolic function, and associated pathologies. An ECG typically shows left atrial abnormality and left ventricular hypertrophy; about 20% of patients have left anterior fascicular block. Septal hypertrophy may produce nonspecific inferior and apical Q waves mimicking myocardial infarction.

Differentiating the disorder from aortic valve stenosis or CAD with papillary muscle dysfunction is important because therapy differs. The murmur must also be differentiated from murmurs due to aortic sclerosis, mitral regurgitation, or mitral valve prolapse, all of which are common among the elderly.

Prognosis and Treatment

Elderly patients have a better prognosis than younger patients, with less likelihood of sudden death.

Treatment of elderly and younger patients is similar. A β-blocker is used most commonly and provides relief of dyspnea and chest pain. Calcium channel blockers with negative inotropic properties (eg, verapamil) and possibly ACE inhibitors (in low doses) may help. Nitroglycerin, diuretics, vasodilators, digoxin, and other positive inotropic drugs may exacerbate outflow obstruction and symptoms.

Patients who have palpitations, presyncope, or syncope (which are less common among elderly than among younger patients) should be monitored for malignant arrhythmias. If patients have syncope, an electrophysiologic study should be performed to determine whether sustained monomorphic ventricular tachycardia can be stimulated. Patients who have monomorphic sustained ventricular tachycardia with symptoms should be considered for an automatic implantable cardioverter-defibrillator.

Myomectomy or an electronic pacemaker can be considered for patients who are very symptomatic and have a significant ventricular outflow gradient refractory to medical therapy.

Antimicrobial prophylaxis against infective endocarditis is indicated before invasive and surgical procedures. ∎

RESTRICTIVE CARDIOMYOPATHY

Myocardial disorders characterized by rigid, noncompliant walls of one or both ventricles (most commonly the left) that resist diastolic filling.

In restrictive cardiomyopathy, increased myocardial stiffness is secondary to infiltrative pathology. Amyloid heart disease is a common cause in the elderly. Other causes include postradiation damage and postoperative pericarditis.

The atria are often dilated, and systolic function, as well as diastolic function, is impaired. Other findings include small ventricles, thickened walls (of both ventricles and of the interatrial septum), a sparkling of the thickened myocardium (seen on an echocardiogram), low QRS voltage and arrhythmias or conduction defects (seen on an ECG), and elevated ventricular filling pressures.

Restrictive cardiomyopathy caused by amyloid heart disease is differentiated from other disorders characterized by age-related amyloid accumulation in the heart. One such disorder is senile cardiac amyloidosis, a separate pathologic entity that is present in 80% of persons > 95. The heart appears normal, but microscopic examination detects amyloid accumulation, usually in the atria. Amyloid accumulation is associated with atrophied myocardial fibers. Two immunologically distinct forms exist: one with only atrial deposits, and the other with ventricular deposits and often with minor extracardiac deposits. Senile cardiac amyloidosis is not characterized by cardiomegaly. Primary amyloidosis, another distinct pathologic entity, is characterized by cardiomegaly. It may also occur in the elderly but is much rarer.

Treatment of restrictive cardiomyopathy is the same for elderly and younger patients. It is directed at ameliorating the primary cause if possible and at optimizing ventricular filling and enhancing diastolic function.

∎ see TABLE 90–1 on page 881

Peripheral arterial problems increase in frequency with age. Atherosclerosis is the most common cause among the elderly. Cigarette smoking and diabetes **1** are the most common exacerbating factors. Because function of the peripheral circulation can be directly scrutinized, a thorough physical examination is the key to evaluation and treatment. Laboratory tests help confirm the diagnosis and quantify the extent of disease.

PERIPHERAL ATHEROSCLEROSIS

(Arteriosclerosis Obliterans)

Occlusion of blood supply to the extremities by atherosclerotic plaques (atheromas).

Etiology and Pathophysiology

Progressive peripheral atherosclerosis is a common, age-related disease; its development parallels that of atherosclerosis in the coronary and cerebral vessels. The pathologic process begins many years before clinical findings are apparent, and the disorder develops slowly and insidiously.

Risk factors for peripheral atherosclerosis include cigarette smoking, diabetes mellitus, hyperlipidemia, hypertension, polycythemia, a family history, hyperhomocysteinemia, age, and, in women, early hysterectomy and oophorectomy. Any disorder that increases the Hct (eg, polycythemia) increases the resistance to blood flow and the shearing force against vessel walls, resulting in intimal injury. This injury promotes atheroma formation. Poorly controlled diabetes mellitus also leads to intimal injury and the buildup of atheromas. High levels of homocysteine directly injure vessel walls. **2**

How smoking damages the arteries is still unclear, but carbon monoxide and the metabolites of smoke components probably are toxic to the intima. Nicotine, a direct arterial vasoconstrictor, decreases distal blood flow. The incidence of limb amputation is 10 times higher in those who continue to smoke after developing arterial occlusion than in those who quit.

Symptoms and Signs

Most patients with peripheral atherosclerosis, including the elderly, have no symptoms. Almost 70% of a vessel's lumen must be occluded before the disease can be clinically recognized.

The cardinal and most specific symptom of peripheral atherosclerosis is intermittent claudication (pain, tightness, or weakness in an

---

1 see page 627   **2** see pages 690 and 852

exercising muscle). Claudication occurs during walking (not during sitting or standing still), forcing a person to halt because walking is too painful, and is relieved in < 5 minutes by rest. The pain is most often described as squeezing and almost always occurs in the calf; if the aortoiliac artery is occluded, pain usually occurs in the hip and buttocks.

The distance at which claudication occurs tends to be constant but may change over time. Cold and windy weather, inclines, and rapid walking may shorten the distance. Using canes or crutches does not improve walking distance, because muscle function is normal until hypoxia occurs.

Less specific symptoms of peripheral atherosclerosis—numbness, paresthesias, coldness, and pain during rest—relate to the foot's cutaneous circulation. Foot or toe numbness that occurs during walking suggests arterial disease and results from maximal vasodilation of muscle arterioles, with stealing of blood flow from the skin.

A sense of coldness that has recently increased, that occurs in only one limb, or that persists after sleep suggests arterial insufficiency. However, a sense of coldness is very common among the elderly and does not necessarily indicate arterial insufficiency; it may be secondary to vasoconstriction instead.

Elderly patients who are relatively sedentary and do not walk far enough to induce claudication may present with foot pain at rest or even gangrene. Foot pain at rest is a dire symptom, indicating that blood flow capacity is reduced to < 10% of normal. The pain is paresthetic and burning, most severe distally, and typically worse at night, preventing sleep.

Gangrene first appears as nonblanching cyanosis (ecchymosis), followed by blackening and mummification of the involved part. In patients with peripheral neuropathy (eg, that due to diabetes), dependent rubor and subsequent gangrene may occur without pain.

Wounds often heal poorly, and the skin is prone to breakdown. Skin breakdown can progress quickly to cellulitis and deeper infections.

In **Leriche's syndrome,** the aortoiliac artery becomes occluded, but the distal vessels are usually patent. Symptoms are hip claudication and impotence secondary to hypotension in the internal iliac arteries. The syndrome is uncommon among the elderly, because they usually have multiple diffuse atherosclerosis and multiple areas of occlusion.

Diagnosis

Absence of peripheral pulses strongly suggests peripheral atherosclerosis. The posterior tibial pulse is always present in healthy persons, although it may be difficult to feel if the patient has edema or prominent malleoli. It is best palpated with the patient supine and the examiner on the same side as the pulse. Meticulous palpation under the medial malleolus is necessary; dorsiflexing and everting the foot slightly may help move the artery into a more superficial position. The dorsalis pedis artery pulse is absent in about 5% of healthy persons. The popliteal pulse is the most difficult to feel; the patient should be supine and relaxed, with the knee slightly flexed. The artery may be located posteriorly, laterally, or medially in the popliteal space. Very deep palpation may be necessary if the patient is obese.

Determination of pulse strength is subjective and depends on the pulse pressure, extremity's girth, patient's age, and examiner's sensitivity. With age, the pulse of arteries that remain patent tends to become more prominent, because the media loses smooth muscle and elastic tissue, predisposing the arteries to ectasia. The upstroke of the pulse wave is more important than the amplitude. Bruits heard over the femoral arteries indicate aortoiliac disease.

Doppler ultrasonography can be used to assess pulses, but it cannot prove that pulsatile flow is adequate. It may detect a signal when the vessel's systolic blood pressure is as low as 30 mm Hg. Thus, the procedure is usually performed with a blood pressure cuff. The pressure at which the Doppler signal disappears is the systolic blood pressure. Blood pressure in the leg is considered low if it is lower than the pressure in the upper extremities or if it decreases during exercise.

Temperature differences between the toes of each foot and changes in skin color are important. To determine whether color changes, the examiner elevates the foot above heart level for 20 seconds and then lowers the foot to the dependent position: Pallor lasting > 30 seconds or rubor (a homogeneous violaceous color) appearing after 20 seconds indicates that normal blood flow capacity is < 10%. Rubor may require 1 to 2 minutes to reach its maximum. It is more pronounced in the toes and extends proximally for various distances. A severely ischemic foot may appear pale even when horizontal. Prolonged pallor and rubor, when associated with pain at rest, are grim signs. Skin ulceration or frank gangrene, particularly of the toes, heels, and lateral malleoli, suggests extensive disease.

A full lipid profile, including total cholesterol, high-density lipoprotein (HDL), low-density lipoprotein (LDL), and triglyceride levels, should be obtained after the patient has fasted.◪ Measuring the homocysteine level is also advisable. If the homocysteine level is borderline, a methionine loading test (ingestion of methionine followed by serial homocysteine measurements) can be performed. If the homocysteine level is high, vitamin B_{12} levels should be measured.

Peripheral atherosclerosis must be differentiated from other disorders that cause similar symptoms. Lumbar and spinal stenosis, very common among the elderly, may produce symptoms similar to claudication. However, the symptoms of stenosis occur at rest as well as during walk-

◪see page 611

ing and are often worse when the patient is sitting, and the pain tends to radiate down the entire extremity. The pain of diabetic neuropathy may be similar to that of atherosclerosis but is generally bilateral and extends above the feet. Diabetic neuropathy, which may coexist with peripheral atherosclerosis, can also cause numbness and paresthesias.

Treatment

Asymptomatic patients: Therapy consists primarily of preventive measures involving foot care (including walking regularly)🔳 and control of risk factors (eg, smoking cessation, weight loss). Patients should be advised to avoid positions that may impair circulation (eg, crossing the legs while sitting). In general, all patients with clinical evidence of atherosclerosis should take folic acid, vitamin B_6 (pyridoxine), and vitamin B_{12} (cyanocobalamin) supplements.

Patients with intermittent claudication: Patients should be taught about foot care 🔳 and advised to walk as much as possible; risk factors should be controlled. As soon as claudication occurs, patients should rest and then continue walking. For a small but significant number of patients who follow these instructions, symptoms abate within the first 3 months. Most patients can adjust to walking long distances with frequent rest stops.

The results of drug therapy for claudication (including vasodilators, pentoxifylline, and cilostazol) are mixed. Pentoxifylline, the first of a new class of drugs approved for treating claudication, decreases blood viscosity and improves red blood cell flexibility, leading to improved blood flow through arterioles and capillaries. In one study, the mean walking distance of patients taking the drug increased by 165 feet (50 meters). Adverse effects are few. However, clinical results have been disappointing, and follow-up studies have not shown increases in muscle blood flow sufficient to prevent claudication. Thus, many experts do not recommend the use of pentoxifylline for claudication.

Early studies suggest that cilostazol produces a mild to moderate increase in walking distance comparable to that produced by pentoxifylline. Because cilostazol is a phosphodiesterase inhibitor, it is contraindicated in patients with heart failure. Cardiovascular toxicity in other patients is also a concern, and the drug should be used with extreme caution.

Because β-blockers increase the longevity of patients with atherosclerotic coronary artery disease and only rarely aggravate intermittent claudication, they should not be withheld from patients who have heart disease and claudication.

The most effective treatment for intermittent claudication is arterial bypass surgery or, for less severe cases, percutaneous transluminal

---

🔳see TABLE 56–2 on page 547   🔳see TABLE 56–2 on page 547 angioplasty. However, bypass surgery and angioplasty are generally reserved for patients who have claudication due to isolated aortoiliac disease and severe symptoms.

Risks of bypass surgery or angioplasty must be weighed against potential benefits. A failed bypass may worsen circulatory impairment if collateral vessels are transected during surgery. Factors such as the patient's general health, lifestyle, and age; the presence of heart disease; and location of the lesions must be considered. Significant coronary artery disease is a contraindication to peripheral artery surgery because heart disease increases the operative mortality rate and because angina, unmasked after a successful bypass, may prevent or mitigate improvement in walking distance.

Angiography to determine the feasibility of surgery should be performed only if surgery is being seriously considered. For surgery to be successful, a major vessel beyond the obstruction must be patent, and distal flow beyond the patent vessel must be good.

The more proximal the lesion, the better the clinical results of bypass surgery and the longer the graft remains patent. In patients with localized aortoiliac disease, the 5-year graft patency rate is > 90%. In patients with femoropopliteal disease, the 5-year patency rate is probably 60 to 70% for bypasses above the knee. Bypasses across the knee into the distal popliteal or proximal tibial arteries have a somewhat lower patency rate. The 5-year patency rate for distal femorotibial grafts is well below 50%, and patency rates are even lower when patients have generalized disease.

When arterial occlusion is bilateral, a femoropopliteal bypass may unmask claudication in the contralateral limb, resulting in only slight clinical improvement. A second operation is necessary to significantly increase claudication-free walking distance.

For aortoiliac and aortofemoral bypass grafts, prosthetic material (Teflon) is used, but for a femoropopliteal bypass, an autologous saphenous vein is preferable because long-term patency rates are higher.

Percutaneous transluminal angioplasty is an alternative to bypass surgery for short stenoses in the aortoiliac and proximal femoral areas. Although it is a relatively simple procedure that can be performed using a local anesthetic, complications (eg, arterial rupture, distal embolization of ruptured atherosclerotic plaques) may require emergency surgery. Therefore, a patient undergoing percutaneous transluminal angioplasty must be able to undergo a full surgical procedure.

Patients with significant foot ischemia: Severe cutaneous ischemia (eg, causing pain at rest, dependent rubor, and tissue loss) is a strong indication for arterial bypass surgery, which may relieve disabling pain and prevent amputation. Patches of dry gangrene, particularly on the toes, should be allowed to demarcate because autoamputation of toes may result in proximal healing. Ischemic ulcers can heal if the surrounding blood flow is adequate; they may respond to pressure relief, debriding agents (eg, collagenase, fibrinolysin with desoxyribonucle-ase, becaplermin gel), and local antiseptic solutions (eg, povidone-iodine applied bid). Soaking the foot in body-temperature water helps infected lesions heal. Pentoxifylline is of uncertain benefit, but it has few adverse effects and can be tried. β-Blockers should be avoided. Elderly patients who do not have tissue loss or pain at rest should not undergo surgery, even if they have florid dependent rubor. For patients with severe heart disease, amputation∎ is sometimes preferable to the risk of bypass surgery.

Lower-risk procedures may be used. A subcutaneous femorofemoral bypass across the lower pelvic area may help save a limb if the disease is unilateral. The graft patency rate with this procedure is almost as high as that with aortofemoral bypass. A subcutaneous bypass from an axil-lary to a femoral artery may help if the disease is bilateral. These grafts often become thrombosed but may be reopened by performing a local thrombectomy within a few days of closure. The 5-year graft patency rate is about 50%.

When a limb is threatened, the presence of stenoses in many areas is not a contraindication to surgery. Bypass of the most proximal occlu-sion often increases collateral flow around more distal occlusions suffi-ciently to salvage the limb. For a short iliac stenosis, angioplasty may be tried before femoropopliteal or femorotibial bypass surgery.

In patients with gangrene, limb salvage after injection of vascular endothelial growth factor into the calf muscle—an experimental approach—has been reported.

SMALL-VESSEL SYNDROME

Cutaneous ischemia or local areas of cyanosis or necrosis in a hand or foot that generally has adequate circulation.

In the elderly, ischemia in a hand or foot that has palpable pulses may be due to cryoglobulinemia, cryofibrinogenemia, disseminated intravascular coagulation, essential thrombocytosis, polycythemia, vas-culitis secondary to drug-induced systemic lupus erythematosus, the phospholipid (anticardiolipin antibody) syndrome, scleroderma, or em-boli from an arterial aneurysm, the heart, or atherosclerotic plaques.

Symptoms, Signs, and Diagnosis

Patients usually present with a cyanotic or gangrenous digit and may have many small lesions on several extremities. Occasionally, cyanosis or dependent rubor affects an entire foot or hand.

∎see page 284

TABLE 93–1.   DIAGNOSTIC CLUES TO CAUSES OF SMALL-VESSEL SYNDROME

Finding	Possible Cause
Use of certain drugs (eg, procain-amide, hydralazine, phenytoin)	Systemic lupus erythematosus
Weight loss and other symptoms of anorexia	Malignancy, leading to cryofibrinogenemia or disseminated intravascular coagulation
Back pain	Multiple myeloma, leading to cryoglobulinemia
Atrial fibrillation and a dyskinetic left ventricular impulse	Emboli possibly originating in the heart
History of myocardial infarction	Ventricular aneurysm
Splenomegaly	Essential thrombocytosis (characterized by digital or cerebral ischemia and sometimes causing abnormal bleeding)
Acute gangrene with fever	Septicemia, leading to cryofibrinogenemia or disseminated intravascular coagulation
Pleural effusion with arthralgias	Systemic lupus erythematosus

In patients with peripheral atherosclerosis and pulseless limbs, sudden worsening of cutaneous ischemia or development of localized cyanosis or necrosis in an otherwise adequately perfused hand or foot may indicate small-vessel syndrome. In such cases, evaluation of the hand is particularly important because severe ischemia is uncommon in the upper extremities, even if atherosclerosis is advanced.

The history and physical examination may provide clues to the cause (see TABLE 93–1). The physical examination should include a search for abdominal, femoropopliteal, and subclavian aneurysms.∎ Popliteal aneurysms shed small emboli and should be considered if ischemia is confined to one foot.

Laboratory evaluation should include a CBC, a platelet count, coagulation screening, and tests for cryoproteins, antinuclear antibodies, lupus anticoagulant, and anticardiolipin antibodies. Lupus anticoagulant, a misnomer, occurs in only 10% of patients with systemic lupus erythematous. In vitro, this anticoagulant and other anticardiolipin antibodies interfere with phospholipid-dependent coagulation tests (eg, partial thromboplastin time) by binding to phospholipids that accelerate the activation of prothrombin by factor Xa. Paradoxically, they cause thrombosis in vivo. An elevated anticardiolipin antibody level or the presence of lupus anticoagulant indicates the antiphospholipid antibody

∎ see pages 934–938

syndrome.∎ Administering normal plasma to such patients does not correct the defect; venous and small arterial thrombi occur in 27% of patients with the lupus anticoagulant.

ECG is indicated if mitral valve disease or ventricular aneurysm is suspected, and ultrasonography of the aorta and popliteal arteries may be necessary to rule out an aneurysm. The diagnosis of atheromatous emboli (due to fracturing of plaques) is reached by exclusion. Occasionally, atheromatous emboli manifest as livedo reticularis (a lacy network of cyanotic-looking superficial vessels on the anterior side of the leg).

Treatment

Underlying disorders should be identified and managed. Aneurysms must be surgically repaired. Long-term anticoagulation therapy with warfarin is indicated for patients with cardiac embolism; antiplatelet drugs, including aspirin, are indicated for patients with atheromatous emboli. Appropriate therapy for patients with the phospholipid syndrome is not established. Warfarin may be effective, but the international normalized ratio (INR) must be > 3.

For all patients with small-vessel syndrome, preventing dehydration, which can further compromise flow, is important.

RAYNAUD'S PHENOMENON

A syndrome of peripheral vasospasm with intermittent cutaneous pallor or cyanosis.

Symptoms, Signs, and Diagnosis

Exposure to cold typically causes blanching, then cyanosis of the hands and feet and sometimes of the ears and nose. An erythematous phase follows when patients enter a warm environment. Episodes can be painless or produce varying degrees of pain, numbness, and cold sensation. Many elderly patients experience only the blanching or cyanotic phase, which may occur even when the ambient temperature is not very cool. Affected persons tend to have cool hands and feet even in a warm environment. If the episodes are severe or of long duration, sclerodactyly may develop.

Bilateral symptoms (affecting both hands) beginning after age 40 usually indicate internal disease, such as hypothyroidism, drug-induced systemic lupus erythematosus, cryoglobulinemia, cryofibrinogenemia, cold agglutinin disease, scleroderma, and the CREST syndrome (calcinosis, Raynaud's phenomenon, esophageal dysfunction, sclerodactyly, telangiectasia). Patients with cold agglutinin disease often have a low-

---

∎ see page 691

grade lymphoma. Unilateral symptoms usually indicate that previous frostbite or a thoracic outlet syndrome is the cause.

Treatment

Generally, treatment of elderly patients with Raynaud's phenomenon should be conservative: Patients should be instructed to wear warm clothing and avoid cold. Smokers should stop smoking.

If Raynaud's phenomenon is caused by scleroderma, treatment should usually be more vigorous, because episodes are associated with reversible but damaging decreases in renal and cardiac blood flow and with impaired myocardial contractility. Nifedipine 10 mg po tid is usually safe and effective. Griseofulvin 250 mg po bid may also help. Ketanserin, a selective 5-hydroxytryptamine$_2$ receptor antagonist, may be beneficial but is not yet available in the USA.

94   PERIPHERAL VENOUS DISEASE

Peripheral venous problems are common among the elderly.

DEEP VEIN THROMBOSIS

The presence of a thrombus in a deep vein.

The incidence of deep vein thrombosis increases with age.

Etiology

Immobilization, prolonged sitting (as may occur during long drives or air travel), or even a relatively sedentary existence can lead to venous stasis and predisposes to thrombosis, because the emptying of veins in the extremities depends entirely on skeletal muscles that pump blood and on one-way venous valves that inhibit retrograde flow. Because incompetent venous valves lead to deep vein thrombosis, which damages the valves, deep vein thrombosis tends to recur. Thrombosis also damages the intima of the vein; such damage may lead to decreased local production of antithrombotic factors (eg, antithrombin III, prostacyclin).

Any condition that increases the Hct increases blood viscosity and results in a higher incidence of clotting. Dehydration, pulmonary disorders, smoking, and polycythemia are common causes of a high Hct in the elderly. The two most common known hypercoagulable states are hyperhomocysteinemia∎ and protein C resistance, which is genetically

∎ see pages 690 and 852

determined and is present in about 15% of the population. ∎ One form of protein C resistance is due to the Leiden gene. In homozygotes, venous thrombosis begins early in life; in heterozygotes, it usually begins after age 30 and may first occur in old age or during immobilization. Deep vein thrombosis occurs in 20 to 25% of patients > 40 after routine surgery and in almost 50% after hip surgery when no prophylaxis is given.

Symptoms and Signs

Deep vein thrombosis usually occurs in the leg, regardless of cause. The hallmark symptom is rapid onset of unilateral leg swelling with dependent edema. Generally, patients first note swelling when they awaken. In ambulatory patients, swelling is maximal at the ankle and lower leg, usually developing over 1 or 2 days. Pain may be present but is usually not severe. Physical examination often reveals pitting edema and a mild to moderate increase in skin temperature over the calf or thigh.

A gap always occurs between the level of thrombosis and the location of edema. With popliteal and lower femoral vein thrombosis, edema occurs only in the lower leg and ankle. With thrombosis in the midfemoral vein area, most or all of the leg is swollen. With upper femoral and external iliac vein thrombosis, the thigh is also swollen. Tenderness, if present, occurs in the calf with femoro-popliteal venous thrombosis and in the medial thigh with iliofemoral venous thrombosis.

Calf vein thrombosis may produce no symptoms or mild tenderness and mild edema. There are four to six deep calf veins. Occlusion of one or two of them is likely to impair venous drainage, because all of them drain into the popliteal vein. Calf vein thrombosis without swelling is common only among sedentary or bedridden patients.

Complications of deep vein thrombosis include venous thromboembolism, particularly pulmonary embolism (which can lead to death within 30 minutes of onset). Unrecognized and untreated deep vein thrombosis can cause long-term morbidity from chronic venous stasis (postphlebitic syndrome) and predispose patients to recurrent venous thromboembolism. Large proximal thrombi may cause chronic severe leg swelling.

Phlegmasia cerulea dolens, a serious form of iliofemoral venous thrombosis, is characterized by massive thigh and calf edema and a cold, mottled foot. Pedal pulses are usually absent, and the leg is very tender. The risk of massive pulmonary embolism is high, even for

∎ see page 690

patients receiving anticoagulation therapy. Foot gangrene also occurs but less often.

Diagnosis

The sudden onset of lower leg swelling in a gravitational distribution without trauma or a precipitating factor suggests deep vein thrombosis. However, laboratory confirmation is needed.

If swelling is absent, comparative measurements of the legs at several levels (just above the ankles is the most important) can usually be used to exclude deep vein thrombosis in ambulatory patients. However, in sedentary or bedridden patients who do not have swelling, calf vein thrombosis can be diagnosed only through laboratory evaluation.

Real-time color Doppler ultrasonography is the procedure of choice for diagnosing deep vein thrombosis above the knee. In symptomatic patients, venous ultrasonography has a sensitivity of 95%, a specificity of 96%, a positive predictive value of 97%, and a negative predictive value of 98%. Ultrasonography can detect clots in the popliteal or femoral vein but can miss clots in the calf veins.

Impedance plethysmography can indirectly detect venous thrombi by recording changes in venous volume when a thigh tourniquet is applied and removed. Plethysmography is reliable only for occlusions above the knee and those of recent onset. The sensitivity and specificity of impedance plethysmography are probably about 75% for thrombi above the knee.

Radiocontrast venography, although rarely needed, is the gold standard for confirmation of deep vein thrombosis. Venography should be considered if clinical suspicion is low but the ultrasonogram is abnormal or if the suspicion is high but the ultrasonogram is normal. In about 25% of these cases, the results of venography and ultrasonography differ. Adverse effects from venography, including allergic reactions and thrombophlebitis, occur in 2% of patients. Venography may be impossible to perform in patients with significant edema. It is contraindicated in patients with significant renal failure (creatinine level > 3 mg/dL [> 265 μmol/L]) and should be used cautiously in those with mild azotemia. Maintaining good hydration—before and 6 to 8 hours after the test—is important.

Radionuclide venography can be performed in patients with severe azotemia or an allergy to contrast material. False-negative results are common, but positive results are generally accurate.

Risk factors (eg, dehydration, estrogen use, heart failure, hip fracture, hypercoagulable states, immobilization or decreased physical activity, malignancy, obesity, polycythemia, thrombocytosis, trauma, venous damage) should be sought unless the cause is clear. All patients with iliofemoral venous thrombosis should have an abdominal diagnostic study (ultrasonography is usually adequate) to rule out extrinsic compression by a tumor or clot in the inferior vena cava. Right iliofemoral venous thrombosis is of particular concern if there is no local problem in the right lower extremity; an abdominal tumor causing compression must be suspected, because the inferior vena cava is located on the right. Thrombosis of the left common iliac vein, which is normally compressed by the right iliac artery, is more likely to be due to conditions other than compression by a tumor.

If a mechanical obstruction is not a risk factor, tests to detect hypercoagulable states◻ are indicated, especially for patients with recurrent and migratory deep vein thrombosis.

Differential diagnosis: The effects of trauma can resemble those of deep vein thrombosis. Traumatic edema should be suspected if edema initially develops during or shortly after walking. Forcefully dorsiflexing the foot during a sudden downward movement can rupture the plantar tendon or injure the gastrocnemius muscle. The resultant swelling tends to be asymmetric and confined; it occurs above the ankle, is very tender, and is often associated with visible ecchymosis.

A popliteal cyst that extends into the calf can cause upper leg swelling and later compress the popliteal vein. Therefore, palpation of the popliteal fossa is important. A popliteal cyst should be suspected if the edema initially develops during physical activity. Ultrasonography can easily confirm or exclude this possibility.

Phlegmasia cerulea dolens may be mistaken for arterial embolism, but misdiagnosis can be avoided by remembering that acute arterial occlusion does not cause edema. Phlegmasia cerulea dolens often indicates occult malignancy.

Prophylaxis

Choice of prophylactic measures depends on the surgical situation.◻

Low-dose heparin is the prophylactic measure most widely used before surgery. The usual dose is 5000 U sc q 8 to 12 h—a dose that rarely results in significant bleeding. Heparin is contraindicated in patients undergoing ophthalmologic or neurosurgical procedures. Aspirin and dextran are not recommended for deep vein thrombosis prophylaxis.

Intermittent pneumatic compression (oscillating) boots applied to the calves are a safer prophylactic measure. A pump rhythmically inflates the boot to 30 to 40 mm Hg, then deflates it, thus keeping the peripheral veins drained. Results are comparable to those of low-dose heparin but without the risk of bleeding. Galvanic stimulation of calf muscles, begun intraoperatively and continued until the patient is ambulatory, is also effective.

Even when other prophylactic measures are taken, patients should be mobilized as quickly as possible and encouraged to move their legs frequently while in bed.

◻ see page 689   ◻ see TABLE 70–3 on page 695

The risk of venous thromboembolism is greatest early in the postoperative period. After orthopedic procedures, prophylaxis should be continued for 10 to 14 days, or longer if the patient has had postoperative complications that delay rehabilitative efforts and ambulation. After general surgery, prophylaxis is indicated; patients with an underlying malignancy or prior venous thromboembolism should be treated longer. In general, prophylaxis should be continued until full ambulation is resumed.

Orthopedic procedures: Deep vein thrombosis is common among the elderly because they commonly undergo high-risk orthopedic procedures, particularly semi-elective or urgent procedures (eg, after a traumatic fracture). If the procedure involves the extremities, the value of low-dose heparin is limited; full-dose heparin or warfarin is effective, but each has a significant risk of bleeding. Hirudin prevents deep vein thrombosis in patients undergoing orthopedic procedures and is useful when heparin-induced thrombocytopenia occurs.

After elective total hip replacement, the incidence of proximal deep vein thrombosis (without prophylaxis after surgery) approaches 25%, and the incidence of fatal pulmonary embolism is 3 to 4%. Prophylaxis reduces the occurrence of venous thromboembolism by 30 to 50%. The most effective regimens include low-molecular-weight heparin (30 mg sc q 12 h) and oral anticoagulants (warfarin dose adjusted to keep the international normalized ratio [INR] between 2.0 and 2.5).

After elective total knee replacement, the incidence of deep vein thrombosis is nearly 60%. Low-molecular-weight heparin and intermittent pneumatic compression boots reduce the incidence of proximal deep vein thrombosis to 5 to 10%. Low-dose subcutaneous heparin is ineffective.

After hip fracture surgery, the incidence of venous thromboembolism (without prophylaxis) is about 50%. A low-intensity oral anticoagulant or low-molecular-weight heparin is the treatment of choice and should be instituted preoperatively if possible. Intermittent pneumatic compression boots may help.

Medical disorders: Prophylaxis for deep vein thrombosis has not been studied extensively in hospitalized patients with medical disorders.

Among patients who have had an acute myocardial infarction and who are not given low-dose heparin, the overall incidence of venous thromboembolism is about 20%; the elderly and patients with complicated infarctions are at greatest risk. Low-dose heparin, low-molecular-weight heparin, or intermittent pneumatic compression boots are recommended as prophylaxis.

Among patients who have had an ischemic stroke that paralyzes a lower extremity, the incidence of deep vein thrombosis is about 30 to 40%. Low-dose heparin or low-molecular-weight heparin reduces the occurrence of deep vein thrombosis by at least 50%. Intermittent pneumatic compression boots are probably beneficial, but supportive data are lacking.

Treatment

The objective is to prevent pulmonary embolism and chronic venous insufficiency.

Anticoagulation therapy:▯ The mainstay of treatment is anticoagulation therapy, beginning with heparin and continuing with warfarin. Heparin is given sc q 12 h, by IV injection q 4 to 6 h, or by continuous IV infusion for at least 4 days. For continuous IV infusion, the patient must first receive a rapid infusion (bolus) of usually 5,000 to 10,000 U. The initial infusion rate is usually about 18 U/kg/h; thereafter, the rate is adjusted according to the partial thromboplastin time, which should be kept between 1.5 and 2.0 times the normal control value. The partial thromboplastin time must be measured daily, because the infusion rate may need to be changed.

Continuous IV infusion offers the most flexibility for adjusting dose. Accurate infusion is critical; inadvertent increases in rate can lead to severe bleeding, and temporary interruptions of the infusion can lead to inadequate anticoagulation within 1 hour. When an IV infusion is restarted, a rapid infusion of 5000 U must generally be given.

Heparin (usually about 240 U/kg) sc q 12 h is as effective as continuous IV infusion. How long therapy should be given is debatable. One recommendation is 4 days for patients with femoropopliteal venous thrombosis and 5 to 7 days for those with iliofemoral venous thrombosis.

For patients receiving heparin, periodic platelet counts should be obtained, usually after 5 days of therapy. If thrombocytopenia develops (incidence is about 1%), heparin should be discontinued. Unexpected embolism, with arterial and venous thrombi, develops in a small proportion of patients with thrombocytopenia.

Low-molecular-weight heparin can be used. The drug is given in a fixed dose, does not require blood monitoring, and has a much lower incidence of heparin-induced thrombocytopenia. Low-molecular-weight heparin (injected sc q 12 h) can be used to treat outpatients with deep vein thrombosis (femoropopliteal area) if they are mentally competent and free of major cardiopulmonary disease.

Warfarin should be started 4 days before heparin is stopped, generally about a day after heparin is begun. A therapeutic level of warfarin must be reached before heparin is stopped. The elderly are more sensitive to warfarin than are younger patients, and doses are usually smaller. The prothrombin time should be kept at 1.2 to 1.5 times the normal control value (INR 2.0 to 2.5). For patients with uncomplicated venous

---

▯ see page 697

thrombosis, at least 3 months of therapy is usually recommended, but patients at high risk of recurrent thrombosis may need extended therapy. Patients with protein C resistance and multiple episodes of venous thrombosis are given long-term warfarin therapy. Patients > 70 (especially women) receiving warfarin therapy are at high risk of hemorrhage. Because many elderly persons with arthritic or neurologic disorders fall frequently, warfarin is generally contraindicated in patients > 80 and frail patients > 70.

Insertion of an inferior vena cava filter (umbrella): The decision to insert an umbrella depends on how likely deep vein thrombosis is to recur, whether pulmonary emboli are present, and where the venous clot is. Tibial vein thrombi, which rarely embolize, can remain untreated in patients at high risk of hemorrhage. For iliofemoral vein thrombi, which embolize often, an umbrella is strongly indicated if patients cannot be given warfarin.

Indications for umbrella insertion include hemorrhage during anticoagulation therapy, bleeding diatheses that are a contraindication to anticoagulation, phlegmasia cerulea dolens, massive pulmonary embolism, and pulmonary embolism that recurs in spite of adequate anticoagulation.

The umbrella acts as a plication device, preventing the occurrence of large pulmonary emboli. The complication rate is low, although occasionally, an umbrella loosens and migrates into another vein or into a pulmonary artery. Pulmonary embolism due to thrombi in the legs is uncommon after umbrella insertion but can occur after a few months, when emboli travel through collateral veins.

Thrombolytic (fibrinolytic) therapy: Patients with severe iliofemoral venous thrombosis and massive edema are at particularly high risk of chronic venous insufficiency and should be considered for thrombolytic therapy (eg, streptokinase, urokinase, tissue plasminogen activator).∎ The risk of bleeding is higher with these drugs than with anticoagulants. The older the patient, the greater the risk of bleeding. The risks of severe bleeding must be weighed against the morbidity of chronic severe leg edema. Contraindications include coagulopathy, recent gastrointestinal bleeding, recent stroke, uremia, history of cerebral hemorrhage, or surgical procedures within the preceding 7 days.

Thrombolytic therapy is unlikely to be effective if thrombi are > 3 days old. Before thrombolytic therapy is started, heparin's effect must be allowed to abate.

To be effective, streptokinase and urokinase must increase the thrombin time to at least twice the normal value; if they do not, they should be discontinued and heparin restarted.

Treatment of underlying disorders: For hyperhomocysteinemia, folic acid, vitamin B_6 (pyridoxine), and/or vitamin B_{12} (cyanocobal-

∎see page 700

amin) supplements may be used. For protein C resistance, long-term therapy with warfarin is used if episodes of venous thrombosis recur. **1**

CHRONIC DEEP VEIN INSUFFICIENCY
(Postphlebitic Syndrome)

A syndrome occurring after thrombosis and caused by destruction of the valves in the deep and communicating veins of the leg and by obliteration of the thrombosed veins.

Chronic deep vein insufficiency almost always results from previous symptomatic or asymptomatic deep vein thrombosis, although most patients cannot recall having had symptoms of that disorder. Rarely, an arteriovenous fistula in the leg causes chronic venous stasis, leading to chronic venous hypertension and eventual valvular incompetence.

Symptoms and Signs

Symptoms include chronic edema, which is generally worse at the end of the day. Hyperpigmentation, stasis dermatitis (scaling and pruritus), and hyperemic ulcers occur around and just above the medial malleolus. Varicose veins may be present. Pain is rare.

If edema is severe and persistent, fibrosis occurs, leading to secondary lymphedema and trapping fluid. The calf becomes permanently enlarged and hard. Ulcers then occur more often and are more difficult to heal.

Prophylaxis and Treatment

Elastic support, usually with elastic stockings, helps prevent edema and ulceration from increasing. A stocking that exerts 30 mm Hg pressure from the toes to just below the knee is usually sufficient. Patients should elevate their legs intermittently during the day and avoid standing still for extended periods. Ambulation should be encouraged. If significant swelling persists overnight, patients should sleep with their legs elevated 3 to 4 inches (8 to 10 cm) above heart level. For severe edema, constrictive stockings powered by pumps can reduce swelling.

For ulcers, elastic support and leg elevation can help; for infected ulcers, topical antimicrobial therapy (eg, povidone-iodine) and warm soaks are indicated. A plaster boot often helps large, clear ulcers heal. Using a boot, although it has to be changed every 1 to 2 weeks, is preferable to limiting ambulation. A boot should not be used if the ulcer shows signs of infection.

1 see page 698

SUPERFICIAL THROMBOPHLEBITIS

Inflammation associated with a thrombosed superficial vein.

In > 90% of cases, superficial thrombophlebitis occurs in varicose veins. Stasis within these incompetent veins leads to clotting.

Symptoms, Signs, and Diagnosis

Superficial thrombophlebitis is a more inflammatory process than is deep vein thrombosis. The usual presenting symptom is pain. Physical examination reveals an area of erythema, warmth, and tenderness overlying a palpable venous cord. Often, many areas of thrombosis occur along the course of a superficial vein.

Superficial thrombophlebitis, especially if below the knee, is usually a self-limited process, and signs of inflammation usually fade within 5 to 10 days. There may be no residual effects, or a nontender cord, representing a permanently thrombosed vein, may remain. Superficial thrombophlebitis rarely leads to pulmonary embolism. However, pulmonary embolism can occur if a clot propagates into the femoral vein as a result of thrombophlebitis of the great saphenous vein spreading toward the inguinal area.

If thrombophlebitis occurs in veins that are not dilated or if it is recurrent and migratory, the patient should be promptly evaluated for an occult neoplasm (especially pancreatic cancer), thrombocytosis, polycythemia, antithrombin III deficiency, collagen vascular disease, the presence of cryoproteins or lupus anticoagulant, protein C and S deficiencies, hyperhomocysteinemia, and protein C resistance.

Prophylaxis and Treatment

Stasis can be prevented with elastic bandages or stockings. For superficial thrombophlebitis below the knee, treatment consists of warm soaks, decreased ambulation, and a nonsteroidal anti-inflammatory drug. For superficial thrombophlebitis in the lower thigh, a short course of heparin may be useful while signs of inflammation are present. If the cord extends to the upper thigh, the great saphenous vein should be ligated at its most proximal point, using a local anesthetic.

VARICOSE VEINS

Dilated, tortuous superficial veins with incompetent venous valves.

Moderate to large varicose veins are common among the elderly. Varicose veins are often primary (affecting only the superficial veins) but may be secondary (due to disorders such as chronic venous insufficiency, which affects deep veins). Primary varicose veins result from primary valvular degeneration, which is often hereditary.

Symptoms and Diagnosis

Varicose veins, overfilled with blood, bulge and become visible, and their capillaries form a network of spider veins, accompanied by purple discoloration. Common sites are the medial thigh and leg and the area behind the knee. Hemorrhoids are a form of varicose veins.◼ Varicose veins occasionally ache or throb. The legs may feel heavy or hot, or they may itch. Severity of symptoms does not necessarily relate to size or severity of the varicosities. Symptoms are worse when standing.

Varicose veins are usually diagnosed by inspection, but their extent can be determined only by palpation with the patient standing.

A tourniquet test can help distinguish primary from secondary varicose veins. When the deep and communicating veins are competent (as occurs with primary varicose veins), compression of the superficial veins by a tourniquet placed above the knee impedes retrograde filling. When the deep veins are totally competent, complete venous filling after tourniquet application requires at least 45 seconds. (Without a tourniquet, all varicose veins would fill rapidly in retrograde fashion.) Primary varicose veins produce no signs of stasis and no evidence of deep and communicating vein incompetence during the test. However, when the deep and communicating veins are incompetent (as occurs with secondary varicose veins), blood flows in a retrograde fashion below the tourniquet and then rapidly fills the superficial veins through the communicating veins.

Treatment

For primary varicose veins, elastic support is the only treatment necessary. The disorder is not dangerous, although it may lead to superficial thrombophlebitis and the veins may bleed easily if traumatized. Venous ligation and stripping have almost no role in the treatment of the elderly. Surgery for primary varicose veins is only cosmetic, and recurrence is common.

For secondary varicose veins, the cause rather than the varicose veins must be treated. If the cause is chronic venous insufficiency, stripping is useless because the pathogenesis of venous insufficiency is related to hypertension in the deep venous system.

◼ see page 1074

Localized dilation of an artery secondary to loss of smooth muscle and elastic tissue in the media.

In the elderly, aneurysms are most likely to occur at branching points (eg, the terminal aorta) or at areas of stress (eg, the popliteal artery) and are almost always of atherosclerotic origin. Systemic hypertension is a major risk factor. When a local dilation develops, blood flow velocity decreases, leading to increased pressure against the arterial wall. The increased pressure results in more dilation and release of elastases in the vessel wall, perpetuating a vicious circle that often terminates in rupture of the artery. Saccular aneurysms are more likely to rupture than fusiform aneurysms because the total wall pressure is applied to a smaller area. Clinical findings and prognosis vary with the aneurysm's location and size.

THORACIC AORTIC ANEURYSMS

About 80% of thoracic aortic aneurysms are secondary to atherosclerosis associated with hypertension. Tertiary syphilis causes about 14%; these aneurysms are always located in the ascending aorta. Other causes include congenital factors, Marfan's syndrome, and blunt trauma to the chest.

Symptoms, Signs, and Diagnosis

Symptoms and signs are related to the site of the lesion. Aneurysms of the **ascending thoracic aorta** rarely cause pain until they rupture. Examination may reveal a loud aortic closing sound and an early decrescendo diastolic murmur of aortic regurgitation secondary to dilation of the aortic ring. The murmur, usually heard best in the aortic area, may be accompanied by a louder systolic murmur. Palpating the chest of a thin patient who is leaning forward may reveal a pulse along the right sternal border.

Although asymptomatic when small, aneurysms of the **transverse thoracic aorta** may cause symptoms and signs of mediastinal compression (hoarseness secondary to compression of the recurrent laryngeal nerve, dysphagia, wheezing, and superior vena cava syndrome) as they enlarge. On chest x-rays, these aneurysms may resemble mass lesions and so can easily be confused with bronchogenic carcinomas and mediastinal neoplasms.

Aneurysms of the **descending thoracic aorta** are generally asymptomatic until very large and can even penetrate the spine without causing pain.

Diagnosis is usually made coincidentally during review of routine chest x-rays. Generally, good posteroanterior and lateral views can distinguish the aorta from other mediastinal structures, and CT can confirm the diagnosis. If an aneurysm seems likely on chest x-ray, contrast CT is recommended to verify its size and location and to distinguish it from a silent aortic dissection. Angiography should be performed only if surgical repair is being considered.

Treatment

Asymptomatic thoracic aortic aneurysms < 8 cm that are not expanding call for a conservative approach. Hypertension should be treated with drugs that do not increase cardiac stroke volume (because the increased volume can stress the aortic wall). β-Blockers (nonvasodilator type) and calcium channel blockers are the drugs of choice; methyldopa, clonidine, and diuretics can also be used. Vasodilators (eg, hydralazine, prazosin, angiotensin-converting enzyme inhibitors) should be avoided.

The decision to perform surgery is based on the aneurysm's size and location, the presence of symptoms, and the patient's general condition. Aneurysms < 5 cm in transverse diameter rarely rupture, but those > 10 cm often do. Pain or compression symptoms suggest an increased likelihood of rupture.

Aneurysmal repair is a high-risk procedure for elderly patients, particularly if they have significant cardiopulmonary disease. Surgery should not be considered for most elderly patients. Rather, they should have chest x-rays every 4 to 6 months.

The transverse thoracic aorta is the most difficult site for surgery because total cardiopulmonary bypass and reanastomosis of the extracranial arteries into the graft are required. Surgery on the descending thoracic aorta is less complicated because only partial cardiopulmonary bypass is required to protect the kidneys and spinal cord. Surgery on the ascending thoracic aorta is of intermediate risk. The risk of surgery on the ascending aorta has been reduced by the sleeve technique, in which a vascular graft is inserted inside the aorta without resection of the vessel. For patients with severe aortic regurgitation, a graft with an attached aortic valve can be inserted.

ABDOMINAL AORTIC ANEURYSMS

Abdominal aortic aneurysms, which are common among the elderly, increase in frequency and size with age. These aneurysms expand much more rapidly than thoracic aortic aneurysms. The distal aorta is the site of the most common and most dangerous atherosclerotic aneurysms. About 98% of abdominal aortic aneurysms are infrarenal in origin, often involving the proximal common iliac arteries. Less than 2% of abdominal aortic aneurysms extend above the level of the renal arteries, affecting the thoracoabdominal portion of the aorta, the celiac axis, the superior mesenteric artery, or the renal arteries. Abdominal aortic aneurysms must be distinguished from aortic dissection. ▇

Symptoms, Signs, and Diagnosis

Aortic aneurysms are almost always silent until they reach or are close to the point of rupture. A rupture usually starts as a small perforation, blocked from leaking for hours or even days by pressure from a retroperitoneal blood clot. If it is diagnosed rapidly, lifesaving surgical repair may be possible. The pain pattern can be misleading. The pain is usually referred to the back and is indistinguishable from general backache. Because the elderly frequently have backache due to other conditions, a symptomatic abdominal aortic aneurysm can be easily overlooked. *No examination for backache in the elderly is complete without palpation of the abdomen for an aneurysm.* Unexplained abdominal or lower back pain with a prominent pulsation should suggest a ruptured aneurysm until proved otherwise. In elderly obese patients, sudden pain suggests the diagnosis, even if a pulsation is undetectable.

Most large abdominal aneurysms can be detected by gentle, thorough palpation of the abdominal aorta, which is an essential component of the physical examination of the elderly. Detecting these aneurysms in asymptomatic patients is imperative because the operative risk is so high after a rupture. Typically, an aneurysm appears as a painless expansile mass that has both lateral and anterior pulsations. However, often only a strong pulse is felt, making it difficult to distinguish a normal aorta from an aneurysm or from generalized ectasia and tortuosity. In patients of normal girth, the normal aortic pulse is generally palpable in the epigastrium, and a strong pulse is normal in thin patients, whereas any pulse may signal an aneurysm in obese patients. About 50% of aneurysms are associated with a bruit.

An aneurysm may be suspected only after an abdominal x-ray is taken for another reason. An anteroposterior view may indicate curvilinear aortic calcification near the midline, but calcification may be better seen in a lateral view, which may outline the aneurysm's calcified anterior and posterior walls.

Ultrasonography is the method of choice for confirming the diagnosis. It is virtually 100% accurate, providing precise information about the aneurysm's size, shape, and location. The likelihood of rupture is directly related to the aneurysm's transverse and anteroposterior diameters and inversely related to its length. Rupture is not likely when the diameter is < 5 cm; when the diameter is larger, the rupture rate rises quickly.

▇ see page 938

If patients have symptoms and signs of a rupturing aneurysm, immediate exploratory laparotomy is indicated. However, if the index of suspicion is low and the onset of pain is recent, contrast CT of the abdomen can be performed. If the aneurysm has already ruptured, retroperitoneal swelling can usually be seen. Diagnosis of rupture is the only advantage CT has over ultrasonography.

Prognosis

The mortality rate associated with unrepaired abdominal aneurysms is high. The 5-year survival rate varies from 14 to 37%. The likelihood that an aneurysm will lead to death is directly related to its size. In one study, the mortality rate was about 25% for patients with an aneurysm < 7 cm in diameter and about 61% for patients with an aneurysm ≥ 10 cm. Data from the 1960s suggest that 1 of 250 persons > 50 years died of a ruptured abdominal aortic aneurysm. This figure may have decreased in recent years because of better diagnostic techniques.

Complications other than rupture occur infrequently. Mural thrombi may embolize to the legs. Rarely, consumption coagulopathy occurs, resulting in thrombocytopenia, elevated thrombin time, fibrin split products in the blood, and a bleeding diathesis. An infection in the aneurysm is even rarer; if it occurs, *Salmonella* sp is most often implicated. Patients with recurrent *Salmonella* septicemia of unknown origin should be evaluated for an aneurysm.

Surgical repair prolongs life. With an experienced surgical team, elective repair has an operative mortality rate of < 3%, even though most patients have other manifestations of atherosclerotic disease. Contraindications to surgery include recent transient ischemic attacks and unstable angina.

Treatment

The operative risk associated with elective aneurysm repair is dramatically lower than the operative risk after rupture. Age should not determine whether elective repair of a large abdominal aortic aneurysm is performed in otherwise healthy elderly patients. Abdominal aortic aneurysms > 5 cm in diameter usually should be repaired. Repair of slightly smaller lesions may be considered, particularly if serial ultrasonograms show progressive enlargement and if patients are otherwise healthy. Patients with small aneurysms can be followed clinically and with ultrasonography every 6 months to 1 year. When the aneurysm is > 4 cm, ultrasonography should be performed every 3 to 4 months.

Angiography is not necessary before repair. During surgery, the aneurysm is opened, a graft is inserted, and then the walls of the aneurysm are closed around the graft. A promising experimental technique, the percutaneous insertion of a collapsed graft with a metallic ring at each end, avoids surgery. The graft is threaded through a femoral artery into the area of the aneurysm and then opened. The rings anchor the graft at each end. If perfected, this technique may allow repair of aneurysms even in very elderly patients with severe heart disease.

Treatment of patients who have both coronary artery disease and an abdominal aneurysm is controversial. Some authorities advocate coronary angiography and bypass surgery as the first intervention, but most reserve this approach for patients with severe heart disease. Most surgeons forgo coronary angiography for patients with little or no angina and a good ejection fraction (as determined by radionuclide left ventricular cineangiography).

The management of patients with significant stable angina is open to question. Thallium scanning of the heart before and after IV injections of dipyridamole is useful. Evidence of blood flow redistribution after dipyridamole administration is well correlated with postoperative myocardial infarction. Conventional submaximal stress tests and 48-hour ambulatory ECG monitoring also can help assess the need for coronary bypass before aneurysm repair.

POPLITEAL ANEURYSMS

The popliteal artery is the second most common site of aneurysms. Knee movements traumatize the artery. In addition, compression of the artery as it leaves Hunter's canal in the lower thigh leads to poststenotic dilation, which is then exacerbated by the development of atherosclerosis. Most lesions are asymptomatic. Patients with a patent aneurysm have pulsatile masses in the popliteal fossa, but an occluded aneurysm may be mistaken for a cyst. Ultrasonography is diagnostic. Other aneurysms should be sought; 50% of patients with a popliteal aneurysm have a popliteal aneurysm in the other leg, and 35% have an abdominal aortic aneurysm.

Thromboembolism—acute or as a series of small emboli to the foot—is the most common complication (16% of patients); it often necessitates amputation. Occasionally, the popliteal pulse disappears and reappears as the thrombus changes position in the aneurysmal sac. Other complications include rupture (in about 10%), popliteal vein compression and thrombosis, and posterior tibial nerve compression with radiating pain or sensory loss in the calf.

Treatment

Patients with occluded aneurysms do not require specific treatment; management is the same as that of peripheral arterial occlusion. ◨ Patent

◨ see page 918

aneurysms, however, are dangerous because of the high risk of rupture and thromboembolism. Surgery is required unless the patient is very debilitated or is expected to die shortly of another cause. Spinal or even local anesthesia can be used, if necessary. The aneurysm is not resected but is bypassed and separated from the circulation by proximal ligation.

FEMORAL ANEURYSMS

Femoral aneurysms have a course similar to that of popliteal aneurysms, can be confirmed by ultrasonography, and require surgical repair.

CAROTID ANEURYSMS

Carotid aneurysms are rare, occur in the midneck area, and manifest as pulsatile masses. Rupture is rare, but these aneurysms are a source of cerebral emboli. Carotid aneurysms must be distinguished from the much more common tortuosity and bending (kinking) of a carotid artery, which lacks clinical consequence. Kinking, usually with a strong pulse just above the clavicle, more often on the right side, is common among the elderly; it requires no treatment. Ultrasonography is useful in distinguishing kinking from aneurysmal dilation but is usually unnecessary. Surgical repair is usually indicated for carotid arterial aneurysms.

AORTIC DISSECTION

A hemorrhage into the media after an initial intimal tear.

Aortic dissection is often inappropriately called a dissecting aneurysm; aortic dissection differs from the localized stretching of the vessel walls that defines a true aneurysm.∎ The tear occurs because of medial necrosis or severe atrophy, often as a result of chronic, sustained hypertension. Dissection secondary to Marfan's syndrome is rare among persons > 55.

The initial intimal tear is almost always just distal to the aortic valve (proximal dissection) or just beyond the left subclavian artery (distal dissection). Proximal dissections are reported more often, but the prevalence of distal dissections may be underestimated because clinical findings can be more subtle.

∎see page 933

Symptoms and Signs

Symptoms vary. Pain may be excruciating, radiating throughout the chest and back; mild and limited to one small area of the back or chest; or totally absent. The clinical findings reflect what the hematoma that forms in the media does: The hematoma may extend distally along the aorta; clot at any point along the aorta; extend distally into any major aortic branch and compress the lumen; become the major blood-flow channel in any aortic branch; reenter the aorta or a branch through a second, more distal intimal tear; or perforate the adventitia at any point.

Distal dissection: The dissection may cause mild or severe back pain, but pain is often absent. The presenting symptom is often related to regional ischemia. Patients may have abdominal pain due to mesenteric ischemia, flank pain and hematuria due to renal infarction, paraplegia due to anterior spinal artery involvement, or leg pain due to iliac artery occlusion. Ischemia may be promptly and spontaneously reversed if the dissecting hematoma reenters the normal lumen; for example, femoral pulses that were missing may suddenly reappear. Symptoms representing many areas of acute ischemia should always suggest a possible aortic dissection.

Spontaneous healing of a dissection usually involves clotting of the hematoma followed by fibrosis around it. However, the aortic wall remains weak, and a true saccular aneurysm can develop. Because the wall has little support, the aneurysm usually expands and soon thereafter ruptures. During acute dissection, rapid expansion of a saccular aneurysm portends imminent rupture. Expansion occurring weeks or months later is generally less dire, although the aneurysm may rupture within days. Patients with a thoracic aortic dissection may present with symptoms of a sudden abdominal aortic aneurysm.

If a distal dissection perforates, the perforation usually occurs near the initial tear, with blood tracking into the left pleural cavity. Frequently, an initial small perforation is sealed off by a clot. A small left pleural effusion on chest x-ray may be the only clue.

Proximal dissection: Because proximal dissections often involve the aortic valve ring, the extracranial arteries, and the pericardium, they are more dangerous than distal dissections. A regurgitation murmur and a loud sound on aortic closure can usually be heard. Less frequently, the dissection produces hemodynamically significant acute aortic regurgitation, which results in low cardiac output, with pulmonary edema and hypotension. Rarely, silent dissection produces chronic aortic regurgitation, and the physician discovers either an asymptomatic diastolic murmur or a murmur and left ventricular failure.

Neurologic symptoms (eg, hemiplegia, aphasia) are common presenting symptoms. The dissection may occlude the innominate and left carotid arteries. If focal neurologic signs are present, the corresponding carotid pulse is usually diminished or absent. A lower blood pressure in the right arm is expected with left hemiplegia, because compression of the innominate artery affects both the subclavian and carotid arteries.

If the false channel is prominent in the transverse aortic wall, findings of mediastinal compression (hoarseness, unilateral external jugular vein distention, and a unilateral Horner's syndrome) can occur. Death often results from rupture of the dissection into the pericardial space.

Diagnosis

Aortic dissection can be a great masquerader, with an onset that can be acute or insidious. Because the diagnosis is easily missed, certain findings should always trigger consideration of this disorder (see TABLE 95–1).

Initially, chest x-ray is important for evaluation of the aortic shadow. The aorta almost always is somewhat prominent, especially in the elderly, so this finding is not specific to dissection. The aortic shadow is usually tortuous and uncoiled because of long-standing hypertension, and sometimes it is very dilated. Aortic calcification not extending to the shadow's borders suggests a false channel and is specific to dissection only if a lateral view shows a lack of calcium in the anterior or posterior wall.

If the index of suspicion is high after clinical evaluation and review of chest x-rays, then MRI, transesophageal echocardiography, or contrast CT is indicated. Transthoracic two-dimensional echocardiography is useful only for proximal dissection. It can usually show the false channel and detect even subclinical degrees of aortic regurgitation. It may also show early mitral valve closure, which indicates acute aortic regurgitation.

CT and MRI can show the false channel and follow the aorta to its bifurcation, revealing cutoff of branches. Both techniques appear to be at least as sensitive as arteriography.

TABLE 95–1. FINDINGS THAT SUGGEST AORTIC DISSECTION

Chest pain, hypertension, and aortic regurgitation
Chest pain radiating to the back
Chest pain with a normal ECG or an ECG showing left ventricular hypertrophy
Chest pain and no femoral or subclavian pulses
Chest pain and the sudden appearance of a pulsatile abdominal mass
Neurologic symptoms with a contralateral weak carotid pulse
Left hemiplegia and hypotension in the right arm
Unilateral jugular vein distention
Symptoms of many areas of ischemia
Limb embolectomy that does not recover a thrombus
Sudden pericardial effusion

Transesophageal echocardiography is a very sensitive and specific method of diagnosing aortic dissection. It detects very small intimal tears from very limited dissections, many of which are asymptomatic. However, it is not as useful as CT and MRI in assessing the abdominal aorta and its branches.

Aortography, usually performed in retrograde fashion through a femoral artery, is rarely needed even for patients about to have surgical repair. Although its ability to distinguish an active from a clotted false channel has prognostic value, the procedure is dangerous because of the risk of perforation.

Treatment

Distal dissection: Patients with an uncomplicated distal dissection can be treated medically. Systemic blood pressure must be lowered to decrease the rising pressure against the aortic wall: *it should be controlled immediately using a titratable drug given by continuous IV infusion.* A sympathetic ganglionic blocker (eg, trimethaphan camsylate) or an α-β-blocker (eg, labetalol) can be used. At the same time, oral therapy with a β-blocker and a diuretic is begun. The dose of oral drugs is increased until the IV infusion is no longer needed. If β-blockers are contraindicated, verapamil can be used. Centrally acting vasodilators (eg, methyldopa, clonidine) have little or no effect on cardiac output and can be used if necessary. Pure vasodilators (eg, prazosin, nitroprusside, hydralazine) and angiotensin-converting enzyme inhibitors (eg, captopril, enalapril) should be avoided because they lead to increased left ventricular contraction—producing increased pressure against the aortic wall—and may do more harm than good.

Surgery must be considered if pain is not reduced within the first few hours of medical therapy and eliminated within the first 2 days. After discharge, patients should be followed weekly for the first month and at least every 3 months afterward. Chest x-rays should be obtained after 1 month and every 3 to 4 months for the first 2 years to look for development of a saccular aneurysm. Mortality rates after 3 and 5 years for patients with uncomplicated distal dissections are about the same, whether these patients are treated medically or surgically. With effective medical or surgical treatment, the likelihood of recurrent dissection is low.

Proximal dissection: If managed only medically, proximal dissections tend to cause serious complications. Perforation rates are high; pericardial tamponade is the most common cause of death. For stable patients, hypertension should first be controlled with IV drugs, and then surgery should be performed. Synthetic grafts can be placed inside the thoracic aorta; this procedure reduces mortality. A graft with an attached aortic valve can be used for patients with severe aortic regurgitation. After graft insertion, the false channel can be obliterated into the true lumen. A distal saccular aneurysm or interference with blood flow through any major distal aortic branch mandates repair at the local site. Thus, a combined thoracoabdominal approach is often necessary.

The small, atypical intimal tears detected only by transesophageal echocardiography should be treated medically.

96   CARDIOVASCULAR SURGERY AND PERCUTANEOUS INTERVENTIONAL TECHNIQUES

Coronary artery bypass grafting, valve replacement, and percutaneous coronary interventions, including percutaneous transluminal coronary angioplasty, are increasingly performed in elderly patients. However, indications, some precautions, as well as any functional outcomes for these procedures are different in elderly patients than in younger patients. In very elderly patients, the goal of surgery is to improve quality of life rather than to prolong life. Although almost all cardiac procedures (even myomectomy, transplantation, and tumor removal) can be performed in selected elderly patients, the morbidity is higher than that in younger patients.

CORONARY ARTERY BYPASS GRAFTING

The most common indication for cardiac surgery is coronary artery disease.[1] More than 50% of patients undergoing coronary artery bypass grafting (CABG) are $\geq$ 65. These elderly patients tend to be sicker than younger patients undergoing this procedure; they are more likely to have unstable angina,[2] a history of heart failure, high-risk coronary artery disease (eg, left main coronary artery stenosis, triple vessel disease), left ventricular dysfunction, and a greater number of coexisting noncardiac disorders. In addition, the proportion of women vs. men who undergo CABG is greater in elderly than in younger populations.

The technique for CABG is similar in younger and elderly patients. Friable tissues, abnormalities of the ascending aorta due to age, severe calcific atherosclerosis, or all three may complicate arterial cannulation or proximal anastomoses. Intraoperative epicardial or transesophageal

---

[1] see page 853   [2] see page 855

echocardiography appears to minimize procedural difficulties and help reduce the risk of atheroembolism, which is a problem in the elderly.

Prognosis

Between 1969 and 1998, mortality rates among elderly patients varied widely from 0 to 21%, probably because patient selection criteria differed, rates increased with age, and results improved over time because of advances in treatment. Overall perioperative mortality rates continue to improve but are still higher for elderly patients than for younger patients. Rates are also higher for those needing urgent or emergency surgery. In addition, perioperative mortality rates are higher for women than for men. Additional predictors of increased mortality are shown in TABLE 96–1.

Increased morbidity leads to longer hospital stays; as a result, the duration of hospitalization increases with age. Stroke, supraventricular arrhythmias, transient psychoses, heart block, pulmonary embolism, postoperative bleeding, respiratory distress, and renal failure occur more frequently in elderly persons than in younger persons. The elderly also have a higher incidence of postoperative psychoses than do younger patients. They also have a tendency toward reduced mobility, requiring that particular attention be given to chest physiotherapy and wound care, especially in patients > 80. However, the absolute duration of hospitalization has declined for all age groups in recent years, and many elderly patients can be rapidly discharged.

The 5-year postoperative survival rate is generally > 80% for patients > 65; the 10-year postoperative survival rate is about 80% for patients < 65 and 65% for those 65 to 74. The 8-year postoperative survival rate is about 55% for patients ≥ 75; however, data are limited. Preoperative left ventricular dysfunction and coexisting disorders strongly affect long-term survival: The 10-year postoperative survival rate is substantially worse for patients ≥ 65 with left ventricular dysfunction than for those with normal left ventricular function.

The 6-year survival rate is better for elderly angina patients treated surgically than for those treated medically, and relief of chest pain is significantly greater for those treated surgically. Among octogenarians, the 3-year survival rate is also better for those treated surgically than for those treated medically. However, the oldest patients who undergo CABG tend to be a select population, which may partially explain this improved outcome. Functional outcome improves significantly only in patients treated surgically. However, among lower-risk elderly patients with mild stable angina but with well-preserved left ventricular function and no left main coronary artery disease, survival rates do not differ between those treated surgically and those treated medically.

Functional outcomes in elderly patients who undergo CABG are generally good. Surgery relieves angina in the elderly equally or possibly more effectively than in younger patients, possibly because levels of physical activity among the elderly are reduced. Postoperative mental health function and health-related quality-of-life measurements appear to be better in patients ≥ 65 than in those < 65. Typically, patients > 70 improve an average of about 1.5 New York Heart Association functional classes. Across all age groups, the symptomatic benefits of CABG tend to be better in men; angina recurs more often in women.

Preoperative Assessment

The severity of angina should be clinically determined; assessing its effect on quality of life may be complicated in the elderly by vagaries of memory, by the masking of symptoms through reduced physical activity, by the occurrence of anginal equivalents (eg, dyspnea, abdominal pain, syncope), and by the presence of coexisting disorders that mimic angina (eg, cervical spine disease, diaphragmatic hernias). Ischemia-induced heart failure and ventricular arrhythmias may also warrant coronary revascularization.

Understanding the patient's desires, motivation, and lifestyle is also important when deciding whether to perform CABG. In this regard, determination of physiologic age as opposed to chronologic age may be helpful. Close attention to coexisting noncardiac disorders is essential. The medical and social histories, physical examination, and routine laboratory tests should provide most of the necessary information.

The efficacy and acceptability of drug therapy must be assessed, because drug-related problems are common in elderly patients.◼ Angiography is needed to assess the potential for adequate revascularization. The presence and severity of left ventricular dysfunction and other cardiac conditions (eg, aortic stenosis, conduction disease) are also important factors to consider when planning therapy.

Postoperative Treatment

In the postoperative intensive care unit, physiologic monitoring and respiratory support may need to be prolonged; thus, the prevention of sepsis is a major goal. Gradual, but steady, resumption of normal activity, mobility, and independence is also a major goal of postoperative treatment.

PERCUTANEOUS CORONARY INTERVENTIONS

Percutaneous coronary interventions (PCIs)—eg, percutaneous transluminal coronary angioplasty (PTCA), coronary stenting, rotational atherectomy, directional atherectomy—are less invasive than CABG and require a shorter recovery time. These benefits are particularly advantageous in elderly patients, especially those with coexisting

◼ see page 62

TABLE 96–1.   INDEPENDENT PREDICTORS OF MORTALITY IN ELDERLY
PATIENTS UNDERGOING CARDIAC PROCEDURES

Procedure	Predictors of Perioperative Mortality	Predictors of Postoperative Mortality
Coronary artery bypass grafting	Left ventricular dysfunction Ejection fraction < 50% Pulmonary rales Prior myocardial infarction Heart failure Increased left ventricular and end-diastolic pressure Emergency surgery Prior coronary artery bypass grafting Class IV angina (angina with minimal activity) or unstable angina Current cigarette smoking Left main coronary artery stenosis Coexisting noncardiac disorders Hypertension	Left ventricular dysfunction Functional impairment due to heart failure Abnormal left ventricular wall motion Increased left ventricular end-diastolic pressure Coexisting noncardiac disorders Peripheral vascular disease
Percutaneous coronary intervention	Extensive coronary artery disease Ejection fraction < 40%	Extensive coronary artery disease Coexisting noncardiac disorders Left ventricular dysfunction

noncardiac disorders that may adversely affect short-term and long-term outcomes.

In the USA, > 50% of PCIs are performed in patients > 65. Elderly patients undergoing PCI are sicker than younger patients undergoing this procedure: They have more extensive coronary artery disease[1] and are more symptomatic, and they more frequently have class III angina (angina with light exercise), class IV angina (angina with minimal activity), or unstable angina.

Prognosis

The technical feasibility of PCI in the elderly is well established. The initial success rate ranges from 92 to 99%, which approximates the success rate for younger patients. The success rate is high even for very old patients.

[1] see page 853

For patients with multivessel coronary disease, the 5-year survival rate with PTCA is similar to that with CABG, although diabetic patients have a better survival rate when treated with CABG. However, most patients undergoing PCI now receive stents, which lower the rate of abrupt vessel closure and restenosis. In addition, antiplatelet glycoprotein IIb/IIIa receptor antagonists (eg, abciximab, tirofiban, eptifibatide) can reduce acute complications of PCI, including mortality, and are now widely used.

Mortality and morbidity rates with PCI are highest for the oldest patients, largely because these patients are frail and have advanced disease. Also, in these patients, complications are more likely to cause death. The hospital mortality rate is < 0.5% for patients < 65 but 2.2 to 4% for patients > 75. The most powerful predictor of mortality (see TABLE 96–1) is diffuse coronary artery disease. Poor left ventricular function and age per se are also independent predictors of periprocedural mortality. The complication rate for elderly patients (9%) is only slightly higher than that for younger patients (6%). Postprocedural renal failure and bleeding complications are more common in elderly patients undergoing PCI than in younger patients.

The overall long-term survival rate after PCI is good, even for patients > 75. The rate (about 85% at 4 years) is comparable with that for younger patients.

Excellent long-term relief of symptoms is achieved in most elderly patients with angina. However, angina patients > 75 who undergo PTCA appear to have higher recurrence rates of symptoms than do younger patients, probably even with stenting. A possible reason for their higher recurrence rates is that these patients are less likely to achieve complete revascularization than are younger patients. Overall, restenosis occurs in 15 to 30% of successful PCI cases and does not appear to be more common in the elderly. Risk of recurrent angina appears to depend largely on the extent of coronary artery disease before PTCA.

Preprocedural Assessment

The decision to perform revascularization and to choose CABG or PCI should not be based principally on age. However, physiologic age and general physical condition are important considerations. The physician must consider the significance of coexisting noncardiac disorders, the patient's ability to tolerate drugs, the patient's activity level and expectations, and the technical feasibility of the revascularization procedure. Enhancing independence and quality of life are important goals of treatment.

Postprocedural Treatment

The postprocedural treatment for elderly patients is similar to that for younger patients. Elderly women in particular have a higher rate of femoral hematomas; important aspects of management include weight adjustment of the heparin dosage, early discontinuation of femoral lines, and meticulous puncture site care.

VALVE REPLACEMENT

The majority of patients undergoing valve replacement are elderly. Valvuloplasty **1** is sometimes an option, especially for patients who may be unable to tolerate more aggressive procedures or who have limited life expectancy.

The most common indication for aortic valve replacement is aortic stenosis **2**, which, in the elderly, is most commonly caused by degenerative (senile) calcification and postinflammatory (primarily rheumatic) aortic valve disease, whose incidence has declined markedly. Although not common among the elderly, aortic regurgitation is another indication. The most common indication for mitral valve replacement is mitral regurgitation **3** or mitral stenosis **4**, which is increasingly caused by degenerative mitral valve disease rather than by rheumatic heart disease.

Age alone does not contraindicate valve replacement or repair. The indications for surgery in the elderly are similar to those in younger patients: the severity of symptoms, the nature of the valve lesion (whether regurgitant or stenotic), the cause of the disorder, and left ventricular function.

Prognosis

Newer techniques have improved the prognosis of valve replacement in the elderly. Although results are comparable among older and younger patients, old age is generally considered a significant risk factor for early mortality and morbidity, partly because of the high incidence of coexisting disorders in elderly patients. However, in many elderly patients, survival and quality of life can be improved with valve replacement or repair.

The overall perioperative mortality rate for aortic valve replacement in elderly patients is 10.5% (range, 5 to 28%), which is higher than that in younger patients. The perioperative mortality rate is higher for those with aortic valve insufficiency than for those with aortic stenosis; it is also higher for those undergoing emergency and urgent operations and for those who have poor left ventricular function, chronic lung disease, peripheral vascular disease, or renal impairment. For elderly patients with aortic stenosis undergoing nonemergency valve replacement in recent years, the perioperative mortality rate is reported to be as low as 4 to 5%, and the surgical mortality rate is 5 to 10%, even if heart failure is present.

---

1 see page 949   **2** see page 864   **3** see page 873   **4** see page 871

The perioperative mortality rate is higher for patients undergoing aortic valve replacement combined with CABG than for those undergoing aortic valve replacement alone (4 to 6% for patients in their mid-70s, 10% for patients in their 80s). The mortality rate for patients undergoing multiple valve replacements is also considerably higher than that for patients undergoing one valve replacement.

The postoperative morbidity rate is higher for elderly patients than for younger patients. Respiratory distress, bleeding, supraventricular arrhythmias, conduction disturbances, delayed wound healing, psychoses, and stroke occur more frequently in elderly patients postoperatively.

Extended long-term survival and symptomatic relief in a symptomatic elderly patient (even in a nonagenarian) with severe valvular heart disease are usually obtained using aortic valve replacement. The long-term survival rate with valve replacement—about 70% at 5 years—appears far superior to that attainable with drug therapy alone. The survival rate for elderly patients undergoing successful operations is similar to that for an age-matched population without valvular disease.

Mitral valve replacement is associated with less complete relief of symptoms and a higher mortality rate than aortic valve replacement, but the mortality rate has improved substantially in recent years. A large percentage of deaths are due to embolic stroke.

Preoperative Assessment

An assessment of the severity of symptoms, coexisting cardiac and noncardiac disorders, and psychosocial factors is important. Coronary angiography is generally performed to identify any significant coronary stenoses for possible revascularization during surgery. In a patient with aortic stenosis, poor left ventricular function does not contraindicate surgery if the mechanical effects of the valve lesion are the primary cause of the patient's symptoms. In a patient with valvular insufficiency, a prolonged delay in surgery may result in irreversible left ventricular dysfunction, with a markedly adverse effect on early and late results.

The choice of a valve warrants a comprehensive preoperative assessment and discussion with the patient, although the final decision often can be made only during the operation. Mechanical prosthetic valves are associated with a high risk of thromboembolism, and anticoagulant therapy is required. In patients with atrial fibrillation or other conditions, anticoagulation may already be necessary; a mechanical valve, with its increased durability, may therefore be a good choice for these patients. Favorable hemodynamic characteristics may warrant the use of certain low-profile mechanical valves (eg, St. Jude Medical, Medtronic-Hall) in specific cases.

Bioprosthetic valves are associated with a lower risk of thromboembolism than mechanical valves are, especially if atrial fibrillation is absent, and they do not require anticoagulant therapy. Bioprosthetic valves (eg, Carpentier-Edwards, Hancock) are generally recommended for patients ≥ 70, for whom the risks of long-term anticoagulant therapy (required for mechanical valves) are higher than those for younger patients. Moreover, bioprosthetic valves do not deteriorate or calcify as rapidly in elderly patients as they do in younger patients.

For patients with coexisting coronary artery stenosis, the question is whether CABG should be performed concomitantly with valve replacement, particularly in patients who do not have angina or prior myocardial infarction. Concomitant CABG increases the operative mortality rate, primarily because more time is required for cardiopulmonary bypass; although this increase has diminished in recent years, no randomized controlled study has compared concomitant surgery with separate procedures. Generally, concomitant CABG should be performed in patients with severely obstructed but operable coronary arteries, even if they do not have angina. However, the decision to perform concomitant CABG should be based on the clinical and hemodynamic status of the patient preoperatively and intraoperatively.

For patients with regurgitation due to coronary artery disease affecting the papillary muscle and the supporting left ventricular wall, CABG and valvuloplasty using an annuloplasty ring are often performed together. Surgical plication or valvuloplasty may be effective when the cause is myxomatous degeneration.

PERCUTANEOUS BALLOON VALVULOPLASTY

For frail elderly patients with aortic stenosis who are not candidates or are high-risk candidates for surgery, balloon valvuloplasty is sometimes performed to relieve symptoms. Also, for mitral stenosis, balloon valvuloplasty is a suitable alternative to surgery for patients with pliable, noncalcified mitral valves.

Prognosis

The mortality rate for balloon aortic valvuloplasty is relatively low: the periprocedural mortality rate is 3%; the 30-day mortality rate is 14%. However, the morbidity rate is relatively high; 31% of patients experience significant complications before discharge, the most common being a need for blood transfusion.

The procedure offers considerable temporary palliation and an acceptable mortality risk even in very ill patients. Even when balloon valvuloplasty is performed in very ill patients who are not surgical candidates, the periprocedural mortality rate is < 5%. The major limitation of balloon aortic valvuloplasty is a very high rate of restenosis. Within 2 years, about 80% of patients have recurrent symptoms leading to a second balloon valvuloplasty, aortic valve replacement, or death. Therefore, patients who are surgical candidates should be treated with surgery.

For mitral stenosis, percutaneous balloon mitral valvuloplasty and surgical commissurotomy for mitral valve stenosis are comparable; they provide similar hemodynamic improvement, symptomatic relief, and intermediate-term symptom-free survival. In patients > 65, the periprocedural mortality rate for percutaneous balloon mitral valvuloplasty is usually ≤ 3%.

The success of balloon mitral valvuloplasty depends heavily on the characteristics of the diseased valve. Results are best when the mitral valve is pliable, noncalcified, and not severely stenotic. However, in elderly patients with mitral stenosis, the mitral valve is most often thickened, nonpliable, and calcified because of long-term rheumatic disease. Only about 45% of elderly patients with mitral stenosis are good candidates for balloon mitral valvuloplasty.

Preprocedural Assessment

Thorough evaluation with echocardiography is critical for proper patient selection for balloon mitral valvuloplasty. Transesophageal echocardiography is advisable to exclude left atrial thrombi for patients in whom the transatrial septal approach is planned. For elderly patients, coronary angiography is also advisable because the presence of coronary artery disease may alter the approach taken. For patients with less pliable mitral valves, surgical mitral valve replacement must be considered as an alternative treatment.

Postprocedural Treatment

Similar to younger patients, elderly patients may quickly regain mobility after balloon valvuloplasty of the mitral or aortic valve. Serial echocardiography can detect complications (eg, pericardial effusions, cardiac tamponade, valvular regurgitation) and allows assessment of the response to therapy.

SECTION 12

KIDNEY AND URINARY TRACT DISORDERS

KID

97   AGING AND THE KIDNEY

Although renal function declines substantially with age, it is usually sufficient for removing bodily wastes and regulating the volume and composition of extracellular fluid. Nevertheless, reduced renal function decreases the elderly person's ability to respond to various physiologic and pathologic stresses. Doses of many drugs excreted primarily by the kidneys (eg, digoxin, aminoglycosides) require adjustment to compensate for decreases in renal function. ∎

∎ see page 59

RENAL ANATOMY AND FUNCTION

Renal blood flow progressively decreases from 1200 mL/minute at age 30 to 40 years to 600 mL/minute at age 80. The primary underlying factor is the decreased renovascular bed. However, the reduction in flow does not simply reflect decreased renal mass because flow per gram of tissue decreases progressively after age 30 to 40. This decrease is due to fixed anatomic changes rather than to reversible vasospasm, as shown by studies with vasoactive agents. Of significance is that cortical blood flow decreases and medullary flow is preserved, a finding consistent with histologic studies that show selective loss of cortical vasculature with age. These vascular changes probably account for the patchy cortical defects commonly seen on renal scans of healthy elderly persons.

A decrease in glomerular filtration rate is the most important functional defect caused by aging. The decrease is measured by creatinine clearance, which is stable until age 30 to 40 and then declines linearly at an average rate of about 8 mL/minute/1.73 m^2/decade in about two thirds of elderly persons without renal disease or not undergoing treatment for hypertension. One third of elderly persons show no decrease in glomerular filtration rate. This variability suggests that factors other than aging may be responsible for the apparent reduction in renal function. For example, increases in blood pressure still within the normotensive range are associated with an accelerated, age-related loss of renal function.

Unless hypertension or marked vascular disease is present, the kidney maintains its relatively smooth contour. With age, however, renal mass progressively declines and renal weight decreases from 250 to 270 grams at about age 30 to 180 to 200 grams at about age 70. The loss of renal mass is primarily cortical, with relative sparing of the medulla. The number of identifiable glomeruli decreases, roughly in accordance with the decrease in renal weight. The proportion of sclerotic glomeruli increases from 1 to 2% between ages 30 and 40 to > 12% after age 70 and is proportionate to the amount of atherosclerosis occurring elsewhere in the body. The glomerular tufts become less lobulated, the number of mesangial cells increases, and the number of epithelial cells decreases, thus reducing the surface area available for filtration. However, glomerular permeability does not change with age.

Several minor microscopic changes occur in the renal tubule with age. Diverticula appear in the distal nephron, reaching a high of about three per tubule by age 90. These diverticula may become retention cysts, which are common in the elderly. Their clinical significance is unknown.

The walls of the large renal blood vessels undergo sclerotic changes with age. The sclerosis does not encroach on the lumen but is augmented when hypertension is present. Smaller vessels appear to be spared—only 15% of elderly normotensive persons have sclerotic changes in the renal arterioles. X-rays show that normotensive persons > 70 have an increasing prevalence of abnormalities (eg, abnormal tapering of interlobar arteries, abnormal arcuate arteries, increased tortuosity of intralobular arteries) similar to that of younger hypertensive persons.

Two age-related patterns of change occur in arteriolar-glomerular units. The first pattern, occurring primarily in the cortical area, is characterized by hyalinization and collapse of the glomerular tuft. The lumen of the preglomerular arteriole becomes obliterated, with a resultant loss in blood flow. The second pattern, occurring primarily in the juxtamedullary area, is characterized by glomerular sclerosis and the development of anatomic continuity between the afferent and efferent arterioles. The end point is shunting of blood flow from afferent to efferent arterioles and loss of glomeruli. Blood flow is maintained to the vasa recta, the medulla's primary vascular supply; these arterioles do not decrease in number with age.

Several proximal tubular functions—maximal excretion of *p*-aminohippurate and iodopyracet and maximal absorption of glucose—parallel the decline in glomerular filtration rate, suggesting that tubular function disappears in entire nephrons with age. The renal threshold for glycosuria, which relates inversely to the degree of splay in reabsorptive capacity of individual nephrons, increases with age. Thus, glucose generally spills into the urine at a higher blood glucose level in an older diabetic patient than in a younger one.

Unless a specific tubular defect exists, the ability to concentrate and dilute urine and to excrete acid also parallels changes in glomerular filtration rate in most persons. Although the renal tubular system responds normally to graded dosages of vasopressin, the maximum ability to concentrate urine decreases. This decrease seems to be due to a relative inability to maintain the solute (osmotic) gradient in the medullary portion of the kidney. The reason for this inability is unclear.

RENIN-ANGIOTENSIN-ALDOSTERONE SYSTEM

Whether estimated by the plasma renin level or renin activity, the basal renin level decreases by 30 to 50% in the elderly despite normal levels of renin substrate. Certain therapies and measures (eg, salt restriction, diuretic administration, upright posture), all designed to augment renin secretion, produce increases in plasma renin concentrations that remain 30 to 50% lower than those observed in younger persons under the same conditions.

The lower renin levels in elderly persons result in 30 to 50% reductions in plasma aldosterone levels; the secretion and clearance rates of aldosterone are comparably reduced. Plasma aldosterone and cortisol responses after corticotropin stimulation are not impaired with age. Therefore, aldosterone deficiency in the elderly is usually a function of the coexisting renin deficiency and is not secondary to intrinsic adrenal changes.

Age-related decreases in renin and aldosterone levels contribute to the development of various fluid and electrolyte abnormalities. For example, elderly persons on salt-restricted diets have a decreased ability to conserve sodium. Decreased angiotensin II production, which also can result from a lack of renin stimulation, has been reported to seriously impair tubular concentrating ability. Together, these conditions contribute to the increased tendency of elderly persons to develop volume depletion and dehydration. Still, the most important cause of dehydration, especially the hypernatremic dehydration that occurs when water loss is greater than sodium loss, is the loss of thirst, which is characteristic in the elderly in response to increased serum osmolality or volume contraction. Loss of thirst is especially important when elderly persons are confronted with an illness that increases demands for or limits the intake of salt and water (eg, an infection).

Age-related decreases in renin and aldosterone also contribute to the elderly's increased risk of hyperkalemia in various clinical settings.∎ Through its action on the distal renal tubule, aldosterone increases sodium reabsorption and facilitates potassium excretion. Aldosterone provides one of the major protective mechanisms in preventing hyperkalemia during periods of potassium challenge. Because glomerular filtration rate (another major determinant of potassium excretion) is impaired in the elderly, plasma potassium levels are likely to become seriously elevated, especially if gastrointestinal bleeding (a major abnormal source of potassium) occurs or if potassium salts are given orally or IV. The tendency toward hyperkalemia is enhanced by acidosis because the aging kidney is slow to correct an increase in acid load, resulting in prolonged depression of serum pH and a shift of potassium out of cells. Potent antagonists of renal potassium excretion (eg, spironolactone, triamterene, most nonsteroidal anti-inflammatory drugs, β-blockers, angiotensin-converting enzyme inhibitors) should be administered cautiously to the elderly. The concomitant administration of these drugs with potassium supplements should be avoided.

▌98▐ RENAL DISORDERS

The most common renal disorders in the elderly are nephrotic syndrome; glomerulonephritis; renal artery stenosis, thrombosis, or embolism; and acute or chronic renal failure.

NEPHROTIC SYNDROME

A condition characterized by severe proteinuria (> 3 g/day), hypoalbuminemia, generalized edema, and susceptibility to infections.

The nephrotic syndrome is as common in the elderly as in young adults but, because edema is characteristic, is often misdiagnosed in the elderly as

---

∎see page 570

heart failure. Membranous nephropathy is the most common histologically diagnosed cause of nephrotic syndrome (35%), followed by minimal change disease (16%) and primary amyloidosis (12%).

Etiology

Nephrotic syndrome is due to a severe, prolonged increase in glomerular permeability for protein and may result from primary glomerular disease or systemic disease affecting the glomerulus (see TABLE 98–1). Causes include diabetic nephropathy, membranous nephropathy, minimal change disease, and amyloidosis.

TABLE 98–1. DISEASES ASSOCIATED WITH THE NEPHROTIC SYNDROME

Primary glomerular diseases
Minimal change disease
Focal segmental glomerulosclerosis
Membranous glomerulonephritis
Membranoproliferative glomerulonephritis
Mesangial proliferative glomerulonephritis
Unusual causes
  IgA nephropathy, rapidly progressive glomerulonephritis, fibrillary
    glomerulonephritis

Secondary renal diseases
Metabolic
  Diabetes mellitus, amyloidosis
Immunogenic
  Systemic lupus erythematosus, Henoch-Schönlein purpura, polyarteritis
    nodosa, Sjögren's syndrome, sarcoidosis, serum sickness, erythema
    multiforme, cryoglobulinemia
Neoplastic
  Leukemia, lymphomas, multiple myeloma, carcinoma (bronchus, breast,
    colon, stomach, kidney), melanoma
Nephrotoxic or drug-related
  Gold, penicillamine, nonsteroidal anti-inflammatory drugs, lithium, street
    heroin
Allergenic
  Insect stings, snake venoms, antitoxins, poison ivy, poison oak
Infectious
  Bacterial—postinfectious glomerulonephritis, vascular prosthetic
    nephritis, infective endocarditis, leprosy, syphilis
  Viral—infection with hepatitis B or C virus, Epstein-Barr virus, herpes
    zoster virus, HIV
  Protozoal—malaria
  Helminthic—schistosomiasis, filariasis
Heredofamilial
  Congenital nephrotic syndrome (Finnish type), Alport's syndrome,
    Fabry's disease
Miscellaneous
  Malignant hypertension, transplant rejection

Diabetic nephropathy: Diabetic nephropathy is the most common cause of nephrotic syndrome in the elderly. Most elderly persons develop diabetic nephropathy from type II diabetes. ◘ Native Americans, Hispanics, and blacks have higher rates of diabetic nephropathy than do whites.

Membranous nephropathy: The etiology of membranous nephropathy includes drugs (eg, nonsteroidal anti-inflammatory drugs [NSAIDs], penicillamine), infections (eg, hepatitis B), and systemic disease (eg, lupus erythematosus). About 10% of cases are associated with carcinoma of the lung, colon, or stomach.

Minimal change disease: The etiology of minimal change disease includes T-cell lymphoma, Hodgkin's disease, malaria, schistosomiasis, and NSAID-induced tubulointerstitial nephritis.

Amyloidosis: In primary amyloidosis, the amyloid fibrils deposited in the glomerular capillary loops are light chains with a composition similar to the Bence Jones protein. Patients with plasma cell dyscrasias (eg, multiple myeloma) develop renal lesions similar to those occurring with primary amyloidosis. The amyloid fibrils of secondary amyloidosis, which are associated with chronic inflammatory diseases (eg, rheumatoid arthritis; chronic bone, lung, and urinary tract infections; inflammatory bowel disease), are composed of a nonimmunoglobulin protein deposited similarly in the glomeruli. However, involvement of other organ systems is different from that occurring in primary amyloidosis.

Symptoms and Signs

Early signs of nephrotic syndrome include frothy urine due to proteinuria, anorexia, malaise, puffy eyelids, retinal sheen, and muscle wasting. Anasarca with ascites and pleural effusions may occur.

Focal edema may present as difficulty breathing (from pleural effusion or laryngeal edema), substernal chest pain (from pericardial effusion), scrotal swelling, swollen knees (from hydrarthrosis), and swollen abdomen (from ascites). Usually, the edema is mobile (eg, detected in the eyelids in the morning and in the ankles after ambulation). Edema may mask muscle wasting. Parallel white lines in fingernail beds may be due to subungual edema.

Patients may be hypotensive, normotensive, or hypertensive depending on the degree of angiotensin II production. Oliguria or acute renal failure may develop because of hypovolemia and diminished renal perfusion.

Diagnosis

Diagnosis is suggested by the clinical features and laboratory findings, especially proteinuria > 3 g/day. Diagnosis should include testing for serum antinuclear antibodies (ANA) and double-stranded DNA; antibodies to specific antineutrophil cytoplasmic autoantibodies (p- and c-ANCA); hepatitis B and C and HIV antibodies; cryoglobulins; and complement.

◘see page 627

Electrophoresis of serum and urine protein and immunoglobulins is also used. Renal biopsy is often needed to make a definitive diagnosis of the underlying cause and should not be avoided because of age alone. In diabetic nephropathy, diagnosis can usually be made clinically from a history of long-standing (15 to 20 years) diabetes mellitus and evidence of diabetic retinopathy; a biopsy is rarely necessary.

Prognosis and Treatment

Prognosis is determined largely by that of the underlying condition. In diabetic nephropathy, once nephrotic-range proteinuria develops, the disease generally progresses to renal failure within 3 to 5 years and eventually requires dialysis.

In diabetic nephropathy, controlling blood pressure slows the rate of deterioration of renal function; the use of angiotensin-converting enzyme inhibitors or angiotensin-II receptor blockers, even in normotensive diabetic patients, promotes efferent arteriolar vasodilatation and decreases glomerular capillary pressure. Intensive efforts to regulate blood glucose levels in young insulin-dependent (type I) diabetics have delayed the onset and slowed the progression of diabetic nephropathy as evidenced by decreased microalbuminuria and macroalbuminuria. It seems reasonable to assume, therefore, that similar aggressive treatment in elderly type II diabetics might produce similar beneficial effects, pending the outcome of new studies. Vigorous treatment of urinary tract infections and avoidance of analgesics (which may cause papillary necrosis), especially in combination, also are warranted.

In membranous nephropathy, the response to corticosteroids and immunosuppressants is variable, but worthy of a trial.

In minimal change disease, the response to corticosteroids and immunosuppressants (eg, cyclophosphamide, chlorambucil) is usually good. Elderly patients tolerate immunosuppressants better than corticosteroids, and the long-term risk of malignancy with immunosuppressants is less of a concern than for younger patients.

In amyloidosis, in most chronic forms of proliferative glomerulonephritis (unless associated with systemic immunologic disease), and in focal sclerosis, there is usually little or no response to corticosteroids and immunosuppressants.

GLOMERULONEPHRITIS

A syndrome characterized pathologically by diffuse inflammatory changes in the glomeruli and clinically by hematuria with red blood cell casts, mild proteinuria, and, often, hypertension, edema, and azotemia.

The important types of glomerulonephritis in the elderly are acute (postinfectious) glomerulonephritis and glomerulonephritis associated with systemic disease or an unknown cause.

Acute (postinfectious) glomerulonephritis: In the past, glomerulonephritis was usually caused by streptococcus; currently, glomerulonephritis is increasingly caused by staphylococcal and gram-negative bacteria. However, streptococcus is still the cause in a greater proportion of elderly patients. Often, these infections occur in immunocompromised persons (eg, alcoholics, diabetics, IV drug abusers).

Symptoms vary considerably by age. In elderly patients, nonspecific symptoms are typical (eg, nausea, malaise, arthralgias, a striking early predilection for pulmonary infiltrates) and suggest worsening of a preexisting illness, especially heart failure. About 75% of elderly persons have renal failure at presentation, with 20% requiring dialysis. Although the prognosis is generally good in younger patients with poststreptococcal disease, it is much less favorable in elderly patients, especially those with renal failure at presentation. The likelihood of progression to chronic glomerulonephritis, which is characterized ultimately by hyalinization of glomeruli, increases with age. Treatment with corticosteroids, immunosuppressants, anticoagulants, and plasmapheresis is generally considered to be of little value and confers a high risk.

Glomerulonephritis associated with systemic disease or an unknown cause: The cause is often an immunologic reaction to a systemic disease (eg, lupus erythematosus, vasculitis, Wegener's granulomatosis) or a primary renal disease of unknown etiology (eg, rapidly progressive [crescentic] glomerulonephritis with or without glomerular immune deposits). Symptoms are similar to those observed with acute postinfectious glomerulonephritis except that onset may be more chronic. Symptoms may also result from the underlying systemic disease (eg, upper and lower respiratory tract symptoms resulting from the necrotizing vasculitis of Wegener's granulomatosis). Diagnosis should include measurements of serum antinuclear antibodies (ANA), serum antibodies to specific antineutrophil cytoplasmic autoantibodies (p- and c-ANCA), serum complement, and serum and urine electrophoresis. In about half of patients with crescentic glomerulonephritis and a positive p-ANCA test but no other evidence of systemic disease, early treatment with high-dose pulse corticosteroid therapy has been shown to stabilize or improve renal function.

RENAL ARTERY STENOSIS, THROMBOSIS, AND EMBOLISM

Partial or total occlusion of the vasculature of the kidney, which can cause renal insufficiency and hypertension.

Renal artery stenosis is common in the elderly and is usually due to atherosclerosis. Although often totally asymptomatic, renal artery stenosis should be considered in an elderly patient with a sudden onset of hypertension, exacerbation of previous well-controlled hypertension, unexplained hypokalemia (eg, from hyperaldosteronism), or an unexplained increase in blood urea nitrogen or creatinine, especially after treatment with an angiotensin-converting enzyme inhibitor. The captopril renogram is the most sensitive screening procedure, but the test can be difficult to interpret when stenosis is bilateral. Unless medical therapy can achieve normotension with stable renal function, percutaneous transluminal renal angioplasty with stent placement is the procedure of choice, even in a very old person.

Renal artery thrombosis may complicate severe aortic and renal arterial atherosclerosis, especially when renal blood flow is reduced because of heart failure or volume depletion. Symptoms may be absent. If renal function previously was good, the only manifestation of unilateral thrombosis may be a small increase in blood urea nitrogen and creatinine levels and a modest increase in blood pressure. In patients with preexisting renal impairment and azotemia, renal artery occlusion may precipitate heart failure, marked hypertension, and renal failure.

Renal ultrasonography is as informative as intravenous urography and is safer. Differential diagnosis includes a coexisting abdominal aortic aneurysm, which may lead to renal artery occlusion by extension of atheroma or dissection.

Prompt revascularization can lead to a substantial return of renal function, and some patients recover even if surgery is delayed by several months.

Renal arterial embolism can occur in any patient with peripheral embolization (eg, from acute myocardial infarction, chronic atrial fibrillation, subacute bacterial endocarditis, aortic surgery, or aortography). Symptoms and signs may vary from essentially none to a full-blown syndrome of severe flank pain and tenderness, hematuria, hypertension, spiking fevers, markedly reduced renal function, and elevated serum lactic dehydrogenase levels.

Small emboli are difficult to detect, because renal scanning shows focal perfusion defects in many apparently healthy elderly patients. Major emboli may be suggested by differential contrast excretion on urography and confirmed by renal scanning and aortography.

Surgery is generally not indicated, and anticoagulant therapy is unlikely to be beneficial. In many cases, even when renal function is impaired, improvement may occur spontaneously over several days to weeks.

Renal cholesterol embolization, which may occur spontaneously or after aortic surgery or angiography in patients with diffuse atherosclerosis, is specific to the elderly. The clinical course varies, with most patients developing progressive renal failure. However, some patients have only moderate impairment and may eventually regain renal function. Definitive diagnosis may be difficult and requires visualization of cholesterol crystals on renal biopsy; diagnosis is often masked by other possible causes of reduced renal function (eg, hypotension, administration of angiographic contrast material). No specific treatment is available.

ACUTE RENAL FAILURE

The clinical conditions that give rise to rapid, steadily increasing azotemia, with or without oliguria (< 500 mL/day).

Acute renal failure (ARF) is more common in the elderly than in younger persons. The prognosis is nearly as favorable; therefore, treatment need not be denied because of age. ARF may be prerenal, renal, or postrenal.

Prerenal ARF results from poor perfusion of the kidneys. Most cases are due to loss of fluids (dehydration, volume depletion), internal redistribution (hypoproteinemia), decreased cardiac output, or certain drugs (diuretics, angiotensin-converting enzyme inhibitors, nonsteroidal anti-inflammatory drugs [NSAIDs]), often in combination. The most important contributor to the high rate of prerenal ARF in the elderly is the loss of thirst regulation compounded by a relative inability to retain salt and a loss of urinary concentrating ability.

Renal ARF may result from a number of renal disorders, including acute tubular necrosis (ATN), acute glomerulonephritis, and acute interstitial nephritis. ATN may be ischemic, nephrotoxic, or pigment-induced. Ischemic ATN is caused by disorders similar to those described for prerenal ARF. Surgical interventions (most notably cardiac and aortic surgery) and infections (sepsis), especially when associated with prolonged hypotension, are the most common causes of ischemic ATN. Nephrotoxic ATN is commonly caused by aminoglycoside antibiotics, although most antibiotics used to treat serious infections have been associated with this entity. Age is a risk factor for aminoglycoside nephrotoxicity; preexisting renal dysfunction and hypovolemia also may contribute. Pigment-induced ATN may be caused by hemoglobin or myoglobin being deposited in the urinary tubules, the latter resulting from rhabdomyolysis. Pigment-induced ATN occurs in all age groups.

Postrenal ARF results from urinary tract obstruction, which is one of the most common causes of ARF in the elderly. Early diagnosis is necessary because the condition is often reversible if the obstruction is relieved early.

Symptoms and Signs

Clinical features in patients with ARF vary depending on the cause, the severity of renal injury, and the speed with which ARF develops. Patients may present with an absent or decreased urine flow and evidence of fluid retention with an unexpected elevation in the blood urea nitrogen and serum creatinine levels. Patients may also present with the symptoms of the underlying cause or with the clinical or biochemical complications of uremia. Nonoliguric renal failure is increasingly being recognized, because use of biochemical monitoring of the severely ill patient and use of therapeutic agents that precipitate renal injury are increasing.

TABLE 98-2.   LABORATORY FINDINGS DISTINGUISHING PRERENAL ACUTE RENAL FAILURE FROM ACUTE TUBULAR NECROSIS

Blood urea nitrogen/creatinine ratio > 20
Fractional excretion of sodium < 1%
Urine osmolality > 500 mOsm/kg H_2O
Urine/plasma creatinine ratio > 40
Urine sodium concentration < 20 mEq/L

Diagnosis

Laboratory findings distinguishing between prerenal ARF and ATN are listed in TABLE 98-2. These findings indicate intact tubular function in a hypoperfused kidney. Another indicator of the prerenal state is the response to treatment with volume repletion (salt and water); elderly patients may have a delayed response to volume expansion.

When oliguria or anuria is present, urinary obstruction should be excluded rapidly, particularly in men with known prostatic hypertrophy or cancer and in women with gynecologic malignancies. The kidney in elderly persons can recover from acute ischemic and toxic insults, although not as rapidly as in younger persons.

Complications and Treatment

Volume overload precipitating acute pulmonary edema, hypertensive crisis, hyperkalemia, and infection are the major complications and causes of death occurring during ARF.

The principles of treatment are the same for elderly as for younger patients. All complications except infection can be successfully managed by supervision of fluid, electrolyte, and nutritional replacement and by early initiation and frequent use of dialysis. Urinary tract infection secondary to bladder catheterization is common. Little is gained from placing a urinary catheter in an oliguric patient; volume status and blood urea nitrogen, creatinine, and potassium levels are better guides to treatment than is urinary output. Infections from IV lines also are common; IV lines should be monitored scrupulously and discontinued as soon as possible.

Fluid and electrolyte replacement and nutritional support: A patient with ARF can lose up to 1 pound of body mass daily from tissue catabolism, even with adequate nutritional support. Because catabolized protein contributes to the serum urea nitrogen increase, calories should be given primarily as carbohydrate. Attempts to keep body weight constant result in gradual expansion of extracellular fluid volume and a consequent increase in blood pressure, with the risk of precipitating heart failure. Overzealous fluid restriction impairs the patient's general condition and central nervous system function and may delay the recovery of renal function. However, when an obstruction causing postrenal ARF is relieved, the patient may experience a remarkable diuresis that requires substantial fluid and electrolyte replacement.

Hyperkalemia becomes a problem primarily when oliguria or anuria is present, when there is excessive tissue catabolism (eg, rhabdomyolysis or inadequate nutritional support), or when there is an exogenous or endogenous source of potassium (eg, gastrointestinal [GI] bleeding, which is often precipitated or aggravated by azotemia, because potassium lysed from red cells is absorbed from the gut). Treatment of hyperkalemia is discussed elsewhere.◻

Acidosis progresses with the duration and degree of renal failure and can potentiate hyperkalemia by shifting potassium out of cells as hydrogen moves in. Infusion of sodium bicarbonate or dialysis can be used to maintain circulating bicarbonate levels > 18 mEq/L.

Other treatment measures: Oral phosphate binding agents can be used to prevent the serum phosphate elevation. The increase in serum phosphate results in precipitation of calcium phosphate, depression of serum calcium concentrations, and an increase in parathyroid hormone secretion (secondary hyperparathyroidism). The physician should increase the dosing interval of drugs excreted partially or totally by the kidney, while recognizing the enhanced sensitivity of elderly uremic patients to psychoactive drugs (eg, hypnotics, antipsychotics).

Dialysis: Hemodialysis, peritoneal dialysis, and ultrafiltration are effective in maintaining homeostasis; complications seem to result more from concurrent cardiovascular disease than from age. Dialysis is best initiated early in patients with ARF. Ultrafiltration therapy (removing excessive water by increasing hydrostatic pressure on the intravascular side of the dialysis membrane and/or decreasing hydrostatic pressure on the dialysate side) can be used to treat pulmonary edema and volume overload unresponsive to diuretics.

CHRONIC RENAL FAILURE

The clinical condition resulting from various pathologic processes that lead to insufficiency of renal excretory and regulatory function.

Chronic renal failure is much more common in the elderly than in younger persons. Although the causes are myriad, some chronic illnesses common in the elderly (eg, diabetes mellitus, hypertension, urinary tract obstruction and hydronephrosis secondary to prostatic hypertrophy or cancer, arterial obstruction secondary to atherosclerosis) can cause or predispose the elderly to chronic renal failure. Long-term use of drugs such as nonsteroidal anti-inflammatory drugs (NSAIDs) and certain analgesics

◻see page 571

(especially in combination) can cause chronic interstitial nephritis and papillary necrosis, resulting in chronic renal failure.

Treatment

Progression of chronic renal failure can sometimes be slowed by dietary modification, antihypertensive therapy, and other renoprotective measures.

Dietary modification: The rate of decrease in renal function in patients with progressing renal disease can be slowed slightly by protein restriction. The benefits of delaying progression of renal disease with a low-protein intake must be weighed against the small declines in various indexes of nutritional status. Protein intake should initially be reduced to 0.7 g/kg of body weight; ultimately, protein intake may need to be reduced to as low as 0.3 g/kg of body weight. Keto acid–amino acid supplementation may be necessary to prevent protein depletion. Salt restriction also may be needed to suppress volume expansion. Restriction of fat intake and lowering of serum cholesterol and triglyceride levels also appear to slow renal deterioration. Reduction of phosphate absorption with the addition of antacids at mealtimes is often necessary to avoid hyperphosphatemia.

Antihypertensive therapy: Patients with diabetic nephropathy benefit from lowering of blood pressure into the normal range. Moreover, angiotensin-converting enzyme inhibitors used not only to control hypertension but also to create lower-than-usual blood pressures have been shown to retard the rate of progression of nondiabetic renal disease.

Dialysis: Long-term maintenance dialysis (hemodialysis or long-term ambulatory peritoneal dialysis) is the mainstay of treatment for patients with chronic renal failure. More than half of all patients receiving chronic dialysis are > 60 years. Most elderly patients do well with dialysis; complications are related more to extrarenal diseases than to age alone. Psychologically, elderly patients often are better able to adapt to chronic dialysis than are younger patients. As soon as a patient is identified as needing hemodialysis, an arteriovenous fistula should be created, because such fistulas tend to mature more slowly in elderly persons.

Renal transplantation: Renal transplantation is increasingly used in persons > 60. Selection criteria should consider the patient's overall health status and severity of extrarenal disease (comorbidity) rather than age. Renal transplantation in elderly persons remains controversial, largely because of a reluctance to allocate a scarce resource (the donor kidney) to an elderly person with a limited life expectancy. Elderly transplant patients matched with dialysis patients by age, underlying diagnosis leading to renal failure, and number of comorbidities have 5-year survival rates of 81% vs. 51%, respectively. Because elderly persons have reduced immunity (immune incompetence), they require less aggressive immunosuppressant therapy, which should make them less susceptible to serious infections.

Treatment of complications: Complications of chronic renal failure, including anemia, hyperphosphatemia, hypocalcemia, hyperparathyroidism, and pruritus, must be treated.

Anemia resulting from chronic renal failure often requires more aggressive treatment in elderly patients than in younger patients because of coexisting heart disease. Red blood cell indices do not provide a reliable estimate of iron deficiency in uremia. Iron deficiency should be excluded by evaluation of serum iron and ferritin levels, and oral iron supplements should be given only if indicated. The management of non-iron deficiency anemia has changed radically with the use of recombinant human erythropoietin. Correction of the anemia results in improved cardiac function, exercise tolerance, central nervous system function, appetite, and sexual function. Erythropoietin (epoetin alfa) usually is started at a dose of 50 to 100 U/kg sc 3 times a week (or IV if the patient is already on hemodialysis) and adjusted downward as necessary to maintain the Hct between 30 and 35%.

Hyperphosphatemia, hypocalcemia, and hyperparathyroidism become problems because phosphate retention begins early in chronic renal insufficiency; phosphate retention stimulates parathyroid hormone hypersecretion and in turn helps to lower the serum phosphate concentrations back within the normal range. Therefore, control of serum phosphate levels is essential for the prevention and treatment of secondary hyperparathyroidism. Calcium carbonate and acetate antacids are the phosphate binders of choice, because toxicity may result from aluminum-containing (bone demineralization, dementia, anemia) and magnesium-containing (respiratory depression) antacids in renal failure patients. More dietary calcium is often needed. When the serum phosphate becomes elevated in the presence of increased parathyroid hormone, phosphate precipitates out with calcium, producing widespread soft tissue calcification and enhanced hypocalcemia.

Hypocalcemia also can result from inadequate vitamin D activity, causing decreased GI absorption of calcium, which in turn stimulates parathyroid hormone release and glandular hypertrophy. Hypocalcemia results from insufficient activity of the 1α-hydroxylase enzyme, which is produced in the proximal tubule of the kidney and is responsible for converting the carrier form of vitamin D_3 (25-OH cholecalciferol) to the metabolically active form of vitamin D_3 (1,25(OH)$_2$ cholecalciferol). The hypocalcemia generally can be corrected by giving 1,25(OH)$_2$ cholecalciferol orally (calcitriol 0.25 to 0.50 µg daily) and ingesting adequate amounts of calcium.

Pruritus [1] can be a major problem in elderly uremic patients, especially if xerosis coexists. In addition to skin moisturizers, ultraviolet treatments are effective and safe. Antipruritic agents (eg, antihistamines, ataractics) are rarely helpful; they also are toxic in the elderly, causing sedation, other central nervous system adverse effects, and anticholinergic adverse effects.

[1] see also page 1245

The involuntary leakage of urine.

Eight to 34% of community-dwelling elderly persons suffer from urinary incontinence; rates are higher in women than in men, and urinary incontinence affects > 50% of elderly patients in hospitals and in nursing homes. Yet, urinary incontinence is abnormal regardless of age, mobility, mental status, or frailty. Moreover, incontinence often causes the affected person to feel embarrassed, isolated, stigmatized, depressed, and regressed; incontinent elderly persons are often institutionalized, because incontinence is a substantial burden to caregivers. Incontinence remains largely a neglected problem despite the fact that it is highly treatable and often curable.

Continence requires input from the central nervous system (CNS) and integrity of lower urinary tract function, as well as adequate mentation, mobility, motivation, and manual dexterity. The role of the CNS is complex and not fully understood. Overall, the CNS integrates control of the urinary tract. The pontine micturition center mediates synchronous detrusor contraction and sphincter relaxation, while higher centers in the frontal lobe, basal ganglia, and cerebellum exert inhibitory and facilitatory effects. Because lower urinary tract function involves so many CNS centers, the impact of diseases such as stroke and dementia, which rarely involve just one center, is often difficult to predict. For example, detrusor overactivity is no more common in demented patients than in those who are cognitively intact.

With age, bladder capacity, contractility, and the ability to postpone voiding decline, and uninhibited bladder contractions become more prevalent. The postvoiding residual volume increases, but probably to ≤ 50 to 100 mL. Urethral length and sphincter strength decline in women, and prostate size increases in most men. Daily ingested fluid is excreted later in the day and into the night. These changes enhance the likelihood of incontinence in an elderly person but alone do not cause it.

Etiology

Incontinence can be categorized by duration of symptoms, by clinical presentation, or by physiologic abnormality. Clinically, however, it is easier to divide the causes into those that are transient and those that reflect intrinsic urinary tract dysfunction (resulting in established urinary incontinence). The former usually reflect problems outside the urinary tract.

Transient incontinence: Transient incontinence is uncommon in younger persons but common in the elderly, in whom it should always be considered. The reversible causes can be recalled using the mnemonic DIAPPERS (misspelled with an extra P): *D*elirium, *I*nfection (symptomatic urinary tract), *A*trophic urethritis and vaginitis, *P*harmaceuticals, *P*sychiatric disorders (especially depression), *E*xcessive urine output (eg, from hyperglycemia), *R*estricted mobility, and *S*tool impaction. Diagnosis and treatment of the underlying cause are necessary. Untreated transient incontinence may become persistent but should not be considered established merely because it is long-standing.

In patients with **delirium,** incontinence abates once the underlying cause of delirium is identified and treated.∎

Symptomatic **urinary tract infection** (UTI) is a cause of transient incontinence, even in young women if dysuria and urgency are so severe that they cannot reach the toilet before voiding. Asymptomatic UTI, which is much more common in the elderly, does not cause incontinence.

Atrophic urethritis and vaginitis in postmenopausal women often cause lower urinary tract symptoms. Atrophic urethritis leads to epithelial and submucosal thinning of the urethral lining, which predisposes to local irritation and loss of the mucosal seal. Incontinence associated with atrophic urethritis is often characterized by urgency and dysuria. Treatment is with topical or systemic estrogen.∎

Alcohol and drug use (see TABLE 99–1) are common causes of transient incontinence in elderly persons.

Other **psychiatric disorders** that cause incontinence have not been well studied; however, they are probably less common in elderly than in younger persons. Initial intervention is directed at the psychiatric disorder, usually severe depression or lifelong neurosis.

Excessive urine output is caused by high fluid intake, diuretic use (including caffeine and alcohol), and metabolic abnormalities (eg, hyperglycemia, hypercalcemia). Nighttime incontinence can be caused or exacerbated by disorders associated with peripheral edema and excess nocturnal excretion, such as heart failure, peripheral venous insufficiency, hypoalbuminemia, and drug use (eg, nonsteroidal anti-inflammatory drugs, dihydropyridine calcium channel blockers).

Restricted mobility can prevent a patient from reaching the toilet and may result from physical limitations, restraint (eg, in a bed or a chair), or more subtle but correctable factors (eg, orthostatic or postprandial hypotension, foot lesions, poorly fitted shoes, impaired vision, fear of falling). If mobility cannot be improved, a urinal or bedside commode may ameliorate or resolve the incontinence.

Impacted stool causes urinary incontinence, especially in elderly patients. The mechanism may involve stimulation of opioid receptors or mechanical disturbance of the bladder or urethra. Patients with impacted stool usually present with symptoms of urge or overflow incontinence and typically have associated fecal incontinence. Removing the impacted stool restores continence.

Established incontinence: If leakage persists after transient causes of incontinence have been addressed, established incontinence due to lower

---

∎see page 350   ∎see also page 1211

TABLE 99-1. DRUGS THAT CAN CAUSE OR WORSEN INCONTINENCE

Type of Drug	Examples	Potential Effects
α-Adrenergic agonists	Nasal decongestants (pseudoephedrine)	Increased prostate tone, urinary retention (in men)
α-Adrenergic blockers	Prazosin, terazosin, doxazosin	Urethral relaxation and stress incontinence (in women)
Alcohol	—	Polyuria, frequency, urgency, sedation, delirium, immobility
Angiotensin-converting enzyme inhibitors	Captopril, benazepril, lisinopril, enalapril	Cough (may precipitate or worsen stress leakage)
Anticholinergics	Antihistamines (1st generation), benztropine, dicyclomine, disopyramide, trihexyphenidyl	Urinary retention and overflow, delirium, fecal impaction
Calcium channel blockers	Nifedipine, diltiazem, verapamil	Decreased detrusor contractility, urinary retention, nocturia from peripheral edema, impaction
Diuretics	Furosemide, bumetanide (not thiazides), theophylline, caffeine	Polyuria, frequency, urgency
Narcotic analgesics	Opioids	Urinary retention, fecal impaction, sedation, delirium
Prostaglandin analog	Misoprostol	Urethral relaxation and stress incontinence
Psychoactive drugs		
Antidepressants (tricyclic)	Amitriptyline, desipramine	Anticholinergic actions, sedation
Antipsychotics	Haloperidol, thioridazine	Anticholinergic actions, sedation, rigidity, immobility
Sedatives and hypnotics (long-acting)	Diazepam, flurazepam	Sedation, delirium, immobility
Vincristine	—	Urinary retention

Adapted from Kane RL, Ouslander JG, Abrass IB: *Essentials of Clinical Geriatrics*. New York, McGraw-Hill, 1989, p. 149.

urinary tract causes must be considered (see TABLE 99–2). Lower urinary tract malfunction generally is similar in elderly and younger persons, although the incidence of specific disorders varies by age.

Detrusor overactivity (involuntary bladder contractions) is the leading urinary tract cause of incontinence in elderly persons regardless of mental status and is also common in younger persons. Frequent and precipitant voiding is characteristic. The urge to void comes on abruptly. The volume of leakage is usually moderate to large, nocturia and nocturnal incontinence are common, sacral sensation and reflexes are preserved, and voluntary control of the anal sphincter is intact. The postvoiding residual volume is generally low; a residual volume of > 50 to 100 mL suggests outlet obstruction (although the residual volume may be nil in early obstruction), a large bladder diverticulum, pooling of urine in a cystocele (in women), or detrusor hyperactivity with impaired contractility (DHIC). A large residual volume is often found in patients with Parkinson's disease, spinal cord injury, or diabetic neuropathy.

Detrusor overactivity in the elderly may coexist with impaired contractility, resulting in DHIC. DHIC is associated with urgency, frequency, a weak flow rate, significant residual urine, and bladder trabeculation and may mimic prostatism in men or stress incontinence in women. Because the bladder contraction is weak in DHIC, urinary retention is common and may interfere with bladder relaxant therapy.

Outlet incompetence is the most common cause of incontinence in younger women and the second most common cause in elderly women. Outlet incompetence manifests as stress incontinence: instantaneous leakage (without bladder contraction) during stress maneuvers such as coughing, laughing, bending, or lifting. It is usually due to pelvic muscle or ligament laxity. A less common cause is intrinsic sphincter deficiency, which is usually due to operative trauma but can result from urethral atrophy; leakage may occur even when standing or sitting quietly. Stress-associated leakage can occur with urinary retention but not as a result of outlet incompetence. Stress incontinence in men is usually due to sphincter damage after radical prostatectomy.

Outlet obstruction is the second most common cause of incontinence in men, but most men with obstruction are not incontinent. Common causes include benign prostatic hyperplasia, prostate cancer, and urethral stricture. In women, outlet obstruction is rare but can occur in those who have had previous surgery for incontinence or who have a large cystocele that prolapses and kinks the urethra when straining to void. In either sex, if secondary detrusor overactivity develops, urge incontinence may result, and if detrusor decompensation supervenes, overflow incontinence may ensue.

Obstruction due to neurologic disease is invariably associated with a spinal cord lesion. Interruptions in pathways to the pontine micturition center (see FIGURE 99–1), where outlet relaxation is coordinated with bladder contraction, cause detrusor-sphincter dyssynergia. Rather than relaxing

TABLE 99-2.   LOWER URINARY TRACT CAUSES OF ESTABLISHED INCONTINENCE

Urodynamic Diagnosis	Some Neurogenic Causes	Some Non-Neurogenic Causes
Detrusor overactivity	Multiple sclerosis Stroke Parkinson's disease Alzheimer's disease	Urethral obstruction or incompetence Cystitis Bladder cancer Bladder stone
Outlet incompetence	Radical prostatectomy* Lower motor neuron lesion (rare)	Urethral hypermobility (types 1 and 2 SUI) Sphincter incompetence (type 3 SUI) Prostate surgery
Outlet obstruction	Spinal cord lesion with detrusor-sphincter dyssynergia (rare)	Prostate enlargement Prostate cancer Large cystocele Anterior urethral stricture After bladder neck suspension
Detrusor underactivity	Disk compression Plexopathy Surgical damage (eg, anteroposterior resection) Autonomic neuropathy (eg, from diabetes mellitus, alcoholism, vitamin B_{12} deficiency)	Idiopathic (common in women) Chronic outlet obstruction

*Other prostate surgery rarely causes neurogenic incontinence.

SUI = stress urinary incontinence.

Adapted from Resnick NM: "Urinary incontinence—A treatable disorder," in *Geriatric Medicine*, ed. 2, edited by JW Rowe. Boston, Little, Brown and Company, 1988, p. 250; used with permission.

when the bladder contracts, the outlet contracts, leading to severe outlet obstruction with severe trabeculation, diverticula, and a "Christmas tree" deformation of the bladder; hydronephrosis; and renal failure.

Detrusor underactivity sufficient to cause urinary retention and overflow incontinence occurs in about 5% of incontinent persons. Causes include injury to the nerves supplying the bladder (eg, by disk compression or tumor involvement) or the autonomic neuropathy of diabetes, Parkinson's disease, alcoholism, and tabes dorsalis. In men with chronic outlet

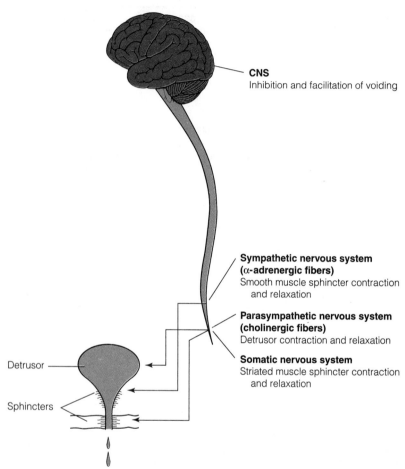

CNS
Inhibition and facilitation of voiding

**Sympathetic nervous system
(α-adrenergic fibers)**
Smooth muscle sphincter contraction
and relaxation

**Parasympathetic nervous system
(cholinergic fibers)**
Detrusor contraction and relaxation

Somatic nervous system
Striated muscle sphincter contraction
and relaxation

Detrusor

Sphincters

FIGURE 99–1.   Normal micturition occurs when bladder contraction is coordinated with urethral sphincter relaxation. The central nervous system inhibits voiding until the appropriate time and coordinates and facilitates input from the lower urinary tract to start and complete voiding. The sympathetic system contracts the smooth muscle sphincter through α-adrenergic fibers from the hypogastric nerve. The parasympathetic nervous system contracts the bladder detrusor muscle through cholinergic fibers from the pelvic nerve. The somatic nervous system contracts the striated muscle sphincter through cholinergic fibers from the pudendal nerve. (Adapted from DuBeau CE, Resnick NM with the Massachusetts Department of Health EDUCATE project collaborators: *Urinary Incontinence in the Older Adult: An Annotated Speaker/Teacher Kit,* 1993; used with permission of the authors.)

obstruction, the detrusor may be replaced by fibrosis, so the bladder fails to empty even when the obstruction is removed. In women, detrusor underactivity is usually idiopathic.

Symptoms of severe detrusor underactivity (eg, urgency, frequency, nocturia) may mimic those of detrusor overactivity, and urinary retention must be excluded before initiating treatment for detrusor overactivity. Less severe degrees of bladder weakness are common in elderly women. Although mild weakness does not cause incontinence, it can complicate treatment if other causes of incontinence also exist.

Functional problems in elderly persons (eg, environment, mentation, mobility, manual dexterity, medical factors, motivation) are often superimposed on lower urinary tract dysfunction. These factors may contribute to established incontinence but rarely cause it.

Symptoms and Signs

Many of the symptoms and signs are specific to the cause of incontinence.

Precipitancy (the abrupt sensation that urination is imminent regardless of the interval and amount of leakage that follows) is a reliable sign of detrusor overactivity. Whether and how much a patient with precipitancy leaks depends on bladder volume, the amount of warning, the accessibility of a toilet, the patient's mobility, and whether the accompanying sphincter relaxation can be overcome. For patients with no warning of imminent urination (often called reflex or unconscious incontinence), an abrupt gush of urine in the absence of a stress maneuver is also almost invariably due to detrusor overactivity.

Urinary frequency (> 7 voids/day) is a nonspecific symptom. Although it may be due to detrusor overactivity, it may instead reflect preemptive voiding habits, overflow incontinence, sensory urgency, a stable but poorly compliant bladder, depression, anxiety, or excessive urine production (eg, due to diabetes, hypercalcemia, or high fluid intake). Conversely, if persons with detrusor overactivity severely restrict fluid intake, they may void infrequently.

Nocturia (urination ≥ 2 times/night) must be placed in context; for example, two episodes may be normal for a person who sleeps 10 hours but not for one who sleeps 4 hours. In general, younger persons excrete most of their daily ingested fluid before bedtime, whereas many healthy elderly persons excrete most of theirs at night. The three major causes of nocturia are excessive urine output, sleep-related difficulties, and bladder and lower urinary tract dysfunction (see TABLE 99–3). The functional bladder capacity, which is defined by the largest single voided volume recorded in the voiding diary (see TABLE 99–4), can provide an important clue: if the volume of most nightly voids is much smaller than functional capacity, the patient has either a sleep-related problem (the patient voids because he is awake anyway) or a bladder problem. Whatever the cause, nocturia is usually treatable.

TABLE 99–3. CAUSES OF NOCTURIA

Excessive urine output
Age-related nocturia
Excess or late intake of fluids or alcohol
Ingestion of diuretic, caffeine, or theophylline
Peripheral edema
    Heart failure
    Hypoalbuminemia
    Peripheral vascular disease
    Drugs (eg, indomethacin, nifedipine)

Sleep-related difficulties
Insomnia
Pain (eg, arthritis)
Dyspnea
Depression
Drugs (eg, caffeine, a short-acting hypnotic such as triazolam)
Alcohol

Bladder and lower urinary tract dysfunction
Small bladder capacity
Detrusor overactivity
Prostate disease
Overflow incontinence
Decreased bladder compliance
Sensory urgency

Adapted from Resnick NM: "Noninvasive diagnosis of the patient with complex incontinence." *Gerontology* 36 (Suppl 2):8–18, 1990.

Obstructive and irritative symptoms are not specific for benign prostatic hyperplasia or bladder outlet obstruction, especially in elderly men. About one third of men referred for prostatectomy because of obstructive symptoms do not have obstruction; instead, they have an overactive detrusor, which will not be improved or may be exacerbated by surgery. Prostatism symptom scores may be used to assess symptom severity but should not be used to screen for or diagnose benign prostatic hyperplasia. All patients or their caregivers should be asked to identify which voiding symptoms are the most bothersome. For example, although a woman may have mixed stress and urge incontinence, the urge component may be more bothersome and should be the focus of the evaluation and treatment. A man with prostatism may be most bothered by nocturia, which may be remedied without treating the enlarged prostate.

Diagnosis

A voiding diary, kept by the patient or caregiver for 48 to 72 hours, is a record of the volume and time of each void and incontinent episode (see TABLE 99–4). The voiding diary is one of the most important components of the evaluation. It provides important clues to the cause of incontinence and helps in devising a therapeutic plan.

Physical examination is important for excluding causes of transient incontinence, detecting serious underlying conditions and causes of established incontinence, and evaluating comorbid disease and functional ability. Neurologic examination helps identify delirium, dementia, stroke, Parkinson's disease, spinal cord compression, and neuropathy (autonomic or peripheral). Additionally, spinal column deformities or dimples suggestive of dysraphism, bladder distention (indicative of bladder weakness or outlet obstruction), and stress incontinence should be explored.

Rectal examination should check for fecal impaction, masses, prostate nodules, sacral reflexes, and symmetry of the gluteal creases. Prostate size, as determined by palpation, correlates poorly with outlet obstruction. The rest of the rectal examination is actually a detailed neuro-urologic examination because the same sacral roots (S2-4) innervate the external urethral sphincter and the anal sphincter. Placing a finger in the patient's rectum, the examiner assesses motor innervation while the patient volitionally contracts and relaxes the anal sphincter. The other hand is placed on the

TABLE 99–4.   SAMPLE VOIDING DIARY OF AN INCONTINENT PERSON

Date	Time	Volume Voided (mL)	Patient Wet or Dry	Approximate Volume of Leakage	Comments
4/5	3:50 PM	240	Wet	Slight	
	6:05 PM	210	Dry		
	8:15 PM	150	Dry		
	10:20 PM	150	Wet	15 mL	Sound of running water precipitated episode
	10:30 PM	30	Dry		Bowel movement
4/6	3:15 AM	270	Dry		
	6:05 AM	300	Dry		
	7:40 AM	200	Dry		
	9:50 AM	?	Dry		
	11:20 AM	200	Dry		
	12:50 PM	180	Dry		
	1:40 PM	240	Dry		
	3:35 PM	160	Wet	Slight	Sound of running water precipitated episode
	6:00 PM	170	Wet	Slight	
	8:20 PM	215	Wet	Slight	
	10:25 PM	130	Dry		

Adapted from DuBeau CE, Resnick NM: "Evaluation of the causes and severity of geriatric incontinence: A critical appraisal." *Urologic Clinics of North America* 18:243–256, 1991.

patient's abdomen to check for abdominal straining, which can mimic sphincter contraction. Many neurologically intact elderly patients cannot volitionally contract the sphincter. However, successful sphincter contraction is evidence against a cord lesion. Innervation can be assessed further by testing the anal wink (S4-5) and bulbocavernosus (S2-4) reflexes. However, the absence of these reflexes (especially the anal wink) is not necessarily pathologic, nor does their presence exclude an underactive detrusor (eg, due to diabetic neuropathy). Finally, afferent nerve supply is assessed by testing perineal sensation.

Pelvic examination should be performed for all incontinent women. Pelvic muscle laxity may cause a cystocele, enterocele, rectocele, or uterine prolapse. Bulging of the anterior wall when the posterior wall is stabilized indicates a cystocele, whereas bulging of the posterior wall indicates a rectocele or enterocele. Unless severe (in which prolapse can kink the urethra and cause obstruction), pelvic floor muscle laxity indicates little about the cause of incontinence. Detrusor overactivity may exist in addition to a cystocele, and stress incontinence may exist without a cystocele.

The vagina should be inspected for signs of atrophic vaginitis, characterized by mucosal erythema, tenderness, friability, petechiae, telangiectasia, or vaginal erosions. Vaginal atrophy (not associated with incontinence) is characterized by loss of rugal folds and a thin, shiny mucosa. A cytologic maturation index showing 100% parabasal cells indicates atrophy but not necessarily atrophic vaginitis.

Stress testing, when performed properly, has a sensitivity and specificity of > 90%. With a full bladder, the patient assumes a position as close to upright as possible, spreads the legs, relaxes the perineal area, and provides a single, vigorous cough. Immediate leakage that starts and stops with the cough constitutes a positive result. A false-negative result may occur if the patient does not relax, the bladder is not full, the cough is not strong, or the test is conducted in the upright position in a woman with a large cystocele. In the last case, the test should be repeated with the patient in the supine position and the cystocele reduced, if possible. Delayed or persistent leakage suggests detrusor overactivity (triggered by coughing) rather than outlet incompetence. Performing the test when the patient has an abrupt urge (possibly reflecting detrusor overactivity) may cause false-positive results.

Observation of voiding provides much information about bladder and urethral function. If observation is not possible, flow rate can be assessed by a uroflow machine (uroflometer) or by a portable audio monitor (such as that used to monitor a baby's room at home). The patient should place a hand on the abdomen to check for straining during urination, especially if stress incontinence is suspected and surgery is contemplated, because straining suggests detrusor weakness that may predispose the patient to postoperative retention.

Postvoiding residual volume can be determined by catheterization or ultrasound. The postvoiding residual volume plus the voided volume provides an estimate of total bladder capacity and a crude assessment of bladder proprioception. Postvoiding residual volume > 50 to 100 mL suggests bladder weakness or outlet obstruction, but smaller amounts do not exclude either diagnosis, especially if the patient strained to void or double voided.

Laboratory Findings

Urinalysis should be performed and blood urea nitrogen and creatinine levels checked. Electrolytes should be measured if the patient is confused, urine culture should be obtained if dysuria is present, and serum concentrations of glucose and calcium (and albumin, to allow calculation of free calcium levels in sick, malnourished patients) should be measured if the voiding record suggests polyuria.

Urine cytology or cystoscopy should be performed if a patient has sterile hematuria, suprapubic or perineal discomfort, or a high risk of bladder cancer (eg, unexplained recent onset of urgency or urge incontinence, exposure to industrial dyes).

If the cause of incontinence cannot be determined, urodynamic evaluation should be considered. Urodynamic evaluation includes various tests (eg, cystometry, uroflowmetry, urethral profilometry) as well as x-ray imaging during bladder filling and emptying. The tests required depend on the clinical question. Although its precise role is debated, multichannel urodynamic evaluation is probably warranted when diagnostic uncertainty may affect therapy, when empiric therapy has failed and other approaches may be tried, or when surgery is being contemplated.

Treatment

Detrusor overactivity treatment begins with simple measures, such as treating peripheral edema, adjusting the timing or amount of fluid ingested, or providing a bedside commode or urinal. However, the cornerstone of treatment is behavior therapy.

Bladder retraining regimens, including techniques to suppress precipitancy, can extend the voiding interval. For example, in a patient who is incontinent every 3 hours, the regimen involves voiding every 2 hours during the daytime and suppressing urgency in between. Patients can suppress urgency by relaxing, standing in place or sitting down (rather than rushing to the toilet), and tightening pelvic floor muscles to prevent leakage. Many also benefit by knowing that the urge will build for a minute or so and then recede, similar to a wave on the beach. Thus, they only need to hold on for a minute or so. Once the patient has maintained daytime urinary control for three consecutive days, the voiding interval can be extended by one half hour and the process repeated until a satisfactory result or continence is achieved. Biofeedback can complement bladder retraining and is helpful for some patients.

In a patient who cannot follow the retraining regimen, a technique of prompted voiding is used. It reduces incontinence frequency by up to 50% in institutionalized elderly patients. The patient is asked at 2-hour intervals about the need to void; a patient who responds yes is escorted to the toilet and given positive reinforcement after voiding (negative reinforcement is avoided). Prompted voiding should not be pursued in those who do not respond.

If the voiding diary reveals nocturia and nocturnal incontinence, the cause should be determined (see TABLE 99–3). Nocturnal diuresis attributable to heart failure lessens with diuretic therapy. Peripheral edema without heart failure may respond to pressure-gradient stockings and daytime leg elevation. Diuresis not due to peripheral edema may respond to a changed pattern of fluid intake or to administration of a rapidly acting diuretic in the late afternoon or early evening. For the patient with detrusor hyperactivity with impaired contractility and uninhibited contractions provoked only at high volumes, catheterization just before bedtime removes the residual urine, increasing functional bladder capacity and often restoring continence and sleep.

Pharmacotherapy can augment behavior therapy but not replace it, because drugs generally do not abolish uninhibited contractions (see TABLE 99–5). The efficacy of each drug in the table is about the same. Drugs with a rapid onset of action (eg, oxybutynin [not the extended-release form]) can be used prophylactically if incontinence occurs at predictable times. Occasionally, combining low doses of two drugs with complementary actions (eg, oxybutynin and imipramine) maximizes benefits and minimizes adverse effects. Some of these drugs can be administered intravesically but only in patients who can catheterize themselves. All bladder relaxant drugs may cause urinary retention. Intentionally inducing urinary retention and using intermittent catheterization may be reasonable for patients whose incontinence (eg, DHIC) defies other remedies and for whom intermittent catheterization is feasible.

Augmentation cystoplasty increases bladder capacity by incorporating a section of intestine or stomach into the bladder. This treatment is reserved for severe cases of intractable detrusor hyperreflexia, especially those associated with a poorly compliant contracted bladder, and is contraindicated in frail patients. Neuromodulation, in which electrodes are implanted around the spinal nerve roots, is a promising new and investigational technique.

Pads and special undergarments may be needed for refractory incontinence. Many products are available, and the choice can be tailored to the patient. Condom catheters can be helpful for some men but often lead to penile skin breakdown and decreased motivation to become dry and may not be feasible for men with a small or retracted penis. New external collection devices may be effective in women. Indwelling urethral catheters are not recommended for detrusor overactivity because they usually exacerbate contractions. If a catheter is necessary (eg, to allow healing of a pressure sore in a patient with refractory detrusor overactivity), a narrow one with a small balloon should be used to minimize irritability and consequent leakage around the catheter. If bladder spasms persist, oxybutynin or tolterodine can be used. Drugs with more potent anticholinergic adverse effects (eg, belladonna suppositories) should be avoided in the elderly.

TABLE 99–5.   DRUGS FOR DETRUSOR OVERACTIVITY

Drug	Mechanism	Dose
Dicyclomine*	Combination smooth muscle relaxant and anticholinergic	30–60 mg/day (10–20 mg po tid)
Diltiazem*	Calcium channel blocker	30–270 mg/day (30–90 mg po 1 to 3 times/day)
Doxepin †	Antidepressant	10–75 mg/day (10–25 mg po 1 to 3 times/day)
Flavoxate*	Smooth muscle relaxant	300–800 mg/day (100–200 mg po 3 to 4 times/day)‡
Imipramine †	Antidepressant	10–100 mg/day (10–25 mg po 1 to 4 times/day)
Nifedipine*	Calcium channel blocker	10–90 mg/day (10–30 mg po 1 to 3 times/day)
Oxybutynin	Combination smooth muscle relaxant and anticholinergic	Short-acting: 7.5–20 mg/day (2.5–5 mg po 3 to 4 times/day) Extended release: 5–30 mg once/day
Propantheline*	Anticholinergic	22.5–150 mg/day (7.5–30 mg po 3 to 5 times/day)§
Tolterodine*	Muscarinic antagonist	2–4 mg/day (1–2 mg po bid)

* The drug is usually given in divided doses.

† Once the best divided daily dose has been determined, the total daily dose may be given once per day.

‡ Some reports of uncontrolled studies suggest that doses up to 1200 mg/day may be effective with tolerable adverse effects; randomized controlled trials do not support the efficacy for any dose.

§ Higher doses are occasionally tolerated and effective; they should be taken on an empty stomach.

Outlet incompetence may be lessened by weight loss in an obese patient, by treatment of precipitating conditions (eg, atrophic vaginitis, coughing), and, in some women, by insertion of a pessary. Pelvic muscle exercises (eg, Kegel's exercises) are often effective, especially if used at the time of stress. Patients must contract the pelvic muscles but not the thigh, abdominal, or buttock muscles; re-instruction is often necessary, and biofeedback is often useful. In women < 75 years, cure rate is 10 to 25% and improvement occurs in an additional 40 to 50%, especially if the patient is motivated, does the exercises as instructed, and receives written instructions and/or follow-up visits for encouragement. Whether women > 75 years can achieve similar success is unknown.

Pessaries, available in many sizes and shapes, ■ may be useful if the patient wishes to defer surgery or is at a high operative risk. Contraceptive

■ see Figure 118–4 on page 1199

diaphragms may ameliorate stress incontinence. Tampons are occasionally useful in elderly women with a narrow introitus. Newer devices, such as urethral inserts or caps, are also becoming available.

Additional nonpharmacologic treatment consists of a toileting and fluid regimen that maintains bladder volume below the leakage threshold. This approach is often appropriate for elderly women, whose sphincter deficiency is more often mild and the result of atrophy.

Pharmacotherapy with an α-adrenergic agonist (eg, sustained-release phenylpropanolamine 25 to 75 mg po bid) may be beneficial, especially when given with estrogen. These drugs may be more effective in women with intrinsic sphincter deficiency. Imipramine 10 to 25 mg po 1 to 4 times daily may be used in patients with stress and urge incontinence and no evidence of postural hypotension.

Surgery to correct urethral hypermobility may be needed if other treatment methods fail or are unacceptable. Anterior colporrhaphy is less likely to cure stress incontinence than are other bladder neck suspension techniques. Many elderly women cannot tolerate a Marshall-Marchetti-Krantz procedure, which entails lengthy abdominal surgery and a prolonged recovery time. An alternative suprapubic procedure, the Burch colposuspension, requires less extensive surgery, corrects anterior vaginal wall laxity, and is highly successful. However, the procedure may exacerbate posterior vaginal wall weakness and cause stranguria (the need to strain to void) and urinary retention in some women with a very weak bladder. Vaginal bladder neck suspensions (eg, Pereyra, Stamey, and Raz procedures) are relatively minor procedures but are often less durable than Burch procedures. A different approach (pubovaginal sling) is often required for intrinsic sphincter deficiency and can also be used in the absence of such deficiency. However, morbidity is higher, and chronic urinary retention is more likely to be precipitated than with procedures usually used to correct urethral hypermobility.

Another treatment for sphincter deficiency, especially for men who have had a prostatectomy, is implantation of an artificial sphincter. With patient selection, about 70% of patients regain continence; of the rest, most use only one or two pads/day, but reoperation or revision may be needed in 20 to 40%. Another approach is periurethral injection of bulking agents. With glutaraldehyde cross-linked bovine collagen, short-term improvement or cure occurs in 50 to 95% of women but much less often in men. Although bulking agents are appealing (injection requires only local anesthesia and little time), success usually involves multiple injections, and long-term data are lacking. Experience with persons > 75 is limited, and urinary retention (often leading to catheterization) is a risk.

In men, if all other interventions fail, a condom catheter, penile clamp, penile sheath (such as a McGuire prosthesis, similar to an athletic supporter), or self-adhesive sheath (especially if lined with a polymer gel or cellulose) may be useful. Some collection devices for women are available. Thin superabsorbent polymer gel pads can more readily absorb the smaller amount of leakage usually associated with stress incontinence. Electrical stimulation, a promising alternative for women, is under investigation.

Outlet obstruction in men is treated with oral α-adrenergic blockers (eg, prazosin 1 to 2 mg bid to qid, terazosin 1 to 10 mg/day, doxazosin 1 to 8 mg/day, or tamsulosin 0.4 to 0.8 mg/day), which relieve symptoms and may improve postvoiding residual volume, outlet resistance, and urinary flow rate. Effects occur within days to weeks.

The 5α-reductase inhibitor finasteride 5 mg/day po decreases prostate size, obstructive events, and the need for transurethral resection of the prostate in glands > 50 g. At least a 3-month trial is necessary to determine if finasteride is effective. Some investigators have suggested combination therapy with an α-adrenergic blocker, but evidence for this approach is equivocal. Recent reports suggest that phytotherapy with saw palmetto may be useful for symptoms of prostatism, but further studies are needed.

Transurethral resection of the prostate or suprapubic or retropubic prostatectomy may be used if bothersome symptoms persist. Alternative approaches (eg, bladder neck incision with bilateral prostatotomy) have made surgical decompression feasible for even the most frail patient.

Urethral stents are promising, but long-term follow-up data are lacking. Adverse effects include stent migration and urinary urgency (usually subsiding after a few weeks to months). Promising new transurethral techniques include microwave hyperthermia, laser therapy, and needle ablation, but long-term data are lacking.

In women, surgery usually is required for a large cystocele, and an outlet suspension procedure should be performed if urethral hypermobility coexists. If the bladder neck is incompetent or the urethral closure pressure is < 10 cm H$_2$O, a different surgical approach may be required. Primary bladder neck obstruction is easily corrected in even the most frail woman. Distal urethral stenosis can be treated with dilation and estrogen. More extensive intervention may be necessary if meatal stenosis is present; alternatively, dilation can be repeated frequently. However, most women who undergo dilation do not have urethral stenosis; they have an underactive detrusor. For these women, dilation is usually not helpful and may be harmful.

Detrusor underactivity is managed by reducing residual volume, eliminating hydronephrosis (if present), and preventing urosepsis. For patients with retention of > 800 mL, an indwelling catheter is used to decompress the bladder for ≥ 7 to 14 days, while potential contributors to impaired detrusor function (eg, fecal impaction, drug adverse effects) are eliminated.

If decompression does not fully restore bladder function, augmented voiding techniques may help: double voiding or implementation of Credé's maneuver (application of suprapubic pressure during voiding) or the Valsalva maneuver. Bethanechol 40 to 200 mg/day po in divided doses is occasionally useful for a patient whose bladder contracts poorly due to an anticholinergic drug that cannot be discontinued (eg, a tricyclic antidepressant). Residual volume should be monitored so that bethanechol can be discontinued if ineffective.

If the detrusor is completely acontractile after decompression, any intervention is likely to be futile, and the patient should undergo intermittent catheterization or have an indwelling urethral catheter placed. Antibiotic or methenamine mandelate prophylaxis against UTI is probably warranted with intermittent catheterization if the patient has frequent symptomatic UTIs or has an abnormal heart valve or an orthopedic prosthesis; such prophylaxis is not useful with indwelling catheterization. If intermittent catheterization is performed in an institutional setting, a sterile rather than clean technique should be used because of the prevalence and virulence of bacteria in such settings.

Nursing and Caregiver Issues

Appropriate care of urinary incontinence is often multidisciplinary. Many diagnostic and therapeutic procedures are often performed by physical therapists, physicians, or nurses. Nurses must also teach patients and caregivers about incontinence. Home health care nurses, nursing home nurses, and hospital-based nurses have partial responsibility for recognizing incontinence and creating care plans.

100 ▬ URINARY TRACT INFECTIONS

Urinary tract infection (UTI) is a common problem in the elderly. Diagnosis, prevention, and treatment can often be complex because clinical manifestations can be atypical and host defenses diminish with age. Common risk factors are listed in TABLE 100–1.

Classification

Bacterial UTIs can be classified according to localization as urethritis (urethra), cystitis (bladder), or pyelonephritis (kidney). In men, prostatitis may mimic or complicate UTI. Alternatively, UTI can be classified by the presence (symptomatic) or absence (asymptomatic) of symptoms, the frequency of its occurrence, the presence or absence of complications, and—especially important in the elderly—whether UTI is associated with catheter use.

Asymptomatic bacteriuria is characterized by $\geq 10^5$ colony-forming units (CFU)/mL without dysuria, urinary frequency, incontinence of recent onset, flank pain, fever, or other signs of infection during the week preceding the time the urine sample was obtained. Small numbers of polymorphonuclear leukocytes (PMNs) are common. Only about 70% of asymptomatic patients with high colony counts in a single urine sample have true bacteriuria as confirmed by the second sample.

TABLE 100-1.   COMMON RISK FACTORS FOR URINARY TRACT INFECTIONS IN THE ELDERLY

Atrophic urethritis
Atrophic vaginal mucosa (atrophic vaginitis)
Benign prostatic hyperplasia
Cancer of the prostate
Catheter use
Chronic bacterial prostatitis
Genitourinary abnormalities (eg, vesicorectal
    fistulas)
Genitourinary calculi
Renal and perinephric abscess formation
Urinary diversion procedures (eg, ileal bladder
    diversion)
Urethral strictures

Sporadic infections are defined as ≥ 3 (or ≥ 2, according to some investigators) episodes of asymptomatic bacteriuria within 1 year. Recurrent infections are classified as either relapse or reinfection UTI. Relapse UTI is defined as an infection in which urine is rendered partially or temporarily sterile by antimicrobial therapy, with the subsequent recurrence of bacteriuria from the uneradicated pathogen, generally within 2 weeks of completion of therapy. Reinfection UTI is defined as an infection that arises ≥ 4 weeks after the previous infection has been cured; the bacterial strain is often different from the strain that caused the successfully treated prior infection.

Complicating factors include urinary calculi, abscess formation, and obstructive uropathy. All UTIs in men are considered complicated whether or not these factors exist.

Epidemiology and Etiology

The prevalence of UTI increases in both sexes with age; the female:male ratio is 2:1 in the elderly. The annual incidence of symptomatic bacterial UTIs is estimated to be as high as 10% in the elderly. However, because many of these infections are recurrent, the percentage of infected patients is lower. Asymptomatic bacteriuria is a common finding in the elderly, especially in women; the estimated cumulative prevalence is 30% in women and 10% in men.

More types of urinary pathogens are isolated from elderly patients with UTI than from younger patients. The severity of any functional disability, nature of underlying illnesses, presence of anatomic or physiologic abnormalities of the genitourinary (GU) tract, and use of indwelling bladder catheters determine the types of organisms and chronicity of bacteriuria. *Escherichia coli* accounts for ≤ 70% of bacteriuria in elderly female outpatients with uncomplicated sporadic cystitis and for about 40% in patients with indwelling bladder catheters, complicated infections, or nosocomial infections. Other Enterobacteriaceae, enterococci, and staphylococci are often found.

Klebsiella sp, especially *K. pneumoniae,* are the second most commonly isolated gram-negative, aerobic pathogens. *Proteus mirabilis, P. vulgaris, P. inconstans,* and *Morganella morganii* are more common in men than in women because these species tend to dominate the normal aerobic preputial flora. They are also commonly isolated from the urine of patients with calculi, because they grow best in an alkaline milieu, and from patients with urogenital tumors. *Proteus* sp, *M. morganii,* and *Providencia* sp are commonly isolated from patients who are chronically catheterized. *Serratia, Enterobacter, Citrobacter, Acinetobacter,* and *Pseudomonas* sp are isolated mainly from patients with nosocomial UTIs.

In patients with recurrent infections, resistant gram-negative bacteria other than *E. coli* and gram-positive bacteria tend to predominate. Of the latter, enterococci, coagulase-negative staphylococci, and group B streptococci are commonly isolated; enterococcal superinfection often results from frequent use of antibiotics that are inactive against these organisms (eg, quinolones, cephalosporins, sulfonamides).

Anaerobes may be rarely isolated from patients with rectovesical fistulas or other abnormal communications between the urinary tract and bowel, which allow anaerobic fecal flora direct access to the urine.

Pathogenesis

In the elderly, the female/male ratio of incidence in UTIs narrows, in part because elderly men often have bladder outlet obstruction due to benign prostatic hyperplasia. Additionally, the relative reduction in the incidence of UTI in elderly women may be due to a decrease in sexual activity, which can introduce bacteria into the bladder. Severe UTIs, particularly those complicated by septicemia originating from the urinary tract, become more common with age, in part because of more frequent bladder catheterization and instrumentation and possibly because of changes in the immune system. Recurrent and complicated infections are also more common because of the higher frequency of predisposing anatomic and pathophysiologic factors, such as prolapse, urolithiasis, and malignancies in the GU tract and uterus.

Bacteria proliferate in stagnant bladder urine, and clinically important bacteriuria becomes established. A large amount of postvoiding residual urine is most common with a neurologic disorder, bladder outlet obstruction, or urethral stricture. A residual urine of 5 to 20 mL is fairly common in otherwise healthy elderly persons. Foreign bodies, most commonly indwelling bladder catheters, also promote bacterial growth. In catheterized patients, clinically important bacteriuria is established within 14 days unless a closed and aseptically handled system is used. ∎ However, recent data suggest that the majority of cases of asymptomatic bacteriuria in the elderly are true infections rather than colonizations. In addition to pyuria, elevated urine and serum antibodies to the implicated uropathogen and measurable urinary interleukin (IL)-6, IL-1a, or IL-8 have been shown to be present in nearly 90% of elderly patients with asymptomatic bacteriuria. The clinical relevance of these observations is unclear.

Symptoms, Signs, and Diagnosis

Many patients are asymptomatic. Symptoms that may occur include dysuria, urinary frequency, incontinence of recent onset, flank pain, and fever. Confusion and delirium are often attributed to UTI, although without high fever or sepsis, uncomplicated UTI is unlikely to cause serious central nervous system dysfunction.

The diversity of potential uropathogens mandates that urine cultures be obtained in all elderly persons with suspected UTI.

Bacteriologic diagnosis of complicated, recurrent UTIs and of asymptomatic bacteriuria is usually based on the concept of clinically important bacteriuria, which for these patients is usually defined as $> 10^5$ CFU/mL in a midstream urine sample after > 4 hours of bladder incubation. For women with uncomplicated symptomatic cystitis, however, the highest diagnostic sensitivity and specificity are achieved when clinically important bacteriuria is defined as $> 10^2$ CFU/mL with pyuria. If the clinical importance of bacteriuria is doubtful (eg, when repeated samples yield more than one bacterial strain) and obtaining culture is critically important, urine may be obtained by bladder puncture (which is better than bladder catheterization because the risk of contamination is minimized). However, bladder puncture may be more difficult to perform in elderly patients, and straight bladder–catheterized specimens often have to suffice.

Rapid tests can provide a semiquantitative determination of bacteriuria. The best is the nitrite test, in which the conversion of nitrate to nitrite by bacteria in the urine is demonstrated by color change on a dipstick. This test has a high degree of sensitivity and specificity but does not demonstrate bacteriuria caused by *Pseudomonas* sp, staphylococci, or enterococci, which are incapable of reducing nitrate to nitrite.

Quantitative urine cultures can be performed in bacteriology laboratories. The urine must be refrigerated if culture and incubation are delayed; however, storage for > 4 to 8 hours should be avoided, because substantial bacterial replication still occurs, even at cold temperatures. Quantitative urine cultures also identify the species involved and determine antibiotic susceptibility. In outpatient clinics, a dip-slide culture (in which an agar-covered slide is dipped in urine and incubated or left at room temperature overnight) may be used. The number of bacteria in the sample is reliably quantified, and gram-negative and gram-positive organisms are differentiated. A positive dip-slide can later be sent to a bacteriology laboratory for identification of species and determination of antibiotic susceptibility. Pyuria (presence of > 10 PMNs/high-power field under light microscopy in the urine) suggests infection rather than colonization.

Recurrent UTIs: In addition to bacteriologic diagnosis, more testing is often necessary, including quantitation of postvoiding residual bladder urine volume and investigation of the architecture of the upper urinary tract via ultrasound or CT in select cases. Urologic consultation may be sought when obstructive uropathy, calculi, abscesses, or GU tract anatomic abnormalities are suspected. Chronic bacterial prostatitis can also result in relapse UTI in elderly men. The diagnosis is suggested when bacterial colony counts from urine or expressed prostate secretion are at least 10-fold greater than counts from the urethral urine sample. Also, the presence of neutrophils in the prostatic secretions substantiates the diagnosis. In relapse UTI, evaluation should include assessment of bladder anatomy and function (ie, postvoiding residual and voiding cystogram or cystoscopy).

Treatment

Asymptomatic bacteriuria: In women, asymptomatic bacteriuria should not be treated unless coexisting conditions increase the risk of symptomatic invasive disease. In untreated asymptomatic bacteriuria, the organisms (especially *E. coli*) lose their virulence and become extremely susceptible to the bactericidal effect of normal human plasma. Large amounts of bacteria in the urine may therefore protect against symptomatic bacteriuria caused by more virulent strains.

In men, asymptomatic bacteriuria should be investigated to exclude complicating factors such as residual urine, calculi, or tumors. While the diagnosis is being determined and causative factors are eliminated, treatment should usually be given.

Cystitis: Most elderly women with uncomplicated lower tract UTI should be treated with antibiotics for 10 days; elderly men are generally treated for 14 days. Abbreviated courses (< 7 days) of treatment for UTI are not recommended for elderly patients because of relatively high rates of failure and relapse. Patients with community-acquired infections can be treated with trimethoprim-sulfamethoxazole (TMP-SMX) or an oral cephalosporin (eg, cephalexin, cefuroxime). When organisms are resistant or when the risk of pyelonephritis is high, a fluoroquinolone (eg, norfloxacin, levofloxacin, ciprofloxacin) can be used. Ampicillin and amoxicillin are generally not preferred because at least 13% of *E. coli* strains are resistant to them. For elderly patients with recurrent, complicated, or nosocomial infections, a fluoroquinolone or TMP-SMX, with ampicillin, is recommended before the cephalosporins; ampicillin adds coverage against sensitive enterococcal isolates.

For patients who have recurrent cystitis or for whom instrumentation of the lower urinary tract is planned, prophylactic treatment may be considered using nitrofurantoin one 50- to 100-mg dose at night (lower doses should be given to patients with markedly reduced renal function) or TMP-SMX 80 to 400 mg (half or full tablet nightly or one tablet 3 times/week). Prophylactic therapy should be avoided in patients with indwelling bladder catheters.

Pyelonephritis: Men and women with infection of the upper urinary tract (eg, presence of urosepsis, flank tenderness, fever > 38.3° C [> 101° F]) should be treated for a minimum of 14 days. Antibiotics for initial oral treatment include fluoroquinolones (eg, norfloxacin, ciprofloxacin, levofloxacin), oral cephalosporins (eg, cefuroxime), and TMP-SMX. For patients with community-acquired infections who have not received previous antibiotic treatment, a 2nd-generation cephalosporin (eg, cefuroxime) covers most pathogens; for patients with nosocomial infections, a 3rd-generation cephalosporin (eg, cefotaxime, ceftazidime, ceftriaxone), aztreonam, or an aminoglycoside is preferred. An alternative is treatment with IV TMP-SMX or a quinolone.

Urosepsis: Urosepsis in elderly persons may give rise to high morbidity and mortality rates. First-line antibiotics for urosepsis include 2nd- and 3rd-generation cephalosporins, quinolones, aztreonam, and aminoglycosides with ampicillin for about 2 weeks. Although the highest recommended initial dose should be used, subsequent doses usually need to be reduced substantially because of decreased renal function in the elderly. Maintenance of fluid and electrolyte balance as well as of adequate blood pressure is critical.

Relapse UTI: Treatment depends on the underlying etiology. Chronic bacterial prostatitis[1] should be treated for a minimum of 4 weeks with drugs such as oral quinolones or TMP-SMX.

Reinfection UTI: Management of uncomplicated reinfection UTI includes hydration and acidification of urine and low-dose suppressive antibiotic therapy.

CATHETER-RELATED BACTERIURIA

Long-term urinary catheterization results in bacteriuria, which may lead to symptomatic UTI and other complications. Avoiding or promptly discontinuing catheter use as soon as possible is recommended.

Catheter-related bacteriuria in the elderly represents the most common nosocomial infection; about 15 to 30% of hospitalized elderly patients with acute conditions undergo urinary catheterization. Indwelling urinary catheterization causes bacteriuria to occur at a rate of 3 to 10% of patients per day; a single in-and-out catheterization may

[1] see also page 1186

cause bacteriuria in as many as 20% of patients. By about 30 days (the conventional cutoff between short- and long-term catheterization), most patients are bacteriuric. At any given time, an estimated 100,000 elderly nursing home residents have long-term indwelling urinary catheters. Bladder calculi can also result in sustained bacteriuria that is difficult to treat even with antibiotics. Development of bacteriuria is facilitated by poorly controlled diabetes mellitus, because increased urine glucose levels provide the substrate for bacterial growth.

Etiology and Pathogenesis

Bacteriuria associated with short-term catheterization usually involves a single uropathogen, most commonly *E. coli*; bacteriuria associated with long-term catheterization is characteristically polymicrobial, usually with two to five isolates, including *E. coli, P. mirabilis, K. pneumoniae, Enterococcus, Providencia stuartii,* and *M. morganii.* Several other bacterial pathogens and yeasts have also been implicated.

Bacteria often gain access into the urinary tract from periurethral colonization by the patient's colonic flora; migration between the catheter and uroepithelium into the bladder and the upper urinary tract may occur. Rarely, uropathogens may be introduced from breaks in the integrity of the closed collection system; furthermore, the bacteria are capable of colonizing the intraluminal surface of the catheter and bag with subsequent proximal migration against the urinary flow into the urinary tract.

Complications

The most common complication of catheter-related asymptomatic bacteriuria is symptomatic infection (which can cause fever, delirium, pyelonephritis, bacteremia, urosepsis, death). In addition, long-term catheterization may give rise to urethritis, urinary calculi, epididymitis, vesicoureteral reflux, chronic pyelonephritis, and chronic tubulointerstitial nephritis with deformed calyces and scarring of the renal parenchyma.

Diagnosis and Prevention

Urine cultures obtained from the lumen of urinary catheters often contain more species than are actually present in the bladder; removal of the catheter and replacement with a new catheter before obtaining cultures are often recommended.

Every attempt must be made to minimize the duration of short-term catheterization and to avoid long-term catheterization. Criteria for the use of long-term catheterization are listed in TABLE 100–2. Maintenance of the integrity of the closed urinary system is also of utmost importance.

The use of bladder irrigation, the addition of antibacterial chemicals in collection bags, the use of silver-coated catheters, and the use of methenamine to reduce bacteriuria have shown equivocal results.

TABLE 100–2.   CRITERIA FOR LONG-TERM CATHETERIZATION USE

Urinary retention that cannot be managed medically or surgically
Fecal or urinary incontinence that results in wound contamination
Terminal illness or severe impairment in which frequent movement causes discomfort
Failure of other treatment modalities combined with a patient preference for catheterization

Treatment

The need to treat asymptomatic bacteriuria in catheterized elderly patients is not supported by current data. Antibiotic use may delay the onset of bacteriuria in short-term catheterization but does not reduce complications; antibiotic use may also promote growth of resistant uropathogens.

Symptomatic UTI associated with short-term and long-term catheterization should be treated with the narrowest spectrum antibacterial drug pending urine culture and sensitivity results. The duration of treatment depends on the clinical scenario; a 7- to 14-day regimen is suggested for most cases. Empiric therapy for symptomatic UTI associated with long-term catheterization (when resistance is not suspected and the patient is not critically ill) should include antibiotics active against likely polymicrobial flora (eg, TMP-SMX or a 2nd- or 3rd-generation cephalosporin). For seriously ill patients, a two-drug combination of ampicillin (to cover enterococci) plus a 3rd-generation cephalosporin, aztreonam, an aminoglycoside, or a quinolone is recommended. Some experts recommend removing and replacing the catheter.

101   URINARY TRACT TUMORS

RENAL TUMORS

The vast majority of renal tumors are malignant adenocarcinomas (historically termed hypernephroma or renal cell carcinoma). Other malignant renal tumors include lymphoma and metastases. Benign solid masses (oncocytoma, angiomyolipoma) of the kidney are uncommon. Tumors of the renal pelvis are categorized separately. ◼

Epidemiology

Renal adenocarcinoma is the 10th most common cancer, accounting for 3% of all malignancies in adults, with a median age at diagnosis of 65

◼ see page 994

years. The male:female ratio is 2:1. Incidence is increasing—sixfold from 1935 to 1989 in men (from 1.6 to 9.6 cases/100,000) and in women (from 0.7 to 4.2 cases/100,000).

No strong risk factors have been identified for the development of renal adenocarcinomas, although obesity and smoking contribute modestly. The strongest risk factors appear to be genetic; multifocal renal adenocarcinomas have a hereditary basis, which is being studied intensively. Several multiorgan syndromes are associated with a high risk of renal malignancies—the most prominent is von Hippel-Lindau disease (an autosomally dominant hereditary disease originating from chromosome 3p, beginning in the teenage years, and characterized by the development of central nervous system hemangioblastomas, renal adenocarcinomas, and other anomalies).

Pathology

Because of the isolated anatomic location of the kidney, renal adenocarcinomas can grow large while remaining clinically silent. Most demonstrate a characteristic hypervascularity. Renal adenocarcinomas have a predilection for vascular invasion and tend to grow intravascularly within the renal vein and into the vena cava. Because these tumor thrombi may extend as far as the right atrium, they present a unique surgical challenge.

Although essentially every organ site can be affected, the most common sites of metastases are the lungs, adrenal glands, liver, and bones (where the lesions are predominantly lytic and prone to pathologic fracture).

Symptoms and Signs

The historic symptom triad of renal adenocarcinoma is hematuria, flank pain, and the presence of a flank mass—most cases with these symptoms are advanced and incurable. Rarely, a patient presenting with heart failure has an underlying renal malignancy as the cause (ie, high-output failure due to a functional arteriovenous fistula). Paraneoplastic disorders are relatively common; hypercalcemia, fever, anemia, weakness, and erythrocytosis occur most often (see TABLE 101–1). A small percentage of tumors secrete inappropriate levels of erythropoietin.

Diagnosis and Staging

Increasingly, localized (not metastatic and not involving the lymph nodes) renal adenocarcinoma is being diagnosed in patients having no symptoms attributable to the tumor; these tumors are often discovered incidentally during imaging evaluation of patients' other complaints.

Gross hematuria is rarely a symptom of renal adenocarcinoma until an advanced stage. Because gross hematuria can occur in patients receiving anticoagulation therapy, it is important to consider renal adenocarcinoma and not to dismiss hematuria as an adverse effect of anticoagulation therapy. Patients with gross hematuria are best evaluated by a urologist. An

TABLE 101–1.   INCIDENCE OF PARANEOPLASTIC DISORDERS ASSOCIATED WITH RENAL ADENOCARCINOMA

Disorder	Incidence (%)
Anemia	20–40
Cachexia/weight loss	30–35
Fever	30
Hypertension	20–25
Hypercalcemia	10–15
Stauffer's syndrome (hypertransaminasemia, elevated alkaline phosphatase, prolonged partial thromboplastin time)	3–6
Amyloidosis	< 5
Erythrocytosis	< 5
Gastrointestinal disturbance	< 5
Neuropathic disorder	< 5

appropriate approach is cystoscopy followed by an upper urinary tract imaging study (usually intravenous urography with tomography).

Microhematuria is problematic. Although the differential diagnosis includes tumors of the kidney, renal pelvis, ureter, bladder, and prostate, the vast majority of cases have a benign or idiopathic etiology. Microhematuria occurs in many patients with nephrosclerosis, benign prostatic hyperplasia, and small clinically insignificant renal arteriovenous malformations. Small, asymptomatic renal stones are another cause of benign microhematuria. The patient's evaluation should be individualized and should consider comorbidities, age, and previous medical history.

Incidental renal masses: The use of imaging studies (eg, ultrasonography, CT, intravenous urography) for evaluation of abdominal complaints or renal colic has significantly increased the incidental discovery of renal masses. Most masses are simple uncomplicated cysts, which become increasingly frequent after age 65. However, because the vast majority of curable (ie, still localized) renal adenocarcinomas are found incidentally, appropriate cost-effective management of these patients is important.

Usually, these incidentally discovered lesions are characterized adequately by imaging studies, without the need for biopsy or exploration. Cysts fulfilling all radiographic criteria of simple uncomplicated lesions (using either dedicated renal ultrasonography or CT) need no further evaluation; however, atypical cysts need further evaluation, as do solid masses, because cystic adenocarcinomas often have an indeterminate image.

The vast majority of solid masses are malignant and require definitive evaluation and treatment. The rare benign solid mass (eg, benign hamartomas [angiomyolipomas]) can be diagnosed by imaging studies alone.

Performing a percutaneous biopsy on a solid renal mass is rarely cost-effective because it is unlikely to change future treatment unless there is evidence of advanced disease. Exceptions are patients with a previous history of another malignancy, multifocal disease, or associated extensive nodal adenopathy suggestive of lymphoma.

A CT (with or without contrast), a plain chest x-ray, and, in some cases, a bone scan are used to stage renal adenocarcinoma. Abdominal MRI rarely provides additional information (unless a tumor thrombus into the renal vein and vena cava is suspected), but MRI is appropriate when use of contrast is precluded (eg, for patients with an allergy to IV contrast or for patients with renal insufficiency).

Prognosis

In most cases of localized renal adenocarcinoma, the 5-year survival rate is > 60%. The natural history of renal adenocarcinoma is far more unpredictable than that of most solid tumors. Disease may recur > 15 years after removal of the original primary lesion. Various host immune factors may contribute to this recurrence.

Metastatic disease has a poor prognosis and is rarely curable. Metastatic recurrence at a remotely distant time is not uncommon.

Treatment

Because renal adenocarcinoma is relatively radioresistant, radiation therapy has little or no role in its treatment.

Localized disease: Surgery is the sole intervention capable of cure. The standard procedure is radical nephrectomy—removal of the whole affected kidney along with adjacent lymph nodes and tissue. In the patient with renal insufficiency or a solitary kidney, partial nephrectomy (a far more complex procedure) may be indicated. For patients with a genetic predisposition and multifocal disease (usually affecting both kidneys), sophisticated renal-sparing surgery is necessary. Laparoscopy is used in extremely carefully selected cases of small incidentally found lesions when the contralateral kidney is healthy.

No consensus exists for monitoring of recurrence or progression after surgery, but most oncologists obtain a chest x-ray and liver function tests (and occasionally a sedimentation rate) every 4 to 6 months. Performing imaging studies, particularly CT, at periodic intervals is controversial and must be individualized based on the patient's estimated prognosis and the tumor's original pathologic stage.

Metastatic disease: Renal adenocarcinoma is resistant to cytotoxic chemotherapeutic drugs. Immunotherapeutic approaches have been used, but few tumors have been cured. Interleukin-2 (IL-2) and α-interferon are two cytokines that produce a low but reproducible response. Although sustained complete responses can occur, few cases are curable. Surgery to resect metastatic disease is highly controversial.

Patients with bony metastasis and substantial cortical destruction (particularly of the long bones) may require preemptive medullary rod placement and local radiation therapy to prevent pathologic fractures, thereby protecting these patients from incapacitation.

BLADDER CANCER

The annual incidence of bladder cancer in the USA is 20 new cases/100,000 persons > 40 years, and the male:female ratio among whites is at least 2:1 (29.6 vs. 7.6 cases/100,000). Racial predisposition is variable and probably geographic.

Various risk factors have been identified (see TABLE 101–2). The strongest risk factor is exposure to heterocyclic organic compounds, particularly arylamines. Bladder cancer was one of the first occupational-related diseases; aniline dye workers contracted bladder cancer at alarmingly high rates. Smoking also confers a significant risk for bladder cancer. Genetic polymorphisms detected at loci of genes whose products are associated with carcinogen metabolism may constitute an additional risk factor. However, there are no strong familial risk factors nor syndromes with a high risk of concurrent bladder cancer. The rare congenital anomaly of bladder exstrophy is associated with development of bladder cancer later in life. In Northern Africa, development of squamous cell carcinoma of the bladder is associated with long-standing schistosomiasis.

Pathology

The vast majority of bladder tumors in the elderly are of epithelial (or urothelial) cell origin, and in the USA and Europe, most are transitional cell carcinomas (TCCs). Bladder tumors can be low grade (noninvasive papillary tumors that grow exophytically within the bladder lumen) or high

TABLE 101–2.   RISK FACTORS ASSOCIATED WITH BLADDER CANCER

Occupational	Manufacturing industries*: Chemical dyes, textiles, tires and rubber, chemicals, petroleum, aluminum processing
	Service industries: Painters, truck drivers, beauticians
Chemical exposure	2-Naphthylamine, benzidine, 4-aminophenyl, nitrosamines
Behavioral	Cigarette smoking
Chronic infection	Schistosomiasis† (primarily in Egypt)
	Genitourinary tuberculosis
	Indwelling catheter†
	Urinary calculi†
Iatrogenic	Cyclophosphamide use
	Long-term phenacetin use
	Pelvic radiation†

* Data are not precise enough to specify which compounds are the causative agents.
† Primarily squamous cell carcinomas.

grade (more insidious sessile [broad-based] tumors that have the propensity for early invasion and metastasis). Bladder cancer often metastasizes to the lymph nodes, lungs, liver, and bone.

Carcinoma in situ (CIS) of the bladder, an unfortunate nomenclature because of the common inference with other organ sites of relative benignity, is a very aggressive, usually multifocal, high-grade cancer that commonly becomes frankly invasive.

Symptoms and Signs

Two clinical presentations are common: gross hematuria and irritated voiding (frequency, dysuria). Painless gross hematuria is an important symptom that should not be ignored even in a patient taking aspirin or warfarin; indeed, a therapeutic anticoagulated state can unmask urinary tract tumors, particularly the ominous, invasive tumors less prone to bleed.

Papillary tumors tend to bleed grossly. Sessile tumors are less prone to manifest as gross hematuria but are still likely to be detectable as microhematuria. Bladder CIS commonly manifests with microhematuria and modest pyuria in patients complaining of urgency, frequency, dysuria, and strangury (pain referred to the urethral meatus at the end of voiding). Bladder tumors should always be considered in patients with urine culture–negative pyuria, especially with concurrent microhematuria.

Diagnosis and Staging

The diagnosis of bladder cancer is made primarily by visual confirmation of proliferative lesions within the bladder during cystoscopy; every patient with gross hematuria, unexplained microhematuria, or persistent irritative voiding symptoms should undergo this procedure. CIS is not a visible proliferation but often appears as epithelial erythema (the result of submucosal neoangiogenesis) and can be diagnosed by endoscopic biopsy.

Urine cytology can be helpful but is inadequate as a screening tool because exfoliated cells from lower-grade tumors are difficult to differentiate from benign epithelia. Mass screening of high-risk patients is controversial because of the low specificity of available laboratory tests. Radiographically, an occasional large tumor can create a filling defect seen on imaging studies using IV contrast, but contrast studies also are insensitive as screening tools for cancer.

Most tumors recognized at the time of office cystoscopy are best staged and treated initially with endoscopic resection (transurethral resection). The tumor is resected to its base; then an additional resection of the base with contained bladder wall muscle is performed to stage the tumor for the possible presence of invasive disease. Biopsy of adjacent suspicious mucosa for CIS is obtained. For low-grade, noninvasive lesions, endoscopic resection is sufficient for staging and treatment. For high-grade (particularly invasive) disease, further staging is needed. Bone scan, abdominal and pelvic CT, and chest x-rays are used to evaluate disease stage. When observed, ureteral obstruction (usually the result of locally invasive cancer at or near the ureteral orifice) is often an ominous sign of locally advanced disease.

Prognosis and Treatment

Recurrent, low-grade disease: Although endoscopic resection is definitive, new lesions subsequently develop within the bladder in > 40% of patients. Monitoring for these new lesions is performed by surveillance cystoscopy every 3 to 6 months. Only a small percentage of patients have gradual worsening of their disease (upgrading and concomitant invasion), thus placing them at some disease-specific risk of death.

Intravesical therapy is used for patients with CIS, and adjuvant postresection intravesical therapy is valuable for patients with multiply recurrent low-grade tumors. Antineoplastic cytotoxic drugs (eg, mitomycin C, thiotepa, doxorubicin) have been used effectively in this setting. An immunotherapeutic approach using intravesical bacille Calmette-Guérin (BCG) is highly effective, particularly for CIS, although it has a higher toxicity profile.

Invasive disease: Mortality rates have decreased substantially for whites and blacks of both sexes with invasive disease—about 24% overall from 1973 to 1996. Early diagnosis and aggressive surgical intervention account for this improvement. The standard of care for invasive, high-grade bladder cancer is complete removal of the bladder and adjacent organs (prostate and seminal vesicles in males; uterus and adnexa in females). Partial cystectomy is rarely appropriate because of the high propensity for multifocal disease throughout the bladder.

Urine excretion is managed by the construction of urinary reservoirs from the intestine. The simplest is the ileal conduit. The ureters are anastomosed to a resected piece of the small bowel, which then tunnels through the abdominal wall to form a stoma; an external appliance is applied ("glued" to the skin) around the stoma. More complex reservoirs provide substantial improvement in quality of life, particularly for patients who object to an external urostomy. A continent reservoir has no external appliance; the patient catheterizes a continent stoma to drain the urine. Another option is construction of an orthotopic reservoir anastomosed to the urethra.

Surgical mortality from cystectomy is now only about 2%. However, for patients who are poor surgical risks, external beam radiation therapy is an option, although it is considered inferior to cystectomy, particularly in patients with concurrent CIS. Complications of radiation therapy include radiation cystitis, bladder contracture, and radiation proctitis; preservation of the bladder has been attempted with systemic IV cisplatin, a chemotherapeutic drug used in this case as a radiosensitizer to improve the therapeutic effect.

Multimodal approaches for invasive bladder cancer are increasingly used, although their effect on survival is still controversial. Treatment with induction (ie, neoadjuvant or presurgical) or adjuvant (ie, immediately postsurgical) chemotherapy is now commonplace.

Metastatic disease: Advanced disease is treated with systemic multi-agent chemotherapy. Use of methotrexate, vinblastine, doxorubicin, and cisplatin (M-VAC) or cisplatin, methotrexate, and vinblastine (CMV) IV combination therapy is standard. However, although response rates exceed 60%, the responses are not durable, and the cure rate is only about 10%. Prolongation of survival has been enhanced by surgical resection, when applicable, after chemotherapy, although this role for surgery is controversial. The increased survival obviously is limited to the subset of patients with potentially resectable disease. Newer combination drug therapies are being explored. Radiation therapy is reserved for palliation, particularly for patients with symptomatic bony metastases; radiation to a neobladder risks serious complications.

RENAL PELVIC AND URETERAL TUMORS

As in the bladder, the preponderance of renal pelvic and ureteral tumors are urothelial transitional cell carcinomas (TCCs). Incidence is considerably lower than in the bladder—such tumors represent only about 4% of all urothelial tumors. However, there is an unexplained predisposition for inhabitants of the Balkans to develop upper urinary tract TCC (Balkan nephropathy); in that population, half of all renal pelvic tumors are TCC. The incidence of concurrent bilateral TCC tumors is 10 times higher than in inhabitants of other geographic areas. The biology of these tumors, including their metastatic behavior, is similar to that of TCC of the bladder.

Symptoms, Signs, and Diagnosis

Hematuria is the most common presenting symptom of renal pelvic and ureteral tumors. Retrograde urography performed in conjunction with cystoscopy remains the most definitive imaging study for characterizing these lesions.

Ureteral tumors uncommonly cause renal colic symptoms (unless a blood clot functions as an intermittently obstructive foreign body); however, retrograde urography commonly shows ureteral tumors as obstructive lesions with varying degrees of hydronephrosis above.

Renal pelvic tumors less commonly cause hydronephrosis (unless the tumor obstructs the ureteropelvic junction). On intravenous urography, a filling defect in the renal collecting system is seen. On CT, the major differential diagnosis is between TCC of the renal pelvis and adenocarcinoma of the renal parenchyma.

Although x-ray imaging of these lesions is critical for initial diagnosis (in contrast with diagnosis of bladder cancer), cytologic or histologic confirmation of the diagnosis is imperative before treatment. Endoscopic catheterization of the ureter for cytologic collections, usually after fluoroscopically controlled endoscopic brushing of the lesion, is usually performed with anesthesia. Miniaturized ureteroscopes permit direct visualization and biopsy of these lesions.

Treatment

Renal pelvic lesions are treated surgically with total nephroureterectomy. Radiation therapy has no role because of the poor tolerance of renal parenchyma to external beam radiation therapy. However, newer techniques permit renal preservation. Low-grade ureteral lesions (and also renal pelvic lesions clearly not contiguous with renal parenchyma) can be fulgurated with laser energy transmitted by fiber through a ureteroscope. Distal high-grade lesions can be managed by partial ureterectomy with reconstruction (including bowel interposition), unless multifocal carcinoma in situ demands total nephroureterectomy. Although the biologic risk and rationale for adjuvant chemotherapy for high-grade invasive disease of the renal pelvis and ureter is similar to that of the bladder, the rarity of this disease has precluded a full evaluation of its clinical effect. Management of metastasis is essentially identical to that of bladder cancer.

URETHRAL TUMORS

Tumors of the female or male urethra are extremely rare. In women, 75% of cases occur after age 50. In men, the peak incidence occurs at age 58. Perhaps the most striking etiologic insight into this disease is the detection of oncogenic forms of human papillomavirus (HPV) within the genome of urethral tumors (in > 60% of tumors in women; 30% in men [but far higher if tumors of just the distal male urethra are analyzed]). Consequently, in women, the urethra is now recognized as one of multiple potential sites of presumed HPV carcinogenesis, although the cervix remains by far the most common site of clinically significant disease.

Urethral tumors invade adjacent structures early in the course of disease and often are not diagnosed until they are locally advanced. Early metastasis affects the external groin nodes or the pelvic (obturator) nodes.

Symptoms, Signs, and Diagnosis

The majority of female patients have a long-standing history of urinary frequency; most have been treated for urethral syndrome—a complex and poorly understood condition of hypersensitivity of the pelvic floor. The development of hematuria and obstructive symptoms or even of frank urinary retention necessitates reevaluation of the woman's voiding problems. A urethral tumor is sometimes first diagnosed by a gynecologist as a vaginal mass.

In men, urethral tumors are extremely insidious. Only occasionally does the patient have hematuria or even bloody urethral discharge. A gradual onset of obstructive voiding symptoms (not unlike prostatism of bladder neck origin) is common. The majority of men present clinically in a manner indistinguishable from that of benign urethral stricture and are dilated routinely without a more extensive assessment. In more advanced cases, a perineal or penile mass is occasionally palpable; in the most extreme cases, a fungating mass with urethral fistulization is encountered.

Cystourethroscopy is the preferred diagnostic procedure. Staging is primarily by CT; MRI can help assess the extent of disease but is more accurate in men.

Treatment

Because of the rarity of these tumors, algorithms of optimal management have not been developed.

In women, small distal lesions generally can be incised and treated with adjuvant radiation therapy, if no gross evidence of nodal involvement is seen. More proximal lesions may be treated with interstitial brachytherapy (insertion of cytotoxic radiation-emitting pellets), but many require total anterior exenteration with wide excision of the anterior vagina (similar to treatment of bladder cancer in women).

In men, total emasculation with cystoprostatectomy and musculocutaneous flap reconstruction of the perineum may be necessary in advanced cases; adjuvant radiation therapy is usually also used in such cases. Chemotherapy has been used in conjunction with these tumors, but its value has not been established. Presence of groin adenopathy may require groin dissection; involvement of pelvic nodes may increase the extent of dissection, and such extended surgery into the pelvis is controversial because of the poor prognosis despite aggressive therapy.

GASTROINTESTINAL DISORDERS

G

102   AGING AND THE GASTROINTESTINAL TRACT

Because of the large functional reserve capacity of most of the gastrointestinal (GI) tract, aging has relatively little effect on GI function. For example, although aging is associated with a reduction in the number of neurons in the myenteric plexus, only subtle changes occur in gut motility under normal conditions. However, aging is associated with an increased prevalence of several GI disorders, including those induced by drugs. Therefore, clinically significant abnormalities in GI function, including reduction in food intake, should be evaluated and not attributed to aging. The presentation of some GI disorders may be atypical in the elderly, possibly reflecting a reduction in visceral perception.

ORAL REGION

Taste sensation decreases with age.∎ Elderly persons demonstrate an impaired ability to identify food by taste. A number of drugs and diseases can also affect taste, and reversible causes of taste impairment must always be considered.

Although dentition may be well preserved in the absence of caries and periodontal disease, poor dentition is a major contributor to impaired chewing and reduced caloric intake. Tooth loss in the elderly has declined dramatically, although in some populations > 60% of the elderly are edentulous.

∎ see page 1025

A modest decrease in saliva production occurs with age.[1] The significance of this change is uncertain, although it has been suggested that susceptibility to esophageal mucosal injury may increase.

ESOPHAGUS

In healthy persons, aging has only minor effects on esophageal motor and sensory function. Upper esophageal sphincter pressure decreases with age (with a delay in swallow-induced relaxation), as does the amplitude of secondary peristalsis; however, lower esophageal sphincter pressure does not seem to change. Cerebral evoked potentials elicited by esophageal balloon distention have a prolonged latency and reduced amplitude in healthy elderly persons compared with younger persons, which indicates a deficit in afferent sensory pathways from the esophagus. However, none of these changes appears to be clinically significant. Previous reports of presbyesophagus (a condition associated with marked abnormalities in esophageal peristalsis) are almost certainly attributable to neurologic or vascular disorders that affect esophageal function.

Gastroesophageal reflux appears to be more common in elderly than in younger persons, even in those who are asymptomatic, possibly because of a reduction in the intra-abdominal length of the lower esophageal sphincter and an increased incidence of hiatus hernia.

Many drugs, including nonsteroidal anti-inflammatory drugs (NSAIDs), potassium chloride, tetracycline antibiotics, quinidine, alendronate, ferrous sulfate, and theophylline, can cause esophageal injury. The elderly are at high risk of pill-induced esophagitis and its complications, particularly when esophageal transit is delayed. Drugs should, accordingly, be swallowed in an upright position, followed by a drink of at least 150 mL.

STOMACH

Although aging has no significant effect on secretion of acid and pepsin by the stomach, conditions that reduce acid production are common. Reductions in basal and stimulated gastric acid secretion that occur with age are now recognized to be attributable to atrophic gastritis.[2] In the absence of atrophic changes in the gastric mucosa, the number of acid-secreting (parietal) cells probably increases with age.

Evidence indicates that aging is associated with a diminished capacity of the gastric mucosa to resist damage, even in healthy persons. A number of factors that may be important in cytoprotection, including

---

mucosal blood flow and gastric mucosal prostaglandin, glutathione, bicarbonate, and mucus secretion, diminish with age. These changes may account for the impaired barrier function of the gastric mucosa and the increased risk of peptic ulcer disease in the elderly,**◻** particularly in association with the use of NSAIDs. Likewise, these changes may contribute to the observation that although most gastric and duodenal ulcers are associated with *Helicobacter pylori* in the elderly, the association appears to be weaker than in younger persons.

Aging is associated with a modest slowing of gastric emptying, which may predispose to anorexia and weight loss by prolonging gastric distention and increasing meal-induced fullness and satiety.

SMALL INTESTINE

Aging has only minor effects on the structure of the small intestine, with some alteration in villus architecture and a reduction in the neuronal content of the myenteric plexus. Aging does not result in major changes in small-intestine motility, transit, permeability, or absorption. Although changes in small-intestine immune function occur, there is no evidence that these changes are clinically important.

Small-intestine bacterial overgrowth**◻** is common among the elderly and is usually associated with malnutrition. Predisposing conditions include hypochlorhydria, diverticulosis, and diabetes mellitus. Bacterial overgrowth may have relatively nonspecific symptoms (eg, anorexia, weight loss) and results in malabsorption of a number of micronutrients, including folate, iron, calcium, and vitamins K and B_6. Bacterial overgrowth is also a cause of diarrhea in the elderly.**◻**

With age, calcium absorption diminishes, even in healthy persons who are vitamin D replete. In such cases, the reduction appears to be due to intestinal resistance to the action of 1,25-dihydroxyvitamin D, not to a reduction in the plasma concentrations of this hormone. Vitamin D deficiency also occurs often in the elderly and is associated with malabsorption of calcium. Malabsorption of calcium is almost certainly a major factor in age-related bone loss in men and women; accordingly, the dietary calcium requirement is higher in the elderly.**◻**

LARGE INTESTINE

Aging does not appear to be associated with major changes in colonic or anorectal motility. Rectal compliance and tone are normal, but the perception of anorectal distention is reduced in the elderly. This

◻ see page 1042   **◻** see also TABLE 111–1 on page 1098   **◻** see page 1085
◻ see page 478

reduction in rectal wall sensitivity may play a role in the pathogenesis of constipation. **1**

Fecal incontinence occurs in up to 50% of nursing home residents. **2** Common causes are constipation with fecal impaction, laxative use, neurologic disorders, and colorectal disorders (eg, traumatic anorectal injury). Fecal incontinence is often associated with diarrhea but should be distinguished from diarrhea when possible. Management should focus on the identification and correction of causes.

The incidence of diverticulosis and colon cancer increases with age; ischemic colitis occurs almost exclusively in the elderly, as a result of the increased prevalence of atherosclerosis. Inflammatory bowel disease, often regarded as a disease of young adults, has a smaller incidence peak in the elderly (8th decade) and may present with complications (eg, toxic megacolon).

PANCREAS

The pancreas undergoes substantial structural changes with age, including a decrease in overall weight, duct hyperplasia, and lobular fibrosis. Surprisingly, these changes do not affect pancreatic exocrine function significantly; pancreatic enzyme and bicarbonate levels decrease only modestly, so that fat and carbohydrate absorption are unaffected by age. Aging is well recognized as a major risk factor for glucose intolerance and type II (non–insulin-dependent) diabetes mellitus. The latter is attributable to decreased insulin secretion (as a result of decreased responsiveness of the pancreatic β cell to glucose) and increased insulin resistance.

LIVER

Age-related changes occurring in the liver are macroscopic, histologic, biochemical, or related to blood flow or stress. The overall survival of transplanted livers is not dramatically different in older and younger patients, and older patients are increasingly undergoing liver transplantations. Evidence suggests that livers from donors ≥ 65 may be viable for transplantation.

Macroscopic changes: The liver becomes brown with age. Increased lipofuscin (a brown pigment) in hepatocytes accounts for much of this change. The brown pigment buildup represents a lifetime accumulation of unexcretable metabolic residue of lipids and proteins and has no known clinical significance. The liver also becomes more

---

1 see page 1080   **2** see page 1092

fibrotic with age. However, the increased capsular and parenchymal fibrosis does not represent cirrhosis.

Hepatic volume decreases by about 17 to 28% between ages 40 and 65. Hepatic weight decreases by about 25% between ages 20 and 70 in men and women.

Histologic changes: Studies of age-related changes in hepatic fine structure have reported disparate results. Although human hepatocytes probably enlarge with age, some studies report no change. Several animal studies confirm that hepatocytes enlarge with age, while others report that they enlarge with maturation but shrink with age.

Although some studies report no significant changes in the nuclei of human hepatocytes with age, other studies report polyploidy, increases in nuclear size, and double nuclei. The number of mitochondria per hepatic volume decreases. However, the number of swollen, vacuolated mitochondria in hepatocytes increases, as does the number of lysosomes and dense bodies.

Biochemical changes: Aging does not alter liver function test results (ie, serum bilirubin, aspartate aminotransferase, alanine aminotransferase, and hepatic alkaline phosphatase levels), which reflect hepatic damage rather than overall hepatic function. The synthesis of clotting factors is also unaffected by age. Although serum bilirubin levels decrease with age, < 0.2% of test results are below the normal range in elderly patients.

Protein synthesis appears to decrease with age, although the degree to which it does so varies widely among various proteins. For example, normally serum protein and albumin levels decrease slightly but remain within the normal range. No sex-related differences are apparent from animal studies.

Protein degradation, including that of some enzymes, appears to decrease with age. Similarly, the accumulation of abnormal proteins with age may reflect a decreased ability of cells to degrade these proteins. A significant increase in the half-life of abnormal hepatic proteins has been observed in mice. The extent to which these abnormal proteins are functional or represent inadequately metabolized "junk" proteins is unclear.

The microsomal enzymes are located in the smooth endoplasmic reticulum of hepatocytes and are responsible for much of the biotransformation of drugs. Enzymatic actions are classified as phase 1 and phase 2 reactions.◨ Phase 1 reactions involve oxidation, reduction, or hydrolysis; they convert the parent drug into more polar metabolites. Phase 2 reactions involve conjugation of the parent drug or metabolite with an additional substrate (eg, glucuronic acid, sulfate), achieving the same result.

◨see also page 57

Phase 1 reactions decrease linearly with age, whereas phase 2 reactions remain essentially unchanged. Most studies suggest that phase 1 enzyme activity per gram of liver tissue is actually preserved and that decreased phase 1 activity results primarily from an age-related decline in hepatic mass. Why phase 2 reactions are relatively preserved despite the decline in hepatic mass is unclear. It may be because of compensatory extrahepatic conjugation.

The older liver may be less responsive to enzyme induction by some agents.

Blood flow: Hepatic blood flow decreases by 35% between ages 40 and 65 largely because of a decrease in splanchnic blood flow. The decreased hepatic blood flow, together with decreased hepatic weight, accounts for decreases in hepatic drug elimination of some compounds in the elderly. ◻

Response to stress: The liver's ability to withstand stress may decrease with age. Many hepatotoxic drugs cause more severe injury in livers of older persons.

Hepatic regeneration is delayed but not greatly impaired with age. In aging rats, the capacity for hepatic regeneration remains intact, but the rate of regeneration decreases. The regulation of regeneration, however, is poorly understood. Some effects are clearly extrahepatic, including decreased serum levels of epidermal growth factor (EGF) and transforming growth factor-α. In elderly persons, hepatocytes seem less able to respond to hepatotropic growth factors (eg, EGF). Studies have demonstrated a decrease in EGF receptors and their binding capacity for EGF. Therefore, delayed hepatic regeneration is clinically important for elderly patients undergoing liver resections—mortality rates resulting from liver resection are higher in patients > 60 than in those < 60. Postoperative morbidity and mortality, however, are usually not due to liver failure but rather to extrahepatic complications of the surgery.

GALLBLADDER

Various age-related changes in bile flow and bile acid secretion occur with age. In animals, basal bile flow and taurocholate (cholyltaurine)-stimulated bile flow decrease. In humans, bile acid synthesis declines, reflecting a significant reduction in the hydroxylation of cholesterol (cholesterol 7 α-hydroxylase). A similar age-related decrease in hepatic extraction of low-density lipoprotein cholesterol from the blood occurs, further elevating serum cholesterol levels. These changes may contribute to the increased incidence of cholelithiasis (gallstones) and coronary artery disease in the elderly.

The prevalence of gallstones increases with age. About 30% of women and 20% of men have cholelithiasis by age 70, and 40% of

◻ see also page 57

women have cholelithiasis by age 80. Most men do not accumulate more stones after age 65. Both stimulated and fasting concentrations of cholecystokinin (a peptide hormone released from duodenal mucosa that contracts the gallbladder and relaxes the biliary sphincter) are higher in elderly persons, which may also partly explain the increased incidence of cholelithiasis in the elderly. However, gallbladder emptying rates and fasting and nonfasting gallbladder volumes do not change with age.

103 ■ ENDOSCOPIC GASTROINTESTINAL PROCEDURES

Viewing the body cavities with tubes is called endoscopy, whether esophagogastroduodenoscopy (gastroscopy or upper intestinal endoscopy) or colonoscopy (endoscopy of the large intestine). Recently, the term endoscopy has been used to refer to upper intestinal endoscopy and not colonoscopy. Although originally considered complementary to a barium x-ray, endoscopy is now often used as the primary tool for evaluating the gastrointestinal (GI) tract. Conventional x-rays cannot identify color changes (eg, in gastritis), bleeding, or vascular malformations. GI endoscopy is particularly valuable in elderly patients because their symptoms may be atypical.

Indications

Endoscopy can be used diagnostically (eg, to visually define and biopsy abnormalities) and therapeutically (eg, to remove stones from the bile duct and to place a stent through a bile duct compressed by a malignant tumor, which may avoid the need for surgery). Endoscopy performed early for GI bleeding may help the physician determine if early surgery is necessary. ■

Procedure

Before endoscopy, food and drink may have to be avoided to allow the stomach to empty, or a purgative may be needed to cleanse the colon. Because transient bacteremia infrequently occurs during endoscopy, patients at high risk of infection—those with valvular heart

---

■ see page 1107

disease (eg, rheumatic heart disease, valvular prosthesis), neutropenia, or a surgical shunt for renal dialysis—should receive antibiotics (usually ampicillin or gentamicin) before the procedure. Most endoscopies are performed while the patient is sedated. Usually, benzodiazepines are given for sedation; doses may need to be reduced by 50 to 75% for elderly patients. During the procedure, the physician or assistant should monitor skin color, pulse, and respirations often. Continuous monitoring of oxygen saturation levels with a pulse oximeter may benefit the elderly patient.

Complications

The elderly usually tolerate endoscopy well, but complications are more common than in younger patients. Not only are older tissues more fragile and more easily traumatized, but elderly patients generally have other medical conditions (eg, heart failure) that may be exacerbated by the preparation or the procedure. Elderly persons may also find aggressive cleansing protocols difficult to tolerate. The current trend is to perform elective examinations on an outpatient basis rather than to admit patients to the hospital. When cathartics are prescribed to cleanse the colon, the patient's hydration needs to be maintained.

ESOPHAGOGASTRODUODENOSCOPY

The goal of esophagogastroduodenoscopy is to visualize the entire upper GI tract (to the second portion of the duodenum).

Indications

Diagnostic indications include obtaining fluid and tissue specimens and exploring upper GI symptoms or abnormalities seen on an upper GI x-ray series. Any pathologic process (eg, ulcer, mass, irregularity) can be characterized by inspection and biopsy. Brush cytology may aid diagnosis in malignant disease.

Esophagogastroduodenoscopy may be used to monitor the healing rate of a gastric ulcer but is usually unnecessary with a duodenal ulcer. Periodic endoscopy and biopsy in Barrett's syndrome, a premalignant process, can detect early evidence of cancer. Esophagogastroduodenoscopy can best identify the site of upper GI bleeding and should be performed as soon as the patient is stable.

Therapeutic indications include dilating esophageal strictures using a dilator threaded over an endoscopically placed guide wire or using a balloon catheter passed through the endoscope. Obstructive esophageal or gastric neoplasms may be vaporized endoscopically with a laser wave guide passed through the gastroscope or with photodynamic therapy in patients who are not surgical candidates. With a more extensive obstructive tumor, enteral nutrition can be reestablished by precisely locating the tumor endoscopically and placing an esophageal stent prosthesis using a guide wire.

The use of esophagogastroduodenoscopy to treat GI bleeding has markedly enhanced the value of this procedure. GI hemorrhage, which is not well tolerated by elderly persons, requires immediate attention; the endoscopic team should be alerted as soon as the patient is first seen. Almost all episodes of upper GI bleeding can be controlled by using endoscopic injection therapy with epinephrine or absolute alcohol or by using a thermal coagulation device. The mortality rate in elderly patients ranges from 6 to 10%.

Sclerotherapy for esophageal varices and injection therapy for bleeding vessels may be performed during the initial diagnostic examination by passing a long, flexible needle-tipped catheter through the endoscope. A new technique, rubber band ligation of varices, can be accomplished rapidly with relatively low morbidity in the elderly. Polyps may be resected using a wire snare loop and an electrocoagulation current to prevent bleeding.

Usually, submucosal lesions cannot be resected endoscopically. Removing foreign bodies such as dentures from the esophagus or stomach may require special maneuvers, including attaching to the tip of the endoscope a shield that folds over sharp objects to prevent esophageal injury during extraction. Foreign bodies smaller than a dime often pass spontaneously and may not require endoscopic removal. Food bezoars can sometimes be broken up with the snare, biopsy forceps, or a strong jet of water.

Percutaneous endoscopic gastrostomy (a nonoperative procedure in which a gastric feeding port is inserted) has largely replaced surgical creation of a feeding gastrostomy. This procedure can be accomplished at the bedside with little risk and is ideally suited for the elderly patient with deglutitive problems.

Contraindications

Absolute contraindications are a recent myocardial infarction and an acute perforated viscus. However, elderly patients with cardiorespiratory disease and dyspnea are at special risk for complications. Even without sedation, these patients have a lowered oxygen partial pressure; with sedation, some are particularly vulnerable to respiratory depression. In these patients, using a small-caliber endoscope and administering additional oxygen during the procedure may help.

Procedure and Complications

For most patients, restricting food and drink for 6 hours before the examination is the only preparation. Those with achalasia or gastric outlet obstruction may have retained food for days and may require lavage to empty the esophagus or stomach. Light sedation with an IV opioid and/or a benzodiazepine may be combined with a local anesthetic applied to the posterior pharynx. After removing the patient's dentures or nonpermanent bridges, the examiner passes the instrument under direct vision through the pharynx to examine the entire esophagus and stomach and the first two portions of the duodenum. An x-ray is not a prerequisite for esophagogastroduodenoscopy because the gastroscope can be passed safely under direct vision even in patients with dysphagia and a possible Zenker's diverticulum. The procedure can be performed in 15 to 30 minutes.

Perforation occurs in 0.03% of patients and death from complications in about 0.006%. Most complications are caused by sedative drugs and include arrhythmias, aspiration, and, rarely, cardiac arrest.

SIGMOIDOSCOPY AND ANOSCOPY

These procedures permit examination of the distal large bowel without extensive preparation or sedation. Disease within the anal canal is best seen with an anoscope—a short tubular instrument with an acutely angulated bevel that allows direct visualization of the canal and the distal rectum. The rigid sigmoidoscope, when passed to its full length of 25 cm, permits inspection of the rectum and distal sigmoid colon. The 60-cm flexible sigmoidoscope permits inspection of the rectum, sigmoid, and most of the descending colon.

Performing a digital rectal examination along with sigmoidoscopy and anoscopy allows the physician to discover and treat precancerous polyps. It is important to discover and remove benign lesions within 6 cm of the anus (the area in which cancer usually requires removal of the rectum and anus), and thus avoid the need for colostomy if the lesions become malignant.

Indications

The flexible sigmoidoscope may be used to evaluate the left side of the colon, where two thirds of neoplasms appear. Rigid or flexible sigmoidoscopy can evaluate the distal colon for suspected disease; either procedure may complement a barium enema. Anoscopy is best suited for visualizing perianal problems (eg, fissures, fistulas, hemorrhoids).

Sigmoidoscopy and anoscopy are valuable for early detection of most colorectal polyps and cancer, which increase in incidence with age and have a predominantly left-sided distribution. For an asymptomatic person, sigmoidoscopy is recommended every 3 to 5 years for patients > 50 years to diagnose adenomas at a stage when their removal will prevent development of colorectal cancer. If polyps are discovered during flexible sigmoidoscopy, they should not be removed because more extensive preparation and complete evaluation of the colon are required.

Contraindications

A recent myocardial infarction contraindicates this procedure. Flexible sigmoidoscopy should not be substituted when indications for colonoscopy (anemia, positive results of a fecal occult blood test, polypectomy) are present.

Procedure and Complications

One or two phosphate enemas cleanse the bowel adequately. Sedation is not required. The patient usually lies on the left side for flexible sigmoidoscopy but assumes the knee-chest position for rigid sigmoidoscopy or anoscopy.

Complications are extremely rare but may include perforation. Air insufflation or instrument looping in the colon may cause cramps and discomfort.

COLONOSCOPY

The goal of colonoscopy is to visualize the entire colon, including the cecal caput. An experienced examiner accomplishes this goal in > 90% of cases, but the inexperienced examiner may achieve total intubation in < 80%.

Indications

Diagnostic indications include evaluating a lower GI symptom such as rectal bleeding or a change in bowel habits.

Colonoscopy is often used as a screening tool in patients without symptoms or signs who are at high risk of colon cancer. No data indicate when to stop screening; opinions range from age 75 to 85 when no other life-limiting disease is present. Surveillance of patients previously found to have polyps or cancer should continue for the rest of their lives, but should be stopped when it appears unlikely that continued follow-up will prolong life expectancy. With colonoscopy, the physician can detect colon cancer early (even when it is in a premalignant stage) and remove polyps before invasive cancer develops. In the past several decades, the trend has been for cancer to develop in the more proximal colon; therefore, a flexible sigmoidoscopy may not be the best procedure when cancer is suspected.

Colonoscopy may be difficult during acute, massive lower GI bleeding,◨ but its use in such cases has been advocated by some investigators. Because 10% of patients admitted to an intensive care unit with suspected colonic bleeding have an upper GI source, esophagogastroduodenoscopy often should precede colonoscopy. This schema provides answers rapidly and efficiently, thereby decreasing the time needed for a diagnosis while providing an opportunity for endoscopic therapy.

◨see page 1111

The source of unexplained GI bleeding or iron deficiency anemia is often determined by colonoscopy because the blood loss often originates in the colon, an area for which x-rays may be inaccurate. However, colonoscopy has a low diagnostic yield when used to identify the cause of chronic abdominal pain. **Therapeutic indications** include removal of colonic polyps. Bleeding sites (eg, arteriovenous malformations) may be treated with electrocoagulation, and volvulus may be decompressed, as may the dilated colon in Ogilvie's syndrome (acute colonic pseudo-obstruction). Laser vaporization of obstructive rectosigmoid neoplasms may provide symptomatic relief. Strictures may be dilated with balloons or bougies. If the stricture is malignant and symptomatic but cancer spread precludes the likelihood of a surgical cure, a self-expanding metal stent can be positioned across the narrow segment via colonoscopy.

Contraindications

Absolute contraindications are fulminant colitis, acute diverticulitis, perforated viscus, and a recent myocardial infarction. Poor colon preparation is a relative contraindication.

Procedure and Complications

The colon must be clean. One or two days of a liquid diet and a cathartic usually suffice. Two oral doses of sodium phosphate or a 4-L electrolyte solution containing polyethylene glycol should be administered. Electrolyte and fluid shifts must be avoided in the elderly patient with cardiovascular and renal instability; the electrolyte solution is safely tolerated. An IV opioid and/or a benzodiazepine generally is given for sedation. General anesthesia is usually unnecessary and undesirable.

During routine colonoscopy, the risk of perforation is about 0.1%, and the risk of bleeding is nil. After polypectomy, perforation occurs in 0.3% of patients and bleeding in 1.5%. Complications from sedative use include arrhythmias, aspiration, and, rarely, cardiac arrest.

ENDOSCOPIC RETROGRADE CHOLANGIOPANCREATOGRAPHY

Endoscopic retrograde cholangiopancreatography (ERCP) enables x-ray visualization of the pancreatic duct and the bile ducts by dye injected through the endoscope.

Indications

Diagnostic indications include determining the cause of jaundice and identifying the site of an obstruction with a high degree of accuracy. The procedure also can demonstrate ductal abnormalities in a nonjaundiced patient when the clinical presentation suggests biliary disease, pancreatic cancer, or pancreatitis. ERCP helps evaluate chronic pancreatitis or pancreatic pseudocyst preoperatively. Magnetic resonance cholangiopancreatography is a noninvasive procedure that may replace diagnostic, but not therapeutic, ERCP. If symptoms, signs, or laboratory tests suggest common bile duct stones, ERCP is indicated to diagnose and remove the stones before laparoscopic removal of the gallbladder, **❶** because exploring the common bile duct during laparoscopic cholecystectomy is difficult. Pressure measurements, which can be performed in highly specialized medical centers, help diagnose dysfunction in the sphincter of Oddi.

ERCP is not indicated for evaluating abdominal pain in the absence of symptoms, signs, or laboratory findings that suggest biliary tract or pancreatic disease, nor is it indicated for evaluating suspected gallbladder disease without evidence of bile duct disease. ERCP has little value diagnostically when pancreatic cancer has already been demonstrated by ultrasound or CT.

Therapeutic indications include removal of stones from the bile duct. In endoscopic sphincterotomy, the muscular fibers at the distal bile duct sphincter are cut to allow the passage of stones that cannot pass spontaneously because of the narrow orifice or large stone size. Emergency sphincterotomy is the procedure of choice for acute gallstone pancreatitis and for stone-induced acute cholangitis. **❷** Large stones may be crushed by a lithotriptor or may be dissolved over several days by chemical instillation via an indwelling nasobiliary tube placed through the sphincterotomy. A benign stricture may be dilated with a balloon. A malignant pancreatic tumor obstructing the bile duct can be relieved by positioning a stent in the common bile duct. With relief of jaundice, the elderly patient will become more comfortable even as the disease advances. Therapeutic ERCP is often used for biliary complications of laparoscopic cholecystectomy (eg, duct obstruction from clips, bile leakage from the cystic duct stump, removal of retained stones). Currently, stones in the gallbladder cannot be treated endoscopically.

Contraindications and Procedure

Absolute contraindications include a recent myocardial infarction and perforated viscus.

The patient should not eat or drink for 6 hours before the procedure to empty the stomach and duodenum. If the patient has recently ingested barium, an x-ray should be obtained to ensure that the barium is not superimposed on the areas of interest. An IV opioid and/or a benzodiazepine is given for sedation.

An endoscope is passed orally to the duodenum. Then under direct vision, a cannula is placed into the ampulla of Vater. Under fluoroscopic

❶ see page 1125   ❷ see page 1126

monitoring, a dye is injected that flows retrograde (or counter) to the normal flow of secretions and makes the common bile duct and its tributaries or the pancreatic duct and its tributaries opaque and visible on an x-ray monitor. Because of the position of the biliary tree, a cholangiogram is more difficult to obtain than a pancreatogram, but an experienced examiner can visualize the desired duct in > 90% of cases. An ultrathin fiberscope, the size of a cannula, which can be passed through the ERCP instrument directly into the ducts for direct intraductal visualization, is under investigation.

Complications

Perforation and drug reactions are rare; other complications of ERCP are pancreatitis, which occurs in < 1% of patients and is usually mild, and infection, which is less common and occurs primarily in patients with duct obstruction. Sphincterotomy has a 1.5% mortality rate and an overall complication rate (including bleeding) of < 10%, which is lower than that of similar surgical procedures.

104 ■ **DENTAL AND ORAL DISORDERS**

Disorders that affect the hard and soft tissues of the oral cavity and their functions (initiation of digestion, production of speech, and provision of host defense).

Dental and oral disorders are common among the elderly. Although most of these disorders are not life threatening, they may have systemic effects and can greatly reduce an elderly person's quality of life. Many of these disorders are not due to aging but are the sequelae of systemic disorders or their treatment (drugs, radiation therapy, and chemotherapy). Poor oral hygiene and inadequate dental care are important factors.

A physician should examine the mouth of elderly patients at each physical examination; dentures must be removed. In addition, all elderly patients should see a dentist every 6 months.

DENTAL CARIES

Decalcification of the tooth's surface (inorganic portion) accompanied or followed by disintegration of the interior (organic portion).

Etiology and Pathophysiology

Dental caries, a major cause of tooth loss, results from dissolution of the tooth surface by bacterial by-products in dental plaque. In the

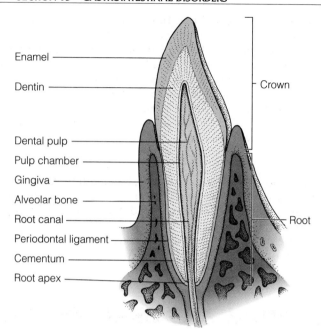

Enamel ——————

Dentin ——————

Dental pulp ——————
Pulp chamber ——————
Gingiva ——————
Alveolar bone ——————
Root canal ——————
Periodontal ligament ——————
Cementum ——————
Root apex ——————

Crown

Root

FIGURE 104–1.   Sagittal section of a mandibular cuspid and surrounding tissue.

elderly, inadequate oral hygiene is a major risk factor for developing caries. Many elderly persons do not obtain sufficient fluoride from their diet and oral hygiene products; this deficiency, combined with salivary hypofunction, ■ increases their susceptibility to caries. Salivary hypofunction, which can be caused by many disorders and drugs, predisposes persons to rapidly developing caries. Other risk factors include having infrequent dental examinations and cleanings and eating soft, carbohydrate-rich foods, with many snacks throughout the day (as elderly persons with compromised dentition tend to do). Ill-fitting removable partial dentures can trap plaque around certain teeth, creating an environment conducive to caries formation.

Two types of caries affect the elderly: coronal caries, which occur on the crown or enamel portion, and root surface caries, which occur on the root or cemental surface (see FIGURE 104–1). Children and young adults are susceptible only to coronal caries. Coronal caries can develop around an existing restoration or on a previously healthy tooth surface. Root surface caries develop in the elderly because many elderly persons lose alveolar (supporting) bone around the teeth, exposing the root surfaces to abrasion, erosion, attrition, demineralization, and caries-

■ see page 1028

causing bacteria. Gingival recession and periodontal pocketing also expose root surfaces.

Symptoms, Signs, and Diagnosis

In the elderly, many caries are asymptomatic until relatively late in their development, when bacteria encroach on the neurovascular supply of the tooth, which is contained in the dental pulp. The elderly are less sensitive to pathogenic and noxious stimuli (eg, caries, extreme temperatures) than are younger persons because with age, the pulp chamber and root canal recede and become filled with mineralized tissue. If untreated, caries progress and penetrate the dental pulp, causing pain and dentoalveolar infection. Dentoalveolar infection can cause bacteremia, facial and pharyngeal infection, and septicemia.

The signs of caries are uniform: Dark brown to black discolorations on any portion of the tooth suggest caries. Early lesions tend to be soft; long-standing lesions become hard. X-rays are helpful in making the diagnosis. Root surface caries are generally more difficult to diagnose than coronal caries, because gingival recession increases the surface area of cementum exposed to oral fluids and covered by bacterial plaque and because dental x-rays are insensitive in showing certain root surface caries.

Prevention and Treatment

Daily use of a toothbrush, floss, and a fluoride dentifrice and mouth rinse can help prevent caries. Elderly persons should have regular professional dental care, including prophylaxis (eg, fluoride rinses, plaque and tartar removal). A dental examination once every 6 months is usually adequate, but patients with a history of rapidly developing caries or with conservatively managed periodontal disease may need examinations more frequently. Elderly persons with diminished dexterity, oral motor or neurologic disorders, or cognitive impairment may need to have professional prophylaxis more often and to learn individualized techniques for oral hygiene. For patients with frequent new or recurrent caries, prescription-strength fluoride dentifrices (0.4% stannous fluoride or 1.0/1.1% sodium fluoride) may help.

Caries should be treated promptly. Many new materials can be used to conservatively restore the affected tooth. If caries are advanced, extraction or root canal therapy is required.

PERIODONTAL DISEASE

Inflammatory, destructive disease of the tooth's supporting structure (gingiva, alveolar bone, and periodontal ligament).

Etiology and Pathophysiology

Periodontal disease, a major cause of tooth loss in the elderly, is caused by bacterial plaque that accumulates and adheres to the teeth.

Bacterial antigens penetrate periodontal tissues, resulting in an inflammatory response and local immunopathologic destruction of connective tissues supporting the tooth.

Infrequent or inadequate oral hygiene, systemic disorders (eg, diabetes, which causes an exaggerated inflammatory response with poor healing), and several drugs can aggravate periodontal disease. Some drugs (eg, cyclosporine, calcium channel blockers, phenytoin) may cause gingival hyperplasia, characterized by enlarged fibrotic, edematous, and erythematous gingivae that tend to bleed readily. Other drugs (eg, antihypertensives, psychoactive drugs, anticholinergics) can reduce the production of saliva, which contains lubricatory and antimicrobial proteins that protect the oral tissues.

Symptoms and Signs

Initially, the gingivae bleed and become edematous—a hallmark of gingivitis. Later, destruction of alveolar bone and the periodontal ligament results in loss of tooth support and in increased tooth mobility; this development is termed periodontitis. Another sign of periodontitis is deep (> 3 mm) periodontal pockets.

Periodontal disease tends to progress slowly and episodically, with frequent asymptomatic periods. The lesions of periodontal disease slowly accumulate over a lifetime.

Prevention and Treatment

Prevention focuses primarily on effective, frequent oral hygiene. After each meal, the teeth should be brushed with a fluoride dentifrice. This measure becomes more important with age because the gingivae tend to recede and more plaque accumulates between teeth. Use of dental floss or interproximal brushes at least once daily is recommended. Electric toothbrushes and irrigation systems are particularly useful for elderly persons with physical or motor impairments. A prescription antimicrobial mouth rinse containing 0.12% chlorhexidine gluconate is particularly useful for persons who have difficulty with oral hygiene because of diminished dexterity. However, regular use can cause taste changes and may stain teeth and composite resin dental restorations. Therefore, use of chlorhexidine twice daily for > 2 weeks should be supervised by a dentist. Professional prophylaxis can remove tenacious stains from teeth, but resin restorations may be permanently discolored.

Local or systemic antibiotics plus periodontal debridement are suggested for aggressive periodontitis. Because both mixed anaerobic and facultative bacteria may cause periodontitis, no single antibiotic is completely suitable. Nevertheless, some elderly patients benefit from short-term oral antibiotic therapy (eg, tetracycline 250 mg qid for 7 to 21 days, doxycycline 100 mg bid for 14 to 21 days, metronidazole 250 mg tid for 5 to 14 days, clindamycin 300 mg qid for 7 to 10 days, amoxi-cillin/clavulanate 250 mg tid for 10 to 14 days). Local-delivery antimicrobial systems may be used to place fibers or gels impregnated with tetracycline, doxycycline, or chlorhexidine into sites of gingival inflammation and periodontal breakdown. Although all of these treatments can arrest inflammation and prevent further tissue breakdown, they do not reverse the bone destruction that has already occurred.

Advanced periodontal disease may require surgical intervention to manage the inflammatory lesion and to restore the normal bony architecture so that oral hygiene can be effectively performed. Wound healing after periodontal surgery is slower in elderly patients than in younger ones, but evidence suggests that long-term healing and regeneration are indistinguishable in the two groups. Nevertheless, surgery may not be indicated in patients with certain confounding systemic conditions (eg, severe immunocompromised or demented states); for such patients, aggressive nonsurgical therapies, as described above, should be used.

BENIGN ORAL MUCOSAL DISORDERS

Various primary and secondary lesions of the oral mucosa, which may appear as erosions, ulcerations, bullae, vesicles, plaques, or tumors.

Little evidence supports the misconception that the oral mucosa of the elderly is pale, thin, atrophic, dry, and readily traumatized. The epithelium atrophies with age, but this atrophy does not appear to be clinically significant. In general, the critical function of the oral mucosa as a barrier against the external environment is well maintained in healthy persons, regardless of age.

Several age-related changes in the oral mucosa, such as varicosities and Fordyce's granules (ectopic sebaceous glands), are not clinically significant. Varicosities in the floor of the mouth, ventral surface of the tongue, and hypopharynx rarely bleed.

STOMATOPYROSIS AND GLOSSOPYROSIS

Burning sensation of the oral mucosa without apparent causative lesions.

Stomatopyrosis (commonly called burning mouth syndrome) is a poorly understood painful chronic intraoral disorder, which is most common among postmenopausal women. Glossopyrosis (burning tongue) is a common form of stomatopyrosis. Proposed causes include ill-fitting dentures; nutritional deficiencies of vitamin B_1, B_2, B_6, or B_{12} or of folic acid; local trauma; gastrointestinal disorders; allergies; salivary hypofunction; and diabetes.

Burning sensations may be constant, gradually increasing throughout the day, or intermittent, without any reliable alleviating agents. Diagnosis of stomatopyrosis is one of exclusion. If oral lesions are present, the diagnosis is not stomatopyrosis. For example, patients with oral candidiasis may have a burning sensation in the mouth, but they do not have stomatopyrosis.

Because stomatopyrosis and glossopyrosis are often idiopathic, treatment can be challenging and frustrating, and referral to a specialist in chronic pain syndromes should be considered. Antidepressants (eg, nortriptyline, clonazepam) given in low doses at bedtime are beneficial. Spontaneous remissions are not uncommon, but exacerbations may occur.

ORAL CANDIDIASIS

Infection of the oral cavity caused by Candida *species (commonly* C. albicans).

Oral candidiasis, a common infection among the elderly, has several forms. Acute pseudomembranous candidiasis (thrush) is characterized by leukoplakic plaques that appear as white patches and that can be scraped away to expose an erythematous base; hyperplastic candidiasis, by confluent leukoplakic plaques that cannot be scraped away; angular cheilitis, by leukoplakic and erosive lesions at the lip commissures; and atrophic candidiasis, by painful erythematous mucosal lesions, frequently located beneath dentures.

Risk factors include salivary gland dysfunction, certain drugs (eg, antibiotics, antineoplastics, corticosteroids, immunosuppressants), diabetes mellitus, and other immunocompromising conditions. Because some factors may be occult, they should be sought when an elderly person presents with oral candidiasis and, if present, managed.

Diagnosis is based on symptoms and signs and can be confirmed by culture, smear, or biopsy. The presence of candidal hyphae in oral smears indicates that the oral mucosal barrier has been breached and that the patient is at risk of systemic infection.

Treatment

Treatment with topical and/or systemic antifungal drugs is required, and an infected denture must be treated. Topical drugs (eg, nystatin oral suspension [100,000 U/mL] 5 mL qid, swished for 5 minutes and swallowed; nystatin pastilles 200,000 U qid; clotrimazole troches 10 mg qid) should be given for 10 to 14 days. Dentures must be kept out of the mouth for long intervals, particularly during sleep. Dentures should be cleaned and soaked for 10 minutes in solutions containing benzoic acid, 0.12% chlorhexidine, or 1% sodium hypochlorite, then rinsed thoroughly. Nystatin-triamcinolone acetonide ointment is effective for angular cheilitis. Patients with refractory candidiasis may require systemic drugs (eg, ketoconazole 200 mg once daily; fluconazole 200 mg immediately, then 100 mg once daily; itraconazole 100 mg bid) for 10 to 20 days.

OTHER BENIGN DISORDERS

There are many causes of benign oral mucosal disorders in the elderly. Local disorders commonly cause such lesions as recurrent aphthous ulcers, burns, and denture sores. Ill-fitting dental prostheses and loss of alveolar bone can cause traumatic lesions, which may be erythematous, hyperplastic, hyperkeratotic, or ulcerative.

Systemic mucocutaneous disorders with oral manifestations (eg, pemphigus vulgaris, cicatricial pemphigoid, lichen planus) are more common among middle-aged and elderly persons than among younger persons. Many drugs can cause oral problems, such as mucocutaneous and pigmented lesions; erythema multiforme; gingival hyperplasia; vesicles, ulcers, and bullae; and xerostomia (see TABLE 104–1). Radiation therapy to the head and neck causes stomatotoxicity and mucositis directly; other disorders (eg, Sjögren's syndrome) cause salivary gland hypofunction, which leads to mucosal disorders. Certain endocrinopathies and nutritional deficiencies can also adversely affect the oral mucosa.

Diagnosis and Treatment

Many benign lesions can be easily recognized by an experienced clinician. If an oral mucosal lesion does not resolve after 3 weeks, a tissue biopsy is required for definitive diagnosis.

For painful lesions (eg, aphthous ulcers, burns, denture sores), palliative topical therapy may help until a definitive diagnosis is established. Diphenhydramine elixir 12.5 mg/5 mL, 0.5% dyclonine elixir, or 2% viscous lidocaine can be combined with sucralfate, an over-the-counter antacid, or attapulgite to produce a topical oral analgesic. These mixtures can be applied with a cotton-tipped applicator directly to well-delineated intraoral ulcerations. Aphthous ulcers and other localized inflammatory lesions may also be treated with topical corticosteroids (eg, triamcinolone 0.025%, clobetasol propionate 0.05%). For generalized stomatitis, 10 mL of one such mixture can be swished for several minutes, then expectorated. Most topical therapies have few systemic adverse effects and thus can be continued for several weeks if necessary. Patients may have to stop consuming spicy or irritating foods and alcoholic beverages and stop using mouth rinses.

Patients with traumatic lesions due to a dental prosthesis should be referred to a dentist for repair or replacement of the prosthesis. Hyperplastic lesions (epulis fissurata) must be surgically removed to enable the patient to wear a denture normally.

TABLE 104–1. DRUGS THAT CAN CAUSE ORAL PROBLEMS IN THE ELDERLY

Oral Problem	Drugs
Mucocutaneous and pigmented lesions	Analgesics (eg, aspirin, NSAIDs) Antiarthritics (eg, gold salts) Antibiotics (eg, chlorhexidine, minocycline) Anticoagulants Antidiarrheal drugs (eg, bismuth) Antimycotics (eg, griseofulvin) Antineoplastics Antipsychotics (eg, phenothiazines)
Erythema multiforme	Analgesics (eg, aspirin, barbiturates, codeine, NSAIDs) Antibiotics (eg, chloramphenicol, ciprofloxacin, clindamycin, dapsone, isoniazid, penicillins, sulfa antibiotics, tetracyclines) Anticonvulsants (eg, carbamazepine, phenytoin) Antihypertensives (eg, diltiazem, hydralazine, minoxidil, verapamil) Antimycotics (eg, griseofulvin) Antireflux drugs (eg, cimetidine) Hypoglycemics (eg, sulfonylurea drugs) Psychoactive drugs (eg, glutethimide, lithium, meprobamate)
Gingival hyperplasia	Anticonvulsants (eg, phenytoin) Antihypertensives (eg, calcium channel blockers) Immunosuppressants (eg, cyclosporine)
Vesicles, ulcers, and bullae	Antiarrhythmics (eg, procainamide, quinidine) Antiarthritics (eg, gold salts) Antibiotics (eg, erythromycin, penicillin) Antihypertensives (eg, ACE inhibitors, chloramphenicol, hydralazine, methyldopa, thiazide diuretics) Antineoplastics Antioxidants (eg, octyl gallate) Chelating drugs (eg, penicillamine) Corticosteroids Dental materials (eg, metals, monomers, resins) Dentifrices (eg, cinnamaldehyde, sodium lauryl sulfate, triclosan) Immunosuppressants

TABLE 104-1. *(Continued)*

Oral Problem	Drugs
Xerostomia	Anticholinergic drugs
	Antidepressants
	Antihistamines
	Antihypertensives (ACE inhibitors, β-blockers, calcium channel blockers, diuretics)
	Antiparkinsonian drugs
	Antipsychotics
	Antireflux drugs
	Anxiolytics (particularly benzodiazepines)
	Diuretics

NSAIDs = nonsteroidal anti-inflammatory drugs; ACE = angiotensin-converting enzyme.

ORAL CANCER

Malignancies of the oral cavity or oropharynx.

In 1999, oral cancer, which represents 3 to 5% of all forms of cancer, was diagnosed in about 30,000 persons and caused almost 9,000 deaths in the USA. About half of the cases occur in persons > 65; the average 5-year survival is only about 50%. The male:female ratio, previously very high, decreased to 2:1 in 1998.

Alcohol use and tobacco use are the strongest risk factors for oral cancer. Pipe smoking and cigar smoking, as well as cigarette smoking, are associated with squamous cell carcinoma. Smokeless (chewing) tobacco appears to be associated with verrucous carcinoma (a highly differentiated variant of squamous cell carcinoma). Other risk factors include age; long-standing leukoplakic lesions (white mucosal plaques) that cannot be scraped away; erythroplakic lesions (flat or eroded, velvety red mucosal patches); ulcerative lesions; dysplasias; and human papillomavirus infection.

Pathology

The oral cavity and oropharynx are the second most common sites of head and neck cancer (the larynx is the most common site). Squamous cell carcinoma accounts for > 90% of oral cancers (as well as head and neck cancers); the remaining cases originate in the salivary glands, lymph nodes, or other tissues. Some oral cancers are metastases from distant sites. Hematologic malignancies may manifest in the mouth before they manifest systemically.

The most common sites of oral cancer are the floor of the mouth, tongue, oropharynx, and lips. Oral cancer in the buccal and labial vestibular areas may be caused by use of smokeless tobacco. Metastatic spread is hematogenous, usually to the lungs, bone, or liver. Oral cancer increases the risk of developing a second primary malignancy (of the mouth, pharynx, larynx, esophagus, or lungs) by up to 33%.

Symptoms, Signs, and Diagnosis

Typically, the main symptom is a sore in the mouth, lips, or throat. Pain and numbness may not be present.

Cancer should be part of the differential diagnosis of many oral lesions. Most intraoral lesions are benign, although clinically they may be easily confused with a malignancy. Conversely, malignant lesions can appear benign. Leukoplakic, erythroplakic, or ulcerated lesions that persist > 3 weeks should be evaluated by a dentist or oral and maxillofacial surgeon and generally should be biopsied. Local induration, fixation, and numbness with lymphadenopathy indicate advanced lesions. Cancer should be considered when a lesion persists 3 to 4 weeks after potential causes of trauma (eg, denture sore, aphthous ulcer, lesion due to cheek biting) have been removed; the lesion must be biopsied, or the patient referred to a specialist. A second primary malignancy should be sought.

Prevention, Prognosis, and Treatment

Prevention consists of abstaining from all tobacco products and limiting use of alcohol. Yearly screening of the head, neck, and oral region is recommended for persons of all ages, because it can detect primary tumors and recurrent or metastatic cancers early, thus improving the chances of survival.

The prognosis depends on the stage of the cancer more than on any other factor. Early-stage oral cancers < 2 cm in diameter that do not involve the lymph nodes and that have not metastasized are easily cured; the 5-year survival rate is > 80%. However, most oral cancers have spread to lymph nodes before they are diagnosed. For patients with advanced oral cancer, the 5-year survival rate is < 20%.

The most common treatment for oral cancer is surgery, with or without radiation therapy, depending on cancer stage. Small tumors with minimal or no lymph node involvement are managed with surgery alone. More extensive cancers are surgically removed, and external beam radiation therapy (60 Gy) is given for about 6 weeks. Chemotherapy is usually reserved for advanced or nonresectable tumors. Advanced nonresectable tumors may shrink after chemotherapy and radiation therapy, but the prognosis is poor.

The immunosuppressive effects of cancer chemotherapy—whether for oral or nonoral cancers—can cause oral problems during or immediately after treatment. Surgery and radiation therapy can cause permanent problems. For example, salivary glands are destroyed if they are exposed to > 25 Gy, and the risk of developing osteoradionecrosis is significantly increased if the mandible is exposed to > 60 Gy.

Dental, periodontal, and oral mucosal problems must be assessed and resolved before definitive treatment, and yearly oral examinations should be performed after treatment. These measures can prevent or minimize treatment-related problems (eg, dental caries, oral mucosal infections, xerostomia, trismus, dysphagia, osteoradionecrosis). Patients should be instructed to abstain from tobacco and alcohol and should be checked for complications due to treatment and for cancer recurrence.

Advanced lesions often cause considerable pain, interfere with eating, and eventually may cause difficulty swallowing. Palliative treatment is required to minimize pain and suffering, maintain nutrition, and maximize quality of life.

ALVEOLAR BONE LOSS

Resorption of the bone that surrounds and provides support for the teeth.

Resorption of alveolar bone (see FIGURE 104–1) results from local factors (eg, periodontitis, mucosal erosion, trauma) rather than from the aging process. Mandibular bone loss, which appears to be correlated with osteoporosis, may accelerate bone resorption due to periodontitis and lead to tooth loss. Once teeth are lost, alveolar bone atrophies quickly.

With resorption of the maxillary and mandibular regions, only a thin crest of edentulous (alveolar) ridge remains. The reduced surface area makes retention of a denture difficult, and pain may result from direct pressure on the mental nerve region. Loss of teeth and supporting bone decreases facial height and results in a tendency toward prognathism, which may damage the patient's self-image. Loss of teeth or improperly fitted dentures may interfere with the patient's ability to eat, limiting dietary selection and compromising nutrition.

Treatment

Fabricating dental prostheses for patients with extensively resorbed alveolar ridges is difficult. Maxillary dentures with a large surface area on the hard palate can usually be adjusted to fit satisfactorily. However, mandibular dentures may be particularly hard to fit and are more likely to be dislodged during speaking and chewing than are maxillary dentures. If fully or partially edentulous patients report increasing difficulty with retaining dentures, endosseous metallic implants (typically titanium) can be surgically placed in maxillas or mandibles to support the dentures.

Dentures must be properly installed and fitted to prevent further bone loss. They must be evaluated at least yearly to ensure proper retention, stability, and mucosal health.

TEMPOROMANDIBULAR JOINT DISORDERS

Disorders of the temporomandibular joint and muscles of mastication.

The temporomandibular joint (TMJ), located between the maxillary glenoid fossa and the condylar process of the mandible, enables articulation of the mandible. TMJ disorders affect mostly women in their 20s, 30s, or early 40s; incidence decreases with age. However, many elderly persons have pain and difficulty chewing because of disorders of the TMJ and associated structures. Temporomandibular disorders include arthritides (eg, TMJ osteoarthritis); displacement of the TMJ disk; and myofascial pain of the masseter, temporal, and pterygoid muscles.

Symptoms, Signs, and Diagnosis

Pain, the most common symptom, can include pain during chewing and jaw movements, otalgia, temporal and neck pain, and pain referred to otherwise healthy teeth. Clinical signs include jaw clicking, popping, and crepitus and a reduction in mandibular range of motion (interincisal distance of < 40 mm). Sharp, debilitating pain suggests an extracranial or intracranial disorder (eg, trigeminal neuralgia, temporal arteritis ◼). Often, osteoarthritis can be detected on the basis of crepitus during mouth opening and degenerative changes seen on panoramic x-rays and CT scans.

Treatment

Treatment should be directed toward providing support to the affected structures and minimizing or eliminating aggravating factors such as teeth clenching or grinding (bruxism). Treatment may consist of an interocclusal appliance, short-term physical therapy, behavior modification, and nonsteroidal anti-inflammatory drugs. A soft diet, muscle relaxants, and moist heat may help.

ORAL MOTOR DISORDERS

Impaired craniofacial muscular function that affects swallowing, chewing, speaking, or facial posture.

Oral motor function declines measurably with age, even in healthy persons. Reduced masticatory muscle performance is common among the elderly and may lead to a tendency to swallow larger food particles than was usually attempted at a younger age. This practice, particularly noticeable in patients using partial or complete dentures, can result in choking or aspiration. Swallowing may be impaired, so that food remains in the mouth longer.

◼see page 506

Most causes of oral motor dysfunction are iatrogenic. For example, certain drugs (particularly those with anticholinergic or diuretic properties), radiation therapy to the head and neck, and chemotherapy can significantly impair salivary gland function, interfering with swallowing. Other drugs—most notably, phenothiazines—can cause tardive dyskinesia. **1**

Changes in motor function are of greater concern in elderly persons with medical disorders. Neuropathies may markedly affect the musculature of the craniofacial region. Stroke is the most common systemic disorder that interferes with swallowing.

Voice and speech change with age**2**; however, the ability to produce speech is not normally impaired with age. Speech abnormalities are more commonly due to systemic disorders that cause muscular, sensory, or neurologic deficits (eg, stroke, Parkinson's disease, multiple sclerosis).

Orofacial posture changes with age. The lower face and lips may droop because of decreased circumoral muscle tone and, in edentulous persons, reduced bone support. This drooping is an aesthetic concern and can lead to drooling or food spills. Closing the lips competently while eating, sleeping, or even resting may become difficult. Often, loss of circumoral muscle tone is first recognized when a person reports excess saliva. However, systemic disorders that cause muscular and neurologic deficits are more likely to affect orofacial posture than is aging per se.

Prevention and Treatment

Evaluation of a patient's drug history may prevent oral motor dysfunction or identify an iatrogenic cause.

Oral motor dysfunction is best managed with a multidisciplinary approach. Coordinated referrals to specialists in prosthetic dentistry, rehabilitative medicine, speech pathology, otolaryngology, and gastroenterology may be needed.

GUSTATORY DYSFUNCTION

Disturbances of taste.

Adequate gustation is essential for enjoying foods and for selecting appropriate foods (eg, foods that are not spoiled). Enjoyment of foods also requires textural sensory cues. Textural sensory function appears to change little if at all with age. Taste function decreases slightly, affecting only a specific quality of taste (ie, sweet, sour, salty, or bitter). However, olfactory function, which contributes to the sensation of flavor, decreases greatly with age, even in healthy persons. **3**

1 see page 447   **2** see page 424   **3** see page 1347

TABLE 104–2.   DRUGS THAT CAN CAUSE GUSTATORY DYSFUNCTION IN THE ELDERLY

Category	Examples
Amebicides and anthelmintics	Metronidazole, niridazole
Anesthetics (local)	Benzocaine, lidocaine, procaine hydrochloride
Anticoagulants	Phenindione
Anticonvulsants	Carbamazepine, phenytoin
Antihistamines	Chlorpheniramine
Antimicrobials	Amphotericin B, ampicillin, bleomycin, cefamandole, ethambutol, griseofulvin, lincomycin, metronidazole, sulfasalazine, tetracyclines
Antineoplastics and immuno-suppressants	Azathioprine, bleomycin, carmustine, doxorubicin, 5-fluorouracil, methotrexate, vincristine
Analgesic, anti-inflammatory, antipyretic, and antirheumatic drugs	Allopurinol, auranofin, colchicine, dexamethasone, gold, hydrocortisone, levamisole, penicillamine, phenylbutazone, salicylates
Antithyroid drugs	Carbimazole, methimazole, methylthiouracil, propylthiouracil, thiouracil
Cholesterol-lowering drugs	Cholestyramine, clofibrate
Antihypertensives and diuretics	Acetazolamide, amiloride and its analogs, captopril, diazoxide, diltiazem, enalapril, ethacrynic acid, nifedipine
Hypoglycemic drugs	Glipizide, phenformin and derivatives
Antiparkinsonian drugs and muscle relaxants	Baclofen, chlormezanone, levodopa
Oral hygiene components	Chlorhexidine gluconate (in mouth rinses), sodium lauryl sulfate
Psychoactive drugs	Lithium, trifluoperazine
Sympathomimetic drugs	Amphetamines, amrinone
Vasodilators	Bamifylline, dipyridamole, nitroglycerin patch, oxyfedrine
Others	Etidronate, germine monoacetate, idoxuridine, iron dextran complex, vitamin D

Systemic diseases (eg, neuropathies, cognitive disorders, upper respiratory infections), oral disorders, and use of some drugs (see TABLE 104–2) may cause gustatory dysfunction. The primary cause may be a systemic disorder (including viral infections) or drug that causes olfactory dysfunction. Taste function may be disturbed by trauma to the 7th (facial), 9th (glossopharyngeal), or 10th (vagus) cranial nerve (which subserve taste sensation to the tongue, soft palate, and oral pharynx); other oral or maxillofacial trauma; dental or alveolar surgery (eg, extractions, periodontal surgery, biopsies); craniomandibular surgery; intraoral infections that produce a purulent discharge; and poor oral hygiene. Poor oral hygiene, particularly of teeth with extensive restorations or of dentures, may result in chronic unpleasant taste sensations and may lead to gingivitis or bacterial and fungal infections, which contribute to gustatory dysfunction.

Symptoms, Signs, and Diagnosis

Many elderly persons report a decreased ability to taste (hypogeusia) or a persistent bad taste in the mouth (dysgeusia); both are due to oral or systemic disorders. Loss of taste (ageusia) is uncommon. In most patients, taste changes occur slowly and insidiously.

Patients should be asked if they can taste the saltiness of a potato chip, the sweetness of ice cream, the sourness of lemon juice, and the bitterness of coffee. Affirmative answers indicate that the deficit is probably olfactory rather than gustatory. If testing of taste function is inconclusive, referral to a chemosensory center for intensive testing may be necessary.

If a patient reports an unpleasant taste that is usually associated with meals or that can be rinsed away with water, the cause may be an oral disorder, including oral trauma and poor oral hygiene.

After local causes have been eliminated, a history of systemic disorders and drug use should be obtained. The patient should be asked about head trauma and upper respiratory infections. A sudden loss of taste may result from a flu-like upper respiratory infection, oral or maxillofacial trauma, or a cranial tumor. If trauma or a tumor is suspected, evaluation must include the 1st (olfactory), 7th, 9th, and 10th cranial nerves. Patients with a sudden change in taste that has no obvious cause should be referred to a neurologist, and MRI or CT of the head should be performed to rule out a cranial tumor.

Prevention and Treatment

Adequate hygiene of teeth, gingival and periodontal tissues, the posterior tongue, and dentures can help prevent gustatory dysfunction.

Causes of altered taste, including oral and systemic disorders and drugs, should be eliminated or controlled. If no cause is identified, there are no established therapies for gustatory dysfunction. Zinc preparations are minimally effective.

Meticulously documenting symptoms and reassuring patients that measurable sensory deficits have been noted often helps. Patients may need counseling and behavior therapy to learn how to live with persistent idiopathic gustatory dysfunction.

XEROSTOMIA

Dry mouth.

Xerostomia is common among the elderly. It may result from salivary gland hypofunction, obstruction, or altered salivary constituents. Adequate production of saliva is essential to oral health. Saliva is necessary to form and move food boluses, to lubricate and maintain the integrity of the oral mucosa, and to prevent demineralization and promote remineralization of teeth. Saliva contains many antimicrobial proteins that control bacterial, fungal, and viral growth. It also buffers acids produced by bacteria, cleanses the mouth after eating, and helps in taste and denture retention.

Generally, saliva production does not decline with age. Parotid gland function remains intact in the elderly. Saliva production by the submandibular and sublingual glands is modestly reduced in healthy elderly persons, but this change is probably not biologically significant.

Etiology

In the elderly, xerostomia can be caused by salivary hypofunction secondary to dehydration. It also results from a variety of iatrogenic causes. It can be an adverse effect of > 400 drugs, many of which are commonly used by the elderly (see TABLE 104–1). Drugs with anticholinergic or diuretic properties are the most common offenders. External beam radiation therapy for head and neck cancer destroys salivary gland tissue and causes long-term xerostomia. Also, cytotoxic chemotherapy for cancer may impair salivary gland function.

In the elderly, the most common salivary gland disorder causing xerostomia is **Sjögren's syndrome**, an autoimmune exocrinopathy affecting mainly postmenopausal women.∎ It has a primary form, which affects only the salivary and lacrimal glands, and a secondary form, which also includes a connective tissue disease (eg, scleroderma, rheumatoid arthritis, thyroiditis).

Other salivary gland disorders that cause xerostomia include duct obstructions (eg, sialoliths, mucoceles), infections (eg, acute or chronic viral or bacterial sialadenitis), and tumors (eg, pleomorphic adenomas, adenoid cystic carcinomas, adenocarcinomas, acinic cell carcinomas). Alzheimer's disease, diabetes, sarcoidosis, cystic fibrosis, and AIDS also may impair salivary gland function.

Patients may experience xerostomia when salivary gland function is normal. These cases may be caused by defective oral sensory receptors or impaired cognition.

∎see page 505

Symptoms, Signs, and Diagnosis

Many elderly patients report xerostomia; usually, it is mild. Typically, patients with true salivary gland hypofunction have difficulty swallowing dry foods and require fluids for swallowing; their lips and mouth are dry during eating and speaking. Signs include an unexpected recent increase in dental caries; the presence of oral fungal infections; and desiccated, ulcerated, erythematous, or furrowed lips and intraoral mucosa. However, the mucosa may appear normal even when the glands are dysfunctional.

Salivary gland status should first be evaluated by oral examination. Enlarged, painful, or tender glands may result from an obstruction, a tumor, an infection, or Sjögren's syndrome. Orifices of the major salivary glands should be palpated to determine patency. Suppuration from the gland orifice indicates acute or chronic sialadenitis, and a specimen should be sent for culture and sensitivity testing (*Staphylococcus aureus* is the most common bacterial cause). Fever and swelling, pain, or erythema over the affected gland suggests sialadenitis.

Retrograde sialography is particularly useful when an inflammatory disorder or obstruction is suspected. Technetium-99m pertechnetate scintigraphy can determine whether acinar parenchymal tissues are functional and whether saliva production is impaired. CT and MRI of the major salivary glands can detect inflammatory disorders, obstructions, and tumors.

If Sjögren's syndrome is suspected, the minor labial salivary glands are biopsied (usually by an oral and maxillofacial surgeon or oral medicine/pathology specialist), and lacrimal gland function is evaluated. Serologic markers of autoimmune disorders (particularly anti–SS-A, anti–SS-B, and antinuclear antibodies and rheumatoid factor) may be present.

Treatment

Drug-induced salivary gland dysfunction is almost always fully reversible. If oral complications are severe, drug doses can be reduced, smaller doses can be given more often, or alternative drugs can be used.

If some secretory function remains, the glands can be stimulated with sugarless candies, mints, or gum. The glands can also be stimulated with the cholinergic drug pilocarpine 5 mg po tid or qid, with the last dose taken before bedtime. This drug should be avoided in patients with heart failure, asthma, a peptic ulcer, a urinary tract obstruction, Parkinson's disease, or angle-closure glaucoma. There is no satisfactory treatment for the autoimmune disorders that cause salivary gland hypofunction.

When gland parenchyma is not functional, patients have no fluid-transporting cells and do not respond to specific salivary or systemic therapy. They require frequent, comprehensive preventive dental care.

For these and other patients with salivary gland disorders, salivary substitutes help limit hard tissue problems (eg, dental caries) but not soft tissue problems (eg, ulcers, fissured tongue, oral yeast infections). For the latter, only palliative therapy is available (eg, with analgesic and antimicrobial elixirs or mouth rinses).

Treatment of sialadenitis consists of rehydration and antibiotics (typically amoxicillin [with or without clavulanic acid] 500 mg po tid for 10 days, depending on culture and sensitivity test results). Occasionally, an abscess requires surgical drainage. Benign and malignant tumors and sialoliths must be surgically removed, and patients must be appropriately followed and treated.

105 ESOPHAGEAL DISORDERS

Most esophageal disorders that occur in elderly patients also occur in younger patients. However, the presentation, complications, and treatment of these disorders may be different in elderly patients than in younger patients. Esophageal bleeding, esophagitis, perforation, Schatzki's ring, and epiphrenic diverticula are discussed in Ch. 112. Esophageal tumors are discussed in Ch. 113.

DYSPHAGIA

The sensation of impaired passage of food from the oropharynx to the stomach.

Dysphagia can occur at any age. It is the most common esophageal disorder in the elderly and is estimated to occur in up to 50% of patients in long-term care facilities.

OROPHARYNGEAL DYSPHAGIA

Difficulty in initiating swallowing or in transferring food from the oropharynx to the upper esophagus.

Etiology

Causes of oropharyngeal dysphagia are listed in TABLE 105–1.

Neurologic disorders may affect neuromuscular function by impairing motor function or sensation. The most common neurologic cause of

TABLE 105–1. CAUSES OF OROPHARYNGEAL DYSPHAGIA

Central nervous system disorders

Amyotrophic lateral sclerosis
Brain stem tumors
Multiple sclerosis
Parkinson's disease
Stroke
Tabes dorsalis
Wilson's disease

Peripheral nervous system disorders

Bulbar poliomyelitis
Metabolic myopathies
Muscular dystrophies
Myasthenia gravis
Peripheral neuropathies

Neuromuscular disorders

Amyloidosis
Metabolic myopathy

Muscular dystrophies
Primary myositis
Systemic lupus erythematosus

Local structural lesions

Cervical osteophyte
Congenital webs
Inflammatory
Neoplastic
Plummer-Vinson syndrome
Postoperative anatomic alterations
Thyromegaly
Zenker's diverticulum

Motility disorders of the upper esophageal sphincter

Abnormal relaxation
Hypertensive upper esophageal
 sphincter

---

oropharyngeal dysphagia in the elderly is a stroke,█ especially a stroke that affects the swallowing center in the midbrain (bilaterally in the reticular substance below the nucleus of the solitary tract) or the anterior cortical areas. Wallenberg's syndrome (a syndrome marked by ipsilateral loss of temperature and pain sensations of the face) may cause dysphagia by impairing the ipsilateral palatal muscles supplied by the lateral area of the medulla resulting from the occlusion of the posterior inferior cerebellar artery. As a result of bilateral multiple cerebral infarctions, pseudobulbar palsy may cause dysphagia by impairing the muscles supplied by the medulla oblongata. Bulbar palsy may also cause dysphagia by paralyzing or weakening the muscles supplied by the medulla oblongata, but bulbar palsy does not occur as a result of cerebral infarctions.

Parkinson's disease, amyotrophic lateral sclerosis, multiple sclerosis, brain tumors, and central nervous system degenerative diseases (eg, Alzheimer's disease) may cause dysphagia by affecting movements of the tongue, pharynx, or upper esophagus.

Muscular disorders (eg, oculopharyngeal muscular dystrophy, myasthenia gravis, Eaton-Lambert syndrome, dermatomyositis, polymyositis)█ may cause dysphagia by inhibiting neuromuscular function.

Upper esophageal sphincter abnormalities also affect neuromuscular function. The cricopharyngeus and some components of the inferior

---

█ see page 397   █ see page 511

pharyngeal constrictor muscle are responsible for the high-pressure zone of the upper esophageal sphincter. Dysphagia can result from a hypertensive upper esophageal sphincter, a hypotensive upper esophageal sphincter (due to amyotrophic lateral sclerosis, myasthenia gravis, or myotonic muscular dystrophy), or incomplete upper esophageal sphincter relaxation (cricopharyngeal achalasia).

Anatomic abnormalities may cause difficult or incomplete passage of food through the esophagus. Head and neck tumors may cause oropharyngeal dysphagia in the elderly. Zenker's diverticulum[1] is associated with premature closure of the upper esophageal sphincter, which increases resistance to the passage of a food bolus and leads to outpouching of the esophageal wall.

Cervical hypertrophic osteoarthropathy[2] may cause dysphagia when the cervical osteophyte (spur) is extraordinarily large or when periesophagitis occurs from rapid expansion of the osteophyte. Osteophyte-induced dysphagia is very rare (only about 75 cases have been reported).

Cervical strictures and esophageal webs[3] can also cause oropharyngeal dysphagia.

Symptoms and Signs

Patients may experience coughing or choking during swallowing, nasopharyngeal regurgitation, changes in speech, or recurrent aspiration. Globus sensation (a subjective sensation of cervical fullness or a "lump in the throat") may occur. Although the physiologic mechanisms underlying globus sensation are unknown, increased pressure or spasm of the upper esophageal sphincter or abnormal hypopharyngeal motility has been suggested. Functional chest pain may occur in patients with high levels of somatic concerns, anxiety, or depression. Obstructive disorders cause dysphagia, especially for solid foods.

Oropharyngeal dysphagia may be intermittent but, when due to neuromuscular disorders, typically progresses. Patients are at high risk of developing aspiration pneumonia.

Diagnosis

A barium swallow is routinely the initial examination and is often accompanied by videofluoroscopy to observe the rapid muscular coordination involved in swallowing. Endoscopy may also be used to assess muscular or anatomic abnormalities. Anatomic evaluation and observation of swallowing allow for an assessment of anatomic structures, uncoordinated movements, and aspiration or spillage.

[1] see page 1036   [2] see page 1037   [3] see page 1038

A sensory deficit should be sought, as it may predispose to oropharyngeal dysphagia and aspiration. Testing the gag reflex is an incomplete assessment of the sensory fibers to the laryngeal and hypopharyngeal mucosa and is an inadequate predictor of aspiration. A fiberoptic endoscopic evaluation of swallowing with sensory testing can determine laryngopharyngeal sensory discrimination thresholds. This newly developed technique can be performed at the bedside and may identify sensory deficits causing aspiration that cannot be identified by barium swallow.

If a head or neck tumor is suspected after clinical assessment, evaluation should include direct laryngoscopy and CT of the head and neck.

If cervical hypertrophic osteoarthropathy is suspected, evaluation should include plain cervical spine films with lateral views and barium videofluoroscopy with food bolus to determine the degree of compression during swallowing.

Treatment

Treatment requires identification of potentially treatable causes. Goals include identifying and maintaining safe swallowing techniques, avoiding aspiration, and providing adequate nutritional support.

For patients with oropharyngeal dysphagia due to untreatable neuromuscular disorders, altering the consistency of food may improve swallowing. Evaluation by a speech therapist may be beneficial, because some patients may be able to improve their swallowing function by changing their head position while eating, performing exercises that improve the ability to accommodate a food bolus in the oral cavity, strengthening and improving the coordination of the tongue, and learning different swallowing techniques.

Depending on the degree of dysphagia, drug treatment for neuromuscular disorders may not completely restore swallowing. For patients with severe dysphagia and recurrent aspiration, gastrostomy tube placement may be necessary.

For patients with oropharyngeal dysphagia due to a stroke, retraining the swallowing muscles may be effective. This rehabilitation is best combined with a videotaped barium swallow to assess the effects of different foods (eg, liquid, semisolid, solid) on swallowing and to evaluate for aspiration.

For patients with oropharyngeal dysphagia due to head and neck tumors, treatment involves surgery, radiation therapy, or chemotherapy as necessary. However, surgery or radiation therapy can result in esophageal stricture.

For patients with oropharyngeal dysphagia due to cervical hypertrophic osteoarthropathy, reassurance and support are usually effective. However, if the dysphagia is unremitting, surgical removal of the osteophyte may be necessary.

TABLE 105–2.   CAUSES OF ESOPHAGEAL DYSPHAGIA

Neuromuscular disorders
Achalasia
Chagas' disease
Diffuse esophageal spasm
Nonspecific motility disorders
Scleroderma (and other collagen
  vascular diseases)

Intrinsic obstruction

Benign tumors
Diverticula

Esophageal rings
Esophageal webs
Foreign body
Malignancy
Strictures (peptic, caustic injury)

Extrinsic obstruction

Cervical osteoarthropathy
Mediastinal abnormalities
Vascular compression

ESOPHAGEAL DYSPHAGIA

Difficulty in swallowing when ingested material cannot be transported from the hypopharynx through the esophagus into the stomach.

Causes of esophageal dysphagia are listed in TABLE 105–2. Neuromuscular causes include achalasia, diffuse esophageal spasm, and progressive systemic sclerosis.◨ Obstructive causes include strictures,◩ esophageal rings and webs◪, and tumors.◫

A less common obstructive cause is an esophageal vascular anomaly, which can cause dysphagia through compression of the esophagus. Dysphagia aortica, which occurs in the elderly, results from esophageal compression by a large thoracic aortic aneurysm or an atherosclerotic, rigid aorta.

Obstructive dysphagia can also result when a foreign body lodges in the esophagus. Some elderly persons may be susceptible to foreign body obstruction because visual acuity may decrease with age and denture wearing can decrease the ability to feel objects in the mouth.

Symptoms and Signs

The sensation is that of food being stuck in the esophagus and of retrosternal discomfort. However, the patient's subjective localization of the site of bolus impaction does not reliably predict the site of the actual problem. For example, impaction in the distal esophagus may produce symptoms in the lower neck.

Diagnosis and Treatment

A barium swallow is often the initial evaluation used. Endoscopy is also used to assess symptoms and to perform diagnostic biopsies. Treatment is tailored to the specific cause of the dysphagia.

◨ see page 506   ◩ see page 1037   ◪ see page 1038
◫ see page 1134

ACHALASIA

A neurogenic esophageal disorder of unknown cause characterized by impaired esophageal peristalsis and a lack of lower esophageal sphincter relaxation.

Achalasia typically occurs in persons aged 20 to 40 years. However, a second peak occurs in the elderly.

In achalasia, lower esophageal resting pressure is increased and intraesophageal pressure is increased relative to gastric pressure. The muscle and nerve components of the esophagus are abnormal. The primary defect appears to be a progressive loss of ganglion cells within the myenteric plexus of the esophageal wall.

Symptoms, Signs, and Diagnosis

All patients with achalasia have dysphagia to solid foods; the majority of patients develop variable degrees of weight loss and dysphagia to liquids. About 60 to 90% of patients regurgitate undigested food into the esophagus shortly after a meal. Regurgitation may cause nocturnal coughing and aspiration. About 30 to 50% of patients have chest pain associated with eating. Elderly patients may have had symptoms for months or years before diagnosis. Complications include weight loss with advanced disease and coughing, bronchospasm, and pneumonia from aspirating esophageal contents.

Achalasia is often suspected from the history. In the early stages of the disease, chest x-ray findings can be normal. In the later stages, chest x-rays can show a dilated esophagus (megaesophagus) with an air-fluid level caused by retained food and saliva. Elderly patients with a long history of achalasia can have a dilated and tortuous esophagus with a "bird-beak" narrowing at the gastroesophageal junction on barium swallow. Esophageal manometry usually shows the motility abnormalities.

Endoscopy can eliminate the possibility of pseudoachalasia, which should be considered when patients are > 50 years, have had dysphagia for < 1 year, and have lost > 15 lb (> 7 kg). Other disorders that can mimic achalasia include malignancy, amyloidosis, sarcoidosis, Chagas' disease, and postvagotomy disturbances. Achalasia must also be differentiated from diffuse esophageal spasm, which more typically affects younger patients.

Treatment

Treatment is directed at relieving symptoms and preventing complications. Various drugs that can decrease lower esophageal sphincter pressure (eg, anticholinergics, amyl nitrite, nitroglycerin, β_2-agonists) have been used, but results have been inconsistent. Anticholinergics are particularly difficult to use in the elderly because of their adverse effects. Isosorbide nitrate (5 to 10 mg po before meals) or nitroglycerin

(0.4 mg sublingually 5 minutes before meals) rapidly decreases lower esophageal sphincter pressure and may lessen dysphagia during meals. However, most patients with achalasia require more definitive treatment. Botulinum toxin, an inhibitor of the release of acetylcholine, can be injected endoscopically into the lower esophageal sphincter. This relatively new treatment appears to approach the success rate of pneumatic dilatation. The most benefit seems to occur in patients > 50. The effects last 6 to 24 months; injection often needs to be repeated.

Mechanical disruption of the lower esophageal sphincter using pneumatic dilatation or surgical myotomy has been the principle method of treatment when drug treatment and botulinum toxin have not been effective. About 60% of patients have a good response with pneumatic dilatation; success rates > 95% have been reported. Elderly patients and patients with a long history of achalasia seem to have the most favorable responses. Twenty to 40% of patients require repeated dilatations. The incidence of immediate complications is 1 to 16%. Perforation occurs in 1 to 13%; in most of these cases, the perforation is small and localized.

Surgical myotomy is indicated when repeated pneumatic dilatations over a relatively short duration are necessary to maintain lower esophageal sphincter patency. Surgical myotomy reduces lower esophageal sphincter pressure more dependably than pneumatic dilatation but causes more complications. A modified Heller's procedure (anterior myotomy of the circular muscle fibers of the lower esophageal sphincter, preserving the sphincter competency) is successful in 80 to 90% of patients. This procedure is increasingly being performed laparoscopically or with video-assisted thorascopic surgery. The most significant complications are gastroesophageal reflux disease (< 10%) and persistence of severe dysphagia (< 10%).

ZENKER'S DIVERTICULUM

An outpouching of the posterior pharyngeal wall immediately above the upper esophageal sphincter.

Zenker's diverticulum may occur because of decreased compliance of the cricopharyngeal muscle with premature closure of the upper esophageal sphincter. It may be asymptomatic, although symptoms may develop if the outpouching becomes large. Symptomatic patients are usually ≥ 50 years. The most common symptoms include dysphagia for solids and liquids, cough, regurgitation of undigested food, recurrent aspiration, bronchitis, halitosis, and recurrent pneumonia. A mass in the left neck may be seen while the patient is eating and may produce esophageal compression, contributing to and worsening the dysphagia.

Zenker's diverticulum is diagnosed by barium swallow. Patients with dysphagia may practice various maneuvers (eg, applying pressure to the neck, coughing repeatedly to empty the diverticulum) to assist swallowing. The treatment for symptomatic patients is cricopharyngeal myotomy with diverticulectomy. Diverticulopexy has been performed for large diverticula, orienting the lumen caudally. Small diverticula are usually not resected.

CERVICAL HYPERTROPHIC OSTEOARTHROPATHY

A disorder characterized by cervical osteophytes.

This disorder occurs in 20 to 30% of the general population, most frequently in the elderly. However, osteophyte-induced dysphagia occurs rarely, most often in persons with diffuse idiopathic skeletal hyperostosis, involving at least four contiguous vertebrae with minimal degenerative disk disease and no apophyseal joint ankylosis. Cervical osteophyte-induced dysphagia occurs when the osteophyte is extraordinarily large or when periesophagitis occurs from rapid expansion of the osteophyte; it can also occur in the cricoid cartilage region (C6), where the esophagus is relatively immobile.

Cervical hypertrophic osteoarthropathy is diagnosed by x-ray. Treatment can include dietary modification (altering meal composition to include softer foods) and surgical intervention.

STRICTURES

A localized narrowing of the esophagus.

Persons with long-standing gastroesophageal reflux disease can develop strictures in the distal esophagus due to acid reflux.

Symptoms, Signs, and Diagnosis

Elderly persons are at risk of developing drug- or injury-induced strictures because they are exposed to irritating drugs, may spend more time in the recumbent position, and are more likely to have motility or anatomic disorders of the esophagus. A wide variety of drugs have been implicated, including doxycycline, tetracycline, clindamycin, emepronium bromide, potassium, iron, alprenolol, quinidine, acetylsalicylic acid, theophylline, nonsteroidal anti-inflammatory drugs (NSAIDs), and alendronate. Injury-induced strictures may result from swallowing caustic (acidic or alkaline) agents. Progressive dysphagia for solids develops. Weight loss rarely occurs in persons with benign strictures, because these persons frequently maintain their good appetites and may alter their diets to include foods and beverages that do not cause symptoms.

Clinical history can suggest the diagnosis. Barium swallow can show clustered ulcers or a stricture of the esophagus, typically at the level of the gastroesophageal junction. The stricture is typically smooth, tapered, and of varying length. An upper endoscopy can show pill fragments and superficial or deep ulcerations with heaped up margins.

An upper endoscopy with biopsy should be performed to exclude Barrett's esophagus (premalignant, metaplastic columnar epithelium in the distal esophagus) or a malignancy.

Treatment

Treatment is aimed at reducing symptoms; acid suppression with proton pump inhibitors reduces concurrent gastric acid–induced injury. Dilatation (with pneumatic or other types of dilator) should be considered, although drug-induced strictures can be difficult to dilate and may require multiple sessions. Occasionally, antireflux surgery is required.

ESOPHAGEAL RINGS AND WEBS

Esophageal ring: A 2- to 4-mm mucosal structure, probably congenital, causing a ringlike narrowing of the distal esophagus at the squamocolumnar junction. Esophageal web: A thin membrane of squamous epithelium that occurs in the upper and mid esophagus.

Lower esophageal mucosal rings involve the mucosa and submucosa. The most common type is Schatzki's ring,∎ which is composed of invaginated mucosa at the gastroesophageal junction, about 3 to 4 cm above the diaphragm. The incidence of esophageal webs increases with age.

Usually, esophageal rings are asymptomatic and may be associated with hiatus hernia. However, patients > 40 years are more commonly symptomatic for uncertain reasons. Nonprogressive, intermittent dysphagia is typical in patients with esophageal rings and webs. The symptoms usually occur when the diameter of the esophagus is decreased to < 12 to 13 mm. Dysphagia may begin when eating meat (referred to as "steakhouse syndrome"), often requiring regurgitation or liquids to expel or swallow the food.

Diagnosis and Treatment

A barium swallow can identify the lesion. Endoscopy can confirm the diagnosis. Symptoms that occur infrequently may be avoided through careful eating habits. Some patients respond to acid suppres-

∎ see page 1113

sion with proton pump inhibitors or H_2 blockers. Others, however, require dilatation, usually with a single large bougie. Electrocautery incision of esophageal rings has also been used.

GASTROESOPHAGEAL REFLUX DISEASE

Reflux of gastric contents into the esophagus.

In the USA, symptoms of gastroesophageal reflux disease (GERD) occur daily in about 7% of adults and monthly in about 44%. GERD occurs more frequently in men than women (2 to 3:1). Incidence in the elderly is uncertain but appears similar to that in younger persons.

Symptoms and Signs

The most common symptom is substernal burning (heartburn), most often after meals or on reclining. Atypical chest pain, which must be differentiated from cardiac pain, can also occur. Esophagitis occurs when the caustic gastric contents remain in contact with the esophageal mucosa long enough to overcome esophageal defense and tissue resistance. Other common symptoms include regurgitation, which causes a bitter or sour taste, and water brash (salivary secretions thought to be stimulated by acid reflux) due to increased salivary secretion. Non-esophageal symptoms can result from mucosal injury of the oropharynx, larynx, or respiratory tract. Oropharyngeal irritation can cause sore throat, earaches, gingivitis, poor dentition, and globus sensation. Laryngeal or respiratory irritation can cause hoarseness, wheezing, bronchitis, asthma, and aspiration pneumonia. Symptoms may be worsened by eating large meals, consuming foods and beverages high in fat or caffeine, using tobacco and alcohol, reclining after eating, and gaining weight.

The clinical course varies. Esophagitis can occur. Strictures can develop at sites of significant recurrent inflammation. Barrett's esophagus, which occurs in 10 to 15% of patients with erosive esophagitis and in up to 40% of patients with peptic strictures, does not worsen symptoms. However, Barrett's esophagus is a premalignant condition for adenocarcinoma. Dysphagia may result due to inflammation, scarring, or malignancy. Hemorrhage can occur due to erosions and ulcerations caused by severe mucosal injury. Rarely, deep esophageal ulcerations can result in perforation.

Diagnosis

Although most diagnostic tests are unnecessary to diagnose GERD or begin treatment, they should be performed in patients with persistent or worsening symptoms or signs suggestive of tissue injury or cancer, including atypical pain, anemia, and weight loss. Early assessment is also important in patients with equivocal symptoms in whom a diagnosis is uncertain.

The most frequently used test for diagnosing GERD is barium swallow. Upper endoscopy is the best method for assessing mucosal injury. Acid perfusion tests require the placement of an esophageal pH probe 5 cm above the lower esophageal sphincter to determine if refluxed acidic contents (confirmed by pH < 4) are present in the esophagus. Continuous intraesophageal pH monitoring records the esophageal pH for 24 hours, which is then correlated with the patient's symptoms. Radionuclide scanning can identify radiolabeled colloid in the area of the esophagus. In the Bernstein acid perfusion test, normal saline and 0.1 N-hydrochloric acid are infused into the esophagus to determine whether atypical chest pain is related to acid reflux. The sensitivity and specificity of these diagnostic tests vary widely.

Treatment

The goal of treatment is to control symptoms and heal any mucosal lesions. Most patients can be empirically managed with lifestyle changes (eg, elevating the head of the bed, reducing the size of meals, decreasing fat and caffeine intake, avoiding the supine position after eating, eliminating tobacco and alcohol use, losing weight if needed) and acid neutralization with antacids. If relief is incomplete, treatment can include sucralfate, H_2 blockers (cimetidine, famotidine, nizatidine, ranitidine), and proton-pump inhibitors (lansoprazole, omeprazole, rabeprazole). Adjunctive therapy with a prokinetic drug (metoclopramide, cisapride) can be used if necessary. Prokinetic drugs should be used with caution in the elderly because of potential neurologic or central nervous system disturbance. Cisapride has been associated with arrhythmias and death.

GERD patients with Barrett's esophagus require aggressive treatment with proton pump inhibitors. Regular endoscopic surveillance is mandatory. High-grade dysplasia dictates elective esophagectomy. Ablation with photodynamic therapy, laser therapy, or electrocauterization has had varying degrees of success and continues to be studied.

A few patients who continue to have symptoms, who have esophagitis that fails to heal, or who develop severe complications may require surgery. Belsey's and Nissen's fundoplication and Hill's posterior gastropexy are the most widely used procedures. They are estimated to be 85% successful, but symptoms recur in about 10% of patients. The morbidity rate is estimated to be 2 to 8%, and the mortality rate is about 1%. The most common complications from surgery are dysphagia and an inability to belch or vomit. Increasingly, Nissen's fundoplication is being performed laparoscopically, which may reduce short-term morbidity and length of hospital stay.

Most gastric disorders that occur in elderly patients also occur in younger patients. However, the presentation, complications, and treatment of these disorders may be different in elderly patients than in younger patients. Hiatus hernia and bleeding in the stomach are discussed in Ch. 112. Stomach tumors are discussed in Ch. 113.

GASTRITIS

Inflammation of the gastric mucosa.

Gastritis can be classified based on the severity of mucosal injury, the site of involvement, or the inflammatory cell type. No classification scheme matches perfectly with the pathophysiology, and a large degree of overlap exists.

Erosive (hemorrhagic) gastritis: This type of gastritis may be caused by use of nonsteroidal anti-inflammatory drugs (NSAIDs), alcohol, ingestion of a corrosive, trauma, radiation therapy, ischemia, bile acids (due to reflux from the duodenum), congestive gastropathy, or sporadic idiopathic gastritis. The diagnosis is usually based on endoscopic appearance. Biopsy is not usually required, except to eliminate the possibility of infection in an immunocompromised patient or to rule out specific gastritis if it is suspected.

Nonerosive (chronic) gastritis: This type of gastritis has four major patterns. It is a histologic diagnosis that cannot be predicted by endoscopic appearance.

Antral gland gastritis (type B) is the most common pattern; it is associated with *Helicobacter pylori* and duodenal ulcers. In some persons, chronic superficial antral gland gastritis associated with *H. pylori* progresses to multifocal atrophic gastritis. However, the mechanism by which gastric atrophy occurs is unclear and is probably multifactorial. As the atrophy progresses, the presence of *H. pylori* decreases, possibly because hypochlorhydria creates an environment that is not conducive to the bacteria.

Fundic (oxyntic) gland gastritis (type A) can be associated with diffuse severe mucosal atrophy and pernicious anemia. Diffuse severe atrophic fundic gland gastritis primarily affects elderly patients, who develop achlorhydria, but with a residual ability to absorb vitamin B_{12}. Patients with pernicious anemia generally have antibodies against parietal cells (90%) and intrinsic factor (60%). Antiparietal cell antibodies also occur in 50% of patients with gastric atrophy without pernicious anemia (but without anti-intrinsic factor antibodies) and in 10 to 15% of normal persons.

In **pangastritis** (coexisting antral gland gastritis and fundic gland gastritis), the fundic gland gastritis is characterized by less severe inflammation than the antral gland gastritis. Pangastritis can result in extensive mucous gland (pseudopyloric) metaplasia and varying amounts of intestinal metaplasia. Nests of parietal cells commonly occur, even in the presence of achlorhydria.

Multifocal atrophic gastritis, which appears to begin near the incisura and extends proximally and distally, is commonly associated with intestinal metaplasia.

Specific (distinctive) gastritis: Specific gastritis may be caused by infections, Crohn's disease, eosinophilia, systemic disorders (eg, sarcoidosis), or physical agents (immunosuppressants, some chemotherapeutic agents [eg, 5-fluorouracil], radiotherapy). Distinctive histologic and sometimes endoscopic features allow a diagnosis or markedly narrow the differential diagnosis.

Treatment

Treatment should be directed at the underlying cause. Factors identified as contributing to the inflammatory process should be eliminated, if possible. Acid neutralization and suppression (with antacids, sucralfate, H_2 blockers, proton pump inhibitors) may be helpful.

PEPTIC ULCER DISEASE

An excoriated segment of the gastrointestinal mucosa, typically in the stomach (gastric ulcer) or first few centimeters of the duodenum (duodenal ulcer), which penetrates through the muscularis mucosae.

In the USA, about 10% of adults have peptic ulcer disease. Although incidence information in the elderly is limited, hospitalization, morbidity, and mortality rates from peptic ulcer disease are higher for the elderly than for the general population.

Gastric ulcers in elderly patients may be located more proximally in the stomach than are those in younger patients. The increasing incidence of chronic gastritis with age, the proximal migration of the pyloric fundic junction, and the use of NSAIDs contribute to their occurrence. High gastric ulcers tend to be large, tend to heal slowly, and may be more prone to recur. They are also associated with a high frequency of complications and death.

Duodenal ulcers are more common than gastric ulcers. Duodenal ulcers may be larger in elderly patients than in younger patients; ulcers > 2 cm are increasingly reported in the elderly. Bleeding from duodenal ulcers occurs more frequently in elderly patients than in younger patients.

Etiology

H. pylori is an important factor in the development of ulcers. The prevalence of *H. pylori* infections increases with age. In the USA, about

50% of adults are seropositive by age 60. The infection affects men and women equally. About 70 to 90% of patients with gastric ulcers and 90 to 100% of patients with duodenal ulcers are infected with *H. pylori.* Despite the apparent association between *H. pylori* infection and peptic ulcer disease, the transmission and pathogenic mechanisms have not been definitively determined. Although almost all patients infected with *H. pylori* develop gastritis, only 15% develop peptic ulcer disease. However, eradication of *H. pylori* is associated with more rapid ulcer healing and a decrease in ulcer recurrence.

Use of NSAIDs increases the incidence of peptic ulcer disease, particularly within the first 3 months. Factors that appear to affect NSAID-induced ulcers in the elderly include a history of ulcer disease and the dose of NSAID. Bleeding tendency may be increased, because an age-related decrease in the sensation of visceral pain results in a delayed diagnosis of peptic ulcer disease. Concurrent use of anticoagulants greatly increases the incidence of upper gastrointestinal bleeding. NSAID use may also predispose elderly patients to large duodenal ulcers; these patients can present without a history of pain or with a history of bleeding and transient pain.

Zollinger-Ellison syndrome, a condition marked by hypergastrinemia and gastric hypersecretion due to a gastrin-producing tumor,◻ can result in peptic ulcer disease that is often persistent, progressive, and poorly responsive to treatment.

Pathogenesis

Presumed pathogenesis involves an imbalance between aggressive and defensive factors. Aggressive factors include acid-induced pepsin-induced mucosal injury and infection by *H. pylori.* Defensive factors include the production of a mucus-bicarbonate barrier, which serves as a barrier for H^+ and pepsin diffusion and protects against mucosal damage, and possibly immunologic and barrier defenses against *H. pylori.* The integrity of the mucus-bicarbonate barrier is prostaglandin-dependent. Elderly patients have decreased prostaglandin concentrations in the stomach and the duodenum. However, these concentrations do not appear to be affected by *H. pylori.* The effect of aging on the immunologic factors that may protect against *H. pylori* have not been elucidated.

Symptoms and Signs

In the elderly, the presentation of peptic ulcer disease is frequently atypical. Classic ulcer symptoms are rare; the characteristic abdominal pain occurs in only about 35% of elderly patients, and abdominal discomfort is absent in about 50% of patients using NSAIDs. Pain, if

◻ see page 1048

present, is often vague and poorly localized. The presentation may be dominated by systemic symptoms related to severe blood loss and anemia.

Dyspepsia (abdominal pain or discomfort associated with bloating, early satiety, distention, or nausea) is the most frequent symptom. However, even dyspeptic symptoms are less common with age. When dyspepsia occurs, it is often localized in the epigastric area, occurs 2 to 3 hours after the evening meal, and is relieved by food or antacids. Nocturnal pain that wakes the patient can be a symptom of peptic ulcer disease.

Complications

Complications occur in about 50% of patients > 70 years. The high mortality rate (up to 30%) may relate to the presence of comorbidity.

Bleeding, the most common complication, occurs in about 10 to 15% of ulcer patients of all ages, most commonly elderly patients. Bleeding is related to increased use of NSAIDs and may be more common in elderly women. Elderly patients with ulcers have more frequent and more severe bleeding than younger patients, require more transfusions, and are more likely to require surgery. About 10 to 20% of patients with bleeding ulcers do not have preceding symptoms. The mortality rate of elderly patients with bleeding ulcers is estimated to be 29 to 60%.

Perforation occurs in about 5 to 10% of ulcer patients. Perforation occurs more frequently with duodenal ulcers than with gastric ulcers. Use of NSAIDs increases the risk of perforated peptic ulcers in patients > 65. The elderly may postpone seeking medical attention because of a lack of symptoms, and diagnosis may be delayed because physical findings are absent. Although most elderly patients with perforated ulcers report abdominal discomfort, about 16% have minimal abdominal pain. Free air may be absent in abdominal x-rays in up to 40% of patients > 60. Most perforations require prompt surgery, which often involves a simple closure.

Gastric outlet obstruction occurs in 2 to 5% of ulcer patients and can result from acute inflammation and edema or scarring near the gastroduodenal junction. Obstruction due to inflammation and edema usually resolves with drug treatment. Obstruction due to scarring may require endoscopic dilatation or surgery. Gastric outlet obstruction typically has a lower mortality rate than other ulcer complications.

Penetration, which is less common than the other complications, is similar to perforation, except that the ulcer crater burrows through the gastric or intestinal wall into an adjacent viscus. Gastric ulcers can penetrate into the pancreas, left lobe of the liver, or colon (causing a gastrocolonic fistula). Duodenal ulcers can penetrate into the pancreas, causing pancreatitis.

Diagnosis

Empiric use of an antiulcer drug as a diagnostic trial may be appropriate in patients with mild or intermittent epigastric symptoms, without systemic complaints or complications. However, in patients > 50, diagnostic tests should be performed because symptoms and complications can be atypical and the risk of gastric malignancy increases. The choice of whether to use x-ray or endoscopy often depends on the expertise available at a particular institution. Endoscopy is the most sensitive and specific test for assessing mucosal abnormalities in the upper gastrointestinal tract, and biopsies and therapeutic intervention can be performed if necessary during the procedure.

Occasionally, benign gastric ulcers may be difficult to differentiate from ulcers due to stomach cancer. Therefore, gastric ulcers must undergo biopsy to eliminate the possibility of malignancy, and the patient should have a repeat diagnostic test after 6 to 8 weeks of therapy to assess healing.

Prognosis

The morbidity and mortality rates from peptic ulcer disease have decreased in the general population. However, the mortality rate has increased significantly in patients > 75; the hospitalization rate due to bleeding and perforation has also increased significantly in these patients.

These increases in morbidity and mortality rates have been attributed to the increased use of NSAIDs among the elderly. However, the introduction of cyclooxygenase (COX-2) inhibitors (eg, celecoxib, rofecoxib) may decrease the incidence and complication rate of ulcer disease. Concurrent use of antiulcer drugs with traditional NSAIDs is not likely to be highly effective.

Treatment

Patients should discontinue use of NSAIDs, alcohol, tobacco, and caffeine. Alcohol may stimulate acid secretion; tobacco and caffeine have been reported to delay healing. Empiric use of antiulcer drugs without diagnostic investigation may be appropriate only in younger patients with mild or intermittent epigastric symptoms and without systemic complaints or complications.

The most effective drugs in ulcer management are those that neutralize acid, inhibit gastric acid secretion, promote healing through stimulation of mucosal defense mechanisms, and promote healing through eradication of *H. pylori*. However, dyspepsia does not consistently improve after *H. pylori* eradication.

Antacids: Antacids neutralize gastric acid, which increases gastroduodenal pH. Various formulations exist; the sodium content is high in some. Calcium carbonate antacids bind dietary phosphorus, which may cause hypophosphatemia. Magnesium-containing antacids have a cathartic effect and can cause diarrhea; these antacids should be used with caution in patients with renal dysfunction because of potential hypermagnesemia and related toxicity. Aluminum-containing antacids can cause constipation, osteomalacia, hypophosphatemia, and related toxicity.

H₂ blockers: H_2 blockers (eg, cimetidine, famotidine, nizatidine, ranitidine) are reversible blockers of histamine-induced acid secretion of gastric parietal cells. They are potent inhibitors of gastric acid secretion and eliminate symptoms and prevent complications of peptic ulcer disease.

H_2 blockers are generally well tolerated; the overall incidence of adverse effects is < 3%. Risk factors for adverse effects include concurrent medical disorders, hepatic or renal disease, and advanced age. Cimetidine has the greatest degree of antiandrogenic effects (eg, gynecomastia, erectile dysfunction) and central nervous system effects (eg, confusion, agitation, anxiety, depression). Clinically significant interaction between H_2 blockers and other drugs may occur because of an alteration in absorption, metabolism, or excretion. Absorption of some drugs may be reduced by the increased gastric pH. Cimetidine inhibits the cytochrome P-450 oxidase system. Ranitidine weakly binds to cytochrome P-450 and appears to have much less potential for significant adverse drug interactions. Famotidine and nizatidine do not affect the cytochrome P-450 oxidase system.

Proton pump inhibitors: Omeprazole, lansoprazole, and rabeprazole suppress gastric acid secretion by specific inhibition of the H^+,K^+-ATPase enzyme system of the gastric parietal cells. The effect is dose-related and inhibits basal and stimulated acid secretion regardless of the stimulus. In the elderly, the elimination rates of omeprazole and lansoprazole are decreased and bioavailability is increased. However, dose alteration does not appear to be necessary. These drugs are well tolerated, and the rates of gastric or duodenal ulcer healing and of adverse effects do not significantly differ in elderly and younger patients. Long-term use (> 5 years) of omeprazole is safe.

Sucralfate: Sucralfate works locally by forming an ulcer-adherent complex that coats the ulcer site and protects it against acid, pepsin, and bile salts. It also creates a barrier to hydrogen ion diffusion, inhibiting the action of pepsin and absorbing bile salts. It is minimally absorbed. Adverse reactions, most frequently constipation, are minor and rarely necessitate drug discontinuation. However, sucralfate should be used with caution in patients with chronic renal failure because of the potential for aluminum absorption and associated toxicity. Sucralfate can bind to several drugs and reduces absorption of quinolone antibiotics, phenytoin, and warfarin.

Misoprostol: Misoprostol, a synthetic prostaglandin E_1 analog, has antisecretory and mucosal protective properties. It is indicated only for prophylactic treatment in patients taking NSAIDs. It helps prevent NSAID-induced damage of the gastric mucosa but has not been shown to prevent duodenal ulcers in patients taking NSAIDs. Dosage is usually the same in elderly and younger persons. Misoprostol causes diarrhea in 13 to 40% of cases and abdominal pain in 7 to 20%. **Anti–*H. pylori* therapy:** In patients with documented *H. pylori* infection, the use of antisecretory drugs combined with antibiotics against *H. pylori* results in more rapid duodenal ulcer healing. No standard therapy for *H. pylori* eradication exists; thus, efficacy, tolerability, compliance, and cost must be considered when selecting a regimen. Triple and quadruple therapy regimens (two or three antibiotics with a proton pump inhibitor) are most effective for eradicating *H. pylori;* eg, oral lansoprazole 30 mg bid, clarithromycin 500 mg bid, and amoxicillin 1000 mg bid for 2 weeks; or lansoprazole 30 mg bid, bismuth subsalicylate 525 mg qid, amoxicillin 500 mg qid, and metronidazole 250 mg qid for 2 weeks. Ranitidine bismuth citrate 400 mg po bid for 4 weeks and clarithromycin 500 mg po tid for 2 weeks may also be effective. Monotherapy is not recommended because of its limited effectiveness and its potential for stimulating antimicrobial resistance. Dual therapy using a proton pump inhibitor and an antimicrobial drug has been used.

Surgery: Surgery is reserved for ulcer patients who are refractory to drug treatment or who have complications.

MÉNÉTRIER'S DISEASE

A disorder in which enlarged gastric rugae affect part or all of the stomach.

This rare idiopathic disease is difficult to define. It most often occurs in patients > 50. A wide variety of symptoms occur, including epigastric pain, weight loss up to 25 kg (55 lb), nausea, vomiting, gastrointestinal bleeding, and diarrhea. Typical findings include enlarged gastric folds (especially in the fundus and body), histologic features of foveolar hyperplasia and glandular atrophy, and an overall increase in mucosal thickness. Hypoalbuminemia occurs in 20 to 100% of patients (depending on at what stage the disease is diagnosed). The amount of basal and stimulated gastric acid secretion is low or normal. Small or moderate increases in serum gastrin levels may be associated with acid hypersecretion.

The natural history of Ménétrier's disease is not well documented. Symptoms may persist for decades. Although a relationship to stomach cancer was initially described, this association is reported to be only 2 to 15%.

Diagnosis

Diagnosis is suggested when barium swallow demonstrates enlarged, nodular folds. Upper endoscopy and endoscopic ultrasound can confirm the x-ray findings. Definitive diagnosis requires biopsy that reveals marked oxyntic gland loss and cystic changes. However, biopsy may not be necessary, especially in patients with typical clinical features occurring over several years.

Treatment

Information about prognosis is limited. No drug therapy has consistently provided beneficial results. Some patients with associated ulcers or erosions may benefit symptomatically from peptic ulcer therapy. *H. pylori,* if found, should be eradicated. Surgery, most commonly subtotal gastrectomy, is advocated for patients who have intractable symptoms or in whom a malignancy cannot be excluded.

ZOLLINGER-ELLISON SYNDROME

A syndrome characterized by marked hypergastrinemia, gastric hypersecretion, and peptic ulceration caused by a gastrin-producing tumor (gastrinoma) of the pancreas or the duodenal wall.

The high output of gastrin from a gastrinoma continuously stimulates the parietal cells to produce acid. The incidence of gastrinomas is unknown, but these tumors are thought to be responsible for about 0.1 to 1% of duodenal ulcers. Onset of Zollinger-Ellison syndrome occurs between ages 30 and 50; about one third of patients with this syndrome are > 60.

Symptoms and Signs

Peptic ulcer disease and its symptoms occur in 90 to 95% of patients; symptoms can be persistent, progressive, and poorly responsive to drug treatment and surgery. Diarrhea occurs in > 30% of patients and may predate ulcer symptoms. Steatorrhea may result from inactivation of pancreatic lipase with a failure to hydrolyze intraluminal triglycerides and from a low pH in the lumen of the small intestine, which can result in insoluble bile acids with decreased formation of micelles. Typically, basal acid output is > 15 mEq/hour.

Diagnosis

Zollinger-Ellison syndrome is suggested by its characteristic clinical findings. Barium radiography can demonstrate prominent gastric rugal folds and duodenal (and occasionally jejunal) folds that may be thickened and dilated. Hypersecretion of gastric acid occurs in > 90% of patients. However, the most sensitive and specific diagnostic test is the demonstration of hypergastrinemia. Patients with gastrinoma typically have serum gastrin levels > 150 pg/mL (> 71.6 pmol/L), with average serum gastrin levels of about 1000 pg/mL (> 477 pmol/L). Provocative tests include the secretin test (the most accurate) and the calcium test. In the secretin test, secretin 2 U/kg is administered over 30 seconds with serum gastrin levels measured 5 minutes before, immediately before, and 2 and 5 minutes after administration, then at 5-minute intervals for a total of 30 minutes. Serum gastrin levels increase by ≥ 200 pg/mL (≥ 95.4 pmol/L), often within 2 minutes and almost universally by 10 minutes. In the calcium test, calcium gluconate infusion at 5 mg/kg/hour is given for 3 hours; serum gastrin levels are measured 30 minutes before and immediately before infusion and at 30-minute intervals thereafter for 4 hours. Serum gastrin levels typically increase by > 400 pg/mL (> 190.8 pmol/L), with maximum levels usually occurring during the final hour of calcium infusion.

Treatment

Some clinicians and investigators would suggest that surgical removal is more desirable than symptom management; cure rates with surgery approach 40%. Preoperative evaluation should include abdominal ultrasound, CT, and selective arteriography to localize gastrinomas and exclude metastases. Surgery is contraindicated in patients with unresectable metastatic disease.

For nonsurgical management, omeprazole is the drug of choice. The initial dose is usually 60 mg/day po, which is adjusted as necessary. Gastric acid production is monitored; the goal is to reduce basal acid output to < 10 mEq/hour in patients who are not surgical candidates, to < 5 mEq/hour in patients with previous gastric resection, and to < 1 mEq/hour in patients with severe gastroesophageal reflux disease (GERD).

Octreotide, a synthetic analog of somatostatin, decreases serum gastrin levels and gastric acid production, but it can be given only parenterally and has no benefit over omeprazole. Chemotherapy with streptozocin and 5-fluorouracil decreases serum gastrin levels in patients with metastatic disease but is usually reserved for patients with liver metastases to relieve symptoms.

GASTRIC VOLVULUS

A disorder in which the stomach twists so as to turn on itself.

This relatively rare condition is more common in elderly persons, in whom the ligaments supporting the stomach are more relaxed than in younger persons. The most common type of gastric volvulus, organoaxial volvulus, involves a rotation of the stomach on its longitudinal axis (from cardia to pylorus). The less common type, mesenteroaxial volvulus, involves a rotation of the stomach on its vertical axis passing through the center of the lesser and greater curvatures. A complete twist of the stomach can result in strangulation of the blood supply, which can lead to gangrene.

Symptoms and Signs

Acute volvulus causes sudden, severe pain localized to the upper abdomen or chest. The upper abdomen can become markedly distended, whereas the lower abdomen remains undistended and soft. Persistent retching with little or no vomitus is common. In complete volvulus, a nasogastric tube cannot be passed. The combination of upper abdominal pain and distention, an inability to vomit, and an impediment to nasogastric tube insertion is known as Borchardt's triad. Chest pain may radiate down the arms and neck and is often accompanied by dyspnea.

Chronic, intermittent gastric volvulus causes mild and nonspecific symptoms, such as epigastric discomfort, heartburn, abdominal fullness or bloating, and borborygmi, especially after meals. Because this is an unusual disorder, these nonspecific symptoms may result in this disorder being underdiagnosed.

Diagnosis and Treatment

Volvulus is usually diagnosed by a plain or contrast x-ray of the abdomen. X-ray of organoaxial volvulus often shows an "upside-down stomach" and double air-fluid levels (fundus and antrum).

The mortality rate is about 15 to 20%. It increases to 40% for cases that require emergency surgery and to about 60% for cases involving strangulation. Treatment is always surgical. In cases of acute strangulation with ischemia or gangrene, or when tube decompression cannot be performed, emergency surgery is necessary. Endoscopic reduction can be used to treat some cases, but it should be considered a temporary measure and is contraindicated in patients who appear to have vascular compromise.

BEZOARS

Concretions of ingested foreign material (animal or vegetable) that remain in the gastrointestinal tract.

The formation of bezoars is usually related to altered gastric physiology with impaired gastric emptying due to vagotomy, antral resection, gastroparesis, or gastric outlet obstruction. Poor mastication, in which food particles are insufficiently broken, and the consumption of large quantities of indigestible solids may also precipitate bezoar formation.

Bezoars most frequently occur in the elderly, especially in elderly diabetic patients, in whom gastric emptying is severely abnormal. An edentulous patient may be at risk because of poor mastication.

Symptoms, Signs, and Diagnosis

A variety of symptoms and signs can occur, including early satiety, nausea, vomiting, and epigastric pain. Complications (eg, localized ulceration and bleeding) have been reported. Physical findings include the presence of a mass, succussion, or evidence of gastrointestinal bleeding from secondary ulceration. Abdominal x-rays may identify the presence of a foreign body. Endoscopy or barium swallow usually confirms the diagnosis.

Treatment

The treatment of bezoars depends on their composition. Prokinetic drugs (eg, metoclopramide, cisapride), manual disruption, and lavage with a large-bore orogastric tube may facilitate passage. However, metoclopramide can cause adverse reactions in the elderly (eg, neurologic or central nervous system disturbances), and cisapride can cause serious cardiovascular reactions (eg, torsades de pointes and other ventricular arrhythmias) when taken simultaneously with certain medications.

Disruption of the bezoar can be performed endoscopically. Instruments inserted through the endoscope into the stomach can break the bezoar into smaller pieces, which can pass spontaneously into the small intestine. Some bezoars must be surgically removed. Dissolution with various enzymes (eg, papain, meat tenderizer, cellulase, acetylcysteine) has had variable results. Recurrence can be prevented by repairing any obstruction, correcting dietary routine, or using a prokinetic drug.

ANGIODYSPLASIA

(Vascular Ectasias)

A syndrome of gastrointestinal mucosal vascular ectasias not associated with cutaneous lesions, systemic vascular disease, or familial syndromes.

Angiodysplasia is found in about 1 to 2% of patients undergoing upper endoscopy. In the elderly, angiodysplasia may occur in the upper and lower gastrointestinal tract.∎ Although gastric and duodenal lesions have occasionally been reported in patients in their 20s, the mean age of patients with upper tract lesions is > 60 years. The etiology is uncertain. The ectasias may be a degenerative process of aging and result from chronic, low-grade obstruction of the submucosal vein or from chronic mucosal ischemia. Brisk or occult gastrointestinal bleeding may occur. Bleeding angiodysplasia is more likely to occur in patients with aortic valve disease, chronic renal failure requiring dialysis, or von Willebrand's disease. The clinical course of untreated lesions is unknown. However, retrospective reviews have suggested that in most persons the course is indolent.

Angiodysplasia is most readily diagnosed by endoscopy. The lesions are typically discrete, flat or slightly raised, and bright red and are often stellate in appearance. Celiac artery and superior mesenteric artery injections may fail to demonstrate the lesions.

Treatment

Gastric and duodenal angiodysplastic lesions are most frequently treated with endoscopic obliteration techniques (eg, electrocautery, heater probe, or multipolar coagulation devices). Argon and neodymium:yttrium-aluminum-garnet (Nd:YAG) lasers have also been used for endoscopic obliteration. Sclerotherapy (sodium tetradecyl sulfate 1.5% 0.5 to 1 mL) obliterates upper tract lesions, but bleeding recurs in half of these patients.

In patients who are not candidates for surgery, transcatheter embolization after selective cannulation of the branches of mesenteric artery has been successful. Selective infusion of vasopressin is less effective than embolization.

Surgical resection has been used to treat bleeding angiodysplasias that have been clearly identified. However, surgery may provide only short-term benefits; bleeding recurs in up to 50% of patients.

Although the causal relationship between aortic stenosis and angiodysplasia has been questioned, several cases have been reported in which bleeding from an angiodysplastic lesion ceased after aortic valve replacement. Estrogen-progesterone therapy (ethinyl estradiol 0.05 mg/day po and norethindrone 1 mg/day; norethynodrel 5 to 10 mg with mestranol 0.075 to 0.15 mg/day po) or conjugated estrogens (0.625 mg/day po) have been used in patients with chronic bleeding, with variable results.

∎ see also page 1057

LOWER GASTROINTESTINAL TRACT DISORDERS

The principal functions of the colon and rectum are storing fecal waste for prolonged periods and expelling it appropriately. Storage is facilitated by adaptive compliance of the intestine and by contractions of colonic smooth muscle, which slow the movement of stool, thereby promoting water absorption and reducing stool volume. Stool moves by relatively infrequent peristaltic contractions. Defecation and continence are maintained by the ability to sense rectal filling and by the coordinated function of the internal and external anal sphincters and the pelvic floor muscles.

Colonic motility and transit in healthy elderly persons are similar to those in younger persons; however, aging is associated with diminished anal sphincter tone and strength and decreased rectal compliance. The latter may increase susceptibility to fecal incontinence in the elderly.

The major symptoms of lower gastrointestinal (GI) disorders are constipation, diarrhea, pain, rectal bleeding, and fecal incontinence. Lower GI disorders that occur more commonly in the elderly than in younger persons are diverticular disease, angiodysplasia, colonic ischemia,[1] antibiotic-associated diarrhea and colitis, fecal incontinence,[2] and constipation.[3] Inflammatory bowel diseases occur in all age groups, but new onset is more likely in the elderly and in persons in their 20s.

DIVERTICULAR DISEASE

Diseases associated with diverticula (acquired sac-like mucosal projections through the muscular layer of the GI tract), which cause symptoms by trapping feces, becoming infected, bleeding, or rupturing.

Diverticula develop in areas where circular smooth muscle has been weakened by the penetration of blood vessels to the submucosa. Usually, diverticula are found in the sigmoid and descending colons and rarely in the rectum.

Aging may lead to structural weakening of colonic muscle and the development of diverticula. In Western countries, diverticular disease occurs in about 50% of persons $\geq$ 65 years and in about 65% of those $\geq$ 80. Diverticula have been found with increasing frequency in Western populations, probably because of increased longevity and insufficient dietary fiber. A low-fiber diet may increase colonic motor activity and intraluminal pressures.

---

[1] see page 1117   [2] see page 1092   [3] see page 1080

Bleeding results from rupture of the penetrating arteriole in its course around the diverticular sac and is usually brisk and painless. The origin of most diverticular bleeding, when known, is the right colon. Although 10 to 20% of patients have persistent hemorrhage, bleeding usually stops spontaneously.

Because diverticula are asymptomatic in most persons and are common in the elderly, other possible causes of nonspecific GI symptoms should be considered before attributing the symptoms to diverticula. For example, colon cancer, inflammatory bowel disease, and ischemia may mimic diverticulitis; a patient with angiodysplasia of the colon may present with brisk, painless bleeding.

DIVERTICULOSIS

Diverticula without inflammation.

Colonic diverticulosis is asymptomatic. Dietary measures aim to prevent complications (eg, diverticulitis, bleeding). However, there is no evidence that such measures prevent complications. Fiber supplements or an increased dietary fiber intake is recommended.

PAINFUL DIVERTICULAR DISEASE

Diverticulosis accompanied by painful spasm or other symptoms.

Painful diverticular disease is characterized by cramps in the left lower abdomen without infection or inflammation. Symptoms are often associated with constipation or diarrhea and tenderness over the affected areas; symptoms increase after eating and may be partially relieved by defecating or passing flatus. Excessive colonic motility is the underlying mechanism producing symptoms. Symptoms of painful diverticular disease are similar to those of irritable bowel syndrome and partial bowel obstruction caused by tumors or ischemia. In contrast with diverticulitis, painful diverticular disease is not characterized by fever, leukocytosis, or rebound tenderness. Treatment aims to reduce symptoms caused by smooth muscle spasm (see TABLE 107–1). Fiber supplements or an increased dietary fiber intake is recommended.

DIVERTICULITIS

Infection arising from colonic diverticula.

The incidence of diverticulitis increases with the duration of diverticulosis. Diverticulitis develops in 15 to 25% of persons with diverticulosis who are followed for $\geq$ 10 years. Diverticulitis is caused by colonic flora (eg, aerobic and anaerobic gram-negative bacilli); the role of enterococci is unknown.

TABLE 107–1.   TREATMENT OF DIVERTICULAR DISEASE*

Measures	Painful Diverticular Disease	Diverticulitis
Diet	Increase fiber	Reduce fiber (or nothing orally)
Bulk laxatives	Probably effective	Not indicated
Analgesics	Nonopioid analgesic (NSAIDs are preferred); if an opioid is needed, choose meperidine over morphine	Nonopioid analgesic (NSAIDs are preferred); if an opioid is needed, choose meperidine over morphine
Antispasmodics†	Propantheline 15 mg po tid Dicyclomine 20 mg po tid Hyoscyamine 0.125–0.250 mg po or sublingually q 4 h Glucagon 2 mg IV (most commonly used to aid diagnosis)	Not indicated
Antibiotics	Not indicated	Oral Amoxicillin and clavulanate 750 mg tid Parenteral (choice) 1. Gentamicin or tobramycin 5 mg/kg/day plus clindamycin 1.2–2.4 g/day or mezlocillin 4 g qid 2. Cefoxitin 4–6 g/day 3. Ampicillin and sulbactam 6–12 g/day 4. Piperacillin sodium and tazobactam sodium 3.375 g q 6 h

* Most of these drugs require dosage adjustments in the elderly, who may have reduced renal or hepatic clearance.

† NOTE: High risk of adverse effects in the elderly.

NSAIDs = nonsteroidal anti-inflammatory drugs.

Modified from Wald A: "Colonic diverticulosis," in *Management of Gastrointestinal Diseases,* edited by SJ Winawer. Published by Wolfe Publishing, an imprint of Times Mirror International Publishers, 1992, Chapter 34, pp. 1–18.

Symptoms, Signs, and Diagnosis

Inflammation begins at the apex of a diverticulum when the opening becomes obstructed with stool. Fever, leukocytosis, or rebound tenderness indicates inflammation, which often remains localized in the adjacent pericolic tissues but may progress to a peridiverticular abscess. Other complications include formation of fistula to the bladder (most common), vagina, or adjacent small intestine; fibrosis and bowel obstruction; perforation with peritonitis; and sepsis. Frank rectal bleeding is not characteristic of diverticulitis.

Distinguishing between painful diverticular disease and diverticulitis is often inaccurate. In an elderly or debilitated patient, the absence of fever, leukocytosis, or rebound tenderness does not exclude diverticulitis.

If diverticulitis, abscess, or extraintestinal complications are suspected (eg, if a palpable mass is detected), a barium enema should usually be delayed by about 1 week to allow some resolution of the inflammatory process. A single contrast study can be performed with precautions to minimize the risk of perforation and extravasation of contrast material. However, abdominal CT or ultrasound provides better definition of colonic wall thickness and extraluminal structures and has supplanted contrast studies for suspected diverticulitis. CT is the most cost-effective study, with additional potential use in the treatment of abscess.

Colonoscopy is less desirable during an acute episode and is best used to exclude tumors or other conditions when other diagnostic tests are inconclusive. When contrast studies fail to identify the bleeding source, colonoscopy is indicated. Before colonoscopy is performed, colon cleansing is necessary; once the patient is stabilized and bleeding has slowed or stopped, balanced electrolyte solutions containing polyethylene glycol are given orally or by nasogastric tube. If bleeding remains brisk or the patient is unstable, selective mesenteric angiography can be used to locate the site of bleeding and to infuse vasoactive substances to control bleeding. If bleeding is intermittent or too slow to be detected by angiography, serial abdominal scans can be used (preceded by injection of technetium-99m–labelled red blood cells).

Treatment

The most important goal is to eliminate bacterial infection (see TABLE 107–1). If diverticulitis is mild, the patient may be treated as an outpatient with oral antibiotics and oral intake restrictions. More acutely ill patients are hospitalized.

Surgery is recommended for patients who fail to respond to medical therapy within 72 hours, for many patients who have had two or more attacks of diverticulitis, for many immunocompromised patients, and for patients whose first attack occurred before age 40. Because of the high risk of recurrences, complications, and increased morbidity, most patients with complicated diverticular disease require surgery even if clinical recovery occurs. The preferred procedure is a one-stage operation in which the diseased segment of bowel is resected and continuity restored by a primary anastomosis. If this procedure is not feasible, a two-stage operation that requires a diverting colostomy should be used.

Before elective surgery, large abscesses often can be drained percutaneously by an interventional radiologist using CT or ultrasound. Surgery may be performed after successful drainage and 2 to 3 weeks of antibiotic therapy.

Emergency surgery is required for generalized peritonitis, persistent high-grade bowel obstruction, or rapid, unremitting GI bleeding. Elderly patients with generalized peritonitis require immediate excision of the perforation site; giving antibiotics and waiting for resolution result in an extremely high mortality.

ANGIODYSPLASIA

(Vascular Ecstasias)

Small clusters of dilated and tortuous veins in the mucosa of the colon and small intestine, which may cause lower GI bleeding.

Angiodysplasia occurs in > 25% of persons ≥ 60 and is an important cause of acute and major lower GI bleeding as well as of slow intermittent blood loss in the elderly. Repeated episodes of low-grade, partial obstruction of submucosal veins are believed to occur when colonic muscles contract or when intraluminal pressure increases, resulting in venous dilation and tortuosity. Mucosal veins drained by the submucosal vein may also be affected. In the final stage of development, the precapillary sphincter becomes incompetent, and a small arteriovenous communication with the ectatic tuft of vessels develops. Angiodysplasia usually develops in the right colon, probably because tension on the bowel wall is greater, as expressed by Laplace's law relating tension to the diameter of the bowel lumen. A causal association between angiodysplasia and aortic stenosis has been questioned after a thorough review of the literature.

Symptoms, Signs, and Diagnosis

Mucosal angiodysplasia is asymptomatic in most persons. Patients usually present with painless, subacute, and recurrent bleeding, which stops spontaneously in the vast majority of cases. Bleeding may be red blood, maroon stools, or melena, or it may be occult. About 10 to 15% of patients have episodes of brisk blood loss.

Diagnosis may be made by colonoscopy or mesenteric angiography. Colonoscopy is preferred because it can exclude other causes of bleeding and can also be used as a therapeutic intervention. Because lesions are small, often multiple, and difficult to see, the colon must be thoroughly cleansed to allow for adequate visualization of the mucosa. Cleansing is usually performed after bleeding has stopped, preferably within 48 hours so that other sources of bleeding (eg, diverticula or ischemia) can be identified. Meperidine should not be used to sedate patients undergoing colonoscopy because it makes identification of ectasias more difficult; if meperidine is required, naloxone can be administered during the procedure to enhance visualization.

Mesenteric angiography is preferred when acute bleeding is brisk. Advanced angiodysplasia is indicated by tortuous, densely opacified clusters of small veins that empty slowly. Arteriovenous communication is indicated by early filling of the vein and is found in most patients evaluated for bleeding. When bleeding is active ($\geq$ 0.5 to 1.0 mL/minute), the contrast medium is extravasated into the bowel lumen, but because bleeding is often intermittent, extravasation is seen in only a minority of patients. However, scintigraphy with technetium Tc-99m–labelled red blood cells may locate a bleeding site. This technique detects active bleeding at rates of 0.05 to 0.1 mL/minute, and the patient can be serially scanned for up to 36 hours if bleeding is intermittent.

Treatment

Conservative treatment with blood or iron replacement as appropriate may be all that is necessary. Diet and the use of laxatives, analgesics, and other drugs are outlined in TABLE 107–1. When bleeding is recurrent, transcolonoscopic electrocoagulation or laser coagulation may be attempted. Difficulties include identifying the ectatic lesions and excluding other causes of blood loss if bleeding has stopped. Also, perforation of the right colon is a recognized hazard of coagulation therapy.

Active, severe bleeding may be controlled quickly by intra-arterial or IV administration of vasopressin 0.2 to 0.6 U/min, which often stabilizes the patient for more definitive treatment. If coagulation therapy is not technically possible or if acute bleeding cannot be controlled, surgery is required. If the right colon is the only identified source of bleeding, a right hemicolectomy is performed. However, after such surgery, bleeding recurs in up to 20% of patients, who then require a more extensive colonic resection or exploratory laparotomy.

Small-bowel enteroscopy may eventually reduce the need for diagnostic laparotomy in patients with recurrent bleeding from obscure sites. For these patients, estrogen-progesterone therapy may decrease transfusion requirements.

INFLAMMATORY BOWEL DISEASE

Inflammatory bowel disease includes ulcerative colitis and Crohn's disease. The age of onset for ulcerative colitis and Crohn's disease is bimodal; the first peak occurs during the 20s, and the second occurs between ages 50 and 80. The reasons for this bimodality are unknown. The prevalence of inflammatory bowel diseases is increasing as more patients with these conditions live longer.

ULCERATIVE COLITIS

A chronic inflammatory process of unknown origin that affects the superficial layers of the colonic wall in a continuous distribution.

Although incidence and prevalence data in the elderly are not precise, ulcerative colitis is probably as common in the elderly as in younger persons, affecting about 128/100,000 persons in the USA and Europe. Histologic examination reveals diffuse ulcerations, epithelial necrosis, depletion of goblet cells, and polymorphonuclear leukocyte infiltration extending from the superficial layers of the colon to the muscularis mucosa. Crypt abscesses are characteristic but not pathognomonic. The inflammatory process invariably involves the rectum and extends proximally for variable distances but not beyond the colon.

Symptoms and Signs

Ulcerative colitis may be classified as mild, moderate, or severe. Symptoms in the elderly are similar to those in younger persons. Most patients have diarrhea with or without blood in the stool, although elderly patients occasionally present with constipation or hematochezia. Systemic manifestations occur during more severe attacks and indicate a poorer prognosis. Although the disease may be less extensive in elderly patients, they present with a severe initial attack more often and have higher mortality and morbidity rates than younger patients.

Extraintestinal manifestations include arthralgias, erythema nodosum, pyoderma gangrenosum, uveitis, and migratory polyarthritis. These conditions occur more often in patients with increased disease activity and less often in patients with ulcerative colitis than in those with Crohn's disease.

Complications

Toxic megacolon, a serious complication of ulcerative colitis, occurs more often in elderly patients than in younger patients. Abdominal x-rays show colonic dilation; patients may be confused and have high fever, abdominal distention, and overall deterioration. Mortality is high.

The risk of developing colorectal cancer increases substantially in all patients beginning about 8 years after the onset of pancolonic disease. However, cancer may develop after many years of even quiescent disease. Therefore, despite some shortcomings in the interpretation of biopsies and in the outcome of surveillance programs, all patients with long-standing ulcerative colitis should have an annual colonoscopy with biopsy to detect mucosal dysplasia, which is considered a premalignant lesion in ulcerative colitis. Biopsies should be taken randomly throughout the colon and in areas that appear suspicious. If high-grade dysplasia is found, proctocolectomy is indicated.

Diagnosis

The diagnosis is made by sigmoidoscopy and rectal mucosal biopsies because the rectum is always involved. The extent of disease is determined by colonoscopy or barium x-ray; both procedures should be avoided in severely ill patients because of the risk of perforation and toxic megacolon. The characteristic findings are diffuse erythema, granularity, and friability of the mucosa without intervening areas of normal mucosa (skip areas). Inflammatory pseudopolyps indicate more severe erosion of the mucosa and must be distinguished from true polyps.

Diseases that may mimic ulcerative colitis, including Crohn's disease, ischemic colitis, radiation coloproctitis, and diverticulitis, must be excluded, particularly in the elderly. In acutely ill patients, stool cultures should be obtained to exclude infectious agents, including *Salmonella, Campylobacter, Shigella,* amebiasis, *Yersinia,* and *Escherichia coli* 0157:H7. *Clostridium difficile*-associated diarrhea and pseudomembranous colitis should be considered in elderly patients, particularly those who recently received antibiotics, were hospitalized, or are institutionalized.

Treatment

Treatment is based on the extent and severity of the disease (see TABLE 107–2). A number of effective drugs (eg, corticosteroids, 5-aminosalicylates [5-ASA], immunosuppressants) can be administered IV, orally, or rectally.

Severe disease: Patients with severe or fulminant disease, including toxic megacolon, should be hospitalized and receive IV hydrocortisone, methylprednisolone, or corticotropin infused in fluids containing enough potassium to avoid hypokalemia. One study suggests that corticotropin is more effective in patients who have not been treated previously with corticosteroids, whereas hydrocortisone may be more effective in those who have. If corticotropin does not produce significant improvement in 2 to 3 days, IV cyclosporine may be tried, but renal function should be closely monitored, especially in the elderly. When improvement is noted, IV therapy should be replaced with oral therapy.

Moderately severe disease: Oral corticosteroids are used to achieve a remission or to sustain one after IV therapy. Therapy consists of prednisone 40 to 60 mg/day initially given in two doses, then in a single morning dose. When the disease is controlled, the prednisone dose should be tapered rapidly to 20 mg every morning; then it can be

TABLE 107–2.   TREATMENT OF ULCERATIVE COLITIS

Indication	Drug	Dosage
Severe disease (patient has previously received corticosteroids)	Methylprednisolone Hydrocortisone	60–80 mg/day IV 300 mg/day IV
Severe disease (patient has not previously received corticosteroids)	Corticotropin	120 U/day IV
Mild to moderate disease (proximal to sigmoid)	Sulfasalazine Mesalamine* Prednisone	2–4 g/day po Varies by formulation 40–60 mg/day po
Active distal disease	Hydrocortisone cream	One application (1% in 30 g) 1–2 times per day
	Hydrocortisone aerosol foam	One application (1% in 10 g) 3–4 times per day
	Mesalamine enema	60 mL (4 g mesalamine) rectally once a day
	Sulfasalazine	4–6 g/day po
	Hydrocortisone retention enema solution	100 mg in 60 mL nightly
Maintenance of remission		
Distal disease	Mesalamine enema	Every night to every 3rd night
Pancolonic disease	Sulfasalazine Olsalazine*	1 g po bid 500 mg po bid

* If sulfasalazine is not tolerated.

tapered by 5 mg/day each week as long as the disease remains quiescent. The corticosteroid dose should be tapered while clinical activity and appropriate laboratory studies are monitored. Long-term corticosteroid therapy risks significant adverse effects related to both the dose and duration of therapy. These drugs may exacerbate diabetes mellitus, heart failure, osteoporosis, and hypertension, which are common in the elderly.

A 5-ASA drug should be given with oral corticosteroids. Sulfasalazine is effective and inexpensive, but its use is limited by adverse effects in up to 30% of patients. The adverse effects, which are often dose-dependent, include nausea, anorexia, headache, and sometimes a generalized rash; in most cases, these effects result from the inactive sulfapyridine carrier rather than the 5-ASA. If adverse effects occur, sulfasalazine should be replaced with a more expensive 5-ASA drug (eg, olsalazine, mesalamine). Diarrhea is a potential adverse effect of all

5-ASA drugs. Treatment should be maintained indefinitely for patients who can tolerate it.

Mild disease: Patients with mild disease may be treated effectively with 5-ASA drugs that can be given orally, by enema in patients with left-sided disease, or by suppositories in patients with limited proctitis. Rectal corticosteroids are also effective in left-sided disease but generally are not more effective than 5-ASA drugs. Because about 60% of a rectal corticosteroid may be absorbed, it is less suitable for maintenance therapy. Several poorly absorbed corticosteroid enema products and corticosteroids that do not affect the adrenal-pituitary-hypothalamic axis are under investigation and appear to be promising.

Maintenance therapy: For patients in remission, long-term maintenance with a 5-ASA drug reduces the frequency of relapses. The usual maintenance dose of sulfasalazine (1 g po bid) produces few or no long-term adverse effects. For patients who cannot tolerate sulfasalazine, olsalazine 500 mg po bid with meals is effective. For those with ulcerative proctitis or left-sided colitis, 5-ASA suppositories and enemas are effective when given every night to every third night. Nonsteroidal anti-inflammatory drugs have been reported to activate quiescent inflammatory bowel disease and should be *avoided* if possible.

Surgery: Surgery is indicated when drug therapy for acute fulminant disease fails, when patients cannot be weaned from long-term corticosteroid therapy, when surveillance studies reveal precancerous colonic lesions, and when drug therapy for chronic ulcerative colitis produces a suboptimal response.

In all age groups, the most common operation for acute fulminant colitis is subtotal colectomy and ileostomy. In elderly patients, proctocolectomy with ileostomy is the procedure of choice when long-term medical therapy fails or when premalignant changes develop. Procedures that avoid ileostomy, such as the ileoanal reservoir, are a good choice for many younger patients. However, the increased morbidity rate associated with this procedure limits its use in the elderly, who are already at greater risk for fecal incontinence because of age-related changes in anal sphincter function.

CROHN'S DISEASE

A chronic inflammatory process of unknown cause that most often affects the terminal ileum or colon and is characterized by transmural inflammation, often with linear ulcerations and granulomas.

The general incidence is 76/100,000 persons in the USA and Europe. Histologic examination reveals transmural inflammation affecting all layers of the bowel and often associated with submucosal fibrosis. Other features that distinguish Crohn's disease from ulcerative colitis are linear ulcerations, fissures, fistulas, discrete mucosal ulcers, granulomas, and skip areas. Unlike ulcerative colitis, Crohn's disease often does not affect the rectum. Although the disease can involve any area of the GI tract from the mouth to the anus, the ileum and colon are most often involved. Crohn's disease confined to the colon (Crohn's colitis) occurs more often in the elderly than in younger persons, and left-sided colitis appears to be prevalent in elderly women.

Symptoms and Signs

The clinical picture in the elderly is similar to that in younger persons and includes diarrhea, fever, abdominal pain, and weight loss. However, elderly patients with Crohn's colitis tend to present more indolently than patients with ileal or ileocolonic involvement. In patients with colorectal involvement, perianal disease, a feature of Crohn's disease, may be an early manifestation characterized by rectal or anal strictures, fissures, fistulas, abscesses, prominent skin tags, or ulcers. The prevalence of extraintestinal manifestations (eg, migratory arthritis, pyoderma gangrenosum, iritis, erythema nodosum) is similar in elderly and younger patients. Common laboratory abnormalities (eg, leukocytosis, hypoalbuminemia, elevated erythrocyte sedimentation rate, abnormalities indicating anemia) vary with the severity of the illness. Rarely, the patient presents with peritonitis caused by bowel perforation, although it is more common with ileal involvement. An elderly patient with peritonitis may present atypically with mild abdominal pain, few abdominal findings, and mental confusion. Uncommonly, a patient with Crohn's colitis presents with massive lower GI bleeding or bowel obstruction.

Diagnosis

Prolonged delays in diagnosis probably occur more often in the elderly.

Because the rectum is often unaffected and the distribution in the colon is often discontinuous, colonoscopy and barium x-ray are the tests of choice. Both procedures can identify the characteristic ulcerations, skip lesions, and areas of colonic narrowing. Barium studies are better able to identify fistulas to adjacent visceral organs, whereas colonoscopy provides better visualization of the mucosa and allows mucosal biopsies to be taken. Biopsies should be taken from affected areas and from mucosa that appears grossly normal. Biopsies help distinguish Crohn's colitis from diseases that mimic it, including diverticulitis, which is common in the elderly, and ischemic colitis, which often occurs in a discontinuous distribution.

CT provides better definition of the colonic wall than colonoscopy and can identify extraintestinal abdominal abnormalities (eg, abscesses in patients with fever or palpable masses). CT and ultrasound may also

TABLE 107–3.   TREATMENT OF CROHN'S DISEASE

Indication	Drug	Dosage
Ileocolonic and colonic involvement	Sulfasalazine	4–6 g/day po
	Mesalamine*	Varies by formulation
	Metronidazole	250 mg po tid
	Prednisone	20–30 mg po bid
	Ciprofloxacin	500 mg po bid
Perianal involvement	Metronidazole	1.5–2 g/day po
	Mercaptopurine	50 mg/day po up to 1.5 mg/kg/day
	or	
	Azathioprine	50 mg/day po up to 2 mg/kg/day
	Ciprofloxacin	500 mg po bid
	Infliximab	5 mg/kg IV at 0, 2, and 6 weeks
Refractory disease	Mercaptopurine	50 mg/day po up to 2 mg/kg/day
	or	
	Azathioprine	50 mg/day po up to 2 mg/kg/day
	Infliximab	5 mg/kg IV
Maintenance of remission	Sulfasalazine	2 g/day po
	Mesalamine*	500 mg/day po
	Mercaptopurine	50 mg/day po
	or	
	Azathioprine	50 mg/day po
	Olsalazine*	500 mg po bid

* If sulfasalazine is not tolerated.

identify renal lithiasis and ureteral obstruction, which occur with increased frequency in Crohn's ileocolitis.

Sexually transmitted diseases and carcinoma should be excluded. Infectious agents should be excluded by appropriate studies.

Treatment

Treatment is based on extent, severity, distribution, and complications. Drug therapy includes all drugs used for ulcerative colitis■; in some patients, selected antibiotics are also useful (see TABLE 107–3).

Ileocolitis and colitis: Patients with mild to moderate disease often respond to sulfasalazine; those who cannot tolerate it may respond to one of the other 5-ASA drugs (eg, olsalazine, mesalamine). Dosages are similar to those used for ulcerative colitis and are listed in TABLE

■ see page 1060

107–3. If the patient responds inadequately and the disease remains mild or moderate, metronidazole 250 mg po tid or ciprofloxacin 500 mg po bid may be tried.

If the disease worsens despite these therapies or if the patient has moderate to severe symptoms, prednisone 20 to 30 mg po bid is given, followed by conversion to a single morning dose when disease activity significantly lessens. After remission is induced, the prednisone dose should be reduced by 5 to 10 mg/week until it is 20 mg/day. Subsequently, the dose should be tapered about 5 mg/day every 3 weeks while clinical activity and laboratory findings such as hemoglobin, white blood cell count, electrolytes, glucose, and albumin are monitored until the patient is weaned.

About 60% of patients who cannot be weaned from oral corticosteroids respond to azathioprine (up to 2 mg/kg/day po) or mercaptopurine (up to 1.5 mg/kg/day po). A therapeutic response may not develop for 6 to 9 months. These drugs may be continued indefinitely, but at least one attempt to discontinue them should be made after 1 year from the time of therapeutic response to determine if remission can be maintained. Other drugs with demonstrated efficacy are methotrexate (25 mg IM/week) and infliximab, an antitumor necrosis factor (5 mg/kg IV). Optimal duration has not been established but is likely to be prolonged.

Perianal disease: Perianal fistulas and abscesses can be debilitating for the patient and frustrating to treat. Although perianal disease often improves with standard therapy for bowel inflammation and control of diarrhea, perianal symptoms may persist in some patients. Short-term success has been reported with metronidazole 1.5 to 2.0 g/day po; however, adverse effects are common at these doses, and relapses occur when the drug is stopped or the dosage is tapered. Ciprofloxacin 500 mg po bid, a more expensive alternative, also has a high relapse rate. If an abscess develops, it should be incised and drained.

Azathioprine, mercaptopurine, or infliximab may be useful in some patients with refractory disease. Infliximab should be given in a dose of 5 mg/kg IV in patients with perianal fistula.

Surgery: Unlike ulcerative colitis, Crohn's disease is not cured by surgery. Therefore, surgery should be reserved for patients who do not respond to drug therapy. If perianal disease does not respond to therapy, the colon may be diverted surgically, but surgery may also fail to heal the disease.

For patients with extensive Crohn's colitis, proctocolectomy with ileostomy is the best surgical option. For elderly patients who are debilitated or malnourished, an initial subtotal colectomy with ileostomy is less debilitating; it also gives the patient an opportunity to gain weight and to improve physically. If a subsequent proctectomy is required, the risk of complications is reduced; if rectal disease is mild or absent, a proctectomy may not be needed. More limited colonic resections may be appropriate if severe disease is localized or if obstructive symptoms are caused by relatively circumscribed bowel involvement.

Patients with small bowel disease may require laparotomy for intestinal obstruction, peritonitis, abscess formation, or occasionally for a suspicion of malignancy. Indications for surgery in elderly patients with Crohn's disease are the same as those for younger patients.

Surgery for ileal disease is generally well tolerated in the elderly, and the prognosis is comparable with that in younger patients. Elderly patients with extensive colitis or severe ileocolitis have higher morbidity and mortality, especially when emergency surgery is needed.

Recurrence rates after surgical resection for Crohn's disease vary; this variation relates in part to the initial site of disease. Proximal extension of distal colonic disease appears to be uncommon in elderly patients, and data suggest that recurrence rates are lower in elderly patients than in younger ones. Mortality rates associated with Crohn's disease do not appear to be significantly higher in the elderly.

ANTIBIOTIC-ASSOCIATED DIARRHEA AND COLITIS

Diarrhea and colonic inflammation that occur during or shortly after the administration of antibiotics or chemotherapy.

The vast majority of cases are caused by a cytotoxin produced by *Clostridium difficile;* this cytotoxin triggers epithelial necrosis and a characteristic inflammatory process. *C. difficile,* the most common agent of nosocomial diarrhea, is acquired most often by elderly patients in hospitals or nursing homes. Nosocomial transmission involving environmental contamination with *C. difficile* and carriage of the organism on the hands of hospital personnel has been documented. Acquisition of *C. difficile* is often asymptomatic, but it may have clinical consequences if elderly patients receive certain antibiotics or chemotherapeutic agents. Other possible risk factors include surgery, intensive care, nasogastric intubation, and length of hospital stay. Some patients have antibiotic-associated diarrhea without evidence of *C. difficile* infection.

Although almost all antibiotics have been implicated, cephalosporins, extended-spectrum penicillins (eg, ampicillin), and clindamycin are implicated most often. Other penicillins and erythromycin are involved less often.

Symptoms and Signs

The disease spectrum ranges from mild diarrhea (with little or no inflammation) to severe colitis often associated with pseudomembranes, which adhere to necrotic colonic epithelium. The typical clinical picture of antibiotic-associated colitis includes watery nonbloody diarrhea, lower abdominal cramps, fever, and leukocytosis. Fever is usually low grade but may be high occasionally. In severe cases, dehydration, hypotension, hypoproteinemia, toxic megacolon, or colonic perforation may occur. When diarrhea occurs without colitis, constitutional symptoms are usually absent. Weight loss and malnutrition are associated with *C. difficile* in the elderly.

Diagnosis

Diagnostic studies are used to define anatomic and histopathologic changes and to identify the causative organism. Certain tests can identify *C. difficile* or its toxin. The tissue culture assay for a cytopathic toxin neutralized by specific antitoxins is the standard; the toxin is present in 95 to 100% of cases of pseudomembranous colitis if three separate stool specimens are examined. However, many hospitals lack the facilities for these assays and must submit stool specimens to reference laboratories. The preferred alternative is an enzyme-linked immunoassay, which yields results comparable to the tissue culture assay. This test has a reported sensitivity of 85% and a specificity of 100%. Stool cultures for *C. difficile* require selective growth media, and inexperienced laboratories have reported difficulties in recovering the organism. Moreover, whether *C. difficile* can be implicated in antibiotic-associated diarrhea without identifying the cytotoxin is controversial.

In general, endoscopy should be performed in severely ill patients who present atypically and require a rapid diagnosis to expedite treatment. In severely ill patients, flexible sigmoidoscopy is usually satisfactory, because the distal colon is involved in most cases. However, changes may be confined to the right colon in up to one third of cases, making colonoscopy necessary when less extensive procedures do not confirm a diagnosis that is strongly suspected. The yellowish gray pseudomembranes are dense and adhere to the underlying colonic mucosa, but the mucosa between the pseudomembranes appears normal. When pseudomembranes are not grossly visible, mucosal biopsies may show characteristic findings. Barium x-rays and CT are less useful. Barium enemas should be performed gently to reduce the risk of colonic perforation.

Treatment

The implicated causative drug should be stopped, if possible. If symptoms persist or the disease is clinically severe, patients should receive metronidazole 250 mg po qid for 7 to 14 days or vancomycin 125 mg po qid for 7 to 14 days. If oral administration is not possible, metronidazole 500 mg IV q 6 h should be given until oral administration is possible. Metronidazole and vancomycin appear to be therapeutically comparable in mild cases, but metronidazole costs substantially less. However, if the patient is seriously ill, oral vancomycin is usually recommended. Fever usually resolves within 24 hours, and diarrhea decreases over 4 to 5 days. A worse prognosis has been reported in patients with a serum albumin < 25 g/L, a fall in albumin > 11 g/L, and persistent toxin in the stools ≥ 7 days after therapy. Prognosis does not seem to be affected by age or sex. Relapse rates average 20 to 25% after successful treatment with either drug. Patients who have one relapse are more likely to have another; this phenomenon cannot be explained by antibiotic resistance but may involve sporulation, which leads to relapse within 4 weeks after successful treatment. Relapses invariably respond to another course of antibiotics. In the 5 to 10% of patients who have multiple relapses, metronidazole or vancomycin in conventional doses should be followed by a 3-week course of cholestyramine or colestipol 4 g tid and/or *Lactobacillus acidophilus* 500 mg po qid, or vancomycin 125 mg po every other day. As an adjunct to antibiotic therapy, *Saccharomyces boulardii*, a nonpathogenic yeast, appears to reduce relapses.

IRRITABLE BOWEL SYNDROME

(Spastic Colon)

A motility disorder of unknown cause characterized by abdominal pain, diarrhea, or constipation.

New-onset irritable bowel syndrome (IBS) is uncommon in elderly persons. The incidence and prevalence in the elderly are not well defined. IBS occurs in about 10 to 20% of persons in the USA, of whom about 10 to 33% seek medical attention. In the USA, more women are diagnosed with this disorder than men (2:1 to 3:1 ratio).

Pathophysiology

Disturbances in intestinal motility may result from physical or psychologic stimuli, although no specific stimulus or response pattern is characteristic. Patients may have an increased motility response in the small and large intestine and more symptoms with various stimuli (ie, food, pentagastrin, cholecystokinin, rectal distention, physical or psychologic stress) when compared with control populations. Patients with IBS also appear to have a lower sensation threshold and pain tolerance to intestinal distention than non-IBS patients.

Foods that increase intestinal gas may exacerbate complaints. Some patients are intolerant of wheat, dairy products, coffee, tea, or citrus fruits, but other studies have not found consistent intolerance to specific foods. Antibiotics, β-blockers, bronchodilators, cardiac drugs, diuretics, and opioids disrupt GI processes and may produce IBS symptoms. Tobacco and alcohol may exacerbate symptoms by altering intestinal motility. Tobacco may also contribute to increased intestinal gas.

Many patients with IBS describe acute episodes of stress preceding the onset of bowel symptoms. In addition, about half of patients have noted that stress can worsen their symptoms. Yet, most patients with IBS do not differ psychologically from the general population.

Diagnosis

Elderly patients with IBS usually have a long history of bowel dysfunction, sometimes beginning in childhood or adolescence. However, if the symptoms have changed, an evaluation should be conducted to eliminate the possibility of concurrent pathologic processes.

The Rome criteria for IBS include continuous or recurrent abdominal pain or discomfort for $\geq$ 3 months that is relieved with defecation. Defecation is irregular or varies $\geq$ 25% of the time and is characterized by two or more of the following: altered stool frequency, altered stool consistency (hard or loose/watery stool), altered stool passage (straining or urgency, feeling of incomplete evacuation), passage of mucus, and bloating or feeling of abdominal distention.

No distinct physical findings occur, although the abdomen may be tender. Laboratory findings are usually normal. However, in the elderly it is prudent to obtain a complete blood count, electrolytes (with vomiting or diarrhea), ESR, urinalysis, and stool testing for blood. Stool should be examined for leukocytes, ova, and parasites and cultured when patients have diarrhea. The selection of other diagnostic tests depends on the primary symptoms (ie, diarrhea vs. constipation), chronicity and severity of symptoms, and associated clinical features. Unnecessary testing should be avoided.

Treatment

Organic disease must be excluded before symptomatic therapy is begun. No drugs have produced consistent results. The physician should educate the patient about the disorder, legitimize the patient's concern about the chronicity of the symptoms, and help the patient to adapt.

Patients with mild or infrequent symptoms tend not to visit their physician often and generally maintain normal activity levels. Foods that can exacerbate symptoms (ie, lactose, fatty foods, alcohol, artificial sweeteners, beans) should be eliminated from the diet, and symptoms should be monitored.

Patients with moderate symptoms that intermittently disrupt activity should record the frequency, duration, and severity of their symptoms and associated factors in a diary for 1 to 2 weeks. Based on this information, the physician may suggest dietary and behavioral modifications. Severe symptoms that impair daily functioning may be treated with drugs. If pain is predominant, anticholinergic (antispasmodic) drugs are most frequently used to decrease intestinal motility. However, these drugs pose a risk to the elderly because of their anticholinergic properties and should be used only when absolutely essential and with close monitoring. Hyoscyamine (0.125 mg po tid to qid before meals) or dicyclomine (10 to 20 mg qid) appears to be most effective for patients with postprandial episodes of pain. If diarrhea is predominant, antidiarrheal drugs can be recommended. Loperamide (2 to 4 mg bid to tid) increases intestinal transit time, facilitates water and ion absorption, and strengthens rectal sphincter tone. If constipation is predominant, fiber (20 to 25 g/day) can be given through diet or as a supplemental bulking agent.

Behavioral interventions (relaxation techniques, hypnosis, therapy) also assist motivated patients with moderate to severe symptoms, especially if the symptoms are associated with stressors.

A small subset of patients with severe symptoms and continuous refractory abdominal pain that does not correlate with intestinal physiology commonly have psychiatric comorbidity. These patients often cannot acknowledge the psychologic contribution to the illness, believe that a serious illness is being overlooked, and often have unrealistic expectations that a cure can be found. They are typically unresponsive to traditional therapy and require a gastroenterologist with expertise in psychoactive drugs and pain relief.

■108■ LIVER AND BILIARY DISORDERS

The liver undergoes several age-related changes,■ but these rarely lead to clinically noticeable changes on their own. However, liver diseases are not rare in the elderly and are becoming more commonly diagnosed. The older liver is more susceptible to drugs and other toxins. The clinical manifestations of liver disorders reflect changes in liver physiology and the elderly person's decreased ability to compensate for various metabolic, infectious, and immunologic insults. Gallstones, gallstone pancreatitis, acute cholangitis, acalculous cholecystitis, retained stones in the common duct, gallbladder fistulas, gallbladder polyps, and jaundice are discussed in Ch. 112. Liver cancer is discussed in Ch. 113.

Symptoms and Signs

In an elderly patient with liver disease, the presentation may be nonspecific and the symptoms and signs ambiguous. Fatigue, malaise,

■ see page 1003

anorexia, and mild weight loss are typical in elderly patients with viral hepatitis, primary biliary cirrhosis, or hepatocellular carcinoma.∎ Hepatic encephalopathy is often initially missed because early symptoms (eg, a disturbance in sleep pattern or mild confusion) may be attributed to dementia.

Prognosis

The complications of end-stage liver disease are the same in elderly and younger patients. However, the prognosis of liver diseases is worse in the elderly because of their diminished capacity to recover from complications and their inability to tolerate the toxic accumulations and other manifestations of liver disease. For example, the complications of cirrhosis and portal hypertension (eg, variceal hemorrhage, ascites, hepatic encephalopathy) portend a dismal clinical outcome in the elderly. An elderly patient may survive a variceal hemorrhage only to die of a myocardial infarction or pneumonia precipitated by the hemorrhage.

VIRAL HEPATITIS

Diffuse liver inflammation caused by specific hepatotropic viruses.

The course of viral hepatitis is often more aggressive in elderly than in younger patients, although the prevalence is lower.

The elderly patient with viral hepatitis may initially be asymptomatic or may present with nonspecific complaints such as nausea, fatigue, and loose stools.

Acute hepatitis A is much less common in the elderly than in younger persons. More than 70% of elderly persons have serologic evidence of previous infection and are therefore immune. Such immunity is even more pronounced in developing countries, where relatively poor hygiene and sanitation practices have previously exposed a high proportion of elderly patients to the virus. Hepatitis A in the elderly often results in a lower serum aminotransferase level and a more prolonged cholestatic course than in younger persons. The risk of death is increased substantially, from 7/10,000 in persons aged 15 to 24, to 400/10,000 in those ≥ 65.

Acute hepatitis B and C are also less common in the elderly than in younger persons. These infections have a more prolonged cholestatic course, and the likelihood that the infection will become chronic is greater. For example, in younger patients with hepatitis B, 5 to 15% of

∎ see page 1149

acute cases become chronic, compared with up to 43% in elderly patients. Treatment of hepatitis C with interferon, whether or not combined with ribavirin, results in poorer clearance of the virus in the elderly compared with treatment in younger persons. This poor clearance is presumably due to the diminished function of the immune system, including a progressive loss of T-lymphocyte activity.◨ Elderly patients infected with hepatitis B are also less likely to respond to lamivudine therapy.

PRIMARY BILIARY CIRRHOSIS

A disease of unknown cause characterized by chronic cholestasis and progressive destruction of intrahepatic bile ducts.

Over 90% of diagnosed cases of primary biliary cirrhosis occur in women aged 50 to 70. In the elderly, characteristic features include osteomalacia, osteoporosis, and dramatically increased serum cholesterol levels. The disease is long-standing and slowly progressive; hence, complications (eg, variceal hemorrhage, ascites) are more likely to occur in patients ≥ 55. The prognosis for elderly asymptomatic patients is the same as that for age-matched controls (ie, the prognosis is good). However, the prognosis is poor for elderly symptomatic patients, because the risk of complications increases.

Treatment in the elderly patient is similar to that in the younger patient and is aimed at symptomatic control of pruritus and malabsorption and prevention of complications. Ursodeoxycholic acid has been shown to improve biochemical abnormalities and, in some patients, may delay the progression to cirrhosis. Corticosteroids are not beneficial and should be avoided, especially because they may accelerate the osteoporosis. Liver transplantation is an option for patients who develop liver failure or intractable complications from portal hypertension.

HEMOCHROMATOSIS

An inherited disorder of iron metabolism in which the homeostasis of iron absorption and accumulation is abnormal.

Iron accumulation, with resultant tissue damage, occurs in the liver, heart, and pancreas. Because of the years required to build up toxic accumulations of iron, hemochromatosis usually manifests with symp-

◨ see page 1354

toms in late adulthood (40% of patients are > 65). Symptoms are nonspecific, especially in the elderly, and include weakness, fatigue, weight loss, joint pain, and those of heart failure. Men are symptomatic more often than are women and are more likely to present with significant liver disease. Cirrhosis may develop, and hepatocellular cancer may occur in a cirrhotic liver.

The diagnosis is suspected by demonstration of increased ferritin levels and transferrin saturation; confirmation requires a liver biopsy and demonstration of increased iron content in the liver.

Phlebotomy is the most effective therapy in the elderly and appears to decrease the risk of liver cancer if started before cirrhosis develops. In patients who cannot undergo phlebotomy because of severe anemia or hypoproteinemia, a chelating agent such as deferoxamine can be used.

109 ◼ ANORECTAL DISORDERS

About 50 disorders can affect the perianal area; pruritus and hemorrhoids are the most common among adults of all ages. Other anorectal disorders include those affecting crypts and papillae (which mark the proximal end of the anal canal) and deep rectal glands, fecal incontinence,◻ and cancer.◻

PRURITUS ANI

Intense chronic itching in the anal region.

Pruritus ani is a common problem with many causes. The most common exogenous causes are using harsh soaps, using sensitizing perfumes or deodorizers, wiping excessively with toilet paper, and wearing synthetic underwear or tight, warm clothing, which promotes sweating. Other causes include fungal diseases (eg, epidermophytosis), parasites (eg, pinworms), psoriasis, and neoplastic disorders (eg, Paget's disease, Bowen's disease). Psychologic factors may also contribute.

Some topical drugs used to treat anal disorders (eg, lidocaine, benzocaine) may produce an intensely pruritic contact dermatitis. Some oral antibiotics suppress normal bowel flora, causing an overgrowth of

◼ see page 1092   ◻ see page 1144

intestinal *Candida* organisms, which leads to pruritus due to perianal candidiasis.

Symptoms and Signs

The hallmark symptom is itching. On physical examination, the perianal area may appear normal, but excoriations from involuntary scratching (during sleep) can often be seen. In advanced cases, secondary bacterial infection may be present, producing edema, erythema, ulceration, and an exudate.

Diagnosis and Treatment

Biopsy of persistent scaly or crusted plaques should be performed to rule out malignancy.

The cause should be determined and corrected. For example, fungal diseases should be treated with over-the-counter topical antifungal powders. Antifungal creams can be used, but they promote excess moisture, which can cause itching. Oral antibiotics should be discontinued, if possible. Patients should not wear synthetic underwear or use perfumes or deodorizers on the perineum. They should be instructed to clean the perianal area gently with moist cotton or hypoallergenic scentless baby wipes after defecation. For mild cases caused by simple irritation, such cleansing followed by application of petroleum jelly can be effective.

The most effective local therapy is 0.5% or 1% hydrocortisone cream. Usually, it is applied only at night, when itching occurs. Severe cases may require application several times a day. The cream is discontinued as soon as itching is controlled. Recurrence is common, but repeated treatment is successful.

Excision of skin tags occasionally helps, but hemorrhoidectomy does not.

HEMORRHOIDS

Abnormally large or symptomatic conglomerates of blood vessels, supporting tissues, and overlying mucous membrane or anorectal skin.

A hemorrhoid is a varicose vein of the anorectal junction. An internal hemorrhoid is the part of the varicosity above the dentate line (involving rectal mucosa); an external hemorrhoid is the distal part, which is covered with anorectal skin (anoderm). Prolapsed internal hemorrhoids extend into the anal canal or through the anus. A thrombosed external hemorrhoid is a localized clot that forms in the vein of an external hemorrhoid or arises from a ruptured hemorrhoidal blood vessel. Combined hemorrhoids include internal and external hemorrhoids.

Hemorrhoids develop because the vena cava and iliac veins have no valves; consequently, erect posture, heavy lifting, and straining can distend the veins. Rarely, hemorrhoids indicate a lesion higher in the colorectum (eg, a left colon or rectal malignancy) or of portal hypertension secondary to intrinsic liver disease.

Symptoms and Signs

Internal hemorrhoids may be asymptomatic in the early stages, but later, they tend to bleed. The bleeding is usually minimal, appearing as bright red blood on stool or on toilet paper. Rarely, significant bleeding occurs: If blood is retained above the sphincter, a large amount can be expelled at one time. Continued blood loss, even in small increments, can lead to anemia. External hemorrhoids may also bleed. Pain occurs only with prolapsed internal hemorrhoids and thrombosed external hemorrhoids (which produce sudden, severe perianal pain). Thrombosed external hemorrhoids may also cause itching.

Diagnosis and Treatment

External hemorrhoids can be diagnosed by inspection and nearly always indicate the presence of internal hemorrhoids. Diagnosis of internal hemorrhoids requires anoscopy, because hemorrhoids are soft and cannot be reliably detected digitally. A thrombosed external hemorrhoid appears as a tense, blue subcutaneous mass. For elderly patients with rectal bleeding, the physical examination should be supplemented with either proctosigmoidoscopy plus a barium enema or total colonoscopy.

For mild hemorrhoids, treatment consists of a soft diet and a bulk producer (eg, psyllium hydrophilic mucilloid). Heavy lifting and straining at stool should be avoided. Sitz baths and suppositories or ointments containing benzocaine or another local anesthetic can relieve symptoms.

For mildly prolapsed or bleeding internal hemorrhoids, rubber bands can be applied snugly around the base of each major hemorrhoid during one or more office visits. The bands should be positioned above the anal canal, or great pain results. Posttreatment discomfort is moderate, and long-term results are good. Rarely, band ligation is complicated by severe perianal sepsis; early symptoms include prolonged pain, fever, and urinary retention.

Sclerotherapy (eg, with quinine urea hydrochloride 5%) has good early results, but later, secondary hemorrhoids tend to develop. Hemorrhoidectomy of secondary hemorrhoids is more difficult.

Cryosurgery and laser therapy are less popular alternatives because the amount of tissue removed is small, thus healing and symptom relief are delayed.

For combined hemorrhoids or internal hemorrhoids with major prolapse, hemorrhoidectomy is the most effective treatment. It can relieve symptoms immediately and has excellent long-term results. For a thrombosed external hemorrhoid, subcutaneous injection of a local anesthetic and evacuation provide immediate relief. A small section of skin should be excised to allow adequate drainage in case of further bleeding. Some small clots resolve without much discomfort, but large ones, if not evacuated, are slow to improve and are painful for many days. Warm sitz baths and analgesics are beneficial.

FISSURES

Longitudinal breaks in the squamous epithelium of the anal canal.

Fissures may be superficial or deep; deep fissures may expose the internal sphincter. An external skin tag (sentinel pile) often forms at the lower end of a chronic fissure (see FIGURE 109–1). The cause may be large or hard bowel movements, rough fecal debris, straining at stool, diarrhea, or trauma to the anal canal caused by rough wiping, foreign bodies (eg, thermometers, enema nozzles), or anoreceptive intercourse.

The main symptom is severe pain, which is aggravated by defecation, persists for several minutes afterward, and subsides until the next bowel movement. Massive bleeding is rare.

Diagnosis and Treatment

Fissures can usually be seen when the buttocks are separated and the patient strains. They usually occur at the posterior midline but occasionally occur at the anterior midline. If the fissure is not visible when the patient strains, anoscopy may be used (although few patients can tolerate the procedure). For some patients, the examination is so painful and causes so much spasm of the sphincter that local or general anesthesia is needed.

For superficial lesions, stool softeners (eg, psyllium hydrophilic mucilloid) and warm sitz baths may accelerate healing. Topical creams or ointments containing local anesthetics or simple protectants may provide relief when applied after bowel movements.

Chronic fissures require surgical intervention. Internal sphincterotomy, a relatively simple procedure using a local, regional, or general anesthetic, is most commonly performed. It relieves pain and allows healing. Division of the lateral anus (lateral sphincterotomy) is necessary, because it is much less likely to result in permanent incontinence than is posterior division. Other procedures pose a higher risk of permanent incontinence.

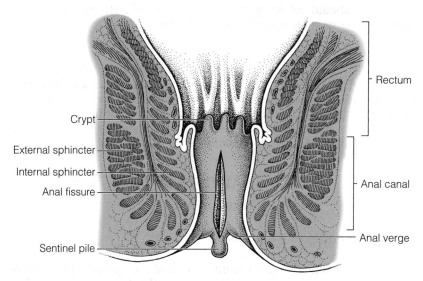

FIGURE 109–1.   Anorectal fissure.

PERIANAL AND ISCHIORECTAL ABSCESSES

Localized collections of pus resulting from infections of the pararectal spaces.

Abscesses may cause substantial tissue destruction. **Perianal abscesses,** the more common type, usually result from inflammation of anorectal crypts or of glands located between the sphincters. These abscesses are located close to the anus and are relatively superficial. Pus tends to track internally into the lower rectum just above the anal canal and externally, forming a tender swelling. The swelling is usually posterior to the midline of the anus but may be anywhere within several centimeters of the anal verge.

Ischiorectal abscesses are located above the anorectal line. They are more difficult to diagnose, are usually larger, and are accompanied by marked systemic symptoms (eg, severe pain, fever). They usually result from a break between the extraperitoneal rectum and the fatty tissue in the fossa; however, the source of infection may lie within the peritoneal cavity. In elderly patients, diverticulitis is the most likely cause.

The cardinal symptom of an ischiorectal abscess is pain. If surgery is delayed, signs of sepsis (eg, chills, fever), local swelling, induration, and tenderness develop, as may life-threatening necrotizing soft tissue infections. Superficial abscesses may rupture spontaneously, but this possibility should not delay surgery. Aerobic and anaerobic organisms similar to those in feces can be cultured from the pus.

Treatment

Surgical drainage should be performed as soon as the abscess is discovered. Antibiotics are given but do not substitute for drainage. Because nearly all abscesses result from a break in the rectal mucous membrane, 25 to 35% of patients may have a persistent fistula after simple incision and drainage. Therefore, a fistula should be sought and repaired during the original operation.

ANAL FISTULA

(Fistula in Ano)

A sinus tract between the rectum and the skin.

Fistulas commonly result from a perianal or ischiorectal abscess caused by inflammation of rectal crypts or glands. Inflammatory diseases (eg, Crohn's disease, tuberculosis, lymphogranuloma) may cause fistulas. Intraperitoneal lesions (eg, diverticulitis, Crohn's disease of the small intestine or colon) may cause fistulas that track into the perineum. Trauma can produce fistulas that track into the vagina.

Symptoms, Signs, and Diagnosis

The main symptom is perirectal pain with pus or blood seen on toilet paper or emanating from an opening on the medial buttock.

Most anal fistulas open near the anus. If the external opening is adjacent to the posterior half of the anus, the tract almost always runs into the rectum exactly in the posterior midline. However, if the opening is adjacent to the anterior half, the tract runs radially into the rectum (Goodsall's rule).

During initial examination, probing the entire tract may be possible, but locating the internal opening is usually difficult until surgery. Because of the many possible causes, microscopic examination of excised tissue is imperative.

Treatment

When the fistula connects with the anorectum just above the anal verge, the tract can be exposed with little risk of damage to the sphincter; this simple procedure is curative. However, when the internal opening is high, a seton (a silk suture or a rubber or polymeric silicone band) should be used to avoid damaging the sphincter and causing incontinence. The seton is passed through the tract into the rectum and is tied. It gradually cuts through the tissues, leading to fibrosis and fixation.

PROCTALGIA FUGAX

Fleeting and intense anorectal pain, occurring at irregular intervals and lasting several seconds to 20 minutes.

Proctalgia fugax occurs in about 13% of adults and is 2 to 3 times more common among women than among men. Incidence in the elderly is unknown. Suggested causes include laxity of the anal sphincter, muscular tenseness proximal to the anal shelf resulting in spasm, and increased contractile activity of the sigmoid colon. Stress and anxiety can precipitate episodes. Many patients have other functional bowel symptoms. The condition is diagnosed by its symptoms.

If episodes are frequent, relaxation training and cognitive behavior therapy may be considered, but their effectiveness has not been established. Drugs have not shown consistent benefit.

RECTAL PROLAPSE AND PROCIDENTIA

Protrusion of part of the rectum through the anus.

Mucosal prolapse involves only the mucosal layer of the rectum. Complete prolapse involves all layers. In procidentia, the most severe form, several inches of rectum may pass through the anus.

Prolapse is common among elderly persons, affecting women more than men. The underlying defect is a long, lax sigmoidorectal mesentery that cannot keep the rectum in position.

Symptoms, Signs, and Diagnosis

The main symptom is protrusion of mucous membrane or the rectum, felt as an anal mass by the patient. Initially, manual reduction is possible, but later, protrusion occurs when the patient stands, causing pain and discharge of mucus and blood from the inflamed mucosa.

During physical examination, the degree of prolapse can be determined by inspecting and palpating the protrusion when the patient is squatting and straining or immediately after the patient has had a bowel movement. In complete prolapse, mucosal folds are circumferential and concentric. When prolapse is subtle, anal manometry and defecography may help in making the diagnosis.

Treatment

Conservative therapy (instruction to avoid straining at stool, lifting, and excessive standing; when necessary, manual reduction) provides temporary relief. However, early surgical repair is necessary, because continued dilation of the anal sphincters leads to fecal incontinence. The weakened muscular ring often remains incompetent despite later attempts at repair. For mucosal prolapse, redundant tissue is excised.

For complete prolapse, conservative therapy may be used, but surgery should not be delayed.

Surgery usually involves transabdominal resection of redundant colon and rectum, coloanal anastomosis, or both. However, surgeons disagree about which specific procedure is best. Complications include intestinal obstruction if the loop is tied too tightly and recurrence if the loop breaks.

Postoperative fecal incontinence is common, particularly among patients with preoperative incontinence. Many surgeons prefer to surgically tighten the sphincter in such patients.

110 ▪ CONSTIPATION, DIARRHEA, AND FECAL INCONTINENCE

CONSTIPATION

A decrease in stool frequency.

Constipation has different meanings to different people, making a precise definition elusive. The medical community usually defines constipation as a decrease in stool frequency; however, patients may also consider constipation as difficult passage of feces, hardness of stool, or a feeling of incomplete evacuation.

Constipation is more common in elderly persons—who report more straining and sensation of anal blockage—than in middle-aged persons. Constipation is the most common gastrointestinal complaint in the elderly, with up to 60% of elderly outpatients reporting laxative use. The overall prevalence of self-reported constipation is 24 to 37%, with women reporting more constipation than men. In the institutionalized elderly, up to 50% self-report constipation and up to 74% use laxatives daily.

Etiology

Age-related changes in anorectal physiology that predispose the elderly to constipation include increased rectal compliance and impaired rectal sensation (such that larger rectal volumes are needed to elicit the desire to defecate). Elderly persons also have reduced resting anal sphincter pressure and decreased maximal sphincter pressure, which predispose to fecal incontinence.∎ Delayed colonic transit, an

---

∎ see page 1092

TABLE 110-1.   CONDITIONS THAT CAN CAUSE OR WORSEN CONSTIPATION

Intestinal disorders	**Myopathic disorders**
Decreased motility	Amyloidosis
Diverticular disease	Dermatomyositis
Hernia	Systemic sclerosis
Inflammation	**Neurologic disorders**
Irritable bowel syndrome	Autonomic neuropathy
Neoplasm	Dementia
Postsurgical abnormality	Multiple sclerosis
Volvulus	Parkinson's disease
	Shy-Drager syndrome
Metabolic disorders	Spinal cord injury
Dehydration	Stroke
Diabetes mellitus	**Medications**
Hypercalcemia	See TABLE 110-2
Hypocalcemia	
Hypokalemia	**Other**
Hyperparathyroidism	Decreased intake of calories, fiber, fluid
Hypoparathyroidism	Fever
Hyperthyroidism	Immobility
Hypothyroidism	Poor access to toilet
Multiple endocrine neoplasia, type II	Weakness

age-related change occurring predominantly in the rectosigmoid region, plays a small role.

Various medical and surgical conditions can cause or worsen constipation (see TABLE 110–1). Medications (see TABLE 110–2), low dietary fiber, and reduced caloric intake are common causes. Functional impairment from immobility, muscular weakness, and neuromuscular disorders make recognition of the need to defecate difficult. Altered mental

TABLE 110-2.   MEDICATIONS THAT CAN CAUSE CONSTIPATION

Analgesics	Anticonvulsants
Nonsteroidal anti-inflammatory drugs	Antihypertensives
Opioids	Calcium channel blockers
Anesthetics	Clonidine
Antacids	Antiparkinson drugs
Anticholinergics	Calcium
Antidepressants (especially tricyclic antidepressants)	Diuretics
Antihistamines	Iron
Antipsychotics	Monoamine oxidase inhibitors
Antispasmodics	Phenothiazines

status or depression may also contribute to constipation. Several factors contributing to constipation can often be identified in a single patient.

Symptoms, Signs, and Complications

Constipation in the elderly is typically divided into two major categories: functional megarectum, which manifests as an enlarged rectum and fecal impaction, and rectosigmoid outlet delay, which manifests as straining and passage of small hard stools. Pelvic floor dysfunction∎ also results in outlet delay. This condition occurs predominantly in elderly women because of pelvic floor laxity and failure of the anorectal angle to open.

About 50% of elderly persons describe their constipation as infrequent defecation, 20% as excessive straining or incomplete evacuation, and 30% as both. Constipation can lead to abdominal discomfort, loss of appetite, and nausea. The belief that constipation can cause mild fever is unproven.

The major complication of constipation in the elderly is **fecal impaction,** which can result in intestinal obstruction, colonic ulceration (also called stercoraceous ulceration), overflow incontinence (leakage of stool around obstructing feces), or paradoxical diarrhea. Fecal impaction is most likely in patients with limited mobility or mental capacity who present with an alteration in bowel habit (eg, reduced frequency, new-onset diarrhea, incontinence). Urinary retention and urinary tract infections also occur with fecal impaction. Excessive straining may have deleterious effects on the cerebral, coronary, and peripheral arterial circulation, resulting in syncope, cardiac ischemia, and transient ischemic attacks. Also, excessive straining can result in hemorrhoids, anal fissures, and rectal prolapse with consequent anal pain and bleeding.

Idiopathic **megacolon** occurs rarely in elderly patients with chronic constipation. Colonic dilatation can be quite marked and predisposes patients to colonic volvulus.▨

Diagnosis

When evaluating a patient with constipation, the first priority is understanding the patient's complaint. Attention should be directed to the patient's beliefs about bowel habits and to psychologic status; misperceptions about normal bowel movement frequency can be identified and corrected.

Appropriate screening for depression and anxiety may uncover previously unrecognized and treatable conditions. Reviewing the patient's history of underlying medical conditions or medications (see TABLES 110–1 and 110–2) may uncover potential contributing factors.

∎ see page 1194   ▨ see page 1124

A physical examination is performed primarily to detect evidence of metabolic, muscular, or neurologic disease. All patients should undergo a rectal examination to evaluate for the presence of perineal lesions, to characterize the stool (ie, small, hard stools, soft stools), and to exclude a low rectal or anal mass. The presence of an empty rectal vault does not exclude the possibility of a higher stool impaction.

Laboratory studies can exclude suspected underlying metabolic conditions, especially hypothyroidism. An abdominal x-ray shows the amount and distribution of stool in the colon; the presence of air fluid levels should prompt surgical consultation.

Colonoscopy or barium enema should be performed in a patient with a recent change in bowel habit to rule out underlying structural lesions (eg, malignancy, stricture). The presence of anemia or heme-positive stool also necessitates an assessment that includes colonoscopy.

In patients with intractable symptoms, assessment of colonic transit and anorectal function may be helpful. Colonic transit can be measured by using radiopaque markers. A capsule containing 24 markers is given at day 0. The patient must avoid laxatives and enemas for the duration of the test. On day 5, a plain abdominal x-ray is taken. If more than five markers remain, colonic transit is delayed. More complex versions of this test (to quantitate segmental colonic transit) are probably unnecessary because drugs to correct these abnormalities are unavailable.

Techniques used to assess anorectal function include defecating proctography and anorectal manometry. Defecating proctography measures defecation dynamics using barium instilled into the rectum. Abnormalities that can be identified include rectoceles, intussusception, prolapse, poorly relaxing puborectal muscle, and excessive perineal descent. Anorectal manometry measures rectal sensation, anal pressures, and expulsion dynamics.

Treatment

Constipation can be treated in most elderly persons with dietary and behavioral changes and judicious use of laxatives and enemas. Agents used to treat constipation are listed in TABLE 110–3.

Dietary approaches begin with adequate hydration, a cornerstone to treating constipation, especially in elderly persons who use diuretics. Food with high residual fiber (eg, bran and other whole grains, vegetables, nuts) is often beneficial and obviates the need for supplemental fiber. Although some people experience bloating and excessive gas initially, these symptoms usually resolve with continued use. When dietary approaches alone do not provide enough fiber (usually 20 g/day are needed), fiber supplementation (eg, methylcellulose, psyllium) is helpful. Because many of these products are high in sugar, they must be selected carefully.

In patients with idiopathic megacolon or other colonic dilatation (eg, bowel obstruction, megarectum), fiber supplementation is not helpful

TABLE 110–3. AGENTS USED TO TREAT CONSTIPATION

Category	Agent	Usual Dose
Fiber	Raw wheat or oat bran	1–6 tbsp in divided doses, mixed with food
	Psyllium	3–6 g
	Methylcellulose	2.4–7.2 g
Osmotic laxatives	Sorbitol 70% solution	15–150 mL po in divided doses
	Lactulose	7.5–90 mL po in divided doses
	Magnesium hydroxide	15–60 mL po at bedtime
	Magnesium citrate	200 mL po
	Polyethylene glycol	200–800 mL po
Stimulant laxatives	Bisacodyl	10–30 mg po
	Cascara sagrada	5 mL po up to 3 times weekly
	Senna	8.6–17.2 mg po daily
Enemas	Sodium biphosphate	One or two enemas weekly
	Tap water	500–1000 mL up to twice weekly
	Oil retention	4 1/2 oz prn, up to once or twice weekly

and should be *avoided*. These patients require a fiber-restricted diet with a regular schedule of laxatives or enemas to minimize fecal retention and impaction. A stool impaction, if present, should be removed before initiating fiber therapy.

Other foods (eg, prunes, melons, other foods with complex carbohydrates) can also help normalize bowel movements.

Behavioral changes include exercise, which strongly stimulates defecation and helps strengthen the abdominal muscles that aid defecation. Patients with constipation should attempt to move their bowels in the early morning, especially after breakfast, when colonic motor activity is highest.

Laxatives are usually recommended if dietary and behavioral changes cannot be achieved or are ineffective. Laxatives should be chosen according to the cause of the constipation. For most persons with chronic constipation, osmotic laxatives are effective and present the lowest risk. Lactulose and sorbitol (from 7.5 to 30 mL daily) are effective and safe. The dose is adjusted to produce a bowel movement daily or every other day. Osmotic laxatives containing magnesium are suitable only for short-term use and for patients without renal insufficiency.

For acute constipation or constipation caused by medications (especially opioids), stimulant laxatives (including senna and cascara) are generally best. They can be taken orally or rectally as a suppository (eg, bisacodyl). However, they may cause abdominal cramping and fluid and electrolyte disturbances, especially if rectal impaction is present. Stimulant laxatives should be used short-term because they can cause dependency.

Stool softeners (eg, docusate sodium) help soften hard stools but provide little relief for constipation. In bed-ridden patients, defecation may be an even more unpleasant experience for patients and caregivers. Mineral oil should generally be reserved for only the most serious cases, because its use can result in aspiration or anal seepage in some patients; long-term use can result in vitamin malabsorption.

Enemas can be used when fecal impaction is present. Plain tap water enemas or sodium phosphate and biphosphate enemas can be used. Soapsuds enemas produce mucosal damage and cramping and should be avoided. Because rectal volumes increase with age, the enema should generally contain about 500 to 1000 mL. After the initial blockage has been removed manually and with enemas, colonic cleansing with polyethylene glycol-electrolyte solutions (which are administered orally or via nasogastric tube) is helpful to remove more proximal colonic stool collections.

Still **other approaches** may be necessary. Patients with refractory constipation may require referral for specialized testing and treatment. Patients with severe slow transit constipation may benefit from subtotal colectomy. Biofeedback may help patients with pelvic floor dysfunction.

DIARRHEA

Abnormal looseness (liquidity) of the stool, which may be accompanied by a change in stool frequency or volume.

Diarrhea is a subjective symptom; some patients experiencing a primary difficulty with fecal continence may describe their condition as "diarrhea." Associated symptoms include urgency, cramping, bloating, and incontinence. Dysentery refers to painful, bloody, low-volume diarrhea. Antibiotic-associated diarrhea is discussed in Ch. 107.

The incidence of diarrhea in the elderly is unknown. The elderly may be more susceptible to infectious diarrhea, because they more often have hypochlorhydria and achlorhydria (eg, from pernicious anemia or gastric acid–suppressing drugs), luminal stasis (eg, from motility disorders or previous surgeries), or decreased mucosal immune function. Diarrhea is a major cause of morbidity and mortality in the elderly. Nursing home outbreaks of *Escherichia coli* O157:H7 infection have

TABLE 110–4.   CAUSES OF DIARRHEA IN THE ELDERLY

Acute
  Diet
  Drugs
  Infections
  Ischemia
Chronic
  Bile acid malabsorption
  Carbohydrate malabsorption (lactose, sorbitol)
  Collagen vascular disease
  Diet
  Drugs
  Endocrine disorders (diabetes, thyroid disease)
  Hormonal disorders (carcinoid, vipoma)
  Impaction
  Infections
  Inflammatory bowel disease
  Malabsorption
  Microscopic colitis (collagenous/lymphocytic)
  Neoplasia
  Radiation colopathy
  Surgery (gastric, small-bowel resection)

been documented with three times the morbidity and mortality than in younger persons. The higher mortality rate (16 to 35%) occurs largely because the elderly are less capable of replenishing their fluid losses and tolerating the intravascular hypovolemia associated with dehydration.

Classification and Etiology

Diarrhea is classified on the basis of duration as acute ($<$ 2 weeks) or chronic ($>$ 4 weeks). There are many causes of diarrhea in the elderly (see TABLE 110–4); however, even in severe cases, a cause cannot be identified in about 25% of patients.

Acute diarrhea: Most diarrhea in the elderly is acute and self-limited. It is usually due to infection (viral, bacterial, or parasitic), a recent drug change, or a food intolerance. Food intolerance may occur when elderly persons eat large amounts of fruits or beans. Acute bloody diarrhea may be caused by ischemia (eg, mesenteric thrombosis or ischemic colitis),**1** diverticulitis,**2** or inflammatory bowel disease.**3**

Viruses responsible for infectious diarrhea include the Norwalk virus–like agents and, less commonly, rotavirus. The exact pathogenetic mechanism is unclear. Diarrhea is caused by Norwalk virus throughout the year; diarrhea due to rotavirus is more common in cooler months.

1 see page 1117   **2** see page 1054   **3** see page 1058

Both viruses are spread easily by the fecal-oral route and have caused epidemic diarrhea in nursing homes.

Toxigenic diarrhea has two forms: food poisoning due to ingestion of food contaminated with preformed bacterial enterotoxin (due to *Staphylococcus aureus*, *Bacillus cereus*, or *Clostridium perfringens*) and infectious gastroenteritis caused by enterotoxin-producing bacteria (*E. coli, Clostridium difficile, Vibrio cholerae, Clostridium botulinum*, or *Vibrio parahaemolyticus*). Invasive diarrhea may be caused by *Shigella, Salmonella, Campylobacter*, or *Yersinia*.

Chronic diarrhea: Diarrhea is classified as secretory (isosmolar to plasma) or osmotic (hyperosmolar to plasma). Chronic diarrhea is categorized as watery, bloody, or fatty.

Secretory diarrhea is caused by agents that trigger intestinal epithelial cells to secrete water and electrolytes into the intestinal lumen. Examples in the elderly are diarrhea secondary to increased secretion of hormones, peptides, or biogenic amines from tumors, including carcinoid tumors, medullary carcinoma of the thyroid, islet cell tumors of the pancreas (eg, vipoma **1** and gastrinoma [Zollinger-Ellison syndrome]), **2** parathyroid adenoma, and small cell carcinoma of the lung; bile acid–induced diarrhea, idiopathic, or after resection of > 100 cm of the distal ileum; postobstructive diarrhea; or diarrhea due to villous adenoma of the distal colon.

Medications are a common cause. Although almost any drug can cause diarrhea, more common offenders include nonsteroidal anti-inflammatory drugs (NSAIDs), magnesium-containing antacids, antiarrhythmics, β-blockers, quinidine, and digoxin.

Microscopic colitis is a cause of chronic persistent watery diarrhea. The etiology is unknown, but the condition is sometimes induced by drugs and may be associated with NSAIDs. Collagenous colitis and lymphocytic colitis may represent different stages of microscopic colitis and can be differentiated based on the histologic appearance. Characteristic changes in both disorders include increased plasma cells and intraepithelial lymphocytes. In collagenous colitis, a distinct subepithelial collagen band is also present. Collagenous colitis has a male:female incidence ratio of about 1:10, whereas lymphocytic colitis has a ratio of about 1:1. Symptoms are crampy abdominal pain and, often, a prolonged chronic watery diarrhea. The colonic mucosa appears grossly normal on colonoscopy.

Small-bowel bacterial overgrowth 3 causes chronic secretory or fatty diarrhea. The diarrhea is often described as fatty because of the deconjugation of bile salts by the bacteria. Predisposing conditions include gastric achlorhydria, prior gastric surgery, and small-bowel diverticulosis.

---

1 see TABLE 113–1 on page 1146   **2** see TABLE 113–1 on page 1146

3 see TABLE 111–1 on page 1098

Patients with long-standing diabetes mellitus can develop diarrhea due to intestinal neuropathy, although constipation is much more common among these patients. Other causes of pseudo-obstruction in which diarrhea may be a presenting symptom include collagen vascular disease (eg, scleroderma), neurologic disorders, primary muscle diseases (eg, muscular dystrophy), and pseudo-obstruction of the small bowel. Less commonly reported causes in the elderly are irritable bowel syndrome**1** and certain infections (eg, giardiasis and, in immunosuppressed patients, microsporidiosis, cryptosporidiosis, and *Mycobacterium avium-intracellulare*); 10% of AIDS patients are elderly, and these infections occur often in AIDS patients.

Osmotic diarrhea results from the ingestion of osmotically active ingredients in certain foods and drugs. In the elderly, osmotic diarrhea is typically caused by the ingestion of poorly absorbable solutes (eg, magnesium sulfate, sodium sulfate), laxatives containing citrate, antacids containing magnesium hydroxide, and some sugars (eg, mannitol, sorbitol, and fructose, which may be found in antacids, chewing gum, diet candy, and fruits).

Disaccharidase deficiencies, especially lactase deficiency, can also cause osmotic diarrhea. About 80% of the world population has primary lactase deficiency. Black Americans and Jews have the highest incidence. The condition begins in childhood and cannot be outgrown.

Osmotic diarrhea also occurs after a gastrectomy or vagotomy, in dumping syndrome, in short-bowel syndrome, and with chronic small-bowel ischemia or small-bowel resection.

Bloody (exudative, inflammatory) diarrhea contains blood and leukocytes; it results from injury and inflammation of the mucosal tissues of the distal ileum and colon. Causes in the elderly include inflammatory bowel disease (ulcerative colitis and Crohn's disease**2**), ischemic colitis,**3** carcinoma of the colon,**4** and radiation colitis.

Several infections may progress to chronic bloody diarrhea (eg, *Campylobacter jejuni, C. difficile, Yersinia enterocolitica,* cytomegalovirus, and *Entamoeba histolytica*).

Fatty diarrhea is due to the maldigestion or malabsorption of dietary fat.**5** Stools are of large volume and malodorous, with floating fat droplets. Pancreatic exocrine insufficiency (especially lipase deficiency) is the prototypic disease causing fat maldigestion. Fat is malabsorbed in the setting of deficient bile salts (biliary tract obstruction, cholestatic liver disease, ileal disease) and small-bowel mucosal disease (eg, gluten-sensitive enteropathy, celiac disease, tropical sprue, giardiasis, Crohn's disease, Whipple's disease). Patients with maldigestion or

---

1 see page 1068   **2** see pages 1059 and 1062   **3** see page 1117
4 see page 1141   **5** see also page 1095

malabsorption often report weight loss despite normal or enhanced food intake.

Diagnosis

Evaluation is indicated for patients with moderate or severe illness when clinical symptoms suggest bacterial infection, for larger volume ($\geq$ 6 stools/24 hours) or bloody diarrhea, and for acute diarrhea lasting > 8 hours.

Diagnosing the cause of diarrhea is challenging. The initial evaluation should first determine whether the patient's problem is diarrhea, fecal incontinence,◻ or fecal impaction with overflow incontinence. Next, to help categorize the diarrhea and narrow the differential diagnosis, the characteristics of the diarrhea are determined. In the elderly, serious diarrhea that leads to dehydration may require hospitalization for further evaluation and treatment.

The history and physical examination provide clues to the etiology and determine the severity of the diarrhea. A temporal relationship should be sought between the onset of diarrhea and the introduction of new drugs. Symptoms from food poisoning usually develop within 6 to 12 hours of ingestion, while symptoms from *Salmonella, Y. enterocolitica,* or *Campylobacter* usually develop 12 to 48 hours after ingestion. Bloody stools suggest significant inflammation or ulceration, as can occur with ischemic colitis or infection with *Shigella, E. histolytica,* or enteroinvasive *E. coli;* patients with a recent history of antibiotic use are at risk for *C. difficile* diarrhea. The presence of atherosclerotic vascular disease, abdominal bruits, and initial painless bleeding suggests colonic ischemia. Significant abdominal tenderness requires prompt evaluation for the underlying etiology.

Initial laboratory tests may include a CBC, biochemical test of electrolytes, renal function, and nutritional parameters (ie, albumin, calcium, phosphorus, total protein). Stool samples are tested for occult blood; white blood cells; qualitative fat (Sudan stain); and, in patients with a recent history of antibiotic use, hospitalization, or institutionalization, *C. difficile* toxin. Stool electrolytes (sodium and potassium) obtained on spot samples of stool are used to calculate an osmotic gap with the following formula: 290 − 2 (Na + K).

Stool cultures are indicated in patients with severe diarrhea and fever, bloody stools, fecal leukocytes, or prolonged illness (> 14 days). Stool samples should be obtained for testing of ova and parasites in patients who travel extensively or live in an endemic area (three fresh samples are required for a 90% sensitivity). When giardiasis is suspected, an

◻see page 1092

enzyme-linked immunosorbent assay for *Giardia* antigen is more sensitive than routine ova and parasitic testing.

When the diagnosis of diarrhea remains obscure, the single most useful test is the quantitative stool collection, typically the 72-hour fecal fat collection. Information can be obtained about total stool weight and the efficiency of fat absorption. Fecal fat concentrations of > 9.5 g/100 g of stool suggest pancreatic insufficiency or biliary steatorrhea.

Flexible sigmoidoscopy may be helpful in some acute cases to evaluate for evidence of pseudomembranes or ischemia.

Secretory diarrhea typically has an osmotic gap of < 50. When the clinical picture suggests a hormone-secreting tumor, serum tests for gastrin, calcitonin, and vasoactive intestinal polypeptide and urine collection for 5-hydroxyindoleacetic acid, metanephrine, or histamine may be helpful.

Osmotic diarrhea has an osmotic gap of > 125. Stool pH of < 5.3 (normal is > 6) supports the diagnosis of carbohydrate malabsorption. In lactase deficiency, the stool pH is usually 4 to 6 with an associated increase in short-chain fatty acids. A lactose-hydrogen breath test reveals breath hydrogen > 20 ppm within 3 hours after lactose ingestion. Measuring magnesium, sulfate, and phosphate in stool water may be necessary in cases of surreptitious laxative abuse, a problem more common in elderly women.

Bloody (exudative) diarrhea (fecal blood and leukocytes) and fatty diarrhea (Sudan stain) require further evaluation. A plain abdominal x-ray may show pancreatic calcification indicating chronic pancreatitis (due to alcohol or familial pancreatitis). A small-bowel follow-through examination may show ileal disease (Crohn's disease) or mucosal thickening (eg, small-bowel lymphoma). Colonoscopy enables direct visualization and biopsy of the colonic mucosa and is the procedure of choice for diagnosing radiation proctopathy, inflammatory bowel disease, and colorectal tumors. Biopsy samples obtained from normal-appearing colonic mucosa can be examined for changes of microscopic colitis.

Upper gastrointestinal endoscopy is helpful in obtaining small-bowel biopsies for suspected mucosal disease (eg, celiac sprue, Whipple's disease■). Small bowel aspirates can be obtained at the same time to evaluate for small bowel bacterial overgrowth and parasites.

Serum tests of antigliadin immunoglobulin (IgA and IgG) antibodies and antiendomysial IgA antibodies are helpful in the diagnosis and treatment of patients with celiac sprue.

In patients with chronic fatty diarrhea, pancreatic exocrine insufficiency can be determined by administrating secretin or cholecystokinin IV and aspirating duodenal contents for bicarbonate and pancreatic enzyme concentration. This test is cumbersome but remains the stan-

---

■ see also TABLE 111–1 on page 1099

dard for assessing pancreatic exocrine function. Although not sensitive in mild and moderate disease, measurement of chymotrypsin or elastase activity in stool samples can also assess pancreatic function.

Treatment

The first management priority for patients with diarrhea is fluid and electrolyte replacement. Patients who can take drugs orally should be given oral rehydration solutions. Elderly patients with symptomatic fluid losses require close monitoring and usually hospitalization. Food poisoning is self-limited, usually of brief symptomatic duration, and is treated using fluid support.

Antibiotic treatment for infectious diarrhea is listed in TABLE 110–5. Empiric antibiotic treatment is indicated for patients with fever, evidence of systemic toxicity, bloody stool, or traveler's diarrhea; the usual drug of choice is a fluoroquinolone for 3 to 5 days. Although treatment can begin immediately, it is helpful to obtain a stool sample for bacterial culture first.

If toxin-producing or invasive bacteria are not suspected, antidiarrheal drugs can be given safely (see TABLE 110–5). Empiric treatment can minimize diarrheal symptoms when the diagnostic evaluation is in progress, when a diagnosis has been made but specific treatment is

TABLE 110–5.   TREATMENT OF DIARRHEA*

Type	Medication	Dose
Nonspecific	Psyllium	3–6 g/day
	Methylcellulose	2.4–4.8 g/day
	Aluminum hydroxide	5–30 mL bid
	Bismuth subsalicylate	15 mL qid
	Loperamide	2–4 mg daily to qid
	Diphenoxylate	2.5–5 mg qid
	Codeine	30–60 mg bid to qid
	Tincture of opium	10 drops, titrating up or down to desired effect
Bile acid	Cholestyramine	4–5 g bid
	Octreotide	50 μg sc, increased as needed
Infectious	Ciprofloxacin	500 mg po bid × 5 days
	Norfloxacin	400 mg po bid × 5 days
	Trimethoprim/sulfamethoxazole DS	160 mg trimethoprim/800 mg sulfamethoxazole po bid × 5 days
	Metronidazole	500 mg po tid × 10–14 days

*Antimicrobial therapy is directed toward the suspected or identified pathogen. Fluoroquinolones are usual empiric therapy for severe diarrhea.

DS = double strength.

unavailable, or when testing fails to reveal a diagnosis. Various prescription drugs and over-the-counter products are available. Soluble fiber (eg, psyllium) adds form to the stool. Synthetic opioids loperamide and diphenoxylate are excellent first-line drugs. Loperamide is generally preferred, because the usual formulation of diphenoxylate incorporates atropine, which can cause significant adverse effects in elderly persons. When the diarrhea cannot be controlled with these drugs, stronger opioids (eg, codeine, tincture of opium) are recommended. Because of its need for injection and increased adverse effects, somatostatin analog is a second-line drug for the treatment of chronic idiopathic diarrhea. When bile acid diarrhea is suspected, cholestyramine may be tried.

Treatment of microscopic colitis consists of removing the offending agent when it is identified and use of antidiarrheal drugs. Clinical improvement is reported with 5-aminosalicylate drugs. Corticosteroids are generally avoided.

FECAL INCONTINENCE

Loss of voluntary control of defecation.

Fecal incontinence is a humiliating regression in bodily function that often causes anxiety, fear, embarrassment, and reclusiveness and can severely impair an elderly person's activity and socialization.

One study suggests that about 5% of the general population are affected. Fecal incontinence more frequently occurs in persons > 65 and is a primary reason for institutionalization of these patients; about 50% of institutionalized patients have fecal incontinence.

Etiology and Pathophysiology

Continence requires rectal and anal sensation to detect rectal filling and to discriminate among fluid, feces, and flatus. The reservoir capacity of the rectum and distal colon permits storing feces for variable periods of time. The coordination of internal and external anal sphincters is critical to blocking unintended defecation. The pelvic floor muscles, especially the puborectal muscle, preserve continence by retarding stool passage. Motivation is also essential to maintaining continence.

With age, contractile strength of the puborectal muscle, rectal elasticity, and external and internal anal sphincter pressures may decrease. Smaller distention volumes can lead to rectal urgency and inhibit anal sphincter tone. Causes of fecal incontinence in the elderly are listed in TABLE 110–6.

Fecal incontinence can result from fecal impaction, usually the result of impaired rectal sensation with flow of liquid stool around the fecal

TABLE 110-6.   CAUSES OF FECAL INCONTINENCE IN THE ELDERLY

Cause	Comment
Fecal impaction	Most common cause in institutionalized elderly patients
Mental or physical functional impairment	—
Decreased rectal reservoir capacity	Caused by aging, radiation, tumor, ischemia, surgical resection
Decreased rectal sensation	Caused by diabetes, megarectum, fecal impaction
Impaired anal sphincter and puborectal muscle function	Caused by trauma, surgery, spinal cord or pudendal lesions, or an unknown cause

mass. These patients do not appropriately contract the striated muscle of the anal sphincter to prevent incontinence. Anal sphincter pressures usually become normal after disimpaction. In patients with global dementia, fecal incontinence may occur after meals or other activities that stimulate the gastrocolonic response, because these patients simply do not suppress the urge to defecate.

In ambulatory, noninstitutionalized elderly patients, fecal incontinence often occurs as a result of decreased contractile strength or impaired automaticity of the puborectal and external anal sphincter muscles. These changes are probably caused by age-related muscle weakness or partial denervation injury from pudendal neuropathy. The cause of pudendal neuropathy is unknown but may include repetitive stretching of the pudendal nerves in elderly women because of chronic constipation and defecatory straining, weaker pelvic floor muscles, and possibly spondylitic compression of nerve roots.

Diagnosis

The history and physical examination give clues to the severity of the problem and determine the integrity of the neuromusculature involved in maintaining continence. Several tests offer objective information useful in defining defects responsible for incontinence.

Anal manometry directly measures the pressure in the anal canal under basal conditions and with squeezing. In general, patients with fecal incontinence have significantly lower basal and squeeze pressures than age- and sex-matched controls, but many have normal sphincter pressures. Anal manometry is most valuable when it demonstrates abnormally low pressures and confirms a sphincter defect.

Manometric testing, which uses an inflatable balloon attached to a manometric catheter, tests rectal sensation, rectal compliance, and anorectal inhibitory reflex. Findings reflect the integrity of the neural pathways mediating sensation (both to consciousness and as a trigger for the anorectal relaxation reflex) and the motor responses.

Electromyography of the puborectal muscle and external anal sphincter assesses motor nerve supply and skeletal muscle responses, but its clinical usefulness is limited because of the discomfort experienced during the test.

Defecography assesses rectal capacity and diameter, anorectal angle (puborectal muscle function), and perineal descent (pelvic floor function). It can readily detect weakness of the puborectal muscle and pelvic floor.

Sigmoidoscopy can assess the mucosa and detect intraluminal lesions (eg, inflammation, melanosis coli due to laxative overuse, tumors, strictures) that may contribute to the symptoms.

Anal ultrasound assesses internal and external anal sphincter integrity by measuring muscle thickness and determining the presence or absence of sphincter disruption.

Treatment

Fecal incontinence can be treated in most patients. Treatment can reduce or eliminate episodes in > 50% of institutionalized patients.

Fecal impaction❚ must be adequately treated. After the colon has been cleared, an immobilized or functionally impaired patient should be placed on a restricted fiber diet and have prophylactic enemas once or twice weekly to prevent recurrent impaction.

In nonconstipated patients without impaction, intervention can include drug therapy, biofeedback, and surgery.

The only drugs that have been evaluated for their effect on fecal incontinence are the opioid antidiarrheals, loperamide, and the combination of diphenoxylate and atropine. In patients with chronic diarrhea, loperamide 4 mg po tid significantly reduces the frequency of incontinent episodes and urgency and slightly increases basal anal sphincter pressure.

When fecal incontinence is associated with impaired reservoir capacity or with neurogenic abnormalities affecting colorectal function, a program of planned regular defecation and fiber restriction to reduce stool volume often reduces incontinence. If incontinence persists, loperamide (maximum 16 mg/day in divided doses) is titrated to decrease stool frequency or eliminate defecation.

Biofeedback is often effective for fecal incontinence due to rectosphincteric abnormalities. A balloon manometry device helps the patient obtain a conscious threshold for sensation of rectal distention and coordinate external anal sphincter contraction with rectal distention. An anorectal manometer attached to a visual display allows the pa-

❚ see page 1082

tient to observe when sphincteric responses are appropriate; the patient subsequently attempts to reproduce the appropriate response. Although some elderly patients have difficulty with this approach because of anxiety and cognitive deficit, this technique has been successful in up to 70% of patients who are motivated, able to understand directions, and have some degree of rectal sensation.

Surgical intervention should be considered in patients who fail to respond to drug therapy and who have a disrupted anal sphincter. Although many surgical procedures have been used, the best procedure has not been determined.

When fecal incontinence is the result of rectal prolapse, resuspension or proctopexy can prevent further prolapse and can be combined with rectosigmoidectomy to restore continence in up to two thirds of patients. However, when prolapse is severe or prolonged, permanent neuropathic sphincter impairment may preclude a good surgical result.

For patients without full-thickness rectal prolapse, surgery should be considered only if conservative treatment has been unsatisfactory, because the available procedures are not easy to perform and may result in complications. The surgical approach should be individualized to suit the specific abnormalities.

▉111▉ MALABSORPTION

A clinical spectrum of symptoms and signs resulting from defective mucosal absorption and excessive excretion of fat, carbohydrates, and proteins, with inadequate absorption of vitamins, minerals, electrolytes, and water.

Although malabsorption generally denotes any defect in the absorptive process, the term strictly refers to the defective mucosal absorption of nutrients. Maldigestion denotes impaired nutrient hydrolysis.

Aging and Digestion

Although small-intestine mucosal surface area is reduced with age, the morphology of the small bowel does not differ from that in younger persons. The digestive and absorptive functions of the gastrointestinal (GI) system do not decline substantially with age. The only age-related defect in intestinal absorption is that of calcium, which is probably due to decreased renal production of 1,25-dihydroxycholecalciferol and reduced intestinal response. Small-intestine motility appears to remain intact with age.

Aging does not significantly affect the structure and function of the exocrine pancreas. The main pancreatic duct may become ectatic and is associated with ductal hyperplasia and intralobular fibrosis. However, such morphologic changes are not known to cause clinical dysfunction; malabsorption and maldigestion only occur when > 90% of pancreatic exocrine function is lost. There are no age-related differences in the pancreatic output of trypsin, chymotrypsin, and lipase after maximal doses of secretin and cerulein.

Etiology

Malabsorption has many causes (see TABLE 111–1). Pancreatic insufficiency, such as occurs with chronic pancreatitis and pancreatic cancer, is the cause of malabsorption in 20 to 30% of cases in the elderly. A significant number of these patients have no history of typical pain or predisposing factors (eg, alcoholism).

About 30% of malabsorption cases in elderly patients are due to anatomic abnormalities (eg, small-intestine diverticulosis, strictures, partial obstruction), which promote stasis of intestinal contents and predispose patients to the bacterial overgrowth syndrome.

Another 20% of patients with malabsorption have bacterial overgrowth syndrome in the absence of anatomic abnormalities. This syndrome occurs when gastric acid secretion is inadequate. Pernicious anemia and vitamin B_{12} deficiency are common, suggesting that gastric atrophy and achlorhydria allow proliferation of gastric and small-intestine bacteria. Intestinal motility disorders may also impair bacterial clearance, which can lead to bacterial overgrowth.

Malabsorption of fat, proteins, minerals, and vitamins often occurs after gastrectomies and small-intestine resections (enterectomy). A gastrectomy with vagotomy can result in rapid gastric emptying and transit through the small intestine. Nutritional deficiencies after a gastrectomy or small-intestine resection result from diminished absorption of iron, calcium, fat, and protein and are related to the extent of the gastrectomy, rapidity of intestinal transit, and the type of anastomosis. As a general rule, one third of the jejunum and ileum may be excised without seriously impairing nutrient absorption. More radical resection is tolerated poorly, and adults who have lost two thirds of the small intestine usually develop severe metabolic problems. After resection of the terminal ileum, absorption of vitamin B_{12} and bile acids is reduced. Resections of more than 100 cm of small intestine result in marked steatorrhea and a depleted bile salt pool. Typically, partial and total colectomy only temporarily diminish the absorption of water and some electrolytes. Total proctocolectomy produces only temporary malabsorption.

Other causes of malabsorption include cirrhosis and biliary tract disease, which can result in impaired micelle formation. Intestinal mucosal abnormalities arising from celiac sprue (the cause in 30% of patients), tropical sprue, Whipple's disease, or Crohn's disease can also cause malabsorption. Obstruction of the intestinal lymphatic system, such as occurs in intestinal lymphangiectasia, results in lipoprotein malabsorption. Infestation with some intestinal parasites (eg, giardiasis, cryptosporidiosis) can rarely lead to malabsorption.

Symptoms and Signs

Often, an elderly patient with a malabsorption syndrome may only have weight loss or failure to maintain body weight, which leads to general debility. Often, symptoms may include diarrhea, greasy stools, abdominal bloating, and gas. Although diarrhea is not always present in persons with malabsorption, chronic diarrhea is the most common GI symptom of malabsorption to prompt an evaluation.

Steatorrhea, which is due to the malabsorption of fat, is suggested by foul-smelling, bulky stools that are difficult to flush. Steatorrhea occurs when > 6% of dietary fat is excreted in the stool. Although physiologic steatorrhea can occur rarely in some conditions, steatorrhea is considered to be the hallmark of malabsorption.

Abdominal bloating and excessive flatus suggest colonic fermentation of maldigested carbohydrates. In advanced malabsorption, severe vitamin and mineral deficiencies occur. Other clinical manifestations include anemia secondary to deficiencies in iron, folate, vitamin B_{12}, or any combination of these micronutrients; easy bruising and bleeding secondary to vitamin K deficiency; muscular weakness and bone pain caused by vitamin D deficiency; and cramps, numbness, and paresthesias suggesting hypocalcemia and hypomagnesemia.

Diagnosis

The clinical features of the malabsorption syndromes are less obvious and more difficult to recognize in the elderly than in younger persons. Occasionally, the syndrome is only suspected when blood tests show deficiency states such as anemia, hypocalcemia, and hypoalbuminemia. Therefore, the physician should maintain a high index of suspicion.

In many cases, the cause may be suggested by a history of lifelong symptoms of diarrhea exacerbated by gluten products, stomach and intestinal operations, use of drugs, or recurrent episodes of abdominal pain.

Steatorrhea should be identified and is usually confirmed by a quantitative 72-hour stool collection. Severe fat malabsorption (fecal fat of ≥ 40 g) almost always indicates pancreatic insufficiency or small-intestine mucosal disease. The D-xylose test ∎ is a good, noninvasive way of differentiating pancreatitis (or another intraluminal etiology) from mucosal disease, especially if the cause is not evident from the clinical data. If severe steatorrhea is accompanied by a normal D-xylose test result, pancreatic disease should be suspected. Often, the combination of history of alcoholism, pancreatic calcifications, and recurrent

∎see page 1102

TABLE 111-1. CAUSES OF MALABSORPTION IN THE ELDERLY

Cause	Risk Factors/ Predisposing Conditions	Presentation	Diagnosis	Specific Treatment
Pancreatic insufficiency	Chronic pancreatitis, pancreatic cancer, heavy alcohol intake, trauma, hyperlipidemia, hyperparathyroidism, pancreas divisum, periampullary tumors, vascular disease, collagen vascular disease	Massive steatorrhea (fecal fat > 20 g/day), epigastric pain usually absent in the elderly	Quantitative stool collection for fat, endoscopic retrograde cholangiopancreatography, secretin test, bentiromide test, serum trypsinogen test	Pancreatic enzyme supplements, a low-fat diet, abstention from alcohol, treatment of any predisposing condition
Bacterial overgrowth syndrome	Achlorhydria, alterations in intestinal anatomy or GI motility due to postsurgical states, diverticulosis, strictures, fistulas, ulcerations, or dilated loops of bowel	May be asymptomatic but patients can have nutrient deficiencies, malnutrition, failure to gain weight, or steatorrhea	Culture of intestinal fluid aspirate, D-xylose breath test	Oral antibiotics (tetracycline 250 mg qid, amoxicillin/clavulanic acid 250–500 mg tid, cephalexin 250 mg qid, metronidazole 250–500 mg tid to qid) usually for 14 days
Short-bowel syndrome	Extensive intestinal resection leading to inadequate absorptive surface	Severe malnutrition, neurologic deficits, diarrhea, or steatorrhea	Based on surgical history	Total parenteral nutrition and parenteral vitamin B_{12} supplementation
Cholestasis	Cirrhosis, hepatitis, drug toxicity, biliary obstruction, pancreatic cancer	Jaundice, dark urine, pale stools, pruritus, steatorrhea, and hypoprothrombinemia	Imaging studies, endoscopic retrograde cholangiopancreatography, liver biopsy	Treatment of the underlying predisposing condition

Celiac sprue	Genetic, immunologically mediated disease	Weight loss, vitamin deficiencies, malnutrition, steatorrhea (10–40 g/day), nonspecific complaints of fatigue and lassitude; anemia in 80%, GI symptoms (diarrhea, flatulence) in 60%	Small-intestine biopsy showing villous atrophy; measurements of endomysial, reticulin, gliadin antibodies; serum xylose and 5-hour urinary xylose excretion (supportive)	Gluten-free diet (no wheat, rye, barley, oats)
Tropical sprue	Travel to tropical or subtropical areas (southern/Southeast Asia, Central and South America, Caribbean Islands)	Sore tongue, diarrhea, weight loss, steatorrhea	Small-intestine biopsy showing subtotal villous atrophy that does not improve with a gluten-free diet	Folic acid (5 mg/day po), vitamin B_{12} (100 µg/month po), and antibiotics (tetracycline 250 mg po qid) for up to 6 mo
Whipple's disease	Infection with *Tropheryma whippelii*	Weight loss, diarrhea, anemia, pleural effusion, polyarthralgia	Lymph node or intestinal biopsy	Oral antibiotics (penicillin 250 mg qid, tetracycline 250 mg qid, chloramphenicol 250 mg qid, trimethoprim-sulfamethoxazole one double-strength tablet bid, or a cephalosporin [eg, ceftriaxone] for 6–12 mo
Crohn's disease	Genetic, unregulated intestinal immune response	Elderly patients with Crohn's colitis tend to present more indolently (see Ch. 107)	See Ch. 107	See Ch. 107

Table continues on the following page.

TABLE 111–1. CAUSES OF MALABSORPTION IN THE ELDERLY (*Continued*)

Cause	Risk Factors/ Predisposing Conditions	Presentation	Diagnosis	Specific Treatment
Intestinal lymphangiectasia	Lymphoma, tuberculosis, sarcoidosis (neoplastic or infiltrative conditions that interfere with the lymphatic flow)	Mild GI symptoms, sometimes severe diarrhea	Small-intestine biopsy	Low-fat diet, medium chain triglycerides
Parasitic infections	IgA deficiency (predisposes to giardiasis), contaminated food and water, immunocompromised state	Usually asymptomatic; sometimes chronic diarrhea, constipation, fever, flatulence, or cramping abdominal pain	Small-intestine aspirate and biopsy (stool samples may be negative)	Treatment targeted to the specific intestinal infection

GI = gastrointestinal.

abdominal pain can make the diagnosis of chronic pancreatitis apparent. If the diagnosis is in doubt, pancreatic insufficiency can be confirmed with the secretin stimulation test or with the bentiromide or pancreolauryl tests.

Other intraluminal causes of malabsorption include inadequate bile salt concentrations from cirrhosis, severe parenchymal liver disease, and cholestasis. If severe steatorrhea is accompanied by an abnormal D-xylose test result, mucosal disease is suggested and an endoscopic biopsy should be performed. However, abnormal results of the D-xylose test can also be caused by bacterial overgrowth. Therefore, an aspirate can be collected during the biopsy to test for bacteria and parasites, particularly if bacterial overgrowth is suspected. If bacterial overgrowth syndrome is documented by culture or breath tests, a barium x-ray should be ordered to look for diverticula, blind loop syndrome, strictures, fistulas, and other anatomic abnormalities.

If no anatomic abnormality that explains the malabsorption is found, pernicious anemia or systemic diseases should be suspected, and a Schilling test is recommended to differentiate between pernicious anemia, pancreatic insufficiency, and bacterial overgrowth.

If pancreatic insufficiency needs to be further documented, pancreatic imaging studies are a reasonable first step. If these are not diagnostic, the patient should be tested for exocrine insufficiency. ▮

Most tests assess malabsorption of fat, which is easier to measure than malabsorption of other dietary components. Confirmation of carbohydrate malabsorption is not helpful once steatorrhea is documented. Because fecal nitrogen is difficult to measure, tests for protein absorption are rarely used.

Blood tests: Although neither sensitive nor specific, some blood tests may be diagnostically helpful. Such tests include a complete blood cell count and peripheral smear; serum levels of iron, ferritin, vitamin B_{12}, calcium, and albumin; and red blood cell (RBC) folate. Microcytic anemia without GI blood loss suggests iron malabsorption. Macrocytic anemia strongly indicates folate or vitamin B_{12} malabsorption. A low RBC folate level confirms folate malabsorption, which is common in mucosal disorders involving the jejunum. A low serum vitamin B_{12} level suggests pernicious anemia, bacterial overgrowth, or terminal ileal disease. A low serum albumin level may indicate poor nutritional intake. Determination of carotene, a precursor of fat-soluble vitamin A, is sometimes helpful. If dietary deficiency can be excluded in the elderly, serum carotene levels of < 0.6 mg/dL indicate mucosal malabsorption.

Tests for steatorrhea: The qualitative Sudan stain is specific for dietary triglycerides and lipolytic metabolites. A stool specimen is examined microscopically after being heated in glacial acetic acid in the pres-

▮see page 1103

ence of Sudan III stain. Multiple orange-red globules indicate steatorrhea. When steatorrhea is < 10 g/24 hours, the estimated false-negative rate is 25%. The correlation between this qualitative test and the quantitative fecal fat test is poor.

The most accurate test for determining steatorrhea is a quantitative fecal fat test, which measures fatty acids from exogenous and endogenous sources. After the patient consumes a daily diet of 100 g of fat for at least 3 days, the total amount of fat in the stool collected during a 72-hour period is measured. Fecal fat > 6 g daily is abnormal. Fecal fat > 40 g daily suggests defective lipolysis (eg, due to pancreatic insufficiency) or massive ileal resection.

The ^{14}C-triolein breath test can confirm fat malabsorption. The patient ingests 60 g of labeled ^{14}C-triolein, a triglyceride that undergoes lipid hydrolysis and is subsequently absorbed and metabolized, releasing CO_2. Breath samples are then analyzed for radioactivity. The results may be erroneous in patients with diabetes mellitus, obesity, hyperlipidemia, thyroid disorders, chronic liver disease, or lung disease, because altered metabolism of triolein or impaired excretion of CO_2 occurs in these conditions.

Tests for mucosal diseases: The D-xylose absorption test is the best noninvasive method for assessing intestinal mucosal integrity. Xylose is a pentose that does not require pancreatic enzymes for digestion. Thus, this test helps differentiate maldigestion from malabsorption. A normal D-xylose test in the presence of steatorrhea indicates pancreatic exocrine insufficiency rather than small-intestine mucosal disease. This test has a reported 98% specificity and 91% sensitivity.

The patient is given an oral dose of 25 g of D-xylose. A venous blood sample is taken 1 hour after ingestion, and urine is collected over 5 hours. A serum level of < 20 mg/dL and a D-xylose level of < 4 g in the urine collection indicate abnormal absorption of the pentose. Falsely low levels can occur in patients with renal diseases, bacterial overgrowth, ascites, portal hypertension, or delayed gastric emptying time.

The Schilling test assesses malabsorption of vitamin B_{12} and can determine whether the deficiency is due to pernicious anemia, pancreatic exocrine insufficiency, bacterial overgrowth, or ileal disease. Controversy exists about the usefulness of this test.∎ In this test, if there is normalization with the addition of pancreatic enzymes, cobalamin malabsorption is secondary to pancreatic insufficiency. Correction after antimicrobial therapy suggests bacterial overgrowth, whereas cobalamin deficiency secondary to ileal disease or ileal resection indicates abnormalities at all stages of absorption.

Endoscopic small-bowel biopsy allows visual assessment of the small-intestine mucosa and can allow directed biopsies if there are areas

∎ see page 686

of patchy involvement. Histologic features may establish a diagnosis of parasitic infection (eg, *Giardia lamblia, Coccidiodes immitis, Cryptosporidia*), amyloidosis, Whipple's disease, mastocytosis, lymphangiectasia, or collagenous sprue. In amyloidosis, deposits of amyloid are seen within the walls of the arterioles in the submucosa. In Whipple's disease, the lamina propria becomes infiltrated with periodic acid-Schiff–positive macrophages. In lymphangiectasia, markedly dilated lamina propria lymphatics are found together with edema and villous distortion. Villous atrophy is characteristic of celiac sprue but may be seen in tropical sprue, Crohn's disease, lymphoma, Whipple's disease, and bacterial overgrowth.

Contrast small-intestine x-rays are not adequately sensitive for evaluating mucosal disease; their usefulness lies in the detection of anatomic abnormalities that predispose to bacterial overgrowth (eg, diverticula, surgically created stagnant loops, strictures, fistulas, ulcerations, dilated small-bowel loops). These x-rays can also demonstrate patchy or distal mucosal disease (eg, Crohn's disease).

Tests for pancreatic insufficiency: The secretin test is the most sensitive test for demonstrating pancreatic exocrine insufficiency. A tube with distal aspiration holes is placed via fluoroscopy in the duodenum at the entrance of the pancreatic duct. Collection of the duodenal aspirate is performed after stimulation of pancreatic secretions by IV administration of secretin alone or with cholecystokinin or cerulein. If cholecystokinin or cerulein is given, the aspirate is measured for trypsin, amylase, or lipase. If secretin alone is given, the aspirate is measured for bicarbonate. Bicarbonate secretion is probably the single most useful measure of exocrine function. Most investigators consider a bicarbonate concentration < 70 mEq/L and a secretion volume < 2 mL/kg of body weight as abnormal. However, this test is invasive, time-consuming, expensive, and unavailable in most hospitals.

Other tests for pancreatic function include the bentiromide test, which measures pancreatic chymotrypsin activity, and the pancreolauryl test, in which oral fluorescein dilaurate is hydrolyzed by pancreatic esterase. Para-aminobenzoic acid and fluorescein are measured in the urine, respectively. Both tests are sensitive for moderate to severe pancreatic insufficiency but are of limited value in mild pancreatic impairment.

The serum trypsinogen test is a simple noninvasive radioimmunoassay blood test that may help diagnose chronic pancreatitis. A serum trypsinogen level of < 20 ng/mL (normal is 20 to 80 ng/mL) is characteristic of pancreatic insufficiency.

Pancreatic calcifications on plain abdominal x-rays suggest chronic pancreatitis. However, calcifications are seen only when severe pancreatic damage has already occurred and are found in only 20 to 30% of patients with pancreatic insufficiency. Ultrasound and CT are useful in imaging the pancreas to exclude pancreatic cancer. Endoscopic retrograde cannulation of the pancreatic duct can demonstrate obstruction, irregularities, and narrowing of the main duct and side branches, which suggest chronic pancreatitis. However, this procedure is invasive and causes pancreatitis in 4% of patients.

Tests for bacterial overgrowth: The diagnosis of bacterial overgrowth is best made with a direct quantitative bacterial count and/or positive aspirate culture. An aspirate is collected from the proximal small intestine, which is normally free of bacteria. An aspirate that contains $> 10^5$ organisms/mL suggests bacterial overgrowth syndrome. Bacteria commonly implicated are coliforms and other aerobic bacteria as well as anaerobic organisms (eg, bacteroides, lactobacilli, clostridia). The same aspirate can also be examined for giardiasis.

Breath tests are sensitive, inexpensive, and generally acceptable to most patients. These tests measure the production of volatile metabolites produced by bacteria after the ingestion of fermentable substrates in a timed breath excretion collection. The acid breath test identifies abnormal bacterial deconjugation of previously administered ^{14}C-glycocholic acid. The glycine residue is metabolized and results in $^{14}CO_2$ in the breath. An early rise of $^{14}CO_2$ within 6 hours indicates small-intestine bacterial overgrowth. However, this test has only a 65% sensitivity. The ^{14}C D-xylose breath test depends on the ability of gram-negative aerobic bacteria to metabolize D-xylose, resulting in $^{14}CO_2$ in the expired air after 60 minutes. This test has an overall sensitivity of 65 to 95%.

Treatment

The main objectives are correcting deficiencies of nutrients, vitamins, and trace minerals and identifying and treating the underlying causes.

Patients with iron deficiency are given supplemental ferrous sulfate or gluconate tablets. Oral folic acid can be given to patients with folate deficiency, and intramuscular vitamin B_{12} injections can be given monthly to persons with cobalamin deficiency. Patients with marked steatorrhea require fat-soluble vitamin and calcium supplementation. A high-protein, low-fat diet and high-calorie dietary supplementation are recommended for patients with severe weight loss. A low-fat diet reduces steatorrhea and bile salt excretion, especially in patients with small-intestine resections. Medium-chain triglycerides, given as a dietary supplement, are preferred because they are hydrolyzed more readily by pancreatic lipase, and micelle formation is not necessary for their absorption. Parenteral nutrition may be considered in patients with severe malnutrition who are unresponsive to oral feeding. However, parenteral nutrition is reserved as the sole source of primary nutrients for persons with conditions in which the temporary avoidance of enteral feeding is necessary. In only rare conditions is long-term parenteral feeding appropriate.

112 ACUTE ABDOMEN AND SURGICAL GASTROENTEROLOGY

Surgical problems of the abdomen are different in many ways in elderly patients compared with those in younger patients. Diagnosis, particularly in emergencies, is more difficult because sensation is not as acute as in younger patients, and pathophysiologic reactions (eg, pain, tenderness, response to inflammation) are not as quick or effective. Thus, minimal symptoms may accompany a potentially fatal intestinal perforation, and the first sign may be free subphrenic gas on a plain abdominal x-ray.

Acute abdomen should be suspected in patients who complain of only minimal abdominal pain. Peritonitis caused by perforation of the sigmoid, stomach, or duodenum may be present even if the patient has only slight abdominal tenderness. Vascular lesions (eg, mesenteric artery thrombosis) also are common. With appendicitis, acute cholecystitis, and strangulated hernias, the interval between onset and gangrene may be only a few hours.

The physical examination is extremely important. Old incisional scars raise the likelihood of intestinal obstruction. An examination of potential hernia sites is essential. Absence of bowel sounds indicates aperistalsis, a serious finding that requires other diagnostic tests be performed expeditiously.

The major indications for emergency surgery are perforation of a viscus, appendicitis, intestinal obstruction, and massive hemorrhage. Acute cholecystitis often requires urgent surgery.

Most elective surgery is for malignant disease. Excluding hernia repairs, > 90% of abdominal procedures involve the colon, gallbladder, and stomach; with effective medical treatment for peptic ulcer disease, operations on the colon and gallbladder now predominate.

Generally, the elderly tolerate a single operation well, provided the offending lesion is removed. However, complications from second or third operations performed soon after the first carry a high mortality rate. Staged procedures should be spaced apart to allow complete recovery. These considerations are particularly important in gastrointestinal (GI) disorders.

GASTROINTESTINAL BLEEDING

Bleeding of the GI tract may manifest clinically as hematemesis (vomiting of blood), melena (passage of black tarry stools), or hematochezia (passage of red bloody stools).

The GI tract has many potential sites of bleeding. The most common sites, in descending order, are the anorectum, stomach, colon, small intestine, and esophagus. Blood that originates in the mouth, the nasopharynx, or the lung can be swallowed and mimic gastric bleeding. The liver, pancreas, and aorta are unusual bleeding sites.

In the elderly, hemorrhoids and colorectal cancer are the most common causes of minor bleeding; peptic ulcer, diverticular disease, and angiodysplasia are the most common causes of major bleeding. Massive GI bleeding is tolerated poorly by elderly patients. Diagnosis must be made quickly, and treatment must be started sooner than in younger patients, who can better tolerate repeated episodes of bleeding.

Resuscitation: While evaluation is being performed, the patient must be adequately resuscitated. Patients who present with bleeding must have adequate IV access (two large-bore IV lines) in anticipation of hemodynamic compromise. While giving large volumes of fluid to elderly patients often frightens clinicians, inadequate replacement is potentially lethal. A Foley catheter should be placed to assess adequacy of resuscitation while awaiting results of renal function tests. It is important to note that, with aging, renal concentrating ability decreases, so that urine output may continue in the face of decreasing intravascular volume until the patient suddenly becomes anuric. Especially for debilitated patients with hypotension or brisk upper GI bleeding, endotracheal intubation may be needed for airway protection.

Diagnosis

The history, physical examination, blood tests, endoscopy, selective arteriography, radionuclide studies, barium contrast studies, and exploratory laparotomy aid in identifying the bleeding site. Often, determining whether bleeding originates in the upper or lower GI tract is difficult. Thus, ongoing diagnostic evaluation and treatment are essential while bleeding continues.

The **history** provides important clinical information. Alcoholism and a previous massive upper GI hemorrhage suggest bleeding caused by esophageal varices in young adults, but in elderly patients, the more likely cause is peptic ulcer disease. If a patient has an aortic aneurysm or an abdominal aortic graft, erosion into the duodenum should be suspected. Massive colonic bleeding is most likely caused by diverticular disease or angiodysplasia. Streaks of red blood on the toilet paper usually indicate hemorrhoids, but polyps and cancer must be ruled out.

Aspirin ingestion may explain GI bleeding. One aspirin tablet can prolong bleeding times for at least 6 days, while a larger dose can cause aspirin-induced gastritis. Nevertheless, the physician should not be influenced too strongly by such a history, because many patients who take aspirin bleed from other causes. Alcohol, anticoagulants, nonsteroidal anti-inflammatory drugs (eg, ibuprofen), and coagulopathies (eg, those associated with metastatic disease or chemotherapy) may cause gastritis or bleeding, and the origin of such bleeding may not be determined by endoscopy or an operation.

Physical examination can help estimate the amount of bleeding. As a rough guide, orthostatic hypotension suggests a 15 to 25% blood loss; shock while recumbent represents at least a 30 to 40% loss. Pulse and blood pressure must be monitored whenever continued or recurrent bleeding is suspected. Hepatomegaly suggests portal hypertension or metastatic disease. Rectal and vaginal examinations are essential. Palpable masses along the course of the colon suggest colon cancer; masses in the left hypogastrium suggest gastric cancer.

Blood tests include serial Hct or hemoglobin levels, red blood cell and platelet counts, and smears for red blood cell, white blood cell, and platelet morphologic studies. Microcytosis can indicate chronic bleeding, even if acute bleeding is superimposed. Determinations of prothrombin time and partial thromboplastin time should be promptly performed routinely; these tests are essential if the patient is taking anticoagulants or has jaundice. Electrolytes, blood urea nitrogen, and creatinine should be measured to assess renal function; results aid in determining whether the patient is significantly fluid-depleted. All patients with bright red blood issuing from the mouth or anus must have adequate blood samples with the blood banking laboratory.

Nasogastric lavage is an essential diagnostic procedure for all patients with bright red bleeding from the mouth or anus. If the nasogastric tube returns bloody fluid, then saline lavage should be performed until the effluent is clear and then endoscopy performed. If the tube returns bilious nonbloody fluid, then the source of bleeding is most likely distal to the ligament of Treitz and colonoscopy should be performed first. If nasogastric lavage is nonbloody but no bile returns, then both colonoscopy and esophagogastroduodenoscopy should be performed.

Endoscopy (including esophagogastroduodenoscopy, anoscopy, rigid sigmoidoscopy, flexible sigmoidoscopy, and colonoscopy∎) can be used diagnostically and therapeutically and should be performed as rapidly as the patient's clinical status allows. The route of first approach (upper or lower) is determined from the results of nasogastric tube lavage. Often, a bleeding lesion in the stomach or duodenum can be controlled by a heater probe, bipolar electrocautery, or epinephrine injection. For colonoscopy, brisk bleeding is usually sufficiently cathartic that no other preparation is needed in the acute setting; however, colonoscopy is most accurate when the patient is bleeding slowly enough to allow a preprocedure polyethylene glycol preparation. For the patient with brisk lower GI bleeding in whom colonoscopy reveals no lesion and no blood in the proximal colon, anoscopy is mandatory; often a bleeding hemorrhoid or a rectal ulcer can be controlled with epinephrine injection and sutures. If bleeding continues and adequate

∎ see also page 1006

endoscopic examination has been performed, the following procedures should be considered.

Selective arteriography is important for identifying the bleeding site (especially in patients for whom endoscopy has not localized the bleeding point) provided blood loss is $\geq$ 0.5 to 1.0 mL/minute. This procedure helps localize lesions in the stomach, small bowel, and colon and may be combined with exploratory laparotomy.

Two types of **radionuclide studies** are generally used in adults. The most common requires withdrawing about 10 mL of blood, labeling red blood cells with a technetium radionuclide, and reinjecting them into the patient. The procedure, which takes about an hour, demonstrates the bleeding site if the loss is $\geq$ 0.1 to 0.5 mL/minute, even if bleeding is intermittent. The second study involves injecting the patient with a prepared sulfur colloid radionuclide. If the patient is bleeding, the bleeding site can be identified in a few minutes. Both methods are less useful with upper GI bleeding because of the amount of background scatter. Technetium scans occasionally demonstrate Meckel's diverticulum because of selective uptake by gastric mucosa, which may be present in the lesion; however, Meckel's diverticulum is a rare cause of bleeding in elderly patients.

Barium contrast studies can be sensitive and specific but should be used only when endoscopy, selective arteriography, and radionuclide studies are unavailable. Barium studies cannot determine whether a structural abnormality is bleeding, and the presence of barium in the GI tract can obscure the findings of the more sensitive and specific studies described above.

Laparotomy should be reserved for treating an identified source of bleeding. However, if endoscopy has adequately excluded a gastric, duodenal, esophageal, or colonic lesion or if angiography indicates a lesion in the small bowel, exploratory laparotomy may be appropriate. Examination of the abdominal viscera, especially the small bowel, can identify many lesions (eg, angiomas, leiomyomas, diverticula). Selective arteriography during exploratory laparotomy might help identify bleeding lesions in the small bowel, allowing resection of the involved segment, but this modality is unlikely to be available to most general surgeons.

Prognosis and Treatment

For patients > 60, the mortality rate is close to zero if patients undergo immediate surgery and is about 15% if they are first treated medically but then require surgery for persistent or recurrent bleeding.

Treating an elderly person who has bleeding other than minor rectal bleeding, tarry stools, or hematemesis as an outpatient is dangerous. Bleeding assumed to be from hemorrhoids or other limited rectal bleeding requiring only diagnostic colonoscopy or barium enema may be treated in an outpatient setting, provided time is not lost in making the diagnosis.

A nasogastric tube may clear bleeding by lavage. For upper GI bleeding, if blood does not clear with lavage, a choice must be made between selective arteriography and immediate exploratory laparotomy; patients with massive GI bleeding can experience cardiovascular collapse in the angiographic suite. Consequently, the operating room is the safest place for a briskly bleeding patient. Once the patient is in the operating room, an attempt at therapeutic endoscopy before laparotomy is acceptable if the patient is stable.

Essentially the same therapeutic choices are applicable whether the bleeding site is in the stomach, duodenum, or colon. The choice depends on the patient's age and cardiovascular status and the rate and quantity of blood loss. Options include expectant treatment by medical measures (eg, intubation, lavage), endoscopy using electrocoagulation or heater probe, selective arteriography with local or peripheral vasopressin or octreotide (a long-acting somatostatin analog) infusion or embolization, and surgery.

When the bleeding site has been identified using selective arteriography, the catheter may be used to inject vasopressin directly. This injection immediately controls bleeding in > 80% of cases. Peripheral vasopressin 0.4 U/minute (or octreotide) is also an option, although caution is necessary because cardiac arrhythmias occur. If the vasopressin infusion fails, embolization with an absorbable gelatin sponge or coils may be attempted. However, there is danger of postembolic necrosis arising in the wall of a viscus or of the liver from a dislodged embolus.

At times, bleeding is so massive that emergency surgery is the only reasonable treatment. If a patient is apparently bleeding from the stomach or the colon but the bleeding site cannot be determined and severe blood loss continues, the only option is to perform a blind gastrectomy or colectomy.

BLEEDING IN THE ESOPHAGUS

Esophagitis∎ may cause slow but persistent bleeding. Treatment with H_2 blockers or proton pump inhibitors usually is very helpful because bleeding results from ulceration due to acid reflux. However, cancer must be excluded by endoscopy and biopsy. Severe bleeding requiring surgery rarely occurs in the elderly.

Varices secondary to portal hypertension are uncommon in the elderly. The initial symptom is usually massive upper GI hemorrhage. When varices occur, the primary treatment is immediate endoscopic sclerotherapy or endoscopic variceal ligation. If this treatment is unavailable, a Sengstaken-Blakemore tube is inserted.

∎see page 1112

BLEEDING IN THE STOMACH

Mallory-Weiss tears usually result from repeated vomiting. They can be identified and often cauterized or hemostatically injected through the endoscope. When necessary, surgery involves suturing the lacerations.

Bleeding ulcers are more likely to be gastric ulcers than duodenal ulcers, and controlling bleeding by conservative measures is less certain in gastric than in duodenal ulcers. The usual operation for intractable gastric ulcer bleeding is partial gastrectomy with or without vagotomy. The usual procedure for duodenal ulcer bleeding is ligation of the bleeding vessel and gastric resection or pyloroplasty and vagotomy.

Anastomotic ulcers may occur just distal to the suture line in patients who had previous peptic surgery even after medical measures stop the bleeding; these ulcers occur commonly when vagotomy or posterior gastroenterostomy is performed. Gastric resection and vagotomy are usually indicated.

Gastritis can cause bleeding **1**; if bleeding is not controlled medically, only a radical subtotal gastrectomy with vagotomy or total gastrectomy achieves hemostasis.

Stress ulcers are similar to gastritis but occur after trauma, surgery, burns, or infections. Nasogastric suction, sucralfate, IV H_2 blockers, proton pump inhibitors, or oral antacids to control gastric pH and IV alimentation are the main medical treatments for bleeding from stress ulcers, gastritis, or peptic ulcer disease. Endoscopic electrocoagulation often is successful. Laser coagulation is dangerous because of the risk of perforation. Nasogastric intubation is necessary to keep the stomach empty, to monitor bleeding, and to administer antacids.

Vascular lesions (cirsoid [racemose] aneurysm, or Dieulafoy's ulcer) are localized arteriovenous malformations and communications in the gastric mucosa. More common in the fundus, they may be impossible to see during endoscopy or surgery unless they are bleeding. If they are bleeding, endoscopic therapy is sometimes possible. Surgically, these lesions require simple oversewing or limited excision; occasionally, a high or total gastrectomy is necessary to achieve hemostasis.

Tumors may cause any type of bleeding. **2** Slow, persistent bleeding is more typical of malignant than benign tumors. Benign leiomyomas often lead to massive bleeding that requires emergency laparotomy.

BLEEDING IN THE SMALL INTESTINE

Diverticular disease can lead to massive bleeding. Meckel's diverticulum of the distal ileum may rarely produce an ulcer of the adjacent normal ileal mucosa, leading to bleeding. Varices secondary to por-

1 see page 1041   **2** see page 1136

tal hypertension at times may involve the small intestine and lead to bleeding. Multiple arteriovenous malformations usually are discovered in children but also may develop later in life.

Tumors, although uncommon in the small intestine, may produce bleeding.**1** Massive bleeding usually results from large leiomyomas. Slow, persistent bleeding is more typical of angiomas.

BLEEDING IN THE COLON

Angiodysplasia and diverticular disease cause massive bleeding and occur with equal frequency in the elderly. Angiodysplasia refers to small (1 to 5 mm in diameter) single or multiple lesions found chiefly in the cecum or ascending colon and resembling submucosal arteriovenous malformations on microscopy.**2** The average age at diagnosis for angiodysplasia and bleeding diverticula is 70 years.

The diagnosis of angiodysplasia can be made by colonoscopy in some cases, and the lesions can be destroyed by electrocoagulation. However, if bleeding is profuse, selective arteriography is the best diagnostic modality. The characteristic angiographic finding in angiodysplasia is an early-filling vein in the region of the ileocecal valve.

Carcinoma of the cecum may first present as anemia. Many tumors are diagnosed on the basis of a positive stool occult blood test. With cancer or a polyp, the amount of visible blood in the stool is usually small.**3**

The exact cause of massive bleeding from the colon cannot be determined in about 10% of cases. In these cases, the surgeon performs a subtotal colectomy; the ileorectal anastomosis is placed within reach of the rigid sigmoidoscope, or < 25 cm from the anal verge (anastomosis just above the sacral promontory usually suffices).

BLEEDING IN THE LIVER AND PANCREAS

Trauma is the cause of bleeding from the liver and pancreas in nearly all cases. Diagnosis is made during abdominal CT with IV contrast (when a blush of arterial bleeding is noted), by selective arteriography (in which case therapeutic embolization is an option), or during exploratory laparotomy (in which bleeding vessels are oversewn).

BLEEDING IN AN AORTIC GRAFT

In elderly patients, a relatively sudden onset of massive GI bleeding can occur months or years after an abdominal aortic aneurysm has been

---

1 see page 1139   **2** see page 1057   **3** see page 1142

excised and replaced with a vascular graft. A fistula between the graft and the small intestine is the most likely cause. Although aortoduodenal fistulas predominate, erosion into any section of the small intestine may occur. Endoscopy to the distal duodenum is usually diagnostic. Arteriography also may be helpful.

Treatment is difficult because infection is common and is a strong deterrent to graft replacement. The usual procedure is to remove the graft and establish an extra-anatomic bypass graft, usually between axillary and femoral arteries.

DISORDERS OF THE LOWER ESOPHAGUS

Lower esophageal disorders that may require surgery include esophagitis, perforation, Schatzki's ring, and epiphrenic diverticula. Esophageal cancer is discussed in Ch. 113.

ESOPHAGITIS

Although acid reflux is by far the most common cause of esophagitis, ▮ bile reflux often occurs after total gastrectomy unless bile diversion has been accomplished by a Roux-en-Y anastomosis or enteroenterostomy. Symptoms depend on the amount of reflux. Pain is most common when the patient lies flat but also may occur when the patient is bent over. Conservative therapy, effective in most cases, includes losing weight, elevating the head at night using at least two pillows, restricting food intake after 6 PM, and taking proton pump inhibitors, H_2 blockers, or antacids before bedtime. Many patients require twice the usual dose of H_2 blockers to control reflux symptoms, because acid suppression must be close to 100%, which can only be achieved using higher doses. However, elderly patients are at greater risk of adverse effects from these drugs, especially when high doses are used or if they have some degree of renal impairment. Intractable esophagitis requires surgery. Laparoscopic Nissen fundoplication is an option for the patient who can tolerate a pneumoperitoneum.

PERFORATION

Iatrogenic injury: Perforation by an endoscope may occur. Perforation is rare with flexible scopes but not with rigid scopes. The perforation is almost always above the diaphragm rather than below it. Overinflation of Sengstaken-Blakemore tubes, balloon dilation for achalasia, and surgery of the upper stomach or esophagus (eg, vagotomy or hiatus hernia repair) may also cause perforation.

▮see page 1039

Pain and fever are the important clinical findings; if they develop after an esophageal procedure, perforation is the probable cause. A chest x-ray probably shows mediastinal emphysema, and, later, extensive subcutaneous emphysema involving the chest, neck, abdomen, and scrotum may occur. *Perforation is an emergency.* A diatrizoate meglumine swallow should be performed immediately; it will nearly always show the perforation. The perforation must be surgically closed immediately and the closure reinforced by the stomach (perforation at the gastroesophageal junction can be repaired by gastric fundoplication), a flap of parietal pleura, or a muscle flap from the chest wall.

Emetic injury: Vomiting when the stomach is full can rupture the distal esophagus, leading to rapid contamination of the left pleural cavity (Boerhaave's syndrome) or peritonitis. Subcutaneous emphysema or complaints of severe pain in the left upper quadrant, chest, or shoulder after vomiting mandate the same emergency diagnostic and therapeutic measures as are required for iatrogenic perforation.

SCHATZKI'S RING

A ring of mucosa and submucosa that causes narrowing at the esophagogastric junction.

Schatzki's rings generally form before old age. However, they tighten with age, occluding passage when the lumen becomes as small as 15 mm. Intermittent dysphagia may occur. When a Schatzki's ring is asymptomatic, dilation with bougies is usually successful. If surgery is necessary, the ring can be broken with a finger inserted into the esophagus, and any associated hernia can be repaired.

EPIPHRENIC DIVERTICULA

These diverticula develop just above the diaphragm and are associated with hyperactivity of the lower esophageal sphincter and often with a sliding hiatus hernia.■ Some may become ≥ 5 cm in diameter. They can retain food and become infected, and cancer may develop in the mucosa. If pain or regurgitation occurs, excision is necessary; if the diverticula are asymptomatic, they probably should be followed up endoscopically. Accompanying distal esophageal spasm is treated with pneumatic dilation.

INTESTINAL OBSTRUCTION

A blockage of the intestinal tract, preventing the passage of intestinal contents.

■ see page 1119

An obstruction may be acute or chronic, mechanical or adynamic, simple or strangulated; it may occur in the small or large intestine. Certain features are common to all types, but the choice of therapy depends on a specific diagnosis.

Adhesions and hernias are the most common lesions of the small intestine causing acute intestinal obstruction; cancer predominates in the colon. Adynamic ileus occurs when the absence of reflex nerve stimulation precludes peristalsis in an otherwise normal bowel. In a simple obstruction, the blood supply to the intestine is not compromised; in a strangulated obstruction, the vessels to a segment are occluded, usually by adhesions or bands.

Symptoms and Signs

Symptoms and signs are highly variable and depend chiefly on the site and cause of the obstruction and the time since onset.

A patient with an acute obstruction characteristically presents with a rapid onset of abdominal cramps, vomiting, distention, and obstipation. Cramps tend to recur about every 3 minutes and are associated with high-pitched bowel sounds caused by peristalsis (borborygmi). Although wide individual variation may exist, crampy pain usually occurs in the epigastrium and periumbilically with small-bowel obstruction and in the lower abdomen with colonic obstruction; cramps may not occur with high jejunal obstruction. Abdominal distention usually occurs and increases. In a simple obstruction, the abdomen is not tender; abdominal tenderness and continuous pain indicate strangulation. Because a simple obstruction can lead to strangulation in as little as 6 hours, every patient with a suspected intestinal obstruction should be hospitalized immediately.

With a small-bowel obstruction, vomiting usually occurs early; it may progress to fecal emesis (a misnomer, given that the etiology is bacterial overgrowth secondary to luminal stasis), which can be distinguished from coffee-ground vomit (caused by upper GI hemorrhage) with a guaiac test. With a large-bowel obstruction, vomiting occurs much later or not at all and is usually preceded by distention and cramps. Initially, scanty diarrhea may occur; complete obstruction is followed by obstipation.

Diagnosis

The abdomen should be inspected for scars from previous abdominal operations and for groin or incisional hernias. The abdomen is auscultated for several minutes to detect bowel sounds and palpated for tenderness or masses. A rectal examination and, in women, a vaginal examination should be performed.

A complete blood cell count, blood chemistry tests, and urinalysis should be performed. An indwelling bladder catheter and central venous pressure line are usually advisable. If the patient has a history of myocardial dysfunction, a pulmonary arterial catheter may be necessary to guide resuscitation.

X-rays are extremely important but should be performed only after a nasogastric tube has been inserted. Plain abdominal films should be taken in the supine and upright positions. Lateral decubitus films sometimes are helpful, particularly in cases of external hernias.

With a typical small-bowel obstruction, a ladderlike pattern of distended intestinal loops appears. With strangulation, however, a mass rather than distended loops may be visible. Distended loops may also be absent in a high jejunal obstruction, particularly if the patient has had a gastric resection.

Obstruction of the ascending colon may resemble a small-bowel obstruction when reflux occurs through an incompetent ileocecal valve. Obstruction of the descending colon leads to distention of the entire proximal large bowel because of gas. A single large gas-filled loop of colon in the midabdomen or left upper quadrant usually results from a cecal volvulus, and a single loop of distended sigmoid usually results from a sigmoid volvulus.∎ If gas appears in the intrahepatic bile ducts, a gallstone obstruction is likely (secondary to cholecystenteric or choledochoenteric fistula).

Colonoscopy or a barium enema is used when the site of an obstruction is unclear. Oral barium may be administered to confirm and better localize small-bowel obstruction but should not be used with a colonic obstruction.

Differential diagnosis of intestinal obstruction includes acute appendicitis,∎ acute cholecystitis,∎ diverticulitis,∎ and pancreatitis.∎ Also, thoracic disease (eg, pneumonia) may cause adynamic ileus.

Treatment

Acute mechanical obstruction requires surgery. Nasogastric intubation and preoperative antibiotics should be started early.

Certain types of intestinal obstruction, including adynamic ileus, early postoperative obstruction, and recurrent obstruction caused by adhesions from previous intra-abdominal surgery, can be treated by GI intubation and IV alimentation. Some surgeons believe that simple obstruction can be treated by intubation, but others believe that surgery is the treatment of choice.

In cases of small-bowel obstruction without evidence of strangulation (ie, audible peristalsis and no abdominal tenderness) but with marked dehydration, several hours may be needed to rehydrate the patient and

---

∎ see page 1124   ∎ see page 1123   ∎ see page 1125
∎ see page 1054   ∎ see page 1131

establish adequate urinary output. A severely dehydrated patient who has advanced strangulation and is in shock may require immediate surgery, thus appropriate and aggressive resuscitation is critical.

ADYNAMIC ILEUS

Adynamic ileus should be suspected in patients with symptoms of obstruction and a history of recent surgery, back injury, severe trauma, or thoracic or renal disease. Peristalsis (and thus bowel sounds) is absent or infrequent, and abdominal x-rays show gas in scattered areas of the small intestine and colon. Treatment consists of nasogastric suction and IV alimentation. Administration of metoclopramide or cisapride usually is not beneficial.

In pseudo-obstruction of the colon, or Ogilvie's syndrome, the colon distends as if obstructed, although there is no mechanical obstruction and a colonoscope can be passed easily. The cause of Ogilvie's syndrome is unknown, although it occurs most often in elderly, debilitated patients with restricted mobility (eg, in an obese elderly patient after a hip replacement). A supine x-ray of the abdomen often shows a dilated proximal colon, but the distention can also involve the splenic flexure and left colon. Colonoscopy, a barium enema, or surgery reveals no obstructing lesion. Usually, advanced colonic ileus can be treated effectively by colonoscopy, which may need to be repeated.

MECHANICAL OBSTRUCTION

Mechanical obstruction may be caused by an impacted gallstone in the terminal ileum; the stone may not appear on x-ray or may appear considerably smaller than it actually is. However, gas in the intrahepatic biliary tree is diagnostic.

Mechanical obstruction may also occur when a patient with false teeth and a partial gastrectomy swallows masses of indigestible fiber. The mass forms an obstructing bezoar in the small intestine. **1** Bezoars also can cause obstruction in patients treated in the intensive care unit with large doses of antacid to prevent bleeding stress ulcers.

Richter's hernia is a nonpalpable, small hernia involving strangulation of only part of the intestinal wall in a small hernial sac.

Fecal impaction **2** is common and rarely produces complete obstruction. More commonly, repeated attempts to evacuate produce small diarrheal stools. If the condition is detected early by rectal examination, the impaction can be removed digitally or with warm mineral oil retention enemas. If the condition is advanced, the patient may require sedation to facilitate complete fecal removal. Fecal impaction high in the

---

1 see also page 1050   **2** see also page 1082

rectum or in the sigmoid can lead to obstruction, perforation, and fecal peritonitis.

Apparent intestinal obstruction accompanied by shock, marked leukocytosis, and variable abdominal tenderness can be caused by mesenteric artery occlusion from thrombosis or embolism. This condition is not a true mechanical obstruction but an ileus caused by aperistalsis. If surgery is performed before infarction of all or most of the small bowel, embolectomy or thrombectomy should be attempted (in a few cases, this may result in survival).

ISCHEMIC SYNDROMES

Ischemic syndromes occur more often in the colon than in the stomach or small intestine, because collateral circulation is not as well developed in the colon.

Colonic ischemia may result in gangrene of the colon—a fulminating, undiagnosable abdominal catastrophe—or a milder version called ischemic colitis—a nongangrenous, spontaneously resolving process that can result in a fibrous colonic stricture. In the stomach and small intestine, acute mesenteric ischemia from arterial occlusion results from a thrombosis or an embolus in the celiac axis or superior mesenteric artery and causes midgut necrosis. If not immediately diagnosed, midgut necrosis almost always causes death. Even with intervention, > 90% of patients die. Less commonly, chronic arterial occlusive disease and acute venous thrombosis can lead to ischemic syndromes. Pain out of proportion to the examination is a hallmark sign of intestinal ischemia; recognizing this pain is key to early diagnosis.

COLONIC ISCHEMIA

Colonic ischemia is common in persons in their 60s and 70s. It is often associated with cardiovascular disorders, including heart failure, myocardial infarction, and pulmonary embolism, and with severe hemorrhage and the postoperative state. Gangrene of the colon commonly occurs in elderly patients in intensive care units with heart failure and sepsis.

The gangrenous form more likely involves the entire colon, with the splenic flexure being most severely affected; in contrast, the milder ischemic (nongangrenous) form more likely involves only a segment of the colon.

Symptoms of a gangrenous colon are generalized abdominal pain (particularly in the left iliac fossa and left hypochondrium), nausea, vomiting, diarrhea, and occasionally frank rectal bleeding. The physical findings suggest an abdominal catastrophe with generalized peritonitis in a patient who is extremely ill. These findings include generalized abdominal tenderness, aperistalsis, and hypotension with cardiovascular collapse. The diagnosis is often confused with perforation of a hollow viscus, fulminant pancreatitis, or mesenteric ischemia. At surgery, the colon is edematous and discolored, with the worst changes at the splenic flexure. A subtotal colectomy is required.

Nongangrenous colitis produces milder symptoms and signs, and an exploratory laparotomy usually is not performed. Acute pain usually occurs in the left iliac fossa; fever and a moderate amount of dark rectal bleeding often occur. On examination, localized left-sided peritonitis suggestive of diverticulitis is found. However, these two conditions can be distinguished based on the degree and quality of the rectal bleeding. The rectal bleeding associated with ischemic colitis usually is bright red, whereas the rectal bleeding associated with diverticulitis is usually occult. Massive rectal bleeding usually occurs in patients with diverticulosis without clinical evidence of diverticulitis. If colonoscopy is performed on a patient with ischemic colitis, the mucosa appears bluish and edematous with mucosal ulcerations and contact bleeding. A barium enema may show thumbprinting, a series of blunt semiopaque projections into the lumen, representing edematous haustra. Treatment is with resuscitation and bowel rest until symptoms abate (usually a few days).

ACUTE MESENTERIC ISCHEMIA

This syndrome is characterized by a sudden onset of severe abdominal colic followed by rectal passage of mucus and blood and circulatory collapse within a few hours. One hallmark is that the severe pain at onset is well out of proportion to the physical findings. However, peritonitis follows promptly with dramatic physical findings and leads to circulatory shock. With the onset of peritonitis, the initial colic is replaced by generalized abdominal pain, ileus, and distention.

None of the simple diagnostic tools specifically identifies acute mesenteric ischemia. The plain abdominal x-ray shows a pattern of ileus with gas-filled loops of edematous small intestine. By the time the diagnostic finding of air in the mesenteric veins appears, irreversible changes have already taken place. Laboratory findings, except for nonspecific leukocytosis, are not helpful in making an early diagnosis. Laparotomy is necessary to make a diagnosis; laparoscopy is *not* recommended.

Without treatment, this abdominal catastrophe commonly leads to death within 48 hours. The key to a successful outcome is very early operative intervention before peritonitis and irreversible shock become established. Unfortunately, in most cases, the presentation is not characteristic, and the diagnosis is made very late.

The only definitive treatment is early surgery that reestablishes blood flow by removing the embolus or bypassing the thrombosis in the visceral vessel. The nonviable intestine is resected. A "second-look" laparotomy should be performed in 24 hours to reevaluate the viability of the remaining intestine. After extensive small-intestine resections, parenteral nutrition is necessary, especially in the elderly. Perioperative management is especially difficult and requires close attention to fluid balance, antibiotic therapy, anticoagulation, and, often, control of metabolic acidosis.

OTHER ISCHEMIC SYNDROMES

Chronic arterial obstruction of the celiac axis or superior mesenteric artery can result in profound weight loss and pain, suggesting abdominal angina. The pain, which is midabdominal or epigastric, often is worse postprandially. These features make this condition indistinguishable from many other more common abdominal conditions (eg, peptic ulcer disease). An arteriogram is diagnostic. Treatment is with aspirin (or another antiplatelet agent). Surgery with vascular reconstruction is used in patients whose disease is segmental rather than diffuse. Endoluminal stents placed by invasive vascular radiologists may also be used.

Acute mesenteric venous thrombosis usually results in death because it is not recognized until the majority of the bowel is infarcted. This disorder should be included in the differential diagnosis of an elderly patient with abdominal distention and pain disproportionate to the examination findings. CT with IV contrast often reveals superior mesenteric vein thrombus. Angiography should follow, with both catheter-based lytic therapy of the superior mesenteric vein and a lytic agent selectively introduced into the superior mesenteric artery. After thrombolysis, the patient must be maintained on an anticoagulant, and a hypercoagulation assessment must be performed. Occasionally, when the diagnosis is made late, a near-total resection of the small intestine allows survival, but it is a particularly devastating procedure in the elderly.

DIAPHRAGMATIC HERNIA

The sliding hiatus hernia is the most common type of diaphragmatic hernia. A portion of the stomach just below the esophagogastric junction and the abdominal esophagus rises into the chest. In paraesophageal hernia, the esophagogastric junction remains in place, but the stomach rises alongside the esophagus. Combinations of sliding and paraesophageal hernias occur.

SLIDING HIATUS HERNIA

A small hiatus hernia can be detected in most elderly persons. Such hernias are almost always asymptomatic, unless the patient has reflux esophagitis. However, mild flatulence or substernal discomfort may occur, and if a Schatzki's ring∎ tightens to a diameter < 11 mm, esophageal obstruction can develop. The diagnosis is based on barium contrast studies, endoscopy, and 24-hour esophageal pH monitoring. The differential diagnosis includes coronary artery disease, esophageal spasm, gallbladder disease, gastritis, peptic ulcer, and functional complaints for which no organic cause can be found. Symptoms that appear suddenly suggest malignant disease, not only of the esophagus but of any abdominal organ. Consequently, an abdominal rather than a thoracic approach is used for repair because an unexpected tumor may be found.

Asymptomatic hernias should not be repaired. Mild complaints are treated by conservative measures, including a bland diet, weight reduction, antacids, and nighttime elevation of the head and chest using several pillows or blocks under the bed supports.

Controversy continues concerning the best surgical procedure for hiatus hernia complicated by esophagitis. Each procedure restores a proper length of abdominal esophagus and strengthens the lower esophageal sphincter. In the Nissen repair, the fundus of the stomach is wrapped around the lower esophagus. In the Belsey repair, a valve is created by suturing the stomach to the anterior surface of the esophagus. In the Hill repair, the part of the stomach at the gastroesophageal junction is anchored to the median arcuate ligament, which lies just anterior to the aorta; a valve is created by anterior sutures through the junction, drawing it back toward the ligament. Laparoscopic Nissen fundoplication has gained wide acceptance during the past few years and is a good option for the patient who has not had previous upper abdominal surgery.

Regardless of the procedure, postoperative recurrences after several years are common, perhaps because of the negative intrathoracic pressure that occurs with every inspiration. Nevertheless, surgery offers great relief for long periods in selected patients. In a few cases, esophagitis is so marked that resection and replacement with a section of jejunum or colon is necessary. In some elderly patients, recurrent strictures at the gastroesophageal junction can be treated by periodic dilation with bougies.

PARAESOPHAGEAL HERNIA

Paraesophageal hernias can be huge, with the entire stomach in the chest. Both the esophagogastric junction and the pylorus may be level with the diaphragm as the gastric fundus rotates upward into the left or right side of the chest. A large gas bubble can be seen on chest x-ray, and the diagnosis is confirmed by barium contrast studies.

∎ see page 1113

Paraesophageal hernias can cause complete pyloric obstruction and gastric incarceration, strangulation, and perforation. Unless the patient is a poor surgical risk, these hernias should be repaired.

HERNIA DUE TO DIAPHRAGMATIC RUPTURE

After an injury to the left side of the chest or the left upper abdominal quadrant, a chest x-ray may show a gas bubble above the diaphragm on the left side, suggesting a diaphragmatic rupture. Barium contrast studies, MRI, or laparoscopy should be performed. If a traumatized patient goes to the operating room for other injuries and a diaphragmatic injury is suspected, laparoscopy is the diagnostic modality of choice. The stomach is the usual organ found to be in the chest, but the colon, spleen, and even other viscera are identified in some cases. Immediate repair is necessary.

INGUINAL HERNIA

Optimal treatment of hernias can be controversial. Obviously, all patients with strangulated inguinal hernias need immediate surgery. Femoral hernias also are prone to strangulation and should be repaired electively, if possible. Many small, direct inguinal hernias and painless, indirect inguinal hernias with relatively large openings do not represent immediate threats. However, the *only* hernias that are safe to simply observe are small, direct, nonpainful hernias that reduce spontaneously when the patient is recumbent. Otherwise, hernias should be repaired, unless surgery is contraindicated.

Often, the operation can be performed using local anesthesia with or without light sedation. Preoperatively, the patient should be led to expect that postoperative pain will be mild to moderate. Postoperative opiate use should be judicious, because the elderly are more sensitive to the disorienting effects of opiate agonists. With current tension-free repair techniques and appropriate analgesia, the elderly patient should expect to return to the activities of daily living within 24 hours after inguinal surgery; however, the patient's functional status, living arrangement, and home support system must be assessed before surgery to ensure postdischarge safety.

DISORDERS OF THE JEJUNUM AND ILEUM

Disorders of the jejunum and ileum may exist alone or with disorders of other viscera (such as gastroenteritis or Crohn's disease). Many of these disorders are treated medically, but some are also treated surgically and must be considered in the differential diagnosis of the surgical abdomen.

Disorders of the jejunum and ileum may be caused by acquired or iatrogenic factors; inflammatory or toxic agents; malabsorption **1**; motility disorders; or tumors. Meckel's diverticulum, the only congenital lesion common in elderly patients, is nearly always an incidental finding, and symptoms are rare in the elderly.

ACQUIRED LESIONS

The most common acquired lesion is diverticulosis, in which sac-like projections of the mucosa protrude through the muscularis of the bowel. **2** These projections are most common in the jejunum of elderly patients. Diverticulosis may be asymptomatic or may be associated with massive bleeding, malabsorption, or inflammation (diverticulitis). In cases of massive bleeding, locating the involved bowel segment is desirable. Selective arteriography, which may be combined with exploratory laparotomy, is the best diagnostic tool. It allows resection of the shortest possible segment of bowel. Perforation is uncommon, but if it occurs, resection and reanastomosis are the procedures of choice.

IATROGENIC LESIONS

The most common iatrogenic lesions are excessive enterectomy, **3** radiation enterocolitis, and blind loop syndrome.

Radiation enterocolitis: The small intestine is damaged by 50 Gy; the colon is slightly more resistant. The symptoms of radiation enterocolitis are indistinguishable from those of chronic intestinal obstruction. Radiation enterocolitis produces bleeding and diarrhea. Conservative therapy usually is indicated at the outset, because some acute symptoms may subside with IV alimentation and restriction of oral intake.

Minor colonic ulceration may be treated with a bland diet and psyllium hydrophilic mucilloid. Surgery to resect bowel is often unsuccessful, because radiation diminishes the intestinal blood supply so that anastomoses tend to heal poorly. Furthermore, because dense pelvic adhesions are likely, dissection is arduous; leakage and fistula formation are occasional sequelae. Thus, resection may be difficult or impossible, and palliative enteroenterostomy may be required. However, in severe cases, resection of the involved segment with reanastomosis may be possible; in other cases, a permanent colostomy may have to be combined with resection of the involved rectum or colon.

Blind loop syndrome: This syndrome develops when a surgeon inadvertently creates a bowel loop in which intestinal contents collect and stagnate. Poor drainage leads to secondary infection and occasionally to deficiency syndromes. It typically occurs with a side-to-side anastomosis but may occur after a gastrectomy in which the terminal ileum rather than the jejunum is erroneously anastomosed to the stom-

---

1see page 1096   **2**see also page 1054   **3**see page 1096

ach. Long afferent loops after a gastric resection and gastrojejunostomy may lead to major dilation of the afferent loop (afferent loop syndrome). In some cases, side-to-side small-intestine anastomosis is followed by marked dilation of the blind ends of the two segments. Typical symptoms include indigestion, gas, cramps, and diarrhea. Antibiotic therapy is not useful. Surgical reconstruction may be needed.

INFECTIVE LESIONS

Diseases that mimic surgical emergencies are common. Acute gastroenteritis with its typical acute onset, nausea, vomiting, and diarrhea can mimic a surgical abdomen. Unusual infections can also mimic a surgical abdomen. These include giardiasis, *Yersinia* infections, and acute amebiasis. Probably the most common and dangerous of all infections is salmonellosis. Patients treated with antibiotics and those receiving immunosuppressants are at particular risk of developing salmonellosis.

Organisms that produce toxins (eg, staphylococci, *Vibrio cholerae*, *Campylobacter* sp, *Clostridium perfringens*) can cause severe enteritis or colitis. One of the most common diseases that can cause a surgeon to be consulted is pseudomembranous enterocolitis from *Clostridium difficile*.

APPENDICITIS

Characteristically, the initial symptom of appendicitis is periumbilical pain, followed by nausea and then by localized pain and tenderness in the right lower quadrant. Low-grade fever and leukocytosis also occur typically. However, in elderly patients, pain more often begins in the right lower quadrant and may not be severe until perforation occurs. Because the blood supply to the appendix is generally decreased in elderly patients, the course of the disease can be fulminant. In some cases, symptoms and signs may be minimal, leading to chronic infection with marked low-grade fever and poorly defined localization of abdominal signs.

In the elderly, appendicitis occasionally occurs in association with colon cancer. Low-grade obstruction can lead to appendiceal distention that mimics true appendicitis.

The treatment is appendectomy. Antibiotics should be given before surgery and continued for at least 48 hours afterward. If perforation has already occurred and peritonitis is spreading, the value of drainage is controversial. Simple drainage is recommended for a localized abscess, and appendectomy should follow in a few weeks. In nearly all other cases, however, the appendix is removed during the initial operation.

If the patient who has had a simple appendectomy fails to recover promptly, the colon should be examined by endoscopy or barium enema.

DISORDERS OF THE COLORECTUM

The most common colorectal disorders requiring surgery in the elderly are cancer, volvulus, diverticular disease, and vascular ectasias. Cancer is discussed in Ch. 113, and diverticular disease and vascular ectasias in Ch. 107. Ulcerative colitis is an uncommon but serious problem and is discussed in Ch. 107.

VOLVULUS

Volvulus arises from a twist of the colon on its mesentery sufficient to produce intestinal obstruction.◾ An unusually long, mobile mesentery in the affected segment or a lack of fixation is needed for the twist to occur. Unless the obstruction is relieved, it progresses proximally and distally because of gas formation within the occluded segment. As a result, the mesenteric vasculature supplying the involved segment is also occluded, and gangrene and perforation can follow.

Volvulus is common in the elderly and is most prevalent in inactive women who have restricted mental capabilities and who live in nursing homes. The combination of an unusually large, long colon and inadequate bowel hygiene is a contributing factor.

Sigmoid volvulus: Volvulus occurs most commonly in the sigmoid. Obstipation, cramps, and marked abdominal distention are the usual complaints. Abdominal x-ray shows a large, distended colon. Distention may be limited to the sigmoid loop but occasionally extends above the liver. A barium enema shows the typical bird-beak deformity at the level of the twist.

Usually, a long rectal tube can be passed through a sigmoidoscope (or colonoscope) beyond the obstruction; this can produce explosive deflation. If deflation is incomplete or gangrene is noted, immediate laparotomy is necessary. The colonoscope is useful in determining if gangrene is present. If deflation occurs, resection of the involved colonic segment is performed electively during the same hospitalization, unless overriding reasons to defer surgery exist. If surgery is not performed, the probability of recurrence is very high.

Cecal volvulus: The cecum is another likely site for volvulus. It produces abdominal cramps, nausea, vomiting, distention, and obstipation. Abdominal x-ray shows a large gas bubble in the midabdomen or the left upper quadrant. Barium enema shows the typical bird-beak deformity in the ascending colon and no reflux into the ileum. *Gangrene supervenes rapidly, so immediate surgery is essential.* If no evidence of gangrene exists, the cecum can be anchored by a cecostomy tube after the twist has been reduced. The alternative for low-risk patients is immediate resection and reanastomosis. When gangrene and

◾see page 1113

perforation with fecal contamination occur in a high-risk patient, resection and the formation of ileal and colonic fistulas are necessary. Intestinal continuity is reestablished later. If fecal contamination is slight or the cecum remains intact, a cecectomy with the ileum anastomosed to the ascending colon or a right colectomy is performed.

DISORDERS OF THE GALLBLADDER AND BILIARY TREE

Disorders of the gallbladder and biliary tree account for about one third of abdominal operations performed in patients > 70. Gallstones (cholelithiasis), cholecystitis, acute cholangitis, and gallbladder cancer are the most important disorders. Cancer of the gallbladder and biliary tree is discussed in Ch. 113.

GALLSTONES

An estimated 25% of persons > 50 develop gallstones. The incidence rises with age; gallstones are found at autopsy in about one third of persons > 70. Gallstones are the indication for nearly all of the > 500,000 cholecystectomies performed annually in the USA (1 in every 500 persons).

The primary symptom of gallstones is biliary colic. Colic, or steady pain, usually is felt in the right subcostal area but often radiates to the right scapula or the right shoulder and, in some cases, is similar to angina. At times, the pain may be felt anywhere in the abdomen. Vomiting may occur but is not repetitive. Usually, slight tenderness occurs in the right upper quadrant. Epigastric distention, gas, and vague dyspepsia occur in so many people that these findings cannot be considered specific for gallbladder disease.

Acute cholecystitis, a complication of gallstones, is characterized by increased local tenderness, fever, and leukocytosis. The gallbladder often is palpable. Migration of a stone into the common duct can lead to jaundice, chills and fever, and gallstone pancreatitis. Pancreatitis is accompanied by more diffuse epigastric tenderness and elevated serum amylase levels.

Ultrasound shows gallstones in > 95% of cases and distended intrahepatic ducts when a patient has a common duct obstruction. However, ultrasound does not visualize the distal common duct adequately, and CT is better for diagnosing pancreatic lesions. Transhepatic cholangiography and endoscopic retrograde cholangiopancreatography are valuable when common duct involvement is suspected.

Treatment

The patient may decide to live with the gallstones. If not, the first surgical choice is cholecystectomy. Laparoscopic cholecystectomy is widely used, although damage to the common duct is more common with this procedure than with open cholecystectomy. Other methods (eg, stone dissolution by chenodeoxycholic acid) are successful in some cases but require continued medication. The recurrence rate for lithotripsy is so high that the procedure has been abandoned. Cholecystectomy combined with common duct exploration (open or laparoscopic) is the preferred operation for common duct stones. Endoscopic papillotomy and basket removal of an obstructing stone from the common duct may be advisable if the patient is very ill or the gallbladder already has been removed.

With acute cholecystitis, antibiotics are given for a longer period but surgery should be performed within 2 or 3 days of the onset. With diabetic patients, glucose levels should be controlled, and surgery should be performed as soon as possible because the danger of perforation is high. In some cases, the pathologic changes at the base of the gallbladder are so great that the surgeon should perform a cholecystostomy, leaving the elective cholecystectomy for later. Another option when the cystic duct is very inflamed and there is no evidence of common bile duct obstruction is to remove the gallbladder and simply drain the gallbladder fossa.

Although asymptomatic gallstones are common in patients > 70, the mortality rate for elective cholecystectomy is estimated at 5%. Therefore, surgery for asymptomatic gallstones in patients > 70 is not advised, and the standard of care in the USA remains surgery only for patients with symptomatic gallstones. Despite previous teachings, even diabetics should not undergo surgery for asymptomatic gallstones.

If an initial attack of biliary colic occurs, a second attack is probable within 2 years in two thirds of patients. The argument for cholecystectomy, therefore, becomes more compelling, and such patients are usually advised to undergo cholecystectomy. However, the diagnosis should be confirmed and symptoms of other diseases (eg, coronary insufficiency) ruled out, especially in elderly patients. In equivocal cases, waiting for at least one more attack before recommending surgery is advisable. Usually, patients have several attacks before surgery is advised.

ACUTE CHOLANGITIS

Acute cholangitis usually results from a stone impacted in the ampulla of Vater, but the syndrome may occur secondary to pancreatic cancer. Other causes (eg, ascending infection after sphincterotomy of Oddi's sphincter, infection secondary to stricture from a previous choledochoduodenostomy or choledochojejunostomy) are rare. In the Far East, Oriental cholangitis results from ascending infection from the intestinal tract by parasites. Patients may develop symptoms of infection as in septic shock. Right upper quadrant pain and tenderness may be present.

Patients in septic shock on admission must be treated vigorously with antibiotics before surgery. Gentamicin 1 to 1.5 mg/kg IV q 8 h (corrected for renal function and blood levels), ampicillin 1 to 2 g IV q 6 h, and clindamycin 600 mg IV q 8 h are recommended (other antibiotic combinations with a similar spectrum and bioavailability are acceptable). Fluid balance must be restored. Emergency operations performed before the patient is stabilized are associated with a high mortality.

Endoscopic sphincterotomy has been valuable in treating Oriental cholangitis and is used widely in the USA and Europe for stones impacted in the distal common duct. Skill in endoscopy is essential because of the hazards of perforation, bleeding, and infection.

MISCELLANEOUS DISORDERS

Gallstone pancreatitis: Patients with gallstone pancreatitis present with symptoms and signs similar to those of acute cholecystitis, except that the pain is more likely to be epigastric and is associated with elevated serum amylase levels and often with increased bilirubin and alkaline phosphatase levels. Initial treatment is conservative, with the patient taking nothing orally and receiving IV alimentation. Typically, pain subsides rapidly, and laparoscopic or open cholecystectomy is performed 5 to 7 days after admission.

Acalculous cholecystitis: This condition is caused by inflammation of the gallbladder resulting from a combination of biliary stasis, bacterial overgrowth, and ischemia in critically ill patients. It tends to occur in patients in intensive care units and in those whose oral intake is poor (eg, because of total IV alimentation). Symptoms are minimal. Unexplained fever and vague abdominal distress warrant ultrasound examination of the gallbladder, which may show edema of the gallbladder wall and increasing distention on successive examinations. Cholecystectomy or cholecystostomy is the usual procedure. Percutaneous cholecystostomy under ultrasound guidance performed by interventional radiologists has become common over the past 10 years.

Retained stones in the common duct: These stones are common, particularly if multiple hepatic duct stones were found during the initial exploration. The surgeon prepares for this possibility in questionable cases by placing a large T tube (No. 14 French) to drain the common duct. The radiologist can extract the stones later. Endoscopic removal also is feasible.

Fistulas: Fistulas can form between the gallbladder and the intestine, allowing gallstones to migrate and cause intestinal obstruction. Patients usually present with signs of distal small-bowel obstruction, often with tenderness over the gallbladder. Abdominal x-ray may show the stone and usually shows gas in the biliary tree. The proper surgical procedure is removal of the stones (if a stone is faceted, then others are present) and cholecystectomy. Cholecystectomy may be deferred if the patient is very ill; it should also be deferred if the gallbladder and porta hepatis are encompassed in a dense phlegmon.

Iatrogenic stricture of the common duct: A major complication of cholecystectomy is damage to the common bile duct. Usually, the problem is manifested very early by protracted biliary drainage; diagnosis is made by fistulogram. Surgical repair is a Roux-en-Y anastomosis of the upper duct to the jejunum. However, a stricture may form at the anastomosis and cause symptoms many years later. Intermittent attacks of pain, fever, and jaundice suggest the diagnosis, which can be confirmed by transhepatic cholangiography. Surgical repair is necessary. For the patient with comorbidities that preclude surgery, a permanent stent can be deployed transhepatically.

Gallbladder polyps: Usually small and filiform, gallbladder polyps have little malignant potential. Many defects shown on ultrasound simulate polyps but actually are small stones. Although of minimal concern when small, a polyp that appears > 1 cm in diameter on repeat ultrasound should prompt cholecystectomy to rule out a malignancy.

Jaundice: The differential diagnosis of jaundice is extensive, and many diagnostic methods are available. The first task is to determine whether jaundice is obstructive. Often, the history is helpful, and the physical examination can give important information. Gastrointestinal causes include cirrhosis, cancer, gallstones, and hepatitis.

Ultrasound determines the presence of gallstones and the size of the intrahepatic and common bile ducts. If necessary, endoscopy follows, providing direct visualization of the lumen of the stomach and duodenum. Endoscopic retrograde cholangiopancreatography (ERCP) ◨ usually can be performed safely, and if required, transhepatic cholangiography can follow. Fine-needle percutaneous biopsy is positive in nearly 80% of patients with pancreatic cancer, although cancer cannot be ruled out by a negative biopsy.

The value of radioisotope scans using dyes (eg, hepato-iminodiacetic acid) that are excreted with the bile is controversial. If the patient has low-grade jaundice and the dye passes through the common duct into the duodenum, obstructive jaundice is unlikely. Some authorities believe that such scans do not reliably detect acute cholecystitis, although others believe that an inability to visualize the gallbladder after giving the dye is a presumptive sign of a blocked cystic duct and, when associated with local tenderness, a presumptive sign of acute cholecystitis. In many cases, establishing a diagnosis is impossible without exploratory laparotomy.

◨ see page 1011

DISORDERS OF THE LIVER

In the elderly, the most common hepatic lesion requiring surgery is metastatic cancer. (Cirrhosis and its complications are more common in younger persons; primary biliary cirrhosis is discussed in Ch. 108.) Because hepatic surgery is not well tolerated in the elderly, heroic measures that might enable long-term survival but that carry a high mortality rate, such as liver transplantation, are not attempted often. Liver tumors are discussed in Ch. 113.

HEPATIC CYSTS

Hepatic cysts may be congenital or acquired. Often, multiple congenital cysts are associated with polycystic disease of the kidney and pancreas. Usually, they are insignificant, and if found during surgery, they can merely be unroofed and left in place. Rarely, a cyst enlarges during periodic follow-up because it is a cystadenocarcinoma; excision is necessary. ▪

Hydatid cysts, the single most important acquired type, are caused by the tapeworm *Echinococcus granulosus* and are common in many parts of the world. Because these cysts develop slowly, symptoms (eg, epigastric pain, liver enlargement, jaundice, anaphylactic reactions) may not be noted for many years. These cysts may be huge and multilocular and are diagnosed by CT or ultrasound. Aspiration should be avoided. Treatment is excision of the entire cyst; care must be taken to avoid spilling daughter cysts or scoleces into the abdomen, and the patient must be treated perioperatively with albendazole. Medical therapy alone and medical therapy plus percutaneous drainage have been studied; in patients who can tolerate laparotomy, surgical excision is the best treatment.

HEPATIC ABSCESSES

Pyogenic abscesses and amebic abscesses of the liver must be differentiated because the treatment differs: pyogenic abscesses must be drained, whereas 75% of amebic abscesses can be treated by medical therapy alone.

Almost 40% of pyogenic hepatic abscesses result from biliary tract obstruction; in another 40% the exact etiology is not discernible. Because of the widespread use of antibiotics, pylephlebitis and secondary abscesses from appendicitis are rare. Diverticulitis and sepsis after hemorrhoidal banding are other known causes of pyogenic abscesses. Aerobic and anaerobic gram-negative bacteria predominate.

Symptoms of hepatic abscesses include upper abdominal pain, chills and fever, and, in many cases, right upper quadrant tenderness and mild

---

▪see page 1145

jaundice. Such symptoms and signs should prompt an abdominal CT, although ultrasound and a radionuclide scan may be helpful. In nearly half the cases, multiple abscesses occur. Aspiration helps establish the bacteria involved.

Treatment of pyogenic abscesses consists of vigorous antibiotic therapy and percutaneous CT-guided drainage. Surgical drainage is now performed only on those that cannot be adequately drained percutaneously or for the patient who needs a laparotomy for other reasons. The cause should be identified and, if possible, treated. For example, cholangitis, a common finding, requires transperitoneal exploration of the biliary tree, cholecystectomy, and T-tube drainage of the common duct.

Amebic abscesses usually respond to metronidazole 500 to 750 mg po tid; metronidazole may also be given IV (500 mg q 6 h). Treatment usually lasts for 5 to 10 days, and an intestinal amebicide is generally given after the metronidazole course. Abscesses that are symptomatic (pain, mass effect) and do not respond to metronidazole, become secondarily infected, or are so large that rupture seems imminent should be aspirated percutaneously. Rupture of the abscess into the peritoneal cavity requires surgery.

DISORDERS OF THE PANCREAS

In the elderly, the most common disorders of the pancreas are traumatic injury, pancreatitis, and cancer. Pancreatic cancer is discussed in Ch. 113.

TRAUMATIC INJURY

Penetrating injuries are diagnosed by exploration of the lesser sac and mobilization of the duodenum at laparotomy.

The most common type of blunt trauma is a steering-wheel injury. At first, the patient may be asymptomatic, but within a few hours epigastric pain and tenderness supervene. Hyperamylasemia is not a reliable marker of injury, having both a high false-negative and false-positive rate. CT with oral and IV contrast is the preferred diagnostic tool. Postoperative endoscopic retrograde cholangiopancreatography (ERCP) is advisable to assess suspected injury of the pancreatic duct and to stent confirmed injuries. Other tests (eg, ultrasound, peritoneal lavage) have not proved helpful.

Surgery is indicated for all suspected pancreatic injuries; the exact procedure depends on what injury is found at surgery. Contusions without evidence of ductal or duodenal injury are drained widely. If the gland has been completely divided or the duct is disrupted, the portion of the gland distal to the injury is resected. Serious injuries involving the head of the pancreas and the duodenum may require pancreatoduodenectomy or temporary defunctioning of the duodenum as a passage for gastric secretions by closing the pylorus with a temporary suture and emptying the stomach by a gastroenterostomy.

Postoperative complications include abscess, pancreatic or duodenal fistulas, persistent pancreatitis, hemorrhage, and pseudocyst formation.

PANCREATITIS

Acute pancreatitis: The major causes in the elderly are alcohol, gallstones, and postoperative inflammation. In elderly patients, gallstones predominate. The mortality rate for acute pancreatitis rises with age—mortality is 6 to 10% for all ages combined.

The patient first notes sudden onset of severe epigastric pain that may radiate to the back or later involve the whole abdomen. Vomiting and epigastric tenderness follow. In severe cases, shock, mild jaundice, and respiratory distress may then develop. Serum amylase levels are elevated early (usually > 1000 U/L) in 95% of cases but may fall thereafter. Serum calcium levels also may fall. Leukocytosis is noted and, if bleeding occurs, Hct is lowered. Hyperglycemia and hypocalcemia are common in severe cases.

Abdominal x-ray sometimes shows a sentinel loop of gas-filled jejunum in the left upper quadrant. Ultrasound is helpful in detecting gallstones but not in evaluating the pancreas; CT is best for evaluating the pancreas.

Differential diagnosis includes perforated peptic ulcer, which may be excluded by endoscopy or by an upper GI series using a diatrizoate meglumine swallow rather than barium. However, strangulating intestinal obstruction or ischemic bowel disease may be more difficult to exclude. Diagnostic laparotomy may be required. Gallstone pancreatitis must also be excluded because it requires surgery.∎ Vascular disease (mesenteric thrombosis or embolism) can lead rapidly to gangrene of the intestine; it mimics acute pancreatitis with pain and leaking toxins.

No laboratory tests can reliably determine the cause of pancreatitis. CT may be helpful and generally shows a relatively normal gland in gallstone pancreatitis and an abnormal gland in severe alcoholic pancreatitis.

Treatment is supportive unless the patient has gallstone pancreatitis. Nasogastric suction, IV alimentation, and fluid replacement are essential. In 85 to 90% of patients, acute pancreatitis is self-limited and conservative measures alone are sufficient. The remainder develop severe disease, resulting in pancreatic necrosis. All patients with severe acute pancreatitis are treated prophylactically with a carbapenem antibiotic (imipenem-cilastatin or meropenem). Those who develop infected necrosis or worsen with nonoperative therapy undergo surgical pancre-

---

∎see page 1127

atic necrosectomy with open or closed drainage. ERCP and endoscopic papillotomy are not used by most surgeons, because there is up to a 20% risk that ERCP will exacerbate preexisting pancreatitis.

The course varies greatly after treatment. Most patients improve rapidly. Patients whose condition worsens require ongoing reevaluations with CT and surgery for the serious complications that can follow.

Chronic pancreatitis: The most severe form of chronic pancreatitis (acute pancreatitis that continues or subsides and recurs) is pancreatolithiasis, in which patients have such severe persistent pain that many become addicted to opioid analgesics. Weight loss, diarrhea caused by loss of enzymes, and diabetes caused by fibrosis of the islets of Langerhans are late complications.

Diagnosis is based on the symptoms and on the secretin test, which is most sensitive. Administration of IV secretin should elicit decreased bicarbonate secretion with or without decreased pancreatic secretions. This test requires ERCP. Other tests that may be helpful are aspartate aminotransferase, lactic dehydrogenase, alkaline phosphatase, serum bilirubin, amylase, glucose, calcium, and phosphate as well as other diagnostic tests—an abdominal x-ray showing pancreatic calcifications is pathognomonic; ERCP and ultrasound can also be helpful.

Surgical treatment consists of pancreaticojejunostomy (anastomosis of a Roux-en-Y loop of the jejunum to the pancreas) when ERCP shows a large, uniformly dilated duct, because obstruction of the ampulla is probable.

Various extirpative procedures may also be required, including distal pancreatectomy when the tail of the gland is involved, Whipple's procedure when only the head is involved, and total pancreatectomy in extreme cases of pancreatolithiasis. Splanchnic nerve resection for pain relief is only occasionally successful. All patients must abstain from alcohol.

PANCREATIC CYSTS

Several types of cysts occur in the pancreas. Congenital cysts are rare but can be found in some cases of polycystic disease. The gland may contain many small cysts from which cystadenocarcinoma can develop. Excision or resection of a portion of the pancreas may be necessary.

Pseudocysts are initiated by extravasation of pancreatic secretions into the lesser peritoneal sac. The fluid collection evokes a surrounding inflammatory process that promotes formation of a pseudocapsule. Pseudocysts may follow trauma, acute pancreatitis, or chronic pancreatitis. The patient complains of left upper quadrant pain and tenderness, and a mass may be palpable. Diagnosis is usually made by CT. Up to 25% of pseudocysts resolve spontaneously within 6 weeks. The majority persist and may cause pain and obstruction, become infected, or evoke bleeding. Percutaneous drainage with a radiologically guided pigtail catheter is often effective at obliterating a pseudocyst. If this fails or if it is not technically feasible, marsupialization of the cyst to the wall of the stomach or small intestine is the treatment of choice. When considering invasive therapy, the physician should verify that the cyst is at least 6 weeks old to ensure that the wall of the cyst has sufficient structural integrity to hold a drain or retain sutures.

DISORDERS OF THE SPLEEN

The main indications for splenectomy are trauma (patients > 55 do not fare well with expectant management of blunt injuries to the spleen), idiopathic thrombocytopenic purpura, massive splenomegaly, disease of adjacent organs (eg, the stomach, pancreas, or colon), and abscesses. Rarely in the elderly, splenectomy is performed for hypersplenism and splenic artery aneurysms, as a staging procedure for Hodgkin's disease, or as a requirement of splenorenal shunt for portal hypertension.

Iatrogenic damage to the spleen commonly results from vagotomy and operations involving the stomach, tail of the pancreas, or colon. Such trauma as well as blunt and penetrating trauma often require splenectomy.

The surgeon decides whether the injury is severe enough to warrant splenectomy or whether simple suturing or hemostasis is possible. Compared with children, elderly patients have a much lower incidence of overwhelming postsplenectomy sepsis. However, elderly patients do not tolerate continued bleeding as well as younger patients do. Therefore, in an elderly patient, unless hemostasis is certain, splenectomy should be performed. If possible, pneumococcal vaccine should be given to unvaccinated persons before splenectomy.

Surgical treatment of gastric cancer often includes splenectomy because of the frequency of splenic lymph node metastases. Other reasons for splenectomy include cancer of the splenic flexure of the colon, which also may invade the spleen; large cysts of the distal pancreas; and splenic artery aneurysms.

Abscesses may form in the spleen secondary to sepsis. For diagnosis, CT is helpful. Many abscesses can be drained by using percutaneous catheters guided by CT scan. When percutaneous drainage fails, surgical debridement and wide drainage are usually effective.

Cancer affects elderly persons more often than younger persons and is second only to heart disease as the leading cause of death in the elderly. Gastrointestinal (GI) tumors account for > 25% of all cancer deaths. The causes of GI cancer remain elusive, and incidence involving specific sites varies enormously worldwide. In the elderly, environmental factors seem to play a much greater role than genetic factors, but clearly genetic factors (eg, DNA hypomethylation, activation of oncogenes, inactivation of tumor suppressor genes, alterations in DNA mismatch repair genes) are important.

Medical decisions regarding GI tumors in the elderly involve consideration of the patient's limited life expectancy, risk of complications from treatment, and overall effects of cancer and its therapy on quality of life. GI endoscopic procedures are discussed in Ch. 103 and end-of-life issues for elderly patients in Ch. 13.

ESOPHAGEAL TUMORS

BENIGN TUMORS

Fewer than 10% of esophageal tumors are benign; leiomyoma is the most common one. Rare tumors include inflammatory polyps, squamous cell papilloma, lymphangioma, granular cell tumor, fibromyxoma, fibrolipoma, and lipoma. Usually asymptomatic, these tumors are often found incidentally on examination for unrelated complaints or at autopsy. Symptomatic tumors may produce dysphagia or upper GI bleeding. Diagnosis often is established by esophagoscopy and biopsy. Endoscopic ultrasound may help. Surgical resection is indicated only when the tumor produces bleeding or obstruction.

MALIGNANT TUMORS

Esophageal cancer accounts for only 4% of all GI cancers in the USA but is more common in China, central Asia, South Africa, and certain Mediterranean countries. It occurs in middle to late adulthood, predominantly in men, and is more common in blacks and in smokers. Mortality rates increase steadily with age, with 66 as the median age at death.

In the last decade, the incidence of esophageal adenocarcinoma has increased dramatically, and esophageal adenocarcinoma is more common than esophageal squamous cell carcinoma in the USA. Esophageal adenocarcinoma has the fastest rate of increase in incidence of any cancer in the USA, excluding skin cancer.

A number of carcinogenic factors and disease states, including chronic thermal injury, achalasia, alcohol, tobacco, and the Plummer-

Vinson syndrome, are associated with esophageal squamous cell carcinoma. An estimated 10% of patients with Barrett's esophagus (an intestinal-type metaplasia that replaces the native squamous cell epithelium of the esophageal mucosa) eventually develop esophageal adenocarcinoma. A strong and probable causal relationship exists between gastroesophageal reflux and esophageal adenocarcinoma.

The middle and lower third of the esophagus are usually involved. Tumors may be infiltrative, ulcerative, or polypoid and may cause a stricture or mass.

Symptoms, Signs, and Diagnosis

The most common symptoms are progressive dysphagia and weight loss; others include odynophagia, hoarseness, recurrent respiratory infections, and hematemesis. Signs appear late in the course of disease and include regional lymphadenopathy, vocal cord paralysis, and pulmonary findings (eg, wheezes, rales). In the elderly, these symptoms and signs may be confused with primary neurologic or pulmonary conditions.

About 50% of patients have advanced disease at diagnosis, which is typically made by barium swallow followed by endoscopy. The upper GI series often shows a stricture or an eccentric or asymmetric mucosal irregularity. Endoscopy provides direct visualization of the lesion and tissue for microscopic examination. The combination of biopsy and brush cytology yields the diagnosis in > 95% of cases. Endoscopic ultrasound and CT are useful for tumor staging, especially in patients considered for curative surgery.

Prognosis and Treatment

The management of the esophageal cancer is determined by the disease stage. Although the overall cure rate for esophageal cancer is only about 5%, selected series show nearly a 25% survival rate in patients with cancer of the distal portion. Because the cure rate is so low, experimental protocols have been designed that combine radiation therapy and chemotherapy using cisplatin and other drugs; in some cases, tumor regression has been remarkable. Nonetheless, aggressive treatment is often not appropriate, especially in elderly persons with significant comorbidities.

Surgical therapy remains the best treatment of limited esophageal tumors. In patients with squamous cell carcinoma, the combination of chemotherapy and radiation therapy before surgery increases the probability of disease-free survival. The benefit of a similar approach in patients with adenocarcinoma is uncertain, although promising. The postoperative mortality rate for elderly patients is comparable with that in younger patients, but the elderly experience a greater incidence of postoperative cardiopulmonary complications.

Endoscopy can be used for palliation in high-risk elderly patients or in those with advanced disease. Dilatation, injection therapy, photodynamic therapy, and placement of an esophageal prosthesis can also provide palliation. Nutritional support may be accomplished by percutaneous endoscopic gastrostomy or jejunostomy tube feedings.

Esophageal cancer is often terminal and leads to a poor quality of life, primarily because patients cannot swallow their own saliva. Therefore, palliative procedures are often offered, even when cure is unlikely.∎ When possible, resection and esophagogastrectomy are preferred. If the tumor cannot be resected, the favored procedure is colonic bypass, in which the esophagus is left in place. Rigid tubes (Celestin's or Souttar's) may be inserted through the tumor, but because these tubes tend to become displaced and cause perforation, they are not often used. Laser therapy or radiation therapy and chemotherapy can debulk obstructing tumors. Gastrostomy allows feeding but does not alleviate dysphagia. Pain should always be treated.

STOMACH TUMORS

BENIGN TUMORS

Fewer than 5% of all stomach tumors are benign. Although leiomyoma is the most common benign stomach tumor in the general population, hyperplastic and adenomatous polyps are also common among the elderly. Hyperplastic polyps are small (usually < 1 cm in diameter), flat lesions that account for about 95% of all gastric epithelial polyps, while the remaining 5% are predominantly adenomatous polyps. Hyperplastic polyps carry no malignant potential, whereas adenomatous polyps do, usually when they are > 2 cm.

The Cronkhite-Canada syndrome, although a rare nonhereditary entity, represents the only nonfamilial GI polyposis syndrome occurring in the elderly. In addition to multiple hyperplastic polyps, the syndrome includes ectodermal changes (eg, increased pigmentation, alopecia, atrophic nails). Diarrhea is common.

Most benign stomach tumors are asymptomatic and are found during examinations performed for unrelated symptoms. The most common presenting finding is anemia from chronic occult bleeding. Less commonly, epigastric pain or acute GI bleeding from tumor ulceration occurs.

In most cases, endoscopy can be used for diagnosis and treatment. If the lesion is submucosal or if its size or location precludes endoscopic resection, surgery may be warranted if significant blood loss or other symptoms have developed.

∎see page 115

MALIGNANT TUMORS

As of 1999 in the USA, about 22,000 new cases and 14,000 deaths from stomach cancer occurred annually, 70% of which affected patients ≥ 65 years. Stomach cancer in the elderly probably develops principally as well-differentiated carcinomas that then progress to poorly differentiated ones with time, in contrast with those of younger patients, most of which emerge in the very early phase as poorly differentiated tumors.

Adenocarcinoma accounts for 95% of all stomach cancers. Gastric adenocarcinoma is more common in blacks and among poor socioeconomic groups; the male:female ratio is 2:1. The worldwide incidence varies dramatically, with low rates in the USA and high rates in Japan, Chile, and Costa Rica. For an unknown reason, overall incidence has decreased worldwide during the past 50 years. *Helicobacter pylori* infection is likely the most important risk factor. This infection is also associated with mucosal-associated lymphoid tissue, a type of low-grade gastric lymphoma. Other risk factors include adenoma, chronic atrophic gastritis with intestinal metaplasia (with or without associated pernicious anemia), adenomatous polyps, stomach remnants after subtotal gastrectomy, and chronic gastric ulcer.

Lymphoma accounts for about 4% of stomach cancers. The stomach is the most common site of primary extranodal lymphoma, accounting for up to 75% of all cases of primary GI tract lymphomas. Gastric lymphoma occurs mainly in men in the 6th decade.

Symptoms and Signs

Stomach cancer is usually asymptomatic in its early stage. The most common presenting symptom is vague epigastric discomfort followed by anorexia, early satiety, hematemesis, melena, and severe abdominal pain as the tumor progresses. If the cardia is involved, dysphagia may occur. If the prepyloric antrum is involved, symptoms of partial or complete gastric outlet obstruction may occur. Patients with gastric lymphoma present with similar symptoms.

No specific signs occur in the early stage. In later stages, nausea, vomiting, dysphagia, weight loss, a palpable mass, and lymphadenopathy in the left supraclavicular region (Virchow's node) may be noted. Liver metastases can present as hepatomegaly. Dermatologic signs include acanthosis nigricans and dermatomyositis.

Diagnosis

An upper GI series is usually the initial test, but lesions are often missed. Endoscopy allows visualization of most lesions, obtains tissue for histologic examination, and yields the diagnosis in > 90% of patients. Stomach cancer is staged using CT and endoscopic ultrasound, which may indicate the depth of invasion. Available tumor markers (eg, carcinoembryonic antigen, fetal sulfoglycoprotein, CA 72-4) provide little help because their sensitivity and specificity are poor. The differential diagnosis includes peptic ulcer and pancreatico-biliary tract disease.

The radiographic appearance of lymphoma may be similar to that of adenocarcinoma, although large gastric folds and evidence of infiltration into the duodenum are more typical of lymphoma than of carcinoma. Endoscopy with multiple directed biopsies combined with brush cytology may confirm the diagnosis, but because the lesions are submucosal, laparotomy may be needed.

Prognosis and Treatment

With adenocarcinoma, the overall 5-year survival rate is < 10%. With early stomach cancer, 5-year survival rates of up to 95% have been reported. With primary gastric lymphoma, the 5-year survival rate approaches 50%. However, the prognosis is adversely affected by age; the 5-year survival rate for patients < 45 with gastric lymphoma is 57%; for those > 65, it is 32%.

Surgery is the only potential curative treatment available for stomach cancer. For distal gastric lesions, adequate resection involves subtotal gastrectomy, whereas total gastrectomy is performed for proximal lesions. Japanese and Western surgeons differ in their approach to lymph node dissection. Although a more radical lymph node dissection increases survival in Japan, it has not been shown to influence survival or prevent local recurrence in Western series. In elderly patients operated on for cure, perioperative morbidity (30 to 40%) and mortality (< 10%) rates are comparable with those obtained in younger patients. Five-year probability of survival after curative surgery for stomach cancer is up to 25%.

Radiation therapy alone is ineffective for adenocarcinoma. Radiation therapy after resection commonly produces good results in patients with gastric lymphoma. Chemotherapy, either as adjuvant therapy after surgery or as treatment for advanced disease, has failed to demonstrate a clear survival benefit in patients with adenocarcinoma. Chemotherapy for gastric lymphoma is much more effective, although perforation can occur during tumor lysis.

Palliative surgery for gastric cancer is difficult and produces higher complication rates than curative surgery. Therefore, palliative surgical procedures, if used at all, should only be performed in patients with few comorbid conditions and good overall function, not in those with advanced metastatic disease. In selected patients with lesions causing distal esophageal or gastric outlet obstruction, palliation has been achieved using endoscopic laser photoablation. Palliative chemotherapy may be an option for patients with advanced stages of gastric adenocarcinoma. One should be mindful of a proclivity to bone metastasis.

Because stomach cancer is often terminal, advance planning for end-of-life issues must be discussed early with elderly patients and their families when appropriate. ◨ The usefulness of treatment must be weighed against the adverse effects it causes. At the end of life, patients are likely to experience nausea, vomiting, pain, and weight loss and should be treated accordingly to control symptoms. ◩

SMALL-INTESTINE TUMORS

BENIGN TUMORS

Benign small-intestine tumors are rare, account for less than 5% of all GI tumors, and usually occur in the 5th, 6th, and 7th decades of life. About 80% of these tumors occur in the jejunum and ileum. Adenomatous polyps are the most common benign tumors, followed by leiomyoma, lipoma, and hemangioma. In the small intestine, as in the rest of the GI tract, adenomatous polyps are premalignant.

Most often, benign tumors are asymptomatic and are found during examination for unrelated symptoms or at autopsy. However, patients may present with recurrent abdominal pain, GI hemorrhage, abdominal mass, or intestinal obstruction. Diagnosis can be made by small-bowel x-ray. When the duodenum or terminal ileum is involved, small-bowel endoscopy may provide visualization and tissue for diagnosis.

Endoscopic or surgical resection is usually the treatment of choice, depending on the tumor's location.

MALIGNANT TUMORS

Cancers of the small intestine account for < 3% of all GI tract cancers and usually occur in the 6th and 7th decades. The most common is carcinoid tumor, followed by adenocarcinoma, lymphoma, and leiomyosarcoma. Lymphoma occurs predominantly in the ileum and is usually of B-cell origin; lymphoma of T-cell origin is associated with adult celiac disease. Leiomyosarcoma is as common as lymphoma.

Symptoms, Signs, and Diagnosis

Whereas most small-intestine cancers are asymptomatic, 60 to 75% of symptomatic small-intestine tumors are malignant. Patients with advanced disease present with abdominal pain resulting from intestinal obstruction, recurrent intussusception, mesenteric thrombosis, perforation, GI hemorrhage, or a palpable abdominal mass. The carcinoid syndrome, which is characterized by diarrhea and flushing, usually occurs when hepatic metastases develop. Lymphoma, especially Hodgkin's disease, may present as malabsorption syndrome with weight loss, diarrhea, malaise, weakness, and edema.

Preoperative diagnosis is generally made with a small-bowel x-ray series and CT. Endoscopy may provide visualization and tissue for diagnosis, and angiography may show vascular malignancies. In carcinoid tumors, urinary 5-hydroxyindoleacetic acid levels may be elevated.

Prognosis and Treatment

The 5-year survival rate for patients with adenocarcinoma is 30%; for those with lymphoma and leiomyosarcoma, it approaches 50%. Survival for patients with carcinoid tumors is commonly > 10 years.

Surgical resection is the usual treatment. Radiation therapy and chemotherapy are potentially effective only for lymphoma. In patients with carcinoid tumors, octreotide is often effective in treating severe flushing and diarrhea. Hepatic arterial chemoembolization with streptozocin or doxorubicin may be considered as palliative treatment in patients with hepatic metastases and preserved liver function.

COLORECTAL TUMORS

BENIGN TUMORS

Benign colorectal tumors are present in up to 75% of persons > 50 years; the incidence increases with age and peaks in the 7th decade. Most benign tumors are polyps, a clinical term without pathologic significance that refers to any mass of tissue arising from a mucosal surface and protruding into the lumen. Predisposing factors to colorectal polyps are similar to those for colon cancer and include age, diet, geographic distribution, family history, and prior tumors.

Adenomatous polyps, the most common colorectal tumors, are found in 50 to 60% of persons > 60 at autopsy. Lesions may be sessile or pedunculated and, depending on the proportion of the villous component, are classified histologically as tubular, tubulovillous, or villous adenomas. Synchronous lesions (more than one at the same time) occur in about 50% of cases. These polyps are true tumors with malignant potential, which increases with size, proportion of villous elements, and degree of dysplasia. The overall risk of malignant change within an adenomatous polyp is about 1 to 2%.

Other benign lesions include hyperplastic and inflammatory polyps, lipomas, hemangiomas, and leiomyomas. Hyperplastic polyps are common benign tumors. They are small, dome-shaped, sessile lesions with no malignant potential. Patients with inflammatory bowel disorders, ischemic colitis, and certain infections (eg, tuberculosis) are especially prone to developing such polyps. Lipomas, the second most common benign colonic tumor, usually occur at or near the ileocecal valve. Incidence peaks in the 7th to 8th decades. Colonic hemangiomas predominantly occur in elderly patients and are a common cause of hemorrhage. The incidence of leiomyomas seems to peak in the 6th decade and declines sharply thereafter.

Symptoms and Signs

Most polyps are asymptomatic and found incidentally during evaluation for another disorder. Rectal bleeding, usually occult and rarely massive, may occur. Large villous adenomas may cause a severe mucoid rectal discharge and diarrhea, which may eventually result in hypokalemia and hyponatremia. Patients with submucosal tumors (eg, lipomas, hemangiomas, leiomyomas) may present with an abdominal mass or abdominal pain from intussusception.

Diagnosis and Treatment

Polyps are usually detected by barium enema or endoscopy. Air-contrast barium enema is far superior to the single-contrast technique, but endoscopy is the most accurate diagnostic procedure. Total colonoscopy should be performed when an adenomatous polyp > 5 mm is found on sigmoidoscopy because additional polyps in more proximal locations are highly likely. The predictive meaning of polyps < 5 mm is uncertain.

Endoscopic polypectomy is the treatment of choice for adenomatous polyps. Surgical excision may be necessary for submucosal tumors or polyps that cannot be removed endoscopically.

When well-differentiated carcinoma is detected in a polyp and no vascular, lymphatic, or stalk invasion exists and a clear resection margin does exist, the only treatment usually needed is endoscopic polypectomy. If these conditions are not met, surgery may be considered, depending on the location of the adenoma and other factors.

For patients with adenomatous polyps, endoscopic surveillance every 3 to 5 years after polypectomy is recommended.

MALIGNANT TUMORS

Colorectal cancer is second only to lung cancer as the most common malignancy among U.S. and Western European men and women. Colorectal cancer is the most common cancer occurring in persons ≥ 65 years. Although early detection and treatment have improved significantly in the last 2 decades, colorectal cancer continues to be the second leading cause of cancer death. About 130,000 new cases occur annually in the USA, and 57,000 deaths from this disease occur annually. Age is a critical risk factor—incidence begins to increase at age 45 and doubles every 5 years thereafter.

Adenocarcinoma constitutes 95% of all colorectal cancers; others include lymphoma, leiomyosarcoma, and carcinoid tumors. Rectal cancer is slightly more common in men, while colon cancer occurs equally in men and women. In addition to age, other predisposing factors for colorectal cancer include a family history of colorectal adenomatous polyps or cancer, inflammatory bowel disease, and a family history of colorectal tumors (ie, cancer or an adenomatous polyp diagnosed before age 60). Inherited disorders (eg, familial adenomatous polyposis, hereditary nonpolyposis colorectal cancer) are also associated with a high incidence of colorectal cancer, but they are rarely the cause in the elderly. Some dietary factors (eg, a diet high in animal fat and refined sugar and low in fiber) have been associated with a higher risk of colorectal cancer, but their causative role is controversial.

The extent of tumor spread is graded by a modified Dukes' classification. Dukes' A lesions involve the mucosa; B lesions extend through the wall but do not involve lymph nodes; C lesions involve lymph nodes; and D lesions have distant metastases. Many modifications of this staging system exist.

Symptoms, Signs, and Diagnosis

Colorectal cancer is asymptomatic in its early stages. In later stages, the location of the tumor influences symptoms. Some evidence indicates that elderly patients are more likely to present with right-sided lesions. Synchronous colorectal lesions appear in about 3.5% of patients. Right-sided lesions are usually large, fungating, bleeding masses that cause iron deficiency anemia, fatigue, and weakness. These tumors usually do not cause obstruction but may grow large enough to be palpable on abdominal examination. Left-sided lesions are usually "napkin-ring," obstructive tumors that cause rectal bleeding, crampy abdominal pain, or altered bowel habits because of the narrower caliber of the left colon. Patients with rectal lesions generally present with stool streaked or mixed with blood. They may also complain of tenesmus or a sensation of incomplete evacuation. Palpable lymphadenopathy, hepatomegaly, or both occur only in the late stages.

Diagnosis is made by barium x-ray or endoscopy. Air-contrast barium enema is usually superior to the single-contrast technique. Sigmoidoscopy can detect lesions in the rectum, sigmoid colon, and distal descending colon, the region where about 50% of cancers occur; colonoscopy allows inspection of the entire colon.

Carcinoembryonic antigen (CEA) levels may be elevated in patients with cancer of the colon, pancreas, breast, lung, prostate, stomach, or bladder as well as in those with benign conditions and thus are nonspecific. An elevated CEA level is especially insensitive for early-stage cancers. However, if the CEA level is elevated before surgery and decreases after it, a subsequent rise may indicate a recurrence.

Preoperative staging of colon cancer should include abdominal CT to rule out liver metastases. In rectal tumors, abdominal-pelvic CT is preferred because it allows a more accurate examination of the pelvis. In these cases, chest x-ray helps determine whether pulmonary metastasis has occurred, and endoscopic ultrasound determines the depth of invasion.

Screening

Annual fecal occult blood testing increases detection of colorectal tumors in an early curable stage and improves overall long-term survival. Sigmoidoscopy as a screening technique also seems to improve prognosis. Because of the marked increase in colorectal cancer prevalence with age, the positive predictive value of both strategies increases in older groups.

Prognosis and Treatment

In patients with adenocarcinoma, the 5-year survival rate is about 90% for patients with Dukes' A lesions, 50 to 80% for those with B lesions, 30 to 40% for those with C lesions, and < 5% for those with D lesions.

Surgery is the mainstay of treatment. When possible, comorbid factors (eg, nutritional deficits, cardiovascular decompensation, pulmonary insufficiency) should be corrected as early as possible.

Cancers of the colon and upper rectum preferably are treated by segmental resection and reanastomosis in a single operation. This procedure is extremely safe in elderly patients; the mortality rate for elective surgery is < 10%. In rectal cancer, the use of preoperative radiation therapy, stapling devices, and newer sphincter-preserving surgical techniques permits extirpation of many lesions without the need for permanent colostomy.

Multiple tumors may require subtotal colectomy. However, because low ileorectal anastomoses may lead to severe diarrhea in elderly patients, an adequate amount of large bowel should be left when possible. Preferably, wide excision of the mesentery and regional lymph nodes is performed concurrently.

Cancers of the middle and lower rectum are more problematic surgically in the elderly because abdominoperineal resection with permanent colostomy (the operation most likely to cure) requires lifestyle changes that may be unsatisfactory to some patients. Fortunately, use of a stapling device permits anastomosis lower than is possible with hand-suturing techniques. However, the anal sphincter can be preserved in only about 5% of lower rectal cancers.

About 25% of patients with colorectal cancer develop hepatic metastases. Surgical resection is indicated when fewer than four nodules affect one single lobe and no evidence of extrahepatic spread exists. Major hepatic resection in patients > 70 can be performed with the same postoperative mortality as in younger patients. When surgery is not indicated, hepatic arterial infusion chemotherapy can be used. Compared with systemic treatment, response rates are higher, but overall survival benefit of this procedure is still poor.

Electrocoagulation also may be effective for small lesions. However, according to one study, when it was used for cancers > 4 cm in diameter, the results were poor.

Adjuvant chemotherapy after surgery with 5-fluorouracil–based regimens modulated by levamisole or leucovorin reduces the probability of recurrence and increases survival in patients with Dukes' B2 or C colon cancer. In rectal tumors, chemotherapy and preoperative or postoperative radiation therapy improve local control and long-term survival. Advanced age is not a contraindication for the use of this type of chemotherapy, but monitoring, supportive care, and patient selection are essential. In addition, a reduced-dose schedule is often necessary to minimize complications. No difference in adverse effects between patients younger and older than 65 has been observed in clinical trials.

In many cases, only palliative procedures are possible, ◨ either initially or when cancer recurs. A colostomy may help relieve unremitting tenesmus. Radiation therapy can ease the pain of recurrent rectal cancer. Laser therapy has been used to reduce inoperable rectal tumors and prevent obstruction.

ANORECTAL TUMORS

Cancer may develop in the perianal skin, the anal canal, or the lower rectum. Epidermoid carcinoma accounts for 2% of colorectal cancers and 90% of anal cancers. The histologic types of anal carcinoma include squamous cell, basal cell, basaloid squamous, and cloacogenic carcinomas. Other malignant tumors include Bowen's disease (intraepithelial squamous cell carcinoma in situ), extramammary Paget's disease, carcinoid tumor, and malignant melanoma. Cloacogenic carcinoma is most prevalent in patients aged 60 to 70. Predisposing factors include human papillomavirus types 16 and 18 or HIV infection, leukoplakia, lymphogranuloma venereum, chronic fistula formation, irradiation of the anal skin, and organ transplantation. The disease spreads by direct extension into soft tissues with early lymphatic dissemination.

Symptoms, Signs, and Diagnosis

Bleeding is the most common symptom. Other common complaints are anal discomfort, constipation, and diminished stool caliber. The presenting feature may be a mass on digital rectal examination, inguinal adenopathy, or perianal dermatitis. Cancer should be considered with all nonhealing ulcers or fistulas, and a biopsy must be obtained.

Treatment

The treatment of choice is local surgical excision. A course of radiation therapy and chemotherapy may be needed to debulk a large tumor

◨see page 115

mass before surgery. Such radiation therapy and chemotherapy may obviate abdominoperineal resection in many patients. Favorable cancers of the lower rectum can be treated with procedures other than proctectomy (eg, local excision, intracavitary radiation therapy, and electrocoagulation). In cases of carcinoma of the anal canal, remarkable local tumor control with chemoradiation therapy has been demonstrated.

Local excision is satisfactory for polypoid rectal tumors that are not fixed, not > 2 cm in diameter, and of low or moderate differentiation.

Fulguration with electrocautery and laser photocoagulation are palliative measures used for selected patients.

PANCREATIC TUMORS

Pancreatic tumors include exocrine and endocrine tumors. The only significant benign exocrine pancreatic tumor is cystadenoma, which usually occurs in the body and tail of the pancreas in middle-aged and elderly women. Surgical resection may be needed for diagnosis and relief of symptoms from a large mass. Endocrine tumors are rare in the elderly and arise from the neuroendocrine cells of the pancreas predominantly in the islets of the pancreatic body and tail. The types and treatment of endocrine tumors are listed in TABLE 113–1.

PANCREATIC CANCER

Pancreatic cancer is the second most common GI cancer in the USA with about 29,000 new cases diagnosed annually, > 20,000 of which occur in patients > 65. The incidence increases with age and is 10 times greater in men > 75 years than in the general population; it is the fifth leading cause of cancer death.

A number of carcinogenic factors and disease states are associated with pancreatic cancer, although their causative role is not fully established. These factors include chronic cigarette smoking, a diet high in animal fat, alcohol, diabetes mellitus, and chronic pancreatitis (idiopathic and hereditary).

Ductal cell adenocarcinoma accounts for 75 to 96% of all cancers arising from the pancreas. Other types include giant cell carcinoma, adenosquamous carcinoma, cystadenocarcinoma, and lymphoma. Giant cell carcinoma, also called carcinosarcoma, is a highly malignant lesion with distant metastases occurring early. Adenosquamous carcinoma occurs predominantly in men, more often in patients with a history of radiation therapy. Cystadenocarcinoma, a low-grade malignancy, has the best prognosis because only 20% of cases have metastasized by the time of surgery. Pancreatic lymphoma accounts for 2% of all non-Hodgkin's lymphomas and may be of B-cell or T-cell origin. Eighty percent of pancreatic lesions occur in the head of the pancreas, and 20% in the body and tail.

TABLE 113-1.   GASTROINTESTINAL ENDOCRINE TUMORS

Type	Characteristics	Treatment
Insulinomas	May be single or multiple; produce insulin and identified by episodes of hypoglycemia (which may progress to coma when severe); are rarely malignant	Removal of all tumor tissue is completely curative
Gastrinomas	Can occur near the ampulla of Vater or the antrum or in the pancreas; cause Zollinger-Ellison syndrome; are malignant in 90% of cases	If not metastatic, complete excision of tumor is curative; if metastatic, large doses of H_2 blockers or proton pump inhibitors should be given; if drugs fail, gastric surgery reduces acid secretion
Glucagonomas	Secrete glucagon; lead to mild diabetes mellitus and severe dermatitis involving lower half of the body; have a high potential for malignancy	Complete removal may not be possible, but debulking may help relieve symptoms; streptozocin can help treat residual tumor
Vipomas	Produce intestinal polypeptide and pancreatic polypeptide; can also be referred to as *W*atery *D*iarrhea, *H*ypokalemia, *A*chlorhydria (WDHA) syndrome; almost 50% are malignant	As much tumor as possible should be resected; streptozocin can help treat residual tumor
Somatostatinomas	Occur rarely and secrete somatostatin; characterized by diabetes, steatorrhea, achlorhydria; can manifest as multiple endocrine neoplasia	As much tumor as possible should be resected; streptozocin can help treat residual tumor

Symptoms and Signs

The clinical features of pancreatic cancer often depend on the location of the lesions. Patients with lesions of the pancreatic head often present with painless jaundice and acholic stools from common duct obstruction or with nausea and vomiting from gastric outlet obstruction. Pruritus may accompany jaundice. The onset of symptoms in patients with lesions of the pancreatic body and tail is more insidious, amounting to little more than weight loss and vague abdominal or back pain.

Symptoms precede diagnosis by about 3 to 6 months. In 70 to 80% of patients with ductal cell adenocarcinoma, advanced stages with locoregional invasion or metastatic spread are present at diagnosis. Other findings include depression, thromboembolic phenomena, GI bleeding from gastric varices secondary to splenic vein thrombosis, polyarthritis, and diarrhea caused by exocrine pancreatic insufficiency. The onset of diabetes mellitus or a worsening of preexisting diabetes warrants an evaluation for pancreatic cancer. Early in the disease, there are no findings on physical examination. Later, jaundice, an epigastric mass, supraclavicular lymphadenopathy, hepatomegaly, or a large, palpable gallbladder may be noted. Painless jaundice and a palpable gallbladder (Courvoisier's sign) combined with acholic stools are highly suggestive of cancer of the pancreatic head.

Diagnosis

Early diagnosis when the tumor is still resectable is unusual and occurs only in patients with cancer of the pancreatic head who present with early jaundice. Abdominal ultrasound may be helpful, but CT is better able to visualize a pancreatic mass and establish its relationship with surrounding tissues. In up to 90% of cases, endoscopic retrograde cholangiopancreatography can detect the tumor with the characteristic findings of ductal irregularity and cutoff. Cytohistologic diagnosis may be performed by fine-needle aspiration biopsy or pancreatic duct brushing. Detection of K-*ras* mutations by DNA amplification from pancreatic aspirates or pancreatic juice may increase the diagnostic use of such techniques. Serologic tumor markers, including CEA and CA 19-9, may be elevated in some cases but are generally not useful clinically.

Assessment of tumor resectability warrants not only a combination of different preoperative radiologic examinations (CT, MRI, and endoscopic ultrasound), but also laparoscopy in some centers when findings are inconclusive.

Prognosis and Treatment

Advanced pancreatic adenocarcinoma has a grim prognosis, with a median survival of 4 months and a 5-year probability of survival of 2%.

Surgery is the only potentially curative therapy for pancreatic cancer. Patients with nonmetastatic, localized, resectable lesions in the pancreatic head may be candidates for pancreatoduodenectomy (Whipple's operation). Although data in the elderly are minimal, mortality and survival rates in patients > 70 seem to be similar to those for younger patients—perioperative mortality rate of 5%, morbidity rate of 45%, and 5-year probability of survival rate of 21%. Therefore, surgery should be considered for the elderly patient with limited disease and appropriately managed comorbid illnesses. However, only 10 to 20% of patients with ductal cell carcinoma fulfill these conditions. For the remainder (and thus the vast majority) of patients, treatment options are less clear. Some elderly patients may do best without any treatment. For other patients, the only procedure that can be performed is a palliative bypass (eg, cholecystojejunostomy or choledochojejunostomy to relieve distal bile duct obstruction or gastrojejunostomy for gastric outlet obstruction); obstructive jaundice can be managed with a biliary stent, placed either endoscopically or radiologically, using transhepatic cholangiography.

Chemotherapy produces little response and no long-term benefit in patients with pancreatic adenocarcinoma. 5-Fluorouracil is the most widely studied drug, is tolerated relatively well in the elderly, and has a response rate of about 15%. Gemcitabine may improve the quality of life by reducing pain medication requirements and improving nutritional status. Nevertheless, there has been no difference in survival when comparing patients who received chemotherapy with those who received only supportive care. Radiation therapy offers minimal benefit, except for palliation of retroperitoneal disease.

Attention must be paid to the treatment of pain in elderly patients. Generally, abdominal pain is treated with analgesics or oral opioids. However, a celiac axis nerve block may be needed for severe, unremitting pain. Pruritus from jaundice may be relieved with antihistamines or cholestyramine 4 g po 1 to 4 times daily. (Cholestyramine is only effective for patients with partial biliary obstruction and is ineffective in completely obstructed patients.) Pancreatic insufficiency can be managed with pancreatic enzymes.

Because many patients present with advanced pancreatic cancer, curative therapy is difficult. Therefore, attention must be paid to patients' quality of life, especially nutritional status and pain relief, along with end-of-life issues. **◻**

LIVER TUMORS

BENIGN TUMORS

Hemangioma, the most common benign liver tumor, is found in about 5% of adults at autopsy. Other benign tumors include adenoma and focal nodular hyperplasia, which are most often associated with oral contraceptive use and do not usually occur in the elderly.

Benign tumors are generally asymptomatic and are found incidentally when a CT or ultrasound is performed for unrelated symptoms. Liver function test results are typically normal. Diagnosis is established by ultrasound, dynamic CT, or MRI. Labeled erythrocyte scintigraphy or angiography may help diagnose vascular lesions. Cytohistologic

---

◻ see also page 115

diagnosis is confirmed by fine-needle biopsy in nonvascular lesions. Therapy for nonvascular tumors usually consists of segmental resection. Hemangiomas usually require no treatment.

MALIGNANT TUMORS

Metastatic carcinoma is by far the most common form of liver cancer. The liver is the most common site of metastasis from other cancers. Hepatic metastases are found at autopsy in 30 to 50% of cancer patients.

Hepatocellular carcinoma is one of the most common cancers worldwide, particularly in areas with a high incidence of viral hepatitis. In the USA, the incidence is 2 per 100,000, but incidence has been increasing over the past 2 decades, significantly among persons 40 to 60. This tumor originates in the hepatocyte and accounts for > 90% of primary adult hepatic cancers. Cholangiocarcinoma (lesions originating in the bile ducts) represents the remaining 5 to 10%. Hepatic malignancies are more common in men than in women and occur between ages 50 and 70.

In most cases, the tumor develops in the setting of cirrhosis, mainly related to hepatitis B and C virus infection. Recently, hepatitis C virus infection has emerged as the leading identifiable risk factor for hepatocellular carcinoma. Therefore, cirrhotic patients constitute the population at risk; the 5-year probability of these patients developing a hepatocellular carcinoma is about 20%. Other predisposing factors include alcohol, tobacco, and aflatoxin exposure.

Symptoms and Signs

Only 20% of cases are asymptomatic at the time of diagnosis. Hepatocellular carcinoma usually presents as decompensated liver disease (ie, ascites, hepatic encephalopathy, jaundice, variceal bleeding) in persons with cirrhosis. Right upper quadrant or epigastric pain and weight loss are also common. Intra-abdominal hemorrhage due to tumor rupture is rare but life threatening.

Physical examination may reveal hepatomegaly, a right upper quadrant mass, ascites, or jaundice. Splenomegaly is less common. Paraneoplastic syndromes associated with hepatocellular carcinoma include erythrocytosis, hypercalcemia, hypoglycemia, hyperlipidemia, porphyria cutanea tarda, and dysfibrinogenemia.

Diagnosis

Liver function test results are usually abnormal, with increased serum bilirubin levels, elevated serum alkaline phosphatase and γ-glutamyl transpeptidase levels, and diminished serum albumin concentration. The serum α-fetoprotein level alone is not useful for early detection.

Diagnosis is often made with a combination of abdominal ultrasound and CT, angiography, and biopsy. Periodic ultrasound seems to be the most adequate screening strategy in high-risk populations (ie, patients with liver cirrhosis) combined with the α-fetoprotein level.

Prognosis and Treatment

Prognosis in patients with hepatocellular carcinoma is determined by the tumor stage and by the liver's functional status. The 5-year survival of selected patients treated by surgical resection or liver transplantation is > 50%.

Surgical resection is usually restricted to patients with solitary tumors without vascular invasion or extrahepatic spread. Extensive lobectomies are contraindicated in cirrhotic patients, and segmentary or subsegmentary resection should be the goal. In the elderly, data regarding liver surgery are limited to major resection for colorectal metastases; thus, it is difficult to infer the results of this procedure in patients with hepatocellular carcinoma associated with liver cirrhosis.

Liver transplantation may be curative for hepatocellular carcinoma, especially when performed in persons with small solitary tumors; the recurrence rate is negligible and survival is similar to patients undergoing transplantation for nonmalignant causes. Nevertheless, most centers will not perform liver transplantation in patients $\geq$ 65, especially with coexisting comorbid illnesses.

Percutaneous hepatic injection with ethanol has gained wide popularity, especially in Japan and Europe. Absolute ethanol is injected through a fine needle into the tumor under ultrasound control, inducing complete necrosis. This procedure is well tolerated and is highly effective for solitary tumors < 4 cm; complications are very rare. In patients with these lesions, the probability of recurrence and survival is almost the same as that obtained by surgical resection. Other options include tumor embolization or chemoembolization, systemic chemotherapy, hormonal manipulation, and immunotherapy. Although some of these treatments have a relatively high antitumor effect, a beneficial effect on survival has not been clearly established.

Like patients with pancreatic cancer, those with liver cancer often present in an advanced stage. Death and dying issues must be addressed for many patients. ▌Attention must be paid to quality of life, especially nutritional status and pain relief.

GALLBLADDER TUMORS

BENIGN TUMORS

Benign gallbladder tumors, including adenomas, cystadenomas, fibroadenomas, adenomyomas, and hamartomas, are found at cholecys-

▌see page 115

tectomy in about 1% of patients. Incidence of benign gallbladder tumors is not higher among the elderly.

MALIGNANT TUMORS

In the USA, gallbladder cancer is the fourth most common GI cancer. The mean age at diagnosis is 76. Women are primarily affected, and workers in rubber and automotive plants are at particularly high risk. Adenocarcinoma accounts for 80% of all gallbladder cancers; squamous cell carcinoma and adenoacanthoma account for the remaining 20%. Gallstones are present in 85% of cases.

Symptoms, Signs, and Diagnosis

Symptoms include intermittent, vague pain in the right upper quadrant or epigastrium. In the late stages, weight loss and jaundice develop. Often a firm, tender mass is palpable. Abdominal ultrasound and CT provide visualization of the tumor. Endoscopic retrograde cholangiopancreatography or percutaneous transhepatic cholangiography is useful for complete evaluation of the biliary tree.

Prognosis and Treatment

Prognosis is related to tumor stage; the majority of patients present with advanced metastatic disease; the 5-year survival rate is only 5%. Death and dying issues must be addressed. ∎

Radical cholecystectomy is the treatment of choice for localized disease. Radiation therapy and chemotherapy are ineffective. Biliary stenting by endoscopic retrograde cholangiopancreatography or percutaneous transhepatic cholangiography may provide limited palliation of a mass that causes obstruction or jaundice.

EXTRAHEPATIC BILE DUCT TUMORS

BENIGN TUMORS

Benign tumors of the bile ducts are rare; papilloma and adenoma are the most common lesions. Symptoms include intermittent jaundice and right upper quadrant pain. The treatment of choice is local excision.

MALIGNANT TUMORS

By far the most common malignant tumor is adenocarcinoma. Bile duct cancer is more common in men; the average age at diagnosis is 60. Tumors of the upper portion of the ducts (50% of all lesions) are intimately related to the liver; those of the middle portion, to the portal vein and hepatic artery; and those of the lower portion, to the pancreas and duodenum.

∎see page 115

Predisposing factors include primary sclerosing cholangitis, *Opisthorchis (Clonorchis) sinensis* infestation, and industrial exposure (in automobile and rubber manufacturing plant workers).

Symptoms, Signs, and Diagnosis

Because of their location, these tumors usually cause symptoms early, with jaundice occurring in almost all patients. Right upper quadrant pain occurs in > 50% of cases. Other symptoms and signs include weight loss, nausea, vomiting, anorexia, fever, chills, and hepatomegaly. If obstruction occurs below the cystic duct, the gallbladder may be palpable (Courvoisier's sign).

Diagnosis is made by ultrasound and CT. Percutaneous transhepatic cholangiography and endoscopic retrograde cholangiopancreatography provide more accurate localization of the tumor. Liver function test results are consistent with extrahepatic obstruction.

Prognosis and Treatment

The 5-year survival rate is only 5%. Tumors in the proximal portion of the bile duct system rarely are operable. Resectable tumors of the central portion of the bile ducts may be treated by local en bloc excision. For resectable tumors of the distal portion, radical resection and pancreatoduodenectomy (Whipple's operation) provide some promising benefit with 5-year survival rates of 20 to 30%, but patients > 70 have a high operative risk.

For the majority of patients with advanced extrahepatic biliary carcinoma, no effective treatment exists. Palliation may be accomplished by dilation and stent insertion either endoscopically or via transhepatic cholangiography perhaps combined with intrabiliary radiation. Death and dying issues must be addressed. ▪

TUMORS OF THE MESENTERY AND PERITONEUM

BENIGN TUMORS

Benign tumors of the mesentery and peritoneum are twice as common as malignant tumors; however, they are still rare. The most common benign tumors are fibromas and lipomas. These tumors often grow large before causing symptoms and are most often found incidentally during routine examination. The most common symptoms are vague abdominal pain and bloating caused by compression or traction of adjacent structures. Intestinal obstruction may occur.

Diagnosis is usually made by x-rays that reveal extrinsic compression of the large or small bowel. Surgical excision is curative.

▪ see page 115

MALIGNANT TUMORS

Malignant tumors of the mesentery and peritoneum, which are rare, include mesothelioma (related to asbestos exposure), fibrosarcoma, and leiomyosarcoma. Symptoms and signs include vague abdominal pain and bloating caused by traction or compression of adjacent structures and intestinal obstruction. Weight loss, anorexia, and weakness can also occur. Patients with mesothelioma have chylous ascites.

Diagnosis is made with an upper GI series, barium enema, and CT, which in combination reveal extrinsic compression or signs of invasion of the small or large bowel and other local structures. Surgery is the only effective treatment for either cure or palliation. However, chemotherapy and radiation therapy may improve results for mesothelioma.

SECTION 14

MEN'S AND WOMEN'S HEALTH ISSUES

MEN/
WOM

▮114▮ SEXUALITY

The quality or state that comprises sexual desire (libido), arousal, function, and activity; physical satisfaction; and emotional intimacy.

A comprehensive survey of sexuality in the elderly has never been done in the USA. The nature and frequency of sexual activity among the elderly are unknown, as is the association between sexual activity and marital status, health status, or any other variable. Available data are from the important but now historic and limited Kinsey studies (1948 to 1949), the physiologic investigations of Masters and Johnson, the Duke Longitudinal Studies, and the Baltimore Longitudinal Study on Aging. Questionnaire surveys of self-reported sexual activity have been conducted by mail (eg, by Consumers Union). The most important conclusion is that sexuality is important to many elderly persons.

The elderly often view sexuality as an expression of passion, affection, admiration, and loyalty; a renewal of romance; a general affirmation of life, especially the expression of joy; and a continuing opportunity for growth and experience. In addition, sexual activity is a means for the elderly to affirm physical functioning, to maintain a strong sense of identity and establish self-confidence, and to prevent anxiety. It remains a mode of pure physical pleasure as well.

However, not all elderly persons have positive attitudes about sexuality. Even healthy elderly persons may internalize the negative stereotypes of elderly persons as desexualized invalids or, at the opposite extreme, as "dirty old men" or "lecherous old women." Some elderly persons show prejudice against other elderly persons and refuse to associate with them, reject an elderly partner, or attempt to appear unreasonably and inappropriately young.

Like all persons, the elderly may experience sexual dysfunction due to boredom, fear, fatigue, grief, or other factors (eg, intrinsically low sexual desire, physical disability). Sexuality in the elderly is particularly affected by problems that are common in this age group: eg, depression, **1** medical disorders, **2** or incapacitation or death of a partner. Partners are in short supply, especially for elderly women, who outlive and outnumber elderly men. Over 50% of elderly women are widows, 7% have never married, and 2% are divorced. Thus, about 60% of elderly women are without a spouse, in contrast to about 20% of elderly men. Elderly persons who have lost their partner may be reluctant to begin dating, an activity abandoned for decades, and feel unfamiliar with dating practices when opportunities arise. How to date and make new and enduring relationships can be challenging.

Negative generational attitudes about masturbation and homosexuality can interfere with sexual expression. Many elderly homosexual persons have not publicly revealed their sexual preference. Although their relationships and sexual problems are generally similar to those of heterosexual persons, homosexual persons may experience additional stress due to a perceived need to hide their sexual orientation. Those who are institutionalized may be particularly vulnerable to loneliness and isolation. Gay-oriented long-term care facilities are virtually nonexistent.

A sexual history is part of the general medical evaluation of all elderly persons. **3** Inquiry about current sexual function and activity is especially important. However, some physicians are uncomfortable discussing sexual issues with elderly persons because of ignorance, personal anxieties, negative stereotypes about the elderly, or objections to expression of sexuality by some elderly persons.

Some patients are misinformed about sexuality, and some may refuse to discuss sexual issues, about which they may harbor feelings of guilt and shame. Even if their sexual dysfunction is obvious, these persons often are unlikely to accept help. However, reassurance and information from a physician may enable some persons to achieve a more positive self-image and to express their sexual needs.

The sexual needs of elderly persons who live in nursing homes and other long-term care facilities deserve respect. These persons may be isolated from their partner, and many have severe neurologic, cardiovascular, or other impairments. As a result, sexuality in these patients may be expressed aggressively or may be accompanied by depression, dementia, or delirium. Staff must strive to understand sexual behavior and provide privacy. Medicaid and the regulations of some states and municipalities establish minimally acceptable guidelines regarding such issues as privacy for institutions.

Interdisciplinary issues: Nurses, social workers, and other health care workers may encounter patients, especially men or demented or

1 see page 310   **2** see page 1159   **3** see page 30

delirious patients, who express their sexuality aggressively. Such health care workers need training in dealing with sexual issues; they may also need to counsel sexually active patients on the appropriate time and place for sexuality and provide them the privacy to do so.

Caregiver issues: Sexual expression or activity by an elderly person may be misunderstood or unwelcomed by family members and caregivers. Family members and caregivers may benefit from information and counseling to better understand that elderly persons have sexual desires and to help the elderly meet such needs when possible (eg, by providing privacy).

AGING AND SEXUAL FUNCTION

With normal aging, persons require more time to become sexually aroused. Although some persons perceive this gradual slowing as a decline in function, others do not consider it an impairment because it merely results in men and women taking more time to achieve orgasm.

Changes in men: In addition to slowing of arousal, elderly men may notice less preejaculatory fluid and less forcefulness at ejaculation. The erection is less firm and shorter-lasting. After orgasm, elderly men take longer than younger men to achieve another erection. Unlike women, who undergo a physiologic climacteric, men often remain fertile throughout life.

Erectile dysfunction [1] is a common concern for many men. Although the incidence of erectile dysfunction increases with age, aging per se is not the cause. Drug treatment helps some men with erectile dysfunction.

Changes in women: Women usually can maintain sexual functioning throughout life unless a medical disorder intervenes. Women tend to be less concerned than men about sexual performance but are more worried about loss of youthful appearance or sexual attractiveness. The frequency of sexual activity for women often relates to the age, health, and sexual functioning of their partner (or the availability of a partner) rather than to their own sexual capacity or desire.

For women, most sexual changes occur during menopause, [2] when estrogen production slows. These changes may include atrophic vaginitis, with dryness of the vaginal mucosa leading to irritation or pain during intercourse. The ability to engage in pleasurable intercourse may be further compromised by age-related shortening and narrowing of the vagina. Less acidic vaginal secretions increase the likelihood of vaginal infections. Cystitis is more common in elderly women than in younger women because of the changes from atrophic urethritis. Decreased estrogen levels can lead to a reduction in clitoral size, stress incontinence, and an increase in facial hair. However, estrogen replacement

[1] see page 1165   [2] see page 1208

therapy[1] prevents or reduces many of these problems, and some women enjoy sexual activity more after menopause because pregnancy is not an issue.

Many women are skeptical about the benefits of estrogen, are concerned about its risks, and may experience "estrogen anxiety." The decision whether to use estrogen should be made by a woman and her physician through careful weighing of the risks and benefits.[2] Nonestrogen measures (eg, water-based vaginal lubricants such as K-Y Jelly) can help prevent or control vaginal dryness and irritation during intercourse.

EFFECTS OF MEDICAL DISORDERS ON SEXUALITY

Several medical disorders common in the elderly can affect sexual functioning, and physicians should discuss sexuality when treating patients with such disorders.

Persons who have had a myocardial infarction and those with angina or heart failure may avoid sexual activity because of concerns about risk to life. However, cardiac death during or after sexual activity is rare, and sexual activity provides an opportunity for mild exercise and release of physical and emotional tension. Cardiac evaluation can generally estimate the risk, and a physician's support and encouragement can greatly help patients for whom sexual activity is safe.

After a **myocardial infarction,** patients are usually advised to avoid sexual activity for 8 to 14 weeks, although no data support such a long abstinence. The duration of abstinence depends primarily on the patient's desire, general fitness, and conditioning. A patient's general fitness for sexual activity can be determined in several ways (eg, stress tests, ability to walk certain distances or up two flights of stairs).

Patients with **angina**[3] may be anxious and require reassurance. Sexual activity should occur in a relaxed atmosphere; it may be best in the late morning, after a full night of sleep. A supine position during intercourse can reduce the level of activity to a level of energy expenditure equivalent to climbing one flight of stairs or walking one city block. Nitroglycerin can be used to prevent or treat angina. However, men who may need to use nitrates cannot use sildenafil to treat erectile dysfunction.

When **heart failure**[4] is managed effectively, the physical exercise and emotional release associated with sexual activity may contribute to a patient's improvement. After an episode of pulmonary edema, patients are usually advised to avoid sexual activity for 2 to 3 weeks or until normal exertion (eg, climbing two flights of stairs) is possible without symptoms.

Patients with serious **arrhythmias,**[5] which can occur after exercise or exertion, may need the reassurance of successfully performing a tread-

[1] see page 1211   [2] see page 1214   [3] see page 855
[4] see page 900   [5] see page 885

mill test to overcome anxiety about engaging in sexual activity. In rare cases, arrhythmias preclude sexual activity. Persons with **hypertension**∎ need not restrict sexual activity. However, untreated hypertension and the use of some antihypertensives increase the prevalence of erectile dysfunction. The effects of hypertension and antihypertensives on sexuality in women are not as well studied as those in men. Antihypertensives should be selected to avoid impairing sexual arousal whenever possible in elderly persons who are sexually active. ∎

Sexual activity has not been shown to cause **stroke** or to increase neurologic deficit after stroke. ∎ Sexual functioning is likely to be affected, but sexual desire is not unless brain damage is severe. Some male stroke patients experience erectile dysfunction; male partners of stroke patients may also experience erectile dysfunction because they fear causing injury during sexual activity. Reassurance and advice by a physician may help the patient and partner. The unaffected side of the body should be the focus of physical stimulation during sexual activity. Patients in whom motor activity is compromised may benefit from the use of pillows, headboards, or overhead chain grips for support during sexual activity.

Men with **diabetes mellitus**∎ experience erectile dysfunction two to five times more often than does the general population, although sexual desire is unaffected. Good control of the diabetes may reestablish potency. However, if the diabetes is already well controlled, erectile dysfunction is likely irreversible.

Hypothyroidism may reduce potency.

The discomforts and disabilities of **osteoarthritis**∎ or **rheumatoid arthritis**∎ may affect sexual function. A program of exercise, rest, and warm baths reduces arthritic discomfort and facilitates sexual performance. Experimenting with sexual positions that do not aggravate joint pain is often helpful. Because osteoarthritis tends to be less severe in the morning and rheumatoid arthritis less severe in the afternoon and evening, sexual activity can be planned for times of the day when pain and stiffness are least severe. Some rheumatoid arthritis patients find that regular sexual activity relieves their pain for 4 to 8 hours, possibly because of hormone production, release of endorphins, or the physical activity involved.

The pain of chronic or recurrent **prostatitis**∎ may decrease sexual desire. Mild prostatitis may cause perineal pain after ejaculation. Therapy for chronic or recurrent prostatitis (eg, antibiotics, warm sitz baths, periodic gentle prostatic massage) may alleviate the problem.

∎see page 833   ∎see page 1163   ∎see page 397
∎see page 624   ∎see page 489   ∎see page 499   ∎see page 1186

Some women experience recurrent episodes of **cystitis** and **urethritis** after intercourse. Although these problems are usually due to the introduction of bacteria into the urethra during thrusting and are exacerbated by mucosal changes caused by atrophic urethritis, the cause may be unclear. Age-related estrogen decline may be a factor. A urologic or gynecologic evaluation is indicated to determine the cause and to plan preventive options or treatment.

About 50% of men with **Peyronie's disease** experience pain during intercourse. When the penis is angled too sharply, penetration may be impossible. However, tumescence is preserved in about 90% of patients, although some pain may occur. Treatment of Peyronie's disease may facilitate intercourse.

Men and women with **chronic renal failure** ◻ may have reduced levels of serum testosterone, although the mechanism is unknown. Patients with chronic renal failure often have diminished libido and erectile dysfunction, especially if testosterone levels are reduced. When the erectile dysfunction is associated with anxiety or depression, psychotherapy and couples counseling can be helpful. Kidney transplantation often restores potency in dialysis patients with erectile dysfunction.

In patients with **Parkinson's disease,** ◻ advanced neurologic involvement may cause erectile dysfunction. Patients with Parkinson's disease are commonly depressed, which may also lead to erectile dysfunction in men and reduced sexual desire in men and women. Sexual drive and performance improve in some men and women treated with levodopa, probably because of greater mobility and an increased sense of well-being; little evidence supports an aphrodisiac effect.

Shortness of breath in patients with **chronic emphysema** and **bronchitis** ◻ hinders physical activity, including sexual activity. Patients may improve sexual activity by resting at intervals, finding the least taxing ways to have sexual contact, and using oxygen.

EFFECTS OF SURGERY ON SEXUALITY

The rate of recovery and return to sexual activity after surgery varies. Thorough explanation of surgical procedures, practical advice, and emotional support before and after surgery can enhance recovery and the return to previous levels of sexual activity.

Candidates for **coronary artery bypass surgery** ◻ may already have sexual dysfunction due to physical symptoms, adverse effects of drug treatment, or fear of sudden death from physical exertion. After surgery, patients are usually advised to avoid sexual activity for a reasonable time (based on the type of sexual activity and the type of surgical inci-

◻ see page 962   ◻ see page 433   ◻ see page 779   ◻ see page 942

sion) to prevent straining the surgical repair. Self-stimulation or mutual masturbation may be a less strenuous alternative to intercourse and usually can be started earlier in the recovery period. Exercise programs to improve cardiac function (eg, increasingly strenuous walking or exercise in a gym) can reassure patients who are afraid to resume sexual activity. The effort involved in having intercourse can be moderated and need be no greater than that required to climb two flights of stairs.

After **hysterectomy,** patients are usually advised to avoid sexual activity for 6 to 8 weeks to allow their surgical wounds to heal. Depression is common and usually lasts a few days to a few months, although some women remain depressed much longer. Hysterectomy per se does not usually impair sexual function. However, women who are highly sensitive to cervical and uterine sensations during orgasm may be aware of the loss. Although oophorectomy decreases testosterone and other androgen levels (as well as estrogen and progesterone levels), its effects on sexuality have not been well studied. However, most women who have had a hysterectomy have also had oophorectomy; most of these women continue to be sexually active, and many, because they are relieved of the fear of pregnancy, become even more sexually active.

Mastectomy may lead some women to feel sexually mutilated. They may lose sexual desire because of embarrassment, concerns about being less feminine, or fear of being less attractive to a partner. Periodic depression is common during the first 1 or 2 years after mastectomy. Rehabilitation programs can help women and their partners deal with the physical, psychologic, and cosmetic concerns of breast surgery. Patients and their partners should be encouraged to share feelings openly and support each other emotionally.

After **prostatectomy,** patients are usually advised to avoid sexual activity for 6 weeks. Transurethral resection of the prostate, the most common form of prostatectomy, may affect potency, and retrograde ejaculation is common. At least 10% of men lose some ability to achieve an erection, although most men return to their presurgery level of sexual functioning. Most erectile dysfunction after transurethral resection of the prostate is psychologic; about 3 to 5% of men develop nonpsychologic erectile dysfunction. Suprapubic or retropubic prostate surgery may result in erectile dysfunction.

Orchiectomy in elderly men is usually performed to treat prostate cancer. Its psychologic effects can be devastating. Counseling before and after surgery is essential. Physiologic erectile dysfunction may occur, but most men can have normal erections.

In men, **removal of the rectum and anus** may result in total erectile dysfunction because of damage to nerves serving the genital organs. In women who undergo this procedure, capacity for sexual arousal and orgasm is usually retained, because essential nerves are further from the surgical site. Sexual activity is possible after colostomy or ileostomy, although the adjustment can be complex. Patients and their partners should be given medical guidance and psychologic counseling. Ostomy support groups are widely prevalent and can provide information and help.

EFFECTS OF DRUGS ON SEXUALITY

Many drugs adversely affect sexuality (see TABLES 114–1 and 114–2). Assessing the effects of drugs on sexuality is difficult in women; in men, sexual dysfunction is more obvious and measurable. In general, drugs that have an adverse effect on sexual desire in men are assumed to have an adverse effect in women as well.

Physicians should inform patients about the possibility of adverse drug effects on sexual function and encourage them to report any problems. Otherwise, patients who attribute their sexual dysfunction to drugs may discontinue the drugs or decrease the doses without informing their physician.

Drugs that dramatically affect sexuality include antipsychotics, which may inhibit erection or the ability to ejaculate, even when the capacity for erection remains; sedative-hypnotics, which can depress sexual arousal in men and women; and some antidepressants, which can inhibit sexual desire. Many antihypertensives, cardiac drugs, and other

TABLE 114–1.   POSSIBLE EFFECTS OF DRUGS ON FEMALE SEXUALITY

Effect	Drug
Increased sexual desire	Androgens, benzodiazepines (antianxiety effect), mazindol
Decreased sexual desire	Some of the drugs that decrease libido in men (see TABLE 114–2) *may* reduce libido in women. The literature on this subject is sparse
Impaired arousal and orgasm	Anticholinergics, clonidine, methyldopa, monoamine oxidase inhibitors, selective serotonin reuptake inhibitors, tricyclic antidepressants
Breast enlargement	Estrogens, penicillamine, tricyclic antidepressants
Galactorrhea (spontaneous flow of milk)	Amphetamines, chlorpromazine, cimetidine, haloperidol, heroin, methyldopa, metoclopramide, phenothiazine, reserpine, sulpiride, tricyclic antidepressants
Virilization (acne, hirsutism, lowered voice, clitoral enlargement)	Androgens, haloperidol

Adapted from Long JW: "Many common medications can affect sexual expression." *Generations* 6:32–34, 1981. Reprinted with permission from *Generations,* Journal of the American Society on Aging, 833 Market Street, Suite 512, San Francisco, California 94103. Copyright 1981, ASA.

TABLE 114–2.   POSSIBLE EFFECTS OF DRUGS ON MALE SEXUALITY

Effect	Drug
Increased sexual desire	Androgens (replacement therapy for deficiency states), baclofen (antianxiety effect), benzodiazepines (antianxiety effect), haloperidol, levodopa (may be an indirect effect due to improved sense of well-being)
Decreased sexual desire	Antihistamines, barbiturates, benzodiazepines (sedative effect), chlorpromazine (10–20% of users), cimetidine, clofibrate, clonidine (10–20% of users), disulfiram, estrogens (therapy for prostate cancer), fenfluramine, glycyrrhiza (licorice), heroin, medroxyprogesterone, methyldopa (10–15% of users), perhexiline, prazosin (15% of users), propranolol (rarely), reserpine, spironolactone, tricyclic antidepressants
Erectile dysfunction	See TABLE 115–1
Impaired ejaculation	Anticholinergics, barbiturates (when abused), chlorpromazine, clonidine, estrogens (therapy for prostate cancer), guanethidine, heroin, mesoridazine, methyldopa, monoamine oxidase inhibitors, phenoxybenzamine, phentolamine, reserpine, selective serotonin reuptake inhibitors, thiazide diuretics, thioridazine, tricyclic antidepressants
Decreased plasma testosterone levels	Barbiturates, corticotropin, digoxin, haloperidol (high doses only), lithium, marijuana, medroxyprogesterone, monoamine oxidase inhibitors, spironolactone
Impaired spermatogenesis (reduced fertility)	Adrenocorticosteroids (eg, prednisone), androgens (moderate to high dose, extended use), antimalarials, aspirin (with abuse or chronic use), chlorambucil, cimetidine, colchicine, co-trimoxazole, cyclophosphamide, estrogens (therapy for prostate cancer), marijuana, medroxyprogesterone, methotrexate, monoamine oxidase inhibitors, niridazole, nitrofurantoin, spironolactone, sulfasalazine, testosterone (moderate to high dose, with extended use)
Testicular disorders Swelling Inflammation Atrophy	Tricyclic antidepressants Oxyphenbutazone Androgens (moderate to high dose, with extended use), chlorpromazine, spironolactone
Penile disorders Priapism Peyronie's disease	Cocaine, heparin, phenothiazine Metoprolol
Gynecomastia (excessive breast enlargement)	Androgens (partial conversion to estrogen), busulfan, carmustine, chlormadinone, chlorpromazine, chlortetracycline, cimetidine, clonidine (rarely), diethylstilbestrol, digitalis and its glycosides, estrogens (therapy for prostate cancer), ethionamide, griseofulvin, haloperidol, heroin, isoniazid, marijuana, methyldopa, phenelzine, reserpine, spironolactone, thioridazine, tricyclic antidepressants, vincristine

drugs cause erectile dysfunction.∎ When drugs that affect sexual functioning cannot be avoided and sexual dysfunction results, patients may benefit from encouragement to explore other forms of intimacy and physical pleasure.

Alcohol, if used excessively, commonly causes sexual dysfunction; however, it is seldom considered a cause by the general public, because moderate use may stimulate desire and reduce inhibitions. Up to 80% of men who drink heavily experience erectile dysfunction. Alcohol's depressant action can also decrease a woman's sexual function. Many of the effects of moderate to heavy drinking are reversible if the drinking is stopped in time. Because alcohol tolerance decreases with age, the elderly are impaired by smaller amounts than younger persons. Persons who drink alcohol regularly should abstain for several hours before sexual activity and should limit themselves to 1.5 oz (45 mL) of hard liquor, 6 oz (180 mL) of wine, or 16 oz (0.5 L) of beer over 24 hours.

▮115 ▮ SEXUAL DYSFUNCTION IN MEN

Testosterone levels diminish with age, as both testosterone production and metabolic clearance decrease. These hormonal alterations lead to loss of libido, decreased muscle strength, alterations in memory, diminished energy and well-being, and possibly osteoporosis. Testosterone appears to influence the frequency of nocturnal erections; however, low testosterone levels do not affect erections produced by erotic stimuli. Indeed, few if any definitive signs or symptoms of androgen deficiency may be apparent in men, in contrast to those seen in women at menopause, when female sex hormone levels fall.

Aging, rather than androgen deficiency per se, is associated with a diminution of sperm quality and quantity, although spermatogenesis does not completely cease.

ERECTILE DYSFUNCTION

(Impotence)

The inability to develop and sustain an erection sufficient for satisfactory sexual intercourse in 50% or more attempts at intercourse.

Once a rarely discussed topic, erectile dysfunction is now a topic of general conversation. Awareness and openness have been driven in

---

∎ see below

large part by the availability of new treatments and the coverage of these treatments by the media.

Erectile dysfunction may occur from time to time at any age for a variety of reasons. However, the incidence of persistent erectile dysfunction increases with age. The prevalence is about 52% among men aged 40 to 70 and even greater among older men. The prevalence is nearly 95% among men > 70 who have certain medical disorders such as diabetes.

Physiology

Penile erection is accomplished through engorgement of the corpora cavernosa, two spongiform, intercommunicative, highly vascular bodies surrounded by a tough, fibrous sheath (the tunica albuginea). The parenchyma of each corpus cavernosum consists of trabecular smooth muscle with a network of endothelial cells that line vascular spaces and helicine arteries. The combination of vascular engorgement and ischiocavernous muscle contraction leads to rigidity. Erection occurs when arterial blood flow into the corpora cavernosa exceeds venous outflow. The pudendal artery supplies blood to the corpora, and blood flow is controlled by relaxation and contraction of arterial smooth muscle, which in turn is under the influence of a variety of neurotransmitters such as nitric oxide, vasoactive intestinal peptide, and neuropeptide Y. When the smooth muscle relaxes, arterial filling occurs.

Venous drainage occurs through venules below the tunica albuginea. Unlike other venous structures, penile venules have no valves; these venules close by compression against the tunica, as the corpora fill with blood.

The T11 through L2 (sympathetic) nerves, S2 through S4 (parasympathetic) nerves, and somatic nerves (sensory and motor) innervate the penis.

Etiology and Pathogenesis

Causes of erectile dysfunction include vascular, neurologic, and endocrine disorders; structural abnormalities of the penis; the adverse effects of drugs; and psychologic disorders. It is most common to have more than one cause of erectile dysfunction (multifactorial etiology).

Vascular disorders: Of all causes of erectile dysfunction, vascular disorders are the most common among the elderly. This is not surprising for a population in whom atherosclerotic disease is prevalent. Arterial insufficiency, excessive venous outflow, or both can affect sexual function. Arterial disease is the most common finding, especially in elderly men with hypercholesterolemia, diabetes, peripheral vascular disease, or hypertension and in those who smoke. Any impairment of the arterial supply to the corpora cavernosa—such as from atherosclerosis, a clot, or loss of distensibility of a vessel wall—can lead to erectile dysfunction. Venous leakage (excessive venous outflow due to inadequate compression of the venous drainage of the corpora cavernosa) also is common with aging.

Neurologic disorders: Penile sensitivity tends to diminish with age and may contribute to erectile dysfunction, as local stimulation plays a role in erectile response. Peripheral and autonomic neuropathy and the alteration of neurotransmitters due to diabetes can cause erectile dysfunction in the elderly. Rarely, the nerves of the penis are impaired because of lumbar disk disease or, more commonly, surgical procedures such as rectal surgery and prostatectomy. Multiple sclerosis, stroke, and other neurologic diseases can also cause erectile dysfunction.

Endocrine disorders: The most common endocrine disorder in older men is the ADAM (*A*ndrogen *D*eficiency in the *A*ging *M*ale) syndrome, which is nontumor-related hypogonadism of aging. Relatively uncommon diseases and disorders associated with primary testicular failure (eg, Klinefelter's syndrome, radiation, chemotherapy, or childhood exposure to mumps) can cause erectile problems. Secondary testicular failure due to pituitary or adrenal tumors or other endocrine disorders (eg, hyperprolactinemia due to chronic renal failure) can cause extremely low testosterone levels and, in rare cases, lead to erectile dysfunction. Hyperthyroidism, hypothyroidism, and Cushing's disease are also possible causes of erectile dysfunction.

Structural abnormalities: Peyronie's disease can make intercourse difficult or contribute to venous leaks, which may lead to erectile dysfunction. The disease is characterized by bands or plaques in the tunica albuginea, which lead to a "deformed" erection. Peyronie's disease is not an uncommon cause of erectile dysfunction in the elderly.

Drugs: About 25% of cases of erectile dysfunction are caused by drugs (see TABLE 115–1), especially antihypertensives (most notably reserpine, β-blockers, guanethidine, and methyldopa), alcohol, cimetidine, antipsychotics, antidepressants, lithium, sedative-hypnotics, leuprolide, and hormones such as estrogen and progesterone. In addition, many drugs can impair sexual function in men, especially elderly men, by altering libido (eg, cimetidine, diazepam), inhibiting ejaculatory function (eg, most tricyclic antidepressants such as amitriptyline, clomipramine, doxepin, nortriptyline), or delaying or inhibiting orgasm (eg, selective serotonin reuptake inhibitors such as fluoxetine). However, trazodone has been found to improve libido and facilitate erectile function, but it does not have a specific therapeutic role in erectile dysfunction. Priapism can be an adverse effect.

Psychologic disorders: Among the elderly, most erectile dysfunction is organic rather than psychologic. Psychologic disorders alone probably account for only 10% of cases. However, psychologic and organic factors are often intermixed. Anxiety over an organic cause often aggravates erectile dysfunction. Depression can cause erectile dysfunction, and erectile dysfunction can worsen depression. Elderly

TABLE 115-1. DRUGS THAT MAY CAUSE ERECTILE DYSFUNCTION

Anticonvulsants	Drugs affecting the CNS (*continued*)
Anti-infective drugs	Levodopa
Cardiovascular drugs	Lithium
Antiarrhythmics	Narcotics
Antihypertensives	Gastrointestinal drugs
Adrenergic blockers (centrally or	Anticholinergics and antispasmodics
peripherally acting)	H₂ blockers
β-Blockers	Metoclopramide
Calcium channel blockers	Miscellaneous drugs
Clonidine	Acetazolamide
Direct vasodilators	Baclofen
Diuretics	Cimetidine
Reserpine	Clofibrate
Drugs affecting the CNS	Danazol
Alcohol	Disulfiram
Anxiolytics and sedative-hypnotics	Estrogens
Antidepressants	Interferon
Antipsychotics	Leuprolide
CNS stimulants	Naproxen
Cocaine	Progesterone

CNS = central nervous system.

Adapted from Stanisic TH, Francisco GE: "Impotence," in *Geriatric Pharmacology,* edited by R Bressler and MD Katz. New York, McGraw-Hill, 1993, p. 272.

men may experience performance anxiety, particularly when having sexual intercourse with a new partner.

Diagnosis

Elderly men may seek help for erectile dysfunction; physicians can make patients feel comfortable by explaining that erectile dysfunction is common and by offering reassurance that effective treatments are available. In private, patients should be asked if they would like to discuss the matter with or without their sexual partner present. It is extremely valuable to have the partner's perspective and to understand the issues that may arise for the partner with resumption of sexual function. Because many men would not otherwise seek medical attention, physicians can use this opportunity to also focus on the management of related disorders (eg, diabetes, hypertension, dyslipidemia, smoking, alcohol abuse). The probability of atherosclerotic disease and the possibility of coronary artery disease should be evaluated.

The physician begins the history by establishing whether the problem does indeed relate to erection, rather than ejaculation, orgasm, or partner-related issues, as well as establishing the setting and frequency with which erectile dysfunction occurs. Assessment should be made as to whether libido is intact. A series of questions can be asked to help assess for androgen deficiency (see TABLE 115–2). Establishing a history of diabetes, hypertension, or vascular disease is also helpful. A review of all medications used, including over-the-counter drugs, and a review of alcohol use are essential. Assessment for depression, anxiety, and psychologic stress should be performed. The physician should also ask about the sexual partner's health or other issues in the patient's relationships that may affect sexual functioning. Establishing the presence of nocturnal or morning erections is not especially helpful in older men, as it does not necessarily predict either functional ability or organic vs. psychologic causes.

The physical examination should include a search for signs of vascular disease (eg, diminished peripheral and femoral pulses, bruits, skin changes), autonomic neuropathy (eg, absent bulbocavernosus and cremasteric reflexes, orthostatic hypotension), and peripheral neuropathy. The genitalia should be thoroughly examined, checking for testicular atrophy and the plaques or bands that signify Peyronie's disease.

Intracavernosal injection of prostaglandin E_1 to assess penile vascular function is not always diagnostically accurate. For example, severe anxiety may override a response to this test. Abnormal penile brachial artery pressure indexes obtained while the patient is supine and after the patient has exercised (eg, bicycling legs in the air for 3 to 5 minutes) can help establish whether vascular insufficiency is a cause. In men without a history of coronary artery disease or stroke, an abnormal penile brachial pressure index predicts an increased risk of myocardial infarction, stroke, or both.

Bioavailable or free testosterone as well as total testosterone levels should be measured, and other tests performed (eg, CBC, fasting blood glucose, thyroid-stimulating hormone level). Measurement of nocturnal penile tumescence is of little value in distinguishing organic from psy-

TABLE 115–2.   QUESTIONNAIRE FOR ASSESSING ANDROGEN DEFICIENCY IN ELDERLY MEN*

1. Is your libido (sex drive) decreased?
2. Do you feel a lack of energy?
3. Is your strength or endurance decreased?
4. Have you lost height?
5. Have you noticed a decreased "enjoyment of life"?
6. Are you sad or grumpy?
7. Are your erections less strong?
8. Have you noticed a recent deterioration in your athletic ability?
9. Do you fall asleep after dinner?
10. Have you noticed a recent deterioration in your work performance?

*A positive response to question 1 or 7 or positive responses to any 3 questions constitutes reason to assess for hypogonadism.

Adapted from Morley JE: "Androgen deficiency in aging men." *Medical Clinics of North America* 83: 1279, 1999.

chologic erectile dysfunction in elderly men and generally should not be performed.

Treatment

The treatment of erectile dysfunction has changed radically in the past few years. The choice of therapy depends on the patient's goals and desires and on the risks of a given option. The least invasive form of therapy should be the first choice in treatment.

Pharmacotherapy: Drugs are available to treat erectile dysfunction and may be used without regard to the cause of dysfunction, although efficacy may differ. **Sildenafil** (50 to 100 mg given 1 hour before a sexual encounter) helps produce erections, but only when the patient is sexually stimulated. Sildenafil has relative selectivity for inhibition of type V phosphodiesterase, which inhibits breakdown of cyclic guanosine monophosphate, resulting in vasodilation. However, inhibition of type III and type VI phosphodiesterase may occur, which can affect cardiac function and vision, especially color vision. Because sildenafil can cause severe hypotension when nitrates are used concurrently, it is contraindicated in patients who take nitrates to relieve angina and in those with significant heart disease. Sildenafil can also cause headaches, flushing, and dyspepsia.

Alprostadil (prostaglandin E_1) can be given by intraurethral pellet or intracavernosal injection with or without papaverine phentolamine. Alprostadil causes vasodilation via smooth muscle relaxation and thus improves blood flow, leading to erection. About 5 to 20 minutes after insertion of the pellet or injection, the patient should initiate sexual activity. Under ideal conditions, an erection can last up to 60 minutes. Common adverse effects include a penile burning sensation and aching. Priapism can occur but is less common when the drug is given by intraurethral pellet. Priapism lasting longer than 4 to 6 hours can result in penile ischemic necrosis and fibrosis.

Drugs such as **yohimbine** have not been shown to be more efficacious than placebo in randomized controlled trials, and use of this drug is not recommended. **Testosterone therapy**◫ may benefit some men whose erectile dysfunction is due to hypogonadism or when libido is at issue.

Nonpharmacologic measures: **Constriction rings,** which are made of rubber, slow venous outflow at the base of the penis and may be useful for men who can obtain erections but cannot sustain them. These devices can be purchased from medical supply houses, pharmacies, or stores that sell sexual paraphernalia. Constriction rings can produce local discomfort and, if too tight, difficulty with ejaculation.

Vacuum tumescent devices increase penile engorgement by creating a vacuum or negative pressure, which draws blood into the penis. These devices consist of a plastic cylinder, placed over the flaccid penis, and a

◫see page 1173

pump mechanism. Once an erection occurs, a wide rubber band or ring (constriction ring) is applied at the base of the penis, and the vacuum device is removed. The band retards venous return and helps sustain the erection for up to 30 minutes. Vacuum devices can produce petechiae and make the tip of the penis slightly cooler than usual.

Permanent penile prostheses or implants may be helpful when erectile dysfunction does not respond to other treatment modalities. A prosthesis produces an erection but does not correct phenomena such as impaired penile sensation. Devices that produce a permanent erection include the Small Carrion semirigid rod prosthesis with a silicone sponge interior and the Flexi-Rod II, a hinged modification of the Small Carrion device that allows the penis to appear more physiologically flaccid when not being used for sexual activity. An inflatable prosthesis (AMS 700 CX) is also available. However, the more complicated the device, the greater the risk of mechanical breakdown and infection. Patients should also be aware that if the prosthesis must be removed, the patient could be left with penile scarring and fibrosis, which may lessen response to other therapeutic options.

Penile revascularization surgery (especially arterial) is relatively experimental and has not been found to have high success rates. With venous disease, ligation surgery may afford benefit in the short run, but < 30% of such operations have an effect that lasts > 5 years.

Patient Issues

When the cause of erectile dysfunction is psychologic, reassurance by the physician or the patient's partner may be helpful. However, some psychologic issues such as depression and anxiety may require psychotherapy, counseling, or medication. Medicare pays 50% of the allowable charges for psychotherapy performed by a physician, psychologist, or social worker.

MALE HYPOGONADISM

Inadequate testicular androgen production resulting in a bioavailable testosterone level < 70 ng/dL (2.4 nmol/L), which can be associated with loss of libido, diminished muscle mass and muscle strength, and altered energy and well-being.

Androgen deficiency in the aging male (ADAM syndrome) is common; at least half of men ≥ 50 have levels of bioavailable testosterone well below those of healthy younger men. Testosterone declines with age (by about 100 ng/dL [3.5 nmol/L] per decade after age 50), but bioavailable testosterone (nonsex hormone–binding globulin [non-SHBG] bound testosterone) as well as free testosterone (non-SHBG, non–albumin-bound testosterone) decline far more dramatically. Sex hormone–binding globulin increases with age.

Although a decreased number of Leydig's cells and decreased testosterone production and clearance rate occur with age, the decline in male hormones is generally not accompanied by the expected rise in luteinizing hormone (LH), suggesting a defect at the level of the hypothalamus or pituitary rather than at the testicular level. Loss of diurnal rhythmicity occurs for LH, testosterone, and bioavailable testosterone with age. Both pulse amplitude and frequency decrease with age. Decreased feedforward stimulation by LH and delayed feedback inhibition by testosterone occur in elderly men. Thus, the majority of elderly men with hypogonadism have secondary, rather than primary, gonadal deficiency. Alterations in gonadotropin-releasing hormone appear to play a key role in the hormonal changes. An age-related increase in prolactin can result in inhibition of gonadotropins at the hypothalamic and pituitary levels.

Relatively rare causes of hypogonadism may include drug use, exposure to toxins, and medical disorders (see TABLE 115–3). With Sertoli cell failure associated with age, follicle-stimulating hormone levels rise, unlike the response to changes in Leydig's cells. Loss of sperm quality and quantity can be noted with age.

Symptoms and Signs

Hypogonadism in elderly men generally has few or nonspecific symptoms or physical findings. The most common symptom is decreased libido, which is directly related to testosterone (and bioavailable testosterone) levels. Although potency is not dependent on testosterone levels, severe impairment of libido causes erectile dysfunction.

TABLE 115–3.   CAUSES OF HYPOGONADISM

Drug use	Medical disorders
Acetate	Acute stress (eg, due to surgery,
Cimetidine	severe burns)
Ethanol	Androgen resistance
Heroin	Chronic renal failure
Ketoconazole	Cirrhosis
Medroxyprogesterone	Collagen vascular diseases
Methadone	Cushing's syndrome
Omeprazole	Diabetes
Ranitidine	Hemochromatosis
Spironolactone	Kallmann's syndrome
	Klinefelter's syndrome
	Mumps orchitis
Exposure to toxins	Myotonic dystrophy
Chemotherapy	Panhypopituitarism/pituitary tumor
Heavy metals	Sarcoidosis
Organic solvents	Testicular trauma
Radiation therapy	Tuberculosis

Male hypogonadism can also lead to fatigue, loss of energy, muscle weakness, and a decreased sense of well-being, which may manifest as depression. Although animal studies suggest that male hypogonadism reduces coronary artery blood flow, the effect in humans is unknown. Muscle mass, which decreases with age (resulting in sarcopenia), can be associated with weakness, immobility, and impaired gait and balance. Muscle mass and balance correlate with the level of bioavailable or free testosterone. Severe prolonged hypogonadism leads to loss of body hair and masculine habitus; small, soft testes; and a loss of scrotal pigmentation and rugae. Bone loss has been associated with hypogonadism; however, an independent non–age-related link of testosterone and bone mass is difficult to demonstrate. It is possible that the lack of substrate (testosterone) for aromatization to estrogen plays a role in osteoporosis in aging men.

Laboratory Findings

Bioavailable testosterone levels < 70 ng/dL (< 2.4 nmol/L) or total testosterone levels < 300 ng/dL (< 10.4 nmol/L) are diagnostic of male hypogonadism. Measuring bioavailable or free testosterone is more sensitive than measuring total testosterone because the sex hormone–binding globulin bound fraction increases with age.

LH levels are normal or low in most hypogonadal men. Dynamic testing with gonadotropin-releasing hormone adds little information, because the response is usually proportional to the basal LH level. A normal prolactin level helps exclude a pituitary tumor as the cause of male hypogonadism. Laboratory findings may show anemia.

Treatment

Male hypogonadism is treated with testosterone therapy. Other androgens, such as dehydroepiandrosterone, are not recommended for therapy. The type and dose of testosterone are somewhat controversial. However, intramuscular formulations are generally preferred. The oral testosterones available in the USA (17-α alkylated compounds) may cause hepatotoxicity, with elevation of hepatic enzymes, and occasionally cholestatic jaundice and hepatic tumors. Oral 17-β testosterone (eg, testosterone undecenoate) has less hepatotoxicity than oral 17-α alkylated compounds, but it is not available in the USA. Thus, testosterone injections—given by a visiting nurse, the patient, or a family member—are a mainstay of treatment. Long-acting esters of testosterone (eg, enanthate, cypionate) are usually given IM in dosages of 200 mg every 2 weeks.

Transdermal testosterone patches (applied to the scrotum or elsewhere) are effective. However, skin rashes and high cost make this modality a second choice.

In most cases, testosterone therapy clearly improves libido, muscle strength, sense of well-being, and mood. Cognitive performance is highly linked to bioavailable testosterone levels, and testosterone therapy has been shown to improve visual spatial memory in middle-aged men. Testosterone therapy stimulates erythropoietin secretion, increasing the Hct. The polycythemia that may occur with testosterone therapy is independent of the baseline erythropoietin level and is neither dose-dependent nor duration-dependent. Use of testosterone may raise the prostate-specific antigen level, but development or exacerbation of obstructive prostatic symptoms is rare. Patients with elevated or borderline levels of prostate-specific antigen probably should not be treated with testosterone until prostate cancer has been ruled out. However, for many patients, the benefit may outweigh the risk, so therapy may be appropriate after careful consideration and with close monitoring. Gynecomastia (due to aromatization to estrogen) and water retention may occur. A negative effect on the lipid profile has not been found with testosterone replacement for hypogonadism in elderly men. Studies showing benefit and safety are continuing to accrue, and the risk/benefit ratio for each patient must be assessed.

116 ■ SEXUAL DYSFUNCTION IN WOMEN

A person's need for intimacy and closeness to another does not end at any age. Sexual function is an important quality-of-life issue for all women and is influenced by many factors, including culture, ethnicity, emotional state, age, previous sexual experiences, medical disorders, ❶ and drug use. ❷ Changes in sexual response associated with normal aging (see TABLE 116–1), medical disorders, incapacitation or death of a partner, or environment (eg, lack of privacy) are problems but not dysfunction per se. The cause of sexual dysfunction is usually multifactorial. Less is known about sexual function in elderly women than in elderly men; the interplay of emotional state, relationship issues, and physiology in women is complex and has not been completely elucidated. Dysfunction can be defined as the persistent impediment to a person's normal pattern of sexual interest, response, or both.

The Sexual History

Sexual function, one of the most important quality-of-life factors, should be assessed as part of the comprehensive care of a patient. It should be evaluated within the context of sexual orientation, psychologic and medical disorders, social situation, drug use (including over-

TABLE 116–1. AGE-RELATED CHANGES IN THE SEXUAL RESPONSE CYCLE IN WOMEN

Phase	Normal Response	Age-Related Change
Desire (libido)	Stimulation of the CNS center by testosterone, other neurotransmitters, sensory stimuli, or memory	No reduction or mild reduction in interest, intensity, frequency, and fantasy
Excitement and plateau	Genital vasocongestion, clitoral engorgement, vaginal lubrication, nipple erection, areolar engorgement, tenting (dilation) of vaginal vault	Reduction and delay in genital vasocongestion, clitoral engorgement, vaginal lubrication, and tenting of vaginal vault; decrease in tactile sensitivity of breasts and genitalia
Orgasm	Pubococcygeal muscle spasms; contractions of the vagina, uterus, rectum, and lower abdomen; increased blood pressure, heart rate, and respiration; multiorgasmic capacity	Reduction in frequency, weaker contractions
Resolution	Reduction in vasocongestion and muscle tension; absent or limited refractory period	More rapid reduction in vasocongestion and muscle tension

the-counter drugs), environmental issues, partner issues, frequency, and satisfaction. Women define normal sexual activity for themselves based on past experiences, self-esteem, presence or absence of medical disorders, and partner issues. Health care practitioners must be careful not to interject their opinion on what constitutes acceptable sexual practice. For example, the continued sexual interest and activity of an 80- or 90-year-old woman, viewed as perfectly normal by her, might be misunderstood by her health care practitioners or others. Because sexual function is often measured only by frequency of intercourse, persons who live alone, have an incapacitated partner, have health problems, are lesbian, or practice masturbation may be erroneously regarded as sexually inactive. In addition, touching, fondling, kissing, holding, and other important components of sexual activity are rarely considered by health care practitioners.

The sexual history can be incorporated into the medical history.∎ Although many physicians lack training in sexual health, they should not avoid this subject because this area of health assessment is becom-

∎see page 30

ing more important for all women, not just older women. The sexual history should address the woman's interest in sex, frequency of spontaneous sexual thoughts and fantasies, frequency of masturbation, self-esteem, attraction to self and others, and past or present relationship issues. The patient's responses help determine whether the problem is situational. Questions should be nonjudgmental; asking "Do you have any problem with your ability to have sex?" or "Are you satisfied with your sex life?" indicates to the patient that the physician is willing to discuss this subject, even if no problem exists. A woman who acknowledges a problem should be further asked about how the problem began and how it affects her sexual activity and response and those of her partner. In both men and women, depression can cause sexual dysfunction, which can in turn cause depression. Thus, an assessment as to whether depression is a component should also be undertaken. Interviewing the partner may provide additional perspective on the nature of the problem.

The sexual history provides an opportunity to reinforce issues related to general health as well as to sexually transmitted diseases. An elderly person who has lost a spouse or long-term partner may not have had to deal with these issues previously and should be reminded about safe sex practices.

DECREASED LIBIDO

Decreased sexual drive.

Libido appears to be testosterone-dependent in both women and men. In women, ovarian hormones and adrenal androgens begin to decrease in the years preceding menopause. A decrease or loss of libido along with a diminished sense of well-being, loss of energy, and loss of bone mass can result.

Causes of decreased libido include low bioavailable testosterone (ie, testosterone not bound to sex hormone–binding globulin), elevated prolactin, and, indirectly, decreased estrogen. Additionally, use of alcohol or drugs may affect sexuality in women.⬛ The literature on the effect of drugs on libido in women is scant; however, anticonvulsants such as carbamazepine, phenytoin, primidone, and phenobarbital and anti-cancer drugs such as tamoxifen may decrease sex drive. Newer antidepressants (eg, selective serotonin reuptake inhibitors) may inhibit libido, arousal, and orgasm. Incontinence can also decrease libido and inhibit arousal.

In evaluating decreased libido in women, as in men, the physician should measure bioavailable testosterone levels rather than total testosterone levels. Sex hormone–binding globulin levels tend to increase with age, and total testosterone levels may not reflect what is actually

---

⬛ see TABLE 114–1 on page 1163

active in the body. Bioavailable testosterone measures the nonsex hormone–binding globulin bound portion of testosterone. Women with decreased libido may benefit from androgen therapy if baseline testosterone levels are low. Most data regarding testosterone use are from studies of women who have undergone oophorectomy; however, testosterone may increase sexual interest and frequency of fantasy even in women with natural menopause. Oral 17α-alkylated testosterone (the only oral form of testosterone available in the USA) may be used in combination with estrogen. Adverse effects of oral 17α-alkylated testosterone include hepatotoxicity, potential long-term increases in cardiovascular risk (even if the lipid profile remains normal), and virilization (eg, hirsutism, acne, lowered voice). Ideally, 17β-alkylated testosterone is used. When giving low-dose intramuscular testosterone enanthate or cypionate (eg, 25 mg every 2 to 4 weeks), the physician should monitor clinical response as well as bioavailable testosterone levels and Hct. Subcutaneous use of testosterone pellets is rare in the USA; long-term use of testosterone has not been established. Duration of treatment depends on response and whether withdrawal of testosterone results in recurrence of problems. Currently, there are no long-term (> 5 years) prospective data on testosterone use in women.

SEXUAL AROUSAL DISORDER

Persistent or recurrent inability to attain or to maintain the response of sexual excitement until the completion of sexual activity.

Sexual arousal disorder may occur during and after menopause, when vaginal lubrication and elasticity decrease because of decreased estrogen levels. Menopausal women who regularly engage in sexual intercourse maintain a greater degree of vaginal lubrication and tissue integrity, even without estrogen replacement therapy, than women who do not.

One cause of sexual arousal disorder is use of certain drugs (eg, anticholinergic drugs, tricyclic antidepressants, many forms of chemotherapy), which may decrease vaginal lubrication. Altered (decreased) cholinergic effect may be involved in some women with diabetes. Pelvic radiation therapy or surgery, stress, and anxiety can also cause loss of lubrication. Although vascular disease is a primary cause of erectile dysfunction in men, its effects in women (eg, decreased vaginal lubrication, decreased clitoral and genital engorgement) are less clear; these effects do not fully explain sexual arousal disorder in women, and therapy with sildenafil directed at improving blood flow to the vagina does not necessarily improve sexual function.

For menopausal women with inadequate lubrication, the use of oral or transdermal estrogen therapy may provide relief. If this approach is contraindicated or inadequate, use of a water-soluble lubricant that simulates natural lubrication or use of an intravaginal estrogen ring may be of benefit. The use of erotic materials (eg, books, movies) or sex toys (eg, vibrators) may enhance arousal.

FEMALE ORGASMIC DISORDER

Persistent or recurrent delay or absence of orgasm (with release of muscular tension) following normal excitement phase of sexual activity that is assessed as adequate in focus, intensity, and duration.

Female orgasmic disorder may occur in women of any age. It can be due to psychologic causes (eg, depression**1**) but may be due to organic causes or to drugs.**2** For women who have undergone a hysterectomy, the loss of uterine contractions may impair the occurrence or intensity of orgasm. For women with cancer who have undergone a hysterectomy with radiation therapy to the pelvis, female orgasmic disorder may be more pronounced; anorgasmia may be accompanied by or caused by decreased libido, vaginal dryness, and dyspareunia. In contrast, sexual function in women who have had severe pain, cramping, and bleeding related to menstrual periods may improve after a hysterectomy.

Evaluation should include questions regarding history of sexual abuse or rape, presence of difficulties in sexual technique (eg, inadequate foreplay), and problems with a partner. Physical examination assists in the evaluation of an organic cause.

Any psychologic or organic disorder should be treated. Discussion with a counselor or partner, engaging in noncoital stimulation, focusing on foreplay and arousal, and ensuring appropriate lubrication may help alleviate female orgasmic disorder.

DYSPAREUNIA

Painful intercourse or pain with attempted intercourse.

About one third of sexually active women > 65 report dyspareunia. Causes include inadequate vaginal lubrication, irritation and dryness of the external genitalia, vulvovaginitis, local trauma (eg, episiotomy scars), urethritis, improper intromission (angle of entry), anorectal disease, altered anatomy of the female genital tract (eg, a retroverted or prolapsed uterus), and even arthritis.

A general medical and sexual history and a physical and pelvic examination usually uncover the cause. Determining if dyspareunia occurs during foreplay, intromission, deep penetration, or certain positions can

1 see page 310   **2** see TABLE 114–1 on page 1163

help in the differential diagnosis. For example, dyspareunia during deep penetration may indicate lesions of the uterus or broad ligament. Management involves treatment of the underlying cause. Because dyspareunia is often caused by atrophic vaginitis, a trial of topical estrogen or an estrogen ring is often warranted. Education and guidance in sexual techniques may also be helpful. For example, dyspareunia in a woman with arthritis of the hips may be alleviated if partners lie on their sides ("spoon fashion") rather than with the woman supine during intercourse to reduce weight and pressure on the hips.

VAGINISMUS

Involuntary painful contraction (spasm) of the lower vaginal muscles.

Vaginismus may relate to dyspareunia. It may be triggered by fear of losing control or of being hurt during intercourse, by a vaginal infection, or by vaginal mucosal irritation. Observation of an involuntary vaginal spasm during pelvic examination confirms the diagnosis, but a pelvic examination may not even be possible in the presence of severe vaginismus.

Painful physical disorders should be corrected. Emotional relaxation techniques and pelvic muscular exercises (eg, voluntary contraction and relaxation of the pubococcygeal and muscles of the introitus) can help reduce muscular spasm. Gradual dilation of the vagina should be performed by the patient, partner, physician, or sex therapist using fingers or a dilator. Intercourse can be attempted after the patient has tolerated insertion of at least 3 fingers or a large dilator without discomfort.

117 ■ MALE GENITAL DISORDERS

DISORDERS OF THE PROSTATE

BENIGN PROSTATIC HYPERPLASIA

(Benign Prostatic Hypertrophy)

Nonmalignant enlargement of the prostate gland with age.

Benign prostatic hyperplasia (BPH) is clinically evident in 50% of men by age 50 and in 80% by age 80. Androgens, particularly dihydrotestosterone, appear to play a major role.

Hyperplasia of the prostate, with subsequent increase in the fibromuscular stroma, results in a narrowing of the urethral lumen as it traverses the prostate (static component). This narrowing creates bladder outlet obstruction. In addition, prostatic smooth muscle tone, mediated through α-adrenergic receptors, creates further bladder outlet obstruction (dynamic component).

Symptoms, Signs, and Diagnosis

Symptoms of bladder outlet obstruction due to BPH include hesitancy, weakness of urinary stream, intermittency, and a feeling of incomplete bladder emptying. The bladder tends to become more irritable, manifested by urinary frequency, nocturia, and urgency. Urinary symptoms may be evaluated using the American Urological Association Symptom Score (see TABLE 117–1).

Initial evaluation should also include a history and digital rectal examination along with urinalysis and measurement of the serum creatinine level. Digital rectal examination may disclose enlargement of the gland, prostatic firmness, or a nodule, which increases the suspicion of prostate cancer.

A blood test to measure serum creatinine should be performed to assess kidney function. A urinalysis that reveals > 4 red blood cells per high-power field in uninfected urine requires intravenous urography and cystoscopy to rule out kidney or bladder cancer. An abdominal ultrasound may help differentiate obstructive from renal causes of an elevated creatinine level. Further diagnostic testing (eg, uroflowmetry, postvoid residuals, more complex urodynamic evaluation) may also be necessary.

Measurement of serum prostate-specific antigen (PSA) ◨ is not part of the diagnostic evaluation of BPH but may help exclude prostate cancer as a cause of urinary tract obstruction.

Treatment

BPH should be treated when symptoms are sufficiently bothersome or when evaluation discloses recurrent urinary tract infection or an increased creatinine level. Absolute indications for treatment, such as refractory urinary retention, are discussed below. Treatment usually starts with drug treatment. However, for patients with urinary retention, surgery may be appropriate initial treatment, because it maximally reduces outflow resistance.

Drug treatment: Drug treatment usually results in minimal objective improvement but significant symptomatic improvement. Selective and uroselective **α-blockers** reduce the dynamic component of obstruction. Selective α-blockers block α_{1a} and α_{1b} subtypes equally. By blocking the α_{1a} receptors of smooth muscle at the bladder neck, these drugs decrease outlet resistance. By blocking α_{1b} receptors, these drugs may cause cardiovascular adverse effects, particularly hypotension. Dose

◨see page 1183

TABLE 117-1.   AMERICAN UROLOGICAL ASSOCIATION SYMPTOM SCORE*
FOR BENIGN PROSTATIC HYPERPLASIA

Over the past 1 month or so	Never	< 20% of the Time	< 50% of the Time	About 50% of the Time	> 50% of the Time	Almost Always
How often have you had a sensation of not emptying your bladder completely after you finished urinating?	0	1	2	3	4	5
How often have you had to urinate again in < 2 hours after you finished urinating?	0	1	2	3	4	5
How often have you stopped and started again several times when urinating?	0	1	2	3	4	5
How often have you found it difficult to postpone urination?	0	1	2	3	4	5
How often has your urinary stream been weak?	0	1	2	3	4	5
How often have you had to push or strain to begin urination?	0	1	2	3	4	5

	None	1 Time	2 Times	3 Times	4 Times	≥ 5 Times
How many times do you most typically get up to urinate between going to bed at night and waking in the morning?	0	1	2	3	4	5

*A score of 0 to 7 indicates mild symptoms, 8 to 19 indicates moderate symptoms, and 20 to 35 indicates severe symptoms.

Adapted from Barry MJ, Fowler FJ, O'Leary MP, et al: "The American Urological Association Symptom Index for benign prostatic hyperplasia." *Journal of Urology* 148:1549, 1992.

titration over several weeks avoids hypotensive episodes. Uroselective α-blockers have at least a 30-times greater affinity for $α_{1a}$ over $α_{1b}$ subtypes. They do not, therefore, require dose titration and have little effect on blood pressure.

Terazosin and doxazosin are selective α-blockers; they are available in titration packs, which may make prescribing easier. The drugs are taken once a day at bedtime, thereby minimizing adverse effects of postural hypotension (in 6 to 8% of cases) and tiredness (in 6 to 10%). Other adverse effects include asthenia (in 6 to 10%) and dizziness (in 5 to 10%). Adverse effects tend to be minor and reversible through dose reduction. Tamsulosin is a uroselective α-blocker. The dosage is 0.4 mg daily, one-half hour after the same meal each day. The incidence of cardiovascular adverse effects is low. In responsive patients, symptoms generally improve within a few days.

The **5-α-reductase inhibitor** finasteride inhibits the conversion of testosterone to dihydrotestosterone. It shrinks overall gland size, thus reducing the static component of obstruction, and decreases obstructive events and the need for surgery in glands > 50 g. A 3-month trial is necessary to determine if finasteride is effective. The adverse effects of finasteride are minimal. About 5% of patients develop sexual dysfunction (ie, decreased libido, decreased ejaculatory volumes, erectile dysfunction). Finasteride also causes a 50% reduction in the serum PSA level; thus, a normal PSA level in men treated with finasteride is one half that of men not treated with this drug.

Minimally invasive therapy: New ablative technologies do not require that patients be hospitalized or given general or regional anesthesia. The effectiveness of these technologies is being evaluated. These technologies use different energies (eg, microwave, radiofrequency, ultrasound) to destroy prostatic tissue. A transurethral device (catheter) is placed after the patient is given local anesthesia or conscious sedation, and the surrounding prostatic tissue is heated to 60 to 100° C (140 to 212° F), causing tissue death. Cystoscopy performed months after an ablative procedure often does not show much obvious visual improvement; however, follow-up over several years has found sustained efficacy using subjective factors (eg, urinary frequency, nocturia).

An intraprostatic stent (a titanium alloy mesh tube) can be placed under local anesthesia inside the prostatic urethra, opening the urethra. Its placement has been suggested for elderly debilitated men poorly able to undergo anesthesia. Unfortunately, if an infection develops within the stent, surgical removal would be necessary. Surgical removal may be traumatic and challenging, requiring regional or general anesthesia.

Surgery: Surgical treatment remains the gold standard for symptomatic BPH. It provides the most reliable and immediate subjective and objective improvement. Surgery is recommended when BPH causes renal insufficiency, recurrent retention, recurrent urinary tract infection, bladder calculi, or gross hematuria. Hydronephrosis or a postvoid residual volume > 500 mL may also require surgical treatment. Open prostatectomy is usually reserved for patients with large prostate glands (> 100 g) or in whom other pathology (eg, a vesical calculus) exists. It requires an abdominal incision and longer convalescence than transurethral approaches. However, subsequent surgery is rarely needed. Transurethral resection of the prostate (TURP) is less invasive than open prostatectomy but requires regional or general anesthesia in an inpatient setting. Its complications include infection, bleeding, and a 20% risk of reoperation within 10 years. Retrograde ejaculation after surgery is usual, whereas impotence or incontinence is rare. Transurethral incision of the prostate (TUIP) is best for patients with glands < 30 g and obstruction at the bladder neck. The complications of TUIP are the same as those of TURP but are significantly less severe and less frequent.

PROSTATE CANCER

Prostate cancer affects about 2% of primary care patients > 50. Adenocarcinoma of the prostate is one of the most common cancers in American men. However, prostate cancer most often runs a protracted course, with other causes of death intervening; thus, most patients die *with* prostate cancer rather than *of* prostate cancer.

Prostate cancer is the second leading cause of cancer death in men after lung cancer. Estimates for the USA in 1998 were that 184,500 men would be diagnosed and 39,200 men would die of prostate cancer. Black men have a significantly higher risk of developing prostate cancer and have a higher mortality from the disease than do white men. The incidence increases with age; > 75% of cancers are diagnosed in men > 65.

Most patients are asymptomatic or have symptoms of obstructive uropathy. A few patients present with symptoms due to distant metastases, such as weight loss, bone pain, or neurologic symptoms.

Screening and Diagnosis

A majority of cases are discovered through screening with digital rectal examination (DRE) and serum prostate-specific antigen (PSA). The decision to screen for clinically localized prostate cancer, particularly in the elderly, is controversial. Screening is based on the hypothesis that early detection allows treatment of the cancer while it is still localized, thereby reducing mortality. However, the hypothesis that early treatment reduces mortality is unproven. Patients with well-differentiated cancer do just as well with or without treatment, and those with poorly differentiated cancers tend to do poorly with or without treatment.

Nonetheless, the American Cancer Society and the American Urological Association recommend annual screening with DRE and PSA for men ≥ 50 years with a life expectancy of ≥ 10 years. Thus, screening men > 75 years is probably not warranted.

DRE is an easy initial screening test for both prostate and rectal cancers. However, cancers diagnosed by DRE are usually already large, and more than half have already extended through the capsule, making cure less likely.

PSA is a serine kinase produced by benign and malignant prostatic epithelial cells. Serum PSA levels < 4 ng/mL are considered normal, levels of 4 to 10 ng/mL have a 25% positive predictive value for prostate cancer, and levels > 10 ng/mL have a 67% positive predictive value. Thus, even at high levels, the test is not specific. Other conditions (eg, benign prostatic hyperplasia, prostatitis, recent prostate biopsy) can also elevate PSA levels. Age-specific upper levels of normal of 4.5 ng/mL for men aged 60 and 6.5 ng/mL for men aged 70 have been suggested to try to reduce the number of biopsies having negative results.

The measurement of free vs. total PSA levels has been suggested to increase specificity further. In general, prostate cancers are associated with less free PSA. Thus, free PSA levels < 15 to 25% are an indication for biopsy. However, no standard percentage has been defined, and the range reflects the individual investigator's conclusions.

Despite low specificity, an abnormal DRE result or elevated PSA level is generally considered an indication for transrectal ultrasound (TRUS)–guided prostate biopsy. Thus, a positive DRE or PSA will statistically lead to a large number of TRUS findings that will prove to be negative.

Prostate cancer is staged using the TNM classification (see TABLE 117–2). It is most commonly graded using the Gleason system, which assesses the microscopic appearance of the prostate gland as a whole (ie, glandular architecture) more so than the individual cells. Grade 1 represents a glandular pattern close to normal, whereas grade 5 corresponds to sheets of cells with little gland formation. The Gleason score is reported as two numbers and their final sum. The first number represents the primary (most common) pattern of the glands, and the second number the secondary (second most common) pattern. A final sum of 2 to 4 is considered well-differentiated; 5 to 7, moderately differentiated; and 8 to 10, poorly differentiated.

Treatment

The treatment of prostate cancer is controversial, particularly in elderly patients.

Watchful waiting involves repeated measurements of serum PSA levels and monitoring of local symptoms. Watchful waiting is probably best for patients > 70 with moderately or well-differentiated, low-volume prostate cancer and a life expectancy of < 10 years. Although watchful waiting has no immediate effect on the quality of life, disease progression and tumor enlargement are possible. Intervention may be required if local symptoms worsen.

TABLE 117–2.   **STAGING OF PROSTATE CANCER**

Stage	Description
T1a	Incidentally found, well-differentiated tumor involving ≤ 5% of resected tissue from transurethral resection of the prostate
T1b	Incidentally found tumor involving > 5% of resected tissue from transurethral resection of the prostate
T1c	Tumor diagnosed because of elevated prostate-specific antigen level
T2a	Palpable tumor involving ≤ 50% of one prostate lobe
T2b	Palpable tumor involving > 50% of one prostate lobe
T2c	Palpable tumor involving both prostate lobes
T3a	Unilateral tumor extension beyond the prostate
T3b	Bilateral tumor extension beyond the prostate
T3c	Tumor invading one or both seminal vesicles
T4a	Tumor involving the bladder neck, external sphincter, or rectum
T4b	Tumor involving additional adjacent organs
N0	No nodal metastases
N1	Metastases in one node < 2 cm in diameter
N2	Metastases in one or more nodes 2 to 5 cm in diameter
N3	Metastases in one or more nodes > 5 cm in diameter
M0	No distant metastases
M1	Distant metastases

Radical prostatectomy involves complete removal of the gland and adnexal structures (eg, seminal vesicles), together with regional lymph nodes. Radical prostatectomy for elderly patients requires careful selection based on life expectancy and comorbid conditions. It is major surgery that requires general anesthesia. Arteriosclerotic cardiovascular disease, pulmonary disease, and renal insufficiency are significant risk factors for anesthesia. In addition, prostate cancer and pelvic surgery predispose elderly patients to thromboembolic events. Complications during or after radical prostatectomy include excessive blood loss, rectal laceration, incontinence, erectile dysfunction, and anastomotic stricture. A nerve-sparing radical prostatectomy may be attempted in a sexually potent man; however, the success rate of preserving potency decreases with age.

Radiation therapy uses conventional external beam, conformational external beam, or interstitial radiation. Conventional external beam radiation uses multiple or rotational fields. Conformational external beam radiation uses computer-guided CT to help precisely localize the treatment area. This technique allows the radiation dose to be increased to > 7000 cGy without an increase in morbidity. Acute adverse effects include radiation proctitis, cystitis, diarrhea, and fatigue. Late adverse effects include chronic proctitis, radiation cystitis, incontinence, erectile dysfunction, and urethral strictures.

Interstitial radiation therapy involves the insertion of radioactive seeds directly into the prostate under ultrasound or CT guidance. Various isotopes are used, including ^{125}I and palladium-103. Long-term data from ultrasound-placed seeds are awaited. Adverse effects include irritative voiding symptoms, urinary retention, rectal urgency, increased bowel movements, rectal bleeding or ulceration, and prostatorectal fistulas.

Hormonal therapy (eg, bilateral orchiectomy, gonadotropin-releasing hormone [GnRH] agonists, estrogen use) is the gold standard for treatment of locally advanced or metastatic prostate cancer. Hormonal therapy cannot cure prostate cancer but provides palliation (eg, decreased symptoms, improved quality of life) for most patients. Different hormonal therapies block different steps of androgen production, secretion, or function. Hormonal therapy suppresses 95% of serum testosterone.

Bilateral simple orchiectomy (ie, castration) is the simplest form of androgen deprivation. However, many patients have significant psychologic difficulty with castration and prefer medical management. GnRH agonists deplete pituitary luteinizing hormone and down-regulating GnRH receptors. They must be injected every 3 to 4 months. They are also expensive; Medicare pays only 80% of the cost. Nonsteroidal antiandrogens (eg, flutamide, bicalutamide, nilutamide) counteract the effect of dihydrotestosterone at the receptor within the prostate cancer cells. These drugs are expensive and must be taken daily. However, they do not cause erectile dysfunction. Ongoing studies are comparing antiandrogen monotherapy with standard hormonal therapy. All hormonal therapy can reduce secondary sex characteristics in men and induce hot flashes and gynecomastia.

PROSTATITIS

Inflammation of the prostate.

Prostatitis affects 1% of primary care patients > 50. Chronic prostatitis has a substantial effect on quality of life because of its relentless, uncomfortable symptoms.

Historically, prostatitis has been classified as acute or chronic bacterial prostatitis, chronic abacterial prostatitis, or prostatodynia. However, a new classification (see TABLE 117–3) is rapidly becoming standard.

TABLE 117–3.   CLASSIFICATION OF PROSTATITIS

Classification	Definition	Description
I	Acute bacterial prostatitis	Acute infection of the prostate
II	Chronic bacterial prostatitis	Recurrent infection of the prostate
III	Chronic abacterial prostatitis, chronic pelvic pain syndrome	No demonstrable infection
IIIA	Chronic inflammatory abacterial prostatitis, inflammatory chronic pelvic pain syndrome	White blood cells in semen, in expressed prostatic secretions, or, after prostatic massage, in urine
IIIB	Chronic noninflammatory abacterial prostatitis, noninflammatory chronic pelvic pain syndrome	No white blood cells in expressed prostatic secretions or, after prostatic massage, in urine
IV	Asymptomatic prostatitis	Incidental finding on pathologic examination

Etiology and Pathogenesis

In cases of acute or chronic **bacterial prostatitis,** an identifiable uropathogen, usually a gram-negative organism, can be localized to the prostate. *Escherichia coli* is identified in about 80% of cases; *Pseudomonas aeruginosa, Serratia, Klebsiella,* and *Proteus* sp in 10 to 15%; and enterococci in 5 to 10%.

In cases of category III **chronic prostatitis,** in which there is no identifiable infection, several etiologic theories have been proposed. For example, in category IIIA chronic prostatitis, etiologic theories include fastidious organisms, an unknown noninfectious agent, chemical irritation from refluxed urine, an autoimmune response, and viruses. In category IIIB chronic noninflammatory abacterial prostatitis, the etiology is thought to be varied, possibly multifactorial. One theory is that bladder neck dysfunction, spasm of the pelvic floor, or both cause turbulent urinary flow in the prostatic urethra, resulting in intraprostatic reflux of urine causing chemical inflammation. The bladder neck dysfunction may result from a disturbance in muscle coordination at the bladder neck secondary to an abnormality in the pelvic sympathetic system, from fibrosis of the bladder neck, or from an acquired functional disorder (psychologic factors, particularly depression and somatization, may be exacerbatory). Some patients with category IIIB chronic prostatitis may also have other disorders (eg, interstitial cystitis, fibromyalgia, back problems).

Symptoms and Signs

The primary clinical feature of prostatitis is suprapubic, perineal, pelvic, scrotal, testicular, penile, or upper thigh pain. (In chronic prostatitis, by definition, the pain must be present for ≥ 3 months.) Urinary symptoms (eg, urgency, frequency, nocturia, dysuria) are primarily irritative. Sexual dysfunction (eg, painful ejaculation, postejaculatory pain, erectile dysfunction) may occur. Patients with acute bacterial prostatitis may present with a high fever, perineal and lower back pain, and severe urinary symptoms.

A comprehensive questionnaire may be used to assess symptom severity and to evaluate treatment efficacy.

Diagnosis

On palpation, the prostate may be tender, swollen, boggy, or firm but is usually unremarkable. A midstream urinalysis should be obtained to rule out infection or hematuria. Although uncommonly used, serial sampling using the Meares-Stamey four-glass test helps determine the site of infection in the urinary tract. A greater concentration of bacteria and white blood cells in samples obtained after prostatic massage is diagnostic for prostatitis. However, prostatic massage should not be performed if acute bacterial prostatitis is suspected, because it increases the risk of septicemia. If initial therapies fail, some patients may require urodynamic studies for evaluation of bladder neck dysfunction. Hydrodistention (in which the bladder is stretched with the patient under anesthesia and then examined for submucosal hemorrhage) can be both diagnostic and therapeutic for patients with IIIB chronic noninflammatory abacterial prostatitis who have interstitial cystitis. Evidence of petechial hemorrhages, submucosal bleeding, or Hunner's ulcers in the bladder epithelium after hydrodistention is diagnostic for interstitial cystitis.

Treatment

Patients with acute bacterial prostatitis should be admitted to the hospital and given intravenous antibiotics (eg, ampicillin, gentamicin). Patients with chronic bacterial prostatitis require 6 weeks of oral antibiotics (eg, doxycycline, co-trimoxazole, fluoroquinolones) to achieve prolonged therapeutic bactericidal levels in the prostatic ducts sufficient to overcome a protective barrier secreted by the bacteria.

In patients with negative results on culture, a reasonable approach is to give antibiotics for 2 weeks; treatment for a further 4 weeks should be given only if improvement occurs. If improvement does not occur, an α-blocker should be given to treat bladder neck dysfunction; the dose is titrated to the dose recommended for benign prostatic hyperplasia.∎ If

∎see page 1180

TABLE 117–4. CAUSES OF BALANITIS

Infectious causes	Noninfectious causes
Candidiasis	Reiter's syndrome (balanitis circinata)
Gonococcal or chlamydial urethritis	Fixed drug eruptions
Chancroid	Contact dermatitis
Trichomoniasis	Psoriasis
Herpes simplex	Lichen planus
Scabies	Seborrheic dermatitis
Primary or secondary syphilis	Lichen sclerosus
	Erythroplasia of Queyrat

effective, the α-blocker should probably be continued for no less than 1 month, although there are no data on how long it should be continued.

Patients with chronic inflammatory or noninflammatory abacterial prostatitis who have interstitial cystitis may benefit from the antihistamine hydroxyzine. A 3-month course of hydroxyzine, an H_1 blocker, starting at 25 mg po at bedtime and increased to 75 mg po at bedtime, followed by reevaluation, improves symptoms in about 30% of patients. However, this drug may produce intolerable anticholinergic adverse effects in the elderly. Hydrodistention may also significantly decrease symptom severity in chronic noninflammatory abacterial prostatitis.

Bladder neck obstruction may require surgical incision of the bladder neck.

DISORDERS OF THE PENIS

With age, the penile sinusoids lose compliance because of increased collagen deposition. Additionally, diseases frequently associated with aging (eg, atherosclerosis, diabetes) may predispose elderly men to erectile dysfunction; with age, men generally have less turgid erections, longer refractory periods, longer latency periods, and loss of forceful ejaculation.∎

BALANITIS

Inflammation of the glans penis.

Balanitis usually occurs in uncircumcised men. Diabetes is a predisposing factor. Causes (see TABLE 117–4), especially candidiasis, should be investigated and the urine tested for glucose. Clinically, the glans is red, often with an exudate on the surface. Balanitis is usually treated with antibiotic creams. Resistant or recurrent balanitis requires circumcision.

∎ see page 1158

Balanitis xerotica obliterans, a genital variation of lichen sclerosus, is due to chronic inflammation. It is characterized by a white discoloration of the tip of the glans penis with associated scarring. In uncircumcised men, the foreskin may become "fused" with the glans penis, making circumcision extremely difficult. The most common complication is meatal stenosis. When this complication occurs, recurrent urethral strictures are common and may require urethral plastic surgery.

CONDYLOMATA ACUMINATA

(Genital Warts; Venereal Warts)

Hyperplastic lesions of the skin or mucous membranes of the genitalia caused by human papillomaviruses.

Condylomata are soft, moist, tiny pink or gray polyps that enlarge, may become pedunculated, and are usually found in clusters, their surface resembling a cauliflower. About 5% of men with condylomata localized at the urinary meatus have urethral involvement. In these patients, the urethra should be evaluated. However, patients with lesions that do not resemble condylomata or balanitis should be referred to a dermatologist. Condylomata can be treated with drugs (eg, topical podophyllin) or laser therapy.

PRIAPISM

A sustained erection that is not associated with sexual arousal and does not subside after orgasm.

Priapism may be primary or secondary to sickle cell disease, neurogenic disorders (eg, spinal cord lesions), metastatic cancer, or drugs (eg, antihistamines; certain antidepressants, especially trazodone). Intracavernosal use of vasoactive drugs (eg, papaverine, prostaglandin) can cause priapism.

Treatment of drug-induced priapism involves aspiration of the corpora and injection of an α-adrenergic agonist (eg, phenylephrine 250 to 500 μg). If this approach fails or if the priapism is not drug-induced, treatment involves aspiration or irrigation of the corpora or use of cavernosal-spongiosal shunts. Any underlying cause should also be treated, if possible.

PENILE CANCER

Penile cancer is rare (0.5% of all malignancies among males) in the USA. It almost exclusively affects men who are not circumcised. Squamous cell carcinoma of the penis is more common (up to 10% of malignancies among males) in countries that do not practice neonatal circumcision. It primarily affects elderly men, although some cases have occurred in men < 50.

Because of the epidemiologic association with neonatal circumcision, one hypothesis suggests that penile cancer is caused by irritation from smegma. Other etiologic possibilities include viral infections (eg, herpes, human papillomavirus).

Squamous cell carcinoma of the penis usually starts as a small erythematous lesion on the foreskin or glans penis, which, if untreated, gradually erodes the penis itself. The lesion spreads to the inguinal lymph nodes, where it may erode the femoral vessels.

Small lesions of the foreskin may be treated with circumcision alone. Small lesions of the glans penis may be treated locally with Mohs' surgery, whereas larger lesions require partial or total penectomy (a margin is left 2 cm proximal to the overt tumor) depending on whether sufficient penis may be retained for voiding. For high-grade tumors or those invading the corpora cavernosa, an inguinal node dissection is performed. Treatment options for metastatic tumors are limited; no chemotherapy regimen has proved effective.

DISORDERS OF THE SCROTUM

Scrotal hernias (ie, direct or indirect inguinal hernias that descend into the scrotum), especially large, neglected ones, are difficult to correct surgically. However, primary surgical repair or secondary repair using autogenous fascia or a plastic mesh may be successful in healthy elderly men without advanced chronic obstructive pulmonary disease or prostatism.

Hydroceles occasionally present de novo in the elderly. Testicular cancer should be ruled out. Large symptomatic hydroceles may be treated with aspiration, which is seldom permanently effective, or surgical excision.

Epididymo-orchitis (inflammation of the epididymis and testis) usually is a temporary sequela of a urinary tract infection, prostatectomy, cystoscopy, or indwelling catheterization. Treatment of this painful condition consists of bed rest, scrotal support, and an antibiotic effective against both gram-negative bacteria and *Chlamydia* sp (eg, tetracycline). These bacterial infections occasionally form abscesses that require surgical drainage.

Testicular cancer is rare in elderly men; however, painless testicular masses should be considered neoplastic until proved otherwise. At a minimum, ultrasound evaluation is indicated. Lymphoma is the most common testicular cancer in the elderly. Of the germ cell tumors, spermatocytic seminomas occur most frequently in the elderly and have a favorable prognosis. Orchiectomy is the only treatment required. Other germ cell tumors, including other seminomas, are usually aggressive and metastasize early.

Although genitourinary symptoms are common in elderly women, these patients often do not report such symptoms to their physician. Thus, the history should specifically seek out common symptoms, such as vaginal itching and burning; pelvic pain, pressure, or protrusion; pain during intercourse; postmenopausal vaginal bleeding; hematuria; and urinary frequency, urgency, or incontinence. Patients should also be asked about their use of estrogen replacement therapy.∎ At the same time, a sexual history is usually appropriate.∎

The **pelvic examination**∎ is difficult in some elderly women. For example, some are embarrassed or uncomfortable. Elderly women with stiff joints and those who lack hip mobility may have difficulty assuming the usual lithotomy position and may find the left lateral position more comfortable. In the left lateral position, the patient lies on the left side with the knees flexed and the right (upward) hip flexed more than the left hip. Many clinicians are unfamiliar performing a pelvic examination with the patient in this position. Nursing homes and many hospitals lack examining rooms and equipment that facilitate such examinations in elderly patients.

The pelvic examination should be performed routinely every 1 to 2 years or whenever postmenopausal vaginal bleeding, pelvic support disorders, urethral caruncles, benign vulvar disorders, fistulas, or pelvic symptoms occur.

The pelvic examination should be performed in three steps: (1) During the external examination, the vulva and external groin area are visually inspected and palpated for ulcerations, inflammation, pigmented lesions, hypertrophic squamous changes, indurations, and nodal enlargement. (2) A speculum is inserted into the vagina and expanded to permit internal visual inspection of the vagina and cervix for atrophy, inflammation, and raised or discolored lesions. A Papanicolaou (Pap) smear is obtained at this time, and microbiology specimens (when indicated) are collected. If the speculum examination is difficult to perform because of vaginal stenosis, a smaller speculum should be used, sometimes with lubrication; once the speculum is inserted, pressure should be exerted toward the rectum. (3) The vaginal walls and cervix are palpated for paravaginal masses and cervical abnormalities; a bimanual examination is performed to assess uterine size and shape, to evaluate pelvic and adnexal structures and the lower rectum, and to detect any adnexal lesions. The deep palpation needed to assess a small uterus and ovaries sometimes causes pain; therefore, extra time, explanation, and gentleness may be required. A stool guaiac test is performed. Further

---

∎ see page 1211   ∎ see page 1174   ∎ see page 35

diagnostic tests may be indicated and may include colposcopy, biopsy, and various imaging modalities (eg, colonoscopy).

A **urologic evaluation** is warranted to evaluate hematuria unaccompanied by evidence of concurrent urinary tract infection or genital atrophy; evaluation is also needed if antibiotic or estrogen treatment does not eradicate hematuria due to infection or genital atrophy. The urologic evaluation may include intravenous urography, renal ultrasonography, urine cytology, and cystourethroscopy. Intravenous urography must be performed with care in elderly patients, who may have a decreased creatinine clearance; hydration helps reduce the risk of renal impairment, but fluid overload and heart failure can occur from overzealous hydration.

POSTMENOPAUSAL VAGINAL BLEEDING

Postmenopausal vaginal bleeding is due to endometrial cancer or atypical adenomatous endometrial hyperplasia in about 20 to 30% of cases (see TABLE 118–1). It may also be caused by estrogen or progesterone use or by genital atrophy secondary to low estrogen levels.

The history should evaluate past and present illnesses, drug use (especially exogenous estrogens), and previous gynecologic problems.

TABLE 118–1.   CAUSES OF POSTMENOPAUSAL BLEEDING

Atrophic vaginitis or cervicitis

Cancer
    Of the cervix
    Of the endometrium (including sarcoma)
    Of the fallopian tube
    Of the ovary
    Of the urethra
    Of the vagina
    Of the vulva

Coagulopathy

Endometrial atrophic bleeding

Endometrial stimulation by endogenous (ie, ovulatory dysfunction, functioning ovarian tumor) or exogenous estrogen

Endometrial or cervical polyps

Endometrial hyperplasia

Gastrointestinal tract lesion

Metastatic cancer to the bladder, urethra, uterus, or vagina

Submucosal fibroid

Urethral caruncle

Urinary tract lesion

Vaginal or vulvar trauma, ulceration, or angioma

Pelvic examination, including a Pap test and bimanual examination, should be performed to rule out trauma, bleeding from atrophic sites, and vulvar, vaginal, or cervical tumors. Most patients are referred to a gynecologist for endometrial biopsy or full fractional dilatation and curettage (D & C). Diagnostic testing can be performed in the physician's office rather than the operating room. For the majority of women at risk of developing endometrial cancer, an attempt at in-office biopsy with a small-caliber (3.1-mm diameter) suction curette is warranted; this procedure has a high sensitivity for detecting endometrial cancer. If cervical stenosis precludes performance of a biopsy, if an inadequate tissue sample is obtained, or if bleeding continues and cannot be explained by biopsy findings, D & C with hysteroscopy is likely to be needed.

Transvaginal ultrasonography is also useful for evaluating postmenopausal vaginal bleeding. If the endometrial thickness is < 4 mm, cancer is unlikely.

Treatment for cancer is discussed in Ch. 72. For women without cancer who are not taking estrogen, estrogen is often started, because the bleeding may be secondary to genital atrophy.∎ For women taking exogenous hormones, the dose of estrogen may need to be lowered or the dose of progesterone increased. Treatment must be individualized, and continued bleeding, if persistent, should be aggressively investigated.

PELVIC SUPPORT DISORDERS

(Pelvic Relaxation Disorders)

Hernia-like protrusions into the vagina by the bladder, rectum, or uterus, caused by weakness of pelvic ligaments, connective tissue, and muscles.

Because women today are living longer, pelvic support disorders are becoming a greater gynecologic health issue. A woman has about an 11% lifetime risk of undergoing surgery for pelvic support disorders and incontinence. Causes of pelvic support disorders are most likely multifactorial; risk factors include trauma during childbirth, increased abdominal pressure secondary to obesity, chronic coughing or straining at stool, estrogen deficiency, and intrinsic connective tissue weakness.

The more common pelvic support disorders include rectoceles, enteroceles, cystoceles, or a combination of these defects. Standardized terminology based on clearly defined anatomic reference points has been developed to permit quantitative, reproducible descriptions of the

∎ see page 1209

degree of severity of pelvic support disorders; this terminology facilitates communication between physicians and enables the progression of these conditions to be accurately followed.

A **rectocele** is a protrusion of the rectum into the vaginal lumen resulting from weakness in the muscular wall of the rectum and the perirectal fascia (see FIGURE 118–1).

An **enterocele** is a herniation of the peritoneum and small bowel and is the only true hernia among the pelvic support disorders. Most enteroceles occur downward between the uterosacral ligaments and the rectovaginal space.

A **cystocele** is a herniation of the urinary bladder through the anterior vaginal wall (see FIGURE 118–1). Cystoceles usually occur when the pubocervical connective tissue weakens or detaches from its lateral or superior connecting points.

Uterine prolapse is generally the result of poor cardinal or uterosacral ligament support. Typically, uterine prolapse is classified as first degree when the cervix descends below the level of the ischial spine, second degree when the cervix descends to but not through the introitus, and third degree when the cervix descends through the introitus.

Procidentia, which involves prolapse of the uterus and vagina, and **total vaginal vault prolapse,** which can occur after hysterectomy, represent eversion of the entire vagina (see FIGURE 118–2).

Symptoms and Signs

Heaviness or pressure in the vaginal area is the most common symptom. A mass may protrude at the introitus. These symptoms almost always occur when the patient is upright; they rarely occur when the patient is supine.

A patient with a rectocele may have difficulty passing stool; manual manipulation may be needed for complete defecation. A patient with an enterocele may experience pelvic fullness, pressure, or pain and lower back pain; the hernia may be palpable in the vagina, particularly on rectovaginal examination. A patient with a cystocele may develop stress or overflow urinary incontinence, ◾ incomplete bladder emptying, or a urinary tract infection.

A patient with uterine prolapse may have lower back or sacral pain while standing, although many patients are asymptomatic. A patient with procidentia may experience lower back pain, sacral pain, discomfort when walking (secondary to the protruding "mass"), and bleeding (secondary to ulceration of the cervix and vaginal mucosa). A patient with total vaginal vault prolapse may experience pain, especially when sitting. Third-degree uterine prolapse or total vaginal vault prolapse may lead to ulceration of the vaginal mucosa and bladder or rectal dysfunction (eg, difficulty voiding, chronic residual urine) that is often

◾ see page 965

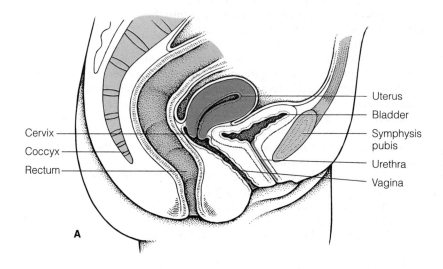

Uterus
Bladder
Symphysis pubis
Urethra
Vagina

Cervix
Coccyx
Rectum

A

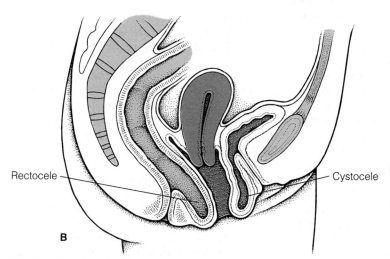

Rectocele

Cystocele

B

FIGURE 118–1.   Sagittal section showing normal anatomy (*A*); cystocele and rectocele (*B*).

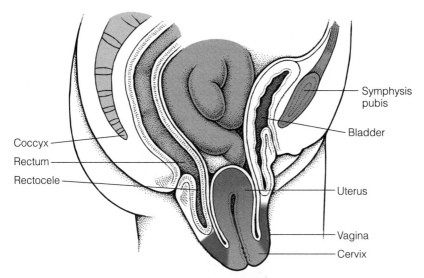

FIGURE 118–2.   Procidentia of the uterus and vagina.

worse after prolonged standing and is presumably due to urethral kinking, and at least two thirds develop stress incontinence when the prolapse is reduced. In some patients, urethral kinking is protective, because it stops urine from leaking when the anterior vagina and bladder protrude.

Diagnosis

Pelvic support disorders are diagnosed by pelvic examination; use of a Sims' speculum facilitates this examination.

Severe prolapse is obvious when the patient is in the dorsolithotomy position. Less severe prolapse may be detected using a Valsalva maneuver, which often reveals a widening of the genital hiatus and an evident rectocele or cystocele. Bimanual examination, including rectovaginal examination, is helpful in palpating a rectocele.

An enterocele is also diagnosed by pelvic examination; the patient performs a Valsalva maneuver while standing, which usually causes the prolapsing small intestine to bulge downward (see FIGURE 118–3). An enterocele may be visually indistinguishable from a rectocele.

If uterine prolapse or total vaginal vault prolapse is suspected, anal sphincter tone and the bulbocavernosus reflex should be assessed. Additional tests include residual urine measurement, urinalysis, urine culture and sensitivity, bladder fill testing, and stress testing with the prolapse reduced. Most patients with severe urinary leakage or symptoms

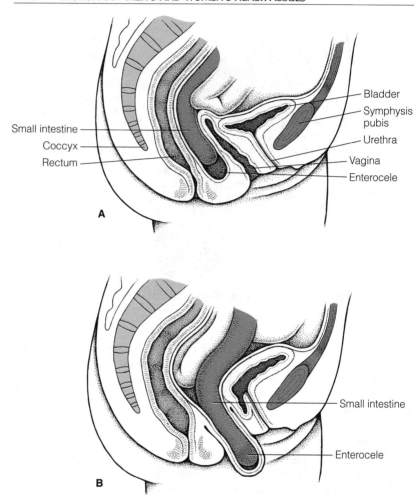

Small intestine
Coccyx
Rectum

Bladder
Symphysis pubis
Urethra
Vagina
Enterocele

A

Small intestine

Enterocele

B

FIGURE 118–3. Posterior enterocele without eversion (*A*); enterocele with eversion (*B*).

and signs of complex bladder dysfunction should undergo full uro-dynamic evaluation.■ Ureteral obstruction and subsequent renal damage are uncommon but should be sought if the patient has an enlarged uterus or a pelvic mass.

■ see page 975

Treatment

Nonsurgical treatment: Nonsurgical treatment includes pelvic muscle (Kegel's) exercises to strengthen the pelvic floor and perineal body for mild cases of rectocele, cystocele, or uterine prolapse; a pessary may help in more severe cases. Pessaries are particularly useful for patients in whom surgery is contraindicated. These devices are made of silicone, plastic, or rubber and have multiple shapes and sizes (see FIGURE 118–4). Pessary choice is determined by the amount of pelvic relaxation, the degree of uterine prolapse, the size of the genital hiatus, and the ease of pessary insertion. Teaching and clinical follow-up are important to ensure that the patient properly inserts and removes the pessary. A patient who plans to leave the pessary in place requires periodic follow-up for removal and cleaning of the pessary and inspection of the vagina. The health of the vaginal tissue is optimized with the use of topical estrogen vaginal cream (if the patient is not taking oral hormone replacement therapy), which helps thicken the vaginal epithelium and prevents ulceration.

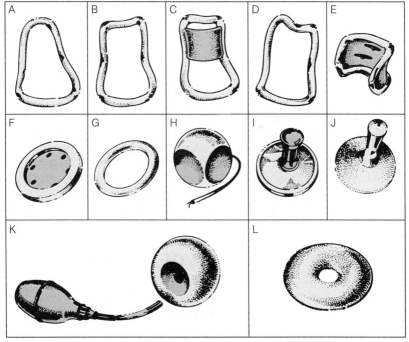

FIGURE 118–4. Types of vaginal pessaries. (A) Smith's; (B) Hodge's; (C) Hodge's with web support; (D) Risser; (E) Gehrung; (F) ring with web support; (G) ring; (H) cube; (I) Gelhorn, rigid; (J) Gelhorn, flexible; (K) Inflatoball; (L) doughnut.

Surgical treatment: Rectoceles are best treated through a vaginal approach with dissection of the rectovaginal space to expose and repair the defect in the rectal wall or pararectal fascia. Enteroceles and cystoceles may be approached transabdominally or transvaginally. Enteroceles are repaired by dissecting and excising the enterocele sac. Cystoceles are repaired by dissecting the vesicovaginal space and plicating the pubocervical fascia to correct its attenuation.

For uterine prolapse, procidentia, or total vaginal vault prolapse, the upper vagina is sutured to a stable structure within the pelvis. Large defects, such as vaginal vault prolapse and procidentia, are best managed by surgeons experienced in repairing these problems.

During surgery, all pelvic support defects should be corrected. Minimal defects that are not repaired are likely to worsen. Any lower urinary tract problems (notably stress incontinence∎) should also be treated.

URETHRAL CARUNCLE

(Prolapsed Urethra)

A nodular mass of erythematous urethral mucosa protruding through the external urethral orifice.

Prolapse of the urethral mucosa most often occurs in children and postmenopausal women. It is caused by redundancy of the mucosa combined with laxity of the periurethral fascia, and it may be aggravated by an increase in intra-abdominal pressure and a relative lack of estrogen.

Patients may be asymptomatic or may present with urethral bleeding, urinary urgency or frequency, or dysuria. Unlike a neoplasm, which generally is firm and nontender, a caruncle is soft and may be tender.

Asymptomatic caruncles generally require no treatment. In a patient who is hypoestrogenic, vaginal estrogen cream may help alleviate symptoms; if symptoms continue, caruncles can be removed using cauterization, laser vaporization or excision, cryotherapy, or surgical excision.

BENIGN DISORDERS OF THE VULVA

Urogenital atrophy due to hypoestrogenism predisposes postmenopausal women to common skin disorders of the vulva. Vulvar pruritus is the primary symptom. Evaluation involves direct examination and, often, biopsy.

∎see page 968

VULVITIS

Various agents (eg, deodorants and soaps used to mask the odor associated with urinary incontinence) can cause superficial irritation and dermatitis, with pruritus, edema, and burning. Treatment involves removal of the cause of irritation and topical use of a corticosteroid cream.

Candidal vulvovaginitis is especially common among elderly women who are diabetic or obese. The most common symptoms are vulvovaginal pruritus and discharge. Candidal vulvovaginitis is diagnosed by physical examination and the use of a wet preparation, in which a cotton-tipped applicator is used to obtain a sample of the discharge from the posterior vaginal fornix. Microscopic examination of the sample reveals the presence of yeast pseudohyphae or spores. Treatment involves use of topical antifungal drugs and, to relieve symptoms, local corticosteroids.

VULVAR NON-NEOPLASTIC EPITHELIAL DISORDERS
(Vulvar Dystrophies)

Lichen sclerosus, a dermatosis of unknown etiology, is characterized by epithelial thinning, edema and fibrosis of the dermis, and labial shrinkage. It typically involves the vulvar vestibule and especially the labia minora, where the affected skin resembles thin, white parchment paper. Vulvar pruritus is the most common symptom. Diagnosis is made by biopsy. A high-potency topical corticosteroid, such as clobetasol propionate cream 0.05%, is applied twice daily for 2 to 3 weeks and then nightly until symptoms and findings subside. The dosage can be tapered to 1 to 3 times weekly depending on response.

Squamous hyperplasia may occur anywhere on the vulva and may be localized to a small area. Squamous hyperplasia produces vulvar pruritus; the skin appears thickened and raised. When squamous hyperplasia affects more than one site, the involved areas are typically asymmetric. The diagnosis is usually one of exclusion. However, biopsy may be necessary to establish the diagnosis. A topical medium-strength corticosteroid, such as triamcinolone acetonide cream 0.1%, is applied twice daily and decreased to once daily until symptoms resolve (usually 2 to 3 weeks). Eliminating local irritants (eg, detergents, dyes, perfumes) and practicing good perineal hygiene (eg, wiping front to back after bowel movements and voiding), with emphasis on keeping the area dry, often cures squamous hyperplasia.

Other dermatoses (eg, lichen simplex chronicus, lichen planus, psoriasis, chronic eczematous dermatitis) can often be diagnosed on clinical grounds alone. However, if the patient has seen other physicians or has been treated previously, biopsy is usually indicated.

FISTULAS

Abnormal communicating tracts between two internal organs or between an internal organ and the external body surface.

Vesicovaginal and ureterovaginal fistulas usually occur in women who have had a hysterectomy for a benign condition. Patients leak urine continuously or intermittently and have some vulvar excoriation and erythema. Vesicovaginal fistulas occasionally occur many years after radiation therapy for gynecologic cancer; patients typically present with total urinary incontinence. In these cases, recurrent cancer is a strong possibility.

A vesicovaginal fistula can be diagnosed by infusing dye colored with water into the bladder and observing the flow of dye into the vagina, where a tampon had been previously placed. It may also be diagnosed by cystoscopy, pelvic examination, or vaginography; a negative test result does not rule out a fistula. A ureterovaginal fistula is diagnosed by intravenous or retrograde urography.

Fistulas caused by hysterectomy are best treated surgically. Those caused by radiation therapy usually require a diversionary procedure (ie, a urinary conduit).

Urethrovaginal fistulas are very rare but may occur after surgery for stress incontinence or urethral diverticula. Postvoiding incontinence is the usual symptom. Diagnosis is made by endoscopy, urethrography, or both, sometimes using a double-balloon catheter to occlude the internal and external urethral orifices. Many fistulas are missed on the first diagnostic attempt. Treatment involves surgical closure of the fistula and often requires interposition of some vascularized tissue (eg, a labial subcutaneous flap).

Colovesical (enterovesical) fistulas in the elderly may be caused by diverticulitis or, less commonly, by malignant neoplasms. Symptoms include lower abdominal pain, cystitis, pneumaturia (ie, passage of gas in the urine), and hematuria. Colovesical fistulas should be sought promptly in a patient who has recurrent or refractory urinary tract infections, especially when multiple bowel flora are cultured from the urine. Diagnosis is often difficult because the fistulas may intermittently seal, making them difficult to find. Diagnostic methods include barium enema, sigmoidoscopy, cystography, and oral ingestion of charcoal with subsequent examination of the urine for charcoal particles.

The treatment of colovesical fistulas caused by diverticulitis depends on the extent and activity of the diverticulitis. In some cases, the involved segment of sigmoid colon can be resected, with immediate reanastomosis and closure of the opening in the bladder. In other cases, a proximal diverting colostomy is safer than immediate resection, because it allows active diverticulitis to subside before the involved segment of colon is definitively repaired and resected. Fistulas caused by

TABLE 118–2.   STAGING OF ENDOMETRIAL CARCINOMA*

Stage†	Definition
IA	Tumor limited to endometrium
IB	Invasion of < 1/2 of the myometrial thickness
IC	Invasion of > 1/2 of the myometrial thickness
IIA	Tumor involvement of only endocervical glands
IIB	Invasion of cervical stroma
IIIA	Invasion of serosa and/or adnexa and/or positive peritoneal cytologic results
IIIB	Metastases to vagina
IIIC	Metastases to pelvic and/or para-aortic lymph nodes
IVA	Invasion of bladder and/or bowel mucosa
IVB	Distant metastases, including intra-abdominal and/or inguinal lymph nodes

*As described by the International Federation of Gynecology and Obstetrics (FIGO), 1988. Endometrial cancer is now surgically staged, so procedures previously used to differentiate stages no longer apply. However, the clinical staging adopted by FIGO in 1971 still applies to a few patients who may be treated primarily with radiation therapy, but use of that staging system should be noted. Ideally, in current staging, width of the myometrium should be measured with the width of tumor invasion.

†For all but stage IVB, the percentage of the tumor with a nonsquamous or nonmorular solid growth pattern is indicated by G1 (≤ 5%), G2 (6–50%), or G3 (> 50%). Notable nuclear atypia inappropriate for the architectural grade raises the grade of a G1 or G2 carcinoma by 1. In serous adenocarcinomas, clear cell adenocarcinomas, and squamous cell carcinomas, nuclear grading takes precedence. Adenocarcinomas with squamous differentiation are graded according to the nuclear grade of the glandular component.

colon cancer usually require excision with proximal diversion and concurrent treatment of the tumor.

ENDOMETRIAL CANCER

Endometrial cancer is the most common gynecologic malignancy in the USA; it is the fourth most common malignancy in women after breast, colorectal, and lung cancer. About 36,000 new cases of endometrial cancer occur per year. Peak incidence occurs in women aged 50 to 60, and the incidence appears to be increasing. Risk factors include obesity, nulliparity, and prolonged use of unopposed exogenous estrogen. **1**

The most common symptom is postmenopausal vaginal bleeding. **2** Diagnosis requires endometrial biopsy, although it is sometimes suggested by Pap smear. Early diagnosis and treatment have made the prognosis for endometrial cancer better than that for other gynecologic

1 see page 1211   **2** see page 1193

malignancies. However, prognosis is influenced by the stage of the tumor (see TABLE 118–2); 5-year survival rates range from 75 to 90% for those with stage I disease to 10% for those with stage IV disease. The combined 5-year survival rate for all stages is about 65%. Older women have a poorer prognosis.

Optimal treatment is hysterectomy, bilateral oophorectomy, and retroperitoneal lymph node dissection in the pelvic and para-aortic areas. Upper vaginal or pelvic radiation therapy, chemotherapy, or both may be required for advanced cancer based on stage, the patient's comorbidities, and the results of a thorough discussion of risks and benefits.

OVARIAN CANCER

Ovarian cancer is the second most common gynecologic malignancy after endometrial cancer. The peak incidence occurs in women in their 50s and 60s. Risk factors include uninterrupted ovulation (ie, no pregnancies or oral contraceptive use) and inherited genetic mutations (*BRCA1* mutations).

Symptoms develop late and are usually nonspecific; vague abdominal or gastrointestinal discomfort is common. As a result, 75% of patients present with stage III or stage IV disease (see TABLE 118–3). Large abdominopelvic masses, ascites, or both may be detected during routine pelvic examination. Ovaries in postmenopausal women are small and normally not palpable; thus, any palpable ovary in a postmenopausal patient suggests ovarian cancer, and prompt evaluation is warranted. If cancer is suggested by pelvic ultrasound, the mass is surgically resected for definitive diagnosis, staging, and treatment.

Initial treatment involves surgical removal of visible tumor. The decision to recommend chemotherapy is based on the tumor stage, the patient's comorbidities, and the results of a discussion of the risks and benefits of therapy. Although chemotherapy may be well tolerated, cure rates for advanced stage disease are low.

Combination chemotherapy is given IV over several months, except to patients with early-stage disease or histologically borderline tumors. Treatment rarely includes radiation therapy. The serum CA 125 marker is useful for monitoring treatment response and disease status in many women, especially those with serous tumors. For patients with recurrent disease, modalities such as new generation chemotherapeutic drugs, monoclonal antibody therapy, and gene therapy are being investigated.

Platinum-based chemotherapy given after surgery results in clinical remission in 70% of patients, with median survival of 3 years. Because most ovarian cancer is diagnosed at an advanced stage, the long-term prognosis is poor. A majority of patients experience a recurrence, and the 5-year survival rate seldom exceeds 20%.

TABLE 118-3.   SURGICAL STAGING OF OVARIAN CANCER*

Stage	Description
I	Limited to the ovaries
IA	Limited to one ovary; no tumor on the external surface, and capsule intact
IB	Limited to both ovaries; no tumor on the external surface, and capsules intact
IC	Stage IA or IB but with tumor on the surface of one or both ovaries, with capsule ruptured, or with ascites or peritoneal washings containing malignant cells†
II	Involving one or both ovaries, with pelvic extension
IIA	Extension and/or metastases to the uterus and/or fallopian tubes
IIB	Extension to other pelvic tissues
IIC	Stage IIA or IIB but with tumor on the surface of one or both ovaries, with capsule rupture, or with ascites or peritoneal washings containing malignant cells†
III	Involving one or both ovaries with histologically confirmed peritoneal implants outside the pelvis and/or positive retroperitoneal or inguinal lymph nodes
IIIA	Grossly limited to the true pelvis with negative lymph nodes, but with histologically confirmed microscopic tumor outside pelvis
IIIB	Involving one or both ovaries with histologically confirmed implants < 2 cm in diameter on abdominal peritoneal surfaces and with negative lymph nodes
IIIC	Abdominal implants > 2 cm in diameter and/or positive retroperitoneal or inguinal lymph nodes
IV	Involving one or both ovaries with distant metastases. If pleural effusion is present, cytologic test results must be positive to signify stage IV. Parenchymal liver metastasis equals stage IV
Special category	Unexplored cases thought to be ovarian cancer

*As described by the International Federation of Gynecology and Obstetrics (FIGO), 1991.

†For stages IC and IIC, knowing whether capsule rupture was spontaneous or caused by the surgeon and whether the source of malignant cells was ascites or peritoneal washings helps determine prognosis.

CERVICAL CANCER

Cervical cancer is the third most common gynecologic malignancy after endometrial cancer and ovarian cancer; it is the eighth most common malignancy among women in the USA. The peak incidence occurs in patients in their 40s or 50s. However, it occurs in women of all ages, including the elderly.

Human papillomavirus (HPV) is thought to play a role in the etiology of cervical cancer. Although HPV is a common component of the biologic flora of the vagina, certain subtypes may have the ability to integrate into the DNA of cervical cells and induce genetic alterations, leading to malignant transformation; HPV types 16 and 18 are present in > 75% of cervical cancers. Prevention strategies that use Pap tests for early detection of HPV types 16 and 18 are being investigated.

Cervical histopathology is classified as mild cervical dysplasia, in which abnormal cells proliferate in the lower third of the epithelium; moderate cervical dysplasia, in which abnormal cells involve the middle third of the epithelium; severe dysplasia (carcinoma in situ), in which a full thickness of epithelium contains abnormal cells; or invasive carcinoma, in which cancer cells penetrate the basement membrane and invade the stroma. About 85% of cervical cancers are squamous cell carcinomas and 15% are adenocarcinomas, although the incidence of adenocarcinomas may be increasing.

Symptoms depend on the stage of the tumor. Some patients have postcoital or postmenopausal vaginal bleeding, although many patients with premalignant or small lesions are asymptomatic. Routine Pap testing is the best screening method. Technologic advances in slide preparation and automated rescreening devices have improved the accuracy rate of the Pap test, so that it can detect about 90% of early-stage neoplasias. In elderly women with no previous history of abnormal Pap smears under routine surveillance and with no outstanding risk factors, the need for frequent Pap tests decreases. Elderly women who have had consistently normal Pap smears need to be tested only every 5 years. Those who have had cancer or dysplasia, regardless of age, should continue to undergo annual Pap tests.

If the Pap test result is positive, colposcopy-directed biopsies and endocervical curettage are used diagnostically; if biopsy results do not exclude invasive carcinoma or if the cervical transformation zone is not visible, subsequent cervical conization may be required. Conization can often be accomplished using diathermy loops under local anesthesia in an office setting.

The combined cure rate for all cervical cancers is 50 to 60%. The cure rate for early-stage cancers treated with radical hysterectomy or radiation therapy approaches 85%. Locally advanced disease is treated with radiation and chemotherapy; the 5-year survival rate in these cases is about 70%. Radiation or chemotherapy can provide palliation for patients with distant metastases; however, the prognosis in these cases is very poor.

VULVAR CANCER

Vulvar cancer, the fourth most common gynecologic malignancy, accounts for about 3 to 4% of all gynecologic malignancies in the USA. The average age at diagnosis is about 70 years, and the incidence increases with age.

Vulvar pruritus is the most common presenting symptom, but many patients are asymptomatic. Lesions may appear erythematous and flat, condylomatous, or ulcerated; discharge or local discomfort is often present.

Vulvar dystrophy and other vulvar lesions∎ must be differentiated from malignant lesions. Premalignant lesions may appear as white patches, brown pigmented areas, or granular red lesions. These lesions and all raised or ulcerated lesions should undergo biopsy. Dystrophic lesions (lichen sclerosus) or inflammatory lesions that do not respond within a few weeks to topical corticosteroid therapy should also undergo biopsy. Flat or slightly raised ulcerative lesions should undergo biopsy if they stain blue when swabbed with toluidine blue or if they turn white when swabbed with 3% acetic acid.

Prognosis is generally good for patients with early-stage lesions. The 5-year survival rate is 80 to 90% if lymph node metastasis is absent and 16 to 30% if lymph node metastasis is present.

Treatment of premalignant and malignant lesions is primarily surgical. Most women, even those who are debilitated, can have skin lesions removed under local anesthesia. Extensive condylomatous or in situ lesions are amenable to treatment with wide local excision or laser therapy. Minimally invasive lesions (< 1 mm) can be treated with partial vulvectomy alone.

Topical therapy with cytotoxic drugs (eg, 5% 5-fluorouracil cream) may be useful for some in situ lesions. Although treatment with 5-fluorouracil cream results in complete response in 50% of cases, it often causes vulvar irritation and painful superficial ulceration.

Radical vulvectomy, with unilateral or bilateral inguinal lymphadenectomy, is required for the staging and treatment of larger or deeply invasive tumors. Radiation therapy occasionally has an adjunctive role; preoperative chemotherapy or radiation therapy may make extensive tumors resectable.

VAGINAL CANCER

Vaginal cancer is relatively rare; it accounts for 1% of gynecologic malignancies in the USA. The average age at diagnosis is 60 to 65 years. Most (95%) vaginal cancer is squamous cell carcinoma, although adenocarcinoma and melanoma may occur.

An early symptom is vaginal bleeding or discharge. Usually, nodules or ulcers develop on the vaginal mucosa; biopsy is necessary for definitive diagnosis.

Prognosis depends on the size and location of the tumor. Five-year survival rates vary from 25 to 48%. Primary treatment usually consists of radiation therapy, although surgery or chemotherapy can be used in

∎ see page 1201

select cases. For example, tumors in the upper third of the vagina near the cervix may be surgically resectable.

119 ■ MENOPAUSE

Permanent cessation of menses due to loss of ovarian function.

In the USA, the average age at which menopause occurs is 51. Thus, on average, women are postmenopausal one third of their life. Despite an increase in the average life expectancy for women in the USA, the average age at menopause is probably unchanged. Prolonged hypothalamic amenorrhea, number of pregnancies, and oral contraceptive use do not influence the age of onset.

With age, ovarian follicles decrease in number, become less responsive to stimulation by gonadotropic hormones, and consequently produce progressively less estrogen. Typically, ovarian function waxes and wanes over several years. This transitional phase is termed perimenopause or the climacteric. Eventually, no estrogen is produced, resulting in menopause.

Symptoms and Signs

Early symptoms and signs of menopause include irregular menstrual cycles, hot flashes, changes in mood and cognition, insomnia, headache, and fatigue. Palpitations, tachycardia, and vertigo may occur. Later manifestations include dry skin, breast changes, genital atrophy with dyspareunia, loss of pelvic muscle tone, urinary incontinence, cystitis, and vaginitis. Osteoporosis and atherosclerosis may develop.

Irregular menstrual cycle: The first manifestation of menopause is often irregular periods. They vary in duration, frequency, and amount of flow but may be regular occasionally. However, unusual bleeding (eg, bleeding that is unusually heavy, that lasts for more than 10 days, or that occurs more frequently than every 3 weeks) should be evaluated to rule out neoplasms.

Hot flashes: Another early manifestation of menopause is hot flashes. About 80% of perimenopausal women report hot flashes. Of these women, 85% are symptomatic for > 1 year, and 25 to 50% are symptomatic for up to 5 years. During perimenopause, hot flashes occur when estrogen levels decrease and cease when estrogen levels increase. They become less frequent and less intense with age, in contrast to other sequelae of menopause (eg, genital atrophy, osteoporosis, atherosclerosis), which progress with age. Hot flashes also occur after surgical menopause or after discontinuation of exogenous estrogen.

Hot flashes are the subjective sensation of intense warmth in the upper body, typically lasting 4 minutes (range, 30 seconds to 5 minutes). A vasomotor flush, the objective counterpart of a hot flash, is a blush that ascends the thorax, neck, and face, followed by profuse sweating. Skin perfusion increases about 1.5 minutes before the sensation and 6 minutes before the peak increase in skin temperature. This increase in skin perfusion causes heat loss with a simultaneous decrease in core body temperature.

A hot flash may follow a prodrome of palpitations or a sensation of pressure in the head and can be accompanied by weakness, faintness, or vertigo.

Insomnia: Perimenopausal women may have difficulty falling asleep, wake often during the night, or wake early. Insomnia is commonly caused by hot flashes but occurs among perimenopausal women whether they have hot flashes or not.

Mood and cognitive changes: Changes in hormone levels during perimenopause may result in moodiness, anxiety, irritability, nervousness, or depression. Perimenopausal symptoms may resemble premenstrual symptoms. Women may become forgetful and less able to concentrate.

Skin changes: The skin may become thinner, less elastic, and drier because collagen production decreases as estrogen levels decrease. The subcutaneous layer of fat also thins. As a result, wrinkles are more likely, and the skin becomes more vulnerable to injury.🔳

Breast changes: Breast tissue requires estrogen for growth. As estrogen levels decrease, the breasts change in size and shape. They become less firm and begin to sag. Fibrous bands may become more prominent.

Genitourinary atrophy: The tissues of the lower vagina, labia, urethra, and bladder trigone are estrogen dependent. As estrogen levels decrease during menopause, the vaginal walls become pale (because of diminished vascularity), thin (usually decreasing to a thickness of only three or four cells), and vulnerable to ulceration and infection. These changes usually occur within several years of the onset of menopause. The epithelial cells contain less glycogen, which, before menopause, was metabolized by lactobacilli to produce an acidic pH, thereby protecting the vagina from bacterial overgrowth. The vagina also loses its rugae, becoming shorter and inelastic. This condition is called **atrophic vaginitis.** Patients with atrophic vaginitis may report symptoms secondary to vaginal dryness (eg, dyspareunia, vaginismus)🔳 or secondary to vaginal ulceration and infection (eg, vaginal discharge, burning, itching, bleeding).

The similar atrophic changes that occur in the urethral epithelium are called **atrophic urethritis.** Patients with atrophic urethritis may develop

---

🔳see also page 1231   🔳see pages 1178 and 1179

dysuria, urgency, frequency, and stress incontinence (partly because thick, well-vascularized urethral mucosa, which is lost during perimenopause, is necessary to provide resistance to urinary flow). Loss of estrogens may also affect the muscles that help maintain continence. Suprapubic pain can occur, even without infection, possibly because the markedly thin urethral mucosa may allow urine to come in close contact with sensory nerves.

Osteoporosis: For about 10 years after menopause, bone loss accelerates by as much as tenfold. Because of this accelerated bone loss, type I (menopausal) osteoporosis (bone density > 2.5 SD below the young adult mean) occurs mainly in women > 60. It is six times more common among women than among men. Osteoporosis leads to fractures.[1]

Atherosclerosis: At menopause, the risk of atherosclerosis increases,[2] although the incidence of atherosclerosis is lower in women than in men at all ages. The increased risk is probably due to decreased estrogen levels, which result in a 6% decrease in high-density lipoprotein (HDL) cholesterol levels and a 5% increase in low-density lipoprotein (LDL) cholesterol levels. Estrogen replacement therapy significantly reduces the incidence of atherosclerosis in postmenopausal women (and increases the survival rate of those with coronary artery disease), possibly in part because it increases HDL cholesterol levels by 16 to 18% and decreases LDL cholesterol levels by 15 to 19%. Only oral (not vaginal or transdermal) estrogens produce these effects on cholesterol levels, possibly because after intestinal absorption, they directly affect lipid metabolism in the liver. Estrogens may also protect against atherosclerosis by promoting vasodilation, preventing platelet aggregation, reducing smooth muscle proliferation, slowing lipoprotein oxidation, and lowering plasma homocysteine levels.

Diagnosis

Menopause can usually be diagnosed clinically. The diagnosis may be confirmed by an elevated level of serum follicle-stimulating hormone. A low level of serum estradiol is not diagnostic, because levels are often low during menses.

A history and physical examination should be sufficient to diagnose hot flashes and exclude other disorders, such as thyrotoxicosis, carcinoid, and pheochromocytoma, that produce similar symptoms.

Atrophic vaginitis may be diagnosed by visual examination of the vaginal tissue, but any atypical lesions should be biopsied. If vaginal discharge is present, cultures for such pathogens as *Neisseria gonorrhoeae, Chlamydia* sp, *Trichomonas* sp, and *Gardnerella* sp (formerly, *Haemophilus vaginalis*) should be obtained. If *Candida* sp is found, the patient should be screened for diabetes, because the low glycogen con-

---

tent of unestrogenized vaginal epithelial cells ordinarily does not support this organism's growth. The diagnosis of atrophic vaginitis may be confirmed by a vaginal cell maturation index, using scrapings from the lateral vaginal wall at the level of the cervix. The exfoliated cells are classified by degree of maturation; a small proportion of superficial cells indicates severe atrophic vaginitis.

Urethroscopy, although rarely needed, shows a pale, atrophic urethra. Cystoscopy may detect the local inflammation of trigonitis.

Treatment

Nondrug treatment such as aerobic exercise, relaxation techniques, meditation, massage, and yoga may help control the effects of hot flashes (eg, fatigue, irritability, depression). However, estrogen replacement therapy is the optimal treatment for all symptoms. [1] Topical (vaginal) estrogen or low-dose oral estrogen replacement therapy may be adequate for managing genital atrophy, but other symptoms of menopause require systemic therapy at standard doses.

An alternative to estrogen replacement therapy is clonidine, a centrally acting α-adrenergic agonist-antagonist, which reduces hot flashes in 30 to 40% of menopausal women. The initial dose of 0.1 mg bid may be increased to 0.2 mg bid if no adverse effects occur and hot flashes persist. Clonidine has a high incidence of adverse effects (eg, postural dizziness, blurred vision), but it is better tolerated by hypertensive patients. If estrogens are inappropriate, synthetic mucopolysaccharides or water-soluble lubricants may relieve dyspareunia associated with genital atrophy.

120 ESTROGEN REPLACEMENT THERAPY

Estrogen replacement therapy, with or without a progestin, has many indications and benefits; eg, it can help relieve symptoms of the climacteric (menopause), [2] including hot flashes. It has a beneficial effect on bone, helps prevent and treat osteoporosis, and may reduce atherosclerosis and coronary artery disease. Estrogen, given systemically or topically, effectively treats atrophic vaginitis, thus helping postmenopausal women maintain sexual function, and atrophic urethritis and the resulting incontinence. Some evidence suggests that estrogen may help prevent Alzheimer's disease. However, estrogen replacement therapy has some adverse effects and risks; [3] it is therefore not suitable for all postmenopausal women.

[1] see below   [2] see page 1208   [3] see page 1214

Before estrogen replacement therapy is prescribed, a history and physical examination (eg, blood pressure, breast and pelvic examinations, a Papanicolaou test) are necessary, and the risks and benefits of the therapy should be fully discussed with the patient. Mammography should be performed (and repeated annually after age 50), because estrogen replacement therapy is contraindicated in patients with known or suspected breast cancer (see TABLE 120–1). An endometrial biopsy should be considered for patients who have a history of abnormal or heavy vaginal bleeding, who are at increased risk of preexisting endometrial hyperplasia, or who experience vaginal bleeding during estrogen and progestin replacement therapy at times other than immediately after withdrawal of progestin. Also, patients should have an annual endometrial biopsy if they are using unopposed estrogens, regardless of whether vaginal bleeding occurs. If adequate tissue cannot be obtained by biopsy, intraoperative dilatation and curettage (D & C) may be necessary.

In the USA, estrogen is usually combined with progesterone replacement therapy as cyclic treatment: For example, conjugated estrogens 0.625 mg are given daily, with medroxyprogesterone acetate 5 mg po given on days 1 through 13 each month. Another estrogen may be substituted for conjugated estrogens or another progestin for medroxyprogesterone acetate.

With this regimen, many patients have withdrawal bleeding between days 11 and 18. To avoid withdrawal bleeding, patients can use continuous rather than cyclic treatment; conjugated estrogens 0.625 or 1.25 mg as needed to control symptoms are given continuously with medroxyprogesterone acetate 2.5 mg/day. Irregular vaginal bleeding usually occurs for the first 3 months but usually stops. Medroxyprogesterone acetate 5 mg/day po may be needed if vaginal bleeding is persistent or if a higher dose of estrogen is necessary. If abdominal bloating and mastalgia occur, norethindrone 0.35 to 1.05 mg/day may be substituted for medroxyprogesterone acetate.

ESTROGENS

Pharmacology

Nonsynthetic (natural) estrogens: Nonsynthetic estrogens may be given orally, vaginally, transdermally, or subcutaneously. In general, conjugated estrogens are twice as potent as estrone preparations (eg, estropipate) because they also contain equine estrogens, which are very potent. In particular, they have a long half-life, in part as a result of their storage in and slow release from adipose tissue.

Conjugated estrogens given orally at 0.3 or 0.625 mg, estropipate 0.625 or 1.25 mg, or micronized estradiol-17β 0.5 or 1 mg is most commonly prescribed. These doses maintain the mean peak serum

TABLE 120-1.   CONTRAINDICATIONS TO POSTMENOPAUSAL USE OF ESTROGEN

Contraindication	Comments
Absolute	
Breast cancer (known or suspected)	Estrogen use may cause exacerbation
Endometrial cancer (known or suspected)	Estrogen use may cause exacerbation
Liver disease (acute)	Estrogen use may worsen liver disease
Thromboembolic disease (active disease or a history of disease related to estrogen use)	Estrogen use may increase the risk of thromboembolism
Vaginal bleeding (undiagnosed)	Preexisting endometrial cancer and hyperplasia must first be excluded
Relative	
Endometriosis (active)	Estrogen use may prevent the postmenopausal involution of endometriosis
Liver dysfunction (chronic)	The liver's impaired ability to metabolize estrogen leads to excessive serum estrogen levels; using smaller or less frequent doses is warranted
Porphyria (acute and intermittent)	Estrogen use precipitates attacks
Thromboembolic disease (a history of disease not related to estrogen use)	Estrogen use increases the risk of thromboembolism
Uterine leiomyomas (symptomatic)	Estrogen use may prevent the postmenopausal involution of uterine leiomyomas

estradiol level at about 30 to 40 pg/mL (110 to 150 pmol/L), similar to that during the early follicular phase of the menstrual cycle, and the estrone level at 150 to 250 pg/mL (555 to 925 pmol/L). These doses are generally effective in relieving menopausal symptoms and preventing osteoporosis. The lowest dose may be used for women who experience adverse effects. However, whether lower doses confer maximal therapeutic benefit is unknown.

Enterohepatic circulation contributes to the prolonged effect of oral estrogens. Thus, patients with altered gut flora (eg, due to antibiotic use) may not sufficiently hydrolyze these conjugates, thereby preventing reabsorption, and may need higher doses. Also, patients given long-term phenytoin have enhanced glucuronidation and therefore excrete estrogens more rapidly; they too may need higher doses.

Because the concentration of oral estrogen is 4 to 5 times higher in the portal than in the general circulation, more estrogen is presented to hepatocytes than to cells of other organs. Thus, the liver is more affected by estrogens given orally than by those given parenterally. Although many of these effects on the liver may be deleterious (eg, stimulating renin-substrate and coagulation factors), some effects may be beneficial (eg, increasing high-density lipoprotein [HDL] cholesterol levels, decreasing low-density lipoprotein [LDL] cholesterol levels).

Vaginally applied estrogens are absorbed and enter the systemic circulation, achieving about one fourth the circulatory level of an equal oral dose. Specifically, vaginal estrogens exert a potent local effect; 0.3 mg of conjugated estrogens given vaginally produces the same degree of epithelial maturation as does 1.25 mg po. Continued use of vaginal estrogen increases blood estrogen levels because of enhanced transfer across a healthier, better vascularized epithelium.

Silastic rings containing estradiol may be placed in the vagina and changed every 3 months; these rings introduce negligible quantities of estradiol into the systemic circulation.

Transdermal estradiol patches 50 μg/24 hours twice weekly provide constant serum levels of estradiol 60 pg/mL (220 pmol/L) and estrone 50 pg/mL (185 pmol/L), which usually reduce menopausal symptoms and prevent osteoporosis. Occasionally, higher doses (eg, 75 μg/24 hours, 100 μg/24 hours) may be needed to control symptoms.

Synthetic estrogens: These chemical derivatives of estradiol are 100 times more potent, on a per-weight basis, than nonsynthetic estrogens in stimulating the production of hepatic proteins. Synthetic estrogens have not been routinely used postmenopausally.

Adverse Effects

Estrogens may cause nausea, mastalgia, headache, and mood changes. They may also cause or aggravate serious disorders.

Endometrial hyperplasia and cancer: Only unopposed estrogen use (ie, without the addition of a progestin) induces endometrial hyperplasia. Unopposed estrogen also increases the risk of endometrial cancer (adenocarcinoma) about fourfold, from 1/1000 to 4/1000 women per year, depending on the dose and duration (minimum, 1 to 2 years). Prescribing estrogen in a reduced dose in a cyclic fashion reduces but does not completely eliminate the increased risk of cancer. Thus, concomitant use of progestins is advised for a patient with an intact uterus.

Progestins can prevent and reverse endometrial hyperplasia; use for 7 days/month significantly reduces the incidence of hyperplasia, and use for 10 to 13 days/month offers even greater protection. Progestins also reduce the incidence of endometrial cancer to below that of women not using estrogen replacement therapy.

Ovarian cancer: Estrogen replacement therapy may increase the risk of endometrioid cancer of the ovary (which accounts for 10 to 20%

of all ovarian cancers), although this effect has not been proved. The effect of progestin use on this risk is unknown.

Breast cancer: Estrogen use may theoretically increase the risk of breast cancer, because breast tumors can be estrogen sensitive, estrogens can induce breast tumors in rats, and women with prolonged endogenous estrogen exposure (eg, due to early menarche, late menopause, or nulliparity) are at increased risk of breast cancer. ◼ However, the association between estrogen replacement therapy and breast cancer is unclear, except for a possible modest increase in risk with use for 10 years or more. Nonetheless, estrogen replacement therapy may not be appropriate for menopausal women at particularly high risk of breast cancer. Whether adding a progestin helps prevent breast cancer has not been determined. The mitotic activity of the breast increases during the luteal phase, when maximum progestin secretion occurs (peak endometrial mitosis occurs during the follicular phase, when progesterone secretion is minimal). Moreover, progestins induce mammary ductal growth in rats. Therefore, the use of progestins in women without an intact uterus is unnecessary and possibly detrimental.

Cholelithiasis: During the first year of use, oral estrogen replacement therapy increases the risk of cholelithiasis by 20%. Cholelithiasis probably occurs because estrogens increase the hepatic excretion of LDL cholesterol and reduce the amount of chenodeoxycholic acid in bile.

Thromboembolic disease: Postmenopausal use of estrogen replacement therapy appears to increase the risk of deep vein thrombosis and pulmonary embolism by about 2.5-fold. Thus, oral estrogen replacement therapy should not be given to a patient with a history of thromboembolic disorders.

Hypertension: Oral estrogen replacement therapy may increase the hepatic production of renin substrate or may stimulate the production of an aberrant form. Estrogen replacement therapy does not usually induce or exacerbate hypertension and may actually lower blood pressure in some women. Moreover, estrogen replacement therapy is not associated with an increased risk of stroke. When blood pressure is increased due to estrogen replacement therapy, it is usually reversible when therapy is discontinued.

Impaired glucose tolerance: Although oral contraceptives can impair carbohydrate metabolism, the doses of estrogen replacement therapy used to treat postmenopausal symptoms do not appear to do so. Postmenopausal women with diabetes who take estrogen replacement therapy show no change, lower glucose levels, or reduced insulin requirements. Indeed, estrogen replacement therapy appears to increase the binding of insulin to its receptor, and in animal models, estrogen replacement therapy improves experimentally induced hyperglycemia.

◼see page 1217

PROGESTINS

Progestins are primarily used postmenopausally to reduce the risk of endometrial hyperplasia due to estrogen replacement therapy. They also help relieve hot flashes and prevent osteoporosis in patients in whom estrogen replacement therapy is contraindicated.

Pharmacology

Oral absorption of progesterone is highly variable, differing as much as threefold among patients. Thus, a dose that is adequate for one patient may be excessive for another. After absorption, oral progestins reach the liver in high concentration and may greatly affect the hepatic metabolism of serum lipoproteins. Progesterone and its derivatives are well absorbed when given vaginally, rectally, or intramuscularly.

Medroxyprogesterone acetate, the most commonly used progestin in the USA, is effective against endometrial hyperplasia and has only minor adverse effects on serum lipid levels. It may be given orally with estrogens; the minimal effective dose is 5 mg po when given as cyclic treatment (days 1 through 13 each month) and 2.5 mg po when given continuously. Alternatively, it may be given as an IM depot formulation, which is well absorbed but has a highly variable duration of action and often causes irregular vaginal bleeding. The usual dose is 50 to 150 mg IM every 1 to 3 months, with the amount and interval depending on bleeding patterns and the effect on symptoms; the 50-mg dose is usually adequate to relieve hot flashes, and the 150-mg dose reduces urinary calcium loss as effectively as conjugated estrogens 0.625 mg.

Micronized progesterone, 200 mg po daily for cyclic treatment and 100 mg po daily for continuous treatment, does not significantly alter serum lipid levels but does prevent endometrial hyperplasia. Megestrol acetate 40 to 80 mg/day po suppresses hot flashes. These high doses are necessary because megestrol acetate has one fourth to one eighth the potency of medroxyprogesterone acetate on a per-weight basis.

19-Nortestosterone derivatives are used in oral contraceptives; they have partial androgenic properties and an adverse effect on serum lipid levels. However, norethindrone (norethisterone) 1 mg/day treats endometrial hyperplasia with no adverse effect on lipid levels. D,L-Norgestrel is not commonly used because it has more potent androgenic properties than norethindrone.

Adverse Effects

Progestins may produce abdominal bleeding, mastalgia, headache, mood changes, and acne. All progestins, particularly the 19-nortestosterone derivatives, adversely affect serum lipid levels, decreasing HDL cholesterol and increasing LDL cholesterol in a dose-dependent manner. Thus, the risk of developing cardiovascular disease may outweigh the benefit of preventing endometrial cancer. Because the protective activity of progestins on the endometrium appears related more to the duration of use (ie, 13 out of 25 days) than to the dose, the lowest effective dose should be used. Because of cardiovascular risk and because progestins have not been proved to protect against breast cancer, these drugs are not recommended for women without an intact uterus receiving estrogen replacement therapy.

121 ■ BREAST CANCER

Breast cancer is a major cause of morbidity and mortality in elderly women. Each year about 50% of the 185,000 new cases of breast cancer in the USA occur in women ≥ 65 years. The risk of developing breast cancer is much greater than that of dying of it: 6.53% of white women and 4.70% of black women ≥ 65 develop breast cancer, but only 1.53% and 1.14%, respectively, die of it (see TABLE 121–1). Breast cancer in men, which also increases in incidence with age (mean age at diagnosis is about 65), accounts for 1% of all new cases.

TABLE 121–1.   WOMEN'S RISK OF DEVELOPING OR DYING
OF BREAST CANCER

Age (yr)	Risk of Developing Breast Cancer (%)		Risk of Developing Invasive Breast Cancer (%)		Risk of Dying of Breast Cancer (%)	
	White	Black	White	Black	White	Black
Birth–110	10.20	7.50	9.80	7.30	3.60	3.00
20–30	0.04	0.07	0.04	0.07	0.00	0.02
20–40	0.49	0.61	0.47	0.61	0.09	0.15
20–110	10.34	7.72	9.94	7.42	3.05	3.11
35–45	0.88	0.80	0.83	0.75	0.14	0.21
35–55	2.53	2.32	2.37	2.16	0.56	0.72
35–110	10.27	7.74	9.82	7.33	3.56	2.98
50–60	1.95	1.74	1.86	1.68	0.33	0.35
50–70	4.67	3.34	4.48	3.28	1.04	0.93
50–110	8.96	6.42	8.66	6.25	2.75	2.14
65–75	3.17	2.10	3.08	1.99	0.43	0.26
65–85	5.48	3.81	5.29	3.66	1.01	0.78
65–110	6.53	4.70	6.29	4.53	1.53	1.14

Adapted from information appearing in Seidman H, Mushinski MH, Gelb SK, Silverberg E: "Probabilities of eventually developing or dying of cancer—United States, 1985." *CA— A Cancer Journal for Clinicians* 35(1):36–56, 1985; used with permission.

The incidence of breast cancer increases up to age 80, plateaus between ages 80 and 85, and then declines. However, the measured decline after age 85 is difficult to interpret and may reflect the inadequacy of epidemiologic data.

Classification and Pathophysiology

Breast cancer may be classified pathologically as noninvasive (in situ) or invasive (infiltrating). The noninvasive carcinomas are generally thought to be antecedents of invasive carcinoma.

Intraductal carcinoma (ductal carcinoma in situ) is the most common noninvasive carcinoma among elderly women. It is generally multicentric, and ≤ 20% recur locally after partial mastectomy. Axillary lymph nodes are involved in < 2% of cases. Lobular carcinoma in situ, often multicentric and involving both breasts, is rare after menopause.

Of the invasive carcinomas, invasive ductal carcinoma is the most common among women of all ages, comprising about 70% of all cases. The incidence of mucinous (colloid) carcinoma, a slow-growing tumor in elderly women, increases with age. The incidence of medullary carcinoma, which is often bilateral, decreases with age. Inflammatory carcinoma of the breast, a very aggressive tumor, is equally prevalent among premenopausal and postmenopausal women.

Paget's disease of the nipple represents spread of a ductal carcinoma to the skin of the nipple; it is usually associated with intraductal carcinoma and less so with invasive carcinoma. A palpable breast lump is present in 50% of cases.

Risk Factors

The major risk factors for breast cancer are listed in TABLE 121–2. The influence of reproductive history, history of estrogen replacement therapy, and abdominal obesity suggest that estrogens play a role in the pathogenesis of breast cancer. An increased prevalence of android obesity among elderly women may partly explain the higher risk of breast cancer with age. Android obesity is defined as a ratio of ≥ 0.71 between the body circumference measured at the waist and at the hips (the "apple" vs. the "pear"). It is associated with an increased concentration of free estrogen.

Use of postmenopausal estrogen replacement therapy◻ for 5, 10, or 15 years is associated with 2, 6, and 12 excess breast cancers diagnosed per 1000 women, respectively. Risk returns to normal 5 years after stopping estrogen replacement therapy. The risk of breast cancer associated with use of oral contraceptives disappears within 10 years after stopping use.

◻see also page 1211

TABLE 121–2.   RISK FACTORS FOR DEVELOPING BREAST CANCER

Increasing age
Personal or family history of breast cancer
History of colon or endometrial cancer in first-degree relatives
Reproductive history
   Early menarche
   Late menopause
   No pregnancies or late first pregnancy (at age ≥ 31)
Diet
   Regular consumption of alcohol
   High-fat diet*
Body size
   Abdominal obesity
Estrogen replacement therapy
Exposure to high doses of ionizing radiation
History of atypical hyperplasia on biopsy for benign breast disease

*Inconclusive evidence.

Symptoms, Signs, and Diagnosis

Breast cancers have the same clinical characteristics in elderly women as in younger women. Cancer is usually suspected when changes are observed on mammography or when a breast lesion is seen or felt. Lesions usually can be felt as firm nodules within the breast. Ulcerations may occur, and lesions within or near the nipple may produce discharge. Sometimes, breast cancer is discovered only after metastatic lesions cause bone fractures, neurologic changes, hypercalcemia, liver failure, or ascites.

When a tumor is detected by physical examination, bilateral mammograms should be obtained to rule out occult lesions. Certain radiographic images, such as speckled calcifications or tissue infiltration, suggest cancer, whereas a cystic appearance suggests a benign process. Even an apparently benign finding on a mammogram requires further evaluation, usually by fine-needle aspiration. This simple and safe procedure, which has 94% sensitivity, allows collection and cytologic examination of cystic fluid and is extremely helpful in planning definitive treatment of breast cancer. A positive result on fine-needle aspiration is diagnostic; a negative result usually should be followed by an open biopsy.

At the time of initial diagnosis, a chest x-ray, a CBC count, and liver enzyme studies are performed. More complex and costly tests should be reserved for specific indications, such as hepatomegaly or abnormal liver enzymes, bone pain and tenderness, nocturnal headache, 6th nerve paralysis, focal neurologic signs, or cranial hypertension.

Breast cancer commonly metastasizes to bone and may cause pathologic fractures, especially in osteoporotic women. Pathologic fractures can cause severe pain, especially when they lead to spinal compression. Bone metastases may also cause profound hypercalcemia, which can be the presenting symptom, most typically in women on bed rest. Breast cancer also frequently metastasizes to the brain, lungs, and liver.

Prevention

The goal of primary prevention is to prevent or halt the carcinogenic process before cancer develops. The goal of secondary prevention is to detect breast cancer at an early and curable stage. ∎

Primary prevention: Chemoprevention is the usual method of primary prevention, and the drugs tamoxifen and raloxifene are promising, although their optimal use is not yet known. For women at high risk of breast cancer (including any woman ≥ 60), taking tamoxifen 20 mg daily for 5 years reduces the incidence of invasive cancer by 49%. The occurrence of osteoporotic fractures also decreases, but the rates of stroke, pulmonary embolism, deep vein thrombosis, and endometrial cancer increase slightly, particularly in women ≥ 50. Hot flushes may limit its use in up to 15% of postmenopausal women. Raloxifene, a selective estrogen receptor modulator, may also reduce the incidence of breast cancer by as much as 45% and does not appear to increase the incidence of endometrial cancer.

Chemoprevention is also recommended for women with a history of invasive or in situ breast cancer, because the risk of developing a new breast cancer increases 0.5 to 1.0% per year. Adjuvant tamoxifen given for 5 years decreases contralateral breast cancer by 47% in all women. Preliminary data suggest that 4-hydroxyphenylretinamide, a retinoid, may provide similar benefit.

Secondary prevention: Elderly women often present with more advanced and symptomatic disease than do younger women. To prevent late diagnosis, health care practitioners should teach elderly women how to examine their breasts and encourage them to perform breast self-examination monthly. However, evidence is lacking concerning the benefit of breast self-examination.

Screening asymptomatic elderly women for breast cancer includes periodic mammography and clinical breast examination. Appropriate screening reduces breast cancer–related mortality among women aged 50 to 75 by 25 to 30%. Regular screening may also benefit women > 75, but this has not been proved. Screening guidelines have been developed by several organizations (see TABLE 121–3). There are no clear data indicating which method of screening is best.

Fewer than 50% of women ≥ 65 have ever undergone mammography, and an even smaller proportion undergo mammography regularly. The participation of elderly women in screening programs is determined mostly by the support of primary care physicians, who are in the

TABLE 121-3.   BREAST CANCER SCREENING GUIDELINES FOR ELDERLY WOMEN

Modality	American Cancer Society	American Geriatrics Society	USPSTF	Comments*
Mammography	Yearly	Every other year	Every other year	Survival results of every-other-year and yearly mammography are comparable
Clinical breast examination	Yearly	Yearly	Yearly	Sensitivity may improve as the breast becomes more atrophic with age; clinical examination may be the most effective way to screen elderly women
Breast self-examination	Monthly	—	—	Value has not been conclusively demonstrated; self-examination requires skill and may be difficult when cognitive function has declined

USPSTF = U.S. Preventive Services Task Force.
*No upper age limit has been established by the American Cancer Society. An upper age limit of 85 years has been established by the American Geriatrics Society, and an upper age limit of 75 years has been established by the USPSTF.

best position to identify and to help patients overcome socioeconomic, cultural, and educational barriers.

Prognosis

It is unclear whether breast cancer in women > 65 has the same or a more indolent clinical course than in younger women. Pure mucinous, pure tubular, pure medullary, and pure papillary carcinomas are associated with longer survival than all other types of intraductal carcinoma.

Tumors found in elderly women are more likely to be well differentiated. Life-threatening hepatic, cerebral, and lymphangitic metastases are less prevalent. In addition, a tumor is more likely to be hormone receptor–rich as a patient ages, a good prognostic sign. Local and regional recurrences appear to decrease with age. However, elderly women often have more advanced, less asymptomatic disease at the time of diagnosis. Stage-specific relative survival is similar to that of younger patients and is worse for patients > 85.

Prognosis is determined by the stage of the disease (see TABLE 121–4) and by different factors within each stage. In the absence of systemic adjuvant therapy, recurrence within 10 years is 24% for node-negative patients and 76% for node–positive patients. Axillary lymph node dissection has therefore become a routine part of staging of invasive breast cancer for tumors > 1 cm, since tumors smaller than this have a < 10% risk of metastatic nodes being present. However, particularly when followed by radiation therapy, axillary node dissection is associated with significant chronic morbidity 1 year after surgery, including lymphedema, decreased grip strength, limitation in shoulder range of motion, shoulder or arm stiffness, pain or numbness, and an increased susceptibility to cellulitis.

In women with **stage I or II disease,** the number of axillary lymph nodes with tumor is the most important prognostic factor. Ten years after diagnosis, 60 to 70% of women with involvement of one to three lymph nodes are alive and free of disease, compared with only 15 to 25% of those with involvement of eight or more lymph nodes. However, 25 to 33% of patients with node-negative breast cancer have recurrent disease. Systemic adjuvant therapy may improve outcomes for these women. However many women are unnecessarily subjected to treatment and its adverse effects, because patients at high risk of disease recurrence cannot be well distinguished from those at low risk. Known prognostic factors for node-negative disease are the size of the primary tumor, negative status of estrogen and progesterone receptors, and a high histologic and nuclear grade (ie, poor differentiation). Plasminogen activator inhibitor type 1 (PAI-1) is a new marker that may indicate a better disease-free and overall survival.

In **stage III disease,** unfavorable prognostic factors include edema, ulceration, fixation to the chest wall, and inflammatory breast cancer.

In **stage IV disease,** the prognosis varies markedly with the metastatic sites: average survival is 3 to 6 months if the patient has liver or lymphangitic lung metastases, 24 months if the patient has nodular lung metastases or pleural effusions, and > 5 years if metastases are limited to bone.

Treatment

Treatment is guided by disease stage, the patient's general condition, and the patient's preferences. In the elderly, frailty, serious comorbidities, and dementia may make aggressive treatment inappropriate. In such cases, palliation might be a better option. Local treatment modalities include partial mastectomy (lumpectomy) or total mastectomy, axillary lymph node dissection, and external beam radiation.

Biopsy of the sentinel lymph node (the first node that receives drainage from the tumor) can decrease the need for axillary lymph node dissection. When the procedure is done by experienced surgeons, the sentinel node is identified in > 90% of patients, the positive predictive value is almost 100%, and the negative predictive value is 95%.

Systemic treatment includes hormonal therapy and cytotoxic chemotherapy (see TABLE 121–5).

Stage 0 breast cancer: Regardless of tumor size, 98% of ductal carcinoma in situ is cured by total mastectomy or partial mastectomy

TABLE 121-4.   STAGING SYSTEM FOR BREAST CANCER

Stage	Primary Tumor	Regional Lymph Nodes	Distant Metastases
0	Carcinoma in situ or Paget's disease of the breast without tumor	No palpable axillary lymph nodes	None
I	Tumor ≤ 2 cm in largest dimension	No palpable axillary lymph nodes	None
II	No evidence of primary tumor	Metastasis to movable ipsi-lateral axillary lymph node(s)	None
	Tumor ≤ 2 cm in largest dimension	Metastasis to movable ipsi-lateral axillary lymph node(s)	None
	Tumor 2–5 cm in largest dimension	No palpable axillary lymph nodes	None
	Tumor 2–5 cm in largest dimension	Metastasis to movable ipsi-lateral axillary lymph node(s)	None
	Tumor > 5 cm in largest dimension	No palpable axillary lymph node(s)	None
IIIA	No evidence of primary tumor	Metastasis to ipsilateral axillary lymph node(s) fixed to one another or to other structures	None
	Tumor ≤ 2 cm in largest dimension	Metastasis to ipsilateral axillary lymph node(s) fixed to one another or to other structures	None
	Tumor 2–5 cm in largest dimension	Metastasis to ipsilateral axillary lymph node(s) fixed to one another or to other structures	None
	Tumor > 5 cm in largest dimension	Metastasis to movable ipsi-lateral axillary lymph node(s)	None
	Tumor > 5 cm in largest dimension	Metastasis to ipsilateral axillary lymph node(s) fixed to one another or to other structures	None
IIIB	Fixation to the chest wall* or skin	Any regional lymph node involvement	None

Table continues on the following page.

TABLE 121–4. **STAGING SYSTEM FOR BREAST CANCER** (*Continued*)

Stage	Primary Tumor	Regional Lymph Nodes	Distant Metastases
	Any size tumor	Metastasis to ipsilateral internal mammary lymph node(s)	None
IV	Any size tumor	Any regional lymph node involvement	Present, including metastases to ipsilateral supraclavicular nodes

*Chest wall includes ribs, intercostal muscles, and the serratus anterior muscle, but not the pectoral muscle.

with radiation therapy. Axillary dissection and systemic adjuvant chemotherapy are not necessary.

Stages I and II breast cancer: The management of localized breast cancer includes local and systemic (adjuvant) treatment. Local treatment involves total or partial mastectomy and axillary lymph node dissection. Total or partial mastectomy may be performed under local anesthetic, with negligible risk even for women ≥ 90. Partial mastectomy is usually followed by postoperative radiation therapy to prevent local recurrence of cancer.

The choice of surgical procedure is the patient's prerogative. Partial mastectomy may be preferable in terms of body image and sexual attractiveness, but the adjuvant postoperative radiation therapy can be inconvenient (it must be given 5 days a week for 7 weeks) and costly. In addition, the benefits and risks of postoperative radiation therapy are unclear for elderly women. Radiation therapy may prevent local recurrences, but it is not known whether it affects survival. Elderly women, however, are less likely to have local recurrences. Radiation therapy may cause toxicity to breast tissue, skin burns, irritation, and heart or lung complications.

Most elderly women choose to use an external prosthesis rather than to have breast reconstruction after mastectomy. Reasons why women elect not to have breast reconstruction include concerns about increased time under anesthesia and increased risk of complications. However, age is not a contraindication to reconstruction. A new prosthesis that adheres to the chest wall and does not require a padded brassiere (and is therefore more comfortable) is being tested in Germany.

Systemic adjuvant treatment is recommended for women with invasive breast cancer and axillary node involvement, invasive ductal or lobular carcinoma ≥ 1 cm in largest diameter, or, with favorable histologic findings, invasive carcinoma ≥ 3 cm in largest diameter because of the high risk of recurrence after local therapy. Tamoxifen prolongs both the disease-free survival and overall survival of postmenopausal patients, even patients ≥ 70 and those whose regional lymph nodes are cancer-free. For women ≥ 70, recurrence is reduced from 42% to 25%. There is no advantage to continuing tamoxifen therapy beyond 5 years.

Women with estrogen receptor–negative (ER−) tumors do not generally benefit from tamoxifen. However, tamoxifen has a similar effect on reducing the incidence of contralateral breast cancer in women with ER− and ER+ tumors. Primary treatment of localized breast cancer with tamoxifen is recommended only for women who cannot or should not undergo surgery.

After treatment, patients with stage I or II breast cancer should be followed up every 3 to 6 months for the first 3 years; every 6 months for the next 2 years; and then annually. These women are at risk of new breast cancer as well as of recurrence of the original tumor. In addition to a general physical examination, patients should undergo clinical breast examination and mammography annually. Additional laboratory and radiologic testing does not improve survival or time to detection of recurrence.

Stage III breast cancer: Locally advanced breast cancer is best managed with a combination of systemic and local therapies. Preoperative systemic treatment with chemotherapy regimens containing doxorubicin or mitoxantrone is the first step. When tumor size is adequately reduced, total or partial mastectomy, radiation therapy, or both may be used. About 50% of patients are alive and disease-free 5 years after treatment. It is unclear whether adjuvant chemotherapy and hormonal therapy after preoperative chemotherapy and regional treatment in locally advanced breast cancer decrease further recurrence or prolong life. In the case of inflammatory breast cancer, hormonal therapy by itself is seldom effective; a combination of chemotherapy and hormonal therapy is advisable.

Stage IV breast cancer: Hormonal therapy is the best treatment for women ≥ 65 with ER+ tumors or tumors whose receptor status is unknown, a long disease-free interval, or metastases only to bone. Antiestrogens are first-line therapy, followed by aromatase inhibitors and progestins. Most practitioners prefer tamoxifen as initial hormonal treatment and use other drugs if the disease progresses or if complications with tamoxifen occur. In about 15% of patients with bone metastases, tamoxifen causes tumor flare-up resulting in hypercalcemia. This transient complication can be managed with IV fluids and furosemide and does not warrant stopping the drug. Patients sometimes respond to a second hormonal treatment after the first becomes ineffective.

For patients with hormone-unresponsive tumors or with life-threatening disease (hepatic or lymphangitic pulmonary spread), chemo-

TABLE 121-5.   SYSTEMIC TREATMENT OF BREAST CANCER

Drug	Complications	Precautions
Hormonal treatment		
Antiestrogens		
Tamoxifen	Deep vein thrombosis;	Use with caution if history of
Toremifene	bone pain, hot flashes;	deep vein thrombosis
	retinal degeneration,	Periodic ophthalmologic and
	endometrial cancer	gynecologic examinations are
		necessary
Progestins		
Megestrol acetate	Increased appetite;	Avoid in obese patients
	weight gain; fluid	Use with caution if history of
	retention; deep vein	deep vein thrombosis
	thrombosis	
Aromatase inhibitors		
Anastrozole	GI symptoms; hot	Avoid if history of deep vein
Letrozole	flashes; deep vein	thrombosis
	thrombosis; pain	
Aminoglutethi-	Hypoadrenocorticism;	Hydrocortisone 100 mg/day for
mide	somnolence; skin rash	2 wk; thereafter, 40 mg/day
		because aminoglutethimide
		inhibits steroid synthesis
Exemestane	Hot flashes, nausea, dizzi-	Use only in tumors that stop
	ness, weakness, periph-	responding to tamoxifen
	eral edema, depression	therapy
Cytotoxic chemotherapy		
CMF		
Cyclophosphamide	Alopecia; myelosup-	Avoid if GFR is $\leq$ 40 mL/min
Methotrexate	pression; mucositis;	Adjust doses of methotrexate
5-Fluorouracil	GI symptoms	and cyclophosphamide to Cr Cl
		HGF for history of neutropenic
		fever
		Hospitalize for diarrhea
		and severe mucositis
		Monitor for hepatic toxicity
CAF or CEF		
Cyclophosphamide	Alopecia; myelosup-	Avoid in patients with heart
Doxorubicin	pression; mucositis;	failure
(Adriamycin)* or	heart failure; nausea	Monitor ejection fraction by
epirubicin	and vomiting	radionucleotide scanning or
5-Fluorouracil		echocardiography
		HGF for history of neutropenic
		fever
		Hospitalize for diarrhea
		and severe mucositis
Capecitabine	Bone marrow suppres-	Monitor for hematologic and
	sion, GI symptoms,	hepatic toxicity
	stomatitis, fatigue,	Hospitalize for diarrhea
	dermatitis, anorexia	

TABLE 121-5. (*Continued*)

Drug	Complications	Precautions
Mitomycin C	Alopecia; myelosuppression; pneumonitis; hemolytic-uremic syndrome	HGF for prophylaxis of neutropenia
Vinca alkaloids		
Vinblastine	Myelosuppression; mucositis; alopecia	HGF for history of neutropenic fever Hospitalize for diarrhea and severe mucositis
Vinorelbine	Neutropenia; mucositis; fatigue; alopecia; GI symptoms	HGF for history of neutropenic fever Hospitalize for diarrhea and severe mucositis
Taxanes		
Paclitaxel Docetaxel	Neutropenia; peripheral neuropathy; severe hypersensitivity; alopecia; GI symptoms; fluid retention	Consider premedication with corticosteroids and diphenhydramine
Monoclonal antibodies		
Trastuzumab	Cardiotoxicity; flu-like symptoms; diarrhea; anemia, leukopenia, but not myelosuppression or alopecia	Monitor for heart failure

*Mitoxantrone (Novantrone) may be substituted (CNF) in a dose of 6 mg/m^2, with reduced risk of alopecia, nausea, and vomiting.

CrCl = creatinine clearance; GFR = glomerular filtration rate; GI = gastrointestinal; HGF = hematopoietic growth factor.

therapy is indicated as first-line therapy. It has a much faster onset of action than hormonal treatment. Women with extensive comorbidity may not be appropriate candidates. Chemotherapy regimens are undergoing rapid change as new drugs and combinations of drugs become available (see TABLE 121–5). The mainstays include CAF (cyclophosphamide, doxorubicin [Adriamycin], 5-fluorouracil) and CMF (cyclophosphamide, methotrexate, 5-fluorouracil). Taxanes (paclitaxel and docetaxel) prolong survival in women with anthracycline-resistant disease. Cytotoxic chemotherapy is usually well tolerated by patients ≥ 70. Randomized clinical trials have included few women with comorbidities or women > 80, thus adverse effects in such women are unknown. Elderly women are more likely to have preexisting heart disease, osteoporosis, and risk factors for delirium and falls (eg, if they become dehydrated) and are more likely to be taking other drugs. Therefore, elderly patients should be closely monitored, and risk factors should be identified and reversed or lessened when possible.

Trastuzumab, a monoclonal antibody that acts against the Her-2/neu oncogene, may be used as monotherapy for women refractory to chemotherapy or with paclitaxel as first-line treatment of metastatic breast cancer. The use of trastuzumab is limited to patients whose tumors overexpress Her-2/neu. The overexpression of Her-2/neu occurs in 20 to 30% of metastatic breast cancers and is associated with aggressive tumors and chemotherapy resistance. When combined with chemotherapy, trastuzumab improves 1-year response rate, median duration of response, and time to progression. The drug is administered intravenously weekly. Adverse effects are milder than those associated with standard chemotherapy, although about 40% of patients develop flu-like symptoms with the first dose. Cardiotoxicity occurs in 7% of patients when the drug is used alone.

Pathologic fractures of long bones may be prevented by prophylactic orthopedic pinning of bones with osteolytic metastases. Patients with lytic lesions develop skeletal complications (eg, pathologic fractures, cord compressions, hypercalcemia) less often and later in their disease when they receive IV pamidronate monthly. Bone pain may be managed with local radiation therapy, pamidronate, and strontium 89. Brain metastases are managed with corticosteroids and radiation therapy.

End-of-Life Issues

Palliative care, which provides physical, emotional, and spiritual relief, must be provided with attempts for curative therapy and becomes the exclusive goal when cure cannot be expected. At all stages of breast cancer, treatment needs to be modified for life expectancy. For patients with metastatic disease for which cure is not attainable, the physician should clarify the goals of care through frequent, clear discussions with the patient and, when appropriate, the family. All should recognize that cognitive impairment alone does not exclude the patient from participating in decision making, because some patients with impaired cognition are able to understand, explain the consequences of, and voice an opinion about certain treatment options. Pain from bony metastases should be treated as described above with nonsteroidal anti-inflammatory drugs, pamidronate, local radiation, and strontium 89 rather than with opioids if possible. Palliative chemotherapy may be useful when the tumor invades vital organs. Other details of palliative care are discussed in Ch. 13.

DERMATOLOGIC AND SENSORY ORGAN DISORDERS

SKN/
SEN

122 ■ AGING AND THE SKIN

Aging leads to many changes in the skin and its appendages (nerves, glands, hair, nails). These changes can be broadly categorized as either intrinsic (true) aging or photoaging. Intrinsic aging results in subtle but important alterations of cutaneous function that are presumed to be due to time alone, whereas photoaging is due to preventable chronic exposure to ultraviolet (UV) radiation superimposed on intrinsic aging. Popular notions of "old skin" often correspond more closely to photoaging than to intrinsic aging. The dramatic differences between photoprotected skin and chronically exposed skin are evident to patients and clinicians alike.

NORMAL CHANGES OF AGING
(Intrinsic Aging)

Structural changes characteristic of aged skin include dryness, roughness, wrinkling, laxity, and increased incidence of neoplasms, both benign and malignant. Functional changes characteristic of aged skin include declines in cell replacement, barrier function, wound healing, immunologic responsiveness, and thermoregulation. (Age-related structural and functional skin changes are summarized in TABLES 122–1 and 122–2.)

Epidermis

Histologically, there is a striking and consistent flattening of the dermal-epidermal junction—a diminished number of interdigitations—which results in a considerably smaller contact surface area between

TABLE 122–1.   STRUCTURAL SKIN CHANGES

Epidermis
  Flattening of dermal-epidermal junction
  Variation in size, shape, thickness, and staining properties of keratino-
    cytes
  Decreased number of Langerhans' cells
  Decreased number of melanocytes

Dermis
  Decreased thickness (atrophy)
  Decreased cellularity and vascularity
  Degeneration of elastin fibers
  Fewer fibroblasts and mast cells
  Decreased number and distorted structure of specialized nerve endings

Subcutaneous fat
  Overall decrease
  Change in distribution

Appendages
  Decreased number and distorted structure of sweat glands
  Loss of hair bulb melanocytes (depigmented hair), decreased number of
    hair follicles (loss of hair), and conversion of terminal to vellus hairs
  Abnormal nail plates

---

the dermis and epidermis. This age-related change probably compromises communication and nutrient transfer between epidermis and dermis, affecting the mechanical, barrier, and immunologic functions of the epidermis. Moreover, epidermal-dermal separation occurs more readily in elderly skin, as manifested by the propensity of elderly skin to tear or blister.

Elderly skin often appears dry and flaky, especially over the lower extremities, at least partly due to a dramatic age-associated decrease in epidermal filaggrin in this area of skin. Filaggrin is a protein required for the binding of keratin filaments into macrofibrils.

Epidermal turnover rates decrease about 30 to 50% between the 3rd and 8th decades. This decrease slows the replacement rate of the stratum corneum. Linear growth rates for hair and nails also decrease, as do healing times for epidermal wound repair.

The number of enzymatically active melanocytes per unit surface area of the skin decreases by about 10 to 20% per decade, probably explaining in part the increased vulnerability to UV radiation in old age. The prevalence of melanocytic nevi also declines, from a peak between ages 20 and 40 to near zero after age 70. An age-associated decline in DNA repair capacity has been found. This decline compounds the loss of melanin protection, thereby increasing the risk of photocarcinogenesis.

Vitamin D production declines with age. One reason may be the 75% decrease in production of 7-dehydrocholesterol, the immediate biosynthetic precursor to vitamin D, between early and late adulthood. Other reasons may include insufficient sun exposure (especially in the institutionalized elderly) and poor intake of dairy products (the dietary source of vitamin D).

Dermis

Loss of dermal thickness averages about 20% in elderly persons overall and is generally greater in photodamaged skin. UV damage produces hyperplastic changes initially, followed by atrophic changes, particularly in fair-skinned persons. These opposing changes probably explain observed variations in the effects of photodamage. In sun-protected skin, there is a relative decrease in cellularity and vascularity. Elderly skin has a 50% decrease in mast cells and a 30% decrease in venular cross-sectional area. Following UV radiation, these decreases are associated with a corresponding decrease in release of histamine (a mast cell product) and other measures of inflammatory response. Basal and peak cutaneous blood flow is reduced by about 60%. Vascular responsiveness is also compromised. The striking involution of dermal vascular beds, which are the vertical capillary loops that occupy the dermal papillae, is thought to account for the pallor, decreased temperature, and impaired thermoregulation found in elderly skin. The decline in vascular supply to the hair bulbs and to the eccrine, apocrine, and sebaceous glands may contribute to their senescence.

Changes in connective tissue stroma are important in dermal structural and functional changes. Dysregulation of collagen synthesis and collagen degradation in the elderly probably contribute to impaired wound healing. Elastic fibers decrease in number and diameter with age. Fragmentation, progressive cross-linkage, and calcification also

TABLE 122-2.   FUNCTIONAL SKIN LOSSES

Barrier function
Cell replacement
DNA repair
Elasticity
Immunologic responsiveness
Inflammatory responsiveness
Mechanical protection
Sensory perception
Sweating and sebum production
Thermoregulation
Vitamin D production
Wound healing

occur. Alterations of mucopolysaccharides may affect skin turgor. Progressive loss of elastic recovery in elderly skin is probably due to these changes.

Subcutaneous Fat

Subcutaneous fat serves two major purposes. First, it acts as a shock absorber, protecting the body from trauma. Second, it plays a role in thermoregulation by limiting conductive heat loss.

The overall volume of subcutaneous fat usually diminishes with age, although the proportion of body fat actually increases until age 70. Fat distribution changes as well; eg, there is a relative decrease in subcutaneous fat on the face and hands but a relative increase on the thighs and abdomen. In some instances, these changes in the elderly can limit the function of subcutaneous fat, such as its ability to diffuse pressure over bony areas (eg, the ischial tuberosities in bedridden patients).

Appendages

Nerves: The density of cutaneous sensory end organs decreases progressively between ages 10 and 90 by about one third. The result is an age-related reduction in sensations of light touch, vibration, corneal sensitivity, two-point discrimination, and spatial acuity. The cutaneous pain threshold increases by about 20%.

Glands: The number of eccrine glands declines by an average of 15% during adulthood. Moreover, decreased output of secretion per gland can result in marked decreases of spontaneous sweating in elderly skin in response to dry heat (by as much as 70% in one study). These changes, compounded by decreased cutaneous vascularity, appear to predispose the elderly to heatstroke.

The apocrine glands decrease in size and function with age. Clinically these changes do not appear to have an effect except possibly a decline in body odor.

The size and number of sebaceous glands do not appear to decrease with age. However, sebum production decreases by about 23% per decade, beginning soon after puberty, probably due to the concomitant decrease in production of gonadal or adrenal androgens, to which sebaceous glands are exquisitely sensitive.

Hair: Hair substantially grays in about 50% of persons by age 50, apparently due to loss of melanocytes.

Hair loss from the vertex and frontotemporal regions (androgenetic alopecia) in men begins between the late teens and the late 20s; by the time they reach their 60s, 80% of men are substantially bald. In women, the same pattern of hair loss may occur after menopause, although it is rarely pronounced. In contrast, diffuse alopecia normally occurs in both sexes with age. However, diffuse alopecia can also result from iron deficiency, hypothyroidism, use of certain drugs (especially anabolic steroids and antimetabolites), chronic renal failure, hypoproteinemia, or severe inflammatory skin disease such as erythroderma. Hair loss with scarring is relatively rare and is associated with disease rather than with aging. It can be caused by deep bacterial or fungal infections; granulomatous disorders such as sarcoidosis, tuberculosis, and syphilis; and inflammatory disorders such as lichen planus and discoid lupus erythematosus. In unusual cases, biopsy of the scalp is indicated to establish the diagnosis.

Excessive or unwanted hair is also common after menopause in women, presumably as a result of the altered estrogen-androgen balance in hormonally sensitive hair follicles. The most common complaint is the appearance of scattered terminal hairs in the beard area. Even men may notice increased hair length in the eyebrows, nares, or ears.

Treatment approaches vary. Topical minoxidil solution can be used to treat physiologic age-associated hair loss. When applied daily to bald or balding areas, it stimulates regrowth in 25 to 30% of patients, particularly in those who begin treatment early. However, < 10% of patients experience cosmetically significant regrowth, and even these patients usually begin to lose hair again within 1 year. Finasteride (a 5α-reductase inhibitor that prevents conversion of testosterone to its active metabolite dihydrotestosterone), in a dose of 1 mg po daily, reduces hair loss in most men and promotes significant regrowth in some with androgenetic alopecia of the vertex. Finasteride is not effective for female androgenetic alopecia. The major adverse effect, occurring in 2% of treated men, is reversible sexual dysfunction, including decreased libido and erectile and ejaculatory dysfunction.

Hair transplantation can be performed with several techniques, including one in which punch grafts from the occipital areas are transplanted to the bald temporal areas. The cosmetic results of this procedure can be enhanced by scalp reduction (excision of bald areas). Hair loss from endocrine, metabolic, inflammatory, or nutritional disorders can be fully reversed by correcting the underlying disorder.

Unwanted hairs can be repeatedly plucked, cut, or dissolved with use of a topical depilatory agent, which breaks the sulfide bonds in the hair shaft. Alternatively, the follicle can be permanently destroyed by electrolysis or by laser.

Nails: The thickness, shape, color, and growth rate of the nails change with age, reflecting changes in the supporting nail bed and germinative matrix. Nails become dry and brittle and flat or concave instead of convex, often with longitudinal ridging. Longitudinal pigment banding is common among blacks, affecting 96% in one study. Nail color may vary from yellow to gray. The lunulae can become poorly defined. Occasionally, the nails become grossly thickened and distorted (onychogryphosis). Yellow thickened nails with distal separation of the nail plate from the nail bed (onycholysis) may indicate a fungal infection (onychomycosis).▮

Lamellar dystrophy manifests as brittle nails with split ends or layering and commonly occurs in middle-aged women and in elderly persons of both sexes.

No effective treatment exists for age-related nail changes. For the patient's safety and comfort, a podiatrist should trim thickened toenails with an electric drill and burrs or a carbon dioxide laser. Wearing gloves while doing housework and laundry protects brittle fingernails. Nails should be kept short, and use of nail polish remover, which dehydrates the nail, should be minimized.

Immunologic Function

Age-related decline of the immune system,▮ specifically of T- and B-lymphocyte function, is thought to compromise the system's two major roles of defense against external insults and internal immunologic surveillance. In the skin, the result is increased susceptibility to infections and increased incidence of neoplasms. Specifically, there is a 20 to 50% reduction of morphologically identifiable epidermal Langerhans' cells between early and late adulthood. These cells are the skin's immune effector cells responsible for antigen presentation. Alterations in the production of interleukins and cytokines by other cells such as keratinocytes may also contribute to immunologic decline.

Percutaneous Drug Absorption

Aging's effect on percutaneous drug absorption is partially dependent on the properties of the topical drug. For example, a hydrophobic substance such as testosterone or estradiol is equally well absorbed by elderly skin and young skin, whereas a hydrophilic substance such as benzoic acid is absorbed less well by elderly skin.

Percutaneous drug absorption is affected in other ways as well. For example, topical preparations are usually prescribed for dermatoses in which the stratum corneum and the skin barrier are already compromised, thereby increasing penetration. Moreover, aging delays the recovery of the stratum corneum's barrier function, which is thought to be related to the slow replacement of neutral lipids. Thus the clinician should always consider the systemic consequences of increased drug absorption (eg, adrenal suppression by topical corticosteroids).

PHOTOAGING

In elderly Americans, most changes in the skin's appearance are the result of chronic UV radiation from sunlight and occur most prominently on exposed areas. This process, known as photoaging, differs

▮ see page 1261   ▮ see page 1351

clinically, histologically, and physiologically from intrinsic aging, although most patients and many physicians do not make the distinction. Elderly persons whose pigmentation or lifestyle protects them from sun damage often look younger than their chronologic age. Some geriatric skin diseases, such as skin cancer, occur almost exclusively in photoaged skin.

Symptoms and Signs

Fine and coarse wrinkling, irregular mottled pigmentation, lentigines (brown macules), roughness, sallowness, and telangiectases characterize photoaged skin. Poorly defined rough, red dysplastic areas of actinic keratoses are associated with more severe damage and a higher risk of skin cancer.∎ The overall picture may be hypertrophic or atrophic, depending on the patient's complexion and the severity of the sun damage. Actinic purpura (also called Bateman's, solar, or senile purpura) appear as nonpalpable ecchymotic areas usually on the extensor forearms of the elderly and are thought to represent extravasation of red blood cells from friable vessels in sun-damaged connective tissue. Thrombocytopenia is often suspected, but platelet function and quantity are not altered. Depigmented stellate pseudoscars on the extremities also indicate photoaging. Cigarette smoking exacerbates the coarse wrinkling of photoaging.

Histologically, photoaged skin changes include epidermal dysplasia and atypia, decreased numbers of Langerhans' cells, and striking dermal elastosis (deposits of abnormal elastic fibers). Loss of immunologic and inflammatory responsiveness is greater than that caused by intrinsic aging alone.

Prevention

Because damage due to photoaging is cumulative, preventive measures are most successful if begun during childhood. However, evidence strongly suggests that avoiding sun exposure and regularly using sunscreen, even after marked actinic damage, achieves considerable clinical improvement.

Patients of all ages should be encouraged to wear hats, keep their shoulders covered, and apply sunscreen before going out, as part of their daily routine. Sunscreens with a sun protection factor (SPF) of ≥ 15 should be applied liberally over all exposed areas and reapplied after swimming or washing. Patients should especially avoid going outdoors unprotected when UV radiation is strongest, around midday. Because sunscreens also block UV-induced vitamin D formation in the skin, elderly patients should be advised to consume vitamin D–fortified milk or vitamin D supplements to safeguard against osteomalacia. Moreover,

∎ see page 1276

cigarette smoking should be discouraged for dermatologic reasons: smoking exacerbates photoaging in a dose-related fashion.

Treatment

Topical tretinoin (all-*trans*-retinoic acid) is useful in treating photoaging. Improvements in global appearance, fine and coarse wrinkling, roughness, mottled hyperpigmentation, and lentigines occur within 4 to 6 months. New capillary formation, collagen synthesis, anchoring fibril formation, and regularization of epidermal melanin distribution and disappearance of premalignant actinic keratoses may also occur.

Initial treatment consists of applying tretinoin cream 0.05% once daily at bedtime. The patient should be warned that mild erythema and peeling (retinoid dermatitis) will occur, although older adult skin is usually less prone to this problem than younger adult skin. If necessary, the regimen can be changed to every other day until tolerance improves. After 8 to 12 months, a maintenance regimen of one to three applications a week may be instituted.

A dermatologist or plastic surgeon may surgically treat photoaging with collagen injections, chemical peels, rhytidectomy (face-lift), and various forms of laser surgery. Before undergoing such elective surgery, elderly patients should be thoroughly screened for cardiovascular, renal, and pulmonary diseases that might increase the risk of complications. Patients should also be advised that the healing time for procedures such as dermabrasion and chemical peels tends to be longer than that for younger adults.

Laser removal of vascular ectasias or benign pigmented lesions is usually very well tolerated, and medical evaluation is rarely indicated before undertaking these procedures.

In general, medical and surgical treatments for photoaging are not covered by third-party payers.

123 ■ COMMON SKIN DISORDERS

Many common skin conditions affect younger and older adults equally. However, certain inflammatory diseases, infections, and neoplasms of the skin increase in prevalence with age. Inflammatory skin reactions that may occur in the elderly include drug-induced eruptions, erythema multiforme, toxic epidermal necrolysis, and anticonvulsant hypersensitivity syndrome (see TABLE 123–1). Benign skin tumors that are common in the elderly include seborrheic keratoses, acrochordons, keratoacanthomas, and cherry angiomas (see TABLE 123–2).

TABLE 123–1. INFLAMMATORY SKIN REACTIONS

Name	Etiology	Symptoms and Signs	Diagnosis	Treatment
Drug-induced eruptions	Most commonly implicated are penicillins, sulfonamides, gold, phenylbutazone, and gentamicin, although any oral drug can be responsible	Skin eruption is usually symmetric, maculopapular, and pruritic. Eruptions typically appear 1 to 10 days after patient starts taking the drug and last until about 14 days after patient stops taking it	Causative agent should be identified. Although some drugs produce fairly characteristic eruptions, the only means of identifying the cause of a given eruption is by temporal association and rechallenge, which is often not intentionally done	Causative agent should be stopped when possible. A lubricant (eg, white petrolatum) may help relieve a dry, itching maculopapular eruption. A topical corticosteroid is often helpful. Acute urticaria may require aqueous epinephrine (1:1000) 0.2 mL sc or IM or the slower-acting but more persistent soluble hydrocortisone 100 mg IV, which may be followed by a short course of an oral corticosteroid
Erythema multiforme	In about 50% of cases, cause appears to be a hypersensitivity reaction to a drug or infectious agent, particularly herpes simplex virus or mycoplasma. In the remaining cases, cause is unknown	Severity varies, from characteristic target lesions with a red periphery, pale edematous interior, and cyanotic center to extensive erosion of the skin with bullae on the mucous membranes in the mouth, pharynx, anogenital region, and conjunctiva (Stevens-Johnson syndrome). Corneal ulceration is common in the severe form	Causative agent should be identified. Skin lesions must be distinguished from bullous pemphigoid, urticaria, and dermatitis herpetiformis; oral lesions, from aphthous stomatitis, pemphigus, and herpetic stomatitis. Hand-foot-and-mouth disease must also be considered	All suspected causative agents should be stopped when possible. Localized eruptions should be treated symptomatically. Patients with severe disease must be hospitalized. Use of systemic corticosteroids is controversial, and some patients, especially those with severe mouth and throat lesions, seem to succumb more readily to fatal respiratory infections if treated with systemic cortico-

Table continues on the following page.

TABLE 123–1. INFLAMMATORY SKIN REACTIONS (*Continued*)

Name	Etiology	Symptoms and Signs	Diagnosis	Treatment
Erythema multiforme (*continued*)				steroids. If herpes simplex precedes recurrent severe erythema multiforme, acyclovir 200 mg po 5 times/day may be administered. Idiopathic recurrent cases have been successfully treated with acyclovir or valacyclovir, presumably because these cases have inapparent viral triggers
Toxic epidermal necrolysis (TEN)	About one third of cases are attributed to a drug reaction—most commonly to sulfonamide, barbiturates, NSAIDs, penicillin, or phenytoin. TEN may represent inappropriate apoptosis	Typically, TEN begins with a painful localized erythema that spreads rapidly. Within erythematous areas, flaccid blisters occur or the epidermis peels off in large sheets with gentle touching or pulling (Nikolsky's sign). Malaise, chills, myalgias, and fever occur. Within 24 to 72 hours, erosion af-	Causative agent should be identified. It may be difficult at first to distinguish TEN from morbilliform drug eruptions or erythema multiforme. Staphylococcal scalded skin syndrome can be differentiated by patient's age, clinical setting, and level of the epi-	Causative agent should be stopped when possible. Patient should be treated in a burn unit, and possible causative agents discontinued. All denuded areas of the dermis should be covered with an antibacterial agent, such as silver sulfadiazine cream. When possible, the area should be covered with a biologic dressing, such as a pigskin xenograft. Close supervision by an

	Clinical picture	Diagnosis	Treatment
	...fects mucous membranes (eyes, mouth, genitals), and the patient may become gravely ill. Mortality approaches 50%. Death is caused by fluid and electrolyte imbalance and resulting multiorgan failure	dermal split seen on biopsy	ophthalmologist is necessary. Use of systemic corticosteroids is common but has not been proved effective and increases the risk of sepsis. Intravenous immune globulin has been used successfully to halt disease progression
Anticonvulsant hypersensitivity syndrome	Usual cause is phenytoin, but other anticonvulsants can produce the same clinical picture. Sulfonamides and allopurinol have been implicated in a similar systemic hypersensitivity syndrome. Clinical picture includes protean cutaneous manifestations, eosinophilia, transaminitis, lymphadenopathy, hepatosplenomegaly, and fever	Causative agent should be identified	Causative agent should be stopped. Alternative non–cross-reacting agents for patients with a strong need for continued anticonvulsant therapy include lamotrigine and gabapentin

NSAID = nonsteroidal anti-inflammatory drug.

TABLE 123–2.   BENIGN SKIN TUMORS

Name	Symptoms and Signs	Treatment
Seborrheic keratoses (seborrheic warts)	Waxy, raised, verrucous lesions that are flesh-colored or pigmented. Can range in size from barely perceptible papules to large plaques. Often, they look as though they were pasted or stuck onto the skin. Dermatosis papulosa nigra is a variant that occurs exclusively in blacks in which the face is studded with numerous small, dark, sometimes pedunculated papules	Lesions may be removed by performing curettage and light cautery or by freezing with liquid nitrogen for 15–20 sec. Sometimes, light freezing of seborrheic keratoses before curettage makes removal easier
Acrochordons (skin tags)	Flesh-colored or pigmented lesions that are soft and often pedunculated. They commonly occur on the neck, axillae, and trunk of middle-aged and elderly people	Lesions may be removed with sharp scissors or a scalpel or by electrocauterization, usually without requiring an anesthetic
Keratoacanthomas	Rapidly enlarging nodules with a smooth outline and a central keratin plug. Left untreated, they usually resolve spontaneously but may leave a scar	Although usually benign, lesions should be managed as well-differentiated squamous cell carcinomas, mainly because they are difficult to differentiate histologically from a malignancy. Lesions are usually removed by curettage and cautery or by excision
Cherry angioma	Small red to violaceous papules usually occurring on the trunk. Lesions begin to appear in early adulthood and are nearly universal by age 30. Tend to increase in size and number with age	Treatment is unnecessary, although unsightly lesions are easily eradicated by pulsed dye laser therapy or electrodesiccation and curettage. For lesions that are not traumatized, bleeding, or otherwise symptomatic, reassurance is the best policy

Management Principles

The elderly patient who presents with a skin condition should be asked about use of potential irritants, such as rubbing alcohol and detergents. The patient's concept of the skin condition and expectations for therapy should also be discussed.

Maximizing compliance: The prescribed treatment regimen should be as simple as possible and should be tailored to the patient's physical capabilities. For example, a patient who has difficulty applying a topical medication because of neurologic impairment or arthritis may need a back scratcher–like applicator for hard-to-reach dematoses. In some situations, the assistance of a visiting nurse may be necessary.

The elderly are 2 to 3 times more likely to experience adverse reactions to antihistamines and corticosteroids, which are frequently used to treat skin disorders. These drugs, therefore, should be prescribed reluctantly and always with clear written instructions. The physician must also consider that regimens that are virtually trouble-free for younger patients, such as adding oil to bathwater, may pose a danger to the elderly.

Choosing the drug formulation: Most dermatologic agents are applied topically in the form of ointments, creams, lotions, powders, soaks, compresses, or gels (see TABLE 123–3). The amount of medication prescribed should suffice for a complete course of therapy or should at least last until the next physician visit. About 30 g of ointment or cream is required to cover the entire body once. The "rule of nines" can be used to estimate the proportion of body surface area involved and hence the amount of the preparation needed for each application (see FIGURE 123–1). The palm of the hand (which represents 1% of body surface) can also serve as a rough guide. Hence, twice-daily applications of an ointment to both palms requires about 4×0.25 g, or 1 g daily, and a 30-g tube or jar should last 1 month. This dosing information should be shared with patients to guide their usage rate.

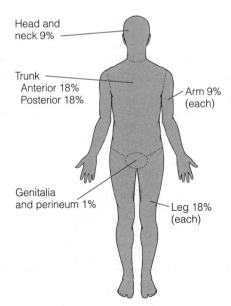

Head and
neck 9%

Trunk
Anterior 18%
Posterior 18%

Arm 9%
(each)

Genitalia
and perineum 1%

Leg 18%
(each)

FIGURE 123–1.   The rule of nines for estimating body surface area.

TABLE 123–3. TYPES OF TOPICAL DERMATOLOGIC FORMULATIONS

Formulation	Description	Indications and Advantages	Disadvantages
Ointments	Greasy preparations containing little water	Appropriate for dry, scaly, irritated skin; soothing; moisturizing; usually deliver active agent efficiently	Promote maceration of weepy or intertriginous lesions; greasiness may be cosmetically unacceptable
Creams	Semisolid emulsions of water in oil	Appropriate for treating exudative conditions and intertriginous areas; often cosmetically appealing to patient	May cause drying or irritation, especially to broken skin; contain preservatives that may cause allergic sensitization
Lotions	Suspensions of fine powder in an aqueous base	Appropriate for exudative lesions; cool and dry the skin; easy to apply to hairy areas	Delivery of active ingredient is somewhat less effective than that by creams or ointments
Powders	Minute porous particles that contain an active drug	Appropriate for moist lesions and intertriginous or difficult-to-reach areas	May be applied unevenly; may not remain at application site
Soaks and compresses	Gauze or other soft material soaked in water, saline, aluminum acetate, or magnesium sulfate solution	Appropriate for highly exudative lesions; soothe and dry weeping lesions; similar to lotions but cause more drying	To avoid overdrying as lesions improve, patients must substitute a cream or lotion or discontinue therapy
Gels	Solid or semisolid phase of a colloidal suspension	Appropriate for oily skin or exudative lesions; evaporation of the volatile phase increases surface concentration of the active ingredient	May be drying or irritating

PRURITUS

(Itching)

An unpleasant sensation that instinctively elicits attempts to scratch or rub.

Pruritus is a common complaint among the elderly and is usually caused by xerosis (dry skin). Other local causes include subtle contact dermatitis, candidal infection, scabies, and pediculosis (see TABLE 123–4). Systemic disorders that cause generalized pruritus in the absence of primary skin lesions (accounting for 10 to 50% of cases) include liver disease, uremia, iron deficiency anemia, lymphomas, leukemias, polycythemia vera, HIV infection, and parasitosis (usually of the gastrointestinal [GI] tract). Less common causes include diabetes mellitus, hyperthyroidism, and solid malignancies. Some drugs (eg, barbiturates) can cause pruritus. Although drug-induced pruritus is usually accompanied by a rash, some drugs (eg, opioids) often do not produce visible clinical findings.

Diagnosis

The history should focus on exacerbating factors, review of systems, and drug history.

In the absence of an obvious skin disease, a systemic disorder (eg, lymphadenopathy, hepatosplenomegaly, jaundice, anemia) should be suspected, particularly when pruritus begins suddenly and is severe and unrelenting. Although the complaint of a hot shower exacerbating pruritus is common regardless of the underlying cause of the pruritus, this symptom may indicate polycythemia vera.

Laboratory tests include a complete blood cell count; ESR; measurement of electrolyte, urea, and thyroid-stimulating hormone levels; and blood glucose and liver function tests. Stool should be tested for blood, ova, and parasites if indicated by history or examination.

Treatment

All patients complaining of pruritus should be treated for xerosis, because even mild dryness can exacerbate pruritus, regardless of cause. Patients should also be advised to avoid very hot baths or showers, rubbing alcohol, and irritants such as harsh detergents. Washing should be done no more than once a day, with soap used only on body folds and dirty areas. The use of opioids or other drugs suspected of causing the pruritus should be discontinued, if possible. Antihistamines and major tranquilizers are often prescribed for pruritus, but they pose danger to the elderly and rarely produce a benefit that justifies the risk. Phototherapy, if not contraindicated, can be tried for pruritus unresponsive to other measures.

TABLE 123-4. PARASITIC SKIN DISEASES

Name	Cause and Mode of Transmission	Symptoms and Signs	Treatment
Scabies	*Sarcoptes scabiei* (a mite): Easily spread by skin-to-skin contact between residents of the same household, nursing home, or other institution	Produces intense pruritus, especially at night. Burrows commonly found in the interdigital webs, the flexor aspects of the wrists, the axillae, and the umbilicus; around the nipples; and on the glans penis and scrotum. Erythematous papules or nodules are common in the same areas	Permethrin 5% cream or lindane 1% cream or lotion is applied to entire body. Patients will need help applying medication. After 24 h, patients should bathe; all clothes and bed linens should be machine-washed in hot water or dry-cleaned. After 7 days, cream or lotion is applied a second time and is also left on the body for 24 h, to kill any newly hatched larvae. All household members and close personal contacts should be treated concurrently. In a nursing home, all clinical staff, patients, and household contacts should be treated, because some infested persons may be asymptomatic. Postscabietic pruritus is treated with topical corticosteroids or, in severe cases, a tapering course of oral corticosteroids
Pediculosis	*Pediculus humanus capitis*: Spread by personal contact or by sharing hairbrushes and head wear	Produces severe scalp itching, often with secondary eczematous changes and impetiginization. Cervical lymphadenopathy may occur	Lindane shampoo 1% is applied to scalp, left in place 4 min, and rinsed off. Patients should then comb hair with fine-tooth comb. Combs and brushes should be soaked in the shampoo for 1 h. Procedure is repeated in 10 days to destroy any remaining nits
	Pediculus humanus corporis: Usually spread by close contact under conditions of poor hygiene	Produces intense generalized pruritus. Often, patient develops an eczematous eruption, severe excoriations, and secondary bacterial infection	Patient's clothing should be boiled, dry-cleaned, or machine-washed with hot water. Seams of clothing should be pressed with hot iron, or clothing can be disinfected with insecticidal powder (eg, DDT 10%, malathion 1%). Because lice do not remain on the host after feeding, treatment is for skin irritation and pruritus only
	Phthirus pubis: Usually spread by sexual contact but can be transferred by clothing or towels	Produces intense itching around genital area	Lindane shampoo 1% is applied to pubic area, left in place for 4 min, then rinsed off. Treatment is repeated in 7 days

XEROSIS

Dryness of the skin.

Dry skin is common in the elderly. The cause is unknown but appears to be related to altered lipid composition of the stratum corneum and to other subtle changes in epidermal differentiation. The HMG-CoA reductase inhibitors (statins) may also produce acquired ichthyosis and severe xerosis.

Symptoms and Signs

Dry skin tends to be itchy and scaly, especially over the lower legs, forearms, and hands. Symptoms are often worse in the winter because of lower humidity both indoors (due to central heating) and outdoors (due to exposure to cold and wind). A complication of xerosis called eczema craquelé, or asteatotic eczema, develops when the stratum corneum (the outermost barrier layer) is compromised by fissures or excoriations, allowing environmental irritants to penetrate the skin and causing inflammation.

Prophylaxis and Treatment

Patients should bathe only once a day and avoid using strong soaps, rubbing alcohol, detergents, and other drying agents whenever possible.

TABLE 123–5.   RELATIVE POTENCIES OF REPRESENTATIVE TOPICAL CORTICOSTEROID PREPARATIONS*

Potency	Compound	Formulation†
Very high	Clobetasol propionate	Cream or ointment 0.05%
	Halobetasol propionate	Cream or ointment 0.05%
High	Betamethasone dipropionate	Cream or ointment 0.05%
	Betamethasone valerate	Ointment 0.1%
	Fluocinolone acetonide	Cream 0.2%
	Halcinonide	Cream or ointment 0.1%
Medium	Betamethasone valerate	Cream 0.1%
	Fluocinolone acetonide	Cream or ointment 0.025%
	Hydrocortisone valerate	Cream or ointment 0.2%
	Triamcinolone acetonide	Cream, ointment, or lotion 0.1% or 0.025%
Low	Hydrocortisone	Cream, ointment, or lotion 2.5% or 1%

* Many equally effective compounds and formulations are not listed.
  † Ointments are more potent than creams containing the same corticosteroid in the same concentration.

Patients should also avoid placing potentially irritating materials (eg, wool) next to the skin. Emollients are helpful if applied frequently and liberally, especially after bathing, when the skin is still moist. Over-the-counter (OTC) emollients differ in cost and quality, but there is no obligate relationship between the two. White petrolatum is an inexpensive and effective emollient. Scented emollients are best avoided because they may irritate dry skin and cause contact sensitization.

Prescription creams and lotions containing urea or an α-hydroxy acid (eg, lactic acid) help remove scales, keep the skin hydrated, and prevent symptoms. A low-potency topical corticosteroid ointment, such as 1 or 2.5% hydrocortisone, is useful in treating inflamed dry skin (see TABLE 123–5). It should be applied to affected areas after bathing and at bedtime. Prolonged use is discouraged because of systemic absorption. A humidifier can help increase humidity during the winter.

ROSACEA

(Acne Rosacea)

A chronic, multiphasic inflammatory disorder, usually beginning in middle age or later, characterized by telangiectasia, erythema, papules, and pustules primarily in the central areas of the face.

Rosacea is most common in persons of Celtic descent. Onset typically occurs between the 4th and 6th decades. The etiology and pathogenesis are unknown, although genetic predisposition, hormonal influences, psychologic factors, GI infections, or *Demodex folliculorum* mites may play a role. A rosacea-like eruption may occur with abuse of topical corticosteroids on the face. Variants include lupoid or granulomatous rosacea, gram-negative rosacea, rosacea conglobata (rosacea fulminans), and persistent edema of rosacea.

Symptoms and Signs

Rosacea is a multiphasic disease characterized by persistent telangiectasia (which may be the principal or only manifestation) and papulopustules of the central face. Comedones and scarring, as observed in acne vulgaris, are notably absent. Episodes of erythema may be triggered by heat, sunlight, alcohol, or hot beverages; the skin may also be sensitive to cosmetic products. Photodamage frequently coexists with rosacea.

Eye involvement of varying severity is common. Eye symptoms include soreness, grittiness, burning, and lacrimation. Blepharitis and conjunctival hyperemia are the most common manifestations, but iritis, episcleritis, superficial punctate keratitis, corneal neovascularization, scarring, thinning, and corneal perforation may also occur.

Rhinophyma, a bulbous hypertrophy of the nose that usually affects men, occasionally manifests at the end-stage of the disease. Not all patients progress through the multiple phases or experience the many manifestations of rosacea.

Treatment

Patients should avoid situations that trigger flushing and vasodilation and should use sun protection. Mild to moderate disease may be treated with topical antibiotics. Metronidazole gel or cream decreases papules but does not significantly alter telangiectasia or erythema. Ketoconazole cream can also be used. Topical erythromycin, clindamycin, and sulfacetamide/sulfur are also effective. Some authorities recommend eliminating *D. folliculorum* mites with crotamiton or lindane cream, especially in resistant cases.

More severe inflammatory disease, including eye involvement, is treated with an oral antibiotic, initially at doses similar to those for acne vulgaris. First-line oral antibiotics include tetracycline 500 mg po bid, doxycycline 100 mg po bid, and minocycline 100 mg po bid, which are continued for ≥ 1 month. Response is usually dramatic. Lower antibiotic doses may also be effective. Second-line oral antibiotics include erythromycin and metronidazole. After control is achieved, the dose is tapered to the smallest effective dose. Many patients require oral maintenance treatment or intermittent courses, each lasting weeks to months. Topical treatment may be given concurrently. Recalcitrant disease can be treated with isotretinoin: the dose ranges from that used to treat acne vulgaris (0.5 to 1 mg/kg/day po in 2 divided doses for 4 to 5 months) to a low dose (0.1 to 0.2 mg/kg/day) to a mini-dose (2.5 to 5.0 mg/day).

Telangiectasia usually responds to pulsed dye laser therapy, a simple outpatient procedure that is widely available. Alternatively, electrocautery may be used.

DERMATITIS
(Eczema)

Superficial inflammation of the skin.

Causes of dermatitis include exposure to irritants or, much less commonly, to allergens (delayed hypersensitivity); genetic factors; and idiopathic factors.

Symptoms, Signs, and Diagnosis

Dermatitis occurs when pruritus, erythema, and edema progress to vesiculation, oozing, crusting, and scaling. Repeated rubbing or scratching may cause the skin to thicken or to develop prominent markings (lichenification). Pruritus is often accompanied by excoriation; papules and lichenified areas may be present. Frequently, the skin is dry with fine scaling.

Diagnosis is generally made clinically. If an allergen is suspected because of recurrent or unresponsive disease, patch testing can be helpful.

Treatment

Patients should avoid any practice or product that might irritate the skin, such as excessive use of soaps and detergents. Clothing made of nonirritating fabrics, such as cotton, is preferred. An emollient can be helpful if used liberally, especially after bathing. A medium-potency corticosteroid ointment may be applied to affected areas 3 times daily to help relieve pruritus and control inflammation. If the skin remains dry, an emollient can be applied between applications of the corticosteroid ointment. Once symptoms are alleviated, the corticosteroid ointment can be used less often or even discontinued, but emollient use should continue.

An antihistamine may reduce pruritus and help the patient sleep. However, in the elderly, antihistamines must be used cautiously because they are strongly anticholinergic; they rarely produce a benefit that justifies the risk.

Phototherapy with ultraviolet B (UVB) or photochemotherapy with psoralens plus ultraviolet A (PUVA) is sometimes effective; however, these therapies are often inconvenient for the patient because supervised treatments at the phototherapy facility are required 2 or 3 times a week for several weeks. Therefore, they are usually considered only after all other treatment options have been tried.

SEBORRHEIC DERMATITIS

A chronic disorder characterized by a scaly, erythematous eruption affecting mainly the face, scalp, and presternal area.

Although seborrheic dermatitis of the scalp (dandruff) is common in all age groups after puberty, involvement of the face and chest is rare before middle age and is most common in the elderly, particularly those with compromised skin care.

Despite its name, seborrheic dermatitis appears to have nothing to do with sebum. A hypersensitivity response to the usually nonpathogenic yeast *Pityrosporum ovale* may play a key role in pathogenesis.

The eyebrows, eyelids (causing seborrheic blepharitis and conjunctivitis), nasolabial folds, and postauricular and beard areas are most commonly affected, but the central chest and interscapular areas can also be affected.

Seborrheic dermatitis of the scalp can be treated with various shampoos containing sulfur, zinc pyrithione, salicylic acid, sulfur, tar, ketoconazole, or a combination of these. If shampooing is inconvenient or physically impossible, the patient can use topical 1% hydrocortisone lotion, especially in severe cases.

Seborrheic dermatitis of the face and trunk can be treated with hydrocortisone 1% cream. Preparations containing ketoconazole, sulfacetamide, sulfur, or salicylic acid are also helpful. Seborrheic blepharitis can be treated with hydrocortisone 1% cream (ophthalmic formulation). If associated conjunctivitis requires intraocular administration of a corticosteroid ointment or suspension, an ophthalmologist may need to monitor intraocular pressure. Warm compresses and gentle cleaning with diluted baby shampoo on a cotton-tipped swab to lid margins facilitates the removal of crust and scales.

LICHEN SIMPLEX CHRONICUS

(Neurodermatitis)

A localized pruritic thickening of the skin resulting from repeated scratching.

Lichen simplex chronicus is common in the elderly. It occurs in patients with pruritus at sites that are readily accessible for scratching, eg, the lateral aspect of the ankle, dorsum of the foot, shin, back of the neck, forearm, and elbows.

Lesions are dry, scaling, well-circumscribed, hyperpigmented, lichenified plaques (thickened skin with accentuated markings) of oval, irregular, or angular shape.

A high-potency topical corticosteroid is often used to control symptoms. A corticosteroid-impregnated tape (eg, with flurandrenolide) can help deliver the medication and provide a mechanical barrier to help break the itch-scratch cycle. When symptoms lessen, the corticosteroid potency can be reduced. Intralesional corticosteroids, such as triamcinolone 5 mg/mL (2 to 5 mg total dose per lesion), are often helpful for more troublesome lesions. Tar-containing preparations may also relieve symptoms.

More extensive lesions at some sites, such as the forearms and legs, can be covered for a week at a time with an Unna's boot (a firm paste bandage). This treatment helps break the itch-scratch cycle and often alleviates symptoms within 1 week.

Phototherapy may be tried when other treatments have failed.

STASIS DERMATITIS

(Gravitational Eczema; Varicose Eczema)

Inflammation associated with venous hypertension in the lower legs.

The pathogenesis is unknown. Stasis dermatitis may be exacerbated by edema, contact dermatitis due to use of topical medications, and scratching. Continued venous hypertension, even in the absence of stasis dermatitis, is a risk factor for venous ulceration.

Affected skin in the lower legs is eczematous and usually is edematous, with hemosiderin pigmentation and dilatation of superficial venules around the ankles. The affected limb must be elevated at least to heart level to facilitate venous return. Compression can be continuous or intermittent and should be increased over days to weeks to 30 to 40 mm Hg of pressure with use of surgical tube stockings and elastic bandages. Compression therapy may need to be continued even if the condition appears to have improved. However, aggressive compression may lead to ischemia in patients with arterial insufficiency, particularly diabetics. Thus, if arterial insufficiency is likely, ankle-brachial indexes and other vascular studies should be performed before initiating compression therapy.

A low- to mid-potency topical corticosteroid (eg, hydrocortisone 1% ointment or triamcinolone 0.1% ointment) may help relieve pruritus, scaling, and inflammation. Any possible contact allergen (eg, bacitracin, neomycin, fragrance) should be avoided.

VENOUS ULCERS

Cutaneous ulceration resulting from venous insufficiency.

Venous ulcers are a major cause of morbidity in elderly patients. Causes include incompetent superficial veins and perforators and postphlebitic syndrome. These factors result in persistent venous hypertension and a corresponding rise in capillary pressure with fibrinogen leakage into the tissues. Pericapillary fibrin cuffs form, limiting the diffusion of oxygen and other nutrients to the skin, predisposing it to ulceration. [1]

Symptoms and Signs

Venous ulcers commonly occur on the medial or lateral aspect of the legs. Edema, hyperpigmentation due to hemosiderin deposition, eczematous changes, and induration often occur on surrounding skin. Distinctive scars composed of sharply demarcated, sclerotic, atrophic, white plaques (termed atrophie blanche) stippled with telangiectasia and surrounded by hyperpigmentation commonly occur in patients with venous insufficiency. Woody induration of the involved areas indicates lipodermatosclerosis, a scarlike process thought to result from tissue hypoxia and increased cellular matrix turnover that often gives the lower leg an inverted champagne bottle appearance.

Basal cell or squamous cell carcinomas [2] sometimes arise in longstanding ulcers.

---

[1] see also page 1261   [2] see pages 1279 and 1280

Diagnosis

Diagnosis is made clinically. All patients with venous ulcers should be evaluated for systemic disorders such as heart failure, hypoalbuminemia, neuropathy, diabetes mellitus, arterial insufficiency, and nutritional deficiencies, which may contribute to the condition. Such evaluation is critical even if there is a clear venous component, because leg ulcers often have multiple etiologies.

Areas suggestive of malignancy require biopsy; if results are positive, referral to a surgeon for definitive treatment is necessary.

Treatment

Reducing edema is the major treatment goal. The patient should be advised to elevate the affected limb whenever possible. Compression stockings and graduated pressure bandages or Unna's boot, applied from toe to knee, effectively reduce limb edema. Diuretics, although widely prescribed, usually do not play a significant role in treatment and may be dangerous in the elderly. Techniques for ulcer dressing and possible debridement are the same as those described for pressure sores. ⬛ Systemic antibiotics do not enhance healing unless cellulitis is present.

If signs of **cellulitis** (erythema, swelling, warmth, lymphangitic streaking) develop around the ulcer, a wound culture should be taken (however, determining whether a positive culture represents colonization or active infection can require considerable clinical acumen). The patient should immediately be given dicloxacillin 250 to 500 mg qid or a 1st-generation cephalosporin for 7 to 10 days. Oral administration is usually appropriate, although rapidly progressive or facial lesions may warrant IV antibiotics initially. If the patient is allergic to penicillin, erythromycin or clindamycin can be substituted. If the wound is infected with *Pseudomonas* sp. (which often produces a fruity smell), frequent applications of compresses with acetic acid 5% reduce the bacterial count. Antibiotic sensitivity of all cultured organisms should be noted, because drug resistance is common.

Patients with venous ulcers and stasis dermatitis are at risk of developing **allergic contact dermatitis** from topical antibiotics or other potential sensitizers applied to the broken skin surface. Chronic, low-grade delayed hypersensitivity reactions (allergic contact dermatitis) may impede ulcer healing and increase local pruritus and edema. Wood alcohols, balsam of Peru, antibiotic ointments (neomycin and bacitracin), wool alcohols (lanolin), and fragrances are among the most commonly implicated allergens. However, all contactants are potential culprits, from the prescribed dressings to OTC products and even articles of clothing. When an allergy is suspected, topical therapy should be discontinued for at least 2 weeks, and the ulcer should be treated

⬛see page 1271

with saline wet-to-dry compresses. If possible, patch testing should be performed. Patients with very deep or nonhealing ulcers may require surgical intervention. Split-thickness skin grafts, pinch grafts, or commercially available cultured allografts may speed healing.

Bed rest and elevation are generally helpful in ulcer therapy, but the benefits of immobilization must be weighed against the risk of deep vein thrombosis and deconditioning.

PSORIASIS

A disorder characterized by well-defined, erythematous plaques covered with a silvery scale.

About 3% of persons with psoriasis first develop the disease after age 60. The cause is unknown, although many drugs, especially β-blockers and lithium, can exacerbate the condition.

Symptoms and Signs

Although psoriasis may occur on any area of the body, the usual sites are the extensor surfaces (especially the knees and elbows), scalp, and buttocks. Psoriatic lesions often appear at sites of trauma, such as surgical scars or scratch marks (Koebner's phenomenon). Nail involvement produces pitting, thickening, "oil-spot" discoloration, and onycholysis (separation of the distal edge of the nail plate from the nail bed).

Guttate psoriasis is a variant characterized by small droplike lesions. It is often associated with a streptococcal pharyngitis (and responds to an antistreptococcal antibiotic). Pustular psoriasis, a rare variant, is characterized by sterile pustules that may be localized to the hands and feet or generalized.

Exfoliative dermatitis can occur with psoriasis, particularly after withdrawal of systemic corticosteroids (therefore systemic corticosteroids should be avoided).

Psoriatic arthritis occurs in a small percentage of elderly persons with psoriasis and typically produces fusiform swelling and tenderness of the distal interphalangeal joints. Other types of arthritis (monarthritis, sacroiliitis, and a seronegative arthritis otherwise indistinguishable from rheumatoid arthritis) can also occur.

Treatment

Treatment of limited plaque psoriasis is usually best managed with a topical regimen. Resistive or extensive disease is best managed with more potent oral drugs or with other modalities, such as phototherapy and photochemotherapy.

Topical drugs: Topical corticosteroids may be used alone or with coal tar or anthralin. Initial short-term use of a potent topical corticosteroid ointment, such as betamethasone dipropionate 0.05% or triam-cinolone acetonide 0.1%, may be needed. As the psoriatic plaques respond to treatment, the frequency of ointment application should be reduced, substituting emollients, until only emollients are used. For small, localized lesions, flurandrenolide-impregnated tape can be applied and left on overnight or the medication can be covered with plastic wrap to increase potency. Systemic corticosteroids should not be used, in part because their withdrawal may cause a flare-up of the psoriasis, including rebound exfoliative dermatitis or conversion to pustular psoriasis.

Calcipotriene (a vitamin D_3 analog) can be used in combination with corticosteroids. Calcipotriene is available as an ointment, cream (preferred for intertriginous areas), and solution (for the scalp). Rarely, because of systemic absorption, calcipotriene causes hypercalcemia. Alternatively, tazarotene (a topical retinoid) can be used in combination with corticosteroids.

Oral drugs: In elderly patients with disabling psoriasis who cannot use topical drugs or who are unresponsive to other treatments, methotrexate, in oral doses as low as 2.5 mg/week, can control psoriasis. Because methotrexate can be toxic in cumulative doses exceeding 1 to 1.5 g/day, close supervision by a dermatologist is recommended; blood counts and hepatic and renal function must be monitored. After a cumulative dose of 1 to 1.5 g, liver biopsy is recommended.

Cyclosporine, in doses of 3 to 5 mg/kg/day, usually controls psoriasis within 8 weeks. Renal toxicity is the major concern—blood pressure, creatinine, and electrolytes must be monitored monthly. Cyclosporine is contraindicated in patients with a history of malignancy.

Systemic retinoids have been used as monotherapy or in combination with psoralens plus ultraviolet A (PUVA), but none are available in the USA. They (eg, acitretin) are contraindicated in patients with prior hepatic insufficiency. Liver function tests and lipids should be monitored regularly. Long-term adverse effects include hyperostosis.

Phototherapy: Phototherapy with ultraviolet B (UVB) in a whole-body treatment cabinet 3 times/week is highly effective for severe, extensive psoriasis. Phototherapy does not produce the adverse effects associated with frequent topical treatment and treats the entire skin surface, thus discouraging new lesions. Regular sun exposure is often as helpful but requires a favorable climate and appropriate sunbathing facilities (tanning parlors do not provide the correct wavelength of light).

Photochemotherapy: Photochemotherapy with PUVA is also useful for treating severe, extensive psoriasis. Typically, methoxsalen 0.6 mg/kg is taken orally 2 hours before exposure to UVA. Topical psoralens can also be combined with UVA for resistant localized disease (eg, palmoplantar involvement) but with a higher risk of severe burns.

BULLOUS DISEASES

BULLOUS PEMPHIGOID

A chronic bullous eruption characterized by tense bullae on normal or erythematous skin.

Bullous pemphigoid occurs predominantly in the elderly. Men and women are equally affected. Autoantibodies directed against a protein on the basal surface of keratinocytes, the bullous pemphigoid antigen, cause the blisters to form.

Symptoms, Signs, and Diagnosis

Pruritus and plaques of erythema often develop before blistering. Tense and intact bullae may be localized or generalized, and mucous membranes are involved in about 50% of cases. The patient usually feels well. Individual bullae heal without scarring while new ones appear.

The clinical presentation is usually characteristic, but confirmatory skin biopsy is recommended. Routine histologic examination reveals subepidermal bullae, and immunofluorescent staining reveals deposits of complement C3 in all patients and IgG along the dermal-epidermal junction in lesional and perilesional skin in many patients. Autoantibodies can be detected in the serum of about 45% of patients with active disease.

The differential diagnosis includes pemphigus vulgaris, dermatitis herpetiformis, erythema multiforme, benign mucosal pemphigoid, and drug-induced eruptions.

Prognosis and Treatment

Bullous pemphigoid is chronic and recurrent. Before the availability of corticosteroids, the disseminated disease was fatal in about 33% of patients as a result of sepsis.

Mild, localized bullous pemphigoid can often be controlled with potent topical corticosteroids; widespread bullous pemphigoid may require hospitalization until the epidermal barrier is restored. Systemic prednisone 40 to 60 mg/day po is needed to control severe disease. The total dose can be given every morning or every other morning to minimize adrenal suppression. After the skin lesions have resolved, the corticosteroid dosage should be decreased by about 50% over 1 month and then tapered more gradually. Patients should be observed for signs of recurrence as the prednisone dosage is reduced. Topical or intralesional corticosteroids may be used for recalcitrant lesions as a supplement to oral therapy.

Elderly patients receiving high-dose corticosteroid therapy should be monitored for corticosteroid-induced diabetes and other corticosteroid complications, including upper GI bleeding, fluid retention, hypertension, and psychiatric disturbances (most commonly hypomania).

Because of the risks of prolonged corticosteroid therapy in the elderly, an immunosuppressant is usually given concomitantly for its corticosteroid-sparing effect—eg, azathioprine 50 to 150 mg/day po, methotrexate 25 to 35 mg/week po or IM, or cyclophosphamide 2 to 3 mg/kg/day po initially, followed by a maintenance dose of 100 mg/day po. Because immunosuppressants require 6 to 8 weeks to become effective, the corticosteroid dosage cannot be reduced immediately. Adverse effects of immunosuppressants include bone marrow suppression and hepatotoxicity.

Patients occasionally respond to a combination of tetracycline and nicotinamide, drugs that have a better long-term safety profile than systemic corticosteroids or immunosuppressants.

After several months of systemic treatment, about 50% of patients with bullous pemphigoid have complete remission and then require no medication.

PEMPHIGUS VULGARIS

A rare, potentially life-threatening condition characterized by intraepidermal bullae on the skin or mucous membranes.

Although the incidence is highest among middle-aged persons, many people with pemphigus vulgaris are elderly.

Histologically, the bullae are intraepidermal; immunofluorescent staining reveals intercellular deposits of complement and immunoglobulin directed against the glycoprotein that forms the intercellular cement.

Symptoms and Signs

Pemphigus vulgaris is characterized by flaccid bullae that rupture easily and leave superficial erosions on the trunk, limbs, and mucous membranes. The surrounding skin looks normal. Many patients present with mouth pain; oral lesions may dominate the clinical picture, especially early in the disease process. Blistering can progress from localized to generalized, and patients are at high risk of secondary infection and sepsis.

Often, applying a lateral force to the skin causes the overlying epidermis to shear off (Nikolsky's sign).

Diagnosis

Diagnosis is suggested clinically. Confirmation requires a Tzanck smear, which involves scraping the base of a vesicle and using a vital stain such as Wright's or Giemsa to highlight nuclei of epidermal cells. In pemphigus, the acantholytic cells typical of pemphigus are unattached and basal cell–like, with large centrally placed nuclei and condensed cytoplasm. Differential diagnosis includes bullous pemphigoid, benign mucous membrane pemphigoid, toxic epidermal necrolysis, drug-induced eruptions, and erythema multiforme.

Prognosis and Treatment

Before the advent of corticosteroids, the disease was always fatal, with a mean survival of about 1 year. The mortality rate is now about 25%, with death usually resulting from complications of therapy. Long-term follow-up and prolonged treatment are required.

Widespread pemphigus may require hospitalization until the epidermal barrier is restored. Usually, prednisone 60 to 100 mg/day po is needed to control the disease. Other details of treatment, including alternative treatments, are as for bullous pemphigoid, including the need for close monitoring of high-dose corticosteroid therapy in elderly patients.◫

Remission may last many months or indefinitely, but some patients require lifelong treatment.

HERPES ZOSTER

An acute eruption caused by reactivation of latent varicella virus in the dorsal root ganglia.

Herpes zoster may occur at any age, but peak incidence is between ages 50 and 70. Herpes zoster usually affects otherwise healthy people, but immunosuppressed persons are at higher risk. The higher incidence among elderly persons may be explained partially by a decrease in cellular immunity—up to 30% of previously immune healthy persons > 60 have no detectable antibodies to varicella zoster. Other factors that predispose persons to a reactivation of varicella virus include use of immunosuppressants or corticosteroids, malignancy, local irradiation, trauma, and surgery. Herpes zoster recurs in about 6% of patients, usually at the same site as the initial episode.

Herpes zoster lesions are infectious until dry crusts appear. A person who has never had varicella may develop it after direct contact with the lesions or with moist contaminated dressings. Usually, only young children are susceptible, although pregnant women (because of risk of teratogenicity) and immunocompromised persons are also vulnerable.

Symptoms and Signs

Prodromal symptoms may include chills, fever, malaise, GI disturbance, and paresthesia or neuralgia along the affected dermatome.

◫ see page 1256

Rarely, prodromal symptoms persist for 5 to 7 days, leading to a variety of misdiagnoses, from herniated disk to acute abdomen. Red papules usually appear along the affected dermatome within 3 days. The distribution of dermatomal herpes zoster infections is 50 to 60% thoracic, 10 to 20% trigeminal, 10 to 20% cervical, 5 to 10% lumbar, and < 5% sacral; 99% of cases are unilateral. These eruptions rapidly develop into grouped vesicles, which vary in size, may be hemorrhagic, and may be extremely painful. The pain, which is an acute neuralgia, may represent a persistence of prodromal neuralgia or arise de novo. After about 5 days, the vesicles begin to dry and crust; gradual healing occurs over the next 2 to 4 weeks. Persistent hyperpigmentation or true scarring may result, particularly in the elderly.

In about 50% of patients with uncomplicated herpes zoster, some vesicles appear outside the affected area. However, if widespread severe dissemination occurs, an underlying lymphoma or other cause of immunodeficiency should be suspected.

In geniculate neuralgia (Ramsay Hunt's syndrome), facial paralysis (usually temporary) occurs, pain develops in the ear on the affected side (with or without deafness, tinnitus, and vertigo), and taste is lost in the anterior two thirds of the tongue. Vesicles appear on the soft palate, fauces, and external auditory meatus on the affected side. Consultation with a neurologist is advisable.

Complications

The major difference between herpes zoster in the elderly and in young adults is the incidence of **postherpetic neuralgia** (variably defined as pain that persists > 30 days or that appears after the eruption has healed), which increases sharply with age to about 40% in persons ≥ 60. The duration and severity of postherpetic neuralgia increase even more markedly with age than does incidence. Other risk factors for postherpetic neuralgia include prodromal neuralgia, severe neuralgia during the acute phase, and ophthalmic herpes zoster. The pain in postherpetic neuralgia is of three types: constant, deep aching or burning pain; spontaneous intermittent lancinating pain; and dysesthetic pain provoked by trivial stimuli (eg, light touch or cold) and often persisting long after the stimulus is removed.

Rare complications of herpes zoster include encephalitis, corneal scarring (when the ophthalmic branch of the trigeminal nerve is involved), motor neuropathies, Guillain-Barré syndrome, and urinary retention (when sacral dermatomes are involved).

Ophthalmic herpes zoster results from involvement of the ophthalmic division of the trigeminal nerve. Lesions on the tip of the nose indicate involvement of the ophthalmic and nasociliary nerves. Conjunctivitis, iridocyclitis, and keratitis may occur. In such cases, an ophthalmologic consultation should be sought. The risk of postherpetic neuralgia is greater with ophthalmic involvement than with involvement of other dermatomes.

Diagnosis

The finding of multinucleate giant cells on a Tzanck smear or biopsy of a vesicle confirms a viral infection. Although not commonly needed, vesicle fluid culture or direct fluorescent antibody analysis can also identify the virus and distinguish it from herpes simplex.

Treatment

Trials of zoster vaccine are underway and offer hope of prevention in the future.

Topical treatment consists of soaking the affected area in Burow's solution (aluminum acetate 5%), diluted 1:20 to 1:40, to remove vesicle crusts, decrease oozing, and dry and soothe the skin. Gauze dressings are soaked in the solution, applied to the affected areas, and loosely bandaged. The dressings are changed every 2 to 3 hours. If impetigo develops, systemic antibiotics should be given.

Oral acyclovir is appropriate if an elderly patient is seen within 3 days of the onset of the eruption. This drug inhibits the development of new vesicles and decreases the duration of viral shedding and discomfort. The effect of acyclovir on the incidence and duration of postherpetic neuralgia is debated, although several controlled trials have demonstrated benefit in otherwise healthy elderly patients. The recommended oral dosage is 800 mg 5 times daily for 10 days. Severely immunocompromised patients should receive IV therapy, 10 mg/kg q 8 h for 7 days. Alternatively, valacyclovir 1 g po tid for 7 days, or famciclovir 500 mg po tid for 7 days, may enhance compliance. The dose of all three drugs must be reduced in patients with moderate to severe renal insufficiency.

A systemic corticosteroid (eg, prednisone 40 to 60 mg/day po), started within a few days to a week of the eruption as monotherapy or combined with acyclovir, appears to reduce the duration of acute neuralgia but may not lower the risk of postherpetic neuralgia more successfully than acyclovir alone. Corticosteroids combined with an antiviral drug are the treatment of choice in patients with geniculate neuralgia.

Analgesia is usually needed. Acetaminophen or aspirin given every 4 hours, or other nonsteroidal anti-inflammatory drugs (NSAIDs), may be sufficient, but some patients require opioids.

Postherpetic neuralgia, once established, is difficult to treat. In addition to simple analgesics, capsaicin cream or lotion may be tried or the anesthetic EMLA patch. Opioids may be tried but are potentially addictive and often insufficient. Drugs used for neuropathic pain (eg, tricyclic antidepressants)▪ are often helpful. Newer drugs for neuropathic

---

▪see also page 393

pain, such as gabapentin, are being studied. Nerve block may be considered in resistant cases.

Isolation: Because varicella virus is teratogenic during early fetal development, pregnant women should avoid contact with herpes zoster patients. Severely immunocompromised persons should also avoid exposure. Ordinarily, however, isolating herpes zoster patients from casual contact with other adults is not necessary.

ONYCHOMYCOSIS

(Tinea Unguium)

A fungal infection of the nails, most often caused by Trichophyton *sp.*

Onychomycosis is caused by dermatophytes, yeast, and nondermatophytic molds, depending on the geographic region and the patient's status. In temperate zones, dermatophytes are most commonly implicated, particularly *Trichophyton* sp.

The nails are yellow and thickened with distal separation of the nail plate from the nail bed (onycholysis). The diseased nail can serve as a reservoir of fungus, which can lead to recurrent tinea pedis, a known risk factor for cellulitis.

Diagnosis of onychomycosis is made clinically and confirmed by a potassium hydroxide preparation, fungal culture, or nail clipping for periodic acid-Schiff staining.

Although not all patients with onychomycosis require treatment, patients with pain, diabetes mellitus, or peripheral vascular disease should generally be treated with itraconazole 200 mg po daily or terbinafine 250 mg po daily. Treatment must continue until the affected nails have grown out, which usually takes 10 to 12 months in the elderly. Because these drugs are retained in the nails, patients can also be treated twice daily for 1 week of each month with comparable cure rates.

124 ■ PRESSURE SORES

(Bedsores; Decubitus Ulcers; Pressure Ulcers)

Ischemic damage and subsequent necrosis of tissues resulting from intense or prolonged pressure.

Pressure sores occur most often among elderly patients who are bedridden, chairbound, or unable to reposition themselves. Pressure sores usually occur below the waist, although they can develop anywhere on the body (eg, in the nares or in the corners of the mouth in patients with nasogastric or endotracheal tubes; between the fingers in patients with rheumatoid arthritis). The elderly have less fat and muscle with which to dissipate pressure. An age-associated decrease in ascorbic acid levels may increase the fragility of vessels and connective tissue and lower the threshold of pressure-induced injury. An age-related decrease in the number of dermal blood vessels may place an elderly person at risk of ischemic injury caused by pressure and shearing forces. All stages of wound healing are affected by aging: the repair rate in elderly skin declines, as measured by cell proliferation, development of wound tensile strength, collagen deposition, wound contraction, and healing of blisters.

Epidemiology

The estimated prevalence among patients in acute care hospitals ranges from 3.5 to 29.5% but is higher in quadriplegic (60%), elderly post–hip fracture (66%), and critical care (41%) patients. The estimated prevalence among nursing home residents is as high as 23%; among home care patients, as high as 12.9%.

Development of a pressure sore increases the cost of medical and nursing care. In the USA, the total cost of pressure sore management in all settings is estimated at $1.335 billion. Complications such as sepsis, chronic infection, cellulitis, and osteomyelitis prolong hospitalization and rehabilitation. Moreover, pressure sores increase the mortality rate in elderly patients.

Etiology and Classification

Risk factors that may lead to the development of pressure sores can be categorized as extrinsic or intrinsic. Patients with certain medical conditions (eg, diabetes mellitus, peripheral vascular disease) are predisposed to developing pressure sores and are thus considered to be at high risk (see TABLE 124–1). Poorly nourished or chronically ill elderly

TABLE 124–1. RISK FACTORS FOR DEVELOPMENT OF PRESSURE SORES

Extrinsic risk factors	**Medical conditions associated with intrinsic risk factors**
Pressure	
Friction	Anemia
Shearing	Infection
Maceration	Peripheral vascular disease
	Edema
Intrinsic risk factors	Diabetes mellitus
Immobility	Stroke
Inactivity	Dementia
Fecal and urinary incontinence	Alcoholism
Malnutrition	Fractures
Decreased level of consciousness	Malignancies
Corticosteroid use	
Smoking	

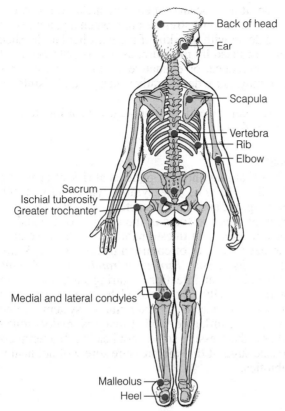

Back of head
Ear
Scapula
Vertebra
Rib
Elbow
Sacrum
Ischial tuberosity
Greater trochanter
Medial and lateral condyles
Malleolus
Heel

FIGURE 124–1.   Common sites of pressure sores. The most common sites are the sacrum, greater trochanters (femur), ischial tuberosities (pelvis), medial and lateral condyles, malleolus (ankle), and heels. Other sites include the elbows, scapulae, vertebrae, ribs, ears, and back of head.

persons are at high risk as well. Persons who are delirious, demented, partially or completely paralyzed, or bedridden are most likely to develop pressure sores.

Pressure is the primary external cause of ischemic damage and tissue necrosis. Normal capillary blood pressure at the arteriolar end of the vascular bed averages 32 mm Hg. When tissues are externally compressed, however, blood pressure may exceed 300 mm Hg, which reduces blood supply to and lymphatic drainage from the affected area. Common pressure points are shown in FIGURE 124–1. Most of them are over bony prominences.

Friction occurs when the skin rubs against another surface (eg, when a patient slides down in bed or is pulled up in bed without a pull sheet), resulting in loss of epidermal cells. **Shearing** occurs when two layers of skin slide on each other, moving in opposite directions and damaging the underlying tissue. It also occurs when skin sticks to a surface and then traction causes it to become stretched (eg, when a patient is sitting up in bed and slides down with the skin of the back held to the sheet by sweat). **Maceration** is caused by moisture, as occurs with perspiration, urinary or fecal incontinence, or exudative wounds. Excess moisture softens the skin and may cause degenerative changes and disintegration of the tissue.

Pressure sores are categorized into four stages according to depth of damage (see TABLE 124–2).

Laboratory Findings

Laboratory values that may indicate patients at risk of or with pressure sores include Hb < 12 g/dL, total lymphocyte count < 1200 μL, serum albumin ≤ 3.5 g/dL, and serum transferrin < 170 mg/dL.

Routine culturing of pressure sores in the absence of clinical symptoms and signs of infection is of questionable value, because all pressure sores are colonized. Growth of common pathogens (eg, *Staphylococcus aureus*, *Escherichia coli*, *Proteus mirabilis*) in such cultures does not necessarily indicate an infection requiring antibiotic therapy. A wound culture and sensitivity test obtained by needle aspiration or biopsy of ulcer tissue is indicated if bacteremia or systemic infection (eg, elevated temperature, inflamed wound margins, malodorous exudate) is suspected or if the pressure sore is not healing. Bacterial counts ≥ 100,000/g of tissue suggest that the pressure sore will not heal without systemic antibiotics.

Prophylaxis

Prevention is the most important factor in managing pressure sores. Identifying risk factors (see TABLE 124–1) and examining the patient's skin, especially over bony prominences, at least daily, are essential for preventing pressure sores. In addition, a validated tool such as the Norton Scale or Braden Scale (see FIGURE 124–2) assesses risk. A preventive regimen that includes the principles of pressure reduction, moisture reduction, and nutritional support should then be initiated.

Pressure reduction: A schedule for repositioning patients should be made based on the degree to which patients are at risk of developing additional pressure sores and the response of the tissues to pressure. Usually, patients with limited bed mobility must be turned at least every 2 hours. A written repositioning schedule should be developed. High-risk patients must be turned from the supine position to the right or left 30° oblique position to relieve pressure on major pressure points. Patients should not be placed in a 90° lateral position, because this position puts intense pressure on the greater trochanter and lateral malleolus. Patients who already have skin breakdown should not be positioned on the pressure sore.

TABLE 124–2.   CLASSIFICATION OF PRESSURE SORES

Stage	Characteristics	Treatment	Comments/ Prognosis
1	Nonblanchable erythema of intact skin, which heralds skin ulceration. In persons with darker skin, skin discoloration, warmth, edema, induration, or hardness may also be indicators	The affected area should be cleaned only with normal saline solution. A liquid barrier, a film dressing, or a hydrocolloid dressing may be used, depending on sore location	This stage is reversible. Symptoms and signs should not be confused with those of reactive hyperemia
2	Partial-thickness skin loss involving the epidermis and/ or dermis. The ulcer is superficial and presents clinically as an abrasion, blister, or shallow crater	The ulcer should be cleaned only with normal saline solution. Skin cleansers and antiseptic agents should not be used because they may be cytotoxic. A film dressing, a hydrocolloid dressing, or a hydrogel dressing may be used. Moist normal saline dressings may be used, although they require more frequent changes and tend to be less comfortable. Dry sterile dressings are not recommended	This stage is reversible
3	Full-thickness skin loss involving damage or necrosis of subcutaneous tissue that may extend down to, but not through, underlying fascia. The ulcer presents clinically as a deep crater with or without undermining of adjacent tissue	The ulcer must be free of infection and necrotic tissue. If signs of infection are present, culture and sensitivity studies should be performed by needle aspiration or tissue biopsy. Until results are known, wound and skin precautions should be taken. Necrotic tissue may be removed by mechanical, surgical, or enzymatic debridement to attain a clean wound base. An exception is a stable heel ulcer with dry eschar and without edema, erythema, fluctuance, or drainage, for which the eschar provides a natural protective cover that should be removed only if complications occur	This stage may be life threatening. Although treated ulcers heal slowly by secondary intention, surgical closure is often needed to shorten hospitalization and rehabilitation
4	Full-thickness skin loss with extensive destruction, tissue necrosis, or damage to muscle, bone, or support-	Irrigation should be performed as described for stage 3. If sinus tracts are present, a catheter attached to an irrigating syringe may be used to direct the flow of irrigant. All exudate and necrotic	Osteomyelitis or septic arthritis in contiguous joints may also occur

Table continues on the following page.

TABLE 124-2.   CLASSIFICATION OF PRESSURE SORES (*Continued*)

Stage	Characteristics	Treatment	Comments/ Prognosis
4 (*cont'd*)	ing structures (eg, tendon or joint capsule). Undermining and sinus tracts may also be present	debris must be removed from narrow pathways. The sore, including crevices and sinuses, should be packed loosely. Gauze, if used, should be kept in one piece to facilitate removal and to ensure that no dressing material is left in the sore. If more than one roll is needed, the rolls should be tied together. Exposed bone should be covered with a wet normal saline dressing, which should be changed every 4 hours to avoid drying and to maintain bone viability. An outer dressing should be applied as for stage 3. Surgical debridement to excise infected or necrotic tissue usually is followed by surgical repair	and may be fatal

The head of the bed should not be elevated $> 30°$ (except when the patient is eating), so that shearing forces are minimized. A pull sheet helps move patients up in bed. The patient's heels are kept off the bed with the use of pillows or foam pads placed under the legs from midcalf to ankle.

Patients should not be seated in a chair for more than 2 hours, because the sitting position creates intense pressure on the ischial tuberosities. Patients seated in a chair must be repositioned at least every hour. A chair that will not allow the patient to slide down avoids friction and shearing forces. A high-density foam or plastic seat cushion or silicone gel pads reduce pressure against bony prominences. However, no cushion uniformly distributes and relieves pressure entirely. (CAUTION: *Pillows and rubber rings [donuts] should not be used because they may cause compression, thus decreasing blood supply to the area.*)

Patients should be taught, if possible, to shift their weight every 15 minutes to help redistribute body weight and promote blood flow to the tissues. Patients are encouraged to perform range-of-motion exercises and to walk at least every 8 hours, if possible, to help prevent contractures, improve circulation, and maintain joint integrity, mobility, and muscle mass.

The appropriate support surface is selected based on the cause of the pressure sore formation, cost, ease of use, maintenance, and patient preference (see TABLE 124–3). No single support surface performs

Patient's Name		Evaluator's Name		Date of Assessment					

SENSORY PERCEPTION Ability to respond meaningfully to pressure-related discomfort	1. *Completely limited:* Unresponsive (does not moan, flinch, or grasp) to painful stimuli, owing to diminished level of consciousness or sedation or limited ability to feel pain over most of body surface	2. *Very limited:* Responds only to painful stimuli; cannot communicate discomfort except by moaning or restlessness or has a sensory impairment that limits the ability to feel pain or discomfort over half of body	3. *Slightly limited:* Responds to verbal commands but cannot always communicate discomfort or need to be turned or has some sensory impairment that limits ability to feel pain or discomfort in 1 or 2 extremities	4. *No impairment:* Responds to verbal commands; has no sensory deficit that would limit ability to feel or voice pain or discomfort					
MOISTURE Degree to which skin is exposed to moisture	1. *Constantly moist:* Skin is kept moist almost constantly by perspiration, urine, etc: dampness is detected every time patient is moved or turned	2. *Moist:* Skin is often but not always moist; linen must be changed at least once a shift	3. *Occasionally moist:* Skin is occasionally moist, requiring extra linen change about once a day	4. *Rarely moist:* Skin is usually dry; linen changes required only at routine intervals					
ACTIVITY Degree of physical activity	1. *Bedfast:* Confined to bed	2. *Chairfast:* Ability to walk severely limited or nonexistent; cannot bear own weight or must be assisted into chair or wheelchair	3. *Walks occasionally:* Walks occasionally during day but for very short distances, with or without assistance; spends most of each shift in bed or chair	4. *Walks frequently:* Walks outside the room at least twice a day and inside room at least once every 2 h during waking hours					
MOBILITY Ability to change and control body position	1. *Completely immobile:* Does not make even slight changes in body or extremity position without assistance	2. *Very limited:* Makes occasional slight changes in body or extremity position but unable to make frequent or significant changes independently	3. *Slightly limited:* Makes frequent though slight changes in body or extremity position independently	4. *No limitations:* Makes major and frequent changes in position without assistance					
NUTRITION Usual food intake pattern	1. *Very poor:* Never eats a complete meal; rarely eats > 1/3 of any food offered; eats ≤ 2 servings of protein (meat or dairy products) per day; takes fluids poorly; does not take a liquid dietary supplement or is NPO or maintained on clear liquids or IV for > 5 days	2. *Probably inadequate:* Rarely eats a complete meal and generally eats only about half of any food offered; protein intake includes only 3 servings of meat or dairy products per day; occasionally takes a dietary supplement or receives less than optimum amount of liquid diet or tube feeding	3. *Adequate:* Eats > 1/2 of most meals; eats a total of 4 servings of protein (meat, dairy products) each day; occasionally refuses a meal, but usually takes a supplement if offered or is on a tube feeding or TPN regimen, which probably meets most of nutritional needs	4. *Excellent:* Eats most of every meal; never refuses a meal; usually eats a total of ≥ 4 servings of meat and dairy products; occasionally eats between meals; does not require supplementation					
FRICTION AND SHEAR	1. *Problem:* Requires moderate to maximum assistance in moving; complete lifting without sliding against sheets is impossible; frequently slides down in bed or chair, requiring frequent repositioning with maximum assistance; spasticity, contractures, or agitation leads to almost constant friction	2. *Potential problem:* Moves feebly or requires minimum assistance; during a move skin probably slides to some extent against sheets, chair, restraints, or other devices; maintains relatively good position in chair or bed most of the time but occasionally slides down	3. *No apparent problem:* Moves in bed and in chair independently and has sufficient muscle strength to lift up completely during move; maintains good position in bed or chair at all times						
				Total Score					

FIGURE 124–2. **The Braden Scale for predicting pressure sore risk.** The patient is evaluated in six categories: sensory perception, moisture, activity, mobility, nutrition, and friction and shear. Pressure sore risk increases as the score decreases: 15–16 = mild risk; 12–14 = moderate risk; < 12 = serious risk. NPO = nothing by mouth; TPN = total parenteral nutrition. Modified from Braden B, Bergstrom N: "Pressure ulcers in adults: Prediction and prevention." *Clinical Practice Guideline,* no. 3, pp. 14–17, May 1992. U.S. Department of Health and Human Services.

TABLE 124-3. SUPPORT SURFACES

Type	Description	Indications	Advantages	Disadvantages
Static support surfaces				
Foam overlay	A high-density, solid 3- to 4-inch foam overlay is less likely than a less dense overlay to be compressed by the patient's weight and may redistribute body weight effectively	For patients whose activity is limited for a short time, such as during surgery or postoperatively	Provides increased support; easy to use; inexpensive	Provides minimal pressure relief; may retain body heat, leading to increased moisture and the potential for maceration; does not reduce shearing forces; is a fire hazard; may emit lethal fumes if ignited
Air or water mattress	An air- or water-filled vinyl mattress placed on top of the bed mattress; distributes the patient's weight evenly over the greatest possible surface	For patients with or at high risk of developing stage 1 or 2 pressure sores	Provides moderate protection against pressure and shearing forces; comfortable; easy to maintain (no pumps required); inexpensive; easy to clean	Minimizes but does not prevent pressure; readily accumulates heat and retains moisture; water mattress weighs 130 to 150 lb when filled
Dynamic support surfaces				
Alternating air mattress	Vinyl air-filled mattress that inflates and deflates small air cells at regular intervals via an electric pump, thus altering points of pressure. Some models have vents that allow air to circulate between the mattress and the patient	For patients with or at high risk of developing stage 1 or 2 pressure sores	Provides moderate protection against pressure and shearing forces; models with vents decrease maceration; lightweight; easy to clean	Minimizes but does not prevent pressure; may be uncomfortable because it feels lumpy; expensive

	Description	Indications	Advantages	Disadvantages
Air-fluidized bed	Mattress uses a high rate of air flow to fluidize fine particulate matter (eg, ultrafine silicone-coated beads). A loose polyester sheet separates the patient from the beads, allowing air to circulate around the skin and allowing body fluids to drain into the bed	For patients with any stage pressure sore, particularly stages 3 and 4; for patients undergoing graft or flap surgery	Supports the patient at subcapillary closing pressures (< 15 to 33 mm Hg); provides maximum protection against pressure, friction, shearing, and maceration; usually considered comfortable	Transferring in and out of bed and turning are difficult; does not easily allow patient to maintain a semi-Fowler's or Fowler's position (causing difficulty with eating and pulmonary problems); weighs about 1800 lb; circulates warm air, which may dehydrate the patient and the wound; turning and range-of-motion exercises are needed to prevent pulmonary and renal complications and flexion contractures; expensive; difficult to adapt for home use
Low-air-loss bed	Air-filled cushions that are fitted onto a hospital bed frame. The cushions are filled to exert the lowest possible pressure for the patient's height, weight, and body type. The distribution of air pressure supports the patient uniformly with minimum pressure on bony prominences	For patients with any stage pressure sore, particularly stages 3 and 4; for patients undergoing graft or flap surgery	Eases patient transfers in and out of bed; provides low pressure; decreases friction and shear; prevents moisture build-up; reduces patient dehydration; allows patient to be placed in the semi-Fowler's position	Expensive

consistently in all situations. Static support surfaces are appropriate for patients who can change position without bearing weight on the pressure sore and without "bottoming out" to the surface beneath it. Dynamic support surfaces are appropriate for patients who cannot change positions without bearing weight on the pressure sore, who bottom out on a static support surface, or whose sore is not healing.

Appropriate adjunctive devices, such as sheepskin, heel and elbow protectors, and trapezes, may help. Sheepskin is not thick enough or dense enough to reduce pressure but may reduce friction. A sheepskin placed at the foot of the bed, for example, may decrease friction against the heels of patients with vascular disease. Similarly, elbow protectors (pads made of sheepskin or a synthetic equivalent) decrease friction and may reduce pressure as well. A trapeze enables patients with upper motor function to move or shift their weight while in bed.

Moisture reduction: The skin must be kept clean and dry. Any moist or irritated area is washed gently with plain water. A small amount of mild soap may be used, although soap removes the skin's natural protective oils, and removing soap residue may mean massaging already damaged tissues. Next, a thin layer of moisturizing lotion is massaged gently around, rather than over, the reddened area or bony prominence. To protect against damage caused by urine and feces, a thin layer of a petroleum-based product is then applied. Heavier agents, such as zinc oxide and aluminum paste, are not recommended, because they are difficult to remove.

Plastic-lined paper bed pads can be covered with a draw sheet or pillowcase so as not to touch the patient's skin, and as few pads as possible should be used. A light dusting of a noncaking body powder applied to the skinfolds helps reduce friction and shearing and absorb moisture.

Incontinence must be evaluated and managed.◻ Absorbent incontinence briefs, indwelling bladder catheters, or condom catheters may be indicated for some patients but are not substitutes for efforts to help a patient regain continence through a bowel or bladder management program.

Nutritional support: Patients who are at risk of developing pressure sores or who already have skin breakdown should be screened for nutritional deficiencies.◻ Clinically significant malnutrition is a risk factor for pressure sore formation and is diagnosed if serum albumin is < 3.5 mg/dL, total lymphocyte count is < 1800/μL, or body weight has decreased more than 15%. Signs of vitamin and mineral deficiencies are also noted during the assessment.

Malnourished patients are started on high-protein, high-calorie oral feedings and oral supplements. Daily vitamin C and zinc supplements are given to patients with vitamin and mineral deficiencies. Functional

◻ see page 965   ◻ see page 598

disabilities affecting nutritional intake (eg, poor dentition, poorly fitting dentures, impaired vision) are identified and modified when possible.

Treatment

Treatment of a pressure sore is based on its stage (see TABLE 124–2). Regardless of stage, prompt treatment is essential, because an untreated pressure sore may worsen and lead to cellulitis, chronic infection, or osteomyelitis. ◙ Pressure, friction, shearing, and maceration must always be reduced. Good nutrition is essential. Total caloric intake should be at least 30 to 35 calories/kg/day, and protein intake should be 1.25 to 1.5 g/kg/day. All patients with pressure sores should receive vitamin C at ≥ 120 mg/day and zinc at 12 to 15 mg/day, although the best dosing of zinc is not known. A single daily high-potency vitamin and mineral supplement is usually recommended.

Effective pressure sore management includes cleansing of the wound initially and with each dressing change; prevention, diagnosis, and treatment of infection; and use of an appropriate dressing. Specific dressings and topical agents are listed in TABLE 124–4.

Debridement: Debridement may be accomplished surgically, mechanically, autolytically, or enzymatically. The method of debridement is selected according to the patient's condition and goals. Surgical debridement is indicated when there is an urgent need for debridement (eg, worsening cellulitis, sepsis). Mechanical, autolytic, or enzymatic debridement or a combination of these may be used when the need for drainage or removal of dead tissue is not urgent. They can also be used for patients who cannot tolerate surgical debridement.

For **surgical debridement,** a scalpel, scissors, or other sharp instrument is used to remove necrotic tissue and thick adherent eschar. Although it is the quickest and most effective method for such removal, surgical debridement increases the risk of hemorrhage, infection, and wound enlargement and usually is more painful than mechanical debridement. Analgesics should be provided as needed and as appropriate.

Mechanical debridement is minimally effective on eschar. Normal saline solution is used to irrigate the wound, cleansing it of purulent drainage or necrotic debris. Aseptic technique is followed with use of a catheter-tipped syringe or high-pressure dental irrigation device. The latter device provides a pulsating stream that both aids debridement and stimulates circulation. A wet-to-dry dressing, consisting of plain loosely woven gauze without cotton filling, moistened with normal saline, is then gently packed into the wound without extending onto the intact skin. The wound should not be packed too tightly, because this inhibits the absorptive capability of the dressing and applies pressure on the area. The dressing is allowed to dry so that loose necrotic tissue and

◙ see page 486

TABLE 124-4. DRESSINGS AND TOPICAL AGENTS FOR PRESSURE SORES

Type	Description	Guidelines for Use	Comments
Liquid barriers	Contain plasticizing agents and alcohol; provide a protective waterproof coating over affected areas; may be sprayed, wiped, or rolled on the skin; generally non-irritating; unaffected by urine, perspiration, or digestive acids; insoluble in water but can be dissolved with a soap solution	1. The skin must be gently cleaned and then rinsed and dried 2. The liquid barrier should be applied and allowed to dry for 1 minute	The patient may feel a momentary sting when the barrier is applied to excoriated skin NOTE: *Tincture of benzoin should not be used on reddened areas.* It becomes sticky when dry, and fragile skin may be inadvertently pulled
Film dressings	Clear, adherent, nonabsorbent polymer-based dressings that are permeable to gases and vapors but not to fluids. Usually left in place for 5 to 7 days, the dressing maintains the wound exudate against the wound surface, promoting epithelial cell migration across the wound	1. The wound and surrounding skin must be cleaned, and the surrounding skin must be dry so that the dressing will adhere 2. The dressing should cover at least a 1-inch margin around the wound 3. The dressing should not be stretched tightly over the wound 4. If excessive exudate threatens to loosen the dressing, the exudate may be aspirated through the dressing with a small-bore needle. The dressing may reseal itself or may need to be patched with another piece of dressing	These dressings work on the principle that healing occurs more quickly in a moist environment Dressings may be cut or overlapped without reducing effectiveness

Hydrocolloid dressings	Opaque, gas-impermeable occlusive dressings made of inert hydrophobic polymers containing fluid-absorbent hydrocolloid particles. When these particles come in contact with wound exudate, they swell, forming a moist gel that promotes cell migration, cleaning, debridement, and granulation	1. The wound and surrounding skin should be cleaned before applying the dressing. The surrounding skin must be dry so that the dressing will adhere 2. The dressing should cover the wound and extend at least 1½ inches beyond its edges 3. The dressing may be left on for up to 7 days unless exudate leakage occurs	These dressings work on the principle that optimal wound healing occurs in a closed, moist environment The dressing is not recommended if signs of infection (elevated temperature, purulent malodorous exudate, inflamed borders) are present The dressing may initially enlarge the wound because of its debriding action
Debriding enzymes	Proteolytic and fibrinolytic agents that act against devitalized tissue; most useful on superficial wound layers. Because these agents must be in contact with the substrate of the wound, they are ineffective on dense, dry eschar. Used as an adjunct to mechanical or surgical debridement	1. All hardened or dry eschar should be removed or crosshatched so that the enzyme can come in contact with the wound substrate 2. Because some preparations become inactive in 24 h, they must be reconstituted for each use	Antibacterials and antiseptics may inhibit the action of some enzymatic agents
Absorption dressings	Hydrophilic beads, grains, or flakes that absorb excess wound exudate and necrotic debris, which may inhibit tissue regeneration	1. Should be reconstituted according to the manufacturer's instructions 2. Should be gently packed into the wound and then covered with a dry outer dressing 3. Usually must be changed once or twice a day	The dressings also keep the wound sufficiently moist to encourage healing and deodorize the wound

Table continues on the following page.

1273

TABLE 124–4. DRESSINGS AND TOPICAL AGENTS FOR PRESSURE SORES (*Continued*)

Type	Description	Guidelines for Use	Comments
Hydrogels	Polymers that absorb wound exudate to form water-soluble gelatinous substances. Semitransparent and nonadhesive, these dressings provide a moist environment for wound healing	1. The dressing may be refrigerated to promote patient comfort 2. After the wound has been gently cleaned with normal saline, the dressing (which should extend 1½ inches beyond the wound edges) is applied directly over the wound 3. If intact, the dressing may be left on for 1 to 3 days	Occasionally, these dressings cause maceration of the surrounding skin
Calcium alginate dressings	Made of natural polysaccharides found in brown seaweed, the dressing is a high-quality textile fiber pad capable of absorbing 20 times its weight in exudate. On contact with exudate, the dressing forms a soft gas-permeable gel, thereby maintaining a moist environment for wound healing	1. After the wound is irrigated with normal saline, the dry dressing is applied 2. If the wound has heavy exudate, the dressing may need to be changed once or twice daily 3. As the wound heals, the dressing may be left on longer, up to several days	As the alginate turns into a gel, it may produce an unpleasant odor of seaweed, which can be controlled by placing a charcoal pad over the outer gauze dressing

wound drainage are absorbed into the dressing and removed with each dressing change (usually every 4 to 6 hours).

An appropriately sized outer dressing is then applied over the packed wound to prevent contamination. This dry sterile dressing may be secured with hypoallergenic tape, Montgomery straps, stockinette, or other materials. The intact surrounding skin should be protected with a liquid barrier or film dressing.

Autolytic debridement involves the use of occlusive or semi-occlusive synthetic dressings to cover a wound and allow the body's own enzymes and moisture to rehydrate and soften devitalized tissue. Enzymes normally found in wound fluids are then better able to digest the tissue. Autolytic debridement is contraindicated if the wound is infected.

For **enzymatic debridement,** topical debriding enzymes (proteolytic and fibrinolytic agents) are used. This method may be used for patients who are not candidates for surgical debridement and for those who have clean wounds and are residents of long-term care facilities or are receiving care at home. Enzymatic debridement is most effective when combined with mechanical or surgical debridement.

Although debridement is often essential, it must eventually be discontinued so that granulation tissue can grow and the wound can heal. After any type of debridement, a moist environment should be maintained to facilitate granulation and wound healing. Either a moist normal saline dressing (changed every 6 to 8 hours) or an absorption, hydrogel, or calcium alginate dressing may be used.

Surgical repair: Musculocutaneous flap procedures are frequently performed, because muscle is a reliable barrier to infection and improves vascularity. However, among patients who are ambulatory, these benefits must be weighed against the loss of functional muscle from the donor site. Extensive pressure sores may require more than one musculocutaneous flap procedure to establish closure.

Postoperative care includes monitoring the patient for infection and keeping pressure off the flap site. Patients who have undergone flap procedures should be placed on an air-fluidized or low-air-loss bed (see TABLE 124–3) for ≥ 2 weeks and gradually increase periods of time sitting or lying on the flap to increase its tolerance to pressure. Recurrence rates for pressure sores after surgical repair are estimated to be between 13% and 56%. Therefore, patients and caregivers must be taught how to reduce risk factors, assess the skin daily, and maintain a healthy diet.

Patient and Caregiver Issues

The interdisciplinary team, usually consisting of the physician, nurses, a dietitian, and rehabilitation specialists, should be involved in teaching the prevention and management of skin breakdown to high-risk patients and their caregivers. This instruction may occur in the acute or long-term care setting or in the patient's home. The main teaching points in the care plan are threefold: keeping pressure off the area of breakdown, cleaning and dressing the wound, and maintaining good nutrition.

Patients and caregivers should learn to examine the skin daily and to note any areas of redness over bony prominences (see FIGURE 124–1). A nurse can help caregivers select the appropriate bed (see TABLE 124–3) and chair support surfaces. Caregivers should be taught how to turn and position bedbound patients every 2 hours, aided by the use of either a written turning schedule developed for the patient or a kitchen timer. Caregivers should also be shown how to support the patient using pillows and foam pads.

Caregivers, and sometimes even patients, can be taught how to clean and dress pressure sores. Clean technique is preferable for patients being cared for in the home setting. Caregivers can be taught how to remove and properly dispose of soiled dressings by placing a disposable plastic bag over the hand, removing the dressing, and inverting the bag for disposal. Saline solution, which is used to clean and irrigate the wound, may be purchased at a drug store or made at home. Cleaning and irrigating the wound should be demonstrated by a health care provider. The patient's physician or nurse recommends the type of dressing to be used for the patient based on the stage of the sore, the ease of use, and cost. Caregivers should also be taught to recognize and report signs and symptoms of infection.

Patients are taught to weigh themselves regularly and report any unplanned gain or loss of $\geq$ 10 pounds occurring within a 6-month period. A dietitian reviews the patient's nutritional status and recommends a diet that will maintain a positive nitrogen balance. Supplemental vitamins and minerals are best taken daily.

125 SKIN CANCERS

PREMALIGNANT LESIONS

Premalignant lesions that are common in the elderly include actinic keratoses, Bowen's disease, and lentigo maligna.

ACTINIC KERATOSES

Premalignant lesions occurring in sun-exposed areas that may give rise to squamous cell carcinomas.

Actinic keratoses are the most common type of premalignant skin lesion. They are caused by ultraviolet light, which induces mutations. Risk factors include older age, fair complexion, blue eyes, and a history of childhood freckling.

Symptoms and Signs

The lesions are scaly sandpaper-like patches, varying in color from skin-colored to reddish-brown or yellowish-black, that occur on sun-exposed areas. Lesions may be single or multiple. They are usually painless but may be slightly tender.

Prognosis and Treatment

A lesion may evolve into a squamous cell carcinoma,◨ but the latent period is long, and the squamous cell carcinoma usually grows very slowly and rarely metastasizes. Patients with actinic keratoses are at high risk of developing other forms of skin cancer as well.

Avoidance of sun exposure leads to regression of early actinic keratoses and may be sufficient therapy for patients with mild disease. Patients with multiple skin lesions should be screened every 6 to 12 months for skin cancer. Patients should be advised to use a broad-spectrum sunscreen with a sun protection factor (SPF) > 15. For only a few lesions, cryotherapy with liquid nitrogen or curettage and light cautery may be used. Particularly for multiple lesions, topical 5-fluorouracil (5-FU) can be used. For facial lesions, a 1 or 2% solution or 1% cream can be used. For lesions on the trunk or limbs, 5% 5-FU cream can be applied. Cream or solution should be applied once or twice a day. Treatment with 5-FU produces progressive erythema and burning and, after 2 to 4 weeks, ulceration followed by reepithelialization over another 2 weeks. Treatment should be discontinued once ulceration occurs. Complete healing usually occurs within 2 months, and the patient has far fewer lesions for months to years thereafter. Pain and burning sensations can be decreased, especially on sensitive areas such as the face, by first applying a 1 to 2% 5-FU solution, then 15 to 20 minutes later applying a medium-potency corticosteroid cream. Patients must be told to avoid the eyes and mucous membranes when applying 5-FU, to follow the directions in the package circular exactly, and to never leave the medication on longer than directed. Tretinoin cream can be combined with 5-FU, especially if lesions appear on more resistant areas such as the trunk or limbs. Masoprocol may be used as an alternative to 5-FU.

BOWEN'S DISEASE

(Squamous Cell Carcinoma In Situ)

Premalignant lesions, often due to arsenic exposure, that may give rise to squamous cell carcinomas.

These lesions predominantly affect the elderly. Sun exposure is a probable contributing cause in many patients, although some patients

---

◨ see page 1280

may have a history of arsenic exposure (either medicinal or occupational). Human papillomavirus (HPV) may also play an etiologic role.

Symptoms and Signs

Lesions consist of persistent, erythematous, scaly plaques with well-defined margins. Lesions can occur anywhere on the skin or mucous membranes and may be single or multiple.

Prognosis and Treatment

Multiple lesions are associated with an increased incidence of internal malignancies and mandate close follow-up. Treatment options include excision, cryotherapy with liquid nitrogen for 15 to 20 seconds, curettage and cautery, and topical 5-fluorouracil.

LENTIGO MALIGNA

(Hutchinson's Freckle)

Premalignant lesions that may give rise to lentigo maligna melanoma.

Symptoms and Signs

These lesions are pigmented macules, often > 1 cm in diameter with an irregular border, occurring mainly on sun-exposed areas, particularly the cheeks and forehead. Lesions characteristically have brown, black, red, and white areas and become more irregularly pigmented over time. Gradually, lesions expand in a prolonged radial (superficial) growth phase. Nodule development, with or without bleeding, signifies invasion and conversion to lentigo maligna melanoma.∎

Prognosis and Treatment

Risk of conversion to melanoma by age 75 is estimated at 1 to 2%.

Patients should undergo regular follow-up examinations for signs of conversion to melanoma. Some authorities suggest cryotherapy or argon laser therapy to decrease the number of abnormal melanocytes and thus, theoretically, to reduce the risk of developing melanoma. However, both of these procedures have a high recurrence rate. Because conversion to melanoma is usually relatively slow, the decision to excise lentigo maligna should be based on several factors, including the size and location of the lesion, which determines the complexity of the procedure required, and the patient's life expectancy and comorbidities.

MALIGNANT TUMORS

Basal and squamous cell carcinomas are the most common malignant skin tumors, accounting for more than 1 million cases per year in the

∎ see page 1282

USA and an estimated 40% of all malignancies. Lifelong environmental exposure to ultraviolet light is the major risk factor, and the annual risk among elderly whites may be 1 to 3% in sunny areas, such as the southwestern USA. Other predisposing factors are exposure to ionizing radiation, exposure to chemical carcinogens (eg, arsenic), and drug- or disease-induced immunosuppression.

Diagnosis is confirmed by biopsy. In general, shave biopsy is adequate for suspected basal and squamous cell carcinomas, whereas excisional biopsy is recommended for pigmented lesions suspected of being melanomas.

BASAL CELL CARCINOMA

A pearly papule that if neglected may evolve into a superficial ulcer, derived from epidermal basal cells, that is generally slow-growing and rarely metastasizes.

Basal cell carcinoma is responsible for about 75% of the more than 1 million skin cancers diagnosed every year in the USA. More than 99% of patients are white; over half are male. About 95% of cases occur in persons between the ages of 40 and 79 years.

Symptoms, Signs, and Diagnosis

More than 90% of lesions occur on the head and neck. The typical basal cell carcinoma (noduloulcerative subtype) has a pearly appearance, rolled edges, and telangiectasia on its surface. As the lesion enlarges, it may develop central ulceration, creating the classic rodent ulcer. Other subtypes include multicentric lesions that appear as a scaly plaque with a typically raised pearly edge (superficial subtype); pigmented basal cell carcinomas, sometimes mistaken for malignant melanoma (pigmented subtype); and solitary flat or slightly depressed indurated lesions that are whitish or yellowish (sclerosing [morpheaform] subtype).

All basal cell carcinomas should be confirmed histologically by biopsy, preferably before starting therapy. Shave biopsy is usually preferred.

Prognosis

If not detected and treated early, the carcinoma may invade deep tissues and destroy bone and cartilage, especially around the eyes, nose, and ears. Basal cell carcinomas rarely metastasize; however, the sclerosing subtype is more likely than other subtypes to recur. About 33% of patients per year develop another primary basal cell carcinoma.

Treatment

The size of the malignancy, depth of invasion, and patient history determine treatment.

Electrodesiccation and curettage can be used to treat small tumors. The procedure has a 95% cure rate, just below that of surgical excision. This method leaves a round depigmented scar, compared with the linear scar left by surgical excision. Cryotherapy can be used to treat small lesions. Usually, two freeze-thaw cycles are used. However, this method has a lower cure rate.

Surgical excision has the highest cure rate. It can be done on an outpatient basis with use of a local anesthetic. Margins of 5 mm are considered desirable. The procedure can be performed with primary closure or skin grafting, which may necessitate the cooperation of a plastic surgeon.

Mohs' surgery is a micrographically controlled surgical technique of staged excision. The entire tissue margins are examined histologically as surgery proceeds, ensuring complete tumor removal and sparing the maximum amount of uninvolved tissue. Mohs' surgery can be used for large, recurrent, or high-risk carcinomas. The sclerosing subtype of basal cell carcinoma, which has a high recurrence rate after conventional surgical excision, probably is best treated with Mohs' surgery.

Radiotherapy can be used when surgery is undesirable or intolerable and when carcinoma has recurred after surgery.

Intralesional interferon and photodynamic therapy using a hematoporphyrin derivative are recent innovations for managing these lesions.

After tumor removal, patients should be followed at least annually for 5 years for recurrence and for new lesions.

SQUAMOUS CELL CARCINOMA

Cancers that arise from the malpighian cells of the epidermis and that have a modest propensity to metastasize.

Squamous cell carcinoma is the second most common skin cancer, with > 200,000 new cases occurring every year in the USA. Squamous cell carcinoma may arise from actinic keratoses or Bowen's disease.∎

These tumors usually occur in sun-exposed areas, although ≤ 25% occur in sites of chronic inflammation or persistent ulceration, such as long-standing lupus vulgaris (cutaneous tuberculosis), chronic venous ulcers, radiodermatitis, or a burn scar (Marjolin's ulcer). Carcinomas arising in areas of chronic inflammation have the highest risk of metastasizing. Fair-skinned people, who have less melanin and thus less protection from the sun, have a higher incidence of squamous cell carcinoma, both solitary and multiple. Tumors range histologically from well-differentiated to poorly differentiated.

∎ see pages 1276 and 1277

Symptoms, Signs, and Diagnosis

Lesions usually occur on sun-exposed areas of skin such as the face or dorsum of the hand. The earliest signs of squamous cell carcinoma are usually erythema and induration. The overlying epidermis may be scaly or hyperkeratotic. In more advanced lesions, ulceration usually occurs, often with crusting. Advanced lesions may become fixed to underlying tissue.

The diagnosis must be confirmed by biopsy. A shave or 3-mm punch biopsy is usually adequate, provided representative viable tissue is obtained.

Prognosis and Treatment

About 2 to 5% of lesions metastasize. Lesions of the vermilion border of the lip, the pinna, and the genitals are more likely to metastasize than those found elsewhere, such as on the face and limbs.

Surgical excision can be used to treat small well-differentiated tumors. At least 5 mm of tissue beyond the tumor borders must be excised. Squamous cell carcinomas that recur in sites previously treated with another modality (eg, radiotherapy) can also be excised surgically.

Cryotherapy is an alternative method for treating multiple small tumors, which are typically found in fair-skinned patients. The tumors, together with a margin of normal tissue, should be frozen; two freeze-thaw cycles should be used. Although cryotherapy is desirable in that it usually does not require anesthesia, healing can be prolonged in elderly patients.

Radiotherapy is generally used for poorly differentiated tumors of the head and neck and for tumors that recur after surgery. Although the cosmetic results of radiotherapy may be inferior to those of surgery, radiotherapy may be preferable for elderly patients in whom surgery is contraindicated. However, multiple treatments are usually necessary, which may present problems for patients with limited mobility. Radiotherapy is not used to treat tumors on the dorsa of the hands because it may leave friable scars.

KAPOSI'S SARCOMA

A multicentric malignant vascular neoplasm affecting the skin and subcutaneous tissues and sometimes affecting other organs.

Classic Kaposi's sarcoma (KS) occurs as an indolent tumor in elderly patients of Central European descent, especially men of Jewish or Italian ancestry. Endemic KS tends to occur in the same areas of equatorial Africa in which Burkitt's lymphoma is prevalent. KS also occurs in immunosuppressed organ-transplant recipients and in AIDS patients, who may develop an aggressive lymphadenopathic form of the disease.

Herpesvirus type 8 appears to have an etiologic role, particularly among immunosuppressed patients.

Symptoms, Signs, and Diagnosis

KS is characterized by one or more purple or dark blue macules that slowly enlarge to become nodules or ulcers. In classic KS, lesions are usually asymptomatic. However, lesions may be painful. In patients with more aggressive forms, symptoms depend on the site of involvement (eg, wheezing may occur from bronchiolar involvement). Diagnosis is made clinically and confirmed by biopsy. On histologic examination, the tumor cells are endothelial; proliferating vessels and connective tissue cells are also present.

Prognosis and Treatment

Classic KS usually runs a relatively benign course, even without treatment. The course of lymphadenopathic (AIDS-related) KS is typically more aggressive and may be fulminant.

Intralesional bleomycin can be used if lesions are symptomatic. Alternatively, simple excision, radiotherapy, or laser ablation can be performed. Generalized progressive lesions causing functional impairment require systemic chemotherapy, such as vinblastine, interferon-α, doxorubicin, daunorubicin, or paclitaxel. Patients with KS are at increased risk of a second primary malignancy and require regular follow-up.

MELANOMAS

Highly malignant skin tumors that readily metastasize.

The incidence of all four types of melanoma increases with age. Superficial spreading melanoma accounts for about 60% of all melanomas and is the most common form in the elderly. Although the overall incidence of this melanoma peaks in middle age, its incidence increases through the 8th decade. Nodular melanoma accounts for about 15% of all melanomas and occurs more commonly among elderly patients. Lentigo maligna melanoma accounts for 5 to 10% of all melanomas and occurs mainly in the elderly; it is an invasive melanoma that arises from lentigo maligna.[◻] The mean age at diagnosis is 67 years. Acral-lentiginous melanoma accounts for 1 to 2% of all melanomas; it is more common among darker-skinned patients.

Symptoms and Signs

Superficial spreading melanoma is a pigmented plaque with an irregular border and variable pigmentation, often with areas of red, white,

◻ see page 1278

black, and brown. Like all melanomas, it is usually asymptomatic. Pruritus and bleeding may occur with advanced lesions.

Nodular melanoma is a darkly pigmented papule (dark brown–black to blue-black) that often enlarges rapidly. Rarely, lesions contain little pigment.

Lentigo maligna melanoma is characterized by nodularity, color change, and/or ulceration occurring in a long-standing lentigo maligna.

Acral-lentiginous melanoma consists of pigmented, usually macular lesions on the nail bed, palms, soles, and fingers.

Diagnosis

Suspicious lesions should be examined clinically by a dermatologist, and a biopsy (optimally, an excisional biopsy) should be performed. After histologic assessment, confirmed cases should be referred immediately to a physician experienced in melanoma management.

In suspected lentigo maligna melanoma, excisional biopsy is often impractical because the lesions are typically > 1 cm and located on the head or neck. Therefore, punch biopsies of areas that are most clinically suspicious are often performed. A nodule, if present, should be included in the specimen.

Prognosis

The rate of progression differs among the melanoma subtypes, but prognosis is always related to tumor thickness at the time of initial excision rather than to histologic type (see TABLE 125–1). Morbidity rates among elderly men are particularly high, probably because of delayed diagnosis. *Because metastatic melanoma is usually fatal, cure depends on early diagnosis and excision while primary tumors are still thin.*

Lentigo maligna melanoma is relatively indolent; however, deeply invasive, neglected lesions have the same poor prognosis as other forms of melanoma of equal thickness.

TABLE 125–1.   PROGNOSIS FOR PATIENTS WITH MELANOMA (ALL TYPES)

Melanoma Depth*	Prognosis
< 0.85 mm	Highly curable; 99% of patients are disease-free at 8 years
0.85–1.69 mm	Low risk of metastasis; 93% of patients are disease-free at 8 years
1.70–3.64 mm	Moderate risk of metastasis; 67% of patients are disease-free at 8 years
≥ 3.65 mm	High risk of metastasis; 35% of patients are disease-free at 8 years

* Measured from skin surface to point of deepest tumor invasion as evaluated in vertical cross sections.

Acral-lentiginous melanoma tends to be diagnosed at a late stage; thus it has usually become deeply invasive before treatment is started.

Treatment

Treatment recommendations depend on the risk category (see TABLE 125–1). If possible, low-risk lesions are excised with 1- to 2-cm margins, and intermediate- to high-risk lesions are excised with 3-cm margins and at least 1 cm of underlying subcutaneous fat. Removal of all palpably enlarged lymph nodes has also been recommended, but prophylactic lymphadenectomy of clinically normal nodes appears to have no benefit. Follow-up is essential; patients should be seen every 6 to 12 months indefinitely.

Traditional treatment of lentigo maligna melanoma consists of a wide local excision, often requiring a skin flap or split-thickness skin graft to repair the defect. Mohs' surgery, which conserves more tissue, has recently been used successfully. However, long-term follow-up is necessary to determine the risk of metastasis with this approach. High-risk patients (those with thick primary lesions but no apparent metastases) may benefit from prophylactic therapy with melanoma vaccines or other immunomodulatory therapy, for which controlled multicenter trials are under way.

Advanced melanoma with metastases is usually incurable and therefore treated palliatively. Surgery (eg, of a solitary brain lesion) can sometimes prolong survival. Radiation combined with corticosteroids may temporarily ameliorate symptoms. Patients with advanced disease limited to a limb may benefit from hyperthermic limb perfusion together with melphalan and tumor necrosis factor. Opioid analgesics for pain control and end-of-life palliative measures may be needed.**1** Patients should be asked to clarify their wishes about end-of-life care in an advance directive.**2**

126 AGING AND THE EYE

Evaluation of age-related ocular symptoms and signs must be based on an understanding of anatomy and physiology of the eye. FIGURE 126–1 depicts the structures that undergo age-related anatomic or physiologic changes. Healthy persons > 65 years should visit an eye doctor once a year. Patients with systemic vascular diseases (eg, diabetes, hypertension), debilitating central nervous system diseases (eg, multiple sclerosis), or chronic eye diseases (eg, glaucoma, macular degener-

1 see page 115   **2** see page 134

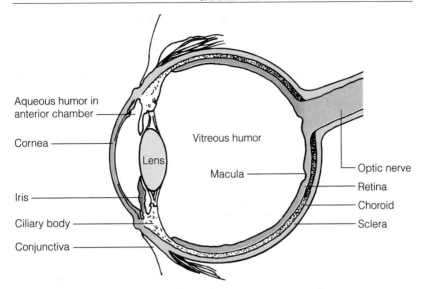

FIGURE 126–1. Structures of the eye that undergo anatomic or physiologic changes with age.

ation) should visit their eye doctor more often. The diagnostic tests used to detect ocular disorders include a visual acuity examination, visual field examination, and ophthalmoscopy.

Sclera

The sclera forms the posterior five sixths of the eyeball. In children, the sclera is opaque, with a slight blue cast where it is thin and the underlying pigment of the chorioid shows through. In adults, the sclera is white; in elderly persons, it may have a yellowish tinge resulting from dehydration and lipid deposits, which should not be confused with jaundice.

Other age-related changes include yellowing or browning due to exposure to ultraviolet light, wind, and dust; more random splotches of pigment, which often occur in dark-complected persons; and a bluish cast due to thinning of the sclera that may occur with some diseases (eg, rheumatoid arthritis).

Conjunctiva

The conjunctiva is a thin mucous membrane that lines the eyelids and the anterior surface of the eyeball. Its goblet cells produce mucin, which lubricates eyelid movements and provides a protective layer to slow evaporation of the tear film. With age, the number of mucous cells decreases, as a result of keratitis sicca (with or without Sjögren's syndrome) or for no specific reason. This change contributes to dry eye condition, which is manifested by a scratchy sensation and chronic irritation, often with increased redness from dilation of blood vessels in the conjunctiva. **1** The increased redness commonly occurs because the conjunctiva is heavily vascularized. Capillaries in the conjunctiva are fragile and burst easily, resulting in a pooling of blood in the space between the sclera and the overlying conjunctiva. Subconjunctival hemorrhages, while alarming in appearance, are benign and resolve without treatment in ≤ 14 days.

Limbus

The limbus marks the junction between the sclera and the cornea. Although it is only 1.5 to 2 mm wide, the limbus contains the trabecular meshwork and the canal of Schlemm, which are important in maintaining correct intraocular pressure.

Aqueous Humor

The aqueous humor lies between the cornea and the lens and exerts an outward pressure on the cornea (intraocular pressure). The aqueous humor must be continuously formed from blood plasma that is filtered through the ciliary body because the aqueous humor is constantly reabsorbed back into the blood after it flows out through the canal of Schlemm in the limbus. Intraocular pressure varies throughout the day, being highest in the morning and lowest in the evening (at the resting level). With age, the value of the resting level of intraocular pressure can rise over time by as much as 25% without damaging vision. The mechanism for this normal increase is unknown, but it may be caused by an increase in the production rate of aqueous humor with age or a partial obstruction of the canal of Schlemm over time. Glaucoma results if the canal becomes completely blocked or the production rate becomes abnormally high. **2** Aqueous humor itself does not change with age.

Vitreous Humor

The vitreous humor is firmly attached anteriorly at the peripheral retina and posteriorly at the optic nerve. The vitreous humor is normally clear, but with age, discrete opacities or structural changes leading to a general haziness may develop. Also, the vitreous humor undergoes liquefaction with age; as a result, normal eye movements produce intermittent tension at the attachment points on the retina. This tugging stimulates the peripheral retina mechanically, causing vertically oriented flashing lights, almost always in the far temporal visual field. **3**

---

1 see page 1312   **2** see page 1295   **3** see page 1291

Cornea

The cornea is transparent and forms the anterior one sixth of the eyeball; it is the most important refractive portion of the eye. Arcus senilis (a deposit of calcium and cholesterol salts appearing as a gray-white ring at the edge of the cornea, 1 to 2 mm inside the limbus) is common in persons > 60 and has no clinical significance. Arcus senilis, which should not be mistaken for a cataract, is on the surface of the eye, not within it.

Corneal sensitivity to touch decreases with age. The threshold to touch doubles between ages 10 and 80, with the largest changes occurring after age 40. The patient does not notice this change; therefore, the cornea should always be examined for asymptomatic changes.

Iris

The iris contains two sets of muscles that work together to regulate pupillary size and reaction to light. With age, these muscles weaken, and the pupil becomes smaller, reacts more sluggishly to light, and dilates more slowly in the dark. Thus, persons > 60 may complain that objects are not as bright (a smaller pupil allows less light to enter the eye), that they are dazzled initially when going outdoors (slow pupillary constriction), and that they experience difficulty when going from a brightly lit environment to a darker one (slow pupillary dilation). If visual acuity is normal, patients need only reassurance that these changes are normal. None of these changes results in decreased visual acuity.

Relative pupillary size and reaction to light, two important clinical signs regardless of the patient's age, can be evaluated in a dimly lit room by shining a penlight obliquely into each eye and observing constriction of the pupil in the illuminated eye (direct response) and the contralateral eye (consensual response). Because pupillary diameter decreases with age, the direct and consensual reactions to light tend to be slower. Both pupils should be the same size when they receive equal light. Unequal pupil size is cause for concern, especially if the pupils were of equal size historically; referral to an eye doctor is indicated. If the pupillary response is sluggish or absent, the patient may be taking a drug (either prescribed or over-the-counter) that causes pupillary constriction or dilation. A drug history should be taken to confirm this suspicion.

Lens

The lens is a transparent, metabolically active mass of proteins and water which, along with the cornea, provides the focusing power of the eye. Lens thickness and surface curvatures are changed by the actions of the ciliary muscle and suspensory ligaments (zonules). The lens continuously grows during life and increases in density and weight. These changes decrease the elasticity of the lens. Between the age of 40 and

50, the lens usually becomes so inelastic that close objects can no longer be brought into focus (presbyopia) without the assistance of corrective lenses.

Retina

The retina is difficult to examine in elderly patients because of their small pupils, increased random eye movements, and lens opacities. The examination is worth any extra effort required because it provides the only opportunity to directly visualize a cranial nerve (the optic nerve), the portion of the retina responsible for the highest level of visual acuity (the macula), and blood vessels (the retinal artery and vein and capillary bed). Recognizing age-related changes in these structures is important.

In general, the retina, which glistens in younger persons, becomes duller with age. The optic nerves tend to have less distinct margins and may appear slightly paler than in younger persons because of a loss of capillaries due to small-vessel disease secondary to atherosclerosis. The macula, which in younger persons usually has a bright central foveal light reflex, may show no foveal reflex in elderly persons. Also, yellowish white spots (drusen) often appear in the macular area, and the retinal layers may become disrupted, resulting in pigmentation showing through and obscuring the view of underlying blood vessels. Unless these macular changes are accompanied by a distortion of edges of objects or a measurable decrease in visual acuity unexplained by other causes, they are not clinically important. The arteries also demonstrate atherosclerotic changes, including slight narrowing and an increased light reflex from thickened vessel walls. The veins may show marked venous indentation (nicking) at the arteriovenous crossings with slight proximal distention.

Lids

With age, the orbicularis oculi muscles (which squeeze the lids shut) decrease in strength, which sometimes results in the lower eyelid falling away from the eyeball (ectropion). Spasm of the orbicularis oculi muscle may cause the lid margin (especially the lower one) to turn in (entropion), bringing the eyelashes in contact with the eyeball and allowing them to rub it with each blink (trichiasis), resulting in chronic irritation.◪ The lids contain many glands that secrete sebum or sweat. These glands drain externally to the skin surface of the lid; they can become blocked and swollen.

Lacrimal Gland and Tear Drainage

Tear production by the lacrimal gland may decrease with age, resulting in fewer tears available to keep the surface of the eye, especially the cornea, well moistened. Abnormalities of the lacrimal system may

◪ see also page 1309

result in decreased or increased tear production.∎ Normal tear production can be measured with the Schirmer test by suspending a 20-mm strip of filter paper from the lower conjunctival sac for 5 minutes. This test is extremely uncomfortable, and in response to the irritation of the filter paper, the patient may produce reflex tears. Thus, care must be taken to distinguish between normal and reflex tearing, recognized as crying. If ≥ 10 mm of the filter paper is wet without crying, then tear production is adequate. If < 10 mm is wet, then tear production is inadequate and the patient should be referred to an eye doctor. Referral is also indicated when the patient complains of excess tears and the punctum of the lower lid is not in contact with the eyeball.

Orbit

With age, there is a loss of periorbital fat, which surrounds and cushions the eyeball. This loss of fat often causes enophthalmos (sinking of the eyeball into the orbit), an asymptomatic condition that often poses a cosmetic problem and may be corrected with surgery.

AGE-RELATED CHANGES IN OCULAR FUNCTION

Age-related changes in ocular function may be divided into two groups: those related to vision (refractive changes, visual acuity, contrast sensitivity, glare, haziness, flashing lights, moving spots, and changes in color vision, dark adaptation, and visual fields), and those related to eye comfort (foreign-body sensation and headache).

Refractive Changes

When a person views an object closer than 2 feet, the ciliary muscles contract, allowing the lens to change shape to provide additional refractive power to focus the near object on the retina, and the pupil constricts. With age, the lens becomes denser and less elastic, and accommodation is lessened. Presbyopia, a universal age-related change in vision beginning in persons in their 40s, is corrected in myopic and hyperopic patients with separate reading or bifocal glasses. Because accommodation is lost progressively from about ages 45 to 65, the reading lens usually must be changed every 2 or 3 years.

Visual Acuity

Uncorrected visual acuity begins to decrease in a normal healthy person around the age of 50. The eye becomes more hyperopic and astigmatic with age. These changes are independent of pupil and lens changes and are thought to be a function of neurologic changes in the visual pathways of the brain rather than of retinal changes. This theory is supported by the fact that with age, visual acuity of fast-moving

∎ see pages 1312 and 1313

objects also declines and perception of moving targets is processed in the brain, not in the retina. Despite these small changes in visual acuity as a result of normal age-related brain changes, in the absence of disease, visual acuity should be at or correctable to 20/20, even in very old persons.

Contrast Sensitivity

Contrast sensitivity (the ability to distinguish extremely fine details [eg, mesh size in a window screen]) decreases with age at middle-spatial and high-spatial frequencies (> 8 cycles/degree). This change was originally thought to be due to the fact that elderly persons have smaller pupils and more lens opacities and, therefore, less light hitting the retina. However, the loss of contrast sensitivity is now thought to be due to a loss of neurons in the visual pathway in the brain rather than to any retinal changes. Functionally, this loss of contrast sensitivity has very little effect on the elderly person's quality of life. Currently, this loss cannot be prevented or reversed.

Glare

Elderly patients often complain of decreased visual perception resulting from glare. As the eye ages, changes in the lens and vitreous humor increase the scattering of light in the ocular media. With an ophthalmoscope, an examiner may be able to distinguish between lens opacities (best seen with a $+10$ lens) and vitreous opacities (best seen with a $+2$ lens).

Opacities appearing in the cortex of the lens are often spokelike; they cause glare but have little effect on visual acuity. Nuclear cataracts cause glare but also have little effect on visual acuity. However, opacities in the central cortex region just beneath the posterior lens capsule (posterior subcapsular lens opacities) tend to scatter light to a greater extent, especially in persons with small pupils. This condition occurs because these opacities are closer to the focal point of the lens through which all light must pass on the way to the retina. Although these opacities may eventually increase in size or density and interfere with visual acuity (posterior subcapsular cataracts), their earliest manifestation is the scattering of light and increased glare, especially in bright light. Sunglasses help reduce glare. Mydriatic drops may also provide relief by causing mild dilation of the pupil, which allows the patient to see around the opacity. Early nuclear opacities may actually improve close vision in the elderly, a phenomenon known as second sight, which results because the eye becomes more myopic and less presbyopic. These patients need to be advised that their vision will eventually deteriorate as their cataracts increase in density and size.∎

∎ see also page 1293

Opacities at the periphery of the lens, although not directly interfering with vision, can also increase the scattering of light passing through the lens, especially at night or in dim light when the pupil is slightly dilated. Thus, it is not unusual for the elderly patient to complain about the glare of oncoming headlights while driving at night. As long as visual acuity is normal, the patient should be advised to avoid looking directly at oncoming headlights and to reduce driving at night. Cataract surgery is elective and the decision to have surgery should be based on two factors: the patient's desire for improved vision and a reasonable likelihood that vision will improve after surgery.∎

Haziness, Flashing Lights, and Moving Spots

Age-related changes in the vitreous humor can create noticeable and disturbing changes in vision, including haziness. Although these changes are not serious, they may upset the patient. Usually, treatment consists of reassurance that these changes are not vision threatening.

Vertically oriented flashing lights may also occur because of age-related changes in the vitreous humor. Unlike the aura in migraine, these flashing lights occur in only one eye at a time. If they are not accompanied by decreased vision or other changes in visual function, they usually need no further evaluation. However, if they persist and the feeling that a veil has descended over the eye or a decrease in the visual field has occurred, the patient should be referred immediately for an ophthalmologic examination to exclude retinal detachment.

In patients with myopia (nearsightedness) or uveitis (generalized eye infections) and in many others in their late 50s and early 60s, opacities appear as lines, spots, or clusters of dots moving slowly across the field of vision. Usually, they move more rapidly with eye movements and become stationary when the eye is not moving. These opacities represent bits of vitreous humor that have coalesced and now float freely in the vitreous cavity (floaters). Although floaters are annoying, they usually have no clinical importance. If an ophthalmoscopic examination shows no retinal detachment, the patient should be reassured and encouraged to ignore the floaters, which can gradually become less noticeable. However, a shower of opacities, often accompanied by flashing lights in the peripheral visual field, requires a prompt referral to rule out retinal detachment.

Color Vision

Color discrimination declines with age. Three classes of cones (short-wavelength [blue], medium-wavelength [green], and long-wavelength [red]) are responsible for normal color vision. With age, all three classes

∎ see page 1294

decline in sensitivity, resulting in a reduction of brightness discrimination. Colors appear to be less bright, and contrasts between colors are less noticeable to the elderly person than to a younger caregiver, possibly resulting in a difference of opinion about appropriate color combinations for apparel. In addition, the lens becomes yellow with age, thus reducing transparency for short wavelengths more than for medium and long wavelengths. In persons > 60, this age-related change results in a reduction in discrimination of blue objects, which often appear gray. This condition can be confirmed with the use of color plates during a routine eye examination. People who use color discrimination in their professions (eg, artists, seamstresses, electricians) need to be alert to these changes and should avoid using blue ink over light blue or gray backgrounds.

Dark Adaptation

Elderly persons invariably note that their ability to function safely in poorly lit environments is reduced. With age, dark adaptation decreases. This decline in sensitivity is due, almost completely, to age-related changes in pupil size and to increasing lens opacity. The resulting loss of light reaching the retina due to reduction of ocular transmittance and pupil miosis accounts for all but a small fraction of the total decrease in dark adaptation with age. The amount of ambient light needed for reading by persons in their 60s is three times that needed by those in their 20s. Therefore, increasing the amount of ambient light in all rooms in the home improves safety and productivity.

Visual Fields

The size of a normal visual field decreases by about 1 to 3° per decade. Thus, for persons in their 70s or 80s, a visual field loss of 20 to 30° may result. This reduction has recently been implicated as a major cause of automobile accidents involving elderly drivers. Because the peripheral retina has fewer neurons than the central retina, equal losses in the two areas have a greater effect on reducing visual acuity in the periphery. To track visual field changes across time for each patient, the examiner should perform visual field tests early in the day, before the patient tires; subsequent tests should be performed at the same time of day to decrease variability in results.

Foreign-Body Sensation

A false foreign-body sensation may be related to a dry eye condition, entropion, chronic fatigue of the eye muscles from lack of sleep, poor health, a latent eye muscle imbalance, excessive close vision, or prolonged computer use. All of these items may lead to incomplete blinking of the eyelids and a decrease in the number of blinks per minute, thus causing the eyeball to dry and a foreign-body sensation to occur. Counseling the patient about these possibilities generally leads to increased blinking, which improves visual comfort and performance, and resolution of the foreign-body sensation. However, a true foreign body must be ruled out.

Headache

In the elderly patient, headache may be due to ocular function. Eye strain can produce tension headaches◻ or direct eye muscle pain. Headache in patients with acute glaucoma is a true ocular emergency and requires immediate attention.

▇127▇ OCULAR DISORDERS

Ocular disorders commonly affecting elderly persons include cataracts, glaucoma, diabetic retinopathy, age-related maculopathy, and certain vascular disorders. Other ocular disorders more common in the elderly include acute diplopia, diabetic ophthalmoplegia, intracranial tumors, some lid disorders, and myasthenia gravis.

CATARACT

An opacity of the lens that reduces visual acuity to ≤ 20/30.

The lens is normally transparent until after age 40, when nonspecific opacities may appear. Because age is the major risk factor for developing cataract, almost anyone who lives long enough will develop it. Other risk factors include smoking, poor nutrition, corticosteroid therapy, a history of atopic dermatitis, and exposure to ultraviolet light (as occurs in sunny climates). The cause of cataract is thought to be oxidative damage to the lens proteins that reduces solubility; eventually, insoluble opacities form in otherwise transparent tissue.

Cataracts are categorized according to their location within the lens. Nuclear cataracts occur in the central part of the lens. Cortical cataracts form more peripherally and are less likely to be visually significant than nuclear cataracts. Idiopathic posterior subcapsular cataracts usually occur at an earlier age and probably have a genetic basis, although corticosteroids should be ruled out as a cause.

Symptoms, Signs, and Diagnosis

The hallmark of all cataracts is painless, progressive loss of vision, but the rate of loss is nonlinear and variable. Both near and far visual acuity should be tested, and refraction should be checked to assess the degree of refractive shift.

◻ see page 1315

When lens opacities first develop, especially in the nucleus, visual acuity is relatively unaffected, but the refractive index and thus the refractive power of the lens increase (ie, the lens shifts toward myopia). This increased refractive power can partially compensate for the loss in accommodation, temporarily correcting presbyopia. Thus, in a person aged 60 to 70, early nuclear lens changes may induce myopia and allow the person to read again without glasses. This condition is referred to as second sight.

An early symptom of posterior subcapsular cataract may be glare from bright lights at night or even during the day—the result of light rays being scattered by the opacities. Over time, however, the lens opacities progress and eventually interfere with vision so that reading becomes difficult, even with glasses.

Lens opacities can be seen easily by observing the red reflex of the retina and choroid with an ophthalmoscope, using a +10 diopter lens in the viewing aperture. A lens opacity appears in silhouette as a black area.

Treatment

About 1.5 million cataract extractions are performed in the USA each year, and about 98% of them involve removal of the lens and placement of an intraocular lens, a plastic prosthetic lens to replace the optical power lost from cataract removal. In most cases, the lens is placed behind the iris (ie, in the posterior chamber). In a small percentage of cases, the lens is placed in the anterior chamber. Posterior chamber placement is considered safer and results in fewer postoperative complications, but anterior chamber placement is easier to perform and may be preferred in some cases. In certain rare cases, the ophthalmologist advises against using an intraocular lens, and correction can be accomplished with glasses or contact lenses. However, the glasses needed are very thick, and elderly persons often have difficulty inserting and removing contact lenses.

In extracapsular cataract extraction, the central portion of the anterior capsule is removed and the lens contents are aspirated so that much of the lens capsule remains intact. This procedure is performed more commonly than intracapsular cataract extraction because it allows for the placement of the intraocular lens in the posterior chamber. In intracapsular cataract extraction, which is rarely the procedure of choice in industrialized countries, the entire lens, including its capsule, is removed.

Cataract surgery is nearly always an elective procedure, requiring justification that the potential benefits outweigh the possible complications and discomfort. Waiting until the cataract matures is no longer considered valid. Surgery can be performed at any stage of cataract maturation; the decision should be based on the degree of the patient's visual disability. If, despite decreased vision, the patient can perform all desired activities, surgery can be postponed. If the patient cannot perform at work, read, drive a car, or watch television, and the surgeon is confident that successful surgery will result in vision of 20/30 or better, surgery should be considered.

Rarely, an advanced cataract may swell, and the capsule may become leaky. Lens material leaking into the anterior chamber may cause secondary glaucoma, which can be readily diagnosed and successfully treated by surgical removal of the cataract and an anterior chamber washout.

If the patient has associated eye disease, cataract extraction should be approached cautiously. Age-related maculopathy, severe diabetic retinopathy, and other retinal diseases jeopardize the prospect for successful cataract extraction. Surgery should be deferred until there is a reasonable prospect that the result will be acceptable to the patient. In many cases, the extent of possible visual improvement can be estimated preoperatively.

Most cataract surgery is performed using local anesthesia. However, consideration should be given to patients with severe respiratory or cardiovascular difficulties that may preclude their lying supine for the 30 to 60 minutes necessary for preoperative preparation and surgery.

Cataract surgery is one of the most successful surgical procedures; postoperatively, about 95% of patients have excellent vision. Patients typically recover rapidly from cataract surgery because of improvements in technique and materials. Most patients have little pain; pain can be controlled with acetaminophen.

Complication rates are low. The most serious complication is expulsive choroidal hemorrhage, which can cause blindness. Other major complications include faulty wound closure with aqueous humor leakage, prolapse of the iris into the corneal wound, and intractable secondary glaucoma. Inflammation of the eye (endophthalmitis), another serious complication that occurs in about 1 in 5000 cases, usually occurs 24 to 48 hours after surgery. Immediate hospitalization and aggressive treatment with IV antibiotics and corticosteroids are needed to prevent eye loss.

GLAUCOMA

Disorders characterized by increased intraocular pressure that can lead to irreversible damage to the optic nerve and impaired vision.

Glaucoma accounts for about 10% of all cases of blindness in the USA. Normal intraocular pressure ranges between 11 and 21 mm Hg; however, this level may not necessarily be healthy for all persons. Increased intraocular pressure occurs because of either increased production or impaired outflow of aqueous fluid. Aqueous fluid is produced constantly in the eye and is drained continuously (see FIGURE

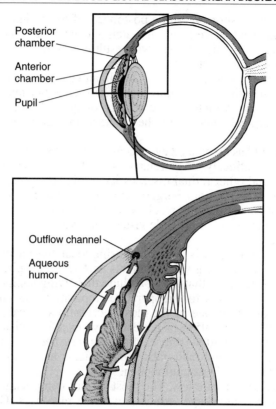

Posterior chamber

Anterior chamber

Pupil

Outflow channel

Aqueous humor

FIGURE 127–1.   Normal aqueous fluid drainage. Aqueous fluid is produced in the posterior chamber, passes through the pupil into the anterior chamber, and then drains through the outflow channels.

127–1). Of the two mechanisms for the pathogenesis of glaucoma, impaired outflow is by far more common. Damage to the optic nerve may result in part from the relationship between the blood pressure within the optic nerve (perfusion pressure) and the intraocular pressure. As long as the perfusion pressure adequately exceeds intraocular pressure, the optic nerve receives sufficient nutrition.

ANGLE-CLOSURE GLAUCOMA

(Narrow-Angle Glaucoma)

Glaucoma associated with a closed anterior chamber angle.

Angle-closure glaucoma accounts for only about 10% of glaucoma cases in the USA, but it is the only type that can be cured. It appears to be more prevalent among Asians.

Pathophysiology

The anterior chamber of the eye is bounded anteriorly by the cornea and posteriorly by the iris and lens. A major risk factor for angle-closure glaucoma is an anatomically shallow anterior chamber, especially at the periphery. The chamber becomes even more shallow with age because the lens continues to thicken throughout life, moving the iris forward. Farsighted persons tend to have smaller eyes and thus may be predisposed to this type of glaucoma in later life.

Elevated intraocular pressure occurs when the pupil margin of the iris presses against the lens, preventing the aqueous fluid from entering the anterior chamber. The fluid is still being produced by the ciliary body epithelium in the posterior chamber, however, and the fluid pushes the midportion of the iris forward, preventing access to the trabecular meshwork of the outflow channels. When these channels are sealed off, intraocular pressure increases to levels as high as 50 to 60 mm Hg in a matter of hours. (The upper limit of the normal range is about 22 mm Hg.)

Drugs with anticholinergic (atropine-like) effects may be dangerous in patients predisposed to angle-closure glaucoma because the drugs produce chronic pupillary dilation.

Symptoms, Signs, and Diagnosis

Angle-closure glaucoma usually presents in one eye, although the other eye is likely to also have a shallow anterior chamber.

In acute glaucoma, the rapid rise in intraocular pressure is accompanied by redness and pain in or around the eye, severe headache, nausea, vomiting, and blurred vision. Patients often see halos around lights as a result of corneal edema. During an acute glaucoma attack, the eye is tender and feels firmer than the other eye. The conjunctiva is injected, and the cornea is hazy or steamy in appearance. As intraocular pressure continues to rise, nausea and vomiting can become so severe that an acute abdomen may be suspected.

Symptoms are more vague in subacute and chronic glaucoma. The potential for angle-closure glaucoma is suspected on slit-lamp examination and best assessed by gonioscopic examination of the angle structures using special corneal contact lenses.

Treatment

Within 48 to 72 hours, depending on the pressure elevation, vision may be irreversibly damaged. *Therefore, an attack of angle-closure glaucoma constitutes an emergency requiring immediate referral to an ophthalmologist.* When an ophthalmologist is unavailable, emergency measures consist of local instillation of one drop of 2% pilocarpine every 5 minutes four to six times along with IV administration of acetazolamide 5 to 10 mg/kg. A topical β-blocker, α_2 agonist, and a corticosteroid may also be effective.

Although intraocular pressure can usually be reduced with drugs, surgical intervention (laser iridotomy) is the only cure. A small opening is made at the base of the iris to allow the pressure to equalize on both sides and to prevent the iris from obstructing the outflow channels. Other procedures are available, but laser iridotomy can be performed in the ophthalmologist's office in only a few minutes. If surgery is performed within the first 24 hours, before permanent adhesions develop between the iris and outflow channels, cure is likely and further attacks will be prevented. The other eye is likely to be predisposed to angle closure, even though it has not undergone an acute attack. Therefore, laser iridotomy is performed on both eyes.

OPEN-ANGLE GLAUCOMA

Glaucoma associated with an anatomically open anterior chamber angle.

Open-angle glaucoma accounts for about 80% of glaucomas in the USA. Unlike angle-closure glaucoma, this type of glaucoma is asymptomatic until very late. It causes a gradual loss of visual fields over years and affects both eyes simultaneously. It occurs about six times more often in black persons, who rarely have angle-closure glaucoma.

In contrast to angle-closure glaucoma, the angle structures in primary open-angle glaucoma appear normal on examination. Indeed, the precise site of resistance to outflow is unknown but is believed to lie in the cells lining the canal of Schlemm (the outflow channel residing in the sclera).

Symptoms, Signs, and Diagnosis

The main outcome—loss of peripheral vision—develops insidiously and is usually unnoticed by patients until advanced. There is generally no pain or other symptoms. Routine intraocular pressure monitoring and ophthalmoscopic examination of the optic nerve head may detect open-angle glaucoma in the absence of symptoms. Although the intraocular pressure usually is > 21 mm Hg in patients with open-angle glaucoma, the intraocular pressure can be within the normal range but still be too high for a particular eye to tolerate. Diagnosis is based on an anatomically normal anterior chamber angle and outflow channels (as viewed by gonioscopy), increased resistance to aqueous humor outflow (as measured by tonography), and a loss of peripheral vision (as measured by quantitative perimetry). With time, optic atrophy (manifest as cupping and pallor of the nerve head) is noted, indicating advanced disease.

When the pressure is > 21 mm Hg but the patient has no visual field defect, the diagnosis is ocular hypertension. The optic nerve usually appears normal. Patients with this condition should be seen at least every 6 months for visual field testing, but treatment is usually not indicated at this stage.

Prevention

Patients > 40 years who are at high risk (eg, black persons, persons who have a parent or sibling with glaucoma, persons receiving long-term corticosteroid therapy) and all patients > 60 should have yearly intraocular pressure measurements and ophthalmoscopic examinations. Measuring pressure alone detects about half the patients with the disease; performing ophthalmoscopy to identify optic nerve head excavation increases the detection rate to about 80%; performing visual field testing further increases the rate.

Intraocular pressure is measured with the applanation tonometer using a topical anesthetic (eg, proparacaine 0.5%). A hand-held electronic applanation device is available to measure intraocular pressure. It is easy to use, portable, and reasonably accurate.

Treatment

Although open-angle glaucoma cannot be cured, it can usually be controlled with topical and systemic therapy. *Whether or not the patient has symptoms, drugs are needed to reduce intraocular pressure to prevent irreversible optic nerve damage and thus the loss of peripheral visual fields.* Various drugs are available for treatment (see TABLE 127–1). Because open-angle glaucoma can be controlled but not cured, treatment is continued indefinitely. A visual field examination should be performed every 6 months. If drugs fail to control progression of the glaucoma, as evidenced by visual field testing, surgery (eg, laser trabeculoplasty or a filtration procedure) is recommended to lower the intraocular pressure to a level at which the disease can be slowed or halted.

Drug treatment for other disorders may have an adverse effect on incipient or recognized glaucoma. If a hypertensive patient with glaucoma is being treated with antihypertensive drugs, the ophthalmologist should monitor the patient's visual fields while the blood pressure is being lowered. The glaucoma drug dose may need to be increased to further reduce the intraocular pressure. Drugs with anticholinergic (atropine-like) effects may be dangerous in patients with open-angle glaucoma because the drugs antagonize the antiglaucoma drugs. A consultation between the patient's personal physician and the ophthalmologist is advised; perhaps a drug can be switched or a dose modified. Other ways to minimize systemic absorption include closing the lids after instillation and occluding the punctum by pressing on the medial aspect of the lids.

TABLE 127–1. DRUGS USED TO TREAT GLAUCOMA

Type	Drug	Comments*
Miotics, direct-acting (cholinergic agonists; topical)	Pilocarpine Carbachol	Less effective as monotherapy than β-blockers; people with darker-pigmented pupils may need higher strengths; pilocarpine may cause brow ache, induced myopia
Miotics, indirect-acting (cholinesterase inhibitors; topical)	Physostigmine Neostigmine Demecarium	Shorter acting, reversible inhibition
	Echothiophate iodide Isoflurophate	Very long acting; irreversible inhibition; can cause cataracts and retinal detachment; should be avoided in patients with narrow-angle glaucoma because of the extreme miosis; echothiophate may cause iris cysts
Carbonic anhydrase inhibitors (oral, IV, topical)	Acetazolamide (oral, IV) Dichlorphenamide (oral) Methazolamide (oral) Dorzolamide (topical) Brinzolamide (topical)	Used as adjunctive therapy; with long-term use, systemic acidosis or kidney stones may occur in predisposed patients; dorzolamide and brinzolamide are selective for carbonic anhydrase-II and may cause blurred vision
Nonselective adrenergic agonists (topical)	Epinephrine Dipivefrin	Often combined with a miotic (dipivefrin is a pro-drug, metabolized to epinephrine); epinephrine may irritate the eye and cause an allergic lid reaction
α_2-Selective adrenergic agonists (topical)	Apraclonidine Brimonidine	Contraindicated in patients taking monoamine oxidase inhibitors; use cautiously in patients with hepatic or renal failure; brimonidine is more α_2-selective than apraclonidine
β-Blockers (topical)	Timolol Betaxolol† Levobunolol Carteolol Metipranolol	Used alone or with other agents; may cause cardiopulmonary symptoms in susceptible persons
Prostaglandin analogs (topical)	Latanoprost (topical)	Increased pigmentation of the iris; possible worsening of uveitis; hypertrichosis
Osmotic diuretics (oral, IV)	Glycerin (oral) Mannitol (IV) Isosorbide (oral)	Used for acute angle closure to break the attack

* Selected adverse effects are noted; others may occur.
† β_1-selective.

SECONDARY GLAUCOMA

Glaucoma caused by a secondary disease process that anatomically or functionally blocks the outflow channels.

Secondary glaucoma accounts for about 10% of glaucomas in the USA. In patients with diabetes mellitus and central retinal vein occlusion, a fibrovascular membrane may grow over and seal off the outflow channels. In patients with uveitis (ocular inflammation), inflammatory cells or debris can obstruct the outflow channels. Ocular tumors may also obstruct the outflow channels, either by direct pressure from the tumor in the anterior chamber angle or by blockage of the channels by the tumor cells.

Patients with secondary glaucoma can present with a red, uncomfortable eye, often chronically painful and usually accompanied by decreased vision. However, some types of secondary glaucoma are asymptomatic.

Treatment

Treatment is directed first at removing the underlying cause (eg, treating uveitis with anti-inflammatory drugs, removing a tumor, or changing medications). Antiglaucoma drugs may also be tried to reduce intraocular pressure (see TABLE 127–1). If these measures fail, surgery is needed to create a new outflow pathway for the aqueous fluid to leave the eye.

DIABETIC RETINOPATHY

Various pathologic retinal changes characteristic of chronic diabetes mellitus.

Diabetic retinopathy is the third leading cause of adult blindness, accounting for almost 7% of blindness in the USA. Diabetic retinopathy is associated primarily with the duration of diabetes mellitus ▪; therefore, as the population ages and diabetic patients live longer, the prevalence of diabetic retinopathy will increase.

Etiology and Pathophysiology

Retinal capillaries have two types of cells: endothelial cells lining the capillary and intramural pericytes (mural cells) embedded in the basement membrane of the capillary.

In **nonproliferative retinopathy,** the first change consistently observed within the retina is a selective loss of pericytes. This cell loss probably involves aldose reductase, an enzyme found in pericytes but not in

▪see page 624

endothelial cells. As glucose levels increase in diabetes, glucose in mural cells is converted by aldose reductase to its sugar alcohol, sorbitol, which is metabolized slowly and diffuses poorly across cell membranes. The sorbitol concentration increases within the pericyte, and water moves down its osmotic gradient into the cell, which swells, eventually ruptures, and disappears.

Because pericytes appear to have contractile properties, their loss results in capillary dilation. The dilated capillaries tend to carry more and more blood because they are wider than adjacent capillaries that still contain a full complement of pericytes. In the dilated capillaries, endothelial cells proliferate and form outpouchings, which become microaneurysms. Meanwhile, the adjacent capillaries carry less and less blood, until eventually they carry none at all, becoming ghost vessels without cellular components. Thus, the area of retina next to clusters of microaneurysms is not perfused.

Eventually, shunt vessels appear between adjacent areas of microaneurysms, and the clinical picture of early diabetic retinopathy with microaneurysms and areas of nonperfused retina is seen. The microaneurysms leak and capillary vessels may bleed, causing exudates and hemorrhages. Once the initial stages of background diabetic retinopathy are established, the condition progresses over a period of years, developing into proliferative diabetic retinopathy and blindness in about 5% of cases.

Proliferative diabetic retinopathy occurs when some areas of the retina continue losing their capillary vessels and become nonperfused, leading to the appearance of new vessels on the disk and elsewhere on the retina. These new blood vessels grow into the vitreous and—because they are friable—bleed easily, leading to preretinal hemorrhages. In advanced proliferative diabetic retinopathy, a massive vitreous hemorrhage may fill a major portion of the vitreous cavity. In addition, the new vessels are accompanied by fibrous tissue proliferation that can lead to traction retinal detachment.

Symptoms and Signs

Usually, little or no evidence of diabetic retinopathy appears until about 3 to 5 years after the onset of diabetes and, in many patients, much later. Symptoms may be subtle (eg, early and minimal visual loss from macular edema, a shower of spots, clouded vision from a small vitreous hemorrhage).

The first signs of nonproliferative diabetic retinopathy are microaneurysms, seen as red spots with sharp margins in the area around the optic nerve and macula. These lesions disappear after 3 to 6 months and are replaced by fresh microaneurysms. The next stage of nonproliferative diabetic retinopathy is marked by the addition of punctate, flame-shaped (linear) or blot-shaped retinal hemorrhages, cotton-wool spots,

TABLE 127–2.   CLASSIFICATION OF DIABETIC RETINOPATHY

Condition	Description
Early nonproliferative diabetic retinopathy	≤ 5 microaneurysms in each eye
Nonproliferative diabetic retinopathy	Multiple microaneurysms, hard exudates, cotton-wool spots, retinal hemorrhages, and intraretinal microvascular abnormalities
Proliferative diabetic retinopathy	New vessels on the disk and elsewhere on the retina, preretinal fibrosis, traction retinal detachment, preretinal hemorrhages, and vitreous hemorrhage

hard exudates, and intraretinal microvascular abnormalities; the last appear as small areas of dilated capillaries. These findings may all be completely asymptomatic.

An important aspect of nonproliferative diabetic retinopathy is the pooling of fluid in the macula, with resulting macular elevation. This macular edema is a major cause of reduced vision in nonproliferative diabetic retinopathy and, if allowed to persist, can result in an irreversible loss of vision.

In proliferative retinopathy, an eye may become blind because of dense vitreous hemorrhage, total traction retinal detachment, or secondary glaucoma resulting from proliferating new vessels obstructing the outflow channels in the anterior chamber angle (see TABLE 127–2).

Diagnosis and Treatment

An annual ophthalmoscopic examination is indicated for all diabetic patients to detect macular edema and evidence of proliferative diabetic retinopathy. Because the onset of type 2 diabetes is often insidious, an examination should be performed as soon as the diabetes diagnosis is made. Diabetic patients should have annual eye examinations. When nonproliferative retinopathy develops, these patients should be examined every 6 months. This interval is decreased to every 4 months when advanced nonproliferative retinopathy is present (increased ischemia, many cotton-wool spots, and other signs of nonperfusion). For those in whom laser treatment would be appropriate, periodic fluorescein angiography should be performed to detect changes when they are most amenable to treatment before advanced retinopathy affects vision.

Laser therapy is beneficial in nonproliferative and proliferative diabetic retinopathy. Focal laser treatment of the leaking microaneurysms surrounding the macular area reduces visual loss in 50% of patients with clinically significant macular edema. In proliferative diabetic retinopathy, panretinal photocoagulation results in several thousand tiny burns scattered throughout the retina (sparing the macular area); this treatment reduces the rate of blindness by 60%. Early treatment of macular edema and proliferative diabetic retinopathy prevents blindness for 5 years in 95% of patients, whereas late treatment prevents blindness in only 50%. Therefore, early diagnosis and treatment are essential.

Blood glucose monitoring and control should be emphasized to all diabetic patients regardless of age because tight control, especially when instituted early in the course of diabetes, slows the development of diabetic complications. Clinical trials have not demonstrated that diabetic retinopathy can be prevented or slowed by limiting sorbitol accumulation with aldose reductase inhibitors. However, more potent inhibitors are being developed and studied.

AGE-RELATED MACULOPATHY

A series of pathologic changes in the macula accompanied by decreased visual acuity.

Immediately beneath the sensory retina lies a single layer of cells called the retinal pigment epithelium. These cells nourish the portion of the retina in contact with them, the photoreceptor cells that contain the visual pigments. The retinal pigment epithelium lies on the Bruch membrane, a basement membrane complex. With age, this membrane thickens and becomes sclerotic.

New vessels may break through the Bruch membrane from the underlying choroid, which contains a rich vascular bed. These vessels may leak fluid or bleed beneath the retinal pigment epithelium and also between the retinal pigment epithelium and the sensory retina. Subsequent fibrous scarring disrupts the nourishment of the photoreceptor cells and leads to their death, resulting in a loss of central visual acuity. This type of age-related maculopathy is called the **wet type** because of the leaking vessels and the subretinal edema or blood. The wet type accounts for only 10% of age-related maculopathy cases but results in 90% of cases of legal blindness (visual acuity of ≤ 20/200) from macular degeneration in the elderly. The **dry type** of age-related maculopathy involves disintegration of the retinal pigment epithelium along with loss of the overlying photoreceptor cells. The dry type reduces vision but usually only to levels of 20/50 to 20/100.

Symptoms, Signs, and Diagnosis

The patient may notice distortion of central vision with objects appearing larger or smaller or straight lines appearing distorted, bent, or without a central segment. If central vision is distorted in only one eye, the patient is unlikely to notice any change in vision. However, if the patient views a grid of fine lines with each eye alternately, distortion can be quickly detected. Therefore, patients considered at high risk for age-related maculopathy (people with many drusen, especially if they are confluent; people who have developed maculopathy in one eye) are given a grid to view each morning. After the onset of distortion, visual acuity may decrease, possibly within days.

In the wet type, a small detachment of the sensory retina may be noted in the macular area, but the definitive diagnosis of a subretinal neovascular membrane requires fluorescein angiography. In the dry type, drusen may disturb the pigmentation pattern in the macular area. Drusen are excrescences of the basement membrane of the retinal pigment epithelium that protrude into the cells, causing them to bulge anteriorly; their role as a risk factor in age-related maculopathy is unclear. Through the ophthalmoscope, they appear as small, rounded, yellow-white areas with indistinct borders.

Treatment

No treatment exists for the dry type. However, laser treatment initially obliterates the neovascular membrane in the wet type and prevents further visual loss in about 50% of patients at 18 months. By 60 months, however, only 20% still have a substantial benefit.

Although patients who have decreased central visual acuity cannot read or drive a car, they can continue to perform many daily activities. Because the remainder of the sensory retina is unaffected, these patients can be assured that they will not become completely blind.

For near-vision tasks (eg, reading and watching television), magnifying lenses and high-intensity lighting matched for daylight are often helpful. A telescopic lens may help the patient identify street signs and perform other visual tasks that facilitate travel. Some optometrists and ophthalmologists specialize in fitting such optical aids.

VASCULAR DISORDERS

Vascular disorders that affect the eyes include central and branch retinal artery and vein occlusion, ischemic optic neuropathy, amaurosis fugax, and occipital lobe stroke.

RETINAL ARTERY OCCLUSION

Blockage of the central retinal artery, producing painless, sudden, unilateral blindness.

The typical cause in elderly patients is an atheroma, usually broken off the carotid artery wall. The atheroma or other embolus occludes the **central retinal artery** in the deeper portion of the optic nerve head and thus cannot be seen. Within an hour after loss of vision, the arterial spasm ceases, and some blood flow is restored to the retina, giving the appearance of a relatively normal retina on ophthalmoscopy. However, within several hours, the retina becomes edematous and gray from the death of retinal ganglion cells. Because the retina in the foveal area contains no ganglion cells, the reddish underlying choroid remains visible, accounting for the characteristic central cherry-red spot surrounded by the gray retina. In 2 to 3 weeks, the cherry-red spot disappears, and as the ganglion cells and their axons die, the optic nerve becomes white, the hallmark of primary optic atrophy.

A **retinal artery branch** may become occluded when an atheroma breaks off and passes through the central retinal artery. The occlusion can usually be seen as a refractile object in the branch and is referred to as a Hollenhorst plaque. This finding indicates embolic activity, usually from the carotid system. The portion of the retina supplied by the occluded vessel loses its function and a visual field defect, which may not affect central vision, results.

Intervention is rarely possible because it is needed within 90 minutes of the occlusion to prevent retinal cell death. Acutely reducing intraocular pressure by paracentesis combined with vasodilators may occasionally induce the embolus to move more peripherally, thus limiting the loss of vision in the affected area.

RETINAL VEIN OCCLUSION

Blockage of the central retinal vein.

Retinal vein occlusion is probably the most common vascular disorder in the eye. Symptoms are similar to those of central artery occlusion—a sudden painless partial or complete loss of vision. About 10% of patients having a **central retinal vein occlusion** in one eye will also develop one in the other eye. Even after the occlusion occurs, some vision remains.

Ophthalmoscopy reveals distended, tortuous veins with massive hemorrhages and edema throughout the retina. The margins of the optic nerve become blurred and the disk swollen. Complete resorption of the hemorrhages and edema may take months or even years. In the elderly patient, the prognosis for vision is poor. Also, about 25% of patients develop a fibrovascular membrane that seals the aqueous humor outflow channels in the anterior chamber, resulting in a painful neovascular glaucoma in 3 to 6 months. If the intraocular pressure remains elevated, blindness results in weeks. Treatment is most often attempted with laser photocoagulation, but its effectiveness is still being assessed.

Branch retinal vein occlusion occurs when a branch of the central retinal vein becomes obstructed, most often the superior temporal branch. The characteristic exudates and hemorrhages are confined to the involved quadrant of the retina, which has an associated visual field defect. Vision is usually unaffected unless the retinal swelling impinges on the macula. The development of neovascular glaucoma is much less common in branch vein occlusion. Laser photocoagulation to treat branch vein occlusion helps preserve vision.

ISCHEMIC OPTIC NEUROPATHY

Insufficient blood supply to the optic nerve, which can cause blindness.

Regardless of the cause, ischemic optic neuropathy is usually only seen in persons > 60. Partial or complete loss of vision occurs suddenly, accompanied by swelling of the optic nerve head and often a hemorrhage or two. A visual field defect may produce a loss of half the visual field with a horizontal demarcation.

Evaluation should be performed urgently, to determine if temporal arteritis is the cause (about 5% of cases). When temporal arteritis is the cause, tenderness along the temporal artery may be noted, as well as headache, jaw pain while chewing, and fever. ∎ Symptoms are almost always accompanied by an elevated erythrocyte sedimentation rate. Generally, prednisone 60 mg/day po should be started as soon as possible, and a temporal artery biopsy should be obtained to look for the typical granulomatous inflammatory changes.

When atheromatosis is the cause, pain is uncommon and decreased vision is soon followed by pallor of the optic disk. The visual loss in the other eye may occur months or years later, and once the ischemic episode has occurred, treatment does not help, although most patients have at least some return of vision. In selected elderly patients with a history of amaurosis fugax suggestive of atheromatosis, long-term anticoagulant therapy may help.

AMAUROSIS FUGAX

(Blackouts)

Transient blindness caused by retinal ischemia.

Amaurosis fugax suggests retinal or optic nerve ischemia caused by carotid artery narrowing, usually at the bifurcation of the common carotid artery. Because atheroma is the major cause of vessel narrowing, patients > 50 are most susceptible. Obstruction of the left carotid artery is six times more common than that of the right. Blackouts present as a dimming of vision in one eye with a slow recovery beginning after 5 to 10 minutes. Clear vision is restored in the reverse order from the onset pattern. Several episodes of blackouts may precede an attack

---

∎see also page 507

of ischemic optic neuropathy, or episodes may occur for years without serious sequelae. Blackouts can be bilateral if associated with low blood pressure.

When a blackout is accompanied by hemiplegia on the side opposite the affected eye (transient ischemic attack), carotid stenosis on the side of the affected eye should be strongly suspected. Early recognition of serious carotid stenosis is important because, without appropriate medical and surgical intervention, many affected patients develop permanent visual loss or hemiplegia.

The aortic arch syndrome may be suspected if increasingly frequent blackouts are related to changes in posture, such as suddenly sitting up or standing.

OCCIPITAL LOBE STROKE

Ischemic vascular lesion of the vertebral-basilar system.

Infarction in one or both occipital lobes may result from local atheromatous disease or emboli in the vertebral-basilar system. An occipital lobe stroke, usually the result of a posterior cerebral artery infarction, is characterized by sudden onset of homonymous hemianopia. Total blindness occurs suddenly, with some vision returning within minutes in the ipsilateral homonymous visual field. Bilateral posterior occlusions usually occur simultaneously. Thrombosis of the basilar artery also produces a bilateral homonymous hemianopia. As with any ischemic stroke, treatment with aspirin or other anticoagulants is indicated. In almost all cases of cortical blindness, some vision returns.

LID DISORDERS

With age, many lesions and tumors may appear on the lids, often at the nasal aspect. They may be clinically significant, as are basal cell carcinomas (see FIGURE 127–2) or squamous cell carcinomas, or merely cosmetically unattractive, as is the yellowish raised area of xanthelasma (see FIGURE 127–3). Because of the possibly aggressive nature of eyelid carcinomas, immediate referral to a dermatologist or ophthalmologist is indicated.

ECTROPION

A condition in which the lower eyelid falls away from the eyeball.

Ectropion leads to an inability of the punctum to drain tears properly from the conjunctival sac into the lacrimal sac (see FIGURE 127–4). Thus, patients complain of excess tear production and tears draining onto the face (epiphora). In addition, with decreased action of the orbic-

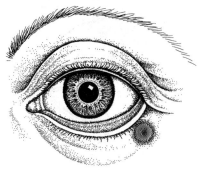

FIGURE 127–2. **Basal cell carcinoma** occurring near the eye usually involves the lower lid. It often appears as a papule with a pearly border and a depressed or ulcerated center.

ular muscles, the lids may not close completely during sleep, resulting in corneal drying and secondary abrasion, redness, and irritation (superficial punctate keratitis).

The definitive treatment of ectropion is surgical. Depending on the degree of laxity and on other factors, any of several lid-tightening procedures can be performed. These usually involve partial excision of the tarsal plate and horizontal shortening of the lid, to bring it into better approximation with the globe.

ENTROPION

A condition in which the eyelid margin turns in, bringing the eyelashes in contact with the eyeball; the eyelashes then rub the eyeball with each blink.

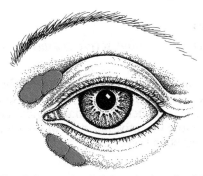

FIGURE 127–3. **Xanthelasma** (a slightly raised, yellowish, well-circumscribed plaque) typically appears along the nasal aspect of one or both eyelids. In some persons, these plaques accompany lipid disorders.

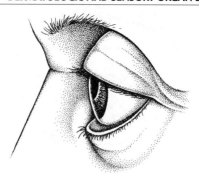

FIGURE 127–4.   **Ectropion of the lower lid margin** means that the punctum of the medial lower lid no longer touches the eyeball and tears cannot drain properly from the conjunctival sac into the lacrimal duct.

Entropion may be caused by spasm of the orbicular muscle, causing the lid margin (especially the lower one) to turn in. With chronic irritation from entropion, corneal and conjunctival scarring may result. Surgery is indicated to prevent scarring.

PTOSIS

Lid droop.

Ptosis may be caused by decreased muscle tone of the levator muscle and thus a decrease in the width of the palpebral fissure (the distance between the margins of the upper and lower lids). There may be disinsertion of the levator muscle into the apex of the tarsus. Another cause of decrease in the size of the palpebral fissure is loss of skin turgor with atrophy and loss of elasticity, which may cause the skin of the upper lid to hang below the lid margin. Excision of the excess skin is indicated only if vision is disturbed.

BLEPHAROSPASM

Bilateral intermittent or constant severe spasms of the orbicular muscles.

Blepharospasm can incapacitate a person; the eyelids shut tightly for periods varying from seconds to minutes. The cause is unknown. The condition often must be treated by partial surgical denervation of the orbicular muscles. More recently, injection of botulinum toxin into the orbicular muscles has been successful.

BLEPHARITIS

Eyelid inflammation that is usually nonspecific but may be caused by staphylococcal infection of the lid margin and follicles.

Blepharitis usually begins in childhood but often becomes more severe in old age. The signs are dilated blood vessels at the lid margins, a loss of lashes, and scaling at the base of the remaining lashes. The most severe cases of blepharitis occur in patients with rosacea. No cure exists, but blepharitis can be controlled by cleaning the eyelid margin, shampooing the scalp often, and if indicated, applying an antibiotic ointment to the lids.

CHALAZION AND STYES

Chalazion: Swelling of the sebum-secreting gland around the eye. Stye: A chalazion that becomes painful.

Chalazia can be painful. They can press on the eye and actually induce astigmatism. As with styes, the treatment for chalazia is hot compresses. Sometimes they need to be incised and drained. Also, in elderly persons, a persistent chalazion-like lesion may actually be sebaceous cell carcinoma. A stye requires treatment. The majority of styes resolve within three days with hot compresses, applied five minutes at a time, twice a day. The heat should unblock the stye and cause the gland to drain on its own. Because most styes are the result of a staphylococcal infection, unresolved styes may need treatment with systemic antibiotics.

MISCELLANEOUS OCULAR DISORDERS

Almost any ocular condition affecting younger persons can affect the elderly. Some are more common in the elderly (eg, acute diplopia, diabetic ophthalmoplegia, intracranial tumors, and myasthenia gravis).

BINOCULAR DIPLOPIA

(Double Vision)

Perception of two images of a single object caused by misalignment of the extraocular muscles.

The **third cranial nerve** innervates the medial, superior, and inferior rectus muscles, the inferior oblique muscle, and the levator muscle and also carries the parasympathetic nerves constricting the pupil and controlling accommodation. A complete third cranial nerve palsy results in ptosis; a divergence of the eye when looking straight ahead; a dilated fixed pupil; and a lack of upward, inward, and downward eye movement. The main causes of isolated third cranial nerve palsy are intracranial aneurysm, trauma, and diabetic neuropathy. An intracranial space-occupying mass is often accompanied by increased intracranial pressure and severe headache. Ophthalmoscopy may show papilledema. Severe eye or forehead pain followed by a third cranial nerve palsy that spares the pupil is usually a manifestation of diabetic neuropathy.[1] Palsy from diabetes mellitus clears spontaneously in 6 to 12 weeks, but palsy from an intracranial aneurysm or trauma requires immediate neurosurgical evaluation and, possibly, therapeutic intervention. As a rule, aneurysms involve the pupil, whereas diabetic neuropathy spares it, but there are exceptions.

The **fourth cranial nerve** innervates the superior oblique muscle, and palsy invariably results from a small hemorrhage in the roof of the midbrain, usually from arteriosclerosis. Bilateral fourth nerve palsies are frequent sequelae of closed-head trauma. Recovery occurs spontaneously after several weeks.

The **sixth cranial nerve** innervates the lateral rectus muscle and, because it has the longest intracranial course, is often affected by meningitis, skull fracture, and increased intracranial pressure. When the nerve is affected by diabetic neuropathy, spontaneous recovery occurs in 6 to 12 weeks.

MYASTHENIA GRAVIS

A disorder characterized by episodic muscle weakness caused by loss or dysfunction of acetylcholine receptors.

Any combination of extraocular muscle palsies, which may vary in severity over days or weeks, along with a normal pupillary response to light and a history of fatigue that waxes and wanes during the day should raise the possibility of myasthenia gravis.[2] An edrophonium chloride (Tensilon) test should help establish the diagnosis, and appropriate treatment can offer relief.

DRY EYES

Dry eyes can result from a number of problems with the tears, lids, or ocular surface. Abnormalities of the goblet cells (mucin-secreting cells that are necessary for surface wetting), the lacrimal glands, or the Meibomian glands (which secrete surface oil that helps stabilize the tear film) can lead to tear problems and dry eye symptoms. Often, more than one abnormality exists.

Artificial tears should be used as needed to relieve symptoms, both as drops during the day and as an ointment during sleep. Moisture-chamber glasses (eg, swimming goggles) may be helpful to maintain humidity. In severe cases, temporary collagen punctal plugs can be placed in the punctum to decrease tear outflow. If disease (eg, Sjögren's syndrome)[3] involves the lacrimal gland, more aggressive surgical inter-

---

[1] see page 627   [2] see also page 520   [3] see page 1028

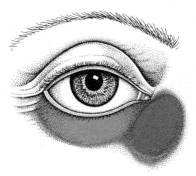

FIGURE 127–5. **Dacryocystitis** due to a chronic, recurrent bacterial infection occludes the punctum, resulting in excessive tearing. Swelling between the lower lid and nose suggests dacryocystitis. Pressure on the sac expresses material through the punctum.

vention (eg, permanent occlusion with plugs or cicatrization) may be indicated.

EXCESSIVE TEARING

Excessive tearing (with an overflow of tears, or **epiphora**) is a frequent complaint. Paradoxically, excessive tearing may be due to extremely dry eyes, according to one theory. In response to extreme dryness, the eyes tear more, diluting the oils normally present in the tears. This loss of oils results in tears that do not adhere to the eyeball and therefore, they spill out onto the cheek rather than be evacuated through the lacrimal system. If extreme dry eye is ruled out, then the cause for epiphora may be the result of an infection. The punctum may be occluded by inflammation from a chronic recurrent bacterial infection, a condition known as dacryocystitis (see FIGURE 127–5), which can be treated with topical or systemic antibiotics. Finally, epiphora may be the result of a loss of contact between the lacrimal punctum and the eyeball (ectropion), causing tears to roll down the face instead of draining properly from the conjunctival sac into the lacrimal system. The condition worsens in cold weather, when tear production increases. If severe ectropion causes excess tearing and a recurrent low-grade inflammation results, surgical correction of the lid is indicated.

PINGUECULA AND PTERYGIUM

Pinguecula: *Accumulations of degenerated collagen at the nasal and temporal junction of the sclera and cornea.* *Pterygium:* *Connective tissue that becomes vascularized and invades the cornea.*

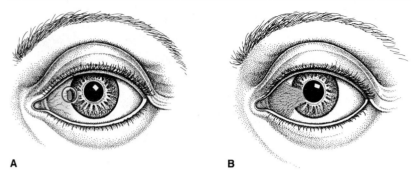

A   **B**

FIGURE 127–6. Pinguecula and pterygium. Pinguecula (A) is tissue accumulation at the nasal or temporal junction of the sclera and cornea. Pterygium (B) is connective tissue that becomes vascularized and invades the cornea.

The conjunctiva can undergo metaplasia and hyperplasia, which leads to pinguecula (see FIGURE 127–6). Pinguecula may be a cosmetic problem (the tissue may be white or yellow) but rarely requires removal. If excised, pinguecula tends to recur.

Conjunctival tissue that grows, vascularizes, and invades the cornea is called a pterygium. If a pterygium continues to grow and reaches the center of the cornea, it can interfere with vision. Pterygia usually occur in persons who spend a lot of time outdoors, especially in dusty and windy environments. At the first sign of corneal involvement, pterygia can be surgically excised.

FUCHS ENDOTHELIAL DYSTROPHY

Degeneration of the endothelial cells lining the inner surface of the cornea.

Fuchs endothelial dystrophy is a serious age-related disorder. Patients may never develop symptoms, and most patients do not know they have this disorder until very late. However, progressive degeneration of the endothelial cells can eventually result in failure to keep the cornea free of extracellular fluid, resulting in pain and corneal edema and producing haze that interferes with vision. Referral to an ophthalmologist is necessary. Diagnosis is made by slit lamp microscopy; corneal transplantation may be required. If a patient is identified as having this disease and surgery (eg, cataract) is contemplated for some reason, then the corneal transplantation may be performed at the same time. It is generally desirable to perform the transplantation before the cornea actually decompensates. Increasing corneal thickness, measured by a pachometer, may indicate a cornea at risk of decompensation.

HEADACHE

Tension headache: Tension headache relates to any cause of increased muscle tone (eg, stress, fatigue, anxiety) that may result in accumulation of lactic acid, which stimulates local pain receptors, resulting in headache. In most cases, the headache is occipital and related to tightness in neck muscles or the masseter muscle. By carefully questioning the patient, the physician should be able to identify the precipitating conditions and invite discussion of strategies needed to alleviate the pain (eg, eliminating the stressor, prescribing muscle relaxants or analgesics).

Temporal arteritis: When a headache has a recent onset and is associated with scalp tenderness, jaw claudication, fatigue, or changes in visual acuity, the physician should suspect temporal arteritis and obtain an erythrocyte sedimentation rate. If the erythrocyte sedimentation rate is elevated or if suspicion is high, prednisone 60 mg/day po should be initiated even before the test results are known, and a temporal artery biopsy should be performed as soon as possible.⬛

Migraine headache: Migraine headaches may occur at any age. However, migraine headaches are rare in the elderly. Indeed, younger persons with migraine headaches usually find that their migraines occur less often with age or stop entirely. The headache is often preceded by an aura of flashing bright lights in a vertical zigzag or picket-fence configuration seen on one side. The aura is caused by marked cerebral vasoconstriction involving vessels of the visual cortex, and the pain results from marked secondary vasodilation and edema (with associated stretching of perivascular nerve endings). The aura is always bilateral and can be seen even when both eyes are closed, but patients will say that it is in one eye. For example, a left-sided aura actually involves the nasal retina of the left eye and the temporal field of the right eye. The aura may be followed by severe, pounding, relentless pain on the opposite side of the perceived aura. The pain is exacerbated by bright lights or movement and can be eased by lying quietly in the dark.

Treatment depends on the frequency of attacks and the presence of comorbid illness. In general, treatment can be classified as prophylactic, abortive, or analgesic (see TABLE 127–3).

Other causes of headache: Other conditions that can cause headache need to be considered. Brain tumors (malignant and benign) and increased intracranial pressure from stroke or other causes tend to produce headaches that continue throughout the night and often wake patients. Other neurologic abnormalities may be found on physical examination. Some drugs, including angiotensin-converting enzyme inhibitors, nitrates, and sildenafil, can cause headaches. However, almost any drug may be the culprit.

⬛ see also page 508

TABLE 127–3. TREATMENT OF MIGRAINE

Drug	Daily Dose/Route	Adverse Effects
Prophylactic		
Amitriptyline	10–150 mg po	Dry mouth, dry eyes, sedation, weight gain, arrhythmias
Methysergide	2–8 mg po	Retroperitoneal fibrosis (drug holiday after 6 mo of use is required)
Propranolol	60–320 mg po	Hypotension, bradycardia, depression, sedation, impotence
Valproate	250 mg–2 g po	Hepatic dysfunction, GI upset, thrombocytopenia, hair loss, weight gain
Verapamil	120–480 mg po	Hypotension, fatigue, constipation
Abortive		
Dihydroergotamine	0.5–1 mg IM/IV	Nausea/vomiting, minor cramps, minor risk of angina
Ergotamine	1 mg po* 2 mg suppository* 1 mg sublingually	Nausea/vomiting, cramping, ergotism, angina
Metoclopramide	10 mg po/IM	Hypotension, sedation, dystonia
Naratriptan	1 or 2.5 mg po (can be repeated 4 h later [maximum 5 mg/24 h])	Similar to those of sumatriptan
Prochlorperazine	10 mg IV/IM 25 mg suppository	Hypotension, sedation, dystonia
Rizatriptan	5 or 10 mg po (as tablets or dissolvable wafers)	Dizziness, sleepiness, fatigue, pain, pressure sensation
Sumatriptan	6 mg sc 25, 50, 100 mg po 5 or 20 mg nasal spray	Flushing, nausea, esophageal spasm, angina
Zolmitriptan	2.5, 5 mg po	Similar to those of sumatriptan
Analgesic†		
Acetaminophen	500–1000 mg po	Hypersensitivity, hepatic toxicity
Aspirin	325–650 mg po	Dyspepsia, GI bleeding, nausea, diarrhea, nephropathy
NSAIDs Indomethacin	50–200 mg po/rectally	Dyspepsia, GI bleeding, nausea, diarrhea, nephropathy
Naproxen	375–1300 mg po	
Opioids	See Ch. 43	Sedation, constipation

*This formulation is combined with 100 mg of caffeine.
†Rebound headache with dose escalation is the major hazard of analgesic use.
GI = gastrointestinal; NSAIDs = nonsteroidal anti-inflammatory drugs.

In the USA, about 10% of the population (24 to 29 million persons) have hearing loss; half of them are ≥ 65 years. About 1 of 3 persons aged 65 to 75 and 1 of 2 > 75 have hearing loss, making hearing loss the most common disability in the elderly. The total cost of hearing loss, including productivity losses, medical care, and related special education, is estimated to be about $56 billion annually.

Hearing loss prohibits persons from easy and effective communication and can socially isolate them from their family members and friends. Hearing loss contributes to psychosocial problems; it can cause or aggravate depression, anxiety, and feelings of inadequacy, contributing to decreased functional ability.

Etiology and Classification

Hearing loss is usually related to aging (resulting in presbycusis) but can be caused by many other conditions (see TABLE 128–1). Hearing loss may be classified as sensorineural, conductive, mixed, central, or retrocochlear.

Sensorineural hearing loss, the most common type of hearing loss in adults, is due to a loss of sensitivity in the inner ear (cochlea) or the 8th cranial nerve. This type includes presbycusis, hearing loss due to noise exposure (estimated to cause half of all hearing loss cases in the USA), and hearing loss due to use of ototoxic drugs (eg, salicylates, cisplatin, streptomycin, gentamicin, quinine, aspirin). Presbycusis has been classified as sensory, neural, metabolic, or mechanical, but these terms are not typically used clinically.

TABLE 128–1.   COMMON CAUSES OF HEARING LOSS

Age-related changes (presbycusis)
Autoimmune disorders
Cerumen impaction
Ear disorders (eg, Meniere's disease, otitis media, otosclerosis)
Foreign bodies in the ear canal
Hereditary factors
Miscellaneous syndromes (eg, Paget's disease, brachio-oto-renal dysplasia syndrome, trisomy 21 syndrome, Waardenburg's syndrome)
Noise exposure
Ototoxic drugs (eg, salicylates, cisplatin, streptomycin, gentamicin, quinine, aspirin)
Perforation of the tympanic membrane
Retrocochlear lesions (eg, acoustic neuroma, meningioma, lesions due to multiple sclerosis, other extra-axial brain stem lesions)
Trauma (eg, a temporal bone fracture due to a motor vehicle accident)

Conductive hearing loss is due to a mechanical or physical blockage of sound—eg, by earwax (cerumen), occlusion of the external auditory canal, perforation of the tympanic membrane, ossicular discontinuity, otitis media with effusion, otosclerosis (otospongiosis), or a foreign body in the ear canal.

Mixed hearing loss includes the presence of both sensorineural and conductive hearing losses. Examples of mixed hearing loss include a noise-induced hearing loss with impacted cerumen, presbycusis with otitis media, and presbycusis with otosclerosis.

Central hearing loss occurs when higher centers of the brain do not perceive sound normally. Central hearing loss can occur in persons with central auditory processing disorders, decreased receptive language abilities after a stroke (receptive aphasia), or various forms of dementia.

Retrocochlear hearing loss is caused by a lesion between the brain and the cochlea (eg, acoustic neuroma [vestibular schwannoma], meningioma, other extra-axial brain stem lesions).

Symptoms and Signs

Hearing loss may affect the hearing threshold (the volume at which a patient can hear sound, expressed in decibels [dB]), discrimination (the ability to differentiate among various speech sounds), or both. Different frequencies of sound (expressed in hertz [Hz]) may be affected. Hearing loss may affect one or both ears. It may affect the ears equally (symmetric) or unequally (asymmetric). Tinnitus∎ often accompanies hearing loss.

Patients with **presbycusis** most commonly report that they can hear but cannot understand. They may say that everyone mumbles. The patient's spouse or partner may report that the patient turns the television up very loud and asks for words to be repeated. Patients may avoid social situations (eg, cocktail parties), religious services, and movie theaters.

Patients with presbycusis have difficulty understanding speech because their hearing is poorest for high-frequency sounds. In English, consonants, which are high-frequency sounds around 3000 and 4000 Hz, provide most of the clarity in speech. Consonant sounds (eg, "s," "sh," "f," "p," "t") are the most important sounds for speech recognition. For example, when "shoe," "blue," "true," "too," or "new" is spoken, many patients with presbycusis can hear the "oo" sound, but most have difficulty recognizing which word was spoken because they cannot distinguish the consonants.

Diagnosis

Screening for hearing loss is strongly recommended for all elderly persons, because they often hide their hearing loss, being embarrassed by it and equating it with aging. Also, those who have few social inter-actions may be unaware of mild hearing loss, placing them at risk of injury and further social isolation.

When hearing loss is suspected, a history should be obtained and an otoscopic examination performed. Tuning fork tests may be useful. Whisper tests and watch-ticking tests are gross measures and therefore are not useful diagnostically. When hearing loss is suspected, a com-plete audiometric evaluation should be performed by an audiologist.

History: The patient is asked about symptoms (eg, pain and tinnitus in either ear, aural drainage, episodic dizziness or vertigo), possible causes of hearing loss (eg, significant noise exposure, previous ear surgery, past and current use of ototoxic drugs), use of hearing aids, and family history of hearing loss and hearing aid use. The patient is also asked when the hearing loss was first noticed, whether it has worsened with time, and whether hearing is about the same in both ears.

Certain symptoms suggest a diagnosis other than presbycusis (which is a diagnosis of exclusion) and require further evaluation by a physi-cian. They include unilateral hearing loss, unilateral tinnitus, recent or sudden changes in hearing, fluctuating hearing loss, and aural pain.

Otoscopic examination: This examination may detect findings that suggest a diagnosis other than presbycusis. They include evidence of a conductive or mixed hearing loss, drainage from an ear, cerumen occlu-sion, anomalies of the ear canal or tympanic membrane (eg, a perfora-tion, tympanosclerosis, a red bulging tympanic membrane, a meniscus, amber fluid, bubbles), blood in the ear, unusual growths or lesions of the pinna or ear canal (eg, a glomus tumor), external otitis, and signs or anatomic abnormalities that suggest a hearing loss due to a hereditary syndrome or a history of medically correctable hearing loss. About 85 to 95% of patients seen by an audiologist do not have such findings.

Tuning fork tests: A patient's ability to hear may be roughly esti-mated in the physician's office; a tuning fork test (most commonly, Rinne's or Weber's test) may be used. Information based on tuning fork tests is limited. Because tuning forks are not calibrated, they have dif-ferent amplitudes when vibrating, potentially leading to erroneous results.

Rinne's test compares hearing by air conduction (the normal route of sound transmission—through the ear canal, tympanic membrane, and ossicles) to hearing by bone conduction. The center prong of a vibrating tuning fork is placed against the patient's mastoid process (for bone conduction). Then the vibrating tuning fork is held an inch in front of the pinna (for air conduction). The patient is asked which presentation is louder. If the mastoid presentation is louder, a conductive or mixed loss is suspected. If the pinna presentation is louder, hearing may be normal or a sensorineural or retrocochlear hearing loss may be present.

Weber's test evaluates hearing by bone conduction only. A vibrating tuning fork is placed on the front teeth, bridge of the nose, or center of the forehead. The patient is asked whether the sound is louder in the left or right ear or if the tone is in the middle. If the sound is louder in the left ear, the patient may have a conductive or mixed hearing loss in the left ear, a neurologically nonfunctional right ear, or a significant sensorineural hearing loss in both ears with better hearing in the left ear than in the right. If the sound is in the middle, hearing is normal or impairment is about the same in both ears.

Audiometry: The audiogram is a standardized tool for recording hearing thresholds at different frequencies (see FIGURE 128–1). It lists the frequencies (pitch) from left (low frequencies) to right (high frequencies) across the x-axis. Although humans can detect frequencies from about 20 to 20,000 Hz, the audiogram records the parts of the spectrum most important to human speech (250 to 8000 Hz, in octaves). Amplitudes (loudness) of sound are displayed from top (soft) to bottom (loud) along the y-axis. The audiogram usually records amplitudes from about −10 to 110 dB.

Typically, the degree of hearing loss is determined by averaging the pure tone hearing thresholds (in decibels) for 500, 1000, and 2000 Hz. The resulting number, the pure tone average, is used to define the degree of hearing loss.

A pure tone average of ≤ 25 dB across the speech frequencies indicates essentially normal hearing in adults. A pure tone average of 26 to 40 dB indicates mild hearing loss; 41 to 70 dB indicates moderate hearing loss; 71 to 90 dB indicates severe hearing loss; and ≥ 91 dB indicates profound hearing loss.

Speech audiometry: Although determining pure tone thresholds is important, patients do not listen to pure tones in their day-to-day lives, and most patients present with problems of speech perception, which pure tone testing does not directly evaluate. Speech audiometry evaluates how well a patient perceives speech sounds. The two standard measures of speech perception are the speech reception threshold and the word recognition score.

The speech reception threshold is the lowest level (in decibels) at which the patient can accurately repeat 50% of a series of two-syllable, balanced (spondaic) words (eg, baseball, railroad, staircase). The speech reception threshold is usually within 5 dB of the pure tone average. Therefore, the speech reception threshold and the pure tone average can be used as checks for each other, validating the threshold responses.

The word recognition score represents the ability of the patient to maximally understand (ie, discriminate, hear clearly, recognize) speech sounds. It is measured by presenting phonetically balanced monosyllabic words (typically, a list of 25) at a comfortable loudness level for the patient. The words are presented using a carrier phrase (eg, "you will say 'boat,'" "you will say 'went'"). The patient's task is to repeat the final word. The score is the percentage of words repeated correctly.

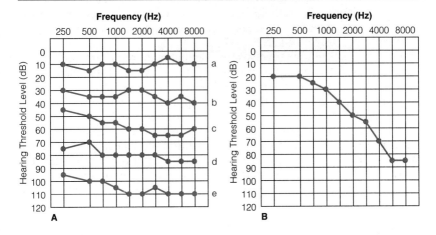

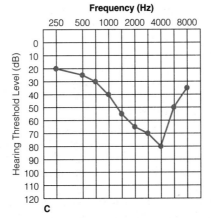

FIGURE 128–1.   Audiograms. Audiogram A shows (a) normal hearing and (b) mild, (c) moderate, (d) severe, and (e) profound hearing loss. Audiogram B shows typical hearing loss with presbycusis, and audiogram C shows typical noise-induced hearing loss.

However, a score of 100% does not necessarily preclude the need for hearing aids. For example, if the score is 100% at a presentation level of 85 dB (which is louder than that of average conversational speech), the patient would almost certainly require and benefit from hearing aids.

Generally, the speech recognition threshold and the word recognition tests are performed using prerecorded cassettes or CD recordings to ensure intertest reliability and to test each patient against the same task. When live voice tests are used, variation in the test signal loudness, accent, timing, and other factors can contaminate the test results to an unknown degree. Nonetheless, live voice tests are sometimes necessary—eg, for patients with Alzheimer's disease and those who have difficulty completing a task.

For patients with presbycusis, the typical audiometric test result is a bilateral mild-to-moderate, high-frequency hearing loss. Hearing is usually best in low frequencies and poorest in high frequencies. Usually, the speech reception threshold is appropriate (within 5 dB of the pure tone average), and the word recognition score is > 80%.

Patients with auditory processing problems or cochlear or neural hearing loss may have a low word recognition score because they do not hear clearly (ie, their auditory system does not faithfully reproduce the clarity of speech, regardless of loudness). Patients with a score below about 70% have difficulty understanding conversational speech without visual cues, despite being able to hear sound.

Treatment

Although physicians diagnose hearing problems and medically and surgically treat appropriate patients, the majority of patients with hearing loss are managed by audiologists. They counsel and advise patients about hearing loss, recommend and fit hearing aids, help manage tinnitus, recommend ways to avoid noise problems, and recommend and supply assistive listening devices for patients requiring them. Audiologists can also provide speech-reading and aural rehabilitation services.

Hearing aids: The primary treatment for patients with hearing loss is hearing aids. In 1998, about 2 million hearing aids were sold in the USA. In 1997, 78% of hearing aids were sold to patients aged 65 to 84.

There are many styles of hearing aids, and patients should choose a style that they will wear without embarrassment. Cosmetics cannot be ignored in the fitting of hearing aids.

Patients with binaural hearing loss generally need binaural hearing aids. About 60% of hearing aid wearers use two aids. Binaural amplification enables the brain to compare and contrast sounds from both ears and to perceive amplitude, spectral, and phase cues, which greatly improve speech recognition in quiet and noisy situations.

If patients with binaural hearing loss wear only one hearing aid, they cannot tell where a sound is coming from, and in difficult situations (eg, noisy ones), they cannot hear speech clearly. Additionally, more amplification is usually required with a monaural unit than with binaural units. A monaural aid is used only if patients have financial constraints, only one ear requiring amplification (the second ear is nonserviceable or normal), or binaural interference (rare).

Realistic expectations are key to successful treatment with hearing aids. Even the best hearing aids do not enable a patient to hear clearly in adverse listening situations, such as those involving poor acoustics (due to high reverberation), a poor signal-to-noise ratio (the intensity of speech in relation to the intensity of competing signals or background noise), excessive background noise, or poor visual contact between speaker and listener (eg, in poor lighting). Even with well-fitted hearing aids, patients usually need redundant and plentiful auditory and visual communication cues during normal discourse to maximize speech perception.

Hearing aids are available in three basic technologies: analog (with traditional circuits), digitally programmable (an analog unit with digitally controllable parameters), and 100% digital (which has analog microphones and receivers, despite its name). Digitally programmable and digital hearing aids are used by about 30 to 40% of hearing aid wearers.

Analog units, the most common and least expensive type, make sound louder but provide the least amount of sound processing. Thus, they may be preferred by patients who need basic amplification at the lowest possible price. Analog units are available in all sizes: behind-the-ear, in-the-ear, in-the-canal, and completely-in-the-canal. They can be manufactured with multiple screw-set controls (potentiometers) to adjust compression ratios and compression knee points (level at which compression is initiated), low- and high-frequency gain (amplification power), maximum output, and other parameters.

Digitally programmable units (digitally controlled analog units) are hybrids that enable the audiologist to control the hearing aid's characteristics with digital accuracy (using a computer) while delivering sound via analog technology. Control of the circuit is vastly improved, and these units can be tuned to the patient's preferences. They are available in all sizes. They vary in price but are generally more expensive than analog units.

Digital units (digital signal processing units) are the most technologically advanced. They may have more computing power than most personal computers, yet they are the size of a pencil eraser and fit inside the ear canal. These units can process speech at > 100 million calculations per second and can use feedback control, directionality, noise reduction, and many processing strategies to maintain a comfortable listening level for all sounds—from very soft to very loud. They are available in all sizes and are the most expensive.

Behind-the-ear hearing aids are the most powerful ear-level units (see FIGURE 128–2). Because the receiver and microphone are separated, gain can be increased with less chance of acoustic feedback (whistling). Because this aid is relatively large, it can accommodate many circuit options (eg, telephone coils, direct audio input, multiple programs, directional microphones, manual switches). Behind-the-ear aids are typically used for patients with moderate, severe, or profound hearing loss.

In-the-ear hearing aids are the most visible and least expensive ear-level aids and the largest of aids worn within the ear (see FIGURE 128–3). By definition, in-the-canal and completely-in-the-canal aids

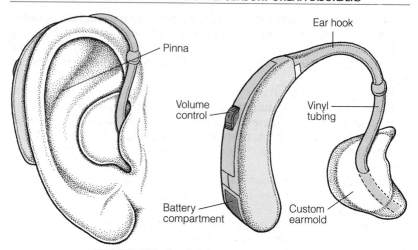

FIGURE 128–2. Behind-the-ear hearing aid.

are also "in the ear," but by convention, only units that occupy the full concha are referred to as in-the-ear aids. In-the-ear aids are ideal for many patients, because they do not go deep into the ear canal. They are sometimes recommended because they are larger than in-the-canal and completely-in-the-canal aids, possibly making them easier to insert and remove. In-the-ear aids are typically used for patients with mild, moderate, or, occasionally, severe hearing loss.

In-the-canal hearing aids are smaller and typically more expensive than in-the-ear aids (see FIGURE 128–3). They are easily inserted and

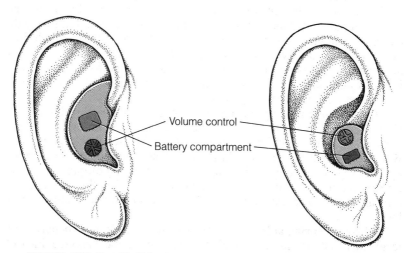

FIGURE 128–3. (*Left*) in-the-ear and (*right*) in-the-canal hearing aids.

removed. In-the-canal aids are typically used for patients with mild or moderate hearing loss.

Completely-in-the-canal hearing aids are the smallest hearing aids (see FIGURE 128–4). A well-fitted aid in an appropriately shaped ear canal is barely visible. These aids fit so deeply into the ear canal that they require a tiny pull string to remove them. Because they are placed so close to the tympanic membrane, they require less sound pressure than traditional hearing aids to yield a similar result. The shape of these aids naturally enhances the response to high frequencies (consonants) where it is most useful, around 3000 Hz. They are often the best choice for patients with mild or moderate hearing loss.

Eyeglass hearing aids are not widely used. If the hearing aid malfunctions, patients must go without their glasses. If glasses are misplaced, the hearing aid is also. Frame styles for these aids are limited.

Body-worn hearing aids resemble personal stereos. The main unit, which is about the size of a deck of cards, is worn in a pocket or on a belt. The receiver is usually a custom-made clear plastic ear mold placed in the ear canal and attached to the main unit by a wire. Body-worn hearing aids are useful for patients with profound hearing loss, because they may provide 85 or 90 dB of gain, often without acoustic feedback. However, body-worn hearing aids are cosmetically unappealing.

Bone conduction hearing aids are excellent for patients with maximal conductive or mixed hearing loss. They may be appropriate for patients with atretic ears, hearing loss due to a hereditary syndrome, or two ears for which surgical treatments are no longer possible (postoperative ears). The bone conduction hearing aid typically consists of a box (sim-

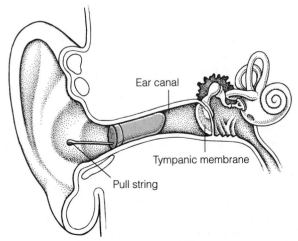

FIGURE 128–4.   Completely-in-the-canal hearing aid.

ilar to the body-worn hearing aid) and wires leading to the receiver, which is a bone conduction oscillator strapped across the head. (The oscillator is much like that used for bone conduction testing.) Bone conduction hearing aids vibrate the skull, and with rare exception, there is no acoustic feedback. Therefore, these aids can overcome the conductive portion of a mixed hearing loss. However, the box and the bone oscillator are cosmetically unappealing.

Cochlear implants: Cochlear implants are appropriate for patients with profound bilateral sensorineural hearing loss who derive little benefit from hearing aids. Accurately predicting which patient will do well with an implant is impossible. However, patients with postlingual hearing loss do much better than those with prelingual hearing loss, and results regarding neural plasticity and successful interpretation of the sounds presented by a cochlear implant are maximized when the procedure is performed as soon as possible after hearing loss occurs.

The cochlear implant is surgically placed in the inner ear, where it electrically stimulates the neural tissue of the inner ear and the 8th cranial nerve. The implant presents an auditory sensation to the patient, but the sensation is not likely to be truly speechlike. The failure rate is < 1%, and some patients have excellent results, including speech recognition while using the telephone. Nonetheless, extensive preoperative counseling regarding realistic expectations and the need for extensive aural rehabilitation is important. Patients must attend rehabilitation sessions regularly.

Assistive listening devices: Various devices can be used to make an auditory signal louder and improve the signal-to-noise ratio. Assistive listening devices are available for persons with every type and degree of hearing loss. They are useful in one-on-one conversations or in movie theaters, in concert halls, at tourist attractions, and in many other venues.

Since 1991, all new telephones are required to be compatible with personal hearing aids. Hearing aids with a telecoil can be set on "T" to receive (through magnetic induction) the signal from the magnetic coil inside the telephone. While the telecoil is activated, the microphone is usually inactivated; therefore, the hearing aid does not concurrently amplify background sounds from the room in which the person is speaking.

Many telephones have a low-high volume switch; others have replacement handsets with modular jacks, which facilitate switching between regular and amplified handsets. Portable telephone amplifiers can be easily attached and removed from the earpiece of most phones. These devices are useful for persons with hearing loss who need access to more than one telephone (home, office, or cell phone) and for those who travel frequently.

Telecommunication devices for the deaf (TDDs) enable persons with a hearing loss to call other TDD users and type their message using an attached keyboard. This system is similar to instant messaging on computers. The typed message is displayed on the recipient's TDD screen or printed on an optional paper scroll. Most states have a free relay service through which persons with normal hearing who wish to contact a person with a hearing loss can call a relay operator who has a TDD.

Some behind-the-ear hearing aids have direct audio input, allowing the hearing aid to be directly coupled to the telephone (or television, radio, or other media source) with special audio boots and cords.

Closed caption decoders are required on new televisions with screens ≥ 13 inches. Closed captioning provides a written transcription of dialogue and sound effects for many television shows.

In **infrared systems,** a transmitter sends signals from the sound source (eg, television, radio) to an infrared receiver in a headset worn by persons with a hearing loss, who can adjust the loudness of the headset to their comfort level. Infrared receivers are portable and can be used in any public arena that has an infrared transmitter. However, infrared systems are ineffective in direct sunlight (some outdoor arenas), and they do not work if light transmission to the receiver is physically blocked.

In **FM systems,** a microphone at the sound source sends signals to a transmitter, which broadcasts the signal via FM radio waves to a receiver worn by persons with a hearing loss. FM systems are portable, can be used indoors and outdoors, and can be used by persons with a wide range of hearing losses. FM systems with attenuated headsets are being increasingly used by persons with normal hearing and central auditory processing disorders.

Assistive listening devices may be used as **alerting systems** for auditory signals in the home and community (eg, telephone, doorbell, door knock, alarm clock, smoke detector, sirens, turn signal on a car). Most devices use a visual signal (eg, strobe light) or tactile signal to represent the auditory signal. For example, a device hooked up to the doorbell can set off a flashing light in the kitchen. One device can be set to flash once for a knock at the door, twice for the telephone, and one long followed by one short flash for the smoke detector.

Ordinary devices, such as portable pagers and e-mail, enable persons with a hearing loss to easily, accurately, and instantly communicate with others.

Other strategies: Hearing dogs can help a small percentage of patients. The dogs are trained to alert patients to various auditory signals in their home, workplace, or community.

Cued speech is a system of brief hand signals used to distinguish various speech sounds that are indistinguishable through speech reading alone. For example, the sounds "p," "b," and "m" look the same on the lips. In cued speech, the speaker makes a discreet gesture at the side of the lips to identify each of the sounds.

Clear speech is simply speech that is well enunciated. Training in clear speech refocuses the speaker on pronouncing each syllable carefully and clearly but without undue exaggeration. With practice, clear speech becomes habitual, making auditory comprehension and speech reading much easier.

Aural Rehabilitation

Most patients lose their hearing gradually and are therefore unprepared for the sudden reintroduction of sounds that occurs with hearing aids. Patients may be distracted by amplification of ordinary sounds, such as the humming of a refrigerator, the turning of newspaper pages, and the sound of their footsteps on the kitchen tile. Almost all patients notice that their own voice takes on a different quality while they are wearing hearing aids.

Most patients benefit from aural rehabilitation. Typically, a small group of age-matched peers meets weekly for instruction and supervised practice in optimizing communication. Patients help set communication goals and receive instruction, hints, and insight regarding making sense of sounds they have not heard for a long time. Time and patience are required, but working with professionals who are experts in maximizing communication makes the process easier and less frustrating.

Sessions almost always include training in speech reading. Patients are taught which sounds are visible on the lips, teeth, and tongue and which are not. The need to notice facial expressions and gestures is stressed, and patients are reminded that context, linguistic redundancy, and familiarity with common English idioms contribute to the understanding of conversations, even when patients cannot hear every word.

Training includes teaching patients to become an advocate for their own needs. Learning to anticipate difficult communication situations and to modify or avoid them gives the patient a sense of control over the listening environment. For example, patients can visit a restaurant during off-peak hours, when it is quieter. They can ask for a booth, which blocks out some extraneous sounds. They can request that specials of the day be written rather than spoken. At the beginning of a telephone conversation, identifying themselves as hearing-impaired may make obtaining information over the telephone easier. In direct conversations, asking the speaker to face them can help greatly.

With age, the walls of the external auditory canal thin, and its skin becomes drier (contributing to itching). Because the number of cerumen glands and the activity of apocrine sweat glands decreases, cerumen becomes drier and more likely to accumulate. The tympanic membrane thickens and widens. Degenerative changes occur in the joints of the ossicular chain but do not seem to affect hearing. Age-related changes in the inner ear cause a decline in auditory and vestibular function. Thus, itching of the canal, cerumen accumulation, tinnitus, hearing loss, and vertigo[1] are common among the elderly. The incidence of other ear disorders such as external otitis, serous otitis media, chronic suppurative otitis media, perforation of the tympanic membrane, cholesteatoma, otosclerosis, and benign tumors is similar in elderly and younger persons. Malignant tumors of the ear tend to be more common among the elderly.

TINNITUS

Perception of a sound in one or both ears without an external stimulus.

In the USA, about 15% of all adults and about 25% of the elderly have tinnitus. For most of them, the tinnitus is brief or is noticeable only in quiet surroundings; consequently, they do not seek medical attention. However, tinnitus is severe in about 1 of 6 affected persons and is disabling in about 1 of 30.

Tinnitus may be subjective (ie, only patients can hear the sound) or objective (ie, it is due to real noise, such as venous hum).

Etiology and Pathophysiology

Most commonly, tinnitus results from hearing loss,[2] and all types of hearing loss (eg, presbycusis, conductive hearing loss due to cerumen accumulation) can cause subjective tinnitus. Because the prevalence of hearing loss increases with age, so does the prevalence of tinnitus.

Tinnitus may also be caused by disorders that do not cause hearing loss and by certain drugs (see TABLE 129–1). Vascular disorders, such as anemia or disorders that disturb blood flow in vessels close to the ear, may cause objective tinnitus by generating detectable sounds (eg, venous hum). Depression, often associated with significant life stress (eg, due to retirement, death of a spouse, or problems with sexual function), may aggravate tinnitus.

The pathophysiology of tinnitus due to hearing loss is unknown, but it may resemble that of phantom limb syndrome, in which sensations are perceived to originate from an amputated limb.[3] Auditory depriva-

---

[1] see page 181   [2] see page 1317   [3] see page 286

TABLE 129–1. CAUSES OF TINNITUS

Cause	Description/Type of Tinnitus	Description/Type of Hearing Loss
Cerumen accumulation obstructing the external auditory canal*	Subjective	Conductive
Cholesteatoma	Subjective	Conductive, rarely sensorineural
Depression*	Subjective; may be an aggravating factor when tinnitus has an organic cause	—
Drugs	Subjective and high-frequency	Sensorineural, symmetric, and high-frequency
Aminoglycosides*	May be only partly reversible	Sensorineural
Antineoplastic drugs*	May be only partly reversible	Sensorineural
Aspirin (in high doses)	Reversible when the drug is stopped	Reversible when the drug is stopped
Loop diuretics*	Reversible when the drug is stopped	Reversible when the drug is stopped
Quinine/chloroquine	Usually transient	Usually transient
Ear surgery	Subjective	—
External otitis	Subjective	Conductive
Foreign body obstructing the external auditory canal	Subjective	Conductive
Head trauma	Subjective, high-pitched, and unilateral or bilateral	Variable, usually high-frequency
Hearing loss, inherited	Subjective and variable	Variable
Hearing loss, noise-induced*	Subjective, typically high-pitched, and bilateral	Sensorineural; early loss at 6 kHz, followed by progressive high-frequency loss
Meniere's disease*	Subjective, usually unilateral, low-frequency, roaring, and fluctuating	—
Myringosclerosis	Subjective	Conductive
Otosclerosis*	Subjective	Conductive

TABLE 129-1. *(Continued)*

Cause	Description/Type of Tinnitus	Description/Type of Hearing Loss
Palatal myoclonus	Subjective or objective and pulsatile; often with repetitive clicking sounds	—
Patulous eustachian tube*	Subjective or objective and pulsatile (patient hears own voice and respiration loudly [autophony])	—
Perforation of tympanic membrane	Subjective	Conductive
Presbycusis*	Subjective, typically high-pitched, and bilateral	Sensorineural; early loss at 6 kHz, followed by progressive high-frequency loss
Serous otitis media*	Subjective	Conductive
Syphilis	Subjective, often unilateral, low-frequency, and roaring (identical to that in Meniere's disease)	—
Tumors, cerebellopontine angle	Subjective, progressive, unilateral, and high-frequency	Sensorineural, progressive, unilateral, and high-frequency
Tumors, glomus	Most commonly unilateral and pulsatile but may be subjective or objective	Conductive
Tympanosclerosis	Subjective	Conductive
Vascular disorders (atherosclerosis*, transmitted cardiac murmurs*, anemia*, arteriovenous malformations or fistulas, intracranial aneurysms, benign intracranial hypertension, vascular neoplasms)	Subjective or objective and pulsatile	Usually normal
Viral infection by herpes zoster (herpes zoster oticus [Ramsay Hunt's syndrome]) and many other viruses	Subjective	Sensorineural

*Common cause among the elderly.

tion, regardless of cause, may lead to the generation of a perceived sensation (tinnitus) by central auditory structures. In support of this theory, tinnitus most commonly affects persons whose hearing loss is acquired. According to another theory, tinnitus resembles the cross talk of telephone wires: Patchy loss of myelin from the auditory nerve results in signals crossing from one auditory fiber to another.

Symptoms and Signs

Tinnitus manifests similarly in elderly and younger patients. It is described as a ringing, hissing, or whistling sound that resembles crickets, bells, or a variety of complex sounds. Tinnitus is usually bilateral, subjective, and continuous. Rarely, patients have objective tinnitus, which often has a pulsatile quality. A few patients may manifest psychotic features (eg, they report hearing music or voices). In most elderly patients, tinnitus is accompanied by symmetric, predominantly high-frequency sensorineural hearing loss with symmetric word recognition.▮ Elderly patients with a long-standing hearing loss may seek care only when tinnitus becomes bothersome.

Diagnosis

The history and physical examination may help determine the cause of tinnitus or suggest additional tests. Examination of the ear may detect a perforated tympanic membrane or middle ear effusion. Tuning fork tests may indicate conductive hearing loss.▮ Auscultation of the precordium, neck, or temporal bone may detect a bruit. The status of hearing, exposure to ototoxic drugs, and history of occupational, military, or recreational noise exposure are determined. The patient should be asked about the onset of tinnitus (acute, subacute, or chronic), its quality (continuous or pulsatile), exacerbating factors (eg, quiet surroundings, stress), alleviating factors (eg, background noise), and effects (eg, insomnia, distraction, interference with normal activities). Determining whether tinnitus is related to depression is sometimes necessary. Clues linking the two include insomnia that the patient relates to the tinnitus, early awakening, and a disproportionately high level of distraction ascribed to the tinnitus.

Blood tests, especially hemoglobin or hematocrit, are required if tinnitus is pulsatile. Other blood tests are useful only if indicated by other symptoms or signs (eg, if anemia or a hyperdynamic state due to hyperthyroidism is suspected or if low-frequency hearing loss suggesting syphilis is detected). If the patient has a carotid bruit and ipsilateral pulsatile tinnitus, ultrasonography of the carotid system may be indicated to rule out arterial obstruction, aneurysms, and vascular neoplasms. If a

---

vascular mass is detected in the middle ear (a glomus tumor or high-riding jugular bulb), high-resolution CT of the temporal bone is required to determine the origin of the mass. When contrast-enhanced CT results are negative in a patient with subjective or objective pulsatile tinnitus, magnetic resonance angiography may be useful. Occasionally, when contrast-enhanced CT or magnetic resonance angiography is unrevealing, cerebral angiography is required.

Audiometry, including pure-tone air and bone thresholds and speech audiometry, should be performed.**1** If sensorineural hearing loss is asymmetric or if tinnitus is considerably worse in one ear, a retrocochlear abnormality (eg, acoustic neuroma)**2** should be sought.

Treatment

Treatment of the underlying disorder may ameliorate the tinnitus.

For patients with tinnitus related to hearing loss, the most effective treatment is usually a well-fitted hearing aid,**3** which, for many patients, significantly reduces tinnitus. Reassuring patients with tinnitus due to bilateral sensorineural hearing loss that no life-threatening underlying disorder exists may alleviate anxiety. Avoiding such stimulants as caffeine and nicotine and avoiding stress and fatigue may help reduce irritability related to the tinnitus.

For patients bothered by tinnitus primarily at night, a white-noise generator at bedside (or a radio tuned to an interband FM frequency) is often effective. Tinnitus maskers, worn in the ear similarly to hearing aids, generate a band of noise corresponding to the patient's tinnitus and are occasionally helpful.

Biofeedback is effective for selected patients who have distressing tinnitus unrelieved by other measures. Patients with tinnitus and depression or anxiety require appropriate counseling and pharmacologic treatment.

OTALGIA

Ear pain.

Otalgia may result from an ear disorder (eg, inflammation of the pinna, external auditory canal, tympanic membrane, or middle ear) or from pain referred along neural pathways, including the trigeminal, glossopharyngeal, vagus, and cervical nerves. Eustachian tube obstruction may cause painful retraction of the tympanic membrane. Malocclusion due to poorly fitting dentures may trigger pain in the temporomandibular joint, which may be referred to the ear. Bruxism (grinding the teeth during sleep or stress) may cause temporomandibular joint

---

1 see page 1320   **2** see page 1341   **3** see page 1322

pain and thus otalgia. More ominously, patients with tumors of the head and neck may present with referred otalgia.

If no otic source for otalgia can be identified, the head and neck—particularly the nasopharynx, hypopharynx, base of the tongue, and tonsillar fossae—must be examined. X-ray evaluation of the skull base may be indicated. Treatment depends on the cause of otalgia.

CERUMEN ACCUMULATION

Accumulation of cerumen (earwax) is more common among the elderly than among younger persons. When cerumen obstructs the external auditory canal or touches the tympanic membrane, it can cause tinnitus, a sensation of aural fullness, and hearing loss. In the elderly, cerumen accumulation may aggravate a preexisting hearing loss, prompting them to seek care for the obstruction earlier than would younger persons.

Cerumen may be rock-hard and, particularly in elderly men, may contain exfoliated hairs. Obstruction of the external auditory canal is obvious during examination. Because the adnexal glands that produce cerumen are located only in the lateral two thirds of the canal, obstruction extending to the medial portion suggests that the patient has used an instrument (eg, cotton-tipped applicator, bobby pin, paper clip), a finger, or a washcloth to force the cerumen medially.

Treatment

Patients with an obstruction can apply hydrogen peroxide, which may atraumatically flush the cerumen from the canal to the external meatus, where it may be wiped away with a washcloth. Patients with recurring cerumen obstructions and an intact tympanic membrane can regularly use small amounts of mineral oil, baby oil, or over-the-counter preparations, which thin cerumen and allow it to flow out of the canal.

If these home remedies are ineffective and the patient seeks treatment, the physician should remove the cerumen as gently as possible. When visualization is good, a cerumen spoon and an aural speculum can be used. For atraumatic removal of hard accumulations, topical therapy with a cerumen softener (eg, mineral or baby oil) for several days to a week may be necessary to avoid injuring the skin of the external auditory canal during removal. Alternatively, the canal can be gently irrigated with warm, soapy water; however, *irrigation is contraindicated if the tympanic membrane is perforated, because an infection may result. Also, irrigation may perforate the tympanic membrane if irrigation is performed too vigorously or if the tympanic membrane has been previously damaged.* Gently directing the water along the canal wall, not at the tympanic membrane, can reduce the risk of perforation.

EXTERNAL OTITIS

(Swimmer's Ear)

A painful infection of the external auditory canal.

External otitis is very common among persons of all ages. It is usually precipitated by damage to the skin of the external auditory canal resulting from immersion in water or from the patient's attempts to remove wax or retained water from the canal. The disorder may result from hearing aid use or, if recurrent, from seborrheic dermatitis. Occasionally, external otitis is due to fungal overgrowth, most commonly by *Aspergillus* and *Candida* sp. Fungal external otitis (otomycosis) can occur without apparent provocation or may follow treatment of bacterial external otitis with antibiotic ear drops.

Symptoms, Signs, and Diagnosis

Symptoms include earache, itching, and swelling of the external auditory meatus. If the swelling completely obstructs the external auditory canal, conductive hearing loss results. Signs include erythema and swelling of the canal, scant watery otorrhea mixed with desquamated debris, and pain when the pinna, tragus, or mastoid tip near the external auditory canal is palpated.

Early in the course of fungal external otitis, itching in the ear is more common than pain. Thick white debris with a velvety appearance or debris with hyphae is characteristic, and edema of the canal skin is less severe than that due to bacterial external otitis.

In elderly patients with diabees, external otitis occasionally progresses (despite treatment with antibiotic ear drops) to **necrotizing (malignant) external otitis,** a potentially life-threatening osteomyelitis of the temporal bone, which produces granulation tissue in the posterior inferior external auditory canal. At first, only acute external otitis may be detected. Immunodeficiency and diabetic angiopathy may promote an invasive process. Once the infection penetrates the external auditory canal epithelium, it spreads along vascular and fascial planes, occasionally resulting in such complications as facial nerve paralysis, lateral venous sinus thrombosis, paralysis of the 9th through 12th cranial nerves, and extension to the contralateral temporal bone through the clivus.

Necrotizing external otitis should be suspected if patients with diabetes do not respond promptly to treatment for routine external otitis or have otalgia disproportionate to clinical findings. Culture and sensitivity testing are performed; *Pseudomonas aeruginosa* is almost always detected. Technetium-99m bone scanning can detect temporal bone osteomyelitis early. Gallium-67 scanning and ESR are used to monitor treatment response. CT of the temporal bone, a secondary test, may show opacification of the mastoid air cell spaces or demineralization of bone, suggesting a more invasive disorder. Granulation tissue should be biopsied to rule out other inflammatory or neoplastic processes.

Treatment

For patients who have recurrent infections, the ear is usually left open to air. During bathing or swimming, water may be prevented from entering the middle ear by inserting a cotton ball impregnated with petroleum jelly. Alternatively, a mixture of alcohol and vinegar can be instilled immediately after bathing. Alcohol helps dry the ear, and vinegar alters the pH, decreasing the risk of infection.

Patients with uncomplicated external otitis and an intact tympanic membrane are given 4 drops of a combination ototopical suspension (polymyxin, neomycin, and hydrocortisone) in the affected ear qid for 7 to 10 days. If the tympanic membrane is perforated, a formulation without neomycin (eg, sulfacetamide sodium-prednisolone, a quinolone solution [such as ofloxacin or ciprofloxacin]) is recommended. Hearing aids should not be used until after the infection resolves.

If swelling of the external auditory canal prevents instillation of antibiotic ear drops, an otic sponge (or an ear wick) should be gently inserted. Antibiotic ear drops applied to the sponge expand it, reducing edema of the canal skin and enabling the drug to reach the deeper regions of the canal. The sponge should be removed within 5 to 7 days. After the swelling resolves, the conductive hearing loss due to swelling also resolves.

For patients with fungal external otitis, the external auditory canal and tympanic membrane are meticulously cleaned under microscopic visualization. Then, 4 drops of clotrimazole (1% solution) are instilled in the affected ear qid for 7 to 10 days.

Patients with necrotizing external otitis must be hospitalized to be given antipseudomonal antibiotics, usually as combination therapy. Several weeks of intravenous antibiotic therapy may be required before switching a patient to oral ciprofloxacin, which is continued for at least 2 weeks after symptoms cease.

SEROUS OTITIS MEDIA

An effusion in the middle ear, usually due to eustachian tube obstruction.

In elderly and younger adults, serous (secretory) otitis media commonly results from temporary eustachian tube dysfunction secondary to a viral or bacterial upper respiratory infection. If unilateral, the disorder may be due to a nasopharyngeal mass.

Symptoms, Signs, and Diagnosis

Symptoms include a sensation of aural fullness and hearing loss without pain. Otoscopic examination detects amber fluid filling the middle ear and causing the malleus handle to appear whiter than usual. An air-fluid level or air bubbles seen through the tympanic membrane after autoinflation of the ear (by blowing the nose), usually accompanied by a bubbling or squealing sound and transient improvement in hearing, suggests improving eustachian tube function and may herald resolution of the effusion. Pneumatoscopy detects sluggish or no movement of the tympanic membrane. A conductive hearing loss is present.

Unilateral serous otitis media in elderly patients (unlike that in young children) requires evaluation for a nasopharyngeal mass, which can obstruct the nasopharyngeal orifice of the eustachian tube. This orifice should be examined with a mirror or fiberscope. CT or MRI may be indicated to look for a more lateral obstruction. The neck must be examined for lymphadenopathy.

Treatment

If the cause is an upper respiratory tract infection or allergy, antibiotics, local vasoconstrictive therapy, or a topical nasal corticosteroid spray may help. Nasal decongestant sprays (eg, oxymetazoline 0.05%) can relieve nasal congestion but should not be used > 5 days in succession. If a nasopharyngeal mass has been excluded, patients with fluid persisting in the middle ear and conductive hearing loss may require myringotomy with aspiration of fluid and possibly insertion of a ventilation tube.

CHRONIC SUPPURATIVE OTITIS MEDIA

A persistent or recurrent middle ear infection, generally associated with a perforated tympanic membrane and intermittent purulent otorrhea.

Chronic suppurative otitis media may complicate a retracted or perforated tympanic membrane that has been stable, or it may cause the ear to drain in elderly persons who have had a quiescent chronic ear infection.

Perforation of the tympanic membrane may be permanent, and the middle ear mucosa may become hypertrophic. In some patients, the inflamed, polypoid hypertrophic mucosa protrudes through the perforation into the external auditory canal as an aural polyp. A cholesteatoma may be present.

Patients usually report ear drainage and hearing loss. Dizziness and facial nerve paralysis are ominous signs suggesting erosion of the labyrinthine bone.

Culture and sensitivity testing of the discharge are performed; generally, *Pseudomonas aeruginosa* and *Staphylococcus aureus* are detected. Under microscopic visualization, polypoid tissue may be gently debrided for biopsy. Tissue must not be avulsed, because its medial attachment may include the stapes or facial nerve. High-resolution CT of the temporal bone with specific bone-imaging settings can show the status of the middle ear and surrounding structures and may be required to exclude an underlying cholesteatoma.

Treatment

Treatment begins with removal of purulent debris under microscopic visualization. Irrigation with a dilute acidic solution (eg, 1:1 distilled vinegar and water) 3 times daily helps remove the remaining debris and restore the canal's normal pH. A topical antibiotic solution should be instilled after each irrigation and in the evening. An ophthalmic preparation containing sulfacetamide sodium-prednisolone or a quinolone solution (eg, ofloxacin, ciprofloxacin) should be used rather than an ototopical preparation containing an aminoglycoside (eg, neomycin), which is potentially ototoxic. Aggressive topical and oral antibiotic therapy, chosen on the basis of culture and sensitivity testing, often heals polypoid tissue. Biopsy of polypoid tissue may accelerate healing. Patients who do not respond to this therapy may require intravenous antibiotics or tympanomastoid surgery. Use of surgery depends on the cause of chronic suppurative otitis media and the patient's general condition.

CHOLESTEATOMA

An enlarging sac of squamous epithelium containing keratin debris located in the middle ear or mastoid.

Cholesteatomas usually result from poor ventilation of the space medial to the pars flaccida (the thin, superior part of the tympanic membrane) leading to retraction of the tympanic membrane. The result is a sac in which keratin debris accumulates. Usually, tufts of keratin debris protrude from the area above the short process of the malleus. Occasionally, cholesteatomas originate from squamous epithelium that grows into the tympanic cavity through a marginal perforation of the tympanic membrane.

Symptoms, Signs, and Diagnosis

Most patients have recurrent ear infections with purulent drainage (ie, chronic suppurative otitis media). However, some patients have few symptoms. Occasionally, the only signs are conductive hearing loss (due to progressive erosion of the ossicular chain) and a tympanic membrane that appears abnormal. Less commonly, progressive erosion of the semicircular canals and the cochlea causes vertigo and sensorineural hearing loss, respectively.

Complications can be grave. A cholesteatoma may erode through the tegmen, allowing an epidural abscess to form. If periphlebitis or thrombophlebitis develops, infection may spread to the brain parenchyma or dural venous sinuses.

High-resolution CT of the temporal bone with specific bone-imaging settings can show the status of the middle ear, mastoid structures, tegmen, and otic capsule.

Treatment

For episodic purulent drainage, oral and ototopical antibiotic therapy is used as in chronic suppurative otitis. Surgery can stop infections and prevent complications; it is almost always recommended unless the patient is in poor health or the cholesteatoma sac can be cleaned of keratin debris in the physician's office.

OTOSCLEROSIS

Formation of spongy bone in the otic capsule due to abnormal bone resorption and new bone formation.

Subclinical otosclerosis (detected only by examination of the temporal bone) occurs in about 7 to 10% of whites and 1% of blacks > 5 years. Otosclerosis tends to be hereditary; 50 to 60% of affected persons have a family history of it. The measles virus has been implicated as a cause.

Generally, otosclerosis is diagnosed before old age. Prevalence increases from about 0.22 per 1000 in persons aged 20 to 30 to 3.53 per 1000 in those ≥ 60. Otosclerosis is a common cause of progressive conductive hearing loss in elderly persons with normal tympanic membranes, and occasionally, when the cochlea is involved, it causes sensorineural hearing loss. Hearing loss becomes clinically significant in about 10% of persons with otosclerosis. Sensorineural hearing loss may be profound in patients, especially elderly ones, with very advanced otosclerosis.

The disorder is characterized by abnormal deposition of bone, predominantly around the rim of the oval window. Eventually, ankylosis of the stapes results. Otosclerosis is suspected when the audiogram shows a Carhart notch (a characteristic notch at 2000 hertz [Hz]).

A hearing aid is an acceptable option for many patients. Surgical bypass of the stapes (stapedectomy or stapedotomy), an outpatient procedure, usually corrects conductive hearing loss. Surgery is recommended for patients who hear a 512-Hz tuning fork louder when it is applied to the mastoid than when it is held 2 to 3 cm from the ear (Rinne's test■). The best candidates for surgery are patients with significant conductive hearing loss, good hearing in the unaffected ear, and good motivation. Elderly patients with mixed hearing loss may benefit from stapedectomy because closing the air-bone gap in an ear with sensorineural loss may bring the hearing threshold to a level more amenable to hearing aid use. Stapedectomy or stapedotomy may help patients with profound sensorineural hearing loss by improving their use of a hearing aid.

NONMALIGNANT TUMORS

GLOMUS TUMORS

(Paragangliomas)

Benign tumors derived from paraganglion tissue (eg, the carotid body).

Among tumors of the middle ear and mastoid (which are rare), glomus tumors are the most common. The first symptom of a glomus tumor in the ear is usually pulsatile tinnitus, followed by conductive hearing loss. Tumors originating in the middle ear (glomus tympanicum) are clinically evident when small; those originating in the jugular vein at the mastoid (glomus jugulare) become clinically evident relatively late and may produce symptoms such as paralysis of the 7th, 9th, 10th, 11th, and 12th cranial nerves. Tumors that infiltrate the labyrinth or 8th cranial nerve cause sensorineural hearing loss. In 1 to 3% of patients, glomus tumors produce catecholamines, which rarely cause intermittent hypertension.

Diagnosis and Treatment

A pulsatile red mass in the middle ear is diagnostic. Tuning fork testing, cranial nerve assessment, and audiometry may detect abnormalities.

Contrast-enhanced CT of the skull base and temporal bone is performed. A glomus tumor must be distinguished from a high-riding jugular bulb, which is of no clinical consequence. Four-vessel cerebral angiography or magnetic resonance angiography is performed to detect occult tumors at other sites, because 7 to 10% of patients with a glomus tumor have multiple tumors.

Treatment depends on the tumor's site of origin and size and the patient's age and general condition. In healthy elderly patients, small tumors confined to the middle ear can be removed relatively easily, resulting in little morbidity. Afterward, the conductive hearing loss and pulsatile tinnitus may resolve. For elderly patients with large tumors,

■ see page 1319

low-dose radiation therapy (2 to 3 Gy) with arteriographic embolization is the primary treatment. The few patients with hypertension due to the tumor must be treated with α- and β-blockers before and after surgery.

ACOUSTIC NEUROMA

(Vestibular Schwannoma)

A benign tumor derived from Schwann cells that sheathe the vestibular nerve.

In the USA, acoustic neuromas are diagnosed in 2000 to 3000 persons each year. Most acoustic neuromas that occur sporadically (ie, that are not part of neurofibromatosis type 2, a hereditary disorder) are diagnosed in persons aged 40 to 60.

Acoustic neuromas most commonly originate in the internal auditory canal. Patients usually report progressive unilateral hearing loss and tinnitus. Often, one ear becomes progressively less useful (eg, for using the telephone). In about one fourth of patients, the unilateral decrease in hearing is sudden. Occasionally, vertigo and disequilibrium develop.

If the tumor grows into the cerebellopontine angle, hearing loss may worsen and vertigo may be gradually replaced by disequilibrium. Large tumors may cause facial numbness (by affecting the 5th cranial nerve) and, eventually, hydrocephalus with visual loss and chronic headache (by collapsing the 4th ventricle).

Diagnosis and Treatment

A typical audiogram shows asymmetric unilateral sensorineural loss with disproportionate loss of word recognition ability. The acoustic reflex may be abnormal or absent. Performance-intensity function testing for phonetically balanced words may detect rollover (a decrease in discrimination as intensity increases).

Additional testing is required to confirm the diagnosis: Contrast-enhanced MRI of the internal auditory canal and posterior fossa is the gold standard. Fast-spin echo T2-weighted MRI is sometimes used. The auditory brain stem response test, which is nonspecific and less sensitive, may not detect small tumors; it is performed only in very elderly or infirm patients when the detection of a small tumor would not affect treatment decisions.

Treatment of elderly patients with an acoustic neuroma is controversial. Tumor size and the patient's age and health must be considered. Very elderly or very infirm patients with a small tumor may be monitored with MRI. Treatment is warranted if the tumor increases in size. Some surgeons recommend complete surgical excision, as for younger patients, but others recommend a palliative subtotal resection. For elderly patients with vertigo, surgical removal may be recommended even if the acoustic neuroma is small. Radiation therapy (eg, with a gamma knife or linear accelerator [LINAC]) is an alternative for selected patients.

PINNAL LESIONS

A variety of systemic disorders, such as gout❶ and rheumatoid arthritis,❷ can cause pinnal lesions. Gouty tophi, which can be confused with rheumatic nodules, occur most commonly on the helix, where they may be painful and occasionally discharge chalk-white material containing sodium biurate. The nodules of rheumatoid arthritis may also be painful and can develop central necrosis. Treatment is directed at the underlying disorder.

Winkler's disease (chondrodermatitis nodularis chronica helicis), a benign disorder particularly prevalent among elderly men, is caused by degeneration of collagen. There is often a history of acute cold exposure or trauma to the ear. Winkler's disease is characterized by tender, firm nodules on the periphery of the pinna and may be confused with squamous or basal cell carcinoma. Intralesional injection of hydrocortisone acetate (25 mg/mm diameter) may provide some pain relief; local excision may be necessary.

PRIMARY MALIGNANT TUMORS

SQUAMOUS CELL CARCINOMA

Squamous cell carcinoma,❸ the most common malignant tumor of the pinna, usually develops when persons are in their 40s or older. The average age at diagnosis is 65. Squamous cell carcinoma is related to sun exposure and local trauma. It appears early as a thickened area of skin or an ulcer. Tumors of the pinna are generally painless; if they extend to the external auditory canal, they may cause a sensation of aural fullness, pruritus, and otorrhea.

Squamous cell carcinoma in the middle ear and mastoid may cause chronic ear infection. Advanced lesions cause deep, boring otalgia, serosanguinous drainage, and cranial neuropathies, including hearing loss.

Diagnosis is made after tissue biopsy and is often delayed because the lesion may closely resemble the granulation tissue of chronic suppurative otitis media. In such cases, the carcinoma may spread beyond the temporal bone or to the intrapetrous carotid artery. The prognosis is then very grave, regardless of treatment.

Treatment

Treatment of tumors confined to the pinna consists of wide local excision. The prognosis is good for patients with small tumors of the

---

❶see page 494   ❷see page 499   ❸see also page 1280

helix but not for patients with tumors near the opening of the external auditory canal.

The treatment of choice for carcinoma of the middle ear and mastoid is en bloc resection of the lesion, followed by radiation therapy. Because the temporal bone is near vital neurovascular structures, surgery frequently results in morbidity and mortality. In elderly patients with advanced carcinoma, surgical risks should be weighed carefully against the pain and debility associated with palliative care.

BASAL CELL CARCINOMA

Basal cell carcinoma, the second most common malignant tumor of the pinna, is most common among elderly patients with a history of sun exposure. It appears as a nodule with pearly, heaped-up borders. Biopsy is required for definitive diagnosis. Basal cell carcinoma confined to the pinna may be managed with wide local excision or Mohs' surgery.

Although generally less aggressive than squamous cell carcinoma, basal cell carcinoma may also involve the external auditory canal, sometimes causing an unrelenting discharge. If it extends to deeper structures, hearing loss and facial nerve paralysis may occur. If the middle ear and facial nerve are not involved, the lateral temporal bone is resected, and the external auditory canal, tympanic membrane, malleus, and incus are removed, followed by radiation therapy. If the middle ear and deeper structures are involved, surgery and radiation therapy or palliative therapy may be appropriate.

METASTATIC TUMORS

The most common primary tumors metastasizing to the temporal bone, in descending order of frequency, are those of the breast, kidney, lung, stomach, larynx, prostate, and thyroid.

Symptoms depend on the location of metastases within the temporal bone. Involvement of the external auditory canal, middle ear, mastoid, or eustachian tube can cause conductive hearing loss and pain; that of the internal auditory canal can cause sensorineural hearing loss, vertigo, and facial paralysis.

Evaluation includes x-ray documentation. The diagnosis is confirmed by biopsy. Treatment depends on the location of the primary tumor and the type of cancer detected.

Nose and throat disorders do not differ in elderly and younger adults. Nasal obstruction, rhinorrhea, epistaxis, and nasal fractures are common among all age groups and can cause bothersome symptoms. However, treatment of elderly patients may differ, partly because drugs routinely prescribed for younger patients with disorders such as nasal congestion and rhinorrhea can cause serious adverse effects in the elderly. Sympathomimetic amines (eg, pseudoephedrine) can cause agitation, confusion, and, more commonly, urinary retention. Most antihistamines are very anticholinergic and thus can cause excessive sedation, hypotension, vertigo, syncope, incoordination, constipation, urinary disturbances (especially in men with benign prostatic hyperplasia), and thickening of nasal secretions.

NASAL OBSTRUCTION

Obstruction due to anatomic changes: With age, the nose gradually changes, largely because of gravitational effects. The tip of the nose droops, and the nose elongates and narrows. The angle between the columella of the nose and upper lip decreases because skin becomes lax and the cartilage of the nasal alae thins and softens. Nasal obstruction may result if the drooping is pronounced or the softened alae close against the septum during inspiration.

Obstruction due to anatomic changes is diagnosed if elevating the tip of the nose with the thumb produces immediate improvement. The nasal airway can be opened further by placing gentle lateral traction on the cheek.

Treatment may involve wearing adherent plastic strips on the nose at night to hold the collapsed nasal airway open. For severe obstruction, surgery to lift the tip, shorten the nasal septum, and tighten the skin may be indicated.

Bilateral obstruction: Seasonal or perennial nasal allergy, as well as anatomic changes, may cause bilateral obstruction. Allergic symptoms may begin when a person moves to a new region of the country. However, for many elderly persons, the symptoms of allergic rhinosinusitis seem to diminish with age.

Bilateral obstruction may also result from bilateral nasal polyps. If the obstruction is associated with unilateral or bilateral hearing loss secondary to serous otitis media, the cause may be a nasopharyngeal tumor (eg, carcinoma, lymphoma, plasmacytoma), which should be ruled out by sinus x-ray.

Occasionally, nasal congestion may be due to hypothyroidism. Nasal congestion may be caused by certain antihypertensives and tricyclic antidepressants. Overuse of nasal decongestant sprays (eg, phenylephrine, oxymetazoline) can cause chronic hypertrophic changes of the turbinates (rhinitis medicamentosa).

For patients with allergies, the mainstay of treatment is antihistamines. However, antihistamines with anticholinergic properties tend to cause sedation, dry mouth, orthostatic hypotension, constipation, urine retention, and confusion in the elderly. Only drugs without anticholinergic properties (eg, astemizole, cetirizine, fexofenadine, loratadine) should be used in the elderly.

Unilateral obstruction: Causes include nasal swelling or polyps secondary to chronic infection in the maxillary or ethmoidal sinuses, particularly in patients who have had maxillary dental abscesses or nasogastric or nasotracheal intubation. If a confused patient has an obstruction with a discharge, the cause may be a foreign body (commonly, a wad of tissue or cotton) pushed into the nose. A unilateral obstruction associated with bleeding may be due to neoplasia involving the sinuses or nose.

Evaluation involves a physical examination, sinus x-rays, and culture; biopsy is indicated if a tumor is suspected. For benign sinus disorders, limited nasal and sinus surgery is usually required. For a malignancy, radiation therapy, surgery, or both are required, depending on biopsy and x-ray findings.

DISORDERS OF THE NASAL MUCOUS MEMBRANE

Nasal dryness: With age, the mucous membrane becomes thinner, the number and size of elastic fibers and the amount of submucosal tissue decrease, and mucus-secreting structures atrophy, resulting in decreased mucus production and nasal dryness. Buffered saline nasal sprays, used as needed, may help.

Rhinorrhea: There are many causes of rhinorrhea, including allergies. In elderly persons, exposure to cold air or intake of certain foods (especially hot or spicy foods) may cause excessive watery, dripping nasal secretions. This effect probably results from age-related changes in the function of parasympathetic vasomotor secretory fibers in the nose. Ipratropium bromide 0.03% nasal spray is effective, although it should be used with caution in patients who have narrow-angle glaucoma or benign prostatic hyperplasia. Anticholinergic antihistamines are dangerous in the elderly and should not be used; antihistamines without anticholinergic properties have no effect on rhinorrhea unless it is caused by allergy.

Epistaxis (nosebleed):   With age, the nasal mucous membrane atrophies and blood vessel walls in the nose thin. As a result, epistaxis is relatively common among the elderly.

Anterior epistaxis may result from ulceration of the mucosa overlying old septal spurs, from deviations (particularly in patients taking anticoagulants, such as daily aspirin for general cardiovascular prophylaxis), or from use of oxygen through nasal cannulas. Posterior epistaxis, the more serious type, is most commonly caused by rupture of a branch of the sphenopalatine artery, located near the posterior tip of the inferior turbinate. Hypertension may play a role. Rarely, a tumor is the cause.

Coagulopathies, if present, should be corrected at least temporarily, so that a thrombus can form and the mucous membrane can heal. Acute anterior epistaxis may be managed with oxymetazoline 0.05% nasal spray, which has long-acting vasoconstrictive properties and no significant systemic effects. It is applied to the bleeding site with cotton; the site is then compressed externally for at least 20 minutes until the bleeding stops. Alternatively, bleeding sites can be cauterized and protected with a petroleum-based ointment until they heal.

For posterior epistaxis, nasal packing is usually needed to control the bleeding, particularly in hypertensive patients. After the nose is anesthetized with a lidocaine-based spray, a vasoconstrictive nasal spray (eg, oxymetazoline 0.05%) is used. Then, an epistaxis balloon is inserted into the nose and expanded with water until the bleeding is controlled. It is left in place for about 5 days. Prophylactic antibiotics are given to prevent sinusitis, and follow-up sinus x-rays should be obtained. Alternatively, a compressed sponge may be placed in the nose and kept moistened with oxymetazoline 0.05% spray. Elderly patients should be hospitalized so that their respiratory status and arterial blood gas levels can be monitored. Gauze packing, although tolerated well by most young patients, should not be used in the elderly. It causes nasal obstruction and often depresses the palate, partially obstructing the oral airway. In the elderly, hypoxia and carbon dioxide retention can result.

If epistaxis persists despite treatment, endoscopic nasal examination and cauterization of the bleeding vessel, transantral ligation of the sphenopalatine artery in the pterygomaxillary space, or angiography with embolization of the internal maxillary and sphenopalatine arteries may be performed. After treatment, a full set of sinus x-rays should be obtained to determine if sinusitis has developed or if the cause of the bleeding was a tumor.

NASAL FRACTURES

Nasal fractures are relatively common among the elderly, who are predisposed to them because of age-related thinning of facial bones. Most fractures result from trauma due to a fall. Fractures produce obvious distortion of the bony nasal framework, accompanied by epistaxis.

Treatment by closed reduction usually suffices: After the nose is anesthetized, the bony fragments are elevated and positioned with a small amount of nonobstructive nasal packing for about 1 week (until the fracture has stabilized). During this period, antibiotics are given to prevent sinusitis.

OLFACTORY DYSFUNCTION

Gustatory function consists of fine taste (eg, distinguishing turkey from chicken), which is an olfactory function, and crude (lingual) taste (eg, distinguishing sweet from sour), which is mediated through the taste buds.∎ The sense of smell and fine taste starts to diminish gradually when persons are in their 50s, because of neural degeneration. However, years of cigarette smoking may accelerate the process. Loss of fine taste does not appear to be related to loss of lingual taste or deficits in cognition. In the elderly, the incidence of a diminished sense of smell (hyposmia) is about 40%.

Abrupt changes in olfactory function can result from influenza or viral infections that affect the olfactory receptors in the superior region of the nose. These changes are often permanent (except when caused by a common cold virus); zinc tablets are a suggested but unproven remedy. Abrupt changes in olfactory function may also result from head trauma, particularly if the cribriform plate is fractured, and from brain tumors in the region of the cribriform plate. A CT scan of the sinuses with coronal views through the cribriform plate can help rule out fractures and tumors.

In the elderly, loss of smell and fine taste may contribute to a lack of interest in eating and maintaining a proper diet and may lead to the harmful, excessive use of salt and sugar to overcome loss of subtle flavors. More hazardous, some patients lose the ability to smell ethyl mercaptan, the malodorous additive to natural gas that makes gas leaks apparent. A few patients report an unpleasant taste in the mouth (dysgeusia) or an unpleasant smell (dysosmia).

SINUSITIS

Inflammation of the paranasal sinuses due to viral, bacterial, or fungal infection or allergic reactions.

Most types of sinusitis begin before old age, commonly in patients with disorders of the respiratory mucosa. In patients with long-standing allergic rhinosinusitis, symptoms generally abate with age. Nonetheless, sinusitis is common among the elderly. Causes include dental

∎see also page 1025

infections, obstruction due to a nasal polyp, and upper respiratory tract infections. In the elderly, a common cause of acute sinusitis is the packing used for treatment of epistaxis.

Symptoms, Signs, and Diagnosis

Symptoms are similar in elderly and younger patients. The area over the affected sinus may be tender and swollen. Facial pain occurs in various sites depending on which sinus is affected. Patients report congestion and may have bad breath, a general feeling of malaise, and yellow or green purulent rhinorrhea. The nasal mucosa is red and swollen, and a purulent exudate may be present. Fever and chills suggest that the infection has spread beyond the sinuses. A malodorous, purulent nasal discharge suggests a dental root abscess that has erupted into a maxillary sinus.

If a patient has nasal or cheek swelling, unilateral or bilateral nasal obstruction, and a purulent or bloody discharge, the cause may be nasal or sinus neoplasia, rather than sinusitis. Sinus x-rays should be obtained, and if indicated, a biopsy should be performed.

The affected sinus appears opaque on x-rays, but CT provides better definition of the extent and degree of sinusitis. If the maxillary sinus is affected, x-rays of the teeth may be needed to exclude a dental root abscess. If an abscess is present, the affected tooth may require extraction.

Treatment

Treatment is aimed at improving drainage and controlling the infection. Inhaling steam (eg, during a hot shower), using a saline nasal wash, blowing the nose, and drinking 6 to 8 glasses of water a day may help. Topical vasoconstrictors (eg, phenylephrine, oxymetazoline) used as a nasal spray may relieve congestion but should not be used > 7 days. Systemic vasoconstrictors (eg, pseudoephedrine) are less effective, can cause adverse effects in the elderly, and should be avoided.

Antibiotics should be given for at least 10 to 12 days if acute bacterial sinusitis is suspected. The initial antibiotic of choice is amoxicillin with or without clavulanate; alternatively, clarithromycin, azithromycin, or cefuroxime may be used. For chronic sinusitis, a broad-spectrum antibiotic should be used for acute flare-ups. Antibiotic therapy is usually effective. If it is not, surgical drainage may be necessary.

ATROPHIC LARYNGITIS

With age, minor salivary gland tissue is lost, and moisture in the larynx decreases. Muscle atrophies, vibratory mass decreases, fibrous tissue support is lost, and squamous metaplasia develops. These changes may cause a chronic tickle in the throat with a constant urge to clear it. In elderly men, a high, trembling, weakened voice may be the first sign of age's effects on the larynx. Voice quality diminishes because the vocal cords bow (due to decreased elasticity and muscle mass), allowing more air to escape with phonation, or because pulmonary volume and expiratory effort decrease.

For chronic tickle, treatment is symptomatic. Lozenges, sugar-free citrus hard candies, or chewing gum can stimulate salivary flow. Patients with a weak voice can be instructed to take a deep breath before they speak; doing so corrects the condition momentarily and confirms the diagnosis. Speech therapy may help. Occasionally, surgical procedures such as injection of collagen preparations into the vocal cords or thyroplasty (insertion of polymeric silicone forms to move the vocal cords toward the midline [medialize]) are performed.

REFLUX LARYNGITIS

Inflammation of the larynx secondary to nocturnal gastric reflux.

Reflux laryngitis secondary to gastroesophageal reflux disease (GERD)▪ is more common among the elderly because they are more likely to have impaired esophageal peristalsis and weakened esophageal sphincter tone. Patients who sleep in the recumbent position may feel a burning sensation in the hypopharynx and larynx; this sensation must be differentiated from angina.

Sleeping with the head elevated often prevents the reflux. If this measure is inadequate, a proton pump inhibitor (eg, omeprazole), an H_2-receptor blocker (eg, famotidine, ranitidine), or a smooth muscle agonist (eg, metoclopramide) may help.

CRICOARYTENOIDITIS

Inflammation of the cricoarytenoid joint.

Cricoarytenoiditis occurs in elderly patients with arthritis. Usually, only those with the severest forms of arthritis have symptoms—chronic pain during swallowing and speaking. Examination of the larynx detects redness and swelling over the arytenoid cartilage. The cricoarytenoid joint eventually becomes fixated, causing the vocal cords to abduct poorly. Respiratory distress can result. Rarely, arytenoidectomy or tracheotomy is required.

▪see page 1039

AGE-RELATED PAIN SYNDROMES

Eagle's syndrome: Elongation of the styloid process and calcification of the stylohyoid ligament, which commonly occur with aging, uncommonly result in intermittent, sharp pain along the distribution of the glossopharyngeal nerve (ie, in the hypopharynx and base of the tongue). Resection of the elongated styloid process is curative.

Carotidynia: Neck pain with carotid bulb tenderness that is intensified by palpation and head movement is characteristic. This disorder is self-limiting but may last for months. Anti-inflammatory analgesics are effective.

Cervical arthritis: Chronic neck and occipital pain often occurs along the distribution of C2 and C3. In the elderly, this pain must be differentiated from atypical angina pectoris (ie, intermittent, intense exercise-related pain in the neck, throat, or jaw). X-rays should be obtained to differentiate cervical arthritis from bone metastases. Analgesics and a cervical collar can relieve the pain.

Trigeminal neuralgia (tic douloureux): This disorder of the trigeminal nerve produces bouts of excruciating, lancinating pain probably caused by compression of the trigeminal nerve root. Pain occurs along the distribution of the trigeminal nerve and usually lasts between a few seconds and 2 minutes. It is often set off by touching a trigger point or by chewing or brushing the teeth.

No clinical signs accompany trigeminal neuralgia, so finding a sensory or cranial nerve abnormality requires searching for a structural cause of the pain. Differential diagnosis includes neoplasm, vascular malformation of the brain stem, a vascular insult, multiple sclerosis, postherpetic pain, and trigeminal neuropathy with Sjögren's syndrome or rheumatoid arthritis. Migraine may produce atypical facial pain.

Carbamazepine 200 mg tid or qid is generally effective, and the benefit is often sustained; liver and hematopoietic functions should be monitored. If carbamazepine is ineffective or produces toxicity, other options include phenytoin 300 to 600 mg/day, baclofen 30 to 80 mg/day, or a tricyclic antidepressant. Peripheral nerve block provides temporary relief. In resistant cases, a craniectomy can be performed to separate pulsating vascular structures (especially arteries) from the trigeminal root in the posterior fossa. Occasionally, a last resort to relieve intractable pain is resection of the 5th nerve fibers between the gasserian ganglion and the brain stem.

SECTION 16

INFECTIOUS DISEASE

131 AGING AND THE IMMUNE SYSTEM

Immune senescence (a progressive dysfunctioning of the immune system) results from loss of some immunologic activities with simultaneous increase of others. Immune senescence leads to an inappropriate, inefficient, and sometimes detrimental immune response. Clinically, immune senescence has been implicated in an increasing number of age-related disorders.∎

Two complementary forms of immunity rid humans of pathogens and cancer cells: natural (innate) immunity and adaptive (acquired) immunity. Natural immunity provides a rapid but incomplete defense against threatening agents until the slower, more definitive adaptive immune response develops. Natural immunity has a relatively rigid structure, whereas adaptive immunity, supported by T and B lympho-

∎ see page 1357

TABLE 131–1. AGE-RELATED CHANGES IN CELLULAR IMMUNITY

Factor	Change
Number of memory T lymphocytes	Increased
Number of naive T lymphocytes	Decreased
Number of CD8⁺ CD28⁻ T lymphocytes	Increased
Number of in vivo activated T lymphocytes	Increased
Number of autoreactive T lymphocytes	Increased
Activation and proliferation	Decreased
Helper and cytotoxic activities	Decreased
Production of interleukin-2	Decreased
Expression of interleukin-2 receptors	Decreased
Production of interleukin-6 and interleukin-10	Increased
Recognition of major histocompatibility complex molecules	Decreased

cytes, is infinitely versatile and adaptable. The age-related changes in cellular (T-lymphocyte–mediated) and humoral (B-lymphocyte–mediated) immunity are listed in TABLES 131–1 and 131–2. Other aspects of the immune response include mucosal immunity and allergic reactivity.

CHANGES IN NATURAL (INNATE) IMMUNITY

The components of natural immunity are dendritic cells, macrophages, natural killer cells, and the complement system.

Dendritic cells: These are the antigen-presenting cells for CD4⁺ T-helper lymphocytes, a crucial step in initiation of the immune response. They take up and process antigen into small peptides, which then complex with newly synthesized class II major histocompatibility complex

TABLE 131–2. AGE-RELATED CHANGES IN HUMORAL IMMUNITY

Factor	Change
Number of antigen-responsive B lymphocytes	Decreased
Number of clonally expanded B lymphocytes	Increased
Number of in vivo activated B lymphocytes	Increased
Number of autoreactive B lymphocytes	Increased
Expression of membrane immunoglobulins	Decreased
Overall production of IgG1, IgG2, IgG3, and IgA	Increased
Overall production of IgM and IgG4	Decreased
Production of high-affinity antibodies	Decreased
Production of antibodies to foreign antigens	Decreased
Production of antibodies to self-antigens	Increased

(MHC) proteins. Whether dendritic cells or other antigen-presenting cells (eg, macrophages) display the class I MHC–peptide complex to CD8+ lymphocytes is unclear. These cells also require the help of CD4+ lymphocytes to proliferate and develop their cytotoxic activity. The antigen–MHC complex is transported to and displayed on the cytoplasmic membrane of the dendritic cell. This complex delivers the first activation signal to CD4+ T-helper lymphocytes. Optimal T-lymphocyte activation also requires signals from other molecules expressed on dendritic cells.

Few studies have examined the effects of aging on dendritic cells. In general, elderly persons have fewer dendritic cells than do younger persons. However, even in the elderly, these cells appear to retain their antigen-presenting capacities: ie, expressing surface molecules and inducing the activation and proliferation of T lymphocytes.

Macrophages: Macrophages are among the first cells that pathogens encounter after traversing the epithelial barrier. Macrophages specialize in phagocytosis and intracellular killing of microorganisms. They demonstrate tumor cytotoxicity and are efficient antigen-presenting cells. Bacteria trigger macrophages to produce numerous chemicals and cytokines, which initiate the acute-phase response, enhance their own microbicidal activity, stimulate the production of cytokines by other cells, and promote the activation of T-helper lymphocytes.

In the elderly, macrophages usually support a normal T-lymphocyte response to specific antigens. The production of cytokines and expression of surface molecules by macrophages are similar in elderly and younger persons. However, the rate of antigen clearance by macrophages decreases notably with age. Also, in elderly persons, the toxicity of macrophages against tumor cells is low, which may contribute to increased cancer susceptibility in this population.

Natural killer (NK) cells: These cells can kill target cells spontaneously (in the absence of any obvious prior activation) and are involved in host resistance to various tumors and infectious diseases.

With age, NK cell activity remains unchanged or increases. Increased activity is usually associated with an increased proportion of cells expressing the NK phenotype.

Complement: The complement system consists of interacting plasma proteins constituting a triggered enzyme system; it appears to be the main soluble effector of natural immunity. Through cytolysis, opsonization, and activation of inflammation, complement efficiently defends against microorganisms.

Healthy elderly persons appear to have slightly lower levels of complement components than do younger persons. Age-related differences are more apparent during the course of bacterial infection: Complement levels increase dramatically in younger persons with acute bacteremia but do not significantly do so in elderly persons.

CHANGES IN ADAPTIVE (ACQUIRED) IMMUNITY

Thymic involution: The thymus is the primary lymphoid organ in which bone marrow–derived T-lymphocyte precursors mature and differentiate into functional T lymphocytes. T lymphocytes that recognize antigens and have a moderate affinity for self-MHC molecules multiply in the thymus and enter the circulation. T lymphocytes that have excessive affinity for self-MHC molecules (> 95% of total T lymphocytes) are negatively selected and are eliminated in the thymus.

Contrary to the belief that thymic involution begins at puberty, the regression of the human thymus starts after birth and continues at a constant rate until middle age. Because the thymus appears to undergo premature aging, thymic involution has been deemed responsible for the age-related decrease in T-lymphocyte–mediated immune response. However, as the multiplication and release of mature lymphocytes become insufficient to compensate for the destruction of mature lymphocytes at the periphery, peripheral lymphoid organs take over the role of the thymus. Once the peripheral T-lymphocyte pool has been established early in life, the thymus may no longer be needed.

The effects of thymectomy in old age are inconsistent and usually mild. Moreover, in studies of aged animals, thymic transplantation or complete structural and functional thymic restoration by growth hormone does not significantly improve immune response.

The thymus produces several immunoregulatory hormones that affect the differentiation of T-lymphocyte precursors and possibly some of the activities of mature B and T lymphocytes. The concentration of thymic hormones decreases with age, and some of these hormones are no longer detected in the plasma of persons > 60. However, whether some aspects of immune senescence may be improved or prevented by supplementation with thymic hormones is unclear.

T-lymphocyte function: CD8+ T lymphocytes respond to class I MHC–antigen complexes and differentiate into cytotoxic effectors, whereas CD4+ T lymphocytes are restricted to class II MHC–antigen complexes and function as helper cells. T-helper lymphocytes promote intracellular killing by macrophages, antibody production by B lymphocytes, and clonal expansion of cytotoxic T lymphocytes.

Alterations of T-lymphocyte activities underlie much of the age-related decrease in protective immune response. Severe age-related defects in T-helper lymphocyte function, demonstrated by a weak allogeneic response, have been well documented. T-lymphocyte cytotoxicity and the proliferative response to mitogens and antigens also decrease significantly in elderly persons. This proliferative defect is attributed in part to the inability of T lymphocytes derived from aged organisms to secrete and respond to the growth factor interleukin-2. T lymphocytes from elderly persons are also hyporesponsive to stimulation mediated by certain co-receptors (eg, CD28 or CD2 surface molecules).

Alteration of T lymphocyte–mediated immunity in the elderly can be partly explained by an age-related decrease in the production of T-helper lymphocytes and cytotoxic precursors and by the different distribution of CD4+ and CD8+ T lymphocytes. Aging also leads to a dramatic increase in the proportion of antigen-experienced memory T lymphocytes with a concomitant decrease in naive T lymphocytes. Although the shift toward memory cells begins early in life, the progressive expansion of cells already committed to particular antigens and functionally different from naive T lymphocytes probably accounts for some aspects of immune senescence. Similar to B lymphocytes, T lymphocytes, especially CD8+ T lymphocytes, can become monoclonally or oligoclonally expanded in most healthy elderly persons. However, clonally expanded CD8+ T lymphocytes lack the CD28 surface molecule, a receptor essential for their optimal activation, which most likely contributes to immune senescence.

Novel or aberrant characteristics of T lymphocytes may appear with age. For example, T lymphocytes from elderly persons sometimes are activated by antigenic peptides that are not presented in association with self-MHC molecules. This finding in the elderly transgresses an essential law of immunology. Enhanced activity of particular T lymphocytes also occurs with age, as demonstrated by the high concentration of interleukin-6 (IL-6) and IL-10 in serum or in cultures of cells from elderly donors.

Understanding of the molecular mechanisms underlying the various defects in T-lymphocyte function is incomplete. Biochemical lesions accumulate along the pathways of signal transmission, activating genes implicated in T-lymphocyte activity. The pathogenesis of the multiplicity of age-related biochemical alterations in T lymphocytes is unexplained, but oxidative stress—a biologic phenomenon implicated in the process of senescence—can interrupt the signalization cascades at different sites and may be common to these various biochemical defects.

B-lymphocyte function: B lymphocytes produce antibodies and display them on the cell surface, where they serve as receptors for antigens. Specific recognition of foreign antigens by surface immunoglobulin receptors is the first step in the induction of humoral immunity. The bound antigen then undergoes endocytosis and is degraded into antigenic peptides and delivered to the plasma membrane in association with class II MHC proteins. T-helper lymphocytes recognize the MHC–antigen peptide complex and stimulate B-lymphocyte proliferation and differentiation into antibody-secreting cells.

With age, humoral immunity is generally impaired quantitatively and qualitatively. The amount of antibody produced in response to most foreign antigens decreases with age. Serum levels of IgM decrease with age, although the significance of this decrease is unknown. Serum levels of IgA and IgG increase, possibly reflecting increased production of antibodies in response to various intrinsic antigens (ie, autoantibodies) or to polyclonal B-lymphocyte activation by bacterial endotoxins.

With age, the number of circulating and antigen-responsive B lymphocytes decreases, but the amount of antibody produced on a per cell basis by responding B lymphocytes does not change. Thus, reduced specific antibody production appears to be due mainly to the presence of nonfunctional cells.

The quality of the humoral response may be more important than the quantity of antibodies produced. With age, B lymphocytes produce less protective antibodies (ie, antibodies that typically bind antigens less well). For example, the serum of elderly persons immunized with pneumococcal vaccine fails to opsonize with pneumococci, despite having a high content of specific antibodies.

Because most B-lymphocyte functions are regulated by T lymphocytes or their products, age-related decreases in humoral immunity due to intrinsic defects of B lymphocytes are difficult to differentiate from those due to T-lymphocyte defects.

Autoimmune reactivity: Although the immune response to exogenous antigens decreases with age, autoimmune reactivity increases. The percentage of autoreactive T and B lymphocytes and the frequency of autoantibodies directed against a wide variety of organ-specific and non–organ-specific antigens increase, indicating an age-related propensity to lose tolerance to self.

Normally, B lymphocytes expressing antibody receptors with high affinity to self are clonally deleted, rendered silent, or switched to a different specificity. With age, subsets of B lymphocytes may escape deletion or may be unable to revise their receptors and to delete their high affinity for self.

Autoimmune antibodies may also result from an immune response against self-molecules that have been altered by age-related processes (eg, oxidation, glycation) or released from anatomic sequestration. Polyclonal B- or T-lymphocyte activation by molecules of microbial origin may also be implicated in the aberrant self-recognition.

CHANGES IN MUCOSAL IMMUNITY

Mucosal immunity provides resistance to infections; resistance to some infections better correlates with the amount of antibodies in external secretions than with serum antibody titers.

The mucosal immune network is structurally and functionally different from the rest of the immune system. Animal studies show that mucosal immunity is preserved with age. However, in humans, aging seems to compromise mucosal immunity to the same extent as it does systemic immunity; the initiation and the regulation of local antibody production are defective.

CHANGES IN ALLERGIC REACTIVITY

Allergy is characterized by the overproduction of IgE antibodies directed at ubiquitous antigens that activate the immune system after inhalation, ingestion, or penetration through the skin. When antigen is reintroduced, IgE-mediated triggering of high-affinity receptors expressed on the surface of mast cells and basophils initiates the release of mediators involved in the allergic cascade. IgE production depends on the presence of IL-4 released by a subpopulation of allergen-activated T lymphocytes.

Although no data are available on the prevalence of allergic reactions in elderly persons, IgE-mediated hypersensitivity reactions are believed to occur less frequently with age, and allergic symptoms tend to diminish. This belief is supported by the observations that serum IgE production decreases with age because of defective IL-4 production and that reactivity to histamine also decreases significantly.

CLINICAL EFFECTS OF IMMUNE SENESCENCE

Immune senescence usually develops insidiously; its effect on health often manifests during intense physiologic stress (eg, surgery, multiple organ failure, protein-energy malnutrition, dehydration). Many chronic illnesses common in old age may adversely affect immune function in elderly persons and should be diagnosed and treated when possible. Genetic and environmental factors also probably play a significant role in the occurrence of immune dysfunction.

The clinical significance of increased autoantibodies in the elderly is unknown. Paradoxically, autoimmune disorders peak in middle age and are less common in elderly persons, which would not be expected considering what is known about decreased tolerance to self with age. On the other hand, autoantibodies may play a role in some of the degenerative diseases of aging.

Because immune senescence results from dysfunction rather than from definitive exhaustion of the immune system, it may theoretically be reversed. Hormonal█ and nonhormonal drug treatment (eg, growth hormone, dehydroepiandrosterone, melatonin, zinc, vitamin E) has shown promising results and may help restore efficient immune function in the elderly.

Infectious diseases: A causal relationship between immune senescence and the reactivation of infectious diseases (eg, herpes zoster, tuberculosis) is clearly established. The incidence of herpes zoster increases fivefold between the ages of 45 and 85 in association with an age-related loss of cellular immunity to the varicella-zoster virus. There

█ see page 655

is also endogenous reactivation of latent Epstein-Barr virus infection in institutionalized elderly patients. Age-related decreases in specific antibody production may partly account for the high incidence and extreme mortality associated with pneumonia, influenza, infectious endocarditis, and tetanus among the elderly. Although the etiology of nosocomial infections is complex, age-related decreases in antibody response probably play some role in the fact that 65% of all nosocomial infections occur in patients > 60. Elderly persons are also more susceptible to parasitic infections, especially those caused by metazoan and protozoan parasites.

However, the risk of infectious diseases attributable to immune senescence is difficult to differentiate from that attributable to the various pathophysiologic structural and functional alterations of different organs, which probably determine the specific location of some infections. For example, an impaired cough reflex, reduced mucociliary clearance, altered microbial flora, and increased colonization of the oropharynx lead to severe respiratory tract infections independent of immune function. The loss of bacteriostatic properties of urine together with reduced kidney ability to acidify urine and incomplete bladder emptying render elderly persons particularly susceptible to urinary tract infections. Age-related changes in the gastrointestinal tract (eg, achlorhydria, diverticula) may predispose to the development of gastrointestinal infection.

Response to immunization: Production of specific antibody is decreased when vaccines containing antigens (eg, tetanus toxoid, hepatitis B virus) are given to elderly recipients who had no prior immunity induced by natural infection. The effect of immune senescence on the antibody response to vaccines in patients with prior immunity induced by natural infection or previous immunization (eg, influenza and pneumococcal vaccines) is difficult to evaluate. As many as 30 to 40% of healthy elderly persons may not develop protective immunity after immunization with influenza vaccine. Pneumococcal vaccines are also less effective among elderly persons than among healthy younger persons.

Cancer: Immune senescence may impair the recognition and elimination of tumor cells, but there is no compelling evidence that failure of immune surveillance contributes to the increased incidence of cancer in the elderly.

Antigen-driven clonal expansion followed by neoplastic transformation may be involved in the aging-related development of chronic lymphocytic leukemia (CLL). CLL is characterized by a clonal outgrowth of B lymphocytes and accompanied by severe immunologic disturbances (eg, hypogammaglobulinemia, autoimmune manifestations).

Monoclonal gammopathy: The frequency of idiopathic paraproteinemia increases from < 1% at age 50 to 20% at age 90. Animal studies have shown an age-related increase in homogenous immunoglobu-lin levels after thymectomy, suggesting that T-lymphocyte dysfunction is involved in the pathogenesis of dysglobulinemia.

Degenerative diseases of aging: Immune senescence may con-tribute to many age-related degenerative diseases that are not ordinarily considered immunologic in etiology.

Autoantibody production tends to increase in the presence of chronic diseases that are prevalent in the elderly and is sometimes associated with organ dysfunction or with a specific disease. For example, high levels of autoantibodies directed toward components of the thyroid, pancreatic, adrenal, and pituitary glands have been associated with the respective hormone deficiency and associated diseases (eg, hypothy-roidism, diabetes, hypopituitarism). Autoimmunity to heparin sulfate proteoglycan has also been associated with vascular disease in the elderly.

This link with specific diseases may explain why the presence of autoantibodies in the elderly is associated with reduced life expectancy. Conversely, the lack of organ-specific autoantibodies (ie, the absence of autoreactivity) after age 80 may represent a survival advantage.

Other altered immunologic activities may be implicated in several pathologic conditions typically associated with aging. For example, activated lymphocytes are found in atheromatous lesions and probably participate in atherosclerosis. The presence of T lymphocytes near neu-ritic plaques indicates that some type of immunologic response occurs in Alzheimer's disease. Also, the association of complement protein with senile plaques suggests that activation of complement pathways may contribute to neuronal cell death in Alzheimer's disease. The age-related increase in IL-6 production, a lymphokine that induces bone resorption, may be involved in the development of osteoporosis and may, if excessive, be part of the pathogenesis of late-life lymphoma, myeloma, and Alzheimer's disease.

132 ■ IMMUNIZATION

By the time most people reach old age, they have been immunized or exposed to many diseases. Nonetheless, they still need immunizations (see TABLE 132–1). Certain immunizations are indicated only in elderly persons; others are not recommended for all elderly persons but are available and appropriate in specific cases.

Active immunization uses vaccines or toxoids; the amount of protec-tion depends on the recipient's immunologic response. The immuno-logic response decreases in most elderly persons; whether the cause is

TABLE 132–1. SOME AGENTS USED FOR IMMUNIZATION IN ELDERLY PERSONS

Agent	Indication	Preparation and Dosage	Comment
Tetanus and diphtheria toxoid	All persons	Bacterial toxoids, given IM q 10 years at mid-decade birthday	See text for details
Influenza vaccine	All persons > 65 All health care providers of and all children living with elderly persons	Inactivated virus, given IM annually	See text for details
Pneumococcal vaccine	All persons ≥ 65 Persons with high-risk conditions, blacks, and Native Americans	23-Valent purified capsular polysaccharides (1 dose IM)	See text for details
Poliovirus vaccine	Travelers to areas where the disease is endemic	Inactivated vaccine (3 doses sc) is used exclusively; live oral vaccine should not be used	Poliovirus has been eradicated from the Western Hemisphere
Hepatitis A vaccine	Travelers to or residents of areas where the disease is endemic Sexually active homosexual men Users of illicit drugs Persons at occupational risk (eg, researchers who work with hepatitis A virus) Persons in whom the consequences of hepatitis A may be especially adverse (eg, those with chronic liver disease) Food handlers	Inactivated vaccine (2 doses IM, given 6 months apart); for travelers making a single trip of < 3 months' duration, immune globulin prophylaxis is just as effective at a lower cost	The vaccine has proven useful in controlling several community-wide outbreaks

Hepatitis B vaccine	Sexually active homosexual men IV drug users Certain institutionalized persons Household or sexual contacts of hepatitis B carriers Health care personnel exposed to blood or blood-contaminated body fluids	Purified hepatitis B surface antigen, given IM in the deltoid region; a 2nd dose is given 1 month later and a 3rd dose is given 6 months later	—
Rabies vaccine	Persons who have been exposed to rabies Veterinarians Animal handlers Persons with occupations or hobbies that expose them to potentially rabid animals Researchers who work with wild rabies virus	Inactivated virus grown in diploid cell cultures (5 doses IM for postexposure prophylaxis, or 3 doses IM for preexposure prophylaxis)	Consultation with the local or state health department is advised for any potential rabies exposure
Rabies immune globulin	Persons who require postexposure prophylaxis	—	Consultation with the local or state health department for use and dosage is advised
Meningococcal vaccine	Travelers to areas where the disease is endemic	Purified polysaccharides (serogroups A, C, Y, W-135) given 0.5 mL IM	In local epidemics or household cases, prophylaxis with rifampin (600 mg q 12 hours for 4 doses) or ciprofloxacin (500 mg) may be given to those intimately exposed; immunity is long-lived

Table continues on the following page.

TABLE 132–1. SOME AGENTS USED FOR IMMUNIZATION IN ELDERLY PERSONS (*Continued*)

Agent	Indication	Preparation and Dosage	Comment
Lyme disease	Persons aged 15 to 70 who engage in activities that result in frequent or prolonged exposure to tick-infested areas Travelers to or residents of areas where the disease is endemic	Three 0.5-mL IM doses, given at 0, 1, and 12 months; the need for booster doses is undetermined	The vaccine acts by eliciting antibodies that kill the spirochete in the tick gut, rather than by any direct bactericidal effect on the human host. The vaccine is not recommended for persons > 70, in whom efficacy has not been established
Varicella vaccine	Use of varicella vaccine in elderly persons to diminish the frequency and/or severity of subsequent herpes zoster is under investigation	—	No recommendations can be made at this time
Typhoid vaccine	Travelers to areas where the disease is endemic	Whole killed *Salmonella typhi* (2 doses sc, given 4 weeks apart) Live attenuated *S. typhi* (4 doses po, given every other day) Purified Vi capsular antigen (1 dose IM)	Because effective alternatives are available, the live attenuated vaccine should not be given to immunocompromised persons
Cholera vaccine	Travelers to areas that require immunization for entry	Whole killed *Vibrio cholerae* (2 doses IM, given 4 weeks apart)	Only marginally effective, immunity lasts for little more than 6 mo
Yellow fever vaccine	Travelers to areas where the disease is endemic	Live attenuated virus (1 dose sc)	This vaccine should be used cautiously in elderly persons; immunocompromised persons usually require a letter from a physician outlining the medical contraindications to the vaccine to obtain a waiver to countries that require it; avoid giving with cholera vaccine

age per se or underlying disease is unclear.∎ For example, elderly nursing home residents produce much lower levels of antibody to influenza or pneumococcal vaccine than do younger persons. Nonetheless, response is sufficient for conferring protection in most elderly persons. However, the need for revaccination is different for some vaccines in the elderly because of waning response.

Vaccines consist of whole killed bacterial cells, wholly or partially purified bacterial proteins or polysaccharides, inactivated viruses or purified viral proteins, or live attenuated viruses. Recombinant technology is increasingly used to produce specific bacterial or viral antigens for use in vaccines.

Toxoids consist of bacterial toxins that have been modified to be nontoxic, although they retain the ability to induce production of antitoxin antibodies.

Passive immunization is used when exposure to a disease has recently occurred or is anticipated. It uses immune globulins, which are usually of human but sometimes of animal origin, or hyperimmune globulins, which are derived from donor pools preselected for a high level of antibody against a specific disease (eg, tetanus, rabies, hepatitis B, herpes zoster). All human plasma entering a donor pool is screened for antibody to the bloodborne viral pathogens HIV, hepatitis B virus, and hepatitis C virus. Furthermore, the purification process used to prepare immune globulins excludes such viruses.

Adverse Effects

Adverse effects do not appear to be different in the elderly than in younger persons. The main type of adverse effect is a hypersensitivity reaction, which occurs because vaccines and toxoids contain specific immunogenic substances. This problem is of particular concern with the use of immune globulins of equine origin (eg, botulism antitoxin, several antivenins), which should be preceded by a skin (prick) test to determine if the patient is allergic or hypersensitive to the product. Hypersensitivity to an agent used in culture media is possible but infrequent. Immunization of elderly persons should be based on risk/benefit considerations. In general, known hypersensitivity to a vaccine component is a *contraindication* to using the vaccine.

Adjuvants, usually consisting of aluminum salts, are sometimes added to vaccines to enhance the immune response. Such adjuvants are believed to be harmless if given IM, but they may produce granulomatous inflammation or even necrosis if given subcutaneously.

Some vaccines (eg, pneumococcal vaccine) produce more local inflammation if given before immunity has waned, but such a reaction is rarely sufficient reason not to give the vaccine when the clinician lacks information on prior immunization.

∎ see page 1358

In general, live attenuated viral or bacterial vaccines should not be given to immunocompromised persons because of the risk of vaccine-induced disease. They should also not be given to persons who have received immune or hyperimmune globulins within the preceding 3 months because the globulins may interfere with the development of subclinical infection, which is the desired response to the vaccine. Several vaccines may be given together without loss of efficacy. For example, influenza and pneumococcal vaccines may be given together, albeit at separate sites.

TETANUS AND DIPHTHERIA TOXOID

Tetanus and diphtheria toxoid for adult use (Td) consists of forma-linized toxoid derived from tetanus and diphtheria toxins. Unlike the vaccine used in children, Td contains no pertussis antigen and a reduced dose of diphtheria toxoid to minimize adverse reactions. Tetanus toxoid alone is recommended for persons who have adverse reactions to the diphtheria toxoid in Td.

Persons who have been primarily immunized need booster doses at 10-year intervals to maintain adequate immunity. Persons who have not been primarily immunized need two IM doses of Td given 1 month apart, followed by the usual booster doses at 10-year intervals. Booster doses of Td have few contraindications; the major one is a neurologic or severe hypersensitivity reaction after a previous dose.

This recommendation for booster doses of Td every 10 years throughout adulthood is controversial. In the USA, most persons who developed tetanus and diphtheria in recent years had never completed the primary immunization series. Once primary immunization is complete and the first 10-year booster dose has been given at age 15, one booster dose at age 50 or 55 may be sufficient to maintain adequate immunity throughout adulthood. However, > 50% of persons > 60 years do not have sufficient levels of antitoxin antibodies to protect against tetanus or diphtheria.

Td can also be used in trauma management; a booster dose is recommended only for a patient with a contaminated or severe puncture wound, in whom > 5 years have elapsed since the last dose. Td is preferred to tetanus toxoid alone because it provides an economical and convenient means of enhancing diphtheria immunity.

INFLUENZA VACCINE

Influenza vaccine contains inactivated influenza virus or viral components. The vaccine is given annually because its composition is changed year to year (as a result of the continuing antigenic drift of influenza viruses) and because immunity is relatively short-lived. Since 1976, the influenza vaccine has been a trivalent product containing the two influenza A strains predominant during recent influenza seasons (H1N1 and H3N2) as well as an influenza B strain. In the USA, elderly persons account for > 80% of all influenza-related deaths.∎ About 90% of these deaths occur in persons with recognized underlying high-risk conditions (eg, chronic pulmonary, cardiac, renal, or metabolic diseases), but some deaths occur in apparently healthy elderly persons. The vaccine should be given IM annually to all persons > 65 and to younger adults with high-risk conditions. To reduce the risk of influenza in the elderly, all health care providers and all children living with elderly persons should be immunized annually. In young adults, influenza vaccines have a protective effect of about 75 to 80% against the influenza virus. The efficacy declines with age, but, even in the elderly, the vaccine is protective and reduces the severity of illness, protects against serious complicating bacterial pneumonia, and reduces mortality.

An increased risk of developing Guillain-Barré syndrome (GBS) was identified with the swine influenza vaccine in 1976. The reason for this unusual association remains unknown, and subsequent use of trivalent influenza vaccines has resulted in no association or only a few additional cases of GBS per year in the USA. Even with this minimally incremental risk, influenza vaccine is highly recommended on a benefit/risk basis.

Although not yet available for use, cold-adapted live attenuated influenza vaccines, given as nose drops or by nasal inhalation, have proved highly effective in children. The optimal usage of these vaccines in adults and the elderly remains to be determined.

PNEUMOCOCCAL VACCINE

Pneumococcal vaccine contains 23 polysaccharides, derived from the 23 pneumococcal capsular types that account for most bacteremic pneumococcal infections in adults in the USA. The attack rate of invasive pneumococcal infection begins to increase at about age 50 and rises sharply at age 65. Blacks and Native Americans of any age are more likely to have underlying high-risk conditions and are more susceptible to invasive pneumococcal infection. Thus, all persons aged 50 to 55, particularly blacks and Native Americans, should be assessed for high-risk conditions that indicate the need for pneumococcal vaccine. Such conditions include sickle cell disease, splenic dysfunction or anatomic asplenia (eg, surgical splenectomy), leukemia, Hodgkin's disease, lymphoma, multiple myeloma, chronic renal failure, nephrotic syndrome, systemic lupus erythematosus, and chronic diseases associated with

∎ see page 767

increased risk of pneumococcal disease (eg, diabetes mellitus, chronic cardiopulmonary disease). The increasing prevalence of antibiotic resistance among strains of *Streptococcus pneumoniae* is another important reason for widespread use of this vaccine. **1**

In the USA, fewer than 40% of adults > 65 have been immunized with pneumococcal vaccine, probably because of conflicting evidence of efficacy in earlier vaccine studies and because of differing perceptions about the importance of pneumococci in causing pneumonia, bacteremia, and death. The vaccine is 70 to 75% effective in healthy elderly patients but less effective in patients with significant underlying disease (eg, cardiopulmonary disease, cancer). Immunization reduces the incidence of disease and may reduce pneumococcal sepsis and mortality in persons who contract pneumonia.

The vaccine is recommended for all persons ≥ 65. Pneumococcal vaccine is given IM only once, rather than annually. If vaccination status is uncertain, it is safer to give the vaccine than not to, although vaccination is likely to cause some local irritation. Persons vaccinated before age 65 should be given a second dose at age 65 if initial immunization occurred > 6 years earlier. Some suggest revaccinating persons > 65 every 6 to 8 years if they have pulmonary, cardiac, or other serious chronic disease.

Recent successes in preventing invasive pneumococcal disease with a protein-conjugated vaccine, formulated for pediatric use, make it likely that a much more immunogenic pneumococcal vaccine will be developed for use in high-risk adults and elderly persons.

133 ■ ANTIMICROBIAL DRUGS

The use of antimicrobial drugs in the elderly does not fundamentally differ from that in younger persons (see TABLE 133–1).

Pharmacokinetics

Age-related changes in pharmacokinetics **2** often require a change in the dose, frequency, and route of administration of antimicrobials, especially for frail elderly persons. For example, a given dose of ciprofloxacin (a fluoroquinolone) achieves peak plasma concentrations that are about twice as high in the elderly as in younger patients. Because elderly persons have less lean body mass and more body fat than do younger persons, water-soluble antimicrobials (eg, aminoglycosides, penicillins, cephalosporins, amphotericin B) achieve higher concentrations in plasma and tissue, and fat-soluble antimicrobials (eg,

Text continues on page 1378.

1 see also page 758   **2** see also page 56

TABLE 133–1. ANTIMICROBIAL DRUGS

Class/Group (Drugs)	Indications	Treatment Considerations
Aminoglycosides (eg, amikacin, gentamicin, kanamycin, neomycin, netilmicin, streptomycin, tobramycin)	These drugs are rapidly bactericidal against staphylococci and gram-negative aerobic bacteria, including *Pseudomonas* sp. Neomycin is used topically for some ear, eye, and skin infections and orally for hepatic coma and for selective decontamination of the large intestine before colorectal surgery. Streptomycin is indicated for tuberculosis and occasionally for endocarditis.	Because plasma half-life is increased in patients with decreased renal function (most elderly persons), the dose should be reduced on the basis of estimated or measured creatinine clearance. Nephrotoxicity is less likely with once-daily than with bid or tid dosing and is usually reversible. Nephrotoxicity may lead to high serum levels of the aminoglycoside and thus to ototoxicity, which is often irreversible. Risk of ototoxicity increases with age and is highest in patients with preexisting hearing deficiencies.
Penicillins		
Penicillin G (benzylpenicillin)	Penicillin G is bactericidal against gram-positive bacteria but is less so against enterococci. It is indicated for borreliosis, infections due to streptococci or meningococci, and most cases of pneumococcal pneumonia (see Ch. 76), even if susceptibility is reduced. For streptococcal endocarditis, penicillin G is combined with an aminoglycoside, which is given for the first week.	Penicillin G has a high degree of safety, although hypersensitivity reactions occur in about 5% of patients. Doses should be adjusted in patients with severe renal impairment to avoid neurotoxicity. Drug fever and hematologic reactions (eg, neutropenia, thrombocytopenia, anemia) may occur with prolonged high doses (eg, for endocarditis) but can be rapidly reversed by stopping treatment.
Penicillin V (phenoxymethyl penicillin)	Activity is almost identical to that of penicillin G. Penicillin V is used as a first-line antibiotic for oral treatment of infections due to β-hemolytic streptococci or pneumococci.	Considerations are the same as those for penicillin G. Because penicillin V is always given orally, life-threatening hypersensitivity reactions are rare.
Penicillinase-resistant penicillins (eg, cloxacillin,	These drugs are active against penicillin G–susceptible pathogens and penicillinase-producing	Considerations are the same as those for penicillin G.

Table continues on the following page.

TABLE 133–1. ANTIMICROBIAL DRUGS (*Continued*)

Class/Group (Drugs)	Indications	Treatment Considerations
dicloxacillin, flucloxacillin [not available in the USA], methicillin, nafcillin, oxacillin	staphylococci. They are indicated for staphylococcal infections (eg, infections in hip and knee prostheses) and staphylococcal and β-hemolytic streptococcal infections (eg, soft tissue infections).	
Aminopenicillins (eg, ampicillin, amoxicillin)	These drugs are more active against gram-negative aerobes, enterococci, and *Listeria monocytogenes* than is penicillin G. These drugs are used mainly for *Haemophilus influenzae* or enterococcal infections. In elderly patients with purulent meningitis, ampicillin is often used empirically with a cephalosporin to cover *Listeria* sp. Because ≥ 15% of *Escherichia coli* strains are resistant, ampicillin and amoxicillin are of limited value in UTIs.	Ampicillin and amoxicillin cause rashes more often than does penicillin G or V. Because oral ampicillin often causes diarrhea, an ampicillin ester or amoxicillin is preferred.
Antipseudomonal penicillins (eg, azlocillin, carbenicillin, mezlocillin, piperacillin, ticarcillin)	These drugs are indicated for severe infections known or suspected to be due to *Pseudomonas* sp. For infections outside the urinary tract, these drugs should be combined with an aminoglycoside to prevent emergence of resistance.	These drugs must be given parenterally, except for carbenicillin indanyl sodium, which may be given orally. Adverse effects are similar to those of ampicillin. Bleeding complications may occur, especially with high doses of carbenicillin and ticarcillin. High doses of carbenicillin may cause hypernatremia in patients with severe renal impairment.
Penicillins plus β-lactamase inhibitors (eg, clavulanate plus ampicillin or ticarcillin; sulbactam plus amoxicillin	These combinations are indicated for lower respiratory tract, urinary tract, soft tissue, and intra-abdominal infections known or suspected to be due to β-lactamase–producing bacteria.	Adverse effects are the same as those of penicillins, but effects on the upper GI tract (eg, vomiting) are more common.

Cephalosporins

1st-Generation injectable cephalosporins (eg, cefazolin, cephalothin, cephapirin, cephradine)	These drugs are indicated for community-acquired (especially gram-positive) infections. They are also used for perioperative prophylaxis. However, newer, cephalosporinase-resistant derivatives (2nd and 3rd generation) are often used instead.	These drugs have a high degree of safety. Hypersensitivity reactions occur less often than with penicillins. Cross-hypersensitivity with penicillins occurs in about 3 to 7% of patients.
2nd-Generation injectable cephalosporins (eg, cefaclor, cefamandole, cefonicid, cefuroxime) and cephamycins (eg, cefoxitin, cefotetan, cefmetazole)	These drugs are indicated for community-acquired infections, especially when the cause is known or suspected to be mixed gram-positive and gram-negative bacteria or when patients are allergic to penicillin. Cephamycins are used mainly for prophylaxis in patients having abdominal or gynecologic surgery.	Cefuroxime and cefoxitin have a high degree of safety. Cefamandole, cefotetan, and cefmetazole may cause hypoprothrombinemia (reversible with vitamin K), especially in the elderly. As with penicillins, prolonged high doses may cause fever or hematologic reactions. Use of these drugs may cause diarrhea (due to *Clostridium difficile* cytotoxin), leading to colitis or pseudomembranous colitis, especially in the elderly. Hypersensitivity reactions are rare, and cross-hypersensitivity with penicillins is unlikely.
3rd-Generation injectable cephalosporins (eg, cefepime, cefmenoxime [not available in the USA], cefotaxime, cefpirome [not available in the USA], ceftazidime, ceftizoxime, ceftriaxone) and cephamycins (eg, cefoperazone, moxalactam [latamoxef])	These drugs are indicated for nosocomial infections due to susceptible gram-negative or gram-positive bacteria (eg, urosepsis, pneumonia). Only cefepime, cefpirome, or ceftazidime should be used for *Pseudomonas* infections. Cefoperazone and moxalactam may be used for infections due to mixed aerobic-anaerobic bacteria. Cefotaxime and ceftriaxone are effective in managing bacterial meningitis due to pathogens other than *Listeria monocytogenes*. Ceftriaxone is effective in managing borreli-	Cephalosporins that are excreted in bile (eg, cefmenoxime, cefoperazone, ceftriaxone) commonly lead to diarrhea or colitis (due to *Clostridium difficile* cytotoxin) in the elderly. Cefoperazone and moxalactam, which have a 3-methylthiotetrazole side chain, may cause hypoprothrombinemia (reversible with vitamin K), especially in the elderly. Ceftriaxone may cause pseudolithiasis in the biliary tree. Other adverse effects are rare.

Table continues on the following page.

TABLE 133–1. ANTIMICROBIAL DRUGS (*Continued*)

Class/Group (Drugs)	Indications	Treatment Considerations
	osis. Many of these drugs, especially ceftazidime, are used as empiric monotherapy in febrile patients with neutropenia.	
Oral cephalosporins (1st-generation: eg, cefadroxil, cephradine, cephalexin; 2nd-generation: eg, cefaclor, cefprozil, cefuroxime, loracarbef; 3rd-generation: eg, cefixime, cefpodoxime, ceftibuten)	These drugs are used mainly in patients with UTIs and in those who are allergic to penicillins. After therapy with an injectable cephalosporin, a 2nd- or 3rd-generation oral cephalosporin may be suitable for follow-up therapy. Patients requiring an oral suspension for a staphylococcal infection should be given oral cephalosporins rather than penicillinase-resistant penicillins, which taste very bitter.	Because these drugs markedly alter normal fecal flora, they may cause diarrhea (due to *Clostridium difficile* cytotoxin), especially in the elderly. If used frequently in hospitalized patients, these drugs may select methicillin-resistant staphylococci. The drugs are generally safe; frequency of adverse effects is about the same as that for penicillins.
Monobactams (only aztreonam is used clinically)	Aztreonam is indicated for nosocomial infections due to gram-negative aerobes. For lower respiratory tract, skin, or soft tissue infections, it should be combined with an antibiotic active against gram-positive bacteria. It is used in patients with hypersensitivity (including anaphylactoid reactions) to other β-lactam antibiotics.	Aztreonam must be given parenterally. Its safety profile is similar to that of an injectable, renally excreted cephalosporin lacking a 3-methylthiotetrazole side chain (eg, cefuroxime). It appears to have no cross-hypersensitivity with other β-lactams.
Carbapenems, or thienamycins (eg, imipenem, meropenem)	Imipenem and meropenem are indicated for infections due to mixed aerobic-anaerobic flora (eg, intra-abdominal infections such as colonic diverticulitis), for empiric treatment of serious nosocomial infections (eg, septicemia), and for empiric monotherapy in febrile patients with neutropenia.	These drugs must be given parenterally. Imipenem, when used with cilastatin, has a high degree of safety. Nausea and seizures may develop if large doses are given rapidly. However, neurotoxicity is rare if dosage recommendations are followed. With meropenem, seizures, nausea, and vomiting occur infrequently.

Macrolides and azalides (macrolides: eg, clarithromycin, erythromycin, roxithromycin [not available in the USA], spiramycin, troleandomycin; azalides: eg, azithromycin)

In the elderly, macrolides are used mainly for *Mycoplasma, Chlamydia, Legionella,* and *Campylobacter* infections. In hypersensitive patients with streptococcal infections, they may be used instead of penicillin G or V. Clarithromycin combined with amoxicillin or metronidazole is recommended for treatment of peptic ulcers due to *Helicobacter pylori* (see Ch. 106). Clarithromycin may be used with other tuberculostatic drugs for atypical mycobacterial infections. Erythromycin, which increases gastric motility, is sometimes given to patients fed through gastric tubes. Azithromycin is indicated for respiratory tract and genital infections.

Upper GI adverse effects (eg, nausea, vomiting) are common, particularly with erythromycin, even if given parenterally. Erythromycin may cause reversible ototoxicity, and erythromycin estolate may cause cholestatic hepatitis. Macrolides and azalides (eg, clarithromycin, erythromycin, azithromycin) that are metabolized via the cytochrome P-450 system may interact with other drugs (eg, astemizole) that are metabolized in the liver.

Nitroimidazoles (eg, metronidazole, tinidazole [not available in the USA])

These drugs should be combined with an antibiotic active against aerobes (eg, an aminoglycoside, a cephalosporin) for systemic bacterial infections. In the elderly, nitroimidazoles are often given orally to manage diarrhea due to *Clostridium difficile*. For this indication, metronidazole is preferred to vancomycin to reduce the risk of emergence of vancomycin resistance, particularly in enterococci. Metronidazole can be used with clarithromycin to manage peptic ulcers due to *H. pylori*.

These drugs cause few serious adverse effects. Metronidazole commonly causes a metallic taste, high doses commonly cause nausea, and overdose may cause neuritis. If taken with alcohol, metronidazole may cause a disulfiram-like reaction. Metronidazole can interact with cimetidine, phenobarbital, coumarin derivatives, disulfiram, and probably tinidazole.

Polymyxins (eg, colistin, polymyxin B)

These drugs are indicated mainly for infections due to multiresistant strains of *Pseudomonas* sp.

Polymyxins are used only parenterally or topically. These drugs (especially at high doses) may cause neurotoxicity, nephrotoxicity, and hypersensitivity reactions and should be used only when no alternative antibiotics are available.

Table continues on the following page.

1371

TABLE 133–1. ANTIMICROBIAL DRUGS (*Continued*)

Class/Group (Drugs)	Indications	Treatment Considerations
Quinolones (nonfluorinated quinolones: eg, cinoxacin, nalidixic acid, pipemidic acid [not available in the USA]; fluoroquinolones: eg, ciprofloxacin, enoxacin, levofloxacin, lomefloxacin, norfloxacin, ofloxacin, pefloxacin [not available in the USA], sparfloxacin, trovafloxacin [not available in Europe])	Nonfluorinated quinolones have no advantages over fluoroquinolones, which are active against more bacteria, including *Pseudomonas* sp. Fluoroquinolones, especially ciprofloxacin, are an oral alternative for infections due to multiresistant gram-negative aerobes (eg, *P. aeruginosa*). Fluoroquinolones can be used to prevent or manage UTIs and enteric bacterial infections. Prophylactic use in patients with neutropenia may lead to resistance. Newer fluoroquinolones, especially grepafloxacin, levofloxacin, and trovafloxacin, can be used in the treatment of community-acquired pneumonia. If identifying the causative organism in elderly patients with pneumonia is difficult, a fluoroquinolone may be used empirically.	These drugs may cause nonspecific neurologic adverse effects (eg, dizziness, headache, dimmed vision, paresthesia), which are dose-dependent, reversible, and, when the drugs are given orally, rare. Some quinolones (eg, nalidixic acid, lomefloxacin) can cause phototoxicity. Nausea and vomiting may occur when the drugs are given orally or IV. Arthralgia develops in a few patients. *Trovafloxacin can cause serious liver toxicity.* Nalidixic acid taken with coumarin derivatives may increase the risk of bleeding; the risk is less with fluoroquinolones. Ciprofloxacin, pefloxacin, and especially enoxacin interact with caffeine and theophylline; adverse effects of theophylline may result. Antacids markedly reduce absorption of all quinolones.
Sulfonamides and trimethoprim (eg, TMP-SMX)	Because of their adverse effects, use of sulfonamides and TMP-SMX should be restricted in the elderly. TMP-SMX is indicated for acute exacerbations of chronic bronchitis and for some serious systemic infections (eg, enteric fever, paratyphoid and *Pneumocystis carinii* infections). Trimethoprim can be used to prevent or treat UTIs.	Sulfonamides frequently cause rashes and rarely cause febrile mucocutaneous syndromes in the elderly. Use of sulfonamides for > 7 days may cause toxic hepatitis. Dose-related, generally reversible hematologic reactions (eg, neutropenia, thrombocytopenia, pancytopenia) can occur, especially in elderly persons taking high doses for ≥ 10 days. Adverse effects of trimethoprim used alone are usually mild and reversible. Rarely, serous meningitis occurs, especially in patients with Sjögren's

Drug	Indications	Adverse effects and comments
		syndrome. Prolonged use of trimethoprim (alone or as TMP-SMX) may cause folate deficiency, which can be prevented by giving folic acid. Hyperkalemia may occur in elderly patients treated with usual doses of TMP-SMX. Sulfonamides may increase the activity of highly protein-bound drugs (eg, coumarin derivatives). Trimethoprim and especially TMP-SMX interact with phenytoin and coumarin derivatives, increasing the risk of adverse effects. TMP-SMX may increase the nephrotoxicity of cyclosporine.
Tetracyclines (eg, chlortetracycline, demeclocycline, doxycycline, methacycline, minocycline, oxytetracycline, tetracycline)	These drugs are indicated for pneumonia due to *Mycoplasma* or *Chlamydia* sp and exacerbations of chronic bronchitis and may be used in the treatment of many skin disorders, including rosacea. Their effectiveness in sinusitis is doubtful.	These drugs may cause diarrhea, candidal overgrowth, induction of resistance in normal flora, bleeding diathesis, and phototoxicity. Tetracyclines rarely cause nephrotoxicity. Demeclocycline can cause diabetes insipidus. Use with antacids reduces absorption of tetracyclines. Dairy products reduce absorption of most tetracyclines. The half-life of these drugs may be reduced when they are taken with carbamazepine, phenytoin, or barbiturates, which induce liver metabolism of tetracyclines.
Other antibiotics Chloramphenicol	Because of its adverse effects, systemic chloramphenicol is generally reserved for life-threatening infections, mainly purulent meningitis, brain abscesses, and enteric fever.	Aplastic anemia with pancytopenia develops in 1 of 5,000 to 100,000 patients, independent of dose; the mortality rate is > 50%. This effect usually occurs shortly after treatment but can occur up to 6 months later. Reversible dose-dependent bone marrow toxicity may develop with prolonged use of large doses. Hematologic

Table continues on the following page.

TABLE 133–1. ANTIMICROBIAL DRUGS (*Continued*)

Class/Group (Drugs)	Indications	Treatment Considerations
Chloramphenicol (*continued*)		adverse effects do not occur with topical preparations (eg, ophthalmic ointment). This drug slows the metabolism of phenytoin. Other drug interactions include increased risk of hypoglycemia with tolbutamide and increased risk of hypoprothrombinemia with dicumarol.
Clindamycin and lincomycin	Clindamycin, which is preferred to lincomycin, is indicated for anaerobic and staphylococcal infections and for life-threatening group A β-hemolytic infections (streptococcal toxic shock syndrome, necrotizing fasciitis). It is also used as a second-line drug for toxoplasmosis.	Antibiotic-associated diarrhea, colitis, or pseudomembranous colitis (due to *Clostridium difficile* cytotoxin) is relatively common among patients treated with clindamycin and is more common among elderly than younger patients.
Ethambutol	This drug is indicated for mycobacterial infections, particularly tuberculosis.	Optic neuritis, usually reversible when treatment is stopped, may occur with high doses. Patients should have baseline and monthly ophthalmologic examinations.
Isoniazid	This drug is indicated for tuberculosis and is generally used with other tuberculostatic drugs (eg, rifampin, ethambutol, pyrazinamide) to prevent emergence of resistance. It is given alone to prevent active tuberculosis in tuberculin-positive persons at high risk (eg, those with renal failure, diabetes mellitus, or immunosuppression).	Adverse effects are dose-dependent. Neuritis, the most common, can be prevented with pyridoxine. Hepatotoxicity occurs idiosyncratically, but the incidence of hepatitis increases with age, and risk is increased in patients who consume alcohol daily or who have alcoholic liver disease. Antacids reduce absorption of isoniazid. In slow acetylators, the metabolism of phenytoin, phenobarbital, and carbamazepine may be inhibited, resulting in drug accumulation.

Nitrofurantoin	This drug is used primarily to prevent or treat bacterial cystitis. It is not indicated for renal cortical or perinephric abscesses.	This drug can produce interstitial pulmonary infiltrates, which cause dyspnea and may result in pulmonary fibrosis if the drug is continued. High doses for > 10 days cause such lung reactions, primarily in elderly women. Deaths have occurred, mainly in patients with concomitant cardiac decompensation. Other adverse effects include nausea, vomiting, brown urine, and skin reactions (more common among elderly than younger patients). Prolonged use of high doses may cause toxic hepatitis.
Rifampin and rifabutin (ansamycin)	Rifampin is used with other tuberculostatic drugs (eg, isoniazid, ethambutol, pyrazinamide) for tuberculosis. Rifampin is also indicated for infections due to methicillin-resistant staphylococci. Rifabutin is used to prevent infections due to atypical mycobacteria in patients with severe immune deficiencies.	The main adverse effect of these drugs is hepatotoxicity. Because these drugs are metabolized in the liver, they may interact with many other drugs, and they may induce liver enzymes that increase their own metabolism.
Vancomycin and teicoplanin	These drugs are indicated for serious gram-positive infections due to enterococci or methicillin-resistant staphylococci. Oral vancomycin is indicated for diarrhea and colitis due to *Clostridium difficile*. Vancomycin, mixed with dialysis fluid, is indicated for peritonitis in patients receiving long-term ambulatory peritoneal dialysis.	These drugs may cause allergic reactions, mainly rashes. If infused rapidly, vancomycin may cause red-neck syndrome (a histamine-like reaction with flushing, headache, and fever). Vancomycin can cause nephrotoxicity and ototoxicity; serum levels should be monitored.

Table continues on the following page.

TABLE 133-1. ANTIMICROBIAL DRUGS (Continued)

Class/Group (Drugs)	Indications	Treatment Considerations
Antifungal drugs		
Amphotericin B and nystatin	These drugs are used topically to treat oral candidal infections. IV amphotericin B is indicated for serious systemic mycoses. Amphotericin B is commonly given during bladder irrigation for treatment of candidal cystitis.	Amphotericin B has many adverse effects; fever, chills, and nausea are common. The dose should be increased slowly over 3 to 5 days, and corticosteroids or antiemetics may be necessary. Nephrotoxicity is common; renal function must be monitored. Using a lipid formulation of amphotericin can minimize adverse effects.
Flucytosine (5-fluorocytosine)	This drug can be used alone or with low-dose amphotericin B for systemic candidal infections due to susceptible strains. It is used with a full dose of amphotericin B for cryptococcal infections, including cryptococcal meningitis.	Topical use should be avoided because it increases risk of resistance. Used in recommended doses, the drug has few adverse effects. Overdosage may cause bone marrow depression.
Imidazoles, or azoles (eg, fluconazole, itraconazole, ketoconazole)	These drugs are indicated for mucocutaneous candidal infections (eg, *Candida* esophagitis). They are used orally to prevent systemic candidiasis in immunosuppressed patients and topically to treat patients with fungal nail bed infections. Fluconazole is indicated for cryptococcal meningitis.	Used topically, these drugs have few adverse effects. Used systemically, they may cause hepatotoxicity and hypersensitivity reactions. Ketoconazole may cause endocrine disorders (eg, gynecomastia, reduced libido). Cimetidine, ranitidine, and antacids reduce absorption of ketoconazole. In transplant patients taking cyclosporine and ketoconazole, risk of nephrotoxicity is increased. Ketoconazole interacts with rifampin, isoniazid, and methylprednisolone. Fluconazole interacts with tolbutamide, coumarin derivatives, cyclosporine, and phenytoin. Itraconazole interacts with many drugs.
Antiviral drugs		
Acyclovir and valacyclovir	Acyclovir is used for prevention and early treatment (within 48 hours of symptom onset) of infections	Used orally, acyclovir and valacyclovir have few adverse effects; used IV, acyclovir may cause

Drug	Indications	Adverse effects
	due to herpes simplex or varicella-zoster viruses. Valacyclovir significantly reduces the incidence of postherpetic neuralgia in immunocompetent patients > 60 with herpes zoster. Acyclovir IV is indicated for severe infections (eg, herpes simplex virus encephalitis, disseminated herpes zoster).	thrombophlebitis. Rapid infusions may markedly increase blood urea nitrogen and serum creatinine levels.
Famciclovir	This drug is indicated for severe genital herpes simplex infections and herpes zoster.	This drug has a high degree of safety, with no specific adverse effects.
Amantadine and rimantadine	These drugs are indicated for prevention and early treatment (within 24 hours of symptom onset) of influenza A infections in elderly patients, especially those with serious underlying disorders (eg, severe cardiac decompensation, pulmonary disorders). Prophylactic use should be considered when influenza A outbreaks occur in nursing homes or other institutions (see Ch. 76).	Both drugs have anticholinergic effects. Amantadine may cause neurotoxicity (especially neuritis) and, rarely, seizures.
Oseltamivir and zanamivir	These drugs, the first of a new class, are indicated for treatment of uncomplicated acute illness due to influenza A or B virus.	Treatment must be started within 48 hours after onset of influenza symptoms.
Foscarnet	This drug is used mainly for systemic cytomegalovirus infections (eg, retinitis, esophagitis). It is also used as a second-line drug for HIV infection.	This drug causes nephrotoxicity, which may be increased when other nephrotoxic drugs (eg, aminoglycosides, cyclosporine) are also used. Serum calcium levels commonly increase.
Ganciclovir	This drug is indicated for prevention and treatment of severe cytomegalovirus infections (eg, retinitis, pneumonitis, esophagitis).	This drug causes bone marrow depression and may cause anemia, neutropenia, and thrombocytopenia. Fever is common. Drugs that reduce renal excretion (eg, probenecid) may slow elimination of ganciclovir.

UTI = urinary tract infection; GI = gastrointestinal; TMP-SMX = trimethoprim-sulfamethoxazole.

chloramphenicol, doxycycline, fluconazole) achieve lower concentrations in elderly persons. Some newer antibiotics (eg, macrolides, azalides, fluoroquinolones) achieve relatively low plasma concentrations, but intracellular concentrations are up to 40 times higher than concurrent plasma concentrations. Because these high concentrations may persist for several days, dosing intervals can be longer and duration of treatment can be shorter.

Protein binding: Plasma albumin concentration decreases slightly with age, although this decrease is usually of little importance. However, disease-related decreases in albumin levels can result in higher concentrations of free drug.

Elimination: Metabolism of antimicrobials seems to be relatively constant with age. However, first-pass metabolism of some drugs (eg, ciprofloxacin) is decreased, possibly leading to increased plasma concentrations. Biliary excretion of antimicrobials is also relatively constant with age. However, half-lives of renally excreted antimicrobials may be markedly prolonged in the elderly, especially if renal excretion is the only mode of elimination (as for aminoglycosides). The increase in plasma half-life is usually moderate unless patients have severe renal impairment (creatinine clearance > 30 mL/minute). For such patients, risk of drug accumulation and adverse reactions is considerable.

Choice of Drug

Elderly persons respond to some antimicrobials differently than do younger persons and sometimes require an alteration in the choice of drug. In addition, the etiology and severity of infection may be different from those in younger persons.

The increased risk of certain infections, especially nosocomial infections, in elderly patients should be considered when choosing an antimicrobial. In patients with symptoms and signs of septicemia, empiric treatment must be accurate because mortality rates can be very high.

134 ■ HUMAN IMMUNODEFICIENCY VIRUS INFECTION

Infection caused by one of two related retroviruses (HIV-1 and HIV-2) resulting in a wide range of clinical manifestations related to defective cellular immunity.

In the USA, an estimated 10% of AIDS cases occur in persons ≥ 50 years; 3% of all AIDS cases occur in patients > 60. AIDS cases are increasing in the over-50 population: From 1990 to 1992, new AIDS cases decreased 3% among persons ≤ 30 but increased 17% among those ≥ 60.

Early in the epidemic, most elderly persons with HIV infection acquired it from blood transfusions; however, transmission by this route has decreased dramatically since the introduction of donor screening procedures. HIV infection in elderly persons is now most commonly transmitted through sexual activity. In the USA, homosexual and bisexual men constitute the largest group (about 35%) of AIDS cases among elderly persons. Heterosexual transmission of HIV has also increased among elderly persons: it accounted for only 6% of AIDS cases among elderly persons in 1988 but for 12% in 1994. Heterosexual high-risk behavior (eg, sex with prostitutes) may be more common among elderly persons living in urban environments.

Most sexually active elderly persons are no longer concerned about contraception and do not perceive themselves as being at risk of HIV infection. They are one sixth as likely as persons in their 20s to use condoms during intercourse.

Pathogenesis

HIV virus belongs to the family of human retroviruses, which contain an enzyme called reverse transcriptase that converts viral RNA into a proviral DNA copy that becomes integrated into the host cell DNA. The hallmark of HIV infection is a profound immunodeficiency resulting predominantly from a progressive decrease in the number of the CD4+ subset of T lymphocytes, referred to as helper or inducer cells. This subset is defined phenotypically by the presence on its surface of a CD4 molecule, which is the cellular receptor for HIV. When the CD4+ T-lymphocyte count decreases below a certain level (usually $< 200/\mu L$ [$< 0.2 \times 10^9/L$]), patients become vulnerable to developing a variety of life-threatening opportunistic infections, such as *Pneumocystis carinii* pneumonia, cryptococcal meningitis, candidiasis, cytomegalovirus, encephalitis, and cancers such as lymphoma and Kaposi's sarcoma.

Symptoms, Signs, and Diagnosis

The clinical manifestations of HIV infection in elderly patients are similar to those in younger patients. Some of the early symptoms of HIV infection (eg, fatigue, anorexia, weight loss, memory problems) are nonspecific and may be attributed to other diseases that are common in old age. As a result, appropriate diagnostic evaluation is often delayed (typically up to 10 months) in some elderly patients. Also, the elderly are one fifth as likely as persons in their 20s to be tested for HIV infection.

HIV infection is diagnosed by the detection of HIV itself, antibodies to HIV, or one of HIV's components. Antibodies to HIV generally appear in the circulation 4 to 8 weeks after infection. The standard screening test for HIV is the enzyme-linked immunosorbent assay (ELISA—sensitivity > 99.5%). A positive ELISA result must be confirmed by the Western blot test, a more specific assay. Testing for p24 antigen, a marker for viral replication, may detect HIV in the early stages of infection. Polymerase chain reaction is a highly sensitive gene amplification technique that may identify HIV in patients with latent infection or no detectable antibody to HIV.

AIDS is diagnosed by a positive serology for the HIV-1 virus and a CD4+ T-lymphocyte count < 200/μL (< 0.2 × 10⁹/L) or by the presence of an AIDS-indicator disease. There is little difference in the initial AIDS-defining diagnosis between younger and older patients; the most predominant AIDS indicator diseases across all age groups are *Pneumocystis carinii* pneumonia (in 75% of all cases) and candidal esophagitis (in 15%). Other AIDS-indicator diseases in the elderly include extrapulmonary cryptococcosis, toxoplasmosis of the brain, cytomegalovirus disease, tuberculosis, recurrent bacterial pneumonia, *Mycobacterium avium* complex infection, and Kaposi's sarcoma. However, an indolent form of Kaposi's sarcoma occurs in elderly men without evidence of HIV infection. Cryptococcal meningitis may have subtle clinical manifestations in elderly patients and few, if any, symptoms. Headaches and lethargy may be the only complaints, and meningeal signs occur in < 30% of cases. In wasting syndrome, another AIDS-indicator disease, weight loss > 10% is accompanied by chronic diarrhea, weakness, and fever unexplained by other causes.

HIV-associated dementia, ▯ also known as HIV encephalopathy, is a neurologic disorder caused by the direct effect of the HIV virus on the central nervous system. Progressive dementia may occur as the HIV infection progresses. Although HIV-associated dementia usually occurs in the later stages of AIDS, it is the presenting symptom in as many as 10% of all cases. HIV-associated dementia occurs more frequently among elderly patients, in whom Alzheimer's disease may be misdiagnosed. HIV-associated dementia, however, differs from Alzheimer's disease in several ways (see TABLE 134–1).

Prevention, Prognosis, and Treatment

Practically no prevention information on AIDS is targeted at elderly persons, although most elderly persons are sexually active. Elderly persons engaging in risky sexual practices should use the same precautions (eg, use of condoms or vaginal barriers, avoidance of exposure to semen) as younger persons. Hormonal changes after menopause make the vaginal lining thinner ▯ and less likely to protect against HIV if a woman has sex with an infected person.

HIV infection progresses more rapidly to AIDS and survival rates are poorer among elderly patients than among younger patients. Cumula-

▯see also page 370   ▯see page 1209

TABLE 134-1.   DIFFERENTIATING HIV-ASSOCIATED DEMENTIA FROM ALZHEIMER'S DISEASE

HIV-Associated Dementia	Alzheimer's Disease
Affects a younger population than Alzheimer's disease does	Affects an older population than HIV-associated dementia does
Is accompanied by motor and spinal cord signs	Is not accompanied by motor or spinal cord signs
Has a rapid clinical course; CT scans may reveal rapidly progressing atrophy	Develops slowly
Is characterized by mild pleocytosis and elevated protein levels on cerebrospinal fluid testing	Produces normal results on cerebrospinal fluid testing
Can be prevented through early and sustained use of high-dose antiretroviral therapy	Cannot be prevented

tive survival rates decrease as age increases. The 1-year survival rate is 80% in younger patients but only 40% in elderly patients.

Why elderly patients with AIDS do worse than younger patients is unclear. Comorbidity, late diagnosis, inadequate treatment, and decreased adherence to antiretroviral therapy may play a role. Of particular interest are age-related changes in the immune system; normally, $CD4^+$ counts do not decrease and may increase. However, at the time of AIDS diagnosis, elderly patients have lower $CD4^+$ counts than younger patients do. This precipitous decrease may be due to impaired T-lymphocyte replacement mechanisms secondary to thymic involution or other age-related hematologic changes.

Aggressive antiretroviral therapy with combination treatment regimens and opportunistic infection prophylaxis, similar to that used in younger patients, is recommended for elderly patients with AIDS. Elderly patients may even require a more aggressive approach to therapy than do younger patients, with earlier use of combination therapies; the elderly appear to respond equally well to combination therapy as younger persons. However, elderly patients are rarely included in clinical trials, and no specific recommendations have been published on the use of antiretroviral therapy in elderly persons. Furthermore, drug toxicities and interactions with drugs used for other conditions are more common in elderly persons.

An interdisciplinary care approach,■ including psychologic and social support, helps manage HIV infection in elderly patients. These patients should be counseled, when appropriate, regarding safe sexual

■see page 74

behavior, and condom use should be emphasized for those who are sexually active.

Long-Term Care

Hospitals and community-based resources provide only a portion of the continued care that AIDS patients require. Long-term care services[1] are increasingly needed for the continued care of AIDS patients, old or young. For example, nursing homes, which traditionally provide skilled nursing care for chronically ill elderly patients, can provide similar care for AIDS patients of all ages. An estimated 10 to 25% of AIDS patients require this type of care, and the number is increasing. However, many nursing homes are reluctant to admit AIDS patients because few personnel are properly trained to care for them, the cost of care is high because of the use of disposable items, and a fear for the safety of other patients and their families may exist.

Personnel who care for AIDS patients in long-term care facilities should follow infection control guidelines. These guidelines are best implemented through general education programs for all personnel, patients, and family members and through on-site training for personnel in the specific units caring for AIDS patients.

End-of-Life Issues

Patients dying of AIDS and their family members often require medical intervention that provides comfort and support.[2] The physician should help elderly AIDS patients and family members cope with the psychologic and spiritual aspects of terminal illness. Physicians must be empathetic and objective. They must acknowledge the patient's pain and suffering and help the patient and family members recognize that dying is a natural progression. Many patients with AIDS or other terminal illnesses prefer to die at home rather than in a hospital or nursing home and elect hospice care.[3]

[1] see page 104   [2] see page 115   [3] see page 90

APPENDIX I

LABORATORY VALUES

Population norms can be established for any physiologic parameter and its laboratory measurement. The normal value for a laboratory measurement is usually defined as its mean value ± 2 SD (which includes 95% of results) in a population of healthy persons. Thus, 5% of results obtained from healthy persons are classified as "abnormal," even though they merely represent variability within a normal population. If each test in a battery of tests is independent, the probability of a healthy person having completely normal results is relatively low (eg, 54% in a battery of 12 tests).

The determination of normal laboratory values in the elderly is complicated by the high prevalence of disease (latent or overt and multisystem) and by age-related physiologic and anatomic changes. In addition, as persons age, they become less like each other. Thus, extrapolating from population norms to individuals is less useful for elderly than for younger persons. With age, organ function declines, but the rate of decline varies from person to person and from system to system within one person. For example, between ages 30 and 70 years, nerve conduction velocity decreases by only about 10%, but renal function decreases on average by nearly 40%. Nonetheless, age-related declines in cardiac, pulmonary, renal, and metabolic function can be correlated with changes in normal laboratory values (see TABLE). Large or sudden changes in function frequently signify a disorder.

Determining the likelihood that an abnormal laboratory test result represents a particular disorder may be difficult in the elderly. Likelihood depends largely on the pretest probability of the disorder (based on clinical findings and prevalence of the disorder) and the operating characteristics of the test (sensitivity, specificity, likelihood ratios). Pretest probability and a test's operating characteristics can be difficult to determine because precise information about prevalence, sensitivity, specificity, and likelihood ratios for the elderly is often unavailable. Inaccurate interpretations tend to lead to excess false-positive results.

Drugs commonly used by the elderly may spuriously alter the results of laboratory tests. For example, isoniazid, levodopa, morphine, vitamin C, nalidixic acid, and penicillin G may lead to false-positive urine glucose results. Levodopa may produce a spurious increase in serum bilirubin and uric acid, also leading to false-positive results.

EFFECT OF AGING ON LABORATORY VALUES

Increased	Decreased
Alkaline phosphatase	Calcium, serum
Cholesterol, serum	Creatine kinase, serum
Clotting factors VII and VIII	Creatinine clearance*
Copper, serum	Dihydroepiandrosterone (DHEA)
Ferritin, serum	1,25-Dihydroxycholecalciferol, serum
Fibrinogen, serum	Estrogen, serum
Glucose, serum (postprandial)	Growth hormone
Immunoreactive parathormone, serum	Insulin-like growth factor I (IGF-I)
Interleukin-6 (IL-6)	Interleukin-1 (IL-1)
Norepinephrine, serum	Iron, serum (minimally)
Parathyroid hormone	Phosphorus, serum
Prostate-specific antigen (PSA)	Selenium, serum
Triglycerides, serum	Testosterone, serum
Uric acid, serum	Thiamine, serum
	γ-Tocopherol (vitamin E), plasma
	Triiodothyronine (T_3)
	Vitamin B_6, serum
	Vitamin B_{12}, serum
	Vitamin C, plasma
	Zinc, serum

*Serum creatinine may be normal, even though creatinine clearance is decreased with age, because creatinine production decreases with age.

AGE-RELATED EFFECTS ON SPECIFIC TESTS

A low **serum albumin** level in healthy elderly persons is usually due to diet. However, low levels may also indicate serious disease, especially when accompanied by undernutrition.

Fasting blood glucose levels increase with age, although values remain within the nondiabetic range. Glucose tolerance decreases gradually with age. However, lack of exercise, obesity, and the use of some drugs may affect glucose tolerance more than aging per se.

The **renal threshold for glucose** decreases with age. Consequently, glucose may be detected in the urine of elderly patients, even when blood glucose is considerably less than 200 mg/dL (11.1 mmol/L).

The **erythrocyte sedimentation rate** (ESR) is not affected by aging per se, but the ESR tends to be higher in the elderly, probably because prevalence of disease is higher. Elevations in ESR usually indicate elevations in serum proteins due to chronic inflammatory activity (including infections), monoclonal gammopathy, or cancer. If elderly patients have an unexplained elevation in the ESR, a monoclonal gammopathy should be sought. This disorder occurs in about 10% of persons aged 62 to 95 who are apparently healthy but in about 35% of those who have an elevated ESR.

The **prostate-specific antigen (PSA)** level increases with age, and it can be increased by benign conditions. Consequently, its value in screening for prostate cancer is debatable.[1] For men with an abnormal prostate detected by rectal examination, PSA may be measured, but this measurement may be less valuable than the ratio of PSA to gland size, and abnormal results are likely to lead to more expensive, invasive tests. An increase in PSA of > 5 to 8% in a year may be highly significant and usually requires rectal ultrasonography and biopsy. Before PSA is measured, patients should be warned about the possibilities of ambiguous and false-positive results.

CBCs and measurement of **thyroid-stimulating hormone** may be useful as screening tests in the elderly because of the high incidence of occult anemia and hypothyroidism.

Protein:creatinine ratios in single-voided urine samples can be used to estimate the magnitude of proteinuria (the incidence of trace proteinuria decreases during a person's 20s, then increases during old age). These spot measurements correlate with determinations of 24-hour urinary protein excretion and are particularly useful in elderly patients when 24-hour specimens are difficult to obtain. Protein:creatinine ratios > 3.0 indicate massive proteinuria (> 3.5 g/24 hour); ratios < 0.2 usually indicate insignificant proteinuria.

Creatinine clearance decreases with age, but serum creatinine remains relatively stable because most elderly persons lose muscle mass as they age. Therefore, when serum creatinine is measured, renal function in the elderly tends to be overestimated, and creatinine clearance should be used to assess renal function, according to the Cockcroft-Gault formula[2]:

$$\text{Creatinine clearance (mL/min)} = \frac{(140 - \text{age [yr]}) \times \text{body wt (kg)}}{72 \times \text{serum creatinine (mg/dL)}}$$

For women, the calculated value is multiplied by 0.85. Creatinine clearance may need confirmation (eg, with timed collections), particularly in patients who are malnourished, who have lost muscle mass, who are severely ill, or who are very elderly.

---

[1] see page 1183   [2] see also page 59

WEIGHTS AND MEASURES

The **milliequivalent (mEq)** expresses the chemical activity, or combining power, of a substance relative to the activity of 1 mg of hydrogen. Thus, 1 mEq is represented by 1 mg of hydrogen, 23 mg of sodium, 39 mg of potassium, 20 mg of calcium, and 35 mg of chlorine. Conversion equations are as follows:

$$mEq/L = \frac{(mg/L) \times valence}{formula\ wt}$$

$$mg/L = \frac{(mEq/L) \times formula\ wt}{valence}$$

(NOTE: formula wt = atomic or molecular wt)

The mEq is roughly equivalent to the **milliosmole (mOsm)**, the unit of measure of osmolality or tonicity. Normally, the body fluid compartments each contain about 280 mOsm/L of solute.

METRIC SYSTEM

Weight
1 kilogram (kg) = 1000 grams (10^3 g)
1 gram (g) = 1000 milligrams (10^3 mg)
1 milligram (mg) = 1000 micrograms (10^{-3} g)
1 microgram (μg) = 1000 nanograms (10^{-6} g)
1 nanogram (ng) = 1000 picograms (pg) (10^{-9} g)

Volume
1 liter (L) = 1000 milliliters (mL)
        = 1000 cubic centimeters (cc)

METRIC–NONMETRIC EQUIVALENTS*

Liquid
30 mL = 1 fluid ounce
250 mL = 8+ fluid ounces
500 mL = 1+ pint
1000 mL = 1+ quart
(1 liter)

Weight
65 mg = 1 grain (gr)
28.35 g = 1 ounce (oz)
1 kg = 2.2 pounds (lb)

Linear
1 millimeter (mm) = 0.04 inch (in)
1 centimeter (cm) = 0.4 inch
2.5 centimeters = 1 inch
1 meter (m) = 39.37 inches

* Conversions are approximate.

HOUSEHOLD NONMETRIC–METRIC EQUIVALENTS*

1 teaspoon (tsp) = 4 mL
1 teaspoon, medical = 5 mL
1 dessert spoon = 8 mL
1 tablespoon (tbsp) = 15 mL   = 1/2 fluid ounce
1 cup = 240 mL = 8 fluid ounces

* Conversions are approximate.

ATOMIC WEIGHTS OF SOME COMMON ELEMENTS*

Element	Atomic Weight	Element	Atomic Weight
Hydrogen (H)	1	Magnesium (Mg)	24
Carbon (C)	12	Phosphorus (P)	31
Nitrogen (N)	14	Chlorine (Cl)	35.5
Oxygen (O)	16	Potassium (K)	39
Sodium (Na)	23	Calcium (Ca)	40

* Weights are approximate.

CENTIGRADE–FAHRENHEIT EQUIVALENTS

Centigrade (°)	Fahrenheit (°)	Centigrade (°)	Fahrenheit (°)
Freezing (water at sea level)			
0	32	Pasteurization (holding),* 30 min at	
		62.8	145.0
Clinical range			
36.0	96.8	Pasteurization (flash),* 15 sec at	
36.5	97.7	71.7	161.0
37.0	98.6		
37.5	99.5	Boiling (water at sea level)	
38.0	100.4	100.0	212.0
38.5	101.3		
39.0	102.2		
39.5	103.1	Conversion	
40.0	104.0	To convert °F to °C, subtract 32,	
40.5	104.9	then multiply by 5/9 or 0.555.	
41.0	105.8		
41.5	106.7	To convert °C to °F, multiply by	
42.0	107.6	9/5 or 1.8, then add 32.	

* According to the FDA Code of Federal Regulations, 1991.

TRADE NAMES OF SOME COMMONLY USED DRUGS

Throughout THE MERCK MANUAL OF GERIATRICS, generic (nonproprietary) names for drugs are used whenever possible. Most prescription drugs have trade names (also called proprietary, brand, or specialty names) to distinguish them as being produced and marketed by a particular manufacturer. In the USA, these names are usually registered as trademarks with the Patent Office, which confers certain legal rights with respect to their use. A trade name may be registered for a product containing a single active ingredient (with or without additives) or two or more active ingredients (combination drugs). A chemical substance marketed by several manufacturers may have several trade names. A drug may be marketed under different trade names in different countries.

Trade names are found in many publications and are used extensively in clinical medicine. For convenience, two tables are included. One lists alphabetically the generic names with their trade names for most drugs mentioned throughout THE MERCK MANUAL OF GERIATRICS, primarily those marketed in the USA. The other lists alphabetically the trade names with their generic name. The tables are not all-inclusive and do not include every trade name for each drug. A few drugs in the table are investigational and may subsequently be approved by the FDA. The inclusion of a drug does not indicate approval of its use for any indication, nor does it imply efficacy or safety of its action. The inclusion of a trade name in the table indicates neither endorsement nor preference by THE MERCK MANUAL OF GERIATRICS.

GENERIC AND TRADE NAMES OF COMMONLY USED DRUGS

Generic Name	Trade Names	Generic Name	Trade Names
Abciximab	REOPRO	Astemizole	HISMANAL
Acarbose	PRECOSE	Atenolol	TENORMIN
Acebutolol	SECTRAL	Atorvastatin	LIPITOR
Acetaminophen	TYLENOL	Atovaquone	MEPRON
Acetazolamide	DIAMOX	Auranofin	RIDAURA
Acetohexamide	DYMELOR	Azathioprine	IMURAN
Acetohydroxamic acid	LITHOSTAT	Azithromycin	ZITHROMAX
		Azlocillin	AZLIN
Acetophenazine	TINDAL	Aztreonam	AZACTAM
Acetylcysteine	MUCOMYST	Baclofen	LIORESAL
ACTH	See Corticotropin	Beclomethasone	BECLOVENT, VANCERIL
Acyclovir	ZOVIRAX	*Belladonna alkaloids	B & O SUP-PRETTES, RESPA-ARM
Adenosine	ADENOCARD		
Albuterol	PROVENTIL, VENTOLIN		
		Benazepril	LOTENSIN
Alendronate	FOSAMAX	Benzonatate	TESSALON
Allopurinol	ZYLOPRIM	Benzquinamide	EMETE-CON
*Alprazolam	XANAX	*Benztropine	COGENTIN
Alprostadil	CAVERJECT	Benzylpenicilloyl polylysine	PRE-PEN
Amantadine	SYMMETREL		
Amifostine	ETHYOL	Bepridil	VASCOR
Amikacin	AMIKIN	Beractant	SURVANTA
Amiloride	MIDAMOR	Beta carotene	SOLATENE
Aminocaproic acid	AMICAR	Betamethasone	CELESTONE, UTICORT, VALISONE
Aminophylline	SOMO-PHYLLIN		
Amiodarone	CORDARONE	Betaxolol	BETOPTIC, KERLONE
*Amitriptyline	ELAVIL, ENDEP	Bethanechol	DUVOID, URECHOLINE
Amlodipine	NORVASC		
Amoxapine	ASENDIN	Bisacodyl	DULCOLAX
Amoxicillin	AMOXIL, LAROTID	Bisoprolol	ZEBETA
		Bitolterol	TORNALATE
Amoxicillin/ clavulanate	AUGMENTIN	Bleomycin	BLENOXANE
		Bretylium	BRETYLOL
Amphotericin B	FUNGIZONE	Bromocriptine	PARLODEL
Ampicillin	OMNIPEN, POLYCILLIN, PRINCIPEN	*Bromodiphen-hydramine	NAUSEATOL
		*Brompheniramine	DIMETANE
Amrinone	INOCOR	Budesonide	RHINOCORT
Anisotropine	VALPIN 50	Bumetanide	BUMEX
Anthralin	ANTHRA-DERM	Bupropion	WELLBUTRIN
Asparaginase	ELSPAR	Buspirone	BuSPAR

GENERIC AND TRADE NAMES OF COMMONLY USED DRUGS (*Continued*)

Generic Name	Trade Names	Generic Name	Trade Names
Busulfan	MYLERAN	Cephalexin	KEFLEX
Butorphanol	STADOL	Cephapirin	CEFADYL
Calcifediol	CALDEROL	Cephradine	ANSPOR,
Calcitonin-human	CIBACALCIN		VELOSEF
Calcitonin-salmon	CALCIMAR	Chenodiol	CHENIX
Calcitriol	ROCALTROL	Chloral hydrate	NOCTEC
Capreomycin	CAPASTAT	Chlorambucil	LEUKERAN
Capsaicin	ZOSTRIX	Chloramphenicol	CHLORO-
Captopril	CAPOTEN		MYCETIN
Carbamazepine	TEGRETOL	*Chlordiazepoxide	LIBRIUM
Carbenicillin	GEOCILLIN	Chlorhexidine	HIBICLENS
Carbidopa-levodopa	SINEMET	Chlormezanone	TRANCOPAL
Carbinoxamine	CLISTIN	Chlorotrianisene	TACE
Carboprost	HEMABATE	*Chlorpheniramine	CHLOR-
*Carisoprodol	SOMA		TRIMETON,
Carmustine	BiCNU		TELDRIN
Carteolol	CARTROL,	Chlorpromazine	THORAZINE
	OCUPRESS	*Chlorpropamide	DIABINESE
Carvedilol	COREG	Chlorthalidone	HYGROTON
Cefaclor	CECLOR	*Chlorzoxazone	PARAFON
Cefadroxil	DURICEF,		FORTE
	ULTRACEF	Cholestyramine	QUESTRAN
Cefamandole	MANDOL	Cidofovir	VISTIDE
Cefazolin	ANCEF,	Cimetidine	TAGAMET
	KEFZOL,	Ciprofloxacin	CILOXAN,
	ZOLICEF		CIPRO
Cefixime	SUPRAX	Cisapride	PROPULSID
Cefonicid	MONOCID	Cisplatin	PLATINOL
Cefoperazone	CEFOBID	Clarithromycin	BIAXIN
Ceforanide	PRECEF	Clemastine	TAVIST
Cefotaxime	CLAFORAN	*Clidinium	QUARZAN
Cefotetan	CEFOTAN	Clindamycin	CLEOCIN
Cefoxitin	MEFOXIN	Clofazimine	LAMPRENE
Cefprozil	CEFZIL	Clofibrate	ATROMID-S
Ceftazidime	FORTAZ,	Clomiphene	CLOMID
	TAZICEF,	Clomipramine	ANAFRANIL
	TAZIDIME	Clonazepam	KLONOPIN
Ceftizoxime	CEFIZOX	Clonidine	CATAPRES
Ceftriaxone	ROCEPHIN	Clopidogrel	PLAVIX
Cefuroxime	CEFTIN,	Clorazepate	TRANXENE
	KEFUROX,	Clotrimazole	LOTRIMIN,
	ZINACEF		MYCELEX
Celecoxib	CELEBREX	Cloxacillin	TEGOPEN

GENERIC AND TRADE NAMES OF COMMONLY USED DRUGS *(Continued)*

Generic Name	Trade Names	Generic Name	Trade Names
Clozapine	CLOZARIL	Diazoxide	HYPERSTAT, PROGLYCEM
Colestipol	COLESTID		
Corticotropin (ACTH)	ACTHAR	Diclofenac	CATAFLAM, VOLTAREN
Cortisol	CORTEF, HYDRO-CORTONE, SOLU-CORTEF	Dicloxacillin	DYCILL, DYNAPEN, PATHOCIL
		*Dicyclomine	BENTYL
Cosyntropin	CORTROSYN	Didanosine	VIDEX
Co-trimoxazole	See Trimetho-prim-sulfa-methoxazole	Diethylpropion	TENUATE, TEPANIL
		Diflunisal	DOLOBID
Cromolyn	CROLOM, INTAL, NASALCROM	Digitoxin	CRYSTODIGIN
		Digoxin	LANOXIN
		Dihydrotachysterol	HYTAKEROL
*Cyclandelate	CYCLOSPAS-MOL	Diltiazem	CARDIZEM, DILACOR
Cyclizine	MAREZINE	Dimercaprol	BAL in oil
*Cyclobenzaprine	FLEXERIL	Dinoprost	PROSTIN F2 ALPHA
Cyclopentolate	CYCLOGYL		
Cyclophosphamide	CYTOXAN	Dinoprostone	PROSTIN E2
Cycloserine	SEROMYCIN	*Diphenhydramine	BENADRYL, NYTOL
Cyclosporine	SANDIMMUNE		
*Cyproheptadine	PERIACTIN	Diphenidol	VONTROL
Cytarabine	CYTOSAR-U	Diphenoxylate with atropine	LOMOTIL
Dacarbazine	DTIC-DOME		
Dactinomycin	COSMEGEN	Dipivefrin	PROPINE
Danazol	DANOCRINE	*Dipyridamole	PERSANTINE
Dantrolene	DANTRIUM	*Disopyramide	NORPACE
Daunorubicin	CERUBIDINE	Disulfiram	ANTABUSE
Deferoxamine	DESFERAL	Divalproex	DEPAKOTE
Delavirdine	RESCRIPTOR	Dobutamine	DOBUTREX
Demeclocycline	DECLOMYCIN	Docusate	COLACE
Desipramine	NORPRAMIN, PERTOFRANE	Donepezil	ARICEPT
		Dopamine	INTROPIN
Desmopressin	DDAVP, STIMATE	Dornase alfa	PULMOZYME
		Dorzolamide	TRUSOPT
Dexamethasone	DECADRON, HEXADROL	Doxazosin	CARDURA
		*Doxepin	SINEQUAN, ZONALON
*Dexchlorphenir-amine	POLARAMINE		
		Doxorubicin	ADRIAMYCIN
Dextromethorphan	BENYLIN DM, DELSYM	Doxycycline	VIBRAMYCIN
*Diazepam	VALIUM	Dronabinol	MARINOL

GENERIC AND TRADE NAMES OF COMMONLY USED DRUGS (*Continued*)

Generic Name	Trade Names	Generic Name	Trade Names
Droperidol	INAPSINE	Flucytosine	ANCOBON
Echothiophate	PHOSPHO-LINE	Fludrocortisone	FLORINEF
		Flunisolide	NASALIDE
Edrophonium	TENSILON	Fluocinolone	SYNALAR
Enalapril	VASOTEC	Fluocinonide	LIDEX
Encainide	ENKAID	Fluoxetine	PROZAC
Enoxacin	PENETREX	Fluoxymesterone	HALOTESTIN
Enoxaparin	LOVENOX	Fluphenazine	PERMITIL, PROLIXIN
Epoetin alfa	EPOGEN, PROCRIT		
		Flurandrenolide	CORDRAN
Ergocalciferol	DRISDOL	*Flurazepam	DALMANE
Ergotamine	ERGOMAR, ERGOSTAT	Flurbiprofen	ANSAID, OCUFEN
Erythromycin	E-MYCIN, ERYTH-ROCIN, ILOSONE	Fluvastatin	LESCOL
		Foscarnet	FOSCAVIR
		Fosinopril	MONOPRIL
		Furosemide	LASIX
Esmolol	BREVIBLOC	Gabapentin	NEURONTIN
Estazolam	PROSOM	Gamma benzene hexachloride	See Lindane
Estrogens, conjugated	PREMARIN		
		Ganciclovir	CYTOVENE
Etanercept	ENBREL	Gemfibrozil	LOPID
Ethacrynic acid	EDECRIN	Gentamicin	GARAMYCIN
Ethambutol	MYAMBUTOL	Glimepiride	AMARYL
Etidronate	DIDRONEL	Glipizide	GLUCOTROL
Etodolac	LODINE	Glyburide	DIABETA, MICRONASE
Etoposide	VePESID		
Etretinate	TEGISON	Gold	MYOCHRY-SINE
Factor IX concentrates	KONYNE 80, PROPLEX T		
		Granisetron	KYTRIL
Famciclovir	FAMVIR	Grepafloxacin	RAXAR
Famotidine	PEPCID	Griseofulvin	FULVICIN, GRIFULVIN V, GRIS-ACTIN
Felodipine	PLENDIL		
Fenfluramine	PONDIMIN		
Fenoprofen	NALFON		
Fentanyl	SUBLIMAZE	Guaifenesin	ROBITUSSIN
Fexofenadine	ALLEGRA	Guanabenz	WYTENSIN
Filgrastim	NEUPOGEN	Guanadrel	HYLOREL
Finasteride	PROSCAR, PROPECIA	*Guanethidine	ISMELIN
		Guanfacine	TENEX
Flavoxate	URISPAS	Halazepam	PAXIPAM
Flecainide	TAMBOCOR	Haloperidol	HALDOL
Fluconazole	DIFLUCAN	Haloprogin	HALOTEX

GENERIC AND TRADE NAMES OF COMMONLY USED DRUGS (Continued)

Generic Name	Trade Names	Generic Name	Trade Names
Hepatitis A vaccine	HAVRIX, VAQTA	Isopropamide	DARBID
		Isoproterenol	ISUPREL
Hepatitis B vaccine	COMVAX, ENGERIX-B, RECOM-BIVAX HB	Isosorbide	ISORDIL, SORBITRATE
		Isotretinoin	ACCUTANE
Hydralazine	APRESOLINE	Isradipine	DYNACIRC
Hydrochloro-thiazide	ESIDRIX, HydroDIURIL, ORETIC	Itraconazole	SPORANOX
		Kanamycin	KANTREX
		Ketoconazole	NIZORAL
Hydrocortisone	See Cortisol	Ketoprofen	ORUDIS, ORUVAIL
Hydromorphone	DILAUDID		
Hydroquinone	ELDOQUIN	Ketorolac	TORADOL
Hydroxychloro-quine	PLAQUENIL	Labetalol	NORMO-DYNE, TRANDATE
Hydroxyproges-terone	DELALUTIN		
		Lactulose	CEPHULAC, CHRONULAC
Hydroxyurea	HYDREA		
*Hydroxyzine	ATARAX, VISTARIL	Lamivudine	EPIVIR
		Lamotrigine	LAMICTAL
*Hyoscyamine	ATROHIST PLUS, DONNATAL, LEVSIN, PROSED	Lansoprazole	PREVACID
		Latanoprost	XALATAN
		Leflunomide	ARAVA
		Levallorphan	LORFAN
Ibuprofen	ADVIL, MOTRIN, NUPRIN	Levamisole	ERGAMISOL
		Levarterenol	See Norepi-nephrine
Idoxuridine	HERPLEX, STOXIL	Levodopa	DOPAR, LARODOPA
Ifosfamide	IFEX	Levothyroxine (T₄)	LEVOXYL, SYNTHROID
Imipenem-cilastatin	PRIMAXIN		
		Lidocaine	XYLOCAINE
Imipramine	TOFRANIL	Lincomycin	LINCOCIN
Indapamide	LOZOL	Lindane	KWELL
Indinavir	CRIXIVAN	Liothyronine (T₃)	CYTOMEL
*Indomethacin	INDOCIN	Liotrix	EUTHROID, THYROLAR
Insulin	HUMALOG, HUMULIN, NOVOLIN	Lisinopril	PRINIVIL, ZESTRIL
Ipratropium	ATROVENT	Lithium	LITHANE, LITHONATE
Iron dextran	IMFERON		
Isoetharine	BRONKOSOL	Lomefloxacin	MAXAQUIN
Isoniazid	NYDRAZID	Lomustine	CeeNU

GENERIC AND TRADE NAMES OF COMMONLY USED DRUGS (*Continued*)

Generic Name	Trade Names	Generic Name	Trade Names
Loperamide	IMODIUM	Methenamine	HIPREX, MANDEL-AMINE
Loratadine	CLARITIN		
*Lorazepam	ATIVAN	Methicillin	STAPH-CILLIN
Losartan	COZAAR		
Lovastatin	MEVACOR	Methimazole	TAPAZOLE
Loxapine	LOXITANE	*Methocarbamol	ROBAXIN
Lypressin	DIAPID	Methotrexate	RHEUMA-TREX
Mafenide	SULFAMYLON		
Maprotiline	LUDIOMIL	Methotrimeprazine	LEVOPROME
Mazindol	MAZANOR, SANOREX	Methoxsalen	OXSORALEN
		Methsuximide	CELONTIN
Mebendazole	VERMOX	*Methyldopa	ALDOMET
Mechlorethamine	MUSTARGEN	Methylphenidate	RITALIN
Meclizine	ANTIVERT, BONINE	Methylprednis-olone	MEDROL
Meclofenamate	MECLOMEN		
Medroxyproges-terone	PROVERA	Methyltestosterone	ORETON
		Methysergide	SANSERT
Mefenamic acid	PONSTEL	Metoclopramide	REGLAN
Megestrol	MEGACE	Metolazone	MYKROX, ZAROXOLYN
Melphalan	ALKERAN		
Menadiol	SYNKAYVITE	Metoprolol	LOPRESSOR
Menotropins	PERGONAL	Metronidazole	FLAGYL
*Meperidine	DEMEROL	Metyrapone	METOPIRONE
Mephenytoin	MESANTOIN	Mexiletine	MEXITIL
*Meprobamate	EQUANIL, MILTOWN	Mezlocillin	MEZLIN
		Mibefradil	POSICOR
Mercaptopurine	PURINETHOL	Miconazole	MICATIN, MONISTAT
Meropenem	MERREM IV		
Mesalamine	ASACOL, ROWASA	Milrinone	PRIMACOR
		Minocycline	MINOCIN
Mesoridazine	SERENTIL	Minoxidil	LONITEN, ROGAINE
Metaproterenol	ALUPENT, METAPREL		
		Misoprostol	CYTOTEC
Metaraminol	ARAMINE	Mitomycin	MUTAMYCIN
*Metaxalone	SKELAXIN	Mitotane	LYSODREN
Metformin	GLUCOPHAGE	Molindone	MOBAN
Methadone	DOLOPHINE	Montelukast	SINGULAIR
Methamphetamine	DESOXYN	Morphine	MS CONTIN
Methandrosten-olone	DIANABOL	Moxalactam	MOXAM
		Nabumetone	RELAFEN
Methdilazine	TACARYL	Nadolol	CORGARD

GENERIC AND TRADE NAMES OF COMMONLY USED DRUGS (*Continued*)

Generic Name	Trade Names	Generic Name	Trade Names
Nafcillin	UNIPEN	Oxacillin	BACTOCILL, PROSTAPH-LIN
Nalbuphine	NUBAIN		
Nalidixic acid	NegGRAM	Oxamniquine	VANSIL
Naloxone	NARCAN	Oxandrolone	OXANDRIN
Naltrexone	REVIA	Oxaprozin	DAYPRO
Nandrolone	DURABOLIN	*Oxazepam	SERAX
Naproxen	ALEVE, ANAPROX, NAPROSYN	*Oxybutynin	DITROPAN
		Oxymetazoline	AFRIN, DURATION
Naratriptan	AMERGE		
Nedocromil	TILADE	Oxymetholone	ANADROL
Nefazodone	SERZONE	Oxytocin	PITOCIN, SYNTOCI-NON
Nelfinavir	VIRACEPT		
Neostigmine	PROSTIGMIN	Paclitaxel	TAXOL
Nevirapine	VIRAMUNE	Pamidronate	AREDIA
Nicardipine	CARDENE	Pancrelipase	PANCREASE, VIOKASE
Niclosamide	NICLOCIDE		
Nicotine	NICORETTE, NICOTROL	Pancuronium	PAVULON
Nifedipine	ADALAT, PROCARDIA	Papaverine	PAVABID
		Paramethadione	PARADIONE
Nimodipine	NIMOTOP	Paramethasone	HALDRONE
Nisoldipine	SULAR	Pargyline	EUTONYL
*Nitrazepam	MOGADON	Paromomycin	HUMATIN
Nitrofurantoin	FURADANTIN, MACRODAN-TIN	Paroxetine	PAXIL
		Penbutolol	LEVATOL
		Penciclovir	DENAVIR
Nitroprusside	NIPRIDE	Penicillamine	CUPRIMINE
Nizatidine	AXID	Penicillin G	BICILLIN, DURA-CILLIN
Norepinephrine	LEVOPHED		
Norfloxacin	NOROXIN		
Nortriptyline	AVENTYL	Penicillin V potassium	PEN-VEE, V-CILLIN K
Nystatin	MYCOSTATIN, NILSTAT		
		Penicilloyl	See Benzyl-penicilloyl polylysine
Octreotide	SANDOSTATIN		
Ofloxacin	FLOXIN		
Olanzapine	ZYPREXA	Pentamidine	NEBUPENT, PENTAM 300
Olsalazine	DIPENTUM		
Omeprazole	PRILOSEC	*Pentazocine	TALWIN
Ondansetron	ZOFRAN	Pentobarbital	NEMBUTAL
Orlistat	XENICAL	Pentoxifylline	TRENTAL
Oseltamivir	TAMIFLU	Pergolide	PERMAX
		*Perphenazine	TRILAFON

GENERIC AND TRADE NAMES OF COMMONLY USED DRUGS (*Continued*)

Generic Name	Trade Names	Generic Name	Trade Names
Phenacemide	PHENURONE	Procyclidine	KEMADRIN
Phenazopyridine	PYRIDIUM	Promazine	SPARINE
Phenelzine	NARDIL	*Promethazine	PHENERGAN
Phenmetrazine	PRELUDIN	Propafenone	RYTHMOL
Phenobarbital	LUMINAL	*Propantheline	PROBAN-THINE
Phenoxyben-zamine	DIBENZY-LINE	Proparacaine	OPHTHAINE, OPHTHETIC
Phensuximide	MILONTIN		
Phentermine	IONAMIN	Propiomazine	LARGON
Phentolamine	REGITINE	*Propoxyphene	DARVON, DOLENE
*Phenylbutazone	AZOLID, BUTAZOLIDIN	Propranolol	INDERAL
Phenylephrine	NEOSYN-EPHRINE	Protriptyline	VIVACTIL
		Pseudoephedrine	AFRINOL, SUDAFED
Phenytoin	DILANTIN		
Phytonadione	KONAKION, MEPHYTON	Pyrantel	ANTIMINTH
		Pyridostigmine	MESTINON
Pindolol	VISKEN	Pyrimethamine	DARAPRIM
Piperacillin	PIPRACIL	Pyrvinium	POVAN
Pipobroman	VERCYTE	Quazepam	DORAL
Piroxicam	FELDENE	Quetiapine	SEROQUEL
Plicamycin	MITHRACIN	Quinacrine	ATABRINE
Pneumococcal vaccine, polyvalent	PNEUMOVAX 23, PNU-IMMUNE 23	Quinapril	ACCUPRIL
		Quinethazone	HYDROMOX
		Quinidine	CARDIO-QUIN, QUINAGLUTE
Pralidoxime	PROTOPAM		
Pramipexole	MIRAPEX		
Pravastatin	PRAVACHOL	Raloxifene	EVISTA
Prazepam	CENTRAX	Ramipril	ALTACE
Praziquantel	BILTRICIDE	Ranitidine	ZANTAC
Prazosin	MINIPRESS	Repaglinide	PRANDIN
Prednisolone	DELTA-COR-TEF, HYDEL-TRASOL	*Reserpine	DIUPRES, DIUTENSEN-R, HYDRO-PRES
Prednisone	DELTASONE, METICORTEN		
		Reteplase	RETAVASE
Primidone	MYSOLINE	Ribavirin	REBETRON, VIRAZOLE
Probenecid	BENEMID		
Probucol	LORELCO	Rifabutin	MYCOBUTIN
Procainamide	PROCAN SR, PRONESTYL	Rifampin	RIFADIN, RIMACTANE
Procaine	NOVOCAIN	Rimantadine	FLUMADINE
Procarbazine	MATULANE	Risperidone	RISPERDAL
Prochlorperazine	COMPAZINE	Ritodrine	YUTOPAR

GENERIC AND TRADE NAMES OF COMMONLY USED DRUGS (*Continued*)

Generic Name	Trade Names	Generic Name	Trade Names
Ritonavir	NORVIR	Terazosin	HYTRIN
Rizatriptan	MAXALT	Terbutaline	BRETHINE, BRICANYL
Rofecoxib	VIOXX		
Ropinirole	REQUIP	Testolactone	TESLAC
Rosiglitazone	AVANDIA	Testosterone	ANDRODERM DELA-TESTRYL, TESTODERM
Salmeterol	SEREVENT		
Salsalate	DISALCID, SALFLEX		
Saquinavir	FORTOVASE	Tetanus immune globulin-human	HYPER-TET
Sargramostim	LEUKINE	Tetracycline	ACHROMY-CIN V, TETRACYN, TETREX
Secobarbital	SECONAL		
Selegiline	ELDEPRYL		
Selenium	SELSUN		
Sertraline	ZOLOFT	Theophylline	ELIXO-PHYLLIN, THEO-DUR
Sibutramine	MERIDIA		
Sildenafil	VIAGRA		
Silver sulfadiazine	SILVADENE	Thiabendazole	MINTEZOL
Simethicone	MYLICON	Thiethylperazine	TORECAN
Simvastatin	ZOCOR	Thioridazine	MELLARIL
Somatrem	PROTROPIN	Thiothixene	NAVANE
Somatropin	HUMATROPE	Thyrotropin	THYTROPAR
Sotalol	BETAPACE	Ticarcillin	TICAR
Spectinomycin	TROBICIN	*Ticlopidine	TICLID
Spironolactone	ALDACTONE	Timolol	BLOCADREN, TIMOPTIC
Stanozolol	WINSTROL		
Stavudine	ZERIT	Tirofiban	AGGRASTAT
Streptokinase	STREPTASE	Tobramycin	NEBCIN, TOBREX
Streptozocin	ZANOSAR		
Sucralfate	CARAFATE	Tocainide	TONOCARD
Sulfamethoxazole	GANTANOL	Tolazamide	TOLINASE
Sulfasalazine	AZULFIDINE	Tolazoline	PRISCOLINE
Sulfinpyrazone	ANTURANE	Tolbutamide	ORINASE
Sulfisoxazole	GANTRISIN	Tolcapone	TASMAR
Sulindac	CLINORIL	Tolmetin	TOLECTIN
Sumatriptan	IMITREX	Tolnaftate	TINACTIN
Suprofen	PROFENAL	Tolpotecan	HYCAMTIN
Tacrine	COGNEX	Torsemide	DEMADEX
Tacrolimus	PROGRAF	Tramadol	ULTRAM
Tamoxifen	NOLVADEX	Trandolapril	MAVIK
Tamsulosin	FLOMAX	Tranylcypromine	PARNATE
Tazobactam	ZOSYN	Trastuzumab	HERCEPTIN
Temazepam	RESTORIL	Trazodone	DESYREL
		Tretinoin	RETIN-A

GENERIC AND TRADE NAMES OF COMMONLY USED DRUGS (*Continued*)

Generic Name	Trade Names	Generic Name	Trade Names
Triacetin	ENZACTIN	Tromethamine	THAM
Triamcinolone	ARISTOCORT, KENACORT, KENALOG	Tropicamide	MYDRIACYL
		Urokinase	ABBOKINASE
		Valacyclovir	VALTREX
Triamterene	DYRENIUM	Valproic acid	DEPAKENE
Triazolam	HALCION	Valsartan	DIOVAN
Triclofos	TRICLOS	Vancomycin	VANCOCIN
Trientine	SYPRINE	Vasopressin	PITRESSIN
Trifluoperazine	STELAZINE	Venlafaxine	EFFEXOR
Triflupromazine	VESPRIN	Verapamil	CALAN, ISOPTIN
Trifluridine	VIROPTIC		
Trihexyphenidyl	ARTANE	Vidarabine	VIRA-A
Trimeprazine	TEMARIL	Vinblastine	VELBAN
Trimethadione	TRIDIONE	Vincristine	ONCOVIN
Trimethaphan	ARFONAD	Vinorelbine	NAVELBINE
*Trimethoben-zamide	TIGAN	Warfarin	COUMADIN
		Zafirlukast	ACCOLATE
Trimethoprim	PROLOPRIM, TRIMPEX	Zalcitabine	HIVID
		Zanamivir	RELENZA
Trimethoprim-sulfamethoxazole	BACTRIM, SEPTRA	Zidovudine	RETROVIR
		Zileuton	ZYFLO
Trimipramine	SURMONTIL	Zolmitriptan	ZOMIG
*Tripelennamine	PBZ	Zolpidem	AMBIEN
*Triprolidine	ACTIFED		
Troglitazone	REZULIN		

*Particularly problematic in the elderly (see TABLE 6–4).

TRADE AND GENERIC NAMES OF COMMONLY USED DRUGS

Trade Name	Generic Name	Trade Name	Generic Name
ABBOKINASE	Urokinase	APRESOLINE	Hydralazine
ACCOLATE	Zafirlukast	ARAMINE	Metaraminol
ACCUPRIL	Quinapril	ARAVA	Leflunomide
ACCUTANE	Isotretinoin	AREDIA	Pamidronate
ACHROMYCIN V	Tetracycline	ARFONAD	Trimethaphan
ACTHAR	Corticotropin	ARICEPT	Donepezil
	(ACTH)	ARISTOCORT	Triamcinolone
ACTIFED	*Triprolidine	ARTANE	Trihexyphen-
ADALAT	Nifedipine		idyl
ADENOCARD	Adenosine	ASACOL	Mesalamine
ADRIAMYCIN	Doxorubicin	ASENDIN	Amoxapine
ADVIL	Ibuprofen	ATABRINE	Quinacrine
AFRIN	Oxymetazoline	ATARAX	*Hydroxyzine
AFRINOL	Pseudoephe-	ATIVAN	*Lorazepam
	drine	ATROHIST PLUS	*Hyoscyamine
AGGRASTAT	Tirofiban	ATROMID-S	Clofibrate
ALDACTONE	Spironolactone	ATROVENT	Ipratropium
ALDOMET	*Methyldopa	AUGMENTIN	Amoxicillin/
ALEVE	Naproxen		clavulanate
ALKERAN	Melphalan	AVANDIA	Rosiglitazone
ALLEGRA	Fexofenadine	AVENTYL	Nortriptyline
ALTACE	Ramipril	AXID	Nizatidine
ALUPENT	Metaproterenol	AZACTAM	Aztreonam
AMARYL	Glimepiride	AZLIN	Azlocillin
AMBIEN	Zolpidem	AZOLID	*Phenylbuta-
AMERGE	Naratriptan		zone
AMICAR	Aminocaproic	AZULFIDINE	Sulfasalazine
	acid	B & O	*Belladonna
AMIKIN	Amikacin	SUPPRETTES	alkaloids
AMOXIL	Amoxicillin	BACTOCILL	Oxacillin
ANADROL	Oxymetholone	BACTRIM	Trimethoprim-
ANAFRANIL	Clomipramine		sulfamethoxa-
ANAPROX	Naproxen		zole
ANCEF	Cefazolin	BAL in oil	Dimercaprol
ANCOBON	Flucytosine	BECLOVENT	Beclomethasone
ANDRODERM	Testosterone	BENADRYL	*Diphenhydra-
ANSAID	Flurbiprofen		mine
ANSPOR	Cephradine	BENEMID	Probenecid
ANTABUSE	Disulfiram	BENTYL	*Dicyclomine
ANTHRA-DERM	Anthralin	BENYLIN DM	Dextromethor-
ANTIMINTH	Pyrantel		phan
ANTIVERT	Meclizine	BETAPACE	Sotalol
ANTURANE	Sulfinpyrazone	BETOPTIC	Betaxolol

TRADE AND GENERIC NAMES OF COMMONLY USED DRUGS (*Continued*)

Trade Name	Generic Name	Trade Name	Generic Name
BIAXIN	Clarithromycin	CENTRAX	Prazepam
BICILLIN	Penicillin G	CEPHULAC	Lactulose
BiCNU	Carmustine	CERUBIDINE	Daunorubicin
BILTRICIDE	Praziquantel	CHENIX	Chenodiol
BLENOXANE	Bleomycin	CHLOROMY-	Chloram-
BLOCADREN	Timolol	CETIN	phenicol
BONINE	Meclizine	CHLOR-	*Chlorphenir-
BRETHINE	Terbutaline	TRIMETON	amine
BRETYLOL	Bretylium	CHRONULAC	Lactulose
BREVIBLOC	Esmolol	CIBACALCIN	Calcitonin-
BRICANYL	Terbutaline		human
BRONKOSOL	Isoetharine	CILOXAN	Ciprofloxacin
BUMEX	Bumetanide	CIPRO	Ciprofloxacin
BuSPAR	Buspirone	CLAFORAN	Cefotaxime
BUTAZOLIDIN	*Phenylbuta-	CLARITIN	Loratadine
	zone	CLEOCIN	Clindamycin
CALAN	Verapamil	CLINORIL	Sulindac
CALCIMAR	Calcitonin-	CLISTIN	Carbinoxamine
	salmon	CLOMID	Clomiphene
CALDEROL	Calcifediol	CLOZARIL	Clozapine
CAPASTAT	Capreomycin	COGENTIN	*Benztropine
CAPOTEN	Captopril	COGNEX	Tacrine
CARAFATE	Sucralfate	COLACE	Docusate
CARDENE	Nicardipine	COLESTID	Colestipol
CARDIOQUIN	Quinidine	COMPAZINE	Prochlorper-
CARDIZEM	Diltiazem		azine
CARDURA	Doxazosin	COMVAX	Hepatitis B
CARTROL	Carteolol		vaccine
CATAFLAM	Diclofenac	CORDARONE	Amiodarone
CATAPRES	Clonidine	CORDRAN	Flurandrenolide
CAVERJECT	Alprostadil	COREG	Carvedilol
CECLOR	Cefaclor	CORGARD	Nadolol
CeeNU	Lomustine	CORTEF	Cortisol
CEFADYL	Cephapirin	CORTROSYN	Cosyntropin
CEFIZOX	Ceftizoxime	COSMEGEN	Dactinomycin
CEFOBID	Cefoperazone	COUMADIN	Warfarin
CEFOTAN	Cefotetan	COZAAR	Losartan
CEFTIN	Cefuroxime	CRIXIVAN	Indinavir
CEFZIL	Cefprozil	CROLOM	Cromolyn
CELEBREX	Celecoxib	CRYSTODIGIN	Digitoxin
CELESTONE	Betamethasone	CUPRIMINE	Penicillamine
CELONTIN	Methsuximide	CYCLOGYL	Cyclopentolate

TRADE AND GENERIC NAMES OF COMMONLY USED DRUGS (*Continued*)

Trade Name	Generic Name	Trade Name	Generic Name
CYCLOSPASMOL	*Cyclandelate	DIDRONEL	Etidronate
CYTOMEL	Liothyronine (T₃)	DIFLUCAN	Fluconazole
		DILACOR	Diltiazem
CYTOSAR-U	Cytarabine	DILANTIN	Phenytoin
CYTOTEC	Misoprostol	DILAUDID	Hydromor- phone
CYTOVENE	Ganciclovir		
CYTOXAN	Cyclophospha- mide	DIMETANE	*Bromphenir- amine
DALMANE	*Flurazepam	DIOVAN	Valsartan
DANOCRINE	Danazol	DIPENTUM	Olsalazine
DANTRIUM	Dantrolene	DISALCID	Salsalate
DARAPRIM	Pyrimethamine	DITROPAN	*Oxybutynin
DARBID	Isopropamide	DIUPRES	*Reserpine
DARVON	*Propoxyphene	DIUTENSEN-R	*Reserpine
DAYPRO	Oxaprozin	DOBUTREX	Dobutamine
DDAVP	Desmopressin	DOLENE	*Propoxyphene
DECADRON	Dexamethasone	DOLOBID	Diflunisal
DECLOMYCIN	Demeclocycline	DOLOPHINE	Methadone
DELALUTIN	Hydroxypro- gesterone	DONNATAL	*Hyoscyamine
		DOPAR	Levodopa
DELATESTRYL	Testosterone	DORAL	Quazepam
DELSYM	Dextromethor- phan	DRISDOL	Ergocalciferol
		DTIC-DOME	Dacarbazine
DELTA-CORTEF	Prednisolone	DULCOLAX	Bisacodyl
DELTASONE	Prednisone	DURABOLIN	Nandrolone
DEMADEX	Torsemide	DURACILLIN	Penicillin G
DEMEROL	*Meperidine	DURATION	Oxymetazoline
DENAVIR	Penciclovir	DURICEF	Cefadroxil
DEPAKENE	Valproic acid	DUVOID	Bethanechol
DEPAKOTE	Divalproex	DYCILL	Dicloxacillin
DESFERAL	Deferoxamine	DYMELOR	Acetohexamide
DESOXYN	Methamphe- tamine	DYNACIRC	Isradipine
		DYNAPEN	Dicloxacillin
DESYREL	Trazodone	DYRENIUM	Triamterene
DIABETA	Glyburide	EDECRIN	Ethacrynic acid
DIABINESE	*Chlorpropa- mide	EFFEXOR	Venlafaxine
		ELAVIL	*Amitriptyline
DIAMOX	Acetazolamide	ELDEPRYL	Selegiline
DIANABOL	Methandro- stenolone	ELDOQUIN	Hydroquinone
		ELIXOPHYLLIN	Theophylline
DIAPID	Lypressin	ELSPAR	Asparaginase
DIBENZYLINE	Phenoxyben- zamine	EMETE-CON	Benzquinamide

TRADE AND GENERIC NAMES OF COMMONLY USED DRUGS (*Continued*)

Trade Name	Generic Name	Trade Name	Generic Name
E-MYCIN	Erythromycin	GLUCOPHAGE	Metformin
ENBREL	Etanercept	GLUCOTROL	Glipizide
ENDEP	*Amitriptyline	GRIFULVIN V	Griseofulvin
ENGERIX-B	Hepatitis B vaccine	GRISACTIN	Griseofulvin
		HALCION	Triazolam
ENKAID	Encainide	HALDOL	Haloperidol
ENZACTIN	Triacetin	HALDRONE	Paramethasone
EPIVIR	Lamivudine	HALOTESTIN	Fluoxyme-sterone
EPOGEN	Epoetin alfa		
EQUANIL	*Meprobamate	HALOTEX	Haloprogin
ERGAMISOL	Levamisole	HAVRIX	Hepatitis A vaccine
ERGOMAR	Ergotamine		
ERGOSTAT	Ergotamine	HEMABATE	Carboprost
ERYTHROCIN	Erythromycin	HERCEPTIN	Trastuzumab
ESIDRIX	Hydrochloro-thiazide	HERPLEX	Idoxuridine
		HEXADROL	Dexamethasone
ETHYOL	Amifostine	HIBICLENS	Chlorhexidine
EUTHROID	Liotrix	HIPREX	Methenamine
EUTONYL	Pargyline	HISMANAL	Astemizole
EVISTA	Raloxifene	HIVID	Zalcitabine
FAMVIR	Famciclovir	HUMALOG	Insulin
FELDENE	Piroxicam	HUMATIN	Paromomycin
FLAGYL	Metronidazole	HUMATROPE	Somatropin
FLEXERIL	*Cyclobenza-prine	HUMULIN	Insulin
		HYCAMTIN	Topotecan
FLOMAX	Tamsulosin	HYDELTRASOL	Prednisolone
FLORINEF	Fludrocortisone	HYDREA	Hydroxyurea
FLOXIN	Ofloxacin	HYDROCORTONE	Cortisol
FLUMADINE	Rimantadine	HydroDIURIL	Hydrochloro-thiazide
FORTAZ	Ceftazidime		
FORTOVASE	Saquinavir	HYDROMOX	Quinethazone
FOSAMAX	Alendronate	HYDROPRES	*Reserpine
FOSCAVIR	Foscarnet	HYGROTON	Chlorthalidone
FULVICIN	Griseofulvin	HYLOREL	Guanadrel
FUNGIZONE	Amphotericin B	HYPERSTAT	Diazoxide
		HYPER-TET	Tetanus immune globulin-human
FURADANTIN	Nitrofurantoin		
GANTANOL	Sulfamethox-azole	HYTAKEROL	Dihydro-tachysterol
GANTRISIN	Sulfisoxazole	HYTRIN	Terazosin
GARAMYCIN	Gentamicin	IFEX	Ifosfamide
GEOCILLIN	Carbenicillin	ILOSONE	Erythromycin

TRADE AND GENERIC NAMES OF COMMONLY USED DRUGS (*Continued*)

Trade Name	Generic Name	Trade Name	Generic Name
IMFERON	Iron dextran	LEVOXYL	Levothyroxine
IMITREX	Sumatriptan		(T$_4$)
IMODIUM	Loperamide	LEVSIN	*Hyoscyamine
IMURAN	Azathioprine	LIBRIUM	*Chlordiaze-
INAPSINE	Droperidol		poxide
INDERAL	Propranolol	LIDEX	Fluocinonide
INDOCIN	*Indomethacin	LINCOCIN	Lincomycin
INOCOR	Amrinone	LIORESAL	Baclofen
INTAL	Cromolyn	LIPITOR	Atorvastatin
INTROPIN	Dopamine	LITHANE	Lithium
IONAMIN	Phentermine	LITHONATE	Lithium
ISMELIN	*Guanethidine	LITHOSTAT	Acetohydrox-
ISOPTIN	Verapamil		amic acid
ISORDIL	Isosorbide	LODINE	Etodolac
ISUPREL	Isoproterenol	LOMOTIL	Diphenoxylate
KANTREX	Kanamycin		with atropine
KEFLEX	Cephalexin	LONITEN	Minoxidil
KEFUROX	Cefuroxime	LOPID	Gemfibrozil
KEFZOL	Cefazolin	LOPRESSOR	Metoprolol
KEMADRIN	Procyclidine	LORELCO	Probucol
KENACORT	Triamcinolone	LORFAN	Levallorphan
KENALOG	Triamcinolone	LOTENSIN	Benazepril
KERLONE	Betaxolol	LOTRIMIN	Clotrimazole
KLONOPIN	Clonazepam	LOVENOX	Enoxaparin
KONAKION	Phytonadione	LOXITANE	Loxapine
KONYNE 80	Factor IX con-	LOZOL	Indapamide
	centrates	LUDIOMIL	Maprotiline
KWELL	Lindane	LUMINAL	Phenobarbital
KYTRIL	Granisetron	LYSODREN	Mitotane
LAMICTAL	Lamotrigine	MACRODANTIN	Nitrofurantoin
LAMPRENE	Clofazimine	MANDELAMINE	Methenamine
LANOXIN	Digoxin	MANDOL	Cefamandole
LARGON	Propiomazine	MAREZINE	Cyclizine
LARODOPA	Levodopa	MARINOL	Dronabinol
LAROTID	Amoxicillin	MATULANE	Procarbazine
LASIX	Furosemide	MAVIK	Trandolapril
LESCOL	Fluvastatin	MAXALT	Rizatriptan
LEUKERAN	Chlorambucil	MAXAQUIN	Lomefloxacin
LEUKINE	Sargramostim	MAZANOR	Mazindol
LEVATOL	Penbutolol	MECLOMEN	Meclofenamate
LEVOPHED	Norepinephrine	MEDROL	Methylpred-
LEVOPROME	Methotrimep-		nisolone
	razine	MEFOXIN	Cefoxitin

TRADE AND GENERIC NAMES OF COMMONLY USED DRUGS *(Continued)*

Trade Name	Generic Name	Trade Name	Generic Name
MEGACE	Megestrol	MYLICON	Simethicone
MELLARIL	Thioridazine	MYOCHRYSINE	Gold
MEPHYTON	Phytonadione	MYSOLINE	Primidone
MEPRON	Atovaquone	NALFON	Fenoprofen
MERIDIA	Sibutramine	NAPROSYN	Naproxen
MERREM IV	Meropenem	NARCAN	Naloxone
MESANTOIN	Mephenytoin	NARDIL	Phenelzine
MESTINON	Pyridostigmine	NASALCROM	Cromolyn
METAPREL	Metaproterenol	NASALIDE	Flunisolide
METICORTEN	Prednisone	NAUSEATOL	*Bromodi-
METOPIRONE	Metyrapone		phenhy-
MEVACOR	Lovastatin		dramine
MEXITIL	Mexiletine	NAVANE	Thiothixene
MEZLIN	Mezlocillin	NAVELBINE	Vinorelbine
MICATIN	Miconazole	NEBCIN	Tobramycin
MICRONASE	Glyburide	NEBUPENT	Pentamidine
MIDAMOR	Amiloride	NegGRAM	Nalidixic acid
MILONTIN	Phensuximide	NEMBUTAL	Pentobarbital
MILTOWN	*Meprobamate	NEO-SYNEPH-	Phenylephrine
MINIPRESS	Prazosin	RINE	
MINOCIN	Minocycline	NEUPOGEN	Filgrastim
MINTEZOL	Thiabendazole	NEURONTIN	Gabapentin
MIRAPEX	Pramipexole	NICLOCIDE	Niclosamide
MITHRACIN	Plicamycin	NICORETTE	Nicotine
MOBAN	Molindone	NICOTROL	Nicotine
MOGADON	*Nitrazepam	NILSTAT	Nystatin
MONISTAT	Miconazole	NIMOTOP	Nimodipine
MONOCID	Cefonicid	NIPRIDE	Nitroprusside
MONOPRIL	Fosinopril	NIZORAL	Ketoconazole
MOTRIN	Ibuprofen	NOCTEC	Chloral hydrate
MOXAM	Moxalactam	NOLVADEX	Tamoxifen
MS CONTIN	Morphine	NORMODYNE	Labetalol
MUCOMYST	Acetylcysteine	NOROXIN	Norfloxacin
MUSTARGEN	Mechloreth-	NORPACE	*Disopyramide
	amine	NORPRAMIN	Desipramine
MUTAMYCIN	Mitomycin	NORVASC	Amlodipine
MYAMBUTOL	Ethambutol	NORVIR	Ritonavir
MYCELEX	Clotrimazole	NOVOCAIN	Procaine
MYCOBUTIN	Rifabutin	NOVOLIN	Insulin
MYCOSTATIN	Nystatin	NUBAIN	Nalbuphine
MYDRIACYL	Tropicamide	NUPRIN	Ibuprofen
MYKROX	Metolazone	NYDRAZID	Isoniazid
MYLERAN	Busulfan		

TRADE AND GENERIC NAMES OF COMMONLY USED DRUGS (*Continued*)

Trade Name	Generic Name	Trade Name	Generic Name
NYTOL	*Diphenhydramine	PHENURONE	Phenacemide
		PHOSPHOLINE	Echothiophate
OCUFEN	Flurbiprofen	PIPRACIL	Piperacillin
OCUPRESS	Carteolol	PITOCIN	Oxytocin
OMNIPEN	Ampicillin	PITRESSIN	Vasopressin
ONCOVIN	Vincristine	PLAQUENIL	Hydroxychloroquine
OPHTHAINE	Proparacaine		
OPHTHETIC	Proparacaine	PLATINOL	Cisplatin
ORETIC	Hydrochlorothiazide	PLAVIX	Clopidogrel
		PLENDIL	Felodipine
ORETON	Methyltestosterone	PNEUMOVAX 23	Pneumococcal vaccine, polyvalent
ORINASE	Tolbutamide		
ORUDIS	Ketoprofen	PNU-IMMUNE 23	Pneumococcal vaccine, polyvalent
ORUVAIL	Ketoprofen		
OXANDRIN	Oxandrolone	POLARAMINE	*Dexchlorpheniramine
OXSORALEN	Methoxsalen		
PANCREASE	Pancrelipase	POLYCILLIN	Ampicillin
PARADIONE	Paramethadione	PONDIMIN	Fenfluramine
PARAFON FORTE	*Chlorzoxazone	PONSTEL	Mefenamic acid
PARLODEL	Bromocriptine	POSICOR	Mibefradil
PARNATE	Tranylcypromine	POVAN	Pyrvinium
		PRANDIN	Repaglinide
PATHOCIL	Dicloxacillin	PRAVACHOL	Pravastatin
PAVABID	Papaverine	PRECEF	Ceforanide
PAVULON	Pancuronium	PRECOSE	Acarbose
PAXIL	Paroxetine	PRELUDIN	Phenmetrazine
PAXIPAM	Halazepam	PREMARIN	Estrogens, conjugated
PBZ	*Tripelennamine		
		PRE-PEN	Benzylpenicilloyl polylysine
PENETREX	Enoxacin		
PENTAM 300	Pentamidine		
PEN-VEE	Penicillin V potassium	PREVACID	Lansoprazole
		PRILOSEC	Omeprazole
PEPCID	Famotidine	PRIMACOR	Milrinone
PERGONAL	Menotropins	PRIMAXIN	Imipenem-cilastatin
PERIACTIN	*Cyproheptadine		
		PRINCIPEN	Ampicillin
PERMAX	Pergolide	PRINIVIL	Lisinopril
PERMITIL	Fluphenazine	PRISCOLINE	Tolazoline
PERSANTINE	*Dipyridamole	PRO-BANTHINE	*Propantheline
PERTOFRANE	Desipramine	PROCAN SR	Procainamide
PHENERGAN	*Promethazine	PROCARDIA	Nifedipine

TRADE AND GENERIC NAMES OF COMMONLY USED DRUGS (*Continued*)

Trade Name	Generic Name	Trade Name	Generic Names
PROCRIT	Epoetin alfa	RESCRIPTOR	Delavirdine
PROFENAL	Suprofen	RESPA-ARM	*Belladonna alkaloids
PROGLYCEM	Diazoxide		
PROGRAF	Tacrolimus	RESTORIL	Temazepam
PROLIXIN	Fluphenazine	RETAVASE	Reteplase
PROLOPRIM	Trimethoprim	RETIN-A	Tretinoin
PRONESTYL	Procainamide	RETROVIR	Zidovudine
PROPECIA	Finasteride	REVIA	Naltrexone
PROPINE	Dipivefrin	REZULIN	Troglitazone
PROPLEX T	Factor IX concentrates	RHEUMATREX	Methotrexate
		RHINOCORT	Budesonide
PROPULSID	Cisapride	RIDAURA	Auranofin
PROSCAR	Finasteride	RIFADIN	Rifampin
PROSED	*Hyoscyamine	RIMACTANE	Rifampin
PROSOM	Estazolam	RISPERDAL	Risperidone
PROSTAPHLIN	Oxacillin	RITALIN	Methylphenidate
PROSTIGMIN	Neostigmine	ROBAXIN	*Methocarbamol
PROSTIN E2	Dinoprostone	ROBITUSSIN	Guaifenesin
PROSTIN F2 ALPHA	Dinoprost	ROCALTROL	Calcitriol
		ROCEPHIN	Ceftriaxone
PROTOPAM	Pralidoxime	ROGAINE	Minoxidil
PROTROPIN	Somatrem	ROWASA	Mesalamine
PROVENTIL	Albuterol	RYTHMOL	Propafenone
PROVERA	Medroxyprogesterone	SALFLEX	Salsalate
		SANDIMMUNE	Cyclosporine
PROZAC	Fluoxetine	SANDOSTATIN	Octreotide
PULMOZYME	Dornase alfa	SANOREX	Mazindol
PURINETHOL	Mercaptopurine	SANSERT	Methysergide
PYRIDIUM	Phenazopyridine	SECONAL	Secobarbital
QUARZAN	*Clidinium	SECTRAL	Acebutolol
QUESTRAN	Cholestyramine	SELSUN	Selenium
QUINAGLUTE	Quinidine	SEPTRA	Trimethoprim-sulfamethoxazole
RAXAR	Grepafloxacin		
REBETRON	Ribavirin	SERAX	*Oxazepam
RECOMBIVAX HB	Hepatitis B vaccine	SERENTIL	Mesoridazine
		SEREVENT	Salmeterol
REGITINE	Phentolamine	SEROMYCIN	Cycloserine
REGLAN	Metoclopramide	SEROQUEL	Quetiapine
		SERZONE	Nefazodone
RELAFEN	Nabumetone	SILVADENE	Silver sulfadiazine
RELENZA	Zanamivir		
REOPRO	Abciximab	SINEMET	Carbidopa-levodopa
REQUIP	Ropinirole		

TRADE AND GENERIC NAMES OF COMMONLY USED DRUGS (*Continued*)

Trade Name	Generic Name	Trade Name	Generic Name
SINEQUAN	*Doxepin	TEGISON	Etretinate
SINGULAIR	Montelukast	TEGOPEN	Cloxacillin
SKELAXIN	*Metaxalone	TEGRETOL	Carbamazepine
SOLATENE	Beta carotene	TELDRIN	*Chlorphenira-
SOLU-CORTEF	Cortisol		mine
SOMA	*Carisoprodol	TEMARIL	Trimeprazine
SOMOPHYLLIN	Aminophylline	TENEX	Guanfacine
SORBITRATE	Isosorbide	TENORMIN	Atenolol
SPARINE	Promazine	TENSILON	Edrophonium
SPORANOX	Itraconazole	TENUATE	Diethylpropion
STADOL	Butorphanol	TEPANIL	Diethylpropion
STAPHCILLIN	Methicillin	TESLAC	Testolactone
STELAZINE	Trifluoperazine	TESSALON	Benzonatate
STIMATE	Desmopressin	TESTODERM	Testosterone
STOXIL	Idoxuridine	TETRACYN	Tetracycline
STREPTASE	Streptokinase	TETREX	Tetracycline
SUBLIMAZE	Fentanyl	THAM	Tromethamine
SUDAFED	Pseudoephe-	THEO-DUR	Theophylline
	drine	THORAZINE	Chlorpromazine
SULAR	Nisoldipine	THYROLAR	Liotrix
SULFAMYLON	Mafenide	THYTROPAR	Thyrotropin
SUPRAX	Cefixime	TICAR	Ticarcillin
SURMONTIL	Trimipramine	TICLID	*Ticlopidine
SURVANTA	Beractant	TIGAN	*Trimethoben-
SYMMETREL	Amantadine		zamide
SYNALAR	Fluocinolone	TILADE	Nedocromil
SYNKAYVITE	Menadiol	TIMOPTIC	Timolol
SYNTHROID	Levothyroxine	TINACTIN	Tolnaftate
	(T_4)	TINDAL	Acetophenazine
SYNTOCINON	Oxytocin	TOBREX	Tobramycin
SYPRINE	Trientine	TOFRANIL	Imipramine
TACARYL	Methdilazine	TOLECTIN	Tolmetin
TACE	Chlorotria-	TOLINASE	Tolazamide
	nisene	TONOCARD	Tocainide
TAGAMET	Cimetidine	TORADOL	Ketorolac
TALWIN	*Pentazocine	TORECAN	Thiethylpera-
TAMBOCOR	Flecainide		zine
TAMIFLU	Oseltamivir	TORNALATE	Bitolterol
TAPAZOLE	Methimazole	TRANCOPAL	Chlormezanone
TASMAR	Tolcapone	TRANDATE	Labetalol
TAVIST	Clemastine	TRANXENE	Clorazepate
TAXOL	Paclitaxel	TRENTAL	Pentoxifylline
TAZICEF	Ceftazidime	TRICLOS	Triclofos
TAZIDIME	Ceftazidime		

TRADE AND GENERIC NAMES OF COMMONLY USED DRUGS (*Continued*)

Trade Name	Generic Name	Trade Name	Generic Name
TRIDIONE	Trimethadione	VIRACEPT	Nelfinavir
TRILAFON	*Perphenazine	VIRAMUNE	Nevirapine
TRIMPEX	Trimethoprim	VIRAZOLE	Ribavirin
TROBICIN	Spectinomycin	VIROPTIC	Trifluridine
TRUSOPT	Dorzolamide	VISKEN	Pindolol
TYLENOL	Acetaminophen	VISTARIL	*Hydroxyzine
ULTRACEF	Cefadroxil	VISTIDE	Cidofovir
ULTRAM	Tramadol	VIVACTIL	Protriptyline
UNIPEN	Nafcillin	VOLTAREN	Diclofenac
URECHOLINE	Bethanechol	VONTROL	Diphenidol
URISPAS	Flavoxate	WELLBUTRIN	Bupropion
UTICORT	Betamethasone	WINSTROL	Stanozolol
VALISONE	Betamethasone	WYTENSIN	Guanabenz
VALIUM	*Diazepam	XALATAN	Latanoprost
VALPIN 50	Anisotropine	XANAX	*Alprazolam
VALTREX	Valacyclovir	XENICAL	Orlistat
VANCERIL	Beclomethasone	XYLOCAINE	Lidocaine
VANCOCIN	Vancomycin	YUTOPAR	Ritodrine
VANSIL	Oxamniquine	ZANOSAR	Streptozocin
VAQTA	Hepatitis A vaccine	ZANTAC	Ranitidine
		ZAROXOLYN	Metolazone
VASCOR	Bepridil	ZEBETA	Bisoprolol
VASOTEC	Enalapril	ZERIT	Stavudine
V-CILLIN K	Penicillin V potassium	ZESTRIL	Lisinopril
		ZINACEF	Cefuroxime
VELBAN	Vinblastine	ZITHROMAX	Azithromycin
VELOSEF	Cephradine	ZOCOR	Simvastatin
VENTOLIN	Albuterol	ZOFRAN	Ondansetron
VePESID	Etoposide	ZOLICEF	Cefazolin
VERCYTE	Pipobroman	ZOLOFT	Sertraline
VERMOX	Mebendazole	ZOMIG	Zolmitriptan
VESPRIN	Triflupromazine	ZONALON	*Doxepin
VIAGRA	Sildenafil	ZOSTRIX	Capsaicin
VIBRAMYCIN	Doxycycline	ZOSYN	Tazobactam
VIDEX	Didanosine	ZOVIRAX	Acyclovir
VIOKASE	Pancrelipase	ZYFLO	Zileuton
VIOXX	Rofecoxib	ZYLOPRIM	Allopurinol
VIRA-A	Vidarabine	ZYPREXA	Olanzapine

*Particularly problematic in the elderly (see TABLE 6–4).

RESOURCES LIST

The following selective list includes mainly national agencies and organizations in the USA; many of them have local chapters. State Administration on Aging (AOA) agencies, listed in the local telephone directory, can provide information about local services for the elderly. The telephone number for state AOA agencies can also be obtained by calling the Eldercare Locator service (800-677-1116), operated by the National Association of Area Agencies on Aging.

The National Institute on Aging provides several helpful booklets related to aging. "Exercise: A Guide from the National Institute on Aging" (Publication No. NIH 98-4258) provides general information about physical activity and exercise and describes an exercise prescription that includes endurance activities, muscle-strengthening activities, balance training, and flexibility training. Patients may obtain a single copy free of charge by calling 800-222-2225 or may access this booklet on the Internet at *http://www.nih.gov/nia/health/general/general.htm.*

AGING (GENERAL)

Administration on Aging
330 Independence Avenue SW
Washington, DC 20201
202-619-7501 (National Aging Information Center);
202-401-7575 (TDD)
http://www.aoa.gov
e-mail: *aoainfo@aoa.gov*;
naic@aoa.gov (National Aging Information Center)

Aging Network Services
Topaz House
4400 East-West Highway, Suite 907
Bethesda, MD 20814
301-657-4329
http://www.agingnets.com
e-mail: *ans@AgingNetS.com*

American Association of Homes and Services for the Aging
901 E Street NW, Suite 500
Washington, DC 20004-2011
202-783-2242
http://www.aahsa.org
e-mail: *info@aahsa.org*

American Association of Retired Persons
601 E Street NW
Washington, DC 20049
800-424-3410
http://www.aarp.org
e-mail: *member@aarp.org*

American Federation for Aging Research
1414 Avenue of the Americas, 18th Floor
New York, NY 10019
212-752-2327
http://www.afar.org
e-mail: *AMFEDAGING@aol.com*

American Geriatrics Society
770 Lexington Avenue, Suite 300
New York, NY 10021
212-308-1414
http://www.americangeriatrics.org
e-mail: *info.amger@ americangeriatrics.org*

American Society on Aging
833 Market Street, Suite 511
San Francisco, CA 94103
415-974-9600
http://www.asaging.org
e-mail: *info@asa.asaging.org*

Children of Aging Parents
1609 Woodbourne Road, Suite 302-A
Levittown, PA 19057
800-227-7294; 215-945-6900

Eldercare Locator
(A service of the National Association
of Area Agencies on Aging)
800-677-1116

Gerontological Society of America
1030 15th Street NW, Suite 250
Washington, DC 20005
http://www.geron.org
e-mail: *mailto:geron@geron.org*

Medicare Hotline
800-633-4227 (800-MEDICAR);
  800-638-6833; 877-486-2048 (TTY)
http://www.medicare.gov

National Alliance of Senior Citizens
1700 18th Street NW, Suite 401
Washington, DC 20009
202-986-0117

**National Asian/Pacific Resource
  Center on Aging**
Melbourne Tower, Suite 914
1511 Third Avenue
Seattle, WA 98101-1626
206-624-1221

**National Association for Hispanic
  Elderly**
Asociacion Nacional Pro Personas
  Mayores
1452 West Temple Street
Los Angeles, CA 90026-1724
213-487-1922

**National Association of Area
  Agencies on Aging**
927 15th Street NW, 6th Floor
Washington, DC 20005
202-296-8130
http://www.n4A.org

**National Association of Professional
  Geriatric Care Managers**
1604 North Country Club Road
Tucson, AZ 85716-3102
520-881-8008
http://www.caremanager.org

**National Caucus and Center on
  Black Aged, Inc.**
1424 K Street NW, Suite 500
Washington, DC 20005
202-637-8400

**National Citizens' Coalition for
  Nursing Home Reform**
1424 16th Street NW, Suite 202
Washington, DC 20036-2211
202-332-2275
http://www.nccnhr.org

National Council of Senior Citizens
8403 Colesville Road, Suite 1200
Silver Spring, MD 20910-3314
301-578-8800
http://www.ncscinc.org

**National Council on Patient
  Information and Education**
666 11th Street NW, Suite 810
Washington, DC 20001
202-347-6711
e-mail: *ncpie@erols.com*

National Council on the Aging
409 3rd Street SW
Washington, DC 20024
800-867-2755; 202-479-1200; 202-
  479-6674 (TDD)
http://www.ncoa.org
e-mail: *info@ncoa.org*

**National Hispanic Council on
  Aging**
2713 Ontario Road NW
Washington, DC 20009
202-745-2521; 202-265-1288
http://www.incacorp.com/nhcoa
e-mail: *nhcoa@worldnet.att.net*

National Indian Council on Aging
10501 Montgomery Boulevard NE,
Suite 210
Albuquerque, NM 87111-3846
505-292-2001
http://www.nicoa.org
e-mail: *dave@nicoa.org*

National Institute on Aging
Public Information Office
Building 31, Room 5C27
31 Center Drive, MSC 2292
Bethesda, MD 20892
800-222-2225; 800-222-4225 (TTY);
301-496-1752
http://www.nih.gov/nia
e-mail: *niainfo@lkacc.com*

Social Security Administration
Office of Public Inquiries
Room 4-C-5 Annex
6401 Security Boulevard
Baltimore, MD 21235
800-772-1213; 800-325-0778 (TTY)
http://www.ssa.gov

United Seniors Health Cooperative
409 Third Street SW, 2nd Floor
Washington, DC 20024
202-479-6973
http://www.ushc-online.org
e-mail: *ushc@erols.com*

**US Department of Health and
Human Services**
200 Independence Avenue SW
Washington, DC 20201
877-696-6775; 202-619-0257
http://www.hhs.gov

ALZHEIMER'S DISEASE

Alzheimer's Association
919 North Michigan Avenue, Suite
1000
Chicago, IL 60611-1676
800-272-3900; 312-335-8700
http://www.alz.org
e-mail: *info@alz.org*

**Alzheimer's Disease Education and
Referral Center**
PO Box 8250
Silver Spring, MD 20907-8250
800-438-4380
http://www.alzheimers.org
e-mail: *adear@alzheimers.org*

ARTHRITIS

Arthritis Foundation
1330 West Peachtree Street
Atlanta, GA 30309
800-283-7800; 404-872-7100
http://www.arthritis.org

**National Institute of Arthritis and
Musculoskeletal and Skin Diseases**
Information Clearinghouse
1 AMS Circle
Bethesda, MD 20892-3675
301-495-4484; 301-565-2966 (TTY)
http://www.nih.gov/niams

BEREAVEMENT
(see Death & Bereavement)

CANCER & OTHER TUMORS

American Cancer Society
National Headquarters
1599 Clifton Road NE
Atlanta, GA 30329
800-227-2345; 404-320-3333
http://www.cancer.org

Cancer Research Institute
681 Fifth Avenue
New York, NY 10022
800-992-2623 (800-99-CANCER)
http://www.cancerresearch.org
e-mail: *cancerres@aol.com*

National Cancer Institute
NCI Public Inquiries Office
Building 31, Room 10A03
31 Center Drive, MSC 2580
Bethesda, MD 20892-2580
800-422-6237 (800-4-CANCER);
300-332-8615 (TTY); 301-435-3848
http://www.nci.nih.gov

Breast:

National Alliance of Breast Cancer Organizations
9 East 37th Street, 10th Floor
New York, NY 10016
800-719-9154; 212-889-0606
http://www.nabco.org
e-mail: *NABCOinfo@aol.com*

Y-ME National Breast Cancer Organization
212 West Van Buren Street
Chicago, IL 60607-3908
800-221-2141; 800-986-9505 (Spanish)
http://www.y-me.org
e-mail: *help@y-me.org*

Prostate:

Prostate Cancer Resource Network
PO Box 966
New Port Richey, FL 34656
800-915-1001; 813-847-1619
http://www.pcrn.org

US-TOO International
930 North York Road, Suite 50
Hinsdale, IL 60521-2993
800-808-7866 (800-80-US TOO);
630-323-1002
http://www.ustoo.com
e-mail: *ustoo@ustoo.com*

Skin:

The Melanoma Research Foundation
PO Box 747
San Leandro, CA 94577
800-673-1290
http://www.melanoma.org
e-mail: *mrf@melanoma.org*

The Skin Cancer Foundation
PO Box 561
New York, NY 10156
800-754-6490
http://www.skincancer.org
e-mail: *info@skincancer.org*

CARDIOVASCULAR DISORDERS
(See also Stroke)

American Association of Cardiovascular and Pulmonary Rehabilitation
7611 Elmwood Avenue, Suite 201
Middleton, WI 53562
608-831-6989
http://www.aacvpr.org
e-mail: *aacvpr@tmahq.com*

American Heart Association
National Center
7272 Greenville Avenue
Dallas, TX 75231-4596
800-242-8721 (800-AHA-USA1);
888-694-3278 (888-MY-HEART, for women's health information)
http://www.americanheart.org

National Heart, Lung, and Blood Institute
PO Box 30105
Bethesda, MD 20824-0105
800-575-9355 (800-575-WELL);
301-592-8573 (information center)
http://www.nhlbi.nih.gov

CAREGIVERS

Family Caregiver Alliance
690 Market Street, Suite 600
San Francisco, CA 94104
415-434-3388
http://www.caregiver.org
e-mail: *info@caregiver.org*

National Family Caregivers Association
10605 Concord Street, Suite 501
Kensington, MD 20895-2504
800-896-3650
http://www.nfcacares.org
e-mail: *info@nfcacares.org*

The Well Spouse Foundation
30 East 40th Street PH
New York, NY 10018
800-838-0879; 212-685-8815
http://www.wellspouse.org

DEATH & BEREAVEMENT

**Association for Death Education
and Counseling**
342 North Main Street
West Hartford, CT 06117-2507
860-586-7503
http://www.adec.org

Choice in Dying
1035 30th Street NW
Washington, DC 20007
800-989-9455; 202-338-9790
http://www.choices.org
e-mail: *cid@choices.org*

Compassion in Dying Federation
PMB 415, 6312 SW Capitol Highway
Portland, OR 97201
503-221-9556
http://www.compassionindying.org
e-mail: *info@compassionindying.org*

**Death With Dignity National
Center**
520 South El Camino Real, Suite 710
San Mateo, CA 94402-1720
650-344-6489
http://www.deathwithdignity.org
e-mail: *info@deathwithdignity.org*

Dying Well Network
PO Box 880
Spokane, WA 99210-0880
509-926-2457
*http://www.ior.com/~jeffw/
homepage.htm*
e-mail: *Rob.Neils@on-ramp.ior.com*

Hemlock Society USA
PO Box 101810
Denver, CO 80250-1810
800-247-7421
http://www.hemlock.org
e-mail: *hemlock@privatei.com*

Hospice Education Institute
190 Westbrook Road
Essex, CT 06426-1510
800-331-1620; 860-767-1620
http://www.hospiceworld.org
e-mail: *hospiceall@aol.com*

Hospice Foundation of America
2001 South Street NW, Suite 300
Washington, DC 20009
800-854-3402
http://www.hospicefoundation.org
e-mail: *hfa@hospicefoundation.org*

National Hospice Organization
1700 Diagonal Road, Suite 300
Alexandria, VA 22314
703-243-5900
http://www.nho.org

DEMENTIA
(see Alzheimer's Disease)

DENTAL DISORDERS

**American Society for Geriatric
Dentistry**
211 East Chicago Avenue, Suite 948
Chicago, IL 60611
312-440-2660
http://www.bgsm.edu/dentistry/foscod

DEPRESSION
(see also Psychiatric Disorders)

**National Depressive and Manic-
Depressive Association**
730 North Franklin Street, Suite 501
Chicago, IL 60610-3526
800-826-3632; 312-642-0049
http://www.ndmda.org
e-mail: *nbunch@ndmda.org*

DIABETES

American Diabetes Association
1701 North Beauregard Street
Alexandria, VA 22311
800-342-2383 (800-DIABETES)
http://www.diabetes.org

National Diabetes Information Clearinghouse
National Institute of Diabetes and Digestive and Kidney Diseases
1 Information Way
Bethesda, MD 20892-3560
301-654-3327
http://www.niddk.nih.gov/health/ diabetes/ndic.htm
e-mail: *ndic@info.niddk.nih.gov*

GASTROINTESTINAL DISORDERS

National Digestive Diseases Information Clearinghouse
National Institute of Diabetes and Digestive and Kidney Diseases
2 Information Way
Bethesda, MD 20892-3560
301-654-3810
http://www.niddk.nih.gov/health/ digest/nddic.htm
e-mail: *nddic@info.niddk.nih.gov*

DISABILITIES & REHABILITATION

National Organization on Disability
910 16th Street NW
Washington, DC 20006
202-293-5960; 202-293-5868 (TDD)
http://www.nod.org
e-mail: *ability@nod.org*

National Rehabilitation Information Center
1010 Wayne Avenue, Suite 800
Silver Spring, MD 20910
800-346-2742; 301-562-2400; 301-495-5626 (TTY)
http://www.naric.com

ELDER ABUSE

National Center on Elder Abuse
1225 I Street NW, Suite 725
Washington, DC 20005
202-898-2586
http://www.gwjapan.com/NCEA
e-mail: *NCEA@nasua.org*

ERECTILE DYSFUNCTION

Impotence World Association
PO Box 410
Bowie, MD 20718-0410
800-669-1603
http://www.impotenceworld.org
e-mail: *info@impotenceworld.org*

HEARING DISORDERS

Alexander Graham Bell Association for the Deaf and Hard of Hearing
3417 Volta Place NW
Washington, DC 20007-2778
202-337-5220 (Voice/TTY)
http://www.agbell.org
e-mail: *agbell2@aol.com*

American Tinnitus Association
PO Box 5
Portland, OR 97207-0005
800-634-8978
http://www.ata.org
e-mail: *tinnitus@ata.org*

Hearing Aid Hotline
National Hearing Aid Society
20361 Middlebelt Road
Livonia, MI 48152
800-521-5247; 313-478-2610

National Association of the Deaf
814 Thayer Avenue
Silver Spring, MD 20910
301-587-1788; 301-587-1789 (TTY)
http://www.nad.org
e-mail: *NADinfo@nad.org*

National Institute on Deafness and Other Communication Disorders
Information Office
31 Center Drive, MSC 2320
Bethesda, MD 20892-2320
800-241-1044; 800-241-1055 (TTY); 301-496-7243; 301-402-0252 (TTY)
http://www.nih.gov/nidcd
e-mail: *nidcdinfo@nidcd.nih.gov*

Self Help for Hard of Hearing People
7910 Woodmont Avenue, Suite 1200
Bethesda, MD 20814
301-657-2248; 301-657-2249 (TTY)
http://www.shhh.org

HOME HEALTH CARE

American Academy of Home Care Physicians
PO Box 1037
Edgewood, MD 21040
410-676-7966
http://www.podi.com/aahcp
e-mail: *aahcp@mindspring.com*

National Association for Home Care
228 Seventh Street SE
Washington, DC 20003
202-547-7424
http://www.nahc.org

National Federation of Interfaith Volunteer Caregivers
One West Armour Boulevard, Suite 202
Kansas City, MO 64111
800-350-7438; 816-931-5442
http://www.nfivc.org
e-mail: *NFIVC@aol.com*

HOSPICES
(see Death & Bereavement)

IMPOTENCE
(see Erectile Dysfunction)

INCONTINENCE

National Association for Continence
PO Box 8310
2650 East Main Street
Spartanburg, SC 29305-8310
800-252-3337 (800-BLADDER);
  864-579-7900
http://www.nafc.org

The Simon Foundation for Continence
PO Box 835
Wilmette, IL 60091
800-237-4666 (800-23-SIMON);
  847-864-3913
http://www.simonfoundation.org

LEGAL ISSUES

American Bar Association Commission on Legal Problems of the Elderly
740 15th Street NW
Washington, DC 20005-1022
202-662-8690
http://www.abanet.org/elderly/home.html
e-mail: *abaelderly@abanet.org*

National Academy of Elder Law Attorneys
1604 North Country Club Road
Tucson, AZ 85716
520-881-4005
http://www.naela.com

National Senior Citizens Law Center
1101 14th Street NW, Suite 400
Washington, DC 20005
202-289-6976
or
3435 Wilshire Boulevard, Suite 2860
Los Angeles, CA 90034
213-639-0930
http://www.nsclc.org

LIVER DISORDERS

American Liver Foundation
75 Maiden Lane, Suite 603
New York, NY 10038
800-465-4837 (800-GO-LIVER)
http://www.liverfoundation.org

MEDIC ALERT

MedicAlert Foundation International
2323 Colorado Avenue
Turlock, CA 95382-2018
800-432-5378 (800-IDALERT)
http://www.medicalert.org

MEN'S HEALTH

American Prostate Society
7188 Ridge Road
Hanover, MD 21076
410-859-3735
http://www.ameripros.org
e-mail: *info@ameripros.org*

Prostatitis Foundation
1063 30th Street, Box 8
Smithshire, IL 61478
888-891-4200
http://www.prostatitis.org

NUTRITION

American Dietetic Association
216 West Jackson Boulevard
Chicago, IL 60606-6995
800-366-1655 (hotline); 800-877-
1600; 312-899-0040
http://www.eatright.org
e-mail: *infocenter@eatright.org*

Food and Nutrition Information Center
Agricultural Research Service
United States Department of Agriculture
National Agriculture Library, Room 304
10301 Baltimore Boulevard
Beltsville, MD 20705-2351
301-504-5719; 301-504-5755
http://www.nal.usda.gov
e-mail: *fnic@nal.usad.gov*

Meals on Wheels Association of America
1414 Prince Street, Suite 202
Alexandria, VA 22314
703-548-5558
http://www.projectmeal.org
e-mail: *mowaa@tbg.dgsys.com*

OSTEOPOROSIS

National Institutes of Health, Osteoporosis and Related Bone Diseases—National Resource Center
1232 22nd Street NW
Washington, DC 20037-1292
800-624-2663 (800-624-BONE);
202-223-0344
http://www.osteo.org
e-mail: *orbdnrc@nof.org*

National Osteoporosis Foundation
1232 22nd Street NW
Washington, DC 20037-1292
202-223-2226
http://www.nof.org

PAIN RELIEF

American Chronic Pain Association
PO Box 850
Rocklin, CA 95677
916-632-0922
http://www.theacpa.org
e-mail: *acpa@pacbell.net*

American Pain Society
4700 West Lake Avenue
Glenview, IL 60025
847-375-4715
http://www.ampainsoc.org
e-mail: *info@ampainsoc.org*

National Chronic Pain Outreach Association
7979 Old Georgetown Road, Suite 100
Bethesda, MD 20814-2429
301-652-4948

National Foundation for the Treatment of Pain
1330 Skyline Drive #21
Monterey, CA 93940
831-655-8812
http://www.paincare.org

PARKINSON'S DISEASE

American Parkinson's Disease Association
1250 Hylan Boulevard, Suite 4B
Staten Island, NY 10305-1946
800-223-2732; 718-981-8001
http://www.apdaparkinson.com
e-mail: *info@apdaparkinson.com*

National Parkinson Foundation
1501 NW Ninth Avenue
Bob Hope Road
Miami, FL 33136-1494
800-327-4545; 305-547-6666
http://www.parkinson.org
e-mail: *mailbox@npf.med.miami.edu*

Parkinson's Action Network
840 Third Street
Santa Rosa, CA 95404
800-820-4726; 707-544-1994
http://www.parkinsonsaction.org
e-mail: *info@parkinsonsaction.org*

Parkinson's Disease Foundation
William Black Medical Building
710 West 168th Street
New York, NY 10032-9982
800-457-6676; 212-923-4700
http://www.pdf.org
e-mail: *info@pdf.org*

United Parkinson Foundation
833 West Washington Boulevard
Chicago, IL 60607
312-733-1893

PSYCHIATRIC DISORDERS

American Association for Geriatric Psychiatry
7910 Woodmont Avenue, Suite 1050
Bethesda, MD 20814-3004
301-654-7850
http://www.aagpgpa.org
e-mail: *main@aagpgpa.org*

National Institute of Mental Health
Public Inquiries
6001 Executive Boulevard, Room 8184, MSC 9663
Bethesda, MD 20892-9663
888-826-9438 (888-8-ANXIETY, for anxiety disorders); 800-421-4211 (for depression); 800-647-2643 (800-64-PANIC, for panic disorder); 301-443-4513
http://www.nimh.nih.gov
e-mail: *nimhinfo@nih.gov*

PULMONARY DISORDERS
(See also Cardiovascular Disorders)

American Lung Association
1740 Broadway
New York, NY 10019-4374
800-586-4872 (800-LUNG-USA); 212-315-8700
http://www.lungusa.org

RENAL AND UROLOGIC DISORDERS

American Urological Association
1120 North Charles Street
Baltimore, MD 21201
410-727-1100
http://www.auanet.org

Interstitial Cystitis Association
51 Monroe Street, Suite 1402
Rockville, MD 20850
301-610-5300
http://www.ichelp.org
e-mail: *icamail@ichelp.org*

**National Kidney and Urologic
Diseases Information
Clearinghouse
National Institute of Diabetes and
Digestive and Kidney Diseases**
3 Information Way
Bethesda, MD 20892-3560
301-654-4415
*http://www.niddk.nih.gov/health/
kidney/nkudic.htm*
e-mail: *nkudic@info.niddk.nih.gov*

National Kidney Foundation
30 East 33rd Street, Suite 1100
New York, NY 10016
800-622-9010; 212-889-2210
http://www.kidney.org
e-mail: *info@kidney.org*

SLEEP DISORDERS

American Sleep Apnea Association
1424 K Street NW, Suite 302
Washington, DC 20005
202-293-3650
http://www.sleepapnea.org
e-mail: *asaa@sleepapnea.org*

**American Academy of Sleep
Medicine**
6301 Bandel Road, Suite 101
Rochester, MN 55901
507-287-6006
http://www.asda.org
e-mail: *info@aasmnet.org*

National Sleep Foundation
1522 K Street NW, Suite 510
Washington, DC 20005
202-347-3471
http://www.sleepfoundation.org
e-mail: *nsf@sleepfoundation.org*

STROKE
(See also Caregivers)

**National Institute of Neurological
Disorders and Stroke**
PO Box 5801
Bethesda, MD 20824
800-352-9424
http://www.ninds.nih.gov

National Stroke Association
96 Inverness Drive East, Suite I
Englewood, CO 80112-5112
800-787-6537 (800-STROKES);
303-649-9299
http://www.stroke.org

THYROID DISORDERS

Thyroid Foundation of America
350 Ruth Sleeper Hall, RSL 350
40 Parkman Street
Boston, MA 02114
800-832-8321; 617-726-8500
http://www.tsh.org
e-mail: *info@tsh.org*

VISION DISORDERS

American Council of the Blind
1155 15th Street NW, Suite 1004
Washington, DC 20005
800-424-8666; 202-467-5081
http://www.acb.org

American Foundation for the Blind
11 Penn Plaza, Suite 300
New York, NY 10001
800-232-5463; 212-502-7600
http://www.afb.org
e-mail: *afbinfo@afb.net*

**American Macular Degeneration
Foundation**
PO Box 515
Northampton, MA 01061-0515
413-268-7660
http://www.macular.org

**Association for Education and
Rehabilitation of the Blind &
Visually Impaired**
4600 Duke Street, Suite 430
PO Box 22397
Alexandria, VA 22304
703-823-9690
http://www.aerbvi.org

The Glaucoma Foundation
116 John Street, Suite 1605
New York, NY 10038
800-452-8266 (800-GLAUCOMA,
    hotline); 212-285-0080
http://www.glaucoma-foundation.org
e-mail: *info@glaucomafoundation.org*

Lighthouse International
111 East 59th Street
New York, NY 10022-1202
800-829-0500; 212-821-9200;
    212-821-9713 (TYY)
http://www.lighthouse.org
e-mail: *info@lighthouse.org*

**National Association for Visually
    Handicapped**
22 West 21st Street, 6th Floor
New York, NY 10010
212-889-3141
http://www.navh.org
e-mail: *staff@navh.org;
    staffca@navh.org* (for western
    states)

National Eye Institute
2020 Vision Place
Bethesda, MD 20892-3655
301-496-5248
http://www.nei.nih.gov

National Federation of the Blind
1800 Johnson Street
Baltimore, MD 21230
410-659-9314
http://www.nfb.org

WOMEN'S HEALTH

**The North American Menopause
    Society**
PO Box 94527
Cleveland, OH 44101-4527
440-442-7550
http://www.menopause.org

Older Women's League
666 11th Street NW, Suite 700
Washington, DC 20001
800-825-3695; 202-783-6686

INDEX

The Third Edition of THE MERCK MANUAL OF GERIATRICS is set in 11-point Times Roman, with text headings set in Friz Quadrata Bold. The index is set in 9-point Times Roman. The original draft was produced using Microsoft Word 97 at the editorial offices of the Merck Manuals Department in Blue Bell, Pennsylvania, and transmitted on disks to Nesbitt Graphics in Glenside, Pennsylvania, where it was electronically assembled into pages using QuarkXpress with Autopage®. The book was printed by web offset on 30-pound paper at National Publishing Company, Philadelphia, Pennsylvania.

NOTES

NOTES